BSAVA Textbook of
Veterinary Nursing
5th edition

Editors

Barbara Cooper CertEd LicIPD DTM HonAssocRCVS RVN
Principal, The College of Animal Welfare, London Road,
Godmanchester, Huntingdon, Cambs PE29 2LJ

Elizabeth Mullineaux BVM&S DVM&S CertSHP MRCVS
Quantock Veterinary Hospital, Quantock Terrace,
The Drove, Bridgwater TA6 4BA

Lynn Turner MA VetMB MRCVS
St David's Farm and Equine Practice, Nutwell Estate,
Lymstone, Exmouth EX8 5AN

Consulting Editor – Equine

Tim Greet CertEO DESTS DipECVS FRCVS
Rossdales Equine Hospital, Cotton End Road, Exning,
Newmarket, Suffolk CB8 7NN

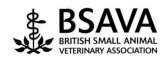
BSAVA
BRITISH SMALL ANIMAL
VETERINARY ASSOCIATION

Published by:

British Small Animal Veterinary Association
Woodrow House, 1 Telford Way,
Waterwells Business Park, Quedgeley,
Gloucester GL2 2AB

A Company limited by Guarantee in England
Registered Company No. 2837793
Registered as a Charity

First Published 1994
Second edition 1999
Third edition 2003
Reprinted 2004
Fourth edition 2007
Reprinted 2008, 2009, 2010 (twice)

Fifth edition Copyright © 2011 BSAVA
Reprinted 2012

Figures 3.2, 3.6, 3.9, 3.11, 3.12, 3.13, 3.14, 3.18, 3.19, 3.20, 3.21, 3.22, 3.23,
3.25, 3.27, 3.30, 3.31, 3.32, 3.33, 3.34, 3.36, 3.38, 3.39, 3.41, 3.43, 3.47,
3.48, 3.49, 3.53, 3.56, 3.57, 3.60, 3.61, 3.69, 3.70, 3.71, 3.72, 3.73, 3.74,
3.76, 3.77, 3.78, 3.79, 3.81, 3.82, 3.87, 3.88, 3.89, 3.90, 3.91, 3.92, 3.93,
3.96, 4.1, 4.4, 4.6, 6.12, 7.48, 10.16, 12.36, 17.8, 17.10, 18.3, 18.5, 18.6,
18.10, 18.19, 18.26, 18.30, 18.76, 19.5a, 19.11, 19.13 and 20.16 were
drawn by S.J. Elmhurst BA Hons (www.livingart.org.uk) and are printed
with her permission.

Front cover main image photographed by Jonathon Bosley.

A catalogue record for this book is available from the British Library.

ISBN   978-1-905319-26-8

Printed in India by Imprint Digital
Printed on ECF paper made from sustainable forests

Contents

Contributors

Wendy Adams RVN
National Dog Health Screening Co-ordinator
Guide Dogs National Breeding Centre
Banbury Road
Bishops Tachbrook
Leamington Spa
Warwickshire CV33 9WF

Davina Anderson MA VetMB PhD DSAS(ST) DipECVS MRCVS
Anderson Sturgess Veterinary Specialists
The Granary
Bunstead Barns
Poles Lane
Hursley
Winchester
Hampshire SO21 2LL

Sally Anne Argyle MVB PhD CertSAC MRCVS
Lecturer, Veterinary Pharmacology and Therapeutics,
Royal (Dick) School of Veterinary Science
The University of Edinburgh
Easter Bush Veterinary Centre
Roslin
Midlothian EH25 9RG

Trudi Atkinson VN DipAS(CABC) CCAB
Accredited Clinical Animal Behaviourist
Bradford-on-Avon
Wiltshire BA15 1NN

Amanda K. Boag MA VetMB DipACVIM DipACVECC FHEA MRCVS
Clinical Director, Vets Now
Penguin House
Castle Riggs
Dunfermline
Fife KY11 8SG

Jan Butler
B & W Equine Group
Willesley Equine Clinic
Byams Farm
Willesley
Tetbury
Gloucestershire GL8 8QU

Sharon Chandler DipAVN(Surg) DipAVN(Med) RVN
Queen's Veterinary School Hospital
University of Cambridge
Madingley Road
Cambridge CB3 0ES

Carole Clarke MA VetMB CVPM MRCVS
Mill House Veterinary Surgery and Hospital
20 Tennyson Ave
King's Lynn
Norfolk PE30 2QG

Barbara Cooper CertEd LicIPD DTM HonAssocRCVS RVN
Principal, The College of Animal Welfare
Headland House
London Road
Godmanchester
Huntingdon
Cambridgeshire PE29 2BQ

Karen Coyne BSc(Hons) PhD
University of Liverpool
Leahurst
Chester High Road
Neston
South Wirral
Cheshire CH64 7TE

Susan Dawson BVMS PhD MRCVS
Head of School
School of Veterinary Science
University of Liverpool
Liverpool L69 7ZJ

Ruth Dennis MA VetMB DVR DipECVDI MRCVS
Centre for Small Animal Studies
Animal Health Trust
Lanwades Park
Kentford
Newmarket
Suffolk CB8 7UU

Jane Devaney RVN REVN
Liverpool University Equine Hospital
Leahurst
Chester High Road
Neston
South Wirral
Cheshire CH64 7TE

Gary England BVetMed PhD DVetMed DVR DVRep DipECAR DipACT FHEA FRCVS
School of Veterinary Medicine and Science
University of Nottingham
College Road
Loughborough
Leicestershire LE12 5RD

Maggie Fisher BVetMed CBiol MSB MRQA DipEVPC MRCVS
Shernacre Enterprise
The Mews Studio
Portland Road
Malvern WR14 2TA

Stuart Ford-Fennah BSc(Hons) RVN
Cave Veterinary Specialists
Georges Farm
West Buckland
Wellington
Somerset TA21 9LE

Vicky Ford-Fennah BSc(Hons) RVN
Langford Veterinary Services
Langford House
Langford
Bristol BS40 5DU

Mary Fraser BVMS PhD CertVD PGCHE FHEA CBiol MIBiol MRCVS
Girling and Fraser Ltd Veterinary Practice
Unit 3 Breadalbane Terrace
Perth PH2 8BY

Isuru Gajanayake BVSc CertSAM DipACVIM MRCVS
Willows Veterinary Centre and Referral Service
Highlands Road
Shirley
Solihull
West Midlands B90 4NH

Robyn Gear BVSc DipECVIM-CA DSAM MRCVS
Veterinary Specialist Group
97 Carrington Road
Mt Albert
Auckland
New Zealand

Simon Girling BVMS(Hons) DZooMed CBiol MSB MRCVS
Head of Veterinary Services
Edinburgh Zoo
134 Corstorphine Road
Edinburgh EH12 6TS

Lucy Goddard DipAVN(Surg) DipAVN(Med) RVN
Davies Veterinary Specialists
Manor Farm Business Park
Higham Gobion
Hertfordshire SG5 3HR

Carol Gray BVMS PGCert MedEd MRCVS
Lecturer in Veterinary Communication Skills,
BVSc Programme Director
School of Veterinary Science
University of Liverpool
Leahurst
Chester High Road
Neston
South Wirral
Cheshire CH64 7TE

Gillian Greet BVSc DVR MRCVS
Newmarket

Tim Greet BVMS MVM CertEO DESTS DipECVS FRCVS
Rossdales Equine Hospital
Cotton End Road
Exning
Newmarket
Suffolk CB8 7NN

Matthew Hanks BVSc MRCVS
Lecturer in Equine Practice and Reproduction
Royal (Dick) School of Veterinary Science
The University of Edinburgh
Easter Bush Veterinary Centre
Roslin
Midlothian EH25 9RG

John Helps BVetMed CertSAM MRCVS
Veterinary Manager, Companion Animal Business Unit
MSD Animal Health
Walton Manor
Walton
Milton Keynes MK7 7AJ

Paula Holmes DipAVN(Surg) RVN
Senior Emergency and Critical Nurse
Queen Mother Hospital for Animals
Royal Veterinary College
Hawkshead Lane
North Mymms
Hatfield
Hertfordshire AL9 7TA

Lynn Irving VN EVN
Rossdales Equine Hospital
Cotton End Road
Exning
Newmarket
Suffolk CB8 7NN

Gemma Irwin-Porter BSc(Hons) VPAC PGCE RVN
Veterinary Nursing, Bridgwater College
Bridgwater
Somerset TA5 2LS

Shailen Jasani MA VetMB DipACVECC MRCVS
Hertfordshire

Andrea Jeffery MSc CertEd DipAVN(Surg) RVN
Programme Director, Veterinary Nursing and Bioveterinary
Science
School of Veterinary Sciences
University of Bristol
Langford House
Langford
Bristol BS40 5DU

Julie Johnson DipAVN(Surg) RVN
Theatre Nursing Supervisor
North Downs Specialist Referrals
The Fresian Buildings 3&4
Brewerstreet Dairy Business Park
Brewerstreet
Bletchingley
Surrey RH1 4QP

Debra Kennedy C-SQP RVN
Royal (Dick) School of Veterinary Science
The University of Edinburgh
Easter Bush Veterinary Centre
Roslin
Midlothian EH25 9RG

Philip Lhermette BSc(Hons) BVetMed CBiol MSB MRCVS
Elands Veterinary Clinic
St John's Church
London Road
Dunton Green
Sevenoaks
Kent TN13 2TE

Susan E. Long BVMS PhD DipECAR MRCVS
Canine Reproduction Referrals
Clarendon Veterinary Centre
2 Clarendon Road
Weston-super-Mare
North Somerset BS23 3EF

Rachel Lumbis BSc(Hons) PGCert(MedEd) CertSAN FHEA RVN
The Royal Veterinary College
Department of Veterinary Clinical Sciences
Hawkshead Lane
North Mymms
Hertfordshire AL9 7TA

Helen Mathie MSc VetPhys BSc(Hons) MCSP HPC ACPAT A
Golland Farm
Golland Lane
Burrington
Devon EX37 9JP

John McGarry MSc PhD
School of Veterinary Science
University of Liverpool
Liverpool L69 7ZJ

Dawn McHugh BA DipAVN(Surg) REVN RVN
Newmarket Equine Hospital
Cambridge Road
Newmarket
Suffolk CB8 0FG

Lucy Middlecote CertEd REVN
Veterinary Nursing Department
Hartpury College
Hartpury
Gloucestershire GL19 3BE

Louise Monsey Cert Ed RVN
Arbury Road Veterinary Surgery
32 Arbury Road
Cambridge CB4 2JE

Helen Moreton BSc(Hons) PhD
Royal Agricultural College
Cirencester
Gloucestershire GL7 6JS

Pam Mosedale BVetMed MRCVS
Chapel-en-le-Frith
Derbyshire

Jo Murrell BVSc PhD DipECVAA MRCVS
School of Veterinary Sciences
University of Bristol
Langford House
Langford
Bristol BS40 5DU

Kate Nichols DipAVN(Surg) RVN
Head ECC Nurse, Queen Mother Hospital for Animals
Royal Veterinary College
Hawkshead Lane
North Mymms
Hatfield
Hertfordshire AL9 7TA

Susan Northwood
Consultant–Veterinary Market
S. J. Northwood Veterinary Consultancy
Crooked Billet Farm
Fullers Hill
Little Gransden
South Cambridgeshire SG19 3BP

Catherine Phillips Cert SAN Cert Ed RVN REVN
Hartpury College
Hartpury
Gloucestershire GL19 3BE

Sophie Pullen BSc(Hons) CertEd RVN
The Royal Veterinary College
Hawkshead Lane
North Mymms
Hatfield
Hertfordshire AL9 7TA

Kendal Shepherd BVSc CCAB MRCVS
Accredited Clinical Animal Behaviourist
16 Church Street
Finedon
Wellingborough
Northamptonshire NN9 5NA

Jenny Smith BSc(Hons) DipAVN(Surgical) RVN
School of Veterinary Medicine and Science
University of Nottingham
Sutton Bonington
Loughborough LE12 5RD

Robyn Taylor RVN
Queen Mother Hospital for Animals
Royal Veterinary College
Hawkshead Lane
North Mymms
Hatfield
Hertfordshire AL9 7TA

Cedric Tutt BVSc(Hons) MMedVet(Med) DipEVDC MRCVS
Cape Animal Dentistry Service
Cape Animal Medical Centre
78 Rosmead Avenue
Kenilworth 7708
Cape Town
South Africa

Sue Vranch VN
Petdent Ltd
Veterinary Dentistry and Oral Surgery Referrals
58 Hampton Lane
Blackfield
Southampton
Hampshire SO45 1WN

Vicky Walsh CertEd RVN
Brentknoll Veterinary Centre
Whittington Road
Worcester WR5 2RA

Angela Wright BSc MSc
Centre for Animal Welfare
Royal Veterinary College
Hawkshead Lane
North Mymms
Hatfield
Hertfordshire AL9 7TA

Alison Young VN
Head Theatre Nurse
Queen Mother Hospital for Animals
Royal Veterinary College
Hawkshead Lane
North Mymms
Hatfield
Hertfordshire AL9 7TA

Foreword

This, the 5th edition of the BSAVA's textbook of veterinary nursing, will be well received by our many veterinary nurses and by practices training future generations. From the first edition of *Animal Nursing,* produced in 1966, this text has grown in step with the development of the veterinary nursing profession in the UK. The book remains clear and focused, however, with excellent illustrations and diagrams as befits a practical and hands-on profession. Producing a new edition of this almost 1000 page textbook is an enormous challenge and the Editors deserve our thanks for their enthusiasm and dedication in producing this superb new edition.

Veterinary nurses are a key part of any practice team, providing nursing care and treatments to pets, as well as helping educate owners as to how better to care for them. Demand for veterinary nurses continues to grow as their skills are increasingly recognized by practices, the pharmaceutical industry, welfare organizations and others. Whilst the majority of nurses are employed in small animal practice, others are employed in farm, equine and a diverse range of referral practices.

Over the years exotic pets have featured increasingly and the standard of knowledge required to treat and care for them has grown accordingly. This edition also includes new equine content, and we are grateful to Tim Greet for assisting the editorial team as a specialist in this field. The Editors of the textbook have integrated the canine, feline, equine and exotic material into this edition so that the student can grasp the essential similarities and differences easily.

The regulation of veterinary nursing has changed with the introduction of the non-statutory Register in September 2007. Since then, RVNs have been required to follow the Guide to Professional Conduct for Veterinary Nurses (currently under review) and to keep up to date through continuing professional development. The RCVS will now investigate complaints concerning an individual nurse's fitness to practice, for example professional misconduct or criminal convictions. I believe that these changes are evidence of the veterinary nursing profession coming of age in this its 50th year.

The British Small Animal Veterinary Association is delighted to be publishing this new edition. In recent years there have been significant changes to the delivery of nurse training in practice; however this new edition remains as core to their training as was the first edition some 46 years ago. This text will be read and referred to by trainee nurses and qualified nurses alike. The Association is supportive of the veterinary nursing profession and the publication of this foundation textbook furthers our mission of promoting excellence in small animal practice through education and science.

Andrew Ash BVetMed Cert SAM MBA MRCVS
President, BSAVA 2011–2012

Preface

This is the fifth edition of the *BSAVA Textbook of Veterinary Nursing*. The new Occupational Standards and the RCVS Level 3 VN Syllabus in September 2010 determined that students study the veterinary nursing of both horses and small animals (including exotic pets) at core level and then opt for either the small animal or equine pathway. This textbook thus covers the core syllabus for small animals and horses plus the syllabus content for those students choosing the small animal option pathway. In accord with this, we have introduced new authors with specialist equine knowledge and experience, and are delighted that Professor Tim Greet has joined us as consulting equine editor.

All chapters have been revised or rewritten. The new chapter on Anatomy and Physiology presents information on exotic pets and equine species in a comparative format in line with current teaching methods. Information on nursing models has been expanded to a stand-alone chapter, with an emphasis on practical applications.

Although not specified in the new syllabus, we have retained and updated the material on small animal behaviour, kennel management and dentistry, as these areas have practical importance for veterinary nurses.

Following reader feedback, self-assessment questions have been introduced at the end of each chapter and it is hoped that students will find these and the new Appendix on Study skills especially useful.

The colour photos, specially commissioned line drawings, tinted tables and highlighted boxes will not only aid students in preparation for exams but will act as a reference source for both students and qualified veterinary nurses in their work, whether in a practice or educational setting.

The work of 57 contributors, in addition to the expertise of the publishing team, has resulted in the production of a contemporary textbook that satisfies the requirement upon us all to deliver high-quality care for both the patient and the client.

Barbara Cooper
Elizabeth Mullineaux
Lynn Turner
August 2011

Related titles from the BSAVA

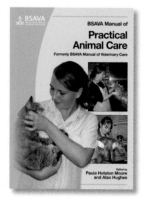

BSAVA Manual of Practical Animal Care
Editors: Paula Hotston Moore and Alan Hughes

- For animal care assistants, veterinary nurses and students
- Replaces *BSAVA Manual of Veterinary Care*

- Practical approach
- Updated and reorganized
- New chapter on Communications skills
- Features Exotic pets
- Illustrated throughout in full colour
- *Published 2007*

Contents: Introduction to the veterinary profession; General care and management of the cat; General care and management of the dog; General care and management of exotic pets and wildlife; Introduction to veterinary care; Management of an animal ward; Use of medicines; Animal first aid; Communicating with clients; Veterinary terminology; Index

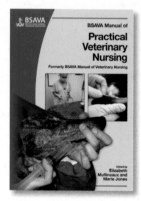

BSAVA Manual of Practical Veterinary Nursing
Editors: Marie Jones and Elizabeth Mullineaux

- For veterinary nurses and students
- Replaces *BSAVA Manual of Veterinary Nursing*

- Practical approach
- Completely reorganized and rewritten
- Includes new elements such as Nursing models
- Geared to the National Occupational Standards
- *Published 2007*

Contents: Responsibilities of the veterinary nurse; Client communication; Practical pharmacy for veterinary nurses; Management of clinical environments, equipment and materials; Management of the inpatient; General principles of veterinary nursing; Triage and emergency nursing; Practical fluid therapy; Medical nursing; Practical laboratory techniques; Diagnostic imaging; Anaesthesia and analgesia; Surgical nursing; Wound management, dressings and bandages; Index

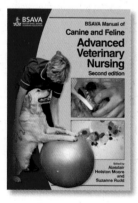

BSAVA Manual of Canine and Feline Advanced Veterinary Nursing, 2nd edition
Editors: Alasdair Hotston Moore and Suzanne Rudd

- For qualified veterinary nurses and those undertaking further qualifications

- Completely revised and updated
- New chapters on Behaviour, Dentistry, Managing nurse-led clinics, Physiotherapy
- Illustrated throughout in full colour
- *Published 2008*

Contents: Advanced nursing practice; Advanced medical nursing; Clinical nutrition; Physiotherapy and rehabilitation; Management of the critical care unit; Advanced fluid therapy; Advanced anaesthesia and analgesia; Advanced surgical nursing; Dentistry; Endoscopy; Advanced imaging; Clinical pathology in practice; Practice administration; Nursing clinics; Behaviour; Index

For information on these and all BSAVA publications please visit our website: www.bsava.com

Chapter 1

Professional responsibilities, regulation and the ethics of veterinary nursing

Sophie Pullen, Angela J. Wright and Barbara Cooper

Learning objectives

After studying this chapter, students should be able to:

- **Interpret the Royal College of Veterinary Surgeons (RCVS) Guide to Professional Conduct for Veterinary Nurses**
- **Describe the legal framework for veterinary nursing practice**
- **Explain the legal and ethical issues surrounding consent to examination and treatment**
- **Explain the principle of duty of care in relation to clients, colleagues and animals**
- **Describe the principles of the Animal Welfare Act 2006**
- **Identify the common ethical issues that arise in veterinary practice**

Introduction

Given the recent changes in regulations that make Registered Veterinary Nurses responsible for their actions, it is imperative to demystify and clarify expectations relating to animal welfare, professional practice, legislation and ethics in situations that may be encountered in practice. Veterinary nurses should not feel intimidated by this new responsibility but embrace it, for it is a positive development, recognizing their skills and professionalism.

In this chapter, a framework is provided, with worked examples, that will allow veterinary nurses to consider any scenario that may be encountered. Occasionally an opportunity to work through a real-life scenario in practice may present itself, for which the given framework can be used. It is advised that the veterinary nurse always acts prudently, establishes the facts and does not over-react. There may be circumstances or relevant information that may not be known to all involved. However, if in doubt student, Listed and Registered Veterinary Nurses should refer to the RCVS or BVNA (if a member) for guidance.

It is essential that veterinary nurses are clear about their role within the profession and the personal responsibilities that they may have within the practice. Decisions they make should be carefully considered, as they are not without consequence. Registered Veterinary Nurses are accountable for their actions and, as a result, they must ensure that the actions they take are responsible and can be justified.

When making a decision, reviewing a case or evaluating an incident, four questions need to be considered:

- Has good animal welfare been promoted?
- Has the animal's welfare been compromised?
- Has the law been adhered to?
- Was the decision made ethical?

To make decisions effectively, veterinary nurses must understand the issues related to each question and how the questions interrelate.

Using an analytical framework, facts can be established (primarily from law, professional practice and animal welfare science). Once this factual information has been gathered, an ethical overview can be considered to help reach a satisfactory course of action or outcome. Each component can be considered in its own right but also interlocks to form an analytical framework (Figure 1.1), from which any situation can be evaluated. A further component to be included, that is integral to veterinary nursing, is **professional conduct**, which is aligned with legislative requirements.

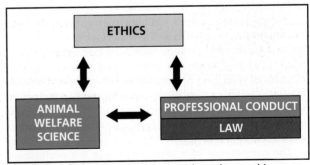

1.1 The components to consider, when making a nursing decision, interlock to form an analytical framework. Professional practice and law are thought of as so closely aligned that they are adjacent. The darker the colour of the component, the greater the degree of certainty regarding the information derived.

Guiding Principles for veterinary nurses

- Animal welfare should be your first consideration in seeking to provide the most appropriate attention for animals committed to your care.
- All animals must be treated humanely and with respect.
- Maintain and continue to develop your professional knowledge and skills.
- Provide emergency first aid and pain relief.
- Report where there are concerns about animal welfare.
- Monitor and review nursing practice with the aim of constantly improving your own nursing care (see Chapter 14 and Appendix 5).
- Foster and maintain a good relationship with clients, earning their trust, respecting their views and protecting client confidentiality.
- Uphold the good reputation of the veterinary nursing profession.
- Ensure the integrity of statements signed by veterinary nurses.
- Foster, and endeavour to maintain, good relationships with your professional colleagues.
- Understand and comply with legal obligations in relation to the supply, administration, safe-keeping and, if a suitably qualified person (SQP) working from registered premises, prescription of veterinary medicinal products (see Chapter 8).
- Familiarize yourself with, and observe, the relevant legislation in relation to veterinary nurses as individual members of the profession and as employers, employees and business owners.
- Respond promptly, fully and courteously to complaints and criticism.

A veterinary nurse must:

- Behave with integrity in all professional appointments. Integrity implies not merely honesty but the need to strive for objectivity in all professional judgements
- Not accept or perform work that they have not been trained to do or are not competent to undertake, unless the veterinary nurse obtains such advice and assistance that will enable them to carry out the work competently
- Conduct themselves with courtesy and consideration towards all with whom they come into contact during the course of performing their work
- Provide suitable nursing care
- Be familiar with the Veterinary Surgeons Act 1966 and the Animal Welfare Act 2006
- Not cause any patient to suffer by carrying out any unnecessary mutilation, excessive restraint or discipline or by failing to assist with the maintenance of adequate pain control and relief of suffering
- Be aware of the exceptions for Listed, Registered and student veterinary nurses in accordance with the Veterinary Surgeons Act 1966 (Schedule 3 Amendment) Order 2002
- Not disclose to any third party any information about a client or their animal either given by the client, or revealed by clinical examination or by post-mortem examination
- Comply with the Data Protection Act 1984. Disclosure of records may be ordered in disciplinary or court hearings, and the RCVS may request copies of case records routinely in the course of investigating a complaint
- Be aware of the exceptions as they apply and the advice notes published by the RCVS from time to time
- Maintain professional competence, including meeting mandatory CPD (continuing professional development) requirements.

The RCVS Guide to Professional Conduct for Veterinary Nurses

The RCVS Guide to Professional Conduct for Veterinary Nurses (RCVS, 2010) identifies the key responsibilities of veterinary nurses to their patients, clients, the public and professional colleagues, as well as their responsibilities under the law. It sets out the fundamental principles and responsibilities that may be applied to veterinary nurses working in all areas of veterinary practice. Failure to observe the Guide may not itself constitute professional misconduct but will be taken into account in assessing the conduct of a veterinary nurse. At the time of writing, the Guide is under review (see www.rcvs.org.uk for updates).

The competence of a veterinary nurse is a professional requirement for the granting of registration (and is therefore assessed by monitoring). Ethical principles are likely to be most commonly applied to the situations in which veterinary nurses work, and experience from other professions has shown it is in this respect that veterinary nurses are likely to need detailed guidance.

Schedule 3 procedures

Veterinary nurses must be familiar with the Veterinary Surgeons Act 1966 and, in particular, the guidance pertaining to Schedule 3 of the Act (amended 2002). Under the Veterinary Surgeons Act 1966, the general rule is that only a veterinary surgeon may practise veterinary surgery.

Veterinary surgery is defined in the Act as the:

- Diagnosis of diseases in, and injuries to, animals including tests performed on animals for diagnostic purposes
- Giving of advice based upon such diagnosis
- Medical or surgical treatment of animals
- Performance of surgical operations on animals.

Schedule 3 of the Act, however, allows anyone to give first aid in an emergency for the purpose of saving life and relieving suffering. This can include the owner of an animal, a member of the owner's household, or an employee of the owner. They may also give it minor medical treatment. There are a number of other exceptions to the general rule, mainly relating to farm animals.

Veterinary nurses may administer first aid and look after animals in ways that do not involve the practice of veterinary surgery. They can also carry out the procedures specified in paragraphs 6 and 7 of Schedule 3 to the Veterinary Surgeons Act 1966 as amended by the Veterinary Surgeons Act 1966 (Schedule 3 Amendment) Order 2002.

Paragraph 6 of the Schedule applies to veterinary nurses whose names are either entered on the List or the Register maintained by the RCVS. Listed nurses may administer 'any medical treatment or any minor surgery (not involving entry into a body cavity)' under veterinary direction. The Schedule does not, however, authorize a veterinary nurse to carry out any of a number of procedures that are specified in Part II of the Schedule. These excluded procedures include the castration of a horse, pony, ass or mule, the castration or spaying of a cat or dog, and a number of other procedures relating to farm animals. The animal must be under the care of a veterinary surgeon and the treatment must be carried out at the veterinary surgeon's direction. The veterinary surgeon must also be the employer of the veterinary nurse or be acting on behalf of the nurse's employer. The directing veterinary surgeon must be satisfied that the veterinary nurse is qualified to carry out the treatment or surgery.

Paragraph 7 of the Schedule applies to student veterinary nurses. A student veterinary nurse is defined as someone enrolled for the purpose of training as a veterinary nurse at an approved training and assessment centre or a veterinary practice approved by such a centre. A student veterinary nurse can administer 'any medical treatment or any minor surgery (not involving entry into a body cavity)' under veterinary direction. Schedule 3 does not, however, allow the student veterinary nurse to castrate a horse, pony, ass or mule, castrate or spay a cat or dog, or carry out certain procedures relating to farm animals. Animals must be under the care of a veterinary surgeon and the treatment must be carried out at the veterinary surgeon's direction. The veterinary surgeon must also be the employer of the student veterinary nurse or be acting on behalf of the nurse's employer. The treatment or minor surgery must be carried out in the course of the student veterinary nurse's training and must be supervised by a veterinary surgeon or a Registered Veterinary Nurse. In the case of surgery, the supervision of a student must be direct, continuous and personal.

The Act does not define 'any medical treatment or any minor surgery (not involving entry into a body cavity)'. It is important, therefore, that veterinary nurses only carry out medical treatment or minor surgery after considering in each individual case whether they are competent to do so, taking into account their training and experience, the nature of the treatment or procedure and the condition of the patient. The directing veterinary surgeon should take the same matters into account in deciding whether the veterinary nurse is qualified to carry out the treatment when giving out directions.

Anaesthesia

Only Listed or Registered Veterinary Nurses and student veterinary nurses enrolled with the RCVS may carry out the maintenance and monitoring of anaesthesia (see Chapter 23).

- A veterinary nurse may induce anaesthesia by the administration of a *specific quantity* of medicine when directed by a veterinary surgeon ▶

  – A veterinary nurse *is not permitted to administer incremental anaesthesia*
- A veterinary nurse may monitor a patient during anaesthesia and recovery
- Maintaining anaesthesia is the responsibility of the veterinary surgeon; however, a suitably trained person may assist by acting as the veterinary surgeon's hands (to provide assistance which does not involve practising veterinary surgery), e.g. by moving the dials on an anaesthetic machine (RCVS, 2010).

Administering medicine incrementally or to effect, to induce and maintain anaesthesia, may only be carried out by a veterinary surgeon.

Consent to treatment

The RCVS Guide to Professional Conduct for Veterinary Surgeons states that the client's informed consent to treatment must be obtained unless delay would adversely affect the animal's welfare (to give informed consent, clients must be aware of the risks).

What is consent?

- Consent is the owner's formal agreement to the medical or surgical course of action proposed, which should ideally also include acknowledgement of an estimate of the associated costs.
- Consent does not have to be written, although it is useful to be able to produce a signed consent form in the event of a dispute.
- If a person who is not the registered owner gives written consent, they should sign the consent form as 'Owner's agent' and state their relationship to the owner.
- Consent must be 'informed'. The owner must understand the nature of the procedure to be undertaken, and the risks and possible side-effects that may ensue.
- Owners must understand what they are signing.
- It is no longer enough to add the catch-all phrase, 'and all other procedures that may be considered necessary', without some explanation as to what they might be. Such procedures will involve additional cost, and possibly additional risk, and the various options should be explained beforehand.
- Consent may include reference to the use of unauthorized drugs. Owners should understand why it is sometimes necessary to use a medication 'off-label' (see Chapter 8) and must give consent for their animal to receive such treatment.

Who can give consent?

If the veterinary nurse is delegated the responsibility of dealing with obtaining consent then they must assume the same responsibilities as a veterinary surgeon in this regard.

- They should be satisfied that the person being dealt with is the owner registered in the clinical records.

- If not the owner, they should be satisfied that the person has the authority to give consent.
- If the animal is presented by one half of a couple (i.e. joint owners), they should be sure that the wishes of the presenting owner are also those of the one who is not present.
- If the animal is presented by the owner of a boarding kennel in the owner's absence, there should be a satisfactory agreement between them that delegates authority to the kennel or cattery owner.
- If the animal is presented by a young person, it must be clear that they are legally competent to give consent. Unfortunately, there is no clear legal ruling on this point. While a minor is defined as someone under 16, and an 18-year-old is an adult, there is a grey area between the two. In such cases it is up to the veterinary surgeon to make a decision, based on their judgement, as to the capability of the client to understand both what they are proposing to do and the consequences.
- If the animal is presented on behalf of an owner by a carer, it must be clear that the carer has the owner's authority to authorize treatment.

Informed consent

Informed consent is an essential part of any contract. It can only be given by a client who has had the opportunity to consider the options for treatment, and has had the significance and risks explained to them. Cost may also be relevant to the client's decision. If any procedure is to be performed by a veterinary student, a veterinary nurse or other member of the support staff, the client should be made fully aware of the fact. Consent can be expressed orally, or in writing, or by implication.

Obtaining consent is a process. The signature of the client on a consent form is the culmination of discussions that should have gone before. Clients should be encouraged to ask questions and be given time to consider the information provided during the process of obtaining consent. Obtaining consent is the responsibility of the veterinary surgeon with the animal under his or her care, although the job may be delegated to the veterinary nurse or other competent staff at the practice. The importance of communicating effectively with clients throughout a case on continuing treatment options, as well as any escalation of fees, is an essential part of maintaining consent. If a client's consent is in any way limited or qualified, contemporaneous notes of this should be made on the clinical records. If the client's consent is in any way limited or qualified or specifically withheld, veterinary surgeons must accept that their own preference for a certain course of action cannot override the client's specific wishes other than on exceptional welfare grounds (RCVS Guide to Professional Conduct for Veterinary Surgeons).

Animal welfare

Promoting good animal welfare is a key element of the veterinary nurses' guiding principles (see above). Before it can be decided whether good welfare has been promoted (or compromised), a working understanding of what is meant by the concept of animal welfare needs to be reached, as it means different things to different people in different contexts.

The science of animal welfare

Animal welfare science is a relatively young discipline but is one of the most comprehensive, drawing on all branches of biology, including behavioural ecology, evolution, ethics, animal behaviour, genetics and neuroscience. As a science it asks three questions (Dawkins, 2006):

1. Is the animal conscious?
2. How can good and bad welfare be assessed?
3. How can science be used to improve animal welfare in practice?

Establishing a **working definition** of animal welfare is essential in order to assess whether an animal's welfare can be considered good or bad, thus enabling, if necessary, recommendations to be made on how to improve it. A variety of definitions for animal welfare have been put forward (Figure 1.2).

Popular definition	The quality of life perceived by the animal: A life worth living
Broom (1986)	The state of the animal as regards its ability to cope with its environment
Dawkins (2004)	Are they healthy? Do they have what they want?
Webster (2005)	Fit and feeling good: Animal welfare is determined by the animal's capacity to avoid suffering and sustain fitness

1.2 Four definitions of animal welfare.

Dawkins' (2004) definition of animal welfare is a useful one to apply when trying to assess welfare definitively. It simply asks two questions:

- Are the animals healthy?
- Do they have what they want?

If the answer to both of these questions is yes, then there is confidence that the animals in question are experiencing good welfare. The first question is relatively easy to answer and is, indeed, the *raison d'être* of the veterinary and veterinary nursing professions. However, at this point it can be realized that a significant number of animals encountered by veterinary nurses will be experiencing a compromised state of welfare by virtue of the fact they are ill and have been brought into the veterinary practice by their owners.

The second question is harder to address and, very importantly, considers the mental state of the animal. It also highlights the importance of animal consciousness, or sentience, as a key to understanding welfare: *if an animal is consciously aware of what it is experiencing, the potential for suffering is increased.* It also raises the issue of whether an animal's **wants** are the most important thing to consider – is it better to consider its **needs**?

Determining wants and needs

In animal welfare science this is carried out by using choice and preference tests. Refining these tests further can allow the animal to illustrate the strength of its preference by how hard it is prepared to work for access to a resource or conditions conducive to performing a desired behaviour (Figure 1.3).

Dogs housed individually in kennels in an animal shelter were given the opportunity to work for three different environmental enrichments:

- Access to a toy
- Contact with another dog
- Contact with a human.

The dogs were trained to press a lever to open a door between them and the enrichment reward. The number of times they pressed the lever was interpreted as a measure of desirability of the particular reward accessed. This was compared to how hard the dogs were prepared to work for a known desirable reward, i.e. food. Results showed that, as expected, the dogs worked hardest to obtain food and that human contact was significantly more important to the dogs in the study than either contact with another dog or access to a toy.

1.3 A preference test for dogs carried out in a dog shelter in Slovenia (Kos, 2005). This kind of information is highly informative and can be used to shape policy for dogs housed in similar environments.

Unfortunately, animals, like humans, do not always choose the best option for their long-term wellbeing. For example, if offered the choice between a salad and a bag of sweets, a person may well choose the sweets even though the salad is considered healthier. The decision that is made is motivated by a different influence, such as taste or a previous pleasurable experience. It is therefore important to distinguish between what an animal wants (its choice) and what it needs to meet requirements for its own physical and mental wellbeing.

Therefore, for the purposes of completing an animal welfare assessment, the second question in the definition above can be refined to:

- Does the animal have what it needs?

Quality of life

The concept of quality of life (QoL) was originally developed in human medicine to assess the potential benefits of treatments to human welfare. Benson and Rollin (2004) discuss animal welfare within this ethical context and outline three different, but overlapping, types of concern about the QoL of animals (Figure 1.4).

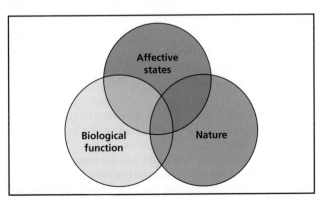

1.4 When considering an animal's quality of life, there are three different, but overlapping, types of concern.

Biological functioning needs little explanation and considers parameters such as normal health, growth, behaviour and development. It is summarized by one of the previously mentioned welfare definitions: *the state of an animal as it attempts to cope with its environment* (Broom, 1986). This is useful, but is it comprehensive enough?

Affective states refer to an animal's emotions or feelings. Particular consideration needs to be given with regard to unpleasant states such as fear, pain, hunger and distress. This assumes that the subjective states of animals can be assessed scientifically by examining an animal's preferences and motivations, linking back to the emphasis on welfare relating to the mental state of animals as well as their biological functioning. Parallels can be drawn between this and the human concept of Maslow's hierarchy of needs (Hagerty, 1999) in which welfare levels increase as the individual's physiological and psychological needs are met. Such effects may even be synergistic.

The last of the interlocking perspectives is the **ability of the animal to lead a natural life**. It is important for an animal to be raised in a manner that suits the needs of the species and allows it to fulfil its full behavioural repertoire (Benson and Rollin, 2004). Allowing animals to live in accordance with their basic nature will allow them to live in an established but adapted manner and to develop physically and mentally as considered to be normal for that species. An inability to meet these needs can seriously affect an animal's welfare. This may well manifest itself in veterinary practice when clients bring in animals with a range of what are considered to be behavioural problems.

Anthropomorphism and anthropocentrism

When considering the needs of animals it is important to remember that human beings can only make an educated guess as to how animals perceive the world. Humans tend to evaluate reality exclusively in terms of their own values and this is called **anthropocentrism**. However, animals interpret the world in different ways. For example, it is easy to forget that vision is not always the primary sense used by animals to interpret the world; e.g. both cats and dogs rely heavily on their sense of smell to inform them of their environment.

Some behaviours are often misinterpreted. For example, it is entirely normal for a cat to bring home a bird or a mouse, yet humans will often see this as an undesirable behaviour and indeed may even be tempted to think the cat has done it maliciously. This is an example of **anthropomorphism**, or the attribution of human characteristics to animals.

It is important always to consider how the animal perceives its environment and to adapt care and conditions accordingly. For example, housing animals of a prey species next to species that would naturally be their predators should be avoided.

Animal welfare legislation

The primary legislation relating to animal welfare in the UK is the **Animal Welfare Act 2006,** which defines acceptable welfare of ALL animals in the United Kingdom. This Act is based on the concept of the Five Freedoms (Figure 1.5; see also Chapter 12), which were first proposed by the Farm Animal Welfare Council in 1979 and initially provided guidelines for an acceptable level of welfare in farmed animals and superseded the 1911 Protection of Animals Act. The content

1. **Freedom from Hunger and Thirst**
   by ready access to fresh water and diet to maintain health and vigour.
2. **Freedom from Discomfort**
   by providing an appropriate environment including shelter and a comfortable resting area.
3. **Freedom from Pain, Injury or Disease**
   by prevention or rapid diagnosis and treament.
4. **Freedom to express Normal Behaviour**
   by providing sufficient space, proper facilities and company of the animal's own kind.
5. **Freedom from Fear and Distress**
   by ensuring conditions and treatment which avoid mental suffering.

1.5   The Five Freedoms.

of the Animal Welfare Act 2006 is considered in greater depth later in this chapter.

Codes of practice for the welfare of a range of companion animals, including cats, dogs, horses and privately owned non-human primates, have been produced by Defra and are a useful reference guide to both veterinary professionals and the general public. These codes also play a role in prosecutions made under the Animal Welfare Act 2006, outlining best practice. If a defendant can demonstrate that they have been following the codes, this will act in their favour. Veterinary nurses will find such codes especially useful when advising clients on best practice for addressing their pets' needs.

To summarize, animal welfare theory comprises three key components: a definition of welfare; the Five Freedoms; and quality of life considerations – all of which interrelate (Figure 1.6).

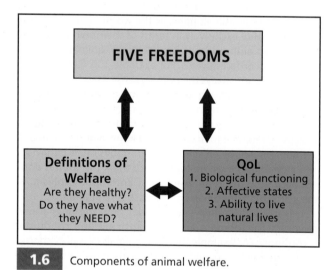

1.6   Components of animal welfare.

Animal welfare in veterinary nursing

The next step is to consider the direct application within the context of veterinary nursing of the two questions:

- Are they healthy?
- Do they have what they need?

It is easy to see how veterinary nursing relates to both the first question and to the physiological components of the second when caring for animals whose welfare is compromised due to illness. For example:

- Giving care during consultations
- Giving care in surgery
- Giving post-surgical care
- Administering medication (and showing clients how to properly medicate their animals at home)
- Advising on duty of care issues, such as dietary and exercise needs.

It is more difficult, perhaps, to see how veterinary nurses can influence the psychological needs of the animals in their care. However, armed with the knowledge of animals' needs derived from animal welfare science, two areas become apparent:

- Care plans (see Chapter 14)
- The behavioural needs of 'problem' animals (see Chapter 11).

Care plans

Care plans are crucial to improving an animal's welfare when it is already compromised. It is important to remember that the welfare of an animal includes its own *perceptions*; as humans, we have to avoid anthropomorphism and anthropocentrism as much as possible, and try to consider the situation from the animal's perspective:

- It has been removed from its own environment and the stability and reassurance that will provide
- It has been removed from familiar people and is now surrounded by strangers
- It may have separation-related problems
- It is now housed in a stark environment full of unfamiliar sights, smells and sounds
- Space is restricted and there is no possibility for retreat
- It may have been restrained and examined, or been given necessary but painful treatments
- Prey species may be housed within sight, smell or sound of predator species.

Any of these will be stressful for the animal and some may not cope very well. Many will be experiencing the adrenaline-driven flight/fight response. In light of this, a well constructed individualized patient care plan is invaluable for addressing the animal's welfare needs during its time in the veterinary nurse's care and minimizing stress to the animal during its time in the practice.

Behavioural needs

Many animals admitted to a veterinary practice exhibit what their owners consider to be problem behaviour. A well informed veterinary nurse will realize that some of these behaviours arise from ill-informed owners keeping animals in a way that is not optimal. This may be due to an owner's overly anthropomorphic perspective.

Advising clients on these issues and the impacts they have on their pets will hopefully improve the long-term welfare of the animals. Through sharing this information with new pet owners, such as at a puppy party, veterinary nurses may be able to prevent such behavioural problems developing in the first place.

Accountability and the law

Veterinary nurses hold a position of responsibility. They are professionally accountable to the RCVS, as well as having a contractual accountability to their employer. They are also accountable to the law for their actions.

When deciding on whether a particular course of action should be taken, it is important to ensure that such action would not break the law. There are many pieces of legislation that affect the veterinary nurse (Figure 1.7), including, for example, those relating to employment and health and safety (see Chapters 2 and 9). Veterinary Nurses should also be aware of their responsibilities as witnesses to fact, as professional witnesses, or as expert witnesses in any civil or criminal proceedings in which they may be involved.

Legislation relevant to veterinary practice includes:

- Veterinary Surgeons Act 1966
- Animal Welfare Act 2006
- Animal Health and Welfare (Scotland) Act 2006
- Veterinary Medicines Regulations 2006
- Health and Safety at Work etc. Act 1974
- Ionising Radiations Regulations 1999
- Control of Substances Hazardous to Health Regulations 2002
- Data Protection Act 1998
- Animals (Scientific Procedures) Act 1986
- Equality Act 2010.

Also other legislation exists pertaining to employment, Inland Revenue, VAT and social security, disease control, animal breeding, public health and zoonoses.

Types of law

A veterinary nurse needs to be mindful of two types of law: **criminal** and **civil**. Each serves a different purpose, and veterinary nurses or veterinary surgeons could be involved in either. They may be called as expert witnesses, often in welfare cases, under criminal law, or prosecuted themselves for not obeying the law (e.g. by practising as a veterinary surgeon when not a registered member of the RCVS). However, if negligence cases were brought by owners against a veterinary practice, this would occur under civil legislation.

Criminal law

The purpose of this type of legislation is **to maintain law and order and protect the public**. The prosecutor can be either the State (the police or Crown Prosecution Service) or, in the case of animal welfare legislation, an organization such as the RSPCA. The case will be heard within a Magistrates' Court or a Crown Court. The case must be proven 'beyond reasonable doubt'. If found guilty, the defendant may be given a conditional discharge, a fine, a community order or a custodial sentence. In addition, the offender may be disqualified from keeping animals. Any of these outcomes will leave the individual with a criminal record, which will have a serious impact on their future.

Civil law

The purpose of this type of law is to uphold the rights of the individual. An individual, referred to as the plaintiff, instigates the case against a defendant if they feel their rights have been affected or they have suffered loss.

The case will be heard in a County Court or a High Court and a judge will decide, on the 'balance of probability', whether the person being taken to court is 'liable' or 'not liable'. If found liable, the defendant will be required to pay damages to the plaintiff and the costs of the plaintiff in bringing the action. Other remedies, such as injunctions, may also be imposed on the defendant by the court.

Year	Legislation
1911	**The 1911 Protection of Animals Act** consolidated existing animal welfare legislation, primarily Martins Act of 1822. It became an offence if a person 'shall cruelly beat, kick, ill-treat, over-ride, over-drive, over-load, torture, infuriate, or terrify any animal, or shall cause or procure, or being the owner, permit any unnecessary suffering to be so caused to any domestic animal'. However, whilst the Act promoted animal welfare a prosecution could only take place once unnecessary suffering had been inflicted.
1966	**The Veterinary Surgeons Act** was established in 1966 to make 'provision for the management of the veterinary profession, for the registration of veterinary surgeons and veterinary practitioners, for regulating their professional education and professional conduct and for cancelling or suspending registration in cases of misconduct; and for connected purposes'.
1991	It was not until 1991 that the Veterinary Surgeons Act was amended to make provision for veterinary nurses. The **Schedule 3 Amendment**, commonly referred to as Schedule 3, was added which allows RCVS listed Veterinary Nurses to administer 'any medical treatment or any minor surgery (not involving entry into a body cavity)' under veterinary direction.
2002	In 2002 Schedule 3 was further amended to allow RCVS-enrolled student veterinary nurses to carry out the same tasks under supervision. Listed or Registered Veterinary Nurses or those enrolled with the RCVS as student nurses should 'act within the remit of Schedule 3 of the Veterinary Surgeons Act and in doing so should only carry out tasks which they are confident and competent in, in accordance with the Act'.
2006	**The Animal Welfare Act 2006** consolidated all welfare legislation created or amended since the 1911 Protection of Animals Act and, significantly, introduced a legal duty of care for pet owners, requiring them to meet the needs of their pets, based upon the Five Freedoms (see Figure 1.5). This permits an improvement notice to be served in circumstances where animals are kept without their needs being met. Such a notice outlines the necessary steps to be taken, within a specified period of time, to prevent the animal from suffering. Should the improvement notice not be acted upon steps can be taken before suffering actually occurs.

1.7 A timeline of legislation.

The role of the RCVS

The role of the RCVS is to maintain the register of veterinary nurses that are deemed fit to practise and to define the standards for the education, clinical practice, and professional conduct of veterinary nurses. This includes:

- Standards for education and training
- Standards for continuing competence
- Powers to investigate professional complaints
- Powers to discipline
- Maintenance of the Register of Veterinary Nurses.

The Guide to Professional Conduct defines the acceptable professional conduct required by the veterinary nurse and confirms the post-registration education and training required to maintain professional competence. Registered Veterinary Nurses are currently required to complete 15 hours/year or 45 hours over 3 years (2 days/year) of relevant continuing education/training based on their individual practice/development/ job role.

Ethics

The word 'ethics' is not new to veterinary nursing – veterinary nurses have been encouraged to think about ethics for a number of years. The RCVS veterinary nursing syllabus published in 1991 required that students be familiar with the 'ethical aspect' associated with areas such as 'working relationships', 'confidentiality of information' and 'the code of conduct'. It was not until the RCVS veterinary nursing syllabus of 2006 that students were asked to explore ethics and morality within the context of veterinary nursing practice by utilizing ethical schools of thought and, as a result, veterinary nurses have begun to identify and explore ethical issues and challenge practice.

Ethics and morality

In simple terms:

- **Morality** tells us if an action is 'right' or 'wrong', or 'good' or 'bad'
- **Ethics** explores the rationale behind the decision.

Example

Many believe that it is 'right' or 'good' that pregnant stray cats are neutered, even though this will cause the death of unborn kittens. At first glance this may seem unreasonable; however, by exploring the reasons behind this decision the procedure seems to become more acceptable:

- Many would argue that adding to the cat population is unacceptable because there are already a large number of stray cats in need of homes. Neutering a pregnant cat not only prevents the birth of more kittens but also stops the cat from having further litters
- However, some may believe that it is 'wrong' or 'bad' to neuter a pregnant cat as this will cause the death of the unborn kittens, which they feel is unacceptable. ▶

- Some may even believe that neutering in general is not justified, e.g. because they feel it causes unnecessary suffering.

From this example it is clear that what one person believes is 'right' or 'good' may seem totally 'wrong' or 'bad' to someone else.

Making choices

Many decisions are made and actions undertaken without much thought. For example, telling the truth about whether a drug has or has not been administered is instinctively the right thing to do.

But how do we know what is a 'right' or 'good' action?

Certain situations may feel 'wrong' or 'bad'. For example, assisting in the treatment of an animal when a participant feels that euthanasia would be in the best interest of the patient as its quality of life is compromised. There are also times when an individual just cannot decide whether something is 'good' or 'bad', 'right' or 'wrong' – a real ethical dilemma!

There are many factors that affect the way humans think and feel. For example, the way a child is raised, peer-group factors, religious beliefs and educational background can all play a part in establishing the way we behave. Through training and the experiences gained in practice, veterinary nurses will continue to develop their views and opinions.

For many years philosophers have been attempting to answer the question of how decisions about 'right' and 'wrong' are made. Theories have been written, rules have been prescribed, and frameworks drawn up. All of these provide useful tools to help with the decision-making process.

Ethical schools of thought

There are many theories; however, several can be grouped under two headings.

- **Non-consequentialism**: Non-consequentialists decide whether an action is 'right' or 'wrong' by examining obligations. They claim that the 'right' thing should be done, whatever the consequences might be. These are known as *deontological* theories. For example, an elderly client who has been with the practice a long time asks the veterinary nurse on duty if she thinks her undershot, bow-legged West Highland White Terrier is a good example of the breed type. The client has clearly asked the veterinary nurse for an opinion; the truth must be told because it is 'wrong' to lie.
- **Consequentialism**: Consequentialists examine the outcome of an action to decide whether it is 'good' or 'bad'. *Utilitarianism* is probably the best known consequentialist theory. Going back to the above example, the veterinary nurse believes that the dog is a poor example of the breed type but would decide that it is better to tell the client that her dog is a good example if the consequences of saying what she actually believes would not produce a 'good' outcome (see below).

Deontology

Deontology is a non-consequentialist theory. Deontologists believe that there are 'rules' that must be followed, no matter what the consequences of the action might be. It is therefore the 'actions' that are 'right' or 'wrong', not the consequences. This is termed the **categorical imperative** (categorical meaning definite or unconditional; imperative meaning crucial or vital).

Immanuel Kant (1724–1804) firmly believed in this theory and offered many reasons why, for example, a person should never lie. Kant stated that in order for an action to be considered 'right', consideration should be given to what would happen if the action were followed by all people at all times, regardless of the situation. If it were concluded that the action should always be carried out, this would make it a 'universal law'. If not, the action should not be carried out. Kant believed that it would not be in the best interests of society for people to lie and therefore that lying should not be a 'universal law', reaching the conclusion that it is 'wrong' to lie.

Example

The practice principal has asked all staff to reduce the amount of disinfectant used by increasing the dilution rate of a disinfectant, stating that this was one of many cost-cutting exercises that needed to be put into place. The veterinary nursing staff argue that by increasing the dilution of disinfectants, the likelihood of hospital-acquired infections would probably increase. The practice principal states that this is a risk that has to be taken.

Using the *categorical imperative* as a way of deciding whether this new protocol should be adopted, a question to ask would be whether it would be acceptable for all veterinary practices around the world to dilute disinfectants, thereby increasing the likelihood of hospital-acquired infections. If it were thought that this would be acceptable, the protocol should be implemented. If not, then a refusal should be given supported by the rationale.

This philosophy is not accepted by all, however. Many philosophers have challenged the idea of 'universal rules'. It is often easy to argue that there are times when a 'rule' may be challenged if a situation demands it. Remembering the earlier example of the West Highland White Terrier, it might be believed that it is 'wrong' to lie but is this a sentiment that should always be followed, especially considering the fact that a lie on this occasion could possibly have an adverse effect on the client?

Philosophers also challenge the idea by arguing that there may be times when two 'universal laws' may conflict, such as in the following scenario. Many philosophers argue that rules cannot be absolute and some deontologists accept that this is sometimes the case and that rules may sometimes need to be prioritized.

Example

Miss B books an appointment as she would like her 3-year-old St Bernard, Tippi, euthanased as she is emigrating to Africa and does not think that Tippi would be able to tolerate the heat. Both the veterinary surgeon and the veterinary nurse discuss the option of re-homing with Miss B; however, she is adamant that she does not want to take up this option. The veterinary nurse suggests that they place Tippi in a kennel to allow Miss B a little more time to decide. Miss B is to call at 4.30pm to confirm whether she still wishes Tippi to be euthanased. At 4.30pm Miss B calls to say that she has not changed her mind. The ▶

veterinary surgeon and veterinary nurse discuss this dilemma and decide that they have two choices:

- To euthanase Tippi as requested
- To re-home Tippi but inform Miss B that he has been euthanased.

If they decide to re-home Tippi and to lie to Miss B they will have broken the 'universal law' stating that 'it is wrong to lie'. However, two conflicting rules could apply in this situation:

- Rule one: 'It is wrong to lie'
- Rule two: 'It is wrong to facilitate the euthanasia of healthy animals'.

NB There are serious legal and professional implications for veterinary surgeons and nurses in not carrying out an owner's request and not telling the truth.

Utilitarianism

Utilitarians believe that a decision should always be taken to ensure that the consequences are the best possible for all involved: 'the greatest good for the greatest number'.

Consider a group of students planning a Friday night out. Four students wish to go to the pub while two want to go to the cinema. Using the utilitarian principle the students should go to the pub. Four students would be satisfied with the outcome whilst two would be dissatisfied, thereby fulfilling the principle of 'the greatest good for the greatest number'. Whilst this outcome may be 'good' for those that wanted to go to the pub it is 'bad' for the people that wanted to go to the cinema. When using this philosophy not everyone 'wins'. Of course, decision-making is not always that simple. It often involves many people with many different ideas. In these situations utilitarians suggest that a cost:benefit analysis is performed.

Example

Imagine a situation where a veterinary surgeon has decided to amputate both hindlimbs from Molly, a 10-year-old Border Collie belonging to Mrs P, a pensioner, in preference to euthanasia. The veterinary nurse is horrified by the prospect but it is clear that the veterinary surgeon is very enthusiastic about the idea and is investigating suitable 'carts' for Molly to use after the operation. A cost:benefit analysis can be performed to identify the 'greatest good for the greatest number'.

Step one: List all the parties that will be affected by the decision:

- Molly – will have to adapt to her new condition
- Mrs P – will need to help and support Molly; there will also be financial costs
- The veterinary surgeon – will be operating on Molly
- The veterinary nurses – will be caring for Molly during her stay at the practice
- Society as a whole – it is not common to see dogs with two legs amputated; what will the public think?
- The practice – effects on its staff and reputation
- The veterinary and veterinary nursing professions – would this procedure be a positive or negative step?

continues ▶

continued

Step two: Identify the potential 'costs' and 'benefits' of the procedure to each of the affected parties.
Let us briefly consider Mrs P and Molly.

Costs
- Mrs P would need to dedicate additional time to looking after Molly. She would also have increased strain placed on her own body as she may have to help Molly in and out of the house and the cart. The operation, which may or may not be successful, is also expensive and Molly is not insured.
- Molly would have to adapt to her new situation. She would not be able to satisfy needs such as chasing play. She may not adapt well to the cart, which she might find painful. When in the cart she would not be able to lie down if she wanted to.

Benefits
- Mrs P would continue to have Molly for companionship.
- Molly would still be alive. She would continue to have the companionship of Mrs P. Molly might respond well to the cart and adapt to her new life very well.

Step three: Once the costs and benefits have been identified for all parties, each needs to be considered.

It is clear from the example of the costs and benefits to Mrs P and Molly that this is not easy. It is difficult to predict the outcome of the operation; e.g. Molly may not take to the cart, or Mrs P may injure herself and be unable to care for Molly, causing additional stress and anxiety.

It can be difficult to weigh up the costs and benefits when people's opinions may differ, some thinking one thing is more important than the other. Animal welfare should be the over-riding concern.

Step four: Make a decision.
There are two options in this scenario:

- Perform the operation to amputate both legs. It may be decided that Mrs P and Molly would benefit more if the operation were performed.

Or

- Do not perform the operation but euthanase Molly. It may be decided that the cost to Molly's quality of life would be too great to allow the procedure to be performed.

From this example it is clear that the decision-making process is not easy. However, the process is useful as it makes people consider all the alternatives. In practice, this is often best achieved as a team, as everyone will have their own thoughts and feelings, ensuring that no cost or benefit is missed and ensuring that it is an unbiased team decision. **The decision is ultimately the owner's, guided by the veterinary surgeon.**

When faced with an ethical dilemma it is important to appreciate that there are often many possible outcomes, some of which are agreeable and others are not. It is essential that, whatever the decision, the veterinary nurse find ways of minimizing the impact of that decision. For example, if it was decided that Molly's operation would go ahead and

she would have two legs amputated, the nurse would need to ensure that:

- A care plan was drawn up to facilitate her recovery (see Chapter 14)
- Mrs P was supported throughout the process
- The correct cart was selected and fitted.

By doing all these things, the impact of the decision would be minimized or 'refined'.

Other schools of ethical thought

Veterinary nurses must be aware of other ethical theories (Figure 1.8) in order to help them appreciate how people may justify their decisions and also to allow them to formulate an argument for or against a decision that needs to be made.

Ethical school of thought	A brief description
Animal rights	The animal rights theory suggests that animals of a certain level are similar enough to people to be given the same privileges of law and ethics that people benefit from. This may be a 'right' to life or a 'right' to freedom from pain, for example. The theory suggests that animals should be considered equal to humans in this 'right' and should have their lives preserved and be pain-free as much as any human. Importantly, the theory also states that animals can never be used as a means to an end, consequently they should not be used in farming or experiments any more than people are farmed or experimented on. It is a very comprehensive theory that affords animals the highest level of protection of any of the suggested theories in this chapter
The four principles of medical ethics	Beauchamp and Childress (2009) developed four principles to help assist with the decision-making process. The best decision should: • Do no harm (referred to as non-maleficence) • Promote good (referred to as beneficence) • Allow parties to make their own decision – act autonomously. This can be challenging in veterinary practice where the client, veterinary surgeon and the animal have a right to autonomy • Treat all in a fair and equal way (referred to as justice)
Feminism and the ethics of care	Gilligan (1982) developed the concept that women think differently from men. This does not suggest that one way of thinking is superior or inferior but does suggest that women may have different insights to men. This may have an impact on the decision-making process and, ultimately, the animal, as different sexes would offer different points of view
Virtue ethics	Mullan (2006) states that 'virtue ethics maintains that it is how we are that is important and that if we are a 'virtuous' or 'morally good' person then we will naturally act correctly in accordance with our character'. This is an important point to consider when we think of how we should act as professional veterinary nurses and what the perceptions of a veterinary nurse are. Consider the headline, 'Woman found guilty of animal abuse'. This is in itself shocking, but consider the headline, 'Veterinary nurse found guilty of animal abuse'; this is much more shocking

1.8 Other ethical schools of thought.

Some representative scenarios

It is suggested that you have a copy of the current RCVS Guide to Professional Conduct for Veterinary Nurses by your side as you read through these.

Scenario 1: Nurse clinics

Lottie, a Registered Veterinary Nurse, has been qualified for a year and has been asked by the practice if she would like to help Imogen, the Head Nurse, run and develop the nurse clinics. Lottie is very excited as she has wanted to do this for a while. She has been focusing her CPD on improving her communication skills and has undertaken a nutrition course run by one of the petfood manufacturers in the hope that the practice would ask her to do this. These clinics are advertised as being delivered by a Registered Veterinary Nurse.

In order to understand how the nurse clinics are run, Lottie decides to watch Imogen in action and arranges to help her one evening. Imogen thinks this is a really good idea and is looking forward to Lottie's help. As the evening progresses, Lottie becomes increasingly concerned. The information and advice that Imogen is giving clients seems to be inaccurate and outdated. Lottie is particularly concerned about the advice given to Mrs W about Midge, a 9-year-old obese Labrador with osteoarthritis. Imogen informs Mrs W that the easiest way to promote weight loss is to reduce by half the amount of food Midge is given (adult maintenance diet) and to walk Midge for one hour each evening.

Lottie questions Imogen about the information she has given Mrs W as she is concerned about the advice, leading her to question whether Imogen has been keeping up with her CPD. If this is the case, she wonders whether Imogen can actually be a Registered Veterinary Nurse and decides to ask her. Imogen states that she does not see the point in paying an annual retention fee and upon further discussion Lottie realizes that Imogen has not been to any CPD events since she qualified 5 years ago.

Issue	Regulatory considerations	Legal considerations	Welfare considerations
Imogen is delivering a clinic that is advertised as being run by a Registered Veterinary Nurse, which Imogen is not. In addition, the advice given is outdated and incorrect	Lottie, as an RVN, has an obligation to animals, clients and other members of staff and, as a result, has to act on this information. The veterinary nursing profession has a vital part to play in terms of education and protection in matters of animal welfare and public health. It is the responsibility of a veterinary nurse to ensure that they continue to be Listed or Registered and not mislead the public	A veterinary nurse is a person whose name is entered in the List of Veterinary Nurses (which incorporates the Register of Veterinary Nurses) maintained by the RCVS. As Imogen's name does not appear on any list, she should not be referred to as an RVN. To do so is misleading the public and other members of staff, who may be unaware that she should not be delivering the clinic advertised as being run by an RVN. It is worth noting that Imogen must not perform any 'Schedule 3' tasks delegated to her. Practices should confirm that a 'veterinary nurse' is listed/registered and continues to be listed/registered	Had Mrs W taken Imogen's advice, Midge's welfare would have been compromised. 1. Incorrect and outdated dietary advice. Correct advice would have been to recommend a specifically formulated weight loss diet, therefore keeping the volume of diet consistent and preventing excessive hunger. 2. Ill-informed advice on exercise regime. Increasing exercise in an old dog with an arthritic condition could cause unnecessary pain and suffering. A general health check should have been performed and the veterinary surgeon asked to examine Midge if it was thought the dog required medication to control pain. Mrs W should have been advised to take Midge for short, frequent walks to reduce excessive strain on the joints and could have suggested non-weight-bearing exercise such as hydrotherapy
Imogen has not undertaken any CPD since qualifying 5 years ago	As Imogen is not a Registered Veterinary Nurse she is not required to undertake any CPD. However, it is clear that, although originally qualified, she is not up to date. She should therefore not have been allowed to deliver a nurse clinic. Veterinary nurses have a responsibility to ensure that they maintain and continue to develop their professional knowledge and skills. CPD is mandatory for all veterinary nurses and should be seen as the continuous progression of capability and competence. The required minimum for an RVN is 45 hours over 3 years, with an average of 15 hours/year. It is recognized that most veterinary nurses will do considerably more than this	There may be contractual issues to resolve, as Imogen may have a contract of employment that requires her to maintain her Registration with the RCVS and hence her CPD	Not applicable

Scenario 2: The cat dental

Stan, a student veterinary nurse, admitted a pedigree cat for a 'dental' during a busy Monday morning surgery. The veterinary nurse was on reception duty in the morning and felt under pressure as there was a queue of people waiting at the desk and a road traffic accident victim was on its way in. Stan knew the owner of the cat as she was often in. He asked her to check the consent form, which had been computer-generated with the owner's and the patient's details, and to sign the form. He then took the cat into the ward.

Later that day the veterinary surgeon asked Stan to perform the dental as they were busy with another patient. They asked Stan to de-scale and polish the teeth and inform them of any problems. Stan had only watched a couple of dentals before and felt unsure of what to do, but felt he did not want to let the veterinary team down. He started the procedure and noticed that some of the teeth needed to be removed. As the veterinary surgeon was busy, Stan decided to attempt to take them out himself. He started the procedure and half way through noticed that the cat's mucous membranes were unusually pale. Unfortunately, the animal nursing assistant, who was monitoring the anaesthetic, had not realized that the oxygen had run out and, despite the veterinary surgeon's best attempt to resuscitate the cat, it died.

Issue	Regulatory considerations	Legal considerations	Welfare considerations
Stan appears to have rushed the consent process	It appears the client was unaware who would be undertaking the procedure. Veterinary nurses should ensure that the client is made aware of any procedures to be performed by a Listed or Registered VN. Although Stan may not have known this when the patient was being admitted, the client should have been contacted prior to the procedure being carried out (RCVS, 2010)	Was the consent informed? Did the client understand the procedure that her cat was going to have?	Not applicable
Stan, a student veterinary nurse, agreed to undertake a procedure that he did not feel confident in doing	'Veterinary nurses should keep within their own areas of competence, save for the requirement to provide emergency first aid.' Stan should have informed the veterinary surgeon that he did not feel competent to undertake the task. As a student he should have been supervised	Not applicable	The welfare of the cat could be compromised
Stan decided to 'have a go' at taking out some rotten teeth	'Veterinary nurses should be familiar with and comply with legislation'	In October 2003 the RCVS Advisory Committee decided that dental procedures beyond routine dental hygiene should be considered more than 'minor surgery' due to the potential complications that can occur. The committee stated that 'dental extractions using instruments should be carried out by veterinary surgeons'	Incorrect action might necessitate a repeat procedure
There was no 'bosun's whistle' on the anaesthetic machine and, as a result, the oxygen ran out without anyone noticing	Stan has a responsibility to 'assist with the maintenance of proper standards in relation to in-patient care and supervision'	Not applicable	The welfare of the cat could be compromised
An animal nursing assistant was monitoring the anaesthetic, a task that had been delegated by a student veterinary nurse	In 2007 the RCVS produced 'Advice Note 19' which provides clear guidelines on the 'Maintenance and monitoring of anaesthesia' and the role of the veterinary nurse. (a) Inducing anaesthesia by administration of a specific quantity of medicine directed by a veterinary surgeon may be carried out by a veterinary nurse or, with supervision, a student veterinary nurse, but not any other person. (b) Administering medicine incrementally or to effect, to induce and maintain anaesthesia may be carried out only by a veterinary surgeon. (c) Maintaining anaesthesia is the responsibility of a veterinary surgeon, but a suitably trained person may assist by acting as the veterinary surgeon's hands (to provide assistance which does not involve practising veterinary surgery), e.g. by moving dials. (d) Monitoring a patient	Not applicable	The welfare of the cat could be compromised

continues ▶

continued

Issue	Regulatory considerations	Legal considerations	Welfare considerations
continued An animal nursing assistant was monitoring the anaesthetic, a task that had been delegated by a student veterinary nurse	during anaesthesia and the recovery period is the responsibility of the veterinary surgeon, but may be carried out on his or her behalf by a suitably trained person. (e) The most suitable person to assist a veterinary surgeon to monitor and maintain anaesthesia is a Veterinary Nurse (listed or registered with the RCVS) or, under supervision, a student veterinary nurse (enrolled as a student with the RCVS)		
The death of the cat	Not applicable	Not applicable	It is believed that an overdose of anaesthesia (as used in euthanasia) does not cause suffering. Assuming the cat was anaesthetized and unconscious throughout the procedure, it was not aware and therefore did not suffer. If 'welfare' is what the animal itself perceives, we can be reassured it has not been affected. However, suffering could have occurred if the cat had regained consciousness at any time during the attempts to revive it

What to do if a dilemma cannot be resolved

Concerns about the standard of care given to animals should, in the first instance, be raised with the veterinary nurse's line manager or employer. An internal solution may well be reached and the issues resolved.

If the veterinary nurse continues to have concerns, the next step is to raise the concern with the professional conduct department at the RCVS for advice. If a formal complaint is brought, the complaints procedure would be followed. It is important to remember that complaints cannot be made anonymously. The RCVS cannot follow up a complaint without the name, and express permission, of the person making the complaint and the name of the individual (or practice) implicated.

Veterinary nurses will have insurance cover under their practice's insurance. Registered Veterinary Nurses working as locums could also take out personal insurance cover.

The role of the BVNA

The British Veterinary Nursing Association (BVNA) is an association dedicated to veterinary nursing and undertakes to represent veterinary nurses.

BVNA Mission Statement

The aim of the British Veterinary Nursing Association is to promote animal health and welfare through the ongoing development of professional excellence in veterinary nursing.

The BVNA undertakes to:

- Represent the veterinary nursing profession and specifically its members
- Develop, provide and monitor continuing professional development for veterinary nurses
- Provide education and training for associated individuals and allied professionals
- Promote the veterinary nursing profession and work proactively with other organizations and professions to shape its future development
- Disseminate advice and guidance to its members.

As the representative body, it can provide assistance in the following ways.

- **Legal helpline:** All BVNA members can access the legal helpline. Legal professionals are available to answer all legal enquiries.
- **Industrial relations service:** This service exists to help members act upon advice provided by the legal helpline. For example, the service helps veterinary nurses to compose letters and assists with issues related to bullying, working hours, etc. The service is run by professionals who specialize in employment law.

Acknowledgements

The authors would like to thank Elizabeth Earle, Andrea Jeffery and Martin Whiting for their assistance with this chapter.

Further reading and references

Beauchamp TL and Childress JE (2009) *Principles of Biomedical Ethics, 6th edn.* Oxford University Press, Oxford

Benson GJ and BE Rollin (2004) *The Well-being of Farm Animals: Challenges and Solutions.* Blackwell, New York

Broom DM (1986) Indicators of poor welfare. *British Veterinary Journal* **142**, 524–526

Dawkins MS (2004) Using behaviour to assess animal welfare. *Animal Welfare* **13**, 3–7

Dawkins MS (2006) A user's guide to animal welfare science. *Trends in Ecology and Evolution* **21**(2), 77–82

Fraser D (1997) Animal welfare, science, and ethics. *Animal Welfare* **6**, 97–106

Gilligan C (1982) *In a Different Voice: Psychological Theory and Women's Development.* Harvard University Press, Cambridge, MA

Hagerty MR (1999) Testing Maslow's hierarchy of needs: national quality-of-life across time. *Social Indicators Research* **46**(3), 249–271

King LA (2003) Behavioural evaluation of the psychological welfare and environmental requirements of agricultural research animals: theory, measurement, ethics and practical implications. *Institute of Laboratory Animal Research* **44**(3), 11

Kos U (2005) Do dogs show preferences for certain types of environmental enrichments? *XIIth International Conference of International Society for Animal Hygiene, Warsaw,* pp. 479–483

Main DCJ *et al.* (2007) Formal animal-based welfare assessment in UK certification schemes. *Animal Welfare* **16**, 233–236

Mullan S (2006) Introduction to ethical principles. In: *Ethics, Law and the Veterinary Nurse,* ed. S Pullen and C Gray, pp. 11–22. Elsevier, UK

Pullen S and Gray C (2006) *Ethics, Law and the Veterinary Nurse.* Elsevier, UK

Rachels J and Rachels S (2006) *Elements of Moral Philosophy.* McGraw-Hill, USA

RCVS (2010) *Guide to Professional Conduct for Veterinary Nurses.* www.rcvs.org.uk [currently under review]

Rollin BE (2003) Assessing animal welfare at the farm and group level: the interplay of science and values. *Animal Welfare* **12**, 433–443

Webster J (2005) *Animal Welfare: Limping towards Eden.* UFAW and Blackwell Scientific, Oxford

Wright B (1994) Ethics in Practice. *Veterinary Practice Nurse* **16**(2), 9–10

Useful websites

Advisory, Conciliation and Arbitration Service (ACAS) (may be able to assist with employment issues and offer free advice): www.acas.org.uk

British Small Animal Veterinary Association (BSAVA): www.bsava.com

British Veterinary Association (BVA): www.bva.co.uk

British Veterinary Nursing Association (BVNA): www.bvna.org.uk

Citizens Advice Bureau: www.citizensadvice.org.uk

Department for Environment, Food and Rural Affairs (Defra): www.defra.gov.uk

Health and Safety Executive (HSE): www.hse.gov.uk

Law Society (for details of solicitors who undertake employment work)**:** www.lawsociety.org.uk

Public Concern at Work (PCAW): www.pcaw.co.uk

Royal College of Veterinary Surgeons (RCVS): www.rcvs.org.uk

RSPCA: www.rspca.org.uk

Self-assessment questions

1. What five questions should be asked when evaluating a nursing incident?
2. What are the implications for a Registered Veterinary Nurse of the Schedule 3 amendment?
3. What can an enrolled student veterinary nurse do as defined by the Veterinary Surgeons Act 1966?
4. What is consent and who can give it?
5. State at least six guiding principles of veterinary nursing.
6. How can an RVN incorporate the Five Freedoms into their nursing care of an inpatient?
7. Who can legally monitor veterinary anaesthesia?
8. How much CPD should a Registered Veterinary Nurse be completing per year?
9. Apply the utilitarian theory to an ethical dilemma.
10. State five ethical dilemmas that may be faced in veterinary practice.
11. Think about each of the following statements. Which theory was used when adopting each of them and how could you formulate arguments to oppose them?
    - 'It is "wrong" to euthanase healthy animals' (a philosophy adopted by some rescue centres)
    - 'The administration of postoperative pain killers is not always essential and may add costs to the client's bill'
12. Evaluate the following three scenarios using the framework given in the chapter. What issues can be identified?
    a. Finley has noticed that another RVN has fallen out with one of the veterinary surgeons and they are now refusing to communicate directly with each other. This is not the first time this has happened; however, this morning Finley sees the RVN administering analgesics to a patient without the permission of the veterinary surgeon. Finley questions the nurse who says that she had emailed the vet about her concerns and he had not replied so in the best interests of the patient she was managing the pain herself.
       Consider: Animal welfare issues, legal implications, professional conduct and ethical perspectives.
    b. Sarah has returned from a week's holiday and has arrived on a late shift. Her first duty is to discharge Lily, a German Shepherd Dog that has been hospitalized for a week following surgery to repair a fractured femur. Sarah discusses the discharge instructions with the owner and then asks the client to take a seat while she goes to get Lily. When she sees Lily, Sarah realizes that the dog is covered in urine and also has patches of urine scalding around her back legs. Upon further examination she finds a decubitus ulcer on the left elbow and notes that Lily appears to be very thin. Sarah asks another veterinary nurse for some information and the nurse says that they have been incredibly busy as they have been short staffed while Sarah was on holiday.
       Consider: Animal welfare issues, legal implications, professional conduct and ethical perspectives.
    c. Maya, an RVN, has assisted the veterinary surgeon all morning and has now been asked to prepare the bill, which she is happy to do. When Maya shows the vet what she has done the vet asks her to add on additional surgical time, which increases the bill significantly. The bill is now higher than the estimate given to the client when the dog was admitted. The client has a strong personality and Maya is worried about informing the client of the elevated price, especially as she feels she cannot personally justify the increase.
       Consider: Animal welfare issues, legal implications, professional conduct and ethical perspectives.

Chapter 2

Principles of health and safety

Pam Mosedale

Learning objectives

After studying this chapter, students should be able to:

- **Describe the aims of effective health and safety practice**
- **Identify the principal risks to health and safety in a veterinary practice**
- **Describe and apply safe principles of practice in relation to a range of situations in veterinary practice**
- **Describe the management and reporting of common risks**
- **Identify provisions of relevant legislation to safe veterinary nursing practice**

The aims of effective health and safety practice

Veterinary practice, as with all areas of work, involves some risks to staff, clients and visitors. The aim of an effective health and safety culture in the veterinary context should be for all staff to consider the risks and possible consequences of all activities in the practice as a top priority and to look sensibly at ways to minimize those risks.

The consequences of *not* considering health and safety include:

- Human costs:
  - Employee injury
  - Employee absence
  - Employee ill health
  - Injury to clients.
- Economic costs:
  - Increased staff costs to cover illness/injuries
  - The cost of criminal proceedings as a result of accidents or injuries
  - Loss of business and professional reputation
  - Legal costs arising from civil cases.

Both employers and employees have a duty to consider health and safety in all their work activities.

The legal framework

The primary piece of legislation covering occupational health and safety in the UK is the **Health and Safety at Work etc. Act 1974** (HSWA). The Act places legal duties on employers, the self-employed and employees. Businesses must assess risks in the workplace, consult with and involve employees, take suitable precautions to avoid risk, and review and revise risk assessments as necessary. Full details can be found on the Health and Safety Executive (HSE) website www.hse.gov.uk.

In addition to the Act, there are also a number of Regulations that require veterinary practices to meet certain legal requirements.

Examples of legal requirements for employers:

- To have employers' liability insurance
- To appoint a competent person to deal with health and safety in the practice
- To have a health and safety policy
- To carry out a risk assessment of practice activities
- To provide a safe and healthy environment for workers, including toilets, washing facilities, drinking water and suitable lighting and temperatures to work in
- To train staff to work safely – this includes self-employed workers
- To consult with staff on health and safety issues and listen to their concerns
- To display a health and safety law poster
- To report certain work-related accidents, ill health and incidents under **The Reporting of Injuries, Diseases and Dangerous Occurrences Regulations 1995** (RIDDOR)
- To keep up to date with changes in health and safety legislation
- To carry out a fire safety risk assessment and implement appropriate fire precautionary and protection measures – this includes raising the alarm and evacuation.

Employees also have a responsibility to take care of their own health and safety, as well as that of others who may be affected by their actions.

- Veterinary nurses and other members of staff in a veterinary practice must cooperate with employers and colleagues on health and safety.
- They must not interfere with or misuse any protective clothing or other equipment provided for the safety of staff.
- They must not put themselves or others at risk by what they do, or fail to do, at work.

The practice should provide all necessary protective clothing, train staff members to do their jobs safely, inform them about any risks involved in their work and provide regular health checks if there is any danger of ill health involved in the work (this includes night work).

Concerns about health and safety issues should be discussed with the employer; if the member of staff is not satisfied, the HSE should be contacted without this having repercussions for the member of staff. Staff members have the right to an uninterrupted rest break of at least 20 minutes if working for more than 6 hours at a stretch. Student veterinary nurses under the age of 18 are entitled to a rest break of 30 minutes when their daily working is more than 4.5 hours.

Health and safety law also applies to farm and equine practitioners working mainly from their vehicles and from home. Self-employed veterinary surgeons or locum nurses also have duties towards their own health and safety and that of others affected by their work.

If the practice is part of the RCVS Practice Standards Scheme (PSS), health and safety arrangements will be checked by PSS Inspectors for core standards practices, general practices and hospitals. Details of the PSS scheme requirements for health and safety can be found in the Practice Standards Scheme Manual on the RCVS website www.rcvs.org.uk.

Health and safety policy

Employers must have a health and safety policy in place, setting out the specific arrangements for managing health and safety in the practice. This should inform staff about the partners' or directors' commitment to health and safety in the practice, and how this will be implemented and monitored. The policy should help ensure that risks to staff, clients and visitors are kept as low as is reasonably practical. It should give the name of the person who has day-to-day responsibility for putting the policy into practice, and delegate responsibilities for certain specific areas such as fire safety, first aid and staff training.

If more than five people are employed (even if temporarily) the health and safety policy must be in writing. It should be brought to the attention of all staff and should direct staff to where they may find more information, for example the findings of the practice risk assessments.

The HSWA requires employers to revise the safety policy whenever there are significant changes in the organization or arrangements, for example:

- The introduction of a new process, such as a new cleaning operation
- Additional responsibilities or transfer of responsibilities
- Change of premises
- Changes in legislation.

Risk assessment

A risk assessment should be performed for any potentially hazardous procedure. Put simply, this is an examination of what in the practice could cause harm to people, so that decisions can be made as to whether enough precautions have been taken or more are needed. A risk assessment should:

- Identify the hazard
- Identify who is at risk as a result of the hazard
- Evaluate the seriousness of the risk – insignificant, minor or major
- Assess the probability of it occurring – unlikely, likely or very likely
- Assess any risk to health
- Assess any risk to the environment
- Identify who is responsible for the task or area
- Identify what control measures are already in place
- Identify what protective clothing or equipment are used
- Assess whether any special procedures are needed for first aid, fire, spillage or storage
- Assess whether current control measures are satisfactory and, if not, identify what additional controls are needed
- Identify when and by whom these will be implemented and the date of the next review
- Be reviewed to make sure it remains up to date.

A risk assessment is not an end in itself. The findings must be implemented and action taken where needed to ensure that the risks are properly managed (Figures 2.1 and 2.2).

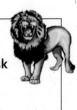

SENSIBLE RISK MANAGEMENT

Remember that Hazard (anything that can cause harm) is not the same as Risk (likelihood harm will occur and its severity)

High Risk   Low Risk

2.1 Sensible risk management. The same hazard does not always present the same risk; it depends on the circumstances and the controls in place. Just because a hazard is present, there is no reason always to fear the worst.

1. Identify the hazards.
2. Decide who may be harmed by each of the hazards and how they may be harmed.
3. Look at how likely it is that harm will occur and how it could be prevented.
4. Record the findings and inform the staff.
5. Review regularly and update if anything changes.

2.2 Risk assessment: five easy steps.

Carrying out a risk assessment

Step 1. Identifying hazards in veterinary practice

A hazard is something that may cause harm. There are some obvious hazards in veterinary practice, such as ionizing radiation, anaesthetic gas pollution and injuries due to bites and scratches from small animals or kicks from horses, and practices are very good at recognizing these. However, there are other hazards associated with activities that are less obvious, such as manual handling, needle-stick injuries and lone working.

A good way to recognize hazards is to ask all staff to walk around the practice and make a list of potential hazards. There are lists in the RCVS Practice Standards Manual of the sort of hazards the practice is expected to have assessed.

Main hazards in veterinary practice are related to:

- Cleanliness/tidiness
- Ionizing radiation
- Handling and restraint of animals
- Manual handling
- Veterinary medicines
- Injection procedures
- Anaesthetic gas pollution
- Slips, trips and falls
- Laboratory procedures
- Chemicals
- Staff security and lone working
- Waste disposal
- Infectious diseases
- Zoonoses
- Risk to pregnant workers
- Stress
- Driving for work
- Transporting animals
- Work equipment
  - Display screen equipment
  - Autoclaves
  - Dental machines
  - Electrical equipment
  - X-ray machine
  - Anaesthetic equipment
  - Laboratory equipment.

Step 2. Deciding who may be harmed and how

For each of the hazards identified, the people that might be harmed should be considered. For example, for anaesthetic gas pollution this will be the veterinary surgeon and veterinary nurse present in theatre during the procedure and also the staff (veterinary nurses and animal care assistants) present in the recovery ward where the animal continues to exhale anaesthetic gases. In equine radiography, the horse owner may be exposed to the radiation hazard as well as the veterinary surgeon if they are assisting with restraining the horse.

There are some groups that may be particularly at risk. These include people with disabilities, young workers and pregnant women.

Young people

If the practice has work experience students or young workers (under 18), their school, college or employer must carry out a risk assessment before the young people start their work placement or job (Figure 2.3). There are some additional factors to consider. The employer must be aware of the young person's inexperience, lack of awareness or perception of danger and physical and/or psychological immaturity, and must take these into account when completing risk assessments. In addition the young person must receive adequate training and supervision during instruction, i.e. until they become confident and proficient. Risks should be reduced to the lowest level reasonably practicable – or removed entirely. Young people should not be exposed to radiation or toxic substances. Students over the minimum school-leaving age (16) and being supervised as part of their course may be exposed to radiation if the risks have been reduced to a minimum. The practice should appoint a person responsible for work experience students during their placement and any special needs should be allowed for.

New mothers and pregnant women

Where new or expectant mothers are employed, the practice must conduct a specific risk assessment, taking into account any advice from their GP or midwife. If risks are identified that cannot be reduced or controlled, the woman must be offered suitable alternative work, or have working conditions or hours adjusted, or be suspended on paid leave, if necessary, to protect the health and safety of mother and child (Figure 2.4).

People with disabilities

Risk assessments should take account of workers with disabilities or long-term health conditions. These assessments need to involve the disabled employees, disability advisors and occupational health professionals where necessary to make any reasonable adjustments to the task involved.

Step 3. Evaluating the risks and deciding on precautions

For each hazard it is necessary to look at the existing controls and compare these with what is necessary to comply with the law. For each hazard identified in the practice, the risk assessment needs to consider whether that hazard can be removed altogether or if exposure to it can be controlled. If it needs to be controlled this can be by:

- Switching to a less hazardous substance, e.g. using an alternative to glutaraldehyde disinfectants
- Preventing access to the hazard, e.g. removing unsafe equipment after electrical testing
- Organizing work to reduce exposure to the hazard, e.g. changing work practices in order that no animal is held for radiography
- Issuing personal protective equipment, e.g. masks and goggles for use when scaling teeth using an ultrasonic scale
- Providing facilities for removal of contamination, e.g. sinks in isolation wards to ensure staff can wash their hands without touching door handles.

These solutions are not always expensive but require thought from the whole practice team.

Note: This assessment must be completed before the young person begins work.	

Name of young person	
Date of birth	
Employment status (e.g. employee/temporary/work placement)	Work placement
Job description	Work placement
Department	
Responsible manager	
Assessor	
Date of assessment	

Hazards associated with the task	Risks to the young worker	Proposed control measures	Residual risks acceptable (✓)
Tiredness	Vulnerable person	Regular rest breaks (30 mins every 4.5 hours) Ensure that young person has something to eat during breaks/lunchtime Regular changes of activities Light duties only Supervision of all activities Training in all areas of work	☐
Fire	Burns, smoke inhalation, collapse, death	Fire evacuation procedures to be communicated on arrival at practice. Fire Warden to show fire exits and location point Fire equipment regularly tested Supervising staff trained as Fire Wardens Regular fire drills	☐
Electricity	Burns, shock, collapse, death	All equipment regularly PAT tested and register maintained Training for equipment Supervision of activities	☐
Lifting	Back injury, muscle strain	Manual handling instructions given during induction Supervision of activities Light loads only Health and Safety online training tool	☐
Visual display screen use	Fatigue, eye strain, headache, dizziness, repetitive strain injury (wrist/arms), back pain	During induction: online training tool on correct positioning/use; supervisor to complete workstation assessment Regular rest breaks and change of activity every 30 mins Direct supervision by clinical coach/qualified VN	☐
Hot water	Scalds	Alert to warning signs Supervision of activities, e.g. coffee making	☐
Animals	Bites, injuries to body	Demonstrate correct handling techniques at induction Supervision of all activities Risk assessment of all activities	☐
Safeguarding	Vulnerability of young person	Young person to complete safeguarding online training activity during initial induction period to raise awareness of what is right and what is not acceptable All activities to be supervised by staff member who has undergone safeguarding training	☐
Falls	Injury to legs, back and other parts of body	All trip hazards to be removed No working at heights Supervision of all activities Wet floor signs used when floors cleaned	☐
Access to buildings	Unable to gain entry	Building has staff cover before and after the start and finish points for young person Supervision of practice centre by qualified staff at all times	☐
RTA	Head injury, broken bones, neck strain, back pain	Seat belt to be worn at all times Only to travel in authorized practice vehicles appropriately insured for staff and student travel Supervision at all times by authorized staff Speed limits to be observed at all times and careful driving employed	☐

Note: Where the young person is a 'child' (i.e. below school leaving age), a copy of this assessment must be given to the parent or guardian.

2.3 An example of a young person risk assessment form.

Date				Job title		Veterinary Nurse	
Hours of work				Assessed by			
Assessment number							

No.	Activity/plant/ materials, etc.	Hazard	Risks to the new or expectant mother/ child	Severity (S)	Likelihood (L)	Risk rating (S x L)	Measures/comments	Result
1	Moving sedated/ anaesthetized dogs to and from kennels.	Strenuous manual handling.	Risk to mother – hormone changes can affect ligaments causing susceptibility to injury or postural problems. Risk to child – prematurity or low birth weight.				Reduce amount of physical lifting/carrying. Use trolleys or stretchers where necessary.	
2	Monitoring anaesthesia.	Exposure to anaesthetic gases.	Anaesthetic gases can affect unborn child.				Avoid if possible. If carried out, efficient anaesthetic gas scavenging. Monitor anaesthetic pollutants in atmosphere. Minimize exposure in recovery wards/kennels.	
3	Assisting with radiography.	Exposure to ionizing radiation.	Damage to unborn child.				Do not include pregnant women in work involving exposure to ionizing radiation unless unavoidable. Amend shifts/duties etc. or find alternative work. Use personal protective equipment aprons, gloves, etc. Wear dosemeters.	
4	Cleaning kennels.	Handling cat/dog faeces.	*Toxoplasma* in cat faeces. Risk of miscarriage in early pregnancy and infection in unborn child in later pregnancy.				Avoid if possible – if carried out wear gloves – hand hygiene.	
5	Dispensing medication.	Active substances in some drugs.	Some drugs teratogenic – can damage unborn child. Some can cause miscarriage.				Wear gloves for all dispensing. Good pharmacy practice. Check COSHH assessment and SPCs for drugs used. Avoid dispensing drugs classified as teratogenic or causing miscarriages.	
6	Standing for long periods.	Tiredness. Dizziness, fainting.	Affects mother.				Amend duties to avoid.	
7	Working long hours, overtime, night shifts.	Tiredness.	Affects mother.				Amend duties to avoid. Can suitable alternative to night shifts be found?	
8	Any specific advice from GP, midwife or health visitor.							

* Key to result: T = Trivial risk   A = Adequately controlled   N = Not adequately controlled   U = Unable to decide. Further information required

2.4 An example of a new and expectant mother risk assessment form. Medical advice should always be sought in addition to the guidance provided.

Step 4. Recording and implementing findings

Practices with fewer than five employees do not have a legal obligation to write down the results of their risk assessments but it is probably sensible to do so. All risk assessments must be regularly reviewed. They should be recorded in a simple form and be easily accessible to all staff.

Step 5. Reviewing and updating risk assessments

Assessments should be reviewed annually, or more frequently if new equipment or working practices are introduced. The principles involved in risk assessments should be used when new practices are designed or new work tasks undertaken. A risk assessment should be carried out for every area of the practice and every task performed by staff.

Task assessments

Every task performed by practice staff should be assessed. Any hazards involved in the task (e.g. chemicals used in the development of radiographs, zoonotic infections when barrier nursing) should be assessed as low (L), medium (M) or high (H) risk.

The staff involved in the procedure and potentially at risk need to be identified and any particularly high-risk group,

for example pregnant women or young workers, need special consideration (see above). The task should be assessed for how staff may be at risk; for instance, unloading a drug order can put the staff involved at risk of back injuries if manual handling issues are not addressed.

Precautions already in use must be assessed, such as the use of masks in dental scaling procedures. Additional precautions that could be introduced to minimize risk further should then be considered, e.g. for dental scaling, goggles could be introduced in addition to masks, and ventilation of the dental area improved (Figure 2.5).

Standard Operating Procedures

This assessment should be considered by all staff involved in the procedure. The results should be recorded in a task assessment and this then used to draw up a **Standard Operating Procedure (SOP)** for the task considered (Figure 2.6). SOPs are written protocols (safe systems of work) for each job within the practice. They should be clear, precise, easy to read and personalized to each practice and each task within the practice. SOPs must be available to all staff and be used in staff induction and training. In some cases, it is a good idea to have laminated copies of SOPs displayed in the appropriate places around the practice, e.g. the SOP for operating equipment should be placed next to the equipment. These SOPs should be working documents, which are re-assessed if work practice or equipment changes.

REFERENCE NO :	RA16	DATE	13/09/11
TASK / ACTIVITY	ULTRASONIC DENTAL SCALING		
HAZARDS	1. Microorganisms in mouth and in aerosols produced could be inhaled by operator. 2. Damage to eyes of operator from debris and teeth. 3. Anaesthetic gases. 4. Electrical equipment – electric shock risk.		
PERSONS INVOLVED	Staff – veterinary surgeons and veterinary nurses.		
LEVEL OF RISK	Low to medium.		
EXISTING CONTROLS	1. Protective clothing (gloves, aprons and masks available); staff training. 2. Protective clothing (goggles available); staff training 3. Anaesthetic scavenging (passive scavenging in place); monitoring of anaesthetic gas pollution carried out annually. 4. SOP for use of machine; PAT testing of electrical equipment carried out.		
CONTROLS NEEDED	1. More ventilation in dental area – install extractor fan. 2. Goggles scratched and mist up easily – source new goggles or face shields.		
ASSESSOR		SIGNATURE	
DATE OF NEXT REVIEW	13/09/12		

2.5 An example of a task risk assessment for dental scaling.

• Anaesthetic gas monitoring and scavenging	• Lone working
• Barrier nursing	• Maintaining a surgically clean environment
• Biosecurity	• Manual handling
• Cleaning floors	• Post-mortem arrangements
• Cleaning kennels	• Packaging and posting laboratory samples
• Clipping and preparing the surgical site	• Radiation protection
• Dental scaling	• Restraint of animals
• Dispensing drugs	• Safe handling of medicines
• Dispensing repeat medication	• Security of animals in transit from branch surgery
• Display screen use	• Spillages
• Driving practice vehicles	• Staff pets
• Electrical equipment inspection	• Staff security
• Examining radiographic protective equipment	• Sterilization of instruments
• Film processing	• Tea, coffee and food preparation
• Fire precautions	• Tidiness
• Home visits	• Unpacking a drug delivery
• Induction of anaesthesia	• Use of autoclave
• Injecting animals	• Use of laboratory equipment
• Isolation procedures	• Visitors

2.6   Examples of tasks in a typical veterinary practice for which an SOP is required.

Area risk assessments

For each room or area of the practice, all the hazards in that area should be considered and listed and the risk from each classified as high (H), moderate (M) or low/negligible (L) (Figure 2.7). All staff members working in the area considered should also be listed and any particular extra risk factors (young person, pregnant, disabled) should be noted. The tasks performed in this area should also be noted and any task assessments already performed and SOPs formulated taken into account when assessing risk levels. Any control measures already in place, such as protective clothing, should be noted.

These factors taken together can be used to draw up **Local Rules** or area SOPs. Staff should be consulted during this process and any extra training needed should be identified. These area assessments or Local Rules should be displayed in the area concerned for staff to refer to. These should be reviewed at least annually.

REFERENCE NO :	RA14		DATE	13/09/11
TASK / ACTIVITY	Practice laboratory.			
HAZARDS	1. Exposure to biological agents. 2. Spillage leading to slips trips and falls. 3. Exposure to chemicals/allergens. 4. Electric shock. 5. Eye strain.			
PERSONS INVOLVED	Staff – veterinary surgeons and veterinary nurses.			
LEVEL OF RISK	Medium – reduced to Low by control measures in place.			
EXISTING CONTROLS	1. Protective clothing (gloves, aprons, etc.); SOP in place (no eating, drinking in lab, etc.); staff training. 2. First Aid kit in place. 3. COSHH assessment results for lab chemicals available; gloves available; extractor fan; staff training. 4. PAT testing of portable machines annually. 5. Good lighting.			
CONTROLS NEEDED	Continued staff training. 2. Spillage kit to be placed in lab. 5. Position of computer screen and keyboard to be assessed.			
ASSESSOR			SIGNATURE	
DATE OF NEXT REVIEW	13/09/12			

2.7   An example of an area risk assessment for a practice laboratory.

Reception and waiting areas

Animals

Animals in the waiting room that are not under control are a hazard to staff, clients and other animals; owners should be asked by staff or by notices to keep their dogs on leads (Figure 2.8) and their cats in baskets.

In equine practice, owners should be asked to try and keep their horses under control after unloading them to protect staff and other clients from injury. Appropriate personal protective equipment (PPE) may be necessary (see later). The practice should provide an area for loading, unloading and examination that is secure to prevent escape of the patient (Figure 2.9).

Visitors

Dealing with members of the public can be a potential hazard in the reception area and the practice should have considered staff security, cash handling, the complaints procedure and any lone working. If necessary, panic buttons and other security measures should be put in place.

Cleaning

Hazards in the waiting room include wet floors and cleaning products used on them; notices can be used to make staff and visitors aware (Figure 2.10). The procedure for cleaning up and disinfection following elimination by animals, and any areas with potential for slips, trips and falls should be assessed.

IT equipment

A risk assessment of display screen equipment should be carried out for the use of computers by receptionists and other staff (Figure 2.11). This should include checks to ensure that the screen is readable, there is no glare from adjacent windows or lights, the keyboard is in a comfortable position, chairs are comfortable and correctly adjusted, and operators have frequent breaks from the screen.

Manual handling

There may be manual handling requirements if food stands have to be restocked with large and heavy bags of pet food (Figure 2.12); staff should be trained to lift safely (see later in chapter), and measures to help, such as trolleys and step stools, should be considered.

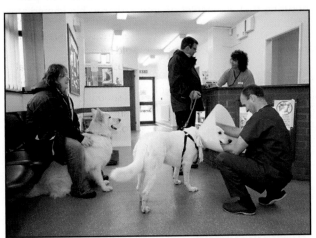

2.8 Waiting room; dogs should be kept on leads. (Photo J. Bosley; ©Quantock Veterinary Hospital)

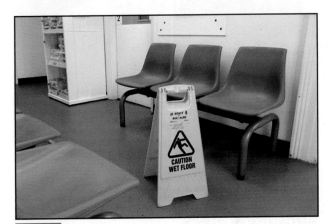

2.10 Wet floor hazard sign.

REFERENCE NO :	RA16	DATE	13/09/11
TASK / ACTIVITY	Loading and unloading of horses.		
HAZARDS	• Horses escaping on to road. • Horses injuring public in car park. • Horse boxes and trailers reversing – danger to people and parked cars.		
PERSONS INVOLVED	• Staff – vets, nurses and grooms. • Horse owners. • Other clients in car park.		
LEVEL OF RISK	Medium.		
EXISTING CONTROLS	• SOP in place – to ensure gates to road closed when loading/unloading horses (not occurring during small animal consultation times). • Staff training.		
FURTHER CONTROLS NEEDED	• Horse boxes to drive to back of building. • Further set of gates for equine area only. • Unloading ramp.		
ASSESSOR		SIGNATURE	
DATE OF NEXT REVIEW	13/09/12		

2.9 Example of a risk assessment for loading/unloading horses.

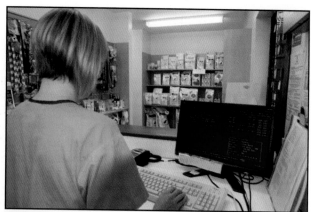

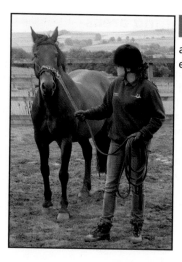

2.13 When handling horses, appropriate protective equipment should be worn.

2.11 Display screen equipment is also subject to risk assessment. (Photo J. Bosley; ©Quantock Veterinary Hospital)

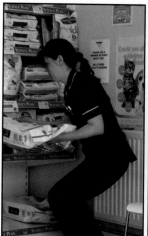
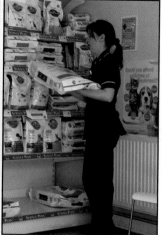

2.12 Lifting requires a straight back

Consulting areas

Animals

Animal handling and restraint is one of the main hazards of the consulting area and must therefore be assessed and staff trained in correct animal restraint procedures. Any equipment required, such as muzzles, gloves, hard hats or nose twitches, should be readily available. For large animal and equine consulting areas it is important to minimize the risk of animals escaping by providing safe loading and unloading areas, with SOPs to ensure that gates are shut, etc., before unloading. PPE should be appropriate for the assessed risks. For example, when trotting up or lungeing horses, staff should wear adequate protective clothing, including hard hats, gloves and suitable footwear (Figure 2.13).

Cleaning

Practice cleaning and disinfection protocols are required. Lists of cleaning tasks to be performed daily, weekly or after each surgery should be kept and updated regularly.

IT equipment

Computer use should be assessed as for reception. In addition, keyboard hygiene should be considered and the use of washable keyboards or keyboard covers introduced. These are important to prevent the spread of infections, including MRSA.

Waste

Waste disposal in the consulting room needs to be considered and an SOP for the disposal of various categories of waste drawn up (see later). Particular attention should be paid to ensuring that all needles go into a 'sharps' bin immediately after use, to avoid needle-stick injuries.

Drugs

Veterinary drug use in the consulting room must be considered, along with the requirements for medicine storage (see Dispensary, below).

Kennels and inpatient areas

Cleaning

Cleaning, disinfection and animal handling must be considered when formulating working practices and Local Rules for the kennels and other inpatient areas.

Infection control

Another hazard to assess in these areas is infection spread from animals either to other animals or to humans (zoonoses). There should be an SOP for the isolation of animals with infections that could be transmitted to other animals or to staff. There should also be an SOP for barrier nursing. This should include details of the area to be used for isolation, the protective clothing to be worn, designated person to be responsible, details of waste disposal, and information on the risks of dangerous pathogens and zoonoses with reference to **Control of Substances Hazardous to Health (COSHH)** information. It is particularly important to have the barrier nursing SOP and equipment used (Figure 2.14) to hand if there is no separate isolation area in the practice. Gloves,

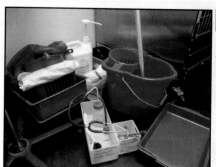

2.14 Equipment ready for use in the isolation facility.

gowns, footbaths, disinfectants and tape to demarcate the area used for isolation should be kept together, available for instant use when the need arises. It is a good idea to have a laminated copy of the SOP displayed or in the isolation kit. A risk assessment of potential zoonotic hazards should be available to all staff.

Dispensary

SOPs should be drawn up for all tasks associated with the storage, handling and dispensing of drugs (Figure 2.15). Staff should be trained using these SOPs before they are allowed to dispense medications.

Gloves should be available in the dispensary, including non-latex gloves for any staff allergic to latex. Any other staff allergies, such as penicillin allergy, should be taken into account when planning tasks.

- Dealing with spillages
- Dispensing protocol
- Disposal of controlled drugs
- Disposal of cytotoxic drugs
- Disposal of out-of-date drugs
- Handling and use of cytotoxic drugs
- Handling veterinary medicines
- Labelling drugs
- Medicine returned by clients
- Placing a drug order
- Receiving and storing Controlled Drugs
- Stock control and expiry date checking
- Temperature monitoring protocols
- Unpacking the drug order delivery
- Using ampoules

2.15 Examples of SOPs required for the dispensary.

Manual handling

Manual handling issues that are involved in unpacking the drug delivery and moving drugs around the building must be addressed. If drugs are kept on high shelves there should be suitable safe equipment to access them (stepstools, etc.); if not, they should be moved to lower shelves.

Spills

A spillage kit should be available in the dispensary and staff trained to use it. The kit should contain gloves, absorbent material (cat litter or sand (Figure 2.16) are suitable) and a laminated copy of the SOP for 'Dealing with spillages'.

The results of the COSHH assessment for all drugs and chemicals used in the practice (see later) should be readily available to staff and easily accessible in the event of a spillage or accident.

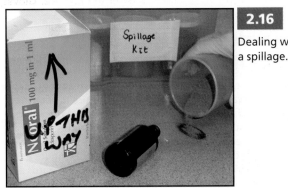

2.16

Dealing with a spillage.

Operating theatre and preparation room

SOPs

It is important to have SOPs in these areas for clipping and preparing animals for surgery and for maintenance of a surgically clean environment. Hazards associated with equipment, e.g. dental scalers, air drills, autoclaves and electrosurgical equipment, must be assessed and clear SOPs produced, and, where appropriate, displayed near to the equipment.

Anaesthetic gases

The risks associated with anaesthetic gases should have been thoroughly assessed. There should be SOPs for filling vaporizers and servicing equipment regularly. There should be a scavenging system in operation, which may be passive, active or using charcoal absorbers. If charcoal absorbers are used there should be a protocol for regular weighing to ensure they are still effective.

Anaesthetic gas monitoring should be performed regularly, preferably annually, but more often if anaesthetic equipment or circuitry is changed, to ensure that readings do not exceed the current Workplace Exposure Limits. These are currently 10 ppm halothane, 50 ppm isoflurane, 60 ppm sevoflurane and 100 ppm nitrous oxide. They are calculated on an 8-hour time-weighted average. These readings are obtained by staff wearing monitoring badges during an operating and recovery session, as there may be significant anaesthetic gas pollution in recovery wards as well as theatres. If a sophisticated active scavenging system is used this should be serviced and tested annually.

Dental scaling

Dental scaling involves hazards to the staff involved both from bacteria from the animals' mouths and from injury caused by dental calculus and teeth during extraction procedures. Good ventilation is important in the dental area, as is the use of protective equipment, goggles, gloves, masks and aprons, which should all be available (Figure 2.17). Staff should be trained to use the equipment safely.

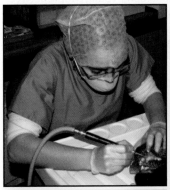 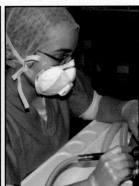

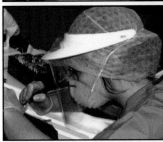

2.17 Personal protective equipment for dental procedures.

Lifting equipment

Any lifting equipment used in equine operating theatres, such as overhead gantry cranes (see Chapter 24), should be strong, stable and suitable for its intended use. It should be positioned to prevent risk of injury, and instructions for its safe use should be available.

Imaging – radiography and ultrasonography

The Ionising Radiation Regulations 1999 (IRR99) require practices to assess the risks of radiography, identifying all hazards with the potential to cause a radiation accident, evaluating the risks, and identifying measures to restrict exposure to radiation of staff and other persons (Figure 2.18). As a result of the risk assessment, Local Rules for radiography should be drawn up and approved by the Radiation Protection Adviser (RPA) appointed by the practice (see Chapter 18).

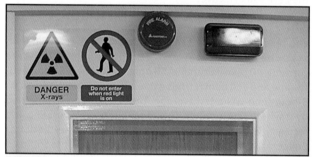

2.18 Controlled area signage for entry to an X-ray room.

All staff involved in radiography should have read and signed the Local Rules. The practice should have informed the HSE of their use of ionizing radiation. Suitable personal protective equipment (PPE) should be provided (Figure 2.19), stored properly and examined at regular intervals. Lead aprons should be stored hung over large-diameter bars to prevent cracking and damage. There should be an SOP for examining PPE approved by the RPA.

Young persons under the age of 18 doing work experience should not be involved in radiography. Young people between 16 and 18 who are on training courses may be involved in radiography provided they are supervised and have suitable training. The maximum exposure limit for these students is lower than for over-18s.

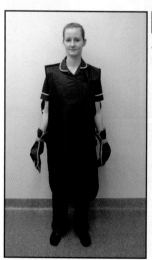

2.19 PPE for radiography, including lead apron and gloves. (Courtesy of E. Mullineaux)

Restraint

No animals should be held unless there are clinical reasons why they cannot be restrained by other means. A range of cradles, sandbags and other positioning aids should be available (see Chapter 18).

For equine radiography, if owners are involved in handling horses during the procedure they should be given the Local Rules to read and have all safety precautions pointed out to them and PPE such as lead aprons made available for their use.

Processing

Film processing facilities should be in well ventilated areas and chemicals should be stored, handled and used according to manufacturers' instructions. COSHH assessment details for these chemicals should be easily available. With the increase in popularity of digital radiography the health and safety implications of processing film are becoming less of an issue for many practices.

Laboratory

Chemicals used in laboratory work should all be included in the practice COSHH assessment and details should be made available to staff. PPE including gloves, aprons and goggles should be to hand. There should be SOPs for the use of all laboratory equipment. No staff should undertake laboratory work until they have been adequately trained and made aware of the risks of handling laboratory specimens and carrying out laboratory work. There should be a sink in the laboratory area. Personnel should not eat or drink in the laboratory.

Handling hazardous substances

Many potentially hazardous substances are encountered in veterinary practice. As noted above, hazard is not the same as risk: hazard is anything that can cause harm whereas risk is the likelihood that harm will occur and its severity. Risk can be minimized by limiting or controlling exposure to hazardous substances. The hazardous substances found in veterinary practices include:

- Medicinal products
- Cleaning agents and disinfectants
- Microorganisms, such as bacteria and viruses (including zoonotic infections)
- Clinical waste
- Animal tissues
- Anaesthetic agents
- Radiographic processing chemicals
- Laboratory chemicals and reagents.

The Control of Substances Hazardous to Health Regulations 2002

Practices are required to make a thorough assessment of the risks to health and safety arising from exposure to veterinary medicines and other hazardous substances used throughout the practice, such as those listed above. As with the risk assessment process, COSHH requires that an assessment is carried out regarding exposure to hazardous substances (Figure 2.20). The purpose of the assessment is to identify the hazards and risks and determine whether control measures are adequate.

Name of assessor	
Date of assessment	

PART 1 – GENERAL INFORMATION
What processes are carried out within the organization? (Define briefly all stages and include cleaning/maintenance procedures.)

At what locations are these processes performed?

What substances are present at these locations (either for use in the processes mentioned or as a product of them) and in what quantity do they exist? (Remember to include all biological substances including microorganisms and all cleaning chemicals.)

Substance	Gaseous (quantity)	Dust (quantity)	Liquid (quantity)	Solid (quantity)

Do all the substances mentioned above have the *supplier's/manufacturer's health and safety information sheets as required by s.6 of the Health and Safety at Work etc. Act 1974, as amended?	Yes ❑	No ❑
Are all products labelled for supply in accordance with the Chemicals (Hazard Information and Packaging for Supply) Regulations 2002?	Yes ❑	No ❑
Are employees trained in the use of all control measures, including personal protective equipment (PPE), associated with their work, and in all emergency procedures?	Yes ❑	No ❑
Are employees trained in respect of the necessary procedures concerning spillage and first aid?	Yes ❑	No ❑
Is adequate information and instruction available to employees regarding the risks and precautions, etc?	Yes ❑	No ❑
Is all information, instruction and training reviewed and amended as appropriate, on a regular basis, and are refresher courses carried out?	Yes ❑	No ❑
Are any changes in conditions or work processes likely which may alter the results of this assessment and necessitate a new assessment?	Yes ❑	No ❑

PART 2 – SPECIFIC INFORMATION
The information in this section must be recorded on a separate checklist for each of the substances identified (in each state) in Part 1.

ASSESSMENT

Substance under assessment, including state and quantity. _____

At what location(s) is this substance present? _____

Is this substance, in the state and quantity specified, considered hazardous?	Yes ❑	No ❑
Will exposure to this substance occur?	Yes ❑	No ❑
Will exposure occur through:		
a. inhalation?	Yes ❑	No ❑
b. ingestion?	Yes ❑	No ❑
c. skin absorption?	Yes ❑	No ❑
Can the exposure be prevented?	Yes ❑	No ❑
Will workplaces/locations other than the ones specified be affected by exposure?	Yes ❑	No ❑

What groups of employees will be affected by exposure? Define job titles.

Will exposure to this substance affect anyone else (other workers, contractors, visitors, etc)?	Yes ❑	No ❑

How often does exposure occur?

Daily	Weekly	Monthly	Other (specify)	

How long does exposure last?

Less than 10 minutes	1 hour	2 hours	4 hours	8 hours

Will Workplace Exposure Limits (WELs) as provided by COSHH Regulations be exceeded? (See HSE Guidance Note EH40.)	Yes ❑	No ❑

2.20 Example of a COSHH assessment form.

continues ▶

CONTROL/MONITORING				
If exposure cannot be prevented are adequate control measures other than personal protective equipment (PPE) available (i.e. local exhaust ventilation, substance substitution, etc)?	Yes	☐	No	☐
Are all control measures (including PPE) tested as required by the COSHH Regulations?	Yes	☐	No	☐
Do control measures meet the approved/recommended standards?	Yes	☐	No	☐
If necessary, is the PPE required approved by the HSE or does it conform to an approved standard?	Yes	☐	No	☐
Are all employees trained in the use of all required control measures?	Yes	☐	No	☐
Are monitoring systems available to ensure all control measures are working effectively?	Yes	☐	No	☐
Is monitoring carried out on a regular basis?	Yes	☐	No	☐
Are records of monitoring control checks and necessary repairs, etc maintained? (To be kept for at least 5 years.)	Yes	☐	No	☐
HEALTH SURVEILLANCE				
Is the substance, as used in the processes determined in this assessment, listed in Schedule 6 of the COSHH Regulations?	Yes	☐	No	☐
Are any of the following conditions, which may necessitate health surveillance and remedial action, apparent:				
• Evidence of dust on surfaces and/or in the air	Yes	☐	No	☐
• Broken, defective or badly maintained control measures/equipment	Yes	☐	No	☐
• Complaints of discomfort	Yes	☐	No	☐
• Reports of previous exposure-related ill health	Yes	☐	No	☐
• Departures from recognized good practice/standards.	Yes	☐	No	☐
Where necessary, is medical surveillance carried out at least every 12 months?	Yes	☐	No	☐
Are health/medical surveillance records maintained as required (personal exposure of identifiable employees – 40 years; other records – 5 years)?	Yes	☐	No	☐

2.20 *continued* Example of a COSHH assessment form.

Drugs and all substances should be classified according to risk, i.e. low, medium or high.

Low- and medium-risk substances can be grouped by therapeutic group, type, route of administration, etc. Standard measures to control exposure can be used for the whole group. Examples of groups include:

- Antibiotics
- Vaccines
- Injectable anaesthetics
- Inhalation anaesthetics
- Steroids
- Disinfectants.

Any specific risks within the groups that may cause longer-term health problems must be identified, such as allergy to penicillin or sensitivity to latex.

High-risk substances must have individual detailed assessments. These substances include:

- Oil-based vaccines
- Cytotoxic drugs (including some creams to treat equine sarcoids)
- Glutaraldehyde disinfectants
- Hormones
- Tilmicosin
- Etorphine.

Measures to control exposure to high-risk substances must be identified to staff. SOPs are likely to be required.

The results of the COSHH assessment must be readily available to all staff so that they are aware of the hazards, risks and precautions to take to prevent harm. They should also be aware of how to access this information so that in the event of an accident or exposure to a hazardous substance they know where to get information about what action to take and can, if necessary, take the product information with them to a doctor. There should be an annual review of the assessment to make sure all information is still current. The results of the COSHH assessment may be stored as hard copy or on a computer, provided there is an SOP on how to access the information.

Drugs

Safety data must be available for all drugs stocked. Drug companies no longer have to supply safety datasheets but many companies still do and some can be found in the National Office of Animal Health (NOAH) datasheet compendium, available from The National Office of Animal Health or their website www.noahcompendium.co.uk.

All veterinary authorized products have summaries of product characteristics (SPCs), available on the Veterinary Medicines Directorate website www.vmd.gov.uk. An authorized product can be found by clicking on the quick link to

Product Information Database. The products are arranged alphabetically and clicking on the chosen product brings up a link to its SPC. All veterinary medicinal products currently authorized in the UK, plus homeopathic products and specified feed additives, including a list of suspended or recently expired products, are on this database.

Summaries of product characteristics of human Prescription Only Medicines (POMs) used under the prescribing cascade can be found at www.emc.medicines.org.uk. Alternatively, copies of the Association of the British Pharmaceutical Industry (ABPI) Compendium of Data Sheets, which are supplied to doctors, pharmacists and nurse prescribers, can be purchased from www.medicines.org.uk.

Cleaners and disinfectants

Disinfectants and cleaning chemicals must have Material Safety Data Sheets (MSDS) under **The Chemicals (Hazard Information and Packaging for Supply) Regulations 2009**, known as **CHIP4**. These regulations require manufacturers to give information about the hazards to their customers. Suppliers usually provide this information on the package itself, generally on the label. Safety datasheet laws have been transferred to the European Registration, Evaluation, Authorisation and Restriction of Chemicals (REACH) regulations and manufacturers no longer have to provide a safety datasheet if there is sufficient safety information available to the user supplied with the product.

Asbestos

Under **The Control of Asbestos Regulations 2006**, owners and tenants with leases that include responsibility for building maintenance must carry out a survey to locate asbestos-containing materials and record their condition, which can then be used to assess risks and decide what action is required (See HSE leaflet INOG223 (rev 3)).

Waste management

Veterinary practices in the course of their work produce various types of waste, and it is important that all waste is stored and disposed of responsibly complying with all relevant legislation. Waste disposal is regulated by the Environment Agency (EA) in England and Wales (www.environment-agency.gov.uk), the Scottish Environmental Protection Agency (SEPA) in Scotland (www.sepa.org.uk) and the Northern Ireland Environment Agency (NIEA) in Northern Ireland (www.ni-environment.gov.uk).

Waste should be kept secure and the practice producing the waste has a legal 'duty of care' to ensure that the person who removes the waste is authorized to carry that type of waste. The contractor should be able to produce evidence that they are authorized but if they cannot, the practice should check with the EA, SEPA or NIEA.

There is also a 'duty of care' to ensure that the waste goes to a site that must be either licensed or exempt from licensing. Each movement of waste must involve a waste transfer note including a description of the waste signed by both parties. The waste transfer notes should be kept for at least 2 years.

There is guidance and a code of practice on 'Waste Management – the duty of care', available from the Department of Food and Rural Affairs (Defra). The British Veterinary Association (BVA), also produces a 'Guide to handling veterinary waste' and a helpful poster. This is available to members and non-members to download from the BVA website www.bva.co.uk and is depicted on page 36 at the end of this chapter. The waste produced needs to be divided into waste streams, all of which are treated differently.

Waste should be divided into hazardous and non-hazardous waste. Under **The Hazardous Waste (England and Wales) Amendment Regulations 2009**, if a practice produces >500 kg of hazardous waste per year it must register with the Environment Agency as a hazardous waste producer. This can be done online, by phone or by post and the practice is then assigned a unique premises code which is valid for 12 months. In Scotland, the term 'Special waste' is used to refer to the equivalent of hazardous waste.

Hazardous waste

- Sharps that are contaminated with blood or pharmaceuticals should be placed into yellow rigid sharps containers (Figure 2.21).
- Cytotoxic and cytostatic pharmaceuticals, plus any equipment used for their administration, protective clothing and animal bedding from animals treated with these agents should be disposed of into rigid yellow containers with a purple lid (Figure 2.21).
- Infectious waste should be placed into yellow bags for high-temperature incineration or orange bags for suitable alternative treatment.
- Photographic (radiographic) chemicals, developer and fixer, should be kept separately and disposed of as hazardous waste or processed to remove the silver and disposed correctly, and with permission from the water authority, into the drain.
- Other hazardous wastes include fluorescent light tubes, low-energy light bulbs and batteries. These must be correctly disposed of.

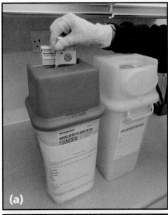

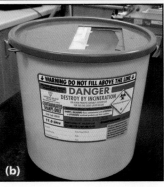

2.21 **(a)** Sharps bins. The bin with the purple lid is for sharps contaminated with cytotoxic or cytostatic pharmaceuticals. The bin with the yellow lid is for sharps contaminated with other pharmaceuticals or blood. **(b)** Container for cytotoxic waste.

Non-hazardous waste

Pharmaceuticals (not cytotoxic or cytostatic)

- Pharmaceuticals should not be removed from their packaging and should be placed into leak-proof containers.
- Solids and liquids should not be mixed together; chemical reactions can cause fires in pharmaceutical disposal bins.
- The contents of the bin should be recorded and list of contents given to the waste disposal contractor.
- Controlled Drugs must be denatured, using denaturing kits that render the drug irretrievable (Figure 2.22), before they can be placed in a pharmaceutical disposal bin.

More information on medicines waste disposal can be found in the *BSAVA Guide to the Use of Veterinary Medicines* which is available to non-members as well as members on the BSAVA website www.bsava.com.

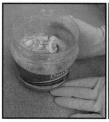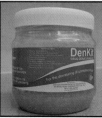

2.22

Denaturing kit for Controlled Drugs.

Offensive waste

- Offensive waste should be placed into a yellow bag with black stripes (tiger striped bag).
- Cadavers can be cremated in a pet crematorium, buried at a pet crematorium or buried at the client's home with the permission of the landowner. If owners wish to bury a horse or other large animal on their own land near a water course they need to contact the Environment Agency for advice. In very rare cases, the body may be deemed hazardous and special arrangements must then be made.

Domestic waste

- Domestic waste can go for landfill or recycling.
- Electrical equipment waste disposal is covered by **The Waste Electrical and Electronic Equipment Regulations 2006** (WEEE Regulations). Practices need to ensure that WEEE is collected separately and is treated and recycled.
- Practices should seek advice from their waste contractor on the appropriate container to be used for each type of waste.

Fire

General fire safety in England and Wales is delivered through compliance with **The Regulatory Reform (Fire Safety) Order 2005** and in Scotland with the **Fire Safety (Scotland) Regulations 2006**. These require employers, building owners and occupiers, as 'responsible persons', to carry out, implement and maintain a fire safety risk assessment. This should cover the risks of fire occurring and the risk to staff and clients in the event of a fire. The fire and rescue authorities are the principal enforcers of this legislation. Responsible persons can either carry out the fire risk assessment themselves or appoint a competent person to assist them. Carrying out the fire safety risk assessment follows the same five steps as discussed earlier in the chapter for general risk assessments.

First, the fire hazards in the premises need to be identified.

Typical fire hazards in veterinary practice include:

- Oxygen cylinders
- Pressurized air cylinders
- Gas cylinders for disbudding irons etc.
- Volatile liquids
- Naked flames such as Bunsen burners
- Dryers
- Cooking equipment.

Secondly, people at risk from these hazards should be identified, particularly those especially at risk such as lone workers, disabled staff or clients. The risks should be evaluated and removed or reduced. Combustible materials such as old record cards, cardboard boxes and packaging, should be removed promptly and not allowed to accumulate. Potentially explosive items, such as oxygen cylinders or gas cylinders, should be stored securely, preferably outside the building. There should be no ignition sources close to combustible materials such as hay and horse bedding.

These hazards and risks should be recorded and from these an emergency plan should be drawn up. The plan should include actions to be taken in the event of a fire (Figure 2.23). Staff should be trained using the plan and instructions.

The fire risk assessment needs to be reviewed regularly and always if there is a change in working practices, such as staff staying overnight or more staff working in the building.

General fire precautions should include suitable fire safety signs, adequate lighting (emergency lighting may be needed), safe escape routes for people with disabilities and suitable fire exit doors

The practice should have an effective fire detection and warning system. This may consist of smoke alarms and a shouted warning or may be an electrical fire detection and alarm system. The system must be adequate to warn people in the premises in all circumstances. Fire alarms and evacuation procedures should be tested regularly. Fire extinguishers, which provide the means of fighting a small fire, should be present and adequately maintained.

If gas or oxygen cylinders are transported in practice vehicles, there should be suitable staff training and a small dry powder fire extinguisher should be carried in the vehicle.

Basic training is required for all staff to ensure that they:

- Understand fire risks
- Know what to do in the event of a fire
- Know how to control fire hazards inherent in their work.

Under The Management of Health and Safety at Work Regulations 1999, training should be provided when:

- A staff member is first recruited
- Increased risks are identified as a result of:
  - Job change or new responsibilities
  - New or altered work equipment
  - New technology
  - New or altered systems of work.

Further details on a fire safety visit can be found at www.fire.gov.uk.

FIRE ACTION

Action on Discovering a Fire:

1. Raise the alarm.

   – Break the glass on one of the fire alarm points throughout the building.
   – Do not be afraid to shout 'FIRE!', to warn all staff and visitors.

2. Attempt to put out the fire using the nearest appropriate extinguisher, BUT ONLY IF:
   a) you have been trained in the use of fire extinguishers,
   b) it is done without risk to yourself,
   c) the alarm has been raised.

3. If it is an electrical fire, the equipment involved should be immediately switched off, provided that no personal risk is involved.

Action on Hearing the Fire Alarm (i.e. a continuous alarm ringing):

1. All staff and visitors must leave the buildings immediately, by the nearest exit route, closing doors behind them, and assemble outside in The Car Park for a roll call.

   – There must be no delays to collect belongings.
   – Staff should escort any clients or visitors in their area to the nearest Fire Exit.
   – If no personal risk is involved animals can also be evacuated (on leads or in baskets).

2. Reception staff must telephone 999 for the fire service and give clear details:

   – State the name of the Practice, proper postal address and telephone number.
   – Tell them it is a veterinary practice with oxygen cylinders present.
   – Give brief details, such as 'Fire in operating theatre'.

3. The Fire Officer or senior person must carry out a roll-call to identify all personnel.

4. No person is to re-enter the building until the all clear is given.

Special Instructions During Surgery:

1. Maintain anaesthesia using continuous intravenous infusion where necessary. The oxygen and anaesthetic machine must be turned off as soon as possible. Animals and equipment for the operation should be moved outside if possible.

2. If necessary the operation should be continued inside and a person should stand by to warn the operators if the fire will put them at risk.

REMEMBER:

- Fire and fumes spread very rapidly, so you must act as quickly as possible.

- Heat and fumes rise; therefore, in obvious fumes or smoke crawl on your hands and knees.

- If fire is spreading rapidly or there is a lot of smoke, personal safety is paramount.

- **If a closed door feels hot do not open it** – the fire is on the other side.

Fire Alarm Points		
Fire Exits		
Fire Extinguishers	Location	Type of Extinguisher
Hose Points		

2.23 Example of a fire action notice.

Practice equipment

All equipment used in the practice should be maintained and serviced according to the manufacturer's directions. For each piece of equipment, any hazards associated with its use should be considered and the risks assessed and minimized if possible. Once this has been carried out, an SOP for the piece of equipment should be written and, where appropriate, displayed alongside the equipment. All staff involved in using the equipment should be trained using the SOP.

For electrical equipment, regular visual inspection and PAT testing is important (see below). For computer equipment, the correct positioning to avoid eye strain and upper limb disorders is important (see below).

Lifting equipment in equine practice, such as hoists and overhead gantry cranes used to lift anaesthetized horses, are covered by **The Lifting Operations and Lifting Equipment Regulations 1998** and must be examined and tested regularly in accordance with the recommendations of a competent person.

Records should be kept of all equipment servicing and testing dates. There should be a system for staff to report any malfunctioning or damaged equipment.

Electrical equipment

The Electricity at Work Regulations 1989 require that employers ensure electrical equipment and installations used at work are safe. Practices should perform a risk assessment to identify any hazards associated with electrical equipment, any risks arising from them and any control measures needed. It is important to check that the equipment is suitable for the job it is being used for, is in good condition and is being correctly maintained.

A quarter of the accidents caused by electrical equipment involve portable electrical appliances. Portable electrical equipment must be checked regularly. It should be visually checked by the user before it is used to ensure that there is no damage to the cable, the plug or the external casing. It should be formally checked by a person trained and appointed to inspect the equipment, and the results recorded. The frequency of the formal visual inspection varies with the type of equipment and environment in which it is used. A combined inspection and test by an electrically competent person, Portable Appliance Testing **(PAT)**, should be carried out at least every 2 years for most equipment. This varies with type of equipment and its use.

Hand-held electrical equipment in regular use, e.g. clippers, needs to be inspected more often than office equipment. Advice should be sought from a competent person regarding the appropriate frequency for a combined inspection and test, as this will vary with the individual circumstances of each practice.

The HSE produces a very useful booklet, 'Maintaining portable and transportable electrical equipment' ref HSG107, which is available to buy in hard copy or to download free from the HSE website www.hse.gov.uk.

A residual current device (RCD) is recommended for portable electrical tools and equipment, particularly in hazardous or wet environments.

The electrical installation of the building should be inspected by a competent person, who will also set the frequency of inspection.

Gas appliances

Gas appliances must be maintained in a safe condition. Advice should be sought from a suitably qualified person regarding the ongoing programme of examination and maintenance.

Visual display units (VDUs)

Computer workstations should be assessed by employers under **The Health and Safety (Display Screen Equipment) Regulations 1992**. These regulations require employers to examine the design of the workstation, the task being carried out and any special needs of individual staff in order to assess and reduce any associated risks. Typical problems can include eye strain, headaches, back, neck and muscular pains from poor posture, and aching arms and wrists from poorly positioned keyboards and desks.

Work should also be planned to ensure that there are regular breaks away from the workstation with changes of activity for staff. Areas for consideration include staff training, provision of adequate lighting, and screen, chair and keyboard position. Incorrect positioning of chairs and keyboards can lead to repetitive strain injury (RSI), now known as upper limb disorder. Steps should be taken to avoid this.

Employees who are covered by the Regulations (those who habitually use VDUs as a significant part of their normal work) can ask their employers to provide and pay for an eye and eyesight test carried out by an optometrist or doctor. The eye test provision does not apply to staff that use VDUs occasionally.

Vehicles

Practice vehicles, like all equipment, should be regularly serviced and checked. If practice ambulances are to be used to transport animals between branch surgeries there must be consideration of the risk of losing animals while transferring them to and from the practice. SOPs should be drawn up on the security of transport, ensuring that all cats are in baskets and that dogs are on safe leads and collars belonging to the practice, in addition to their own. The van should be unloaded and loaded in a secure area if possible. There should also be SOPs on the driving of practice vehicles so that, for example, mobile phones are not used when driving. Security of vehicles also needs to be considered.

For large animal and equine veterinary surgeons working from their vehicles there should be SOPs for waste disposal. Sharps should always be put directly into a sharps container after use. Temperatures must be monitored if drugs are stored in the car, and the security of drugs and equipment needs to be considered.

Biosecurity of vehicles going on to farm and equine premises is important, as is the cleanliness and biosecurity of any protective clothing.

Visits and staff security

For small animal house calls, particularly out of hours, it is important to look at hazards to staff, including driving, animals that are difficult to handle, visiting certain areas late at night, security and lone working. The risks arising should be assessed and practice SOPs for visits drawn up, which may include always having two members of staff on a visit and informing a third party before and after the visit.

For farm and equine visits, security must also be considered, but other hazards exist, including the presence or absence of animal handling facilities on the premises, and biosecurity.

It is also important to make a risk assessment of any staff working by themselves in the practice. As far as possible, lone working should be avoided and the rota designed to ensure there two staff are present at the end of surgeries and also that staff are not locking up alone. Where lone working cannot be avoided, for example with call outs to the surgery at nights and weekends, the same precautions should be taken as for house visits, and the use of panic buttons and alarms considered.

Manual handling

Manual handling includes lifting, carrying, putting down, pushing, pulling, moving or supporting a load by hand or using other bodily force. Veterinary work involves a lot of manual handling of animals, equipment, drugs and food. Back problems as a result of poor manual handling techniques are common throughout the veterinary profession. It is important that practices look to identify any hazardous manual handling involved in their day-to-day work.

The **Manual Handling Operations Regulations 1992** require that hazardous manual handling must be avoided where reasonably practicable, that practices assess the risks from any hazardous manual handling where it cannot be avoided, and take action to reduce these risks. The Regulations do not set specific weight limits for lifting and carrying but do ask practices to assess the hazards and risks of manual handling. Setting weight limits can be too simple an approach and does not take into account other factors involved, such as individual capability. An ergonomic approach to manual handling is based on looking at a whole range of factors: the task, the load, the working environment and, in particular, the individual's capability. With an ergonomic approach, practices may try to fit the job to the person rather than fitting the person to the job.

Each lifting task should be assessed by considering whether the load is heavy, sharp or easy to grasp. For example, if the drugs order is in a box that is too big or heavy, it may be better split into two smaller boxes. It may be possible to modify the height and the distance the load has to be lifted through, as well as the frequency of the task and the degree of twisting involved. It is important that the environment where the task is performed is dry and clean, with a non-slip floor if possible.

For each potentially hazardous manual handling task, the practice should examine whether they can avoid it completely; for example, no longer storing heavy boxes on high shelves, and thereby avoiding the need to lift. If the task cannot be avoided, the risk of injury should be reduced as far as is reasonably practicable. Mechanical assistance can be used to reduce the risk; for example if animals are normally carried from the preparation room to the operating theatre, the practice could consider using a trolley as an induction table. This may then be wheeled through into theatre, thus avoiding the need to carry the patient. Planning work to avoid unnecessary moves of equipment or the patient is an important part of the manual handling risk assessment. Where

appropriate, the use of trolleys, stretchers, hoists and mechanical lifting equipment should be considered.

For each manual handling task that cannot be avoided, the practice must look at the task, the load, the working environment, the individual's capability and any other factors. The staff should then be trained for this specific task and the use of any lifting equipment fully explained.

The HSE produces Manual Handling Assessment Charts for lifting operations, carrying operations and team handling. These are available on the HSE website, as are many useful free information leaflets about manual handling.

Where manual handling tasks cannot be avoided, staff should receive training in safe manual handling techniques, either in house or from external training agencies. Good handling technique, however, is not a substitute for other risk-reduction steps, such as mechanized handling.

Guidelines for manual handling:

- Always assess the load before attempting to lift
- If in doubt ask for assistance
- Make sure the area is clear and that you can obtain the correct foot position
- Stand square on to the object about to be lifted
- Keep your back straight and bend at the knees
- Get a good grip and trial lift
- Lift with your thigh muscles
- Move your feet, do not twist
- Move/walk smoothly to the lowering position
- Lower the load, bending at the knees
- Position the load down, making sure not to trap fingers or hands.

Workplace behaviour

Stress and bullying

Work-related stress is a significant cause of illness, staff absence, increased staff turnover and human error. This stress occurs where work demands on an individual exceed that individual's ability to cope. The HSE publishes advice on work-related stress which can also be found on their website www.hse.gov.uk.

The HSE also has advice for managers at all levels on how to try to reduce stress in their team. An effective practice policy on stress should contain a statement of intent:

- The health, safety and welfare policy of the practice
- Details of the organizational structure and responsibilities
- A description of the systems and procedures in place to eliminate, minimize, control or treat stress in the workplace.

The policy should be regularly reviewed to incorporate changes within the practice and changes in legislative requirements relating to work-related stress.

Training is considered an important part of tackling stress.

Bullying and harassment can also be significant sources of stress. Bullying at work includes malicious gossip, excluding people, assigning unachievable or pointless tasks, or undervaluing work performed. Practices should draw up a bullying and harassment policy and promote a culture where it is not tolerated.

Help for veterinary staff experiencing work or other stress can be found at www.vetlife.org.uk.

Alcohol and drugs misuse

Alcohol misuse is believed to be a significant cause of accidents and lost productivity in the workplace. Drug use is also a growing concern. Those practices that have developed policies to deal with issues sympathetically, fairly and consistently are best prepared. Drug and alcohol misuse may result in reduced workplace performance, damaged client relations and resentment amongst employees who have to 'carry' a colleague whose work declines due to their substance misuse. Substance misuse will also increase the risk of an accident at work.

An employer needs to define the following when developing a policy:

- Alcohol, drug and/or substance misuse
- Who the policy applies to – usually all staff
- Who implements the policy
- How the practice expects employees to ensure that their alcohol or drug consumption does not affect work
- Whether the rules apply in all circumstances.

This may include:

- A statement assuring that any problems will be treated in strict confidence
- A description of the support available
- A commitment to providing information on alcohol and drug misuse
- Details of the circumstances in which disciplinary action will be taken.

Reporting accidents

As a result of considering health and safety, assessing hazards and risks in the practice, the incidence of accidents should be reduced. However, despite all precautions accidents will still occur.

First Aid

The practice should have a suitably stocked first aid box (Figure 2.24) as required by **The Health and Safety (First Aid) Regulations 1981**. There should also be a first aid box in every practice vehicle. Employers must nominate a staff member to take charge if someone is injured or falls ill. This 'appointed person' is responsible for calling an ambulance and for restocking the first aid box. Appointed persons should not administer first aid unless trained to do so. A first aider is someone who has been trained in first aid and holds a current First Aid at Work certificate. This is awarded when the person has successfully completed an HSE approved first aid course.

Accident book

The practice is required by law to have an accident book, which must meet the requirements of the Data Protection Act. It must record the date and time of any accident or occurrence, the full name and address of the person involved and the injury or condition suffered, where the accident happened and a brief description of the circumstances.

Records should be removed from the book, stored securely and kept for at least 3 years. The duty to report accidents falls on employers and the self-employed and covers everyone at work, including visitors and members of the public.

	Expiry date		Dates checked†					
Guidance card	N/A	N/A						
20 individually wrapped, sterile adhesive dressings (assorted sizes)								
2 sterile eye pads, with attachment								
4 individually wrapped triangular bandages (preferably sterile)								
6 safety pins	N/A	N/A						
6 medium-sized individually wrapped sterile unmedicated wound dressings (12 cm x 12 cm)								
2 large sterile individually wrapped unmedicated wound dressings (18 cm x 18 cm)								
1 pair of disposable gloves								
Other equipment required, specify								
Checked by (initials)								
† Please mark * next to items when replaced or renewed								

2.24   Example of a first aid box contents checklist.

Reporting of Injuries, Diseases and Dangerous Occurrences Regulations 1995

If any injury or work-related illness keeps a person off work or unable to do their normal job for more than 3 days it must be reported under the **RIDDOR regulations**. Examples of what should be reported under RIDDOR include:

- Death
- Major injuries, such as broken arms or legs
- Amputation injuries
- Any injury where a person is away from work and unable to do their normal job for more than three days
- Certain cases of work-related disease
- Poisoning
- Electric shock.

Incidents should be reported to the Incident Contact Centre (ICC) within 10 days. The ICC can be contacted by phone or fax or online at www.riddor.gov.uk.

Useful websites and resources

BSAVA: www.bsava.com
- BSAVA Guide to the Use of Veterinary Medicines
- BSAVA Health and Safety (members only)

BVA: www.bva.co.uk
- BVA Good Practice Guide to Handling Veterinary Waste poster and related web pages
- BVA Good Practice Guide to Veterinary Medicines
- Guidance Notes for Safe Use of Ionising Radiations in Veterinary Practice (IRR 1999)

Environment Agency: www.environment-agency.gov.uk

Fire and Rescue Services: www.fire.gov.uk

HSE: www.hse.gov.uk
- Health and safety law, what you need to know
- Risk management – five steps to risk assessment
- Maintaining portable and transportable electrical equipment
- Stress management
- RIDDOR forms

National Office of Animal Health: www.noah.co.uk

Northern Ireland Environment Agency: www.ni-environment.gov.uk

Office of Public Sector Information: www.opsi.gov.uk

RCVS: www.rcvs.org.uk
- RCVS Practice Standards Manual 2010
- Summary report of recent HSE Inspections in Yorkshire Scottish Environmental Protection Agency: www.sepa.gov.uk

Veterinary Medicines Directorate: www.vmd.gov.uk

Self-assessment questions

1. Classify the following wastes as hazardous or non-hazardous:
    a) Out-of-date drugs
    b) Hypodermic needles contaminated with blood
    c) Waste X-ray developing chemicals
    d) The cadaver of a cat killed in a road accident
    e) Horse manure.
2. What factors should a fire risk assessment consider?
3. What does PAT stand for? How often should PAT testing be carried out?
4. What are the weight limits for lifting and carrying for men and for women?
5. What are the common health problems associated with long periods of working at a computer?
6. What are the five easy steps to risk assessment?
7. How often should risk assessments be reviewed?
8. What does COSHH stand for?
9. Name three high-risk substances often found in a veterinary practice.
10. Are young people between the ages of 16 and 18 allowed to assist with radiographic procedures?

BVA Good Practice Guide to Handling Veterinary Waste ▶

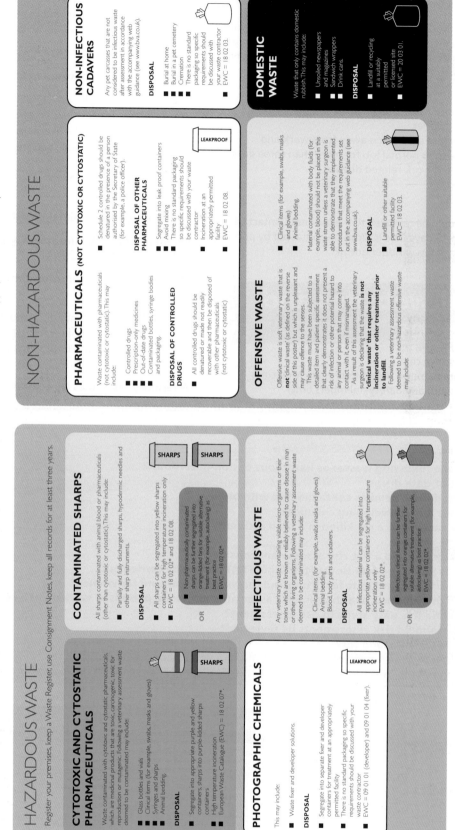

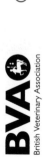

Waste streams in veterinary practice. (©BVA 2008 and reproduced with their permission)

Chapter 3

Anatomy and physiology

Mary Fraser and Simon Girling

Learning objectives

After studying this chapter, students should be able to:

- **Recognize the terminology relating to anatomy and physiology**
- **Identify anatomical landmarks of the skeleton and soft tissues of dogs, cats, exotic species and horses**
- **Demonstrate an understanding of normal anatomy and physiology of body systems**
- **Describe the body systems and how they relate to each other**
- **Compare normal form and function with that seen in disease processes.**

Term	Description
Cranial (anterior)	Towards the head
Caudal (posterior)	Towards the tail
Lateral	Towards the side of the animal
Medial	Towards the middle of the animal
Ipsilateral	On the same side
Contralateral	On the opposite side
Dorsal	Near the back
Ventral	Near the underside of the animal
Palmar	The back or under surface of the front foot
Plantar	The back or under surface of the back foot
Rostral	Towards the nose
Proximal	Applies to limbs near the body
Distal	Applies to limbs near the toes
Superficial	Near the outside of the animal
Deep	Near the centre of the animal

3.1 Directional terminology.

- Median/mid-sagittal plane – a line which divides the body into right and left halves
- Sagittal/paramedian plane – any line parallel to the median plane
- Dorsal plane – parallel to the back of the animal
- Transverse plane – perpendicular to the long axis of the animal.

Introduction

This chapter describes the anatomy and physiology of a wide range of species commonly encountered in veterinary practice: dogs, cats, horses, small mammals, birds and reptiles. The anatomy of the digestive tract of ruminants has also been included for comparison. In each section basic generic anatomy is described, usually with the dog as a reference model; this is followed by consideration of the *major* anatomical differences between species or groups.

Terminology

- Anatomy – the physical structure of the body.
- Physiology – the way in which body systems work.

When describing the anatomy of animals, directional terms are used to provide more information about the structure and position of organs and tissues (Figure 3.1). Sectional planes are also used to describe the location of parts of the animal (Figure 3.2):

Body fluid

Approximately two-thirds of the body is made up of water. This varies between different species and is affected by both the age of animal, with younger animals having a greater percentage of water than older animals, and how fat or thin the animal is. Thinner animals have a higher percentage of water than fatter animals.

Of the 60% bodyweight made up of water, approximately two-thirds is in the intracellular fluid and one-third in extracellular fluid (Figure 3.3). **Intracellular fluid** is the fluid

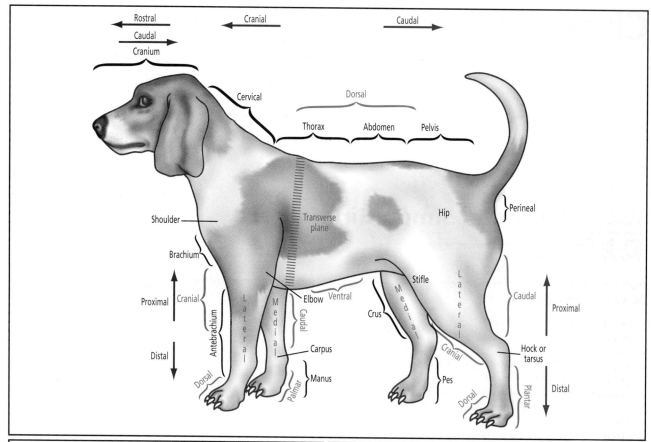

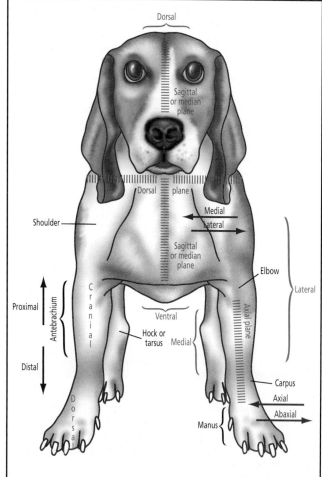

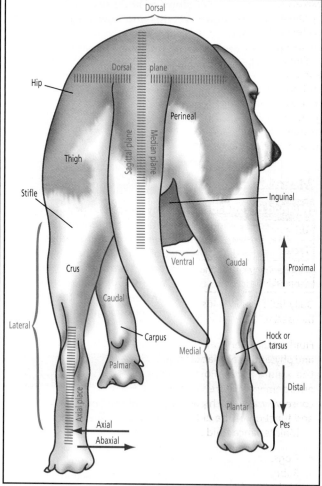

3.2 Anatomical planes and directions.

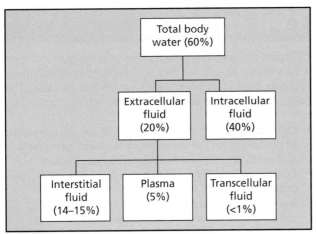

3.3 Distribution of fluid in the body. Percentages are of bodyweight

found inside the individual cells of the body. **Extracellular fluid** is the fluid found outside the cells, including:

- Interstitial fluid (fluid found around cells) – roughly three-quarters of extracellular fluid
- Plasma – roughly one-quarter of extracellular fluid
- Transcellular fluid (such as lymphatic fluid, synovial fluid and cerebrospinal fluid) – very small amount of extracellular fluid.

The volume of fluid in the body is maintained within constant limits by controlling the amount taken in and the amount excreted. The term **homeostasis** describes the method used by the body to maintain parameters within narrow limits. Water content, body temperature and electrolyte content are all maintained by homeostasis.

Fluid is taken into the body via food and water. Water is also produced from the breakdown of food products; this is an important source of water for many arid area-dwelling species. Fluid is lost from the body via the urinary tract, gastrointestinal tract, respiration and sweating. Water lost through the skin as sweat and from the respiratory tract is often termed **insensible fluid loss**.

Maintenance fluid requirements

Method of fluid loss	Volume of fluid lost
Urine	20 ml/kg/day
Faeces	10–20 ml/kg/day
Respiration and sweating (insensible losses)	20 ml/kg/day

Daily fluid loss in dogs, cats and horses. These values can be used to determine maintenance fluid requirements.

Fluid requirements are influenced by both metabolic rate and physiological adaptations to the environment in which the animal lives. For example, reptiles often live in environments where water is scarce and have evolved to conserve water, with particular reference to the structure and function of the kidneys (see below).

Maintenance fluid requirements are as follows:

- Dogs, cats, horses: 50–60 ml/kg/day
- Rabbits and small mammals: 100 ml/kg/day
- Birds: 50 ml/kg/day
- Reptiles: 25 ml/kg/day

Electrolytes

Fluid in the body is not just made up of water; it consists of minerals dissolved in water (solution). **Electrolytes** are solutions containing free ions (such as sodium, potassium and chloride), which conduct electricity, and can have either a positive or a negative charge. Ions with a positive charge are known as **cations**; ions with a negative charge are known as **anions** (Figure 3.4). The number of electrolytes present determines the concentration of the solution (i.e. the higher the level of electrolytes, the greater the concentration).

Type of fluid	Cations	Anions
Intracellular	Potassium Magnesium Sodium	Phosphate Bicarbonate Chloride
Extracellular	Sodium Potassium Magnesium Calcium	Chloride Bicarbonate Phosphate

3.4 Distribution of electrolytes in body fluid.

Diffusion and osmosis

Electrolytes and water are not static but can move from one body compartment to another by diffusion, osmosis or active transport.

- **Diffusion** – a passive process whereby electrolytes pass from a solution of high concentration to a solution of low concentration (Figure 3.5).
- **Osmosis** – the passive movement of water molecules from a solution of low concentration to a solution of high concentration across a semi-permeable membrane (Figure 3.5).
- **Active transport** – the movement of electrolytes against an osmotic gradient. Cells use energy to transport electrolytes across a cell membrane, enabling them to move from a solution of low concentration to a solution of high concentration.

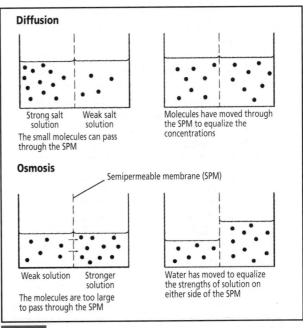

3.5 Diffusion and osmosis.

In the body different fluids can be separated by a **semi-permeable membrane**. This means that water, but not all electrolytes, can move passively across the membrane. If a solution has a high concentration of electrolytes, then it has a low concentration of water. Conversely, if a solution has a low concentration of electrolytes, then it has a high concentration of water. Water molecules move across a semi-permeable membrane from a solution of low electrolyte concentration, to a solution of high electrolyte concentration, until the solutions on either side of the semi-permeable membrane have the same equilibrated concentration. This process is called osmosis.

The pressure with which water molecules are drawn across the semi-permeable membrane is known as the **osmotic pressure**. Where fluids on either side of a semi-permeable membrane have the same osmotic pressure as plasma then they are called **isotonic**. Where a fluid has a higher osmotic pressure than plasma, it is described as **hypertonic**. Where a fluid has a lower osmotic pressure than plasma, it is referred to as **hypotonic**. A hypotonic fluid will lose water to a hypertonic fluid until both fluids are isotonic, assuming that the permeability of the membrane does not change.

Electrolytes also exert an **osmotic force** on water molecules, preventing them from moving. Thus, if there is a high concentration of electrolytes then less water will be able to leave the solution.

Acid–base balance

The terms acidity and alkalinity refer to the concentration of hydrogen ions present within a solution and are expressed as a pH.

- Where the pH is <7, the solution is termed **acidic**.
- Where the pH is >7, the solution is termed **alkaline**.
- Where the pH is 7, the solution is termed **neutral**.

In order for the body to function properly, it needs to be kept within a narrow pH range. The normal pH of blood is 7.4 and the body strives to maintain this level.

Maintaining blood pH

When animals are ill (e.g. with diarrhoea or vomiting), the blood pH changes due to a loss of hydrogen or bicarbonate ions. Loss of hydrogen ions as a result of acute vomiting episodes leads to metabolic alkalosis. Loss of bicarbonate ions from the gut as a result of severe diarrhoea often leads to metabolic acidosis (see Chapter 22). Therefore, the body has mechanisms in place to maintain a pH of 7.4, including:

- **Respiration** – carbon dioxide forms carbonic acid (a weak acid) when dissolved in water. If the pH of blood falls and becomes more acidic, an increased respiratory rate will increase the excretion of carbon dioxide, thereby reducing the concentration of carbonic acid in the blood. This is why animals in metabolic acidosis have increased respiration rates
- **Sodium and hydrogen ion exchange** – in the distal convoluted tubules of the kidneys, hydrogen rather than sodium ions can be excreted into the urine to increase the pH of blood
- **Buffers** – these are substances which can maintain the pH in the presence of increased or decreased levels of hydrogen ions; they include bicarbonate.

Cell structure

All organs of the body are made up of cells. The basic structure is the same for all cells, but they can have specialized structures or forms depending upon their location and function. The basic cell is comprised of the following structures (Figure 3.6):

- **Cell membrane** – the outer covering of the cell composed of phospholipid. The cell membrane is semi-permeable and controls entry and exit of materials/molecules
- **Cytoplasm** – the fluid within the cell which contains the organelles
- **Nucleus** – the control centre of the cell. The nucleus contains DNA (deoxyribonucleic acid) in the form of chromosomes. The **nucleolus** forms part of the nucleus and contains RNA (ribonucleic acid). It is also responsible for the manufacture of ribosomes.

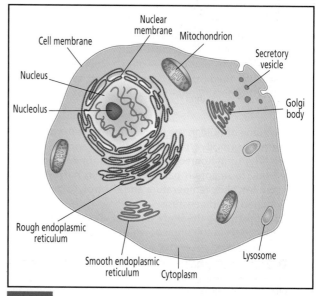

3.6 The structure of a cell.

Organelles

Organelles are smaller structures located within the cytoplasm of the cell and include:

- **Centrosome** – involved in cell replication and comprise two **centrioles**
- **Mitochondria** – produce energy for the cell by aerobic respiration
- **Ribosomes** – responsible for protein synthesis and are often attached to the rough endoplasmic reticulum
- **Rough endoplasmic reticulum** (RER) – synthesis and transport of proteins in conjunction with the attached ribosomes
- **Smooth endoplasmic reticulum** (SER) – synthesis and transport of lipids
- **Golgi body/apparatus** – consists of flattened membrane sacs. Involved in the production of lysosomes, secretory granules and plasma membrane. Responsible for the transport and modification of substances such as glycoproteins
- **Lysosome** – collection of digestive enzymes in membrane sacs. Forms part of the defence mechanism of the cell.

Cell division

Cells reproduce by a process of division. Two types of division can take place, **mitosis** and **meiosis**.

Mitosis (Figure 3.7) is the process by which most cells in the body divide: one parent cell divides into two identical daughter cells. The daughter cells have exactly the same number of chromosomes as the parent cell. There are five stages to mitosis:

- Interphase – cells are at rest and there is no division

- Prophase – chromosomes become apparent
- Metaphase – chromosomes line up along the middle of the cell
- Anaphase – chromatids separate
- Telophase – separation into two new cells.

Meiosis (see Chapter 4, Figure 4.5) is the process whereby one parent cell divides to produce four daughter cells. The daughter cells have half the number of chromosomes of the parent cell. This type of division takes place in the gonads (ovaries and testicles) to produce ova (eggs) or sperm.

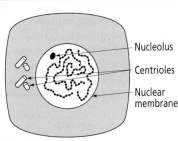

A Interphase
Cell has normal appearance of non-dividing cell condition: chromosomes too threadlike for clear visibility.

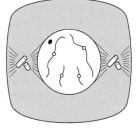

B Early prophase
Chromosomes become visible as they contract, and nucleolus shrinks. Centrioles at opposite sides of the nucleus. Spindle fibres start to form.

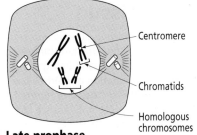

C Late prophase
Chromosomes become shorter and fatter – each seen to consist of a pair of chromatids joined at the centromere. Nucleolus disappears. Prophase ends with breakdown of nuclear membrane.

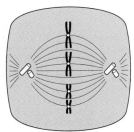

D Early metaphase
Chromosomes arrange themselves on equator of spindle. Note that homologous chromosomes do not associate.

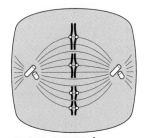

E Late metaphase
Chromatids draw apart at the centromere region. Note that the daughter centromeres are orientated toward opposite poles of the spindle.

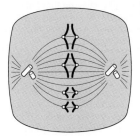

F Early anaphase
Spindle fibres contract and pull the chromatids apart, moving them to the opposite ends of the cell.

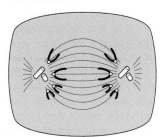

G Late anaphase
Chromosomes reach their destination.

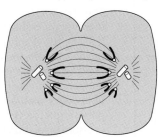

H Early telophase
The cell starts to constrict across the middle.

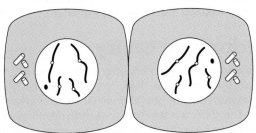

I Late telophase
Constriction continues. Nuclear membrane and nucleolus reformed in each daughter cell. Spindle apparatus degenerates. Chromosomes eventually regain their threadlike form and the cells return to resting condition (interphase).

Note that the daughter cells have precisely the same chromosome constitution as the original parent cell.

3.7 Cell reproduction: mitosis. (Redrawn after M.B.V. Roberts (1986) *Biology: a functional approach, 4th edn*, Nelson)

Basic tissue types

Where similar cells are found in the one location, they are described as a tissue. The three types of tissue found in the body are:

- **Epithelial** – tissue which provides protection, absorption and secretion (e.g. squamous epithelium of the skin)
- **Connective** – tissue consisting of fibroblasts, fibres and a glycosaminoglycan matrix (e.g. bone and cartilage)
- **Muscle** – tissue which undergoes contraction and relaxation (e.g. skeletal, smooth and cardiac muscle).

Epithelial tissue

Epithelial tissue is found lining the outside of the animal (skin surface), the gastrointestinal tract, respiratory tract, reproductive tract and urinary tract, and lining the thoracic and abdominal cavities. The function of epithelial cells is to provide protection for underlying structures. Epithelial tissue can be classified depending on the appearance of the cells under a light microscope (Figure 3.8).

Type of epithelium	Description/function
Simple squamous	Outer layer of cells. Composed of a single sheet of very thin, flat cells. The sheet of cells is thin and delicate, and is found in areas where diffusion occurs (e.g. alveoli of lungs, lining blood vessels, glomerular capsule)
Simple cuboidal	Cells have a square appearance. This type of epithelium is found lining many of the glands and their ducts, and also lining parts of the kidney tubules
Simple columnar	Cells are tall and rectangular. This type of epithelium is found lining the intestine, allowing the absorption of soluble food material
Ciliated	Cells are usually columnar in shape. Cilia or elongated structures, which can move, are present on the free surface of the cells. This type of epithelium lines tubes and cavities where materials must be moved (e.g. respiratory tract, oviducts)
Stratified	Layers of cells make it tough. It has a protective function. It is found in areas that are subjected to friction (e.g. oesophagus, mouth, vagina). In areas where it is subject to considerable abrasion, the cells are infiltrated with a tough protein called keratin, as seen in the epidermis of the skin
Transitional	Layers of cells which can stretch. A modified form of stratified epithelium. Found in structures that must be able to stretch (e.g. bladder, urethra)
Glandular	This type of epithelium has interspersed secretory cells, which secrete mucus/materials into the cavity or space they are lining. Folding of glandular epithelium results in the formation of a gland

3.8 Classification of epithelial tissue.

Connective tissue

Connective tissue can be fibrous or loose, depending on the specific cells and materials present. The basic structure of connective tissue comprises cells (fibroblasts, macrophages, mast cells, plasma cells, leucocytes), fibres (collagen, reticular fibres, elastic fibres) and a glycosaminoglycan matrix.

The main connective tissue types in the body are:

- Areolar (loose connective) tissue
- Dense connective tissue
- Reticular tissue
- Adipose (fat) tissue
- Cartilage
- Bone
- Nervous tissue.

Muscle

The main feature of muscle tissue is that it can contract and relax, either voluntarily as in the case of **skeletal muscle**, or involuntarily as in the case of **smooth muscle** and **cardiac muscle**. Skeletal muscle is found in association with the skeleton and is responsible for movement of the animal; cardiac muscle is found in association with the heart; and smooth muscle is found in the internal organs, including the gastrointestinal tract, respiratory tract, urinary tract and reproductive tract.

Body cavities

Anatomically, the body can be divided into different compartments:

- Thorax
- Abdomen
- Pelvic cavity
- Mediastinum
- Coelom (birds and reptiles).

The body cavities are lined with connective tissue known as serosa. The lining of the cavity is known as parietal serosa; the lining of organs is known as visceral serosa.

Thoracic cavity

The thoracic cavity is the space bound by the ribcage and diaphragm; cranially it is bound by the thoracic inlet, caudally by the diaphragm, dorsally by the vertebrae, ventrally by the sternum and laterally by the ribs. The thoracic cavity is lined by a serous membrane known as the **parietal pleura**, and where it covers the surface of the lungs, it is known as **pulmonary pleura** (Figure 3.9). Between the lungs and the parietal pleura is the **pleural space**, which has a negative pressure in relation to atmospheric pressure. It is this negative pressure which keeps the lungs inflated. In addition, there is a very small amount of fluid in the pleural space, known as **pleural fluid**, which enables the lungs to move freely against the ribcage during inspiration and expiration.

Abdominal cavity

The abdominal cavity is defined cranially by the diaphragm, caudally by the pelvic opening, dorsally by the vertebrae and ventrally/laterally by the abdominal muscles. The organs within the abdomen are lined by a serous membrane known as the **peritoneum**. This membrane comprises a single layer of cells, which produce a very small amount of **peritoneal fluid**, to allow free movement of the organ surfaces against one another.

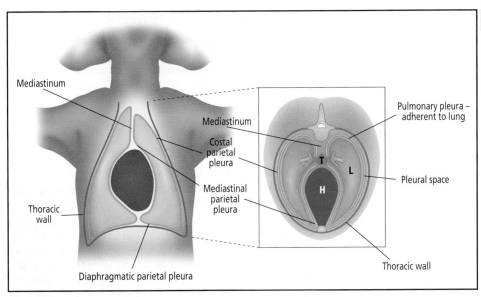

3.9 Thoracic cavity and serous membranes. H = heart; L = lungs; T = trachea. (Reproduced from the *BSAVA Manual of Canine and Feline Thoracic Imaging*)

The part of the peritoneum that covers the abdominal organs is known as the **visceral peritoneum**; the **parietal peritoneum** is the part that covers the abdominal wall. The folds of peritoneum which connect the parietal to the visceral part and suspend the small intestine are known as the **mesentery**. Along the greater and lesser curvatures of the stomach, the serosa is continuous with a very thin connective tissue known as the **omentum**. The omentum has a lacy appearance due to the fat found therein.

Pelvic cavity

The pelvic cavity is not physically separated from the abdomen and therefore is purely an anatomical term rather than a truly separate cavity. Cranially the pelvic cavity is defined by the pelvic inlet, caudally by the pelvic outlet, dorsally by the pelvic bones and laterally by the muscles around the pelvic girdle.

Mediastinum

The mediastinum is the space in the anterior chest between the lungs, which contains the thymus, heart, aorta, trachea, oesophagus and various nerves and other blood vessels.

Coelom

In mammals, the diaphragm separates the thorax from the abdomen. However, birds and reptiles do not possess a true diaphragm and therefore the terms thorax and abdomen cannot be accurately used when describing these species. The one cavity is instead known as the **coelom** or **coelomic cavity**.

Skeletal system

The skeleton has a number of different functions:

- To act as a **framework** for other structures to attach to
- To enable **movement**
- To **protect** softer tissues and organs within the body
- To play a part in **haemopoiesis** (production of blood cells)
- To **store minerals** such as calcium and phosphorus.

Bone
Structure

Bone is a living organ, which undergoes change throughout the life of the animal. It consists of cells, collagen and glycoproteins. The main mineral in bone is calcium hydroxyapatite, thus bone is a reservoir of calcium for the body. The principal cells found in bone are:

- **Osteoblasts** – immature cells which can synthesize osteoid (the bone matrix)
- **Osteocytes** – mature cells which maintain bone structure
- **Osteoclasts** – cells which can break down and remodel bone.

There are two main forms of bone: **compact** and **cancellous**.

Compact bone

This is found in areas that are prone to stress, such as the outer surfaces (cortices) of bones. It has a dense and regular structure almost entirely made of mineralized matrix. Compact bone comprises concentric circles of matrix called **lamellae**, which are arranged around a central canal (**Haversian canal**) that contains blood vessels, nerves and loose connective tissue (Figure 3.10). Gaps in the matrix are called **lacunae** and contain osteocytes. The whole system is known as the **Haversian system** or **osteon**.

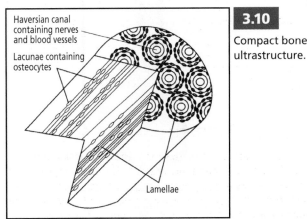

3.10 Compact bone ultrastructure.

Haversian canal containing nerves and blood vessels

Lacunae containing osteocytes

Lamellae

Cancellous bone

This is more commonly found in vertebrae, flat bones and at the ends of long bones. Cancellous bone (also known as spongy bone) comprises **trabeculae** (interconnected 'bars' of bone) with spaces in between. This means that cancellous bone is not as strong as compact bone.

Types

- **Long bones** (such as the femur and humerus) consist of an outer cortex of bone and a central medullary cavity which contains bone marrow. The outer part of the bone is covered in a connective tissue layer known as the **periosteum**. The blood supply to the bone enters at the periosteum and then branches to supply the bone tissue. Long bones have a central shaft known as the **diaphysis** and at each end an **epiphysis** (Figure 3.11). The area between the diaphysis and the epiphysis, which contains the **epiphyseal growth plate**, is known as the **metaphysis** and is an area of transition important in bone growth (see below).
- **Short bones** (such as the carpus) only have one section and develop from one centre of ossification. **Sesamoid** bones are a type of short bone.
- **Flat bones** (such as the bones of the skull) stretch out in two directions as they grow.
- **Irregular bones** – do not fit easily into the other categories, as they are variable in shape. The bones of the pelvis and spine are in this category.
- **Pneumatic bones** – these bones are found in birds. The medullary cavity is largely replaced by air and is connected to the air sacs. The function is to make the skeleton lighter as an adaption to flight.

Growth and development

In the very young animal the skeleton is predominantly cartilage. As the animal grows the amount of bone present increases as the cartilage is converted to bone. Bone development can take place by:

- Intramembranous ossification
- Endochondral ossification.

Intramembranous ossification

This is where bone is laid down to replace fibrous connective tissue. This occurs in the development of the bones of the skull, maxilla and mandible.

Endochondral ossification

This is where the initial hyaline cartilage is gradually replaced by osteocytes and calcium hydroxyapatite. This occurs in the long bones, vertebrae and pelvis in the following way:

1. The outline structure of the bone is formed first of cartilage.
2. Osteoblasts replace cartilage with bone:
   a. Primary ossification centres appear in the **diaphysis** of bones
   b. Secondary ossification centres appear at the ends (**epiphyses**) of bones (Figure 3.12).
3. The primary ossification centre in the diaphysis and the secondary centre in the epiphysis meet at a thick band of cartilage, known as the **epiphyseal growth plate**. The epiphyseal growth plate can be seen as a radiolucent 'gap' in the bone on radiographs of juvenile animals. This is an area of weakness and can be easily damaged through trauma.
4. The epiphyseal growth plate produces new cartilage cells on the epiphysis side of the plate, thus elongating the bone at either end.

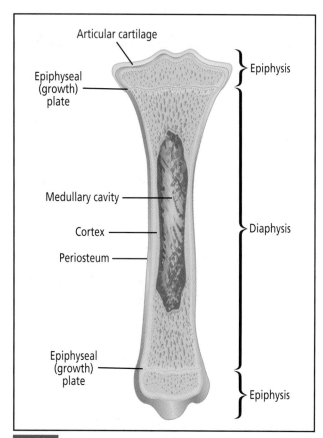

3.11 Structure of a long bone.

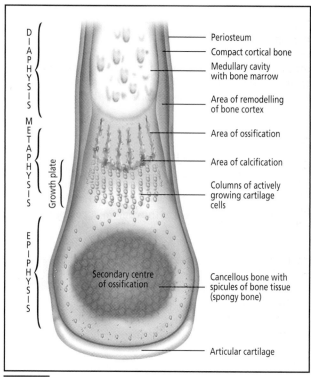

3.12 Endochondral ossification of a long bone.

5. The cartilage cells on the side of the epiphyseal growth plate nearest the diaphysis are steadily converted to bone as they are ossified by **osteoblasts**.
6. **Osteoclasts** remodel the interior of the diaphysis and create the medullary cavity.
7. Once the bone has reached its final length, the cartilage cells stop dividing and all cartilage is ossified, thereby 'closing' the growth plate.

Physiology

Bones are living tissue which are constantly remodelling. They act as source of calcium which can be added to, or utilized as the body needs (e.g. during lactation or egg laying in birds and reptiles). **Parathyroid hormone**, **calcitriol** and **calcitonin** control the amount of calcium present in bone (with help from the accessory hormone vitamin D3; see also 'Endocrine system').

Parathyroid hormone (PTH)

This is released by cells within the parathyroid gland and increases the activity of osteoclasts to break down bone and release calcium into the circulation. PTH inhibits the activity of osteoblasts, thus reducing calcium deposition in bone. PTH also increases the rate of excretion of inorganic phosphate by the kidneys, resulting in a drop in serum phosphate and leading to an increase in the release of both calcium and phosphate from bone. PTH works alongside and stimulates the production of **calcitriol (1,25-dihydroxycholecalciferol)** from the kidney.

Vitamin D3 and calcitriol

Vitamin D3 (hydroxycholecalciferol) is the inactive precursor of calcitriol (1,25-dehydroxycholecalciferol). Calcitriol promotes intestinal absorption of calcium, increases renal tubular resorption of calcium and stimulates osteoclast activity.

Calcitonin

This has the opposite effect to PTH and calcitriol. It decreases the activity of osteoclasts, thereby reducing the amount of calcium released from bone. It also increases the activity of osteoblasts, resulting in calcium deposition in bone. Calcitonin inhibits calcium absorption from the intestine.

Cartilage

Structure

Cartilage is a similar substance to bone, but without the mineralization, and so is softer. It is predominantly composed of collagen produced by chrondrocytes. The type of collagen present varies between the different types of cartilage according to the functions that it is required to perform.

Types

The three different types of cartilage found in the body are:

- Hyaline cartilage
- Fibrocartilage
- Elastic cartilage.

Hyaline cartilage

This is the most common form of cartilage. It is bluish white in appearance and is found between the epiphysis and diaphysis of growing long bones, at the articular surfaces of moveable joints, the walls of the respiratory tract (from the nose to the bronchi) and at the ventral ends of the ribs.

Fibrocartilage

This has a structure somewhere between that of hyaline cartilage and dense connective tissue. It is found in intervertebral discs, the pubic symphysis and at the attachment points of ligaments and tendons. It is very strong in tension.

Elastic cartilage

This contains elastic fibres, which allow the cartilage to bend more than hyaline cartilage. It is found in the auricle of the ear, the external auditory canal, the Eustachian tube and epiglottis.

Skeleton

The skeleton in most vertebrate species is organized into three main portions:

- The **axial** skeleton consists of the skull, spine and pelvis
- The **appendicular** skeleton comprises the limbs, which attach to the axial skeleton
- The **splanchnic** skeleton is composed of those bones not attached to the appendicular or axial skeleton such as the os *penis* in the dog and cat.

The basic skeleton of the dog is shown in Figure 3.13, of the horse in Figure 3.14 and of a bird in Figure 3.15.

Terminology

Before examining the skeleton, it is useful to be aware of the terminology used to describe bones:

- **Condyle** – a rounded protuberance at the end of a bone
- **Crest** – a raised area of bone
- **Foramen** – a hole or opening within a bone
- **Fossa** – a depression within a bone where another structure is found
- **Groove** – a depression in a bone
- **Medullary cavity** – the centre of long bones, often where bone marrow is found
- **Periosteum** – the outer covering of bones
- **Process** – a thin, elongated projection
- **Sinus** – a narrow, hollow cavity
- **Spine** – the central part of a bone
- **Trochanter** – a prominent area of the femur that lies behind the head of the femur
- **Tubercle** – a small elevation on the surface of a bone
- **Tuberosity** – the area of the tubercle where tendons attach.

Axial skeleton

The axial skeleton is made up of the skull, vertebral column, ribs and sternum.

Skull

The skull consists of: an upper section called the **cranium,** which houses the brain; the **maxilla** (the upper jaw and nasal chambers); the **mandible** (the lower jaw); and the

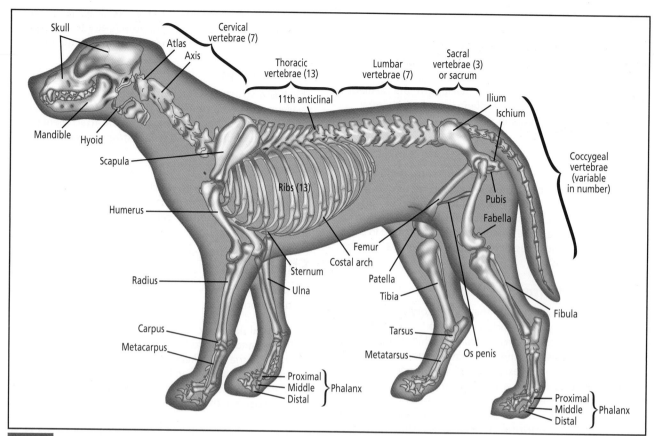

3.13 Skeleton of the dog.

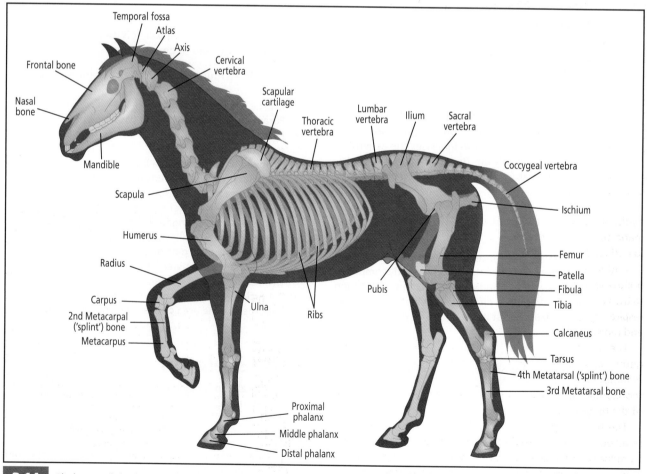

3.14 Skeleton of the horse.

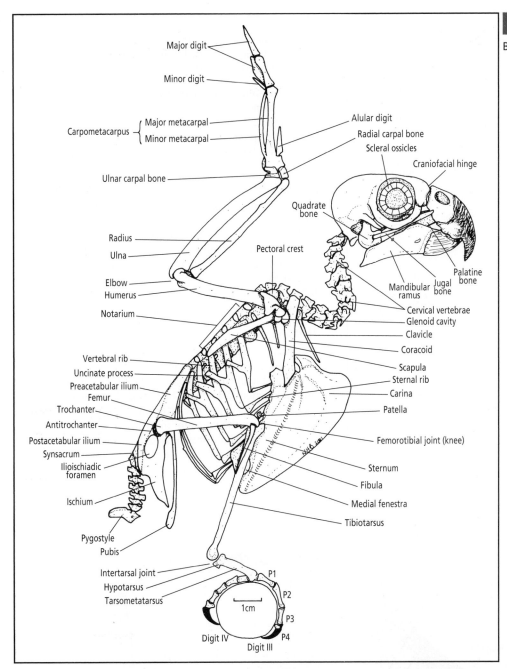

3.15 Skeleton of a bird. (© Nigel Harcourt-Brown)

Labels in figure:
Major digit
Minor digit
Major metacarpal
Carpometacarpus
Minor metacarpal
Ulnar carpal bone
Alular digit
Radial carpal bone
Scleral ossicles
Craniofacial hinge
Quadrate bone
Radius
Ulna
Pectoral crest
Elbow
Humerus
Notarium
Palatine bone
Mandibular ramus
Jugal bone
Cervical vertebrae
Glenoid cavity
Clavicle
Coracoid
Vertebral rib
Uncinate process
Preacetabular ilium
Femur
Trochanter
Antitrochanter
Postacetabular ilium
Synsacrum
Ilioischiadic foramen
Ischium
Scapula
Sternal rib
Carina
Patella
Femorotibial joint (knee)
Sternum
Fibula
Medial fenestra
Tibiotarsus
Pygostyle
Pubis
Intertarsal joint
Hypotarsus
Tarsometatarsus
P1
P2
P3
P4
1cm
Digit IV
Digit III

hyoid apparatus. These areas, particularly the cranium, are made up of many different bones (Figure 3.16) which are joined together by 'sutures'.

Within the maxilla of the skull are the sinuses. These are hollow spaces which lighten the skull and provide resonance to the vocal chords. The sinuses are also attached to the upper respiratory tract and provide an area where air can be warmed and moistened.

The mandible consists of two halves, which are held together by connective tissue in the midline rostrally at the mandibular symphysis. Each mandible consists of a **body** (horizontal part) and a **ramus** (vertical part), which forms part of the hinge joint of the jaw.

The hyoid apparatus (Figure 3.17) comprises a series of small bones, which together suspend the tongue and larynx from the skull. Small holes known as foramina (singular: foramen) are present in the skull through which blood vessels and nerves pass.

Area of the skull	Composite parts
Cranium	Foramen magnum Frontal Occipital Orbit Parietal Sphenoid Temporal Tympanic bulla Zygomatic arch
Maxilla (upper jaw and nasal chambers)	Incisive Nasal Palatine
Mandible (lower jaw)	Alveoli (areas of tooth attachment) Condylar process Coronoid process Horizontal ramus symphysis Mandibular symphysis Vertical ramus

3.16 Parts of the skull.

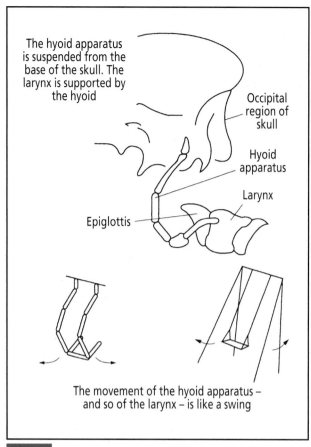

The hyoid apparatus is suspended from the base of the skull. The larynx is supported by the hyoid

Occipital region of skull

Hyoid apparatus

Larynx

Epiglottis

The movement of the hyoid apparatus – and so of the larynx – is like a swing

3.17 Hyoid apparatus.

Dogs and cats

The normal skull of the dog and cat is shown in Figures 3.18 and 3.19. In dogs the wide range of breeds has resulted in three basic skull shapes:

- **Dolicocephalic** – long, narrow head (collies, Wolfhounds)
- **Mesocephalic** – medium sized head (normal; German Shepherd Dogs, setters)
- **Brachycephalic** – short, wide head (Staffordshire Bull Terriers, Pekingese).

In dogs and cats (and other carnivores) the orbit is not a complete bony circle. The orbit is completed by a ligament, which connects the zygomatic process of the frontal bone to the zygomatic arch.

The main sinuses in dogs and cats are the **frontal sinus** and the **maxillary sinus**. The frontal sinus is found under the frontal bone and is divided into lateral, medial and rostral parts. The maxillary sinus is a large lateral diverticulum of the nasal cavity (located beneath the nasal and maxillary bones).

Horses

The normal skull of the horse is shown in Figure 3.20. The ocular bony orbit in horses (and other herbivores) is complete. The caudal skull has a prominent occipital ridge to which the nuchal ligament attaches. The ramus of the mandible is significant in order to provide attachment for the major muscles of mastication, the masseter muscles.

The horse has a complex system of sinuses (Figure 3.21). The frontal sinus is continuous with the dorsal conchal sinus and together they form the conchofrontal sinus. This sinus

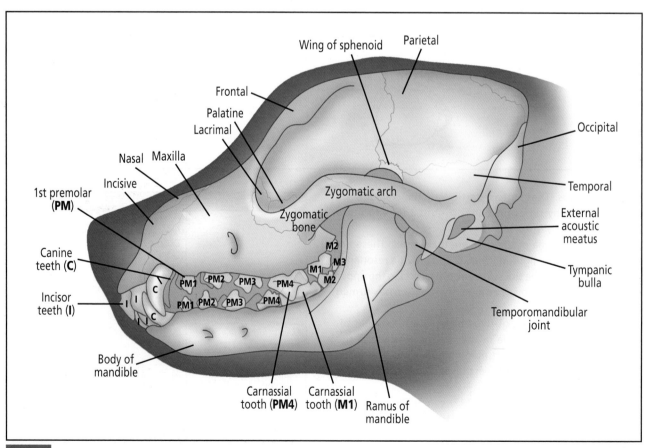

3.18 Lateral view of a dog skull showing tooth position.

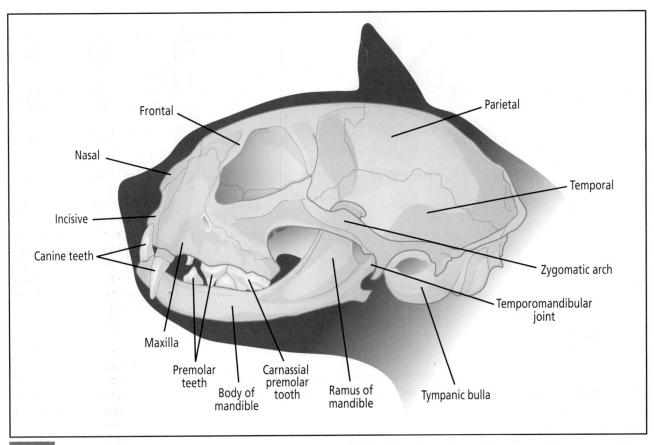

3.19 Lateral view of a cat skull showing tooth position.

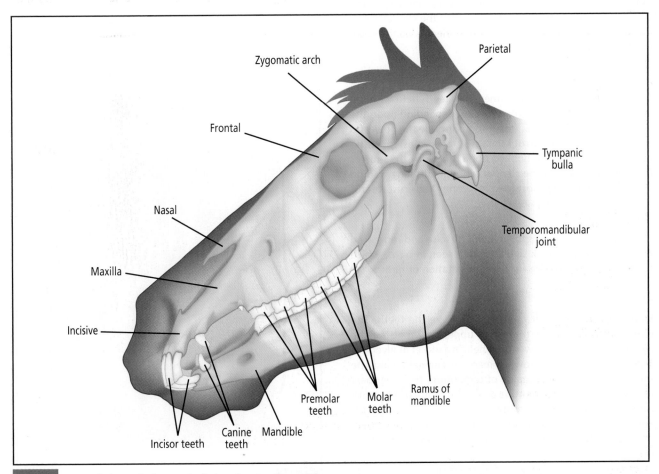

3.20 Lateral view of a horse skull showing tooth position.

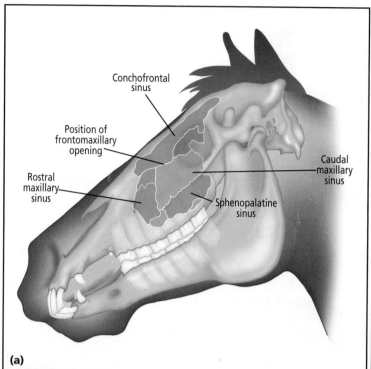

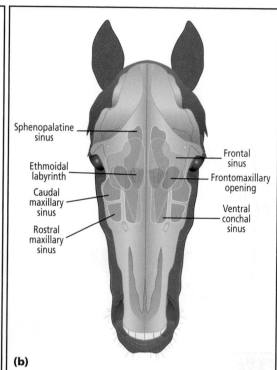

3.21 Location of the sinuses in the horse. **(a)** Lateral view. **(b)** Dorsoventral view.

communicates with the caudal maxillary sinus through the frontomaxillary opening. The rostral and caudal maxillary sinuses are separated by an oblique bony septum. The rostral maxillary sinus and the medial chamber of the caudal maxillary sinus communicate with the middle meatus via the nasomaxillary opening.

Birds

The avian skull has a beak (rather than teeth held within a jaw). The beak varies between species, depending upon the type of food the bird eats. Adaptations include the powerful crushing beak of the parrot family (Psittaciformes) for cracking seeds and nuts, the hooked ripping beak of the raptors for tearing flesh, and the slender long bill of many wading birds used for probing soft mud for worms and crustaceans.

Reptiles

Chelonians (such as the spur-thighed tortoise and red-eared terrapin) possess a beak similar to that seen in birds, which forms a shearing surface for biting vegetation or flesh.

Dentition

Embedded in the maxilla and mandible are the teeth. The basic tooth structure is that of an upper **crown** above the level of the gum and a lower **root**, held in a socket or **alveolus**. The outer part of the crown is made of **enamel**, whilst the outer part of the root is made of **cementum**. The inner part of the tooth is made of **dentine** and in the centre of the tooth is the **pulp cavity**, which contains blood vessels, lymphatics and nerves (Figures 3.22 and 3.23). Teeth differ in shape, depending on their location within the mouth and function (Figure 3.24).

In most mammals, two sets of teeth are produced. The first set of teeth, which are seen in the young animal and are

known as **deciduous** or milk teeth, are shed before adulthood. The deciduous teeth are replaced by larger and more robust teeth, known as **secondary** teeth.

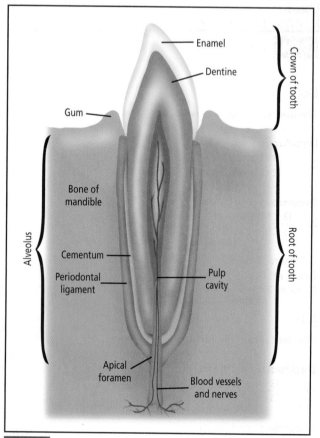

3.22 The structure of an incisor.

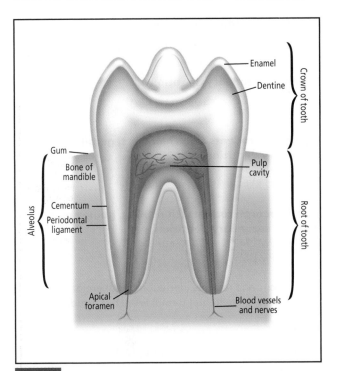

3.23 The structure of a molar.

Tooth	Function
Incisor	Nibbling of food, grooming
Canine	Piercing of food (e.g. for holding on to prey items)
Premolar	Shearing of food
Molar	Shearing and grinding of food (these teeth are flatter than premolars)

3.24 Functions of teeth.

Dogs

The dental formula for dogs is as follows:

Deciduous dentition

$$2x \quad \frac{i3 \ c1 \ pm3}{i3 \ c1 \ pm3} \quad = 28 \text{ teeth}$$

Secondary dentition

$$2x \quad \frac{I3 \ C1 \ PM4 \ M2}{I3 \ C1 \ PM4 \ M3} \quad = 42 \text{ teeth}$$

Where: C = canine; I = incisor; M = molar; PM = premolar. Deciduous teeth are signified by lower case letters (see Chapter 27 for further information).

Cats

The dental formula for cats is as follows:

Deciduous dentition

$$2x \quad \frac{i3 \ c1 \ pm3}{i3 \ c1 \ pm2} \quad = 26 \text{ teeth}$$

Secondary dentition

$$2x \quad \frac{I3 \ C1 \ PM3 \ M1}{I3 \ C1 \ PM2 \ M1} \quad = 30 \text{ teeth}$$

Horses

The dental formula for the horse is as follows:

Deciduous dentition

$$2x \quad \frac{i3 \ pm3}{i3 \ pm3} \quad = 24 \text{ teeth}$$

Secondary dentition

$$2x \quad \frac{I3 \ C1 \ PM3(4) \ M3}{I3 \ C1 \ PM3 \ M3} \quad = 40 \ (42) \text{ teeth}$$

The entrance to the mouth is small in horses. Canine teeth are present in both sexes, but they generally only erupt above the gum level in males. In addition, the first premolar ('wolf tooth') often fails to erupt and when it does it is generally vestigial and confined to the maxilla. The rest of the premolars form a continuous rank of teeth with the molars.

Horses can be aged according to the dental wear of the incisors (Figure 3.25) and the eruption of teeth. Deciduous central incisors are all erupted by 6 months. Secondary central incisors erupt at 2.5 years, second incisors by 3.5 years and

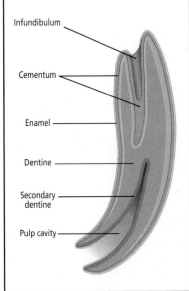

3.25 Occlusal tooth surfaces can be used for assessing approximate age in horses, as the teeth are progressively worn down with age.

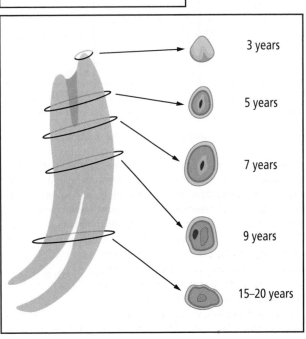

third incisors by 4.5 years. At approximately 5 years of age when all the secondary teeth have erupted, a horse is often said to have a 'full mouth'.

The original oval occlusal surface of the incisors becomes progressively round and then triangular. The enamel on the occlusal surface continues to erode and the central depression (cup), which often becomes stained with food material, wears out in the central incisors by 6 years and by 8 years in all incisors. At 11 or 12 years of age when the cups are absent from all upper and lower incisors a horse is said to be 'smooth mouthed'. However, it is now accepted that ageing horses by their teeth is an inexact science in anything but the youngest animals.

Ruminants

The dental formula for ruminants is as follows:

Deciduous dentition

$$2x \ \frac{pm3}{i3 \ c1 \ pm3} \ = 20 \ teeth$$

Secondary dentition

$$2x \ \frac{PM3 \ M3}{I3 \ C1 \ PM3 \ M3} \ = 32 \ teeth$$

Ruminant dentition has some unusual features. There are no upper incisors; the lower incisors cut on to a dental pad. In addition, the lower canines have migrated rostrally and function as fourth 'incisors'. For this reason they are referred to as 'incisor 4' from here on. As with horses, cattle and sheep can be aged according to the eruption of the incisor teeth (Figures 3.26).

Species	Tooth	Deciduous eruption	Secondary eruption
Cattle	Incisor 1	Birth–2 weeks of age	18–24 months
	Incisor 2	Birth–2 weeks of age	24–30 months
	Incisor 3	Birth–2 weeks of age	36–42 months
	Incisor 4	Birth–2 weeks of age	42–48 months
Sheep	Incisor 1	Before birth–1 week of age	12–18 months
	Incisor 2	Before birth–1 week of age	21–24 months
	Incisor 3	Before birth–1 week of age	27–31 months
	Incisor 4	Birth–1 week of age	36–48 months

3.26 Average eruption dates of incisor teeth in cattle and sheep.

The incisors are separated from the premolars by a gap devoid of teeth known as the **diastema**. The premolars and molars are arranged as a continuous arcade of teeth (cheek teeth; similar to the rabbit). The occlusal surfaces are ridged and interlock with the opposing teeth, but because the maxilla is wider than the mandible, lateral movement of the mandible is required to allow mastication to occur.

Small mammals

The dental formulae of various small mammals are as follows:

Ferrets – deciduous dentition

$$2x \ \frac{i1 \ c1 \ pm3}{c1 \ pm3} \ = 18 \ teeth$$

Ferrets – secondary dentition

$$2x \ \frac{I3 \ C1 \ PM3 \ M1}{I3 \ C1 \ PM3 \ M2} \ = 34 \ teeth$$

Rabbits – secondary dentition

$$2x \ \frac{I2 \ PM3 \ M3}{I1 \ PM2 \ M3} \ = 28 \ teeth$$

Myomorph rodents (rats, hamsters, gerbils, mice) – secondary dentition

$$2x \ \frac{I1 \ M3}{I1 \ M3} \ = 16 \ teeth$$

Hystricomorph rodents (chinchillas, guinea pigs, degus) – secondary dentition

$$2x \ \frac{I1 \ PM1 \ M3}{I1 \ PM1 \ M3} \ = 20 \ teeth$$

In rabbits and rodents, deciduous teeth are often shed *in utero* and so these dental formulae are not listed.

Reptiles

Lizards possess fine simple peg-like teeth in four rows (two in the maxilla and two in the mandible). Depending upon the species, these teeth may be shed and replaced throughout life (e.g. iguanids who have **pleurodont dentition**) or the lizard may have just one set of teeth for the whole of its life (e.g. agamids and chameleons who have **acrodont dentition**). Some species have hollow teeth and venom glands (e.g. Gila monster).

Snakes possess fine simple curved teeth in six rows (average: four rows in the maxilla and two rows in the mandible). Some of the teeth are adapted into fangs with venom glands. The teeth are often shed and regrow during the course of the snake's life. The teeth point caudally to encourage swallowing of prey.

Vertebral column

The vertebral column is formed from a variety of different vertebrae: cervical, thoracic, lumbar, sacral and coccygeal. The basic structure of a vertebra consists of a **body, transverse processes**, a **spinous process** and a **vertebral foramen** (Figure 3.27). However, there are regional differences in the shape of the vertebrae (Figure 3.28).

- The first two **cervical vertebrae** are the **atlas** and **axis**:
  - The **atlas** is the first cervical vertebra and allows the head to nod. It articulates with the occipital condyles of the skull. It comprises two lateral wings with little or no body. These wings are joined dorsally and ventrally to surround the vertebral canal with a dorsal and ventral arch.
  - The **axis** is the second cervical vertebrae and allows a rotating or shaking movement of the head. It has a prominent dorsal spinous process. It also possesses a prominent ventral cranial projection from the body of the vertebra known as the odontoid process or 'dens'.
  - The remaining cervical vertebrae are more box-like in character.
- The **thoracic vertebrae** have a tall spinous process and very short transverse processes.
- The **lumbar vertebrae** have a short spinous process but enlarged transverse processes. This allows the lumbar muscles to attach to the vertebrae.

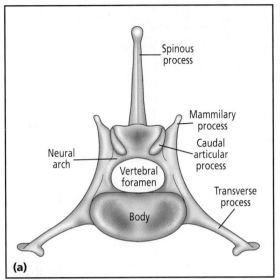

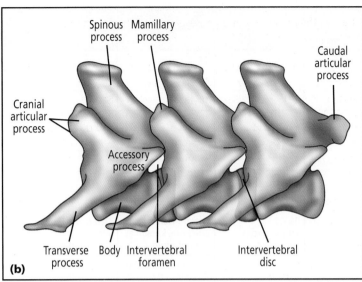

3.27 **(a)** Basic lumbar vertebra (caudal view). **(b)** Part of the vertebral column showing three lumbar vertebrae (left lateral view).

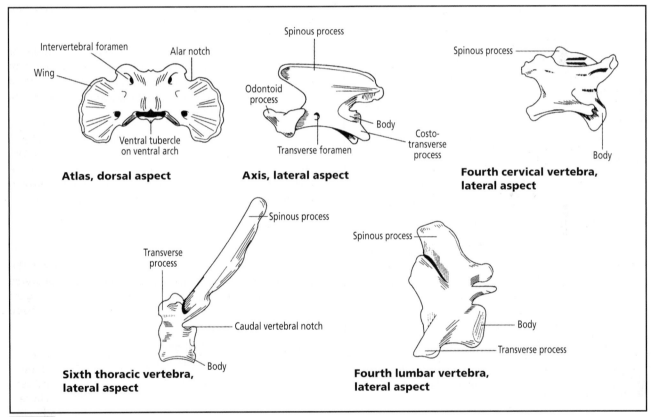

3.28 Regional differences in the vertebrae.

- The **sacral vertebrae** are fused in the dog and cat into the **sacrum**.
- The **coccygeal vertebrae** have very small transverse and spinous processes, making them almost cuboid in shape.

In addition, the number of different vertebrae (or the **vertebral formula**) varies between species (Figure 3.29).

Between the bodies of the vertebrae are **intervertebral discs** (see Figure 3.27b). These have two main parts: the **nucleus pulposus** and the **annulus fibrosus**. Intervertebral discs have a shock absorber effect, minimizing damage to the bones whilst allowing some flexibility and 'give' to the spinal column.

Ribs and sternum

The basic rib structure (Figure 3.30) consists of a bony part, which articulates with the thoracic vertebrae dorsally at the **head** of the rib, also known as the **body**. Ventrally, the lower half of the rib comprises cartilage known as **costal cartilage**. The area where the bone meets the cartilage is the **costochondral junction**.

Species	Type of vertebra				
	Cervical	*Thoracic*	*Lumbar*	*Sacral*	*Coccygeal*
Dog	7	13	7	3	20–23
Cat	7	13	7	3	20–23
Horse	7	18–19	5–6	5	18
Ferret	7	15	5(6)	3	18
Rabbit	7	12–13	7	4	15–16
Guinea pig	7	13	6	3–4	4–6
Rat	7	13	6	4	27–31
Hamster	7	13	6	4	7–14
Birds	11–25 Large species variations	Often fused into one bone known as the notarium	Often one mobile lumbar vertebra. The rest are fused into the synsacrum	Fused together to form the roof of the pelvis known as the synsacrum	Large species variations. The last few vertebrae are fused together to form the pygostyle
Reptiles	Large species variations. Generally box-like	Chelonians: may be fused into the shell Lizards and snakes: mobile and box-like	Chelonians: may be fused into the shell Lizards and snakes: mobile and box-like	Chelonians: may be fused into the shell Lizards: may be fused to the roof of the pelvis or mobile	Large species variations Chelonians: may be few in number Lizards: significantly greater in number than chelonians

3.29 Vertebral formulae for different species.

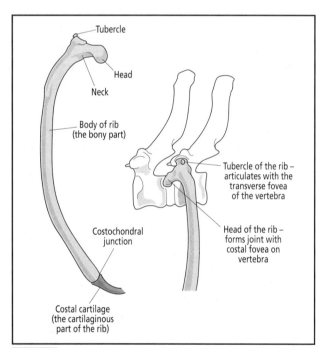

Tubercle

Head

Neck

Body of rib (the bony part)

Costochondral junction

Costal cartilage (the cartilaginous part of the rib)

Tubercle of the rib – articulates with the transverse fovea of the vertebra

Head of the rib – forms joint with costal fovea on vertebra

3.30 Structure of a rib and rib articulation.

The ribs from the left and right sides meet ventrally at the **sternebrae**. The most cranial sternebra is known as the **manubrium**, and the most caudal sternebra is known as the **xiphoid**, the process of which can be felt protruding from the end of the sternum. Ribs 1–8 articulate with the sternum. Ventrally each rib curves cranially to touch the rib in front at its junction with the sternum.

Dogs and cats

In dogs and cats ribs 9–12 curve cranially to touch the rib in front but do not touch the sternum, thus forming the **costal arch**. However, rib 13 does not curve cranially and the ventral point can be felt at the end of the ribcage; this is called the 'floating rib'.

Birds

These animals possess a **keel** bone over the sternum. This varies in prominence, being more important in species that are strong fliers as it provides the surface area for the attachment of the flight muscles.

Appendicular skeleton

The appendicular skeleton comprises the limbs, which are attached to the vertebral column via the pectoral and pelvic girdles. For this reason snakes do not have an appendicular skeleton, with the exception of the occasional vestige of the pelvis in some *Boa* species.

Forelimbs

The forelimb consists of the clavicle, scapula, humerus, radius, ulna, carpus, metacarpus and phalanges.

Clavicle

The clavicle is the collarbone, which is present to varying degrees in different animals (e.g. in dogs it is made of cartilage rather than bone and is not obvious on radiographs, whereas in cats it is fully formed and visible on radiographs).

Scapula

The scapula is a flat bone, which attaches to the body via muscles, not a joint. It consists of a cranial and caudal surface separated by a **spine**. The distal part of the spine is known as the **acromion**. In the dog the acromion comprises one part, whereas in the cat it is split into two sections. The distal end of the scapula articulates with the humerus.

Humerus

The humerus is a simple bone comprising a head, which articulates with the scapula, and a **greater tubercle**, which makes up the shoulder. Distally there is a hole in the humerus known as the **olecranon fossa**, which is where the ulna articulates with the humerus to form the elbow joint.

Radius and ulna

The lower part of the forelimb consists of the radius and ulna, which lie alongside each other. The radius is a short bone without any distinctive features. The ulna is longer than the radius and can be felt as the point of the elbow at the **olecranon**. The ulna articulates with the humerus where the **anconeal process** of the ulna fits into the **olecranon fossa** of the humerus. Distally the ulna tapers to a point known as the **styloid process**. Thus, the radius provides most of the proximal articular surface of the carpus.

Carpus

The carpus is made up of a number of different bones (Figure 3.31). Proximally there are three carpal bones: the **radial** and **ulnar**, which articulate with the radius and ulna, respectively, and the **accessory carpal bone**, which can be felt to protrude laterally. Distal to this is another row of carpal bones, which articulate between the first row of carpal bones and the metacarpal bones. However, these **distal carpal bones** are only present next to the first four metacarpal bones. The fifth metacarpal bone articulates with the ulnar carpal bone.

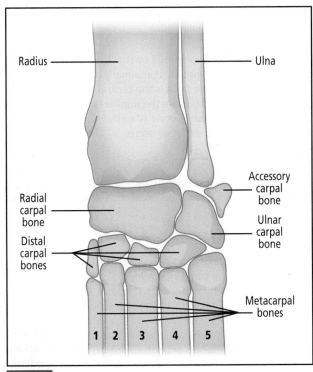

Radius — Ulna

Radial carpal bone

Distal carpal bones

Accessory carpal bone

Ulnar carpal bone

Metacarpal bones

1 2 3 4 5

3.31 Structure of the left carpus.

Metacarpus and phalanges

Metacarpal bones are long and thin and join the carpus to the digits. The digits comprise smaller bones known as phalanges. The first digit is made up of two phalanges (the dew claw) and the other digits are made up of three phalanges. These are known as the proximal, middle and distal phalanges. The most distal phalange is modified to allow the nail to grow at the ungual process.

Horses

The ulna of the horse fuses with the radius distally. There are usually seven carpal bones:

- Proximal row: radial, ulnar and intermediate with an accessory carpal bone projecting palmarly (not involved in weight bearing)
- Distal row: second, third and fourth carpal bones.

However, in some individuals there may also be a first carpal bone in the distal row, which is small, pea-shaped and not physically connected to the other carpal bones, but embedded in the carpal ligament palmar to the second carpal bone. The carpus is often incorrectly referred to as the knee in the horse.

There are only three metacarpal bones in the horse and the third metacarpal bone bears the majority of the animal's bodyweight. The second and fourth metacarpal bones are reduced to palmar situated 'splint' bones that fuse to the third metacarpal. The section of the forelimb represented by the metacarpal bones is referred to as the **cannon bone**.

The third metacarpal bone articulates distally with the first phalanx. This joint is referred to as the **metacarpophalangeal joint** or **fetlock**, which articulates with the middle phalanx, which in turn articulates with the distal phalanx. The distal phalanx is hoof-shaped. Thus, the horse has only one digit per limb. Two large proximal sesamoid bones, which provide support for the flexor tendons of the lower limb, are located over the palmar aspect of the fetlock. The distal sesamoid bone, commonly referred to as the **navicular bone**, is located over the palmar aspect of the distal interphalangeal joint. The section of lower forelimb between the fetlock and hoof is referred to as the **pastern**. The hoof is described in detail later (see Figure 3.96).

Small mammals

In ferrets, rabbits and most rodents the clavicle is present and obvious on radiographs. The scapula in small animals varies slightly between species; rabbits have a markedly hooked suprahamate process. In chinchillas, guinea pigs, hamsters and gerbils there are only four digits in the forelimbs.

Birds

The clavicles are well developed in birds and fused together to form the furcula or wishbone, which creates a spring-like effect to counteract the compressive forces generated on the downbeat of the wings. Birds also possess a **coracoid** bone, which projects ventrally from the shoulder joint to the keel bone and acts as a strut or support for the shoulder, allowing it to cope with the stress of rapid wing movements during flight.

The forelimbs are adapted to form wings, which results in a reduction in the overall number of bones. The scapulae are flattened and lie across the lateral surface of the ribcage. Each of the scapulae forms a shoulder joint with the humerus, the clavicle and the coracoid bones.

The radius is the smaller of the antebrachial bones in the bird. The secondary flight feathers attach directly to the periosteum of the stouter and more caudally placed ulna. The carpal bones are reduced to one major and one minor carpal bone. There are only three metacarpal bones: a vestigial first metacarpal bone known as the **alula** or 'bastard wing' (equivalent to the bird's thumb), and the major and minor metacarpal bones. The digits are similarly reduced to a single phalanx representing the first (minor) digit and two phalanges representing the major digit, which forms the tip of the wing. The primary feathers attach to the periosteum of the metacarpal bones and phalanges.

Reptiles

Lizards and chelonians possess well developed clavicles, although in the latter these are located within the ribcage. In addition, chelonians have a coracoid bone that projects dorsally from the shoulder joint to the inside of the dorsum of the carapace, which acts as a supporting strut for the shell and shoulder joint. The forelimbs in lizards and chelonians usually have five digits, although there is some species variation.

Hindlimbs

The hindlimb consists of the pelvis, femur, tibia, fibula, tarsus, metatarsus, phalanges, patella and fabellae.

Pelvis

The hindlimbs attach to the vertebral column via the pelvis. The pelvis is made up of a number of different bones, which are fused together (Figure 3.32). Dorsally and cranially the **ilium** can be felt lying alongside the vertebral column. Ventrally the left and right sides of the pelvis meet at the **pubis**. Caudally the **ischium** can be felt on either side of the tail. Ventrally there is a large hole in either side of the floor of the pelvis known as the **obturator foramen**. The hindleg attaches to the pelvis via the **acetabulum** formed at the junction of the ilium, ischium and pubis.

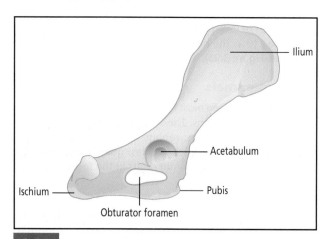

3.32   Structure of the pelvis.

Femur

The femur is the most proximal bone of the hindlimb. Structurally it is similar to the humerus. The round **head** articulates with the acetabulum of the pelvis (ball and socket joint). Laterally the **greater trochanter** can be felt on the proximal femur protruding alongside the hip joint. Distally the femur has a groove known as the **trochlea**, which forms part of the **stifle** (equivalent to the human knee joint).

Tibia and fibula

Distal to the stifle, making up the lower part of the leg, are the tibia and fibula. The tibia is the main weight-bearing bone, forming most of the distal articular surface of the stifle joint. Lateral to the tibia is the fibula, which is a long, thin bone. Distally the tibia and fibula articulate with the **tarsus** (or **hock**).

Tarsus

The tarsus is similar to the carpus in that it comprises rows of smaller bones (Figure 3.33). The tibia and fibula articulate

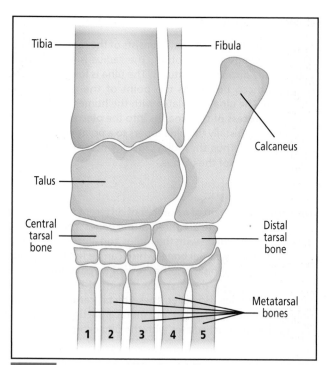

3.33   Structure of the left tarsus.

with the **talus** in the proximal tarsus. Lateral to the talus is the **calcaneus**, which projects proximally to form the point of the hock. Distal to the talus is the central tarsal bone. Distal to the central tarsal bone are the smaller tarsal bones I, II and III. Lateral to this is tarsal bone IV (distal tarsal bone), which is larger than the other tarsal bones.

Metatarsus and phalanges

The metatarsal bones and phalanges of the hindlimb are similar to the metacarpal bones and phalanges of the forelimb.

Patella and fabellae

Sesamoid bones are found near to joints. Most are found in tendons, but some can be found in ligaments. The function of these bones is to protect the tendons. The **patella** (knee cap) is the largest sesamoid bone in the body. It is found on the cranial surface, and makes up the largest part, of the stifle. It sits in the trochlea of the femur and moves every time the knee is straightened or bent. Caudal to the stifle, smaller sesamoid bones known as **fabellae** can be found in the tendons of the gastrocnemius muscle.

Horses

The fibula of the horse is much reduced and fuses with the tibia proximally. The tarsus is a compound joint. The bones in the tarsus are:

- Proximal row: the calcaneus (to which the Achilles tendon attaches at the point of the hock) and the talus
- Intermediate row: a central tarsal bone
- Distal row: fused first and second tarsal bones and separate third and fourth tarsal bones.

Proximally the distal tibia articulates with the trochlea of the talus. The next joint is the proximal intertarsal (technically the talo-centro-calcaneal) joint where the talus and the calcaneus articulate with the third and fourth tarsal bones. The centrodistal joint articulates the central tarsal bone with the first, second and third tarsal bones. The tarsometatarsal joint articulates the first, second, third and fourth tarsal bones with the second, third and fourth metatarsal bones. There are three joint cavities in the tarsus: one for the tarsocrural and proximal intertarsal joints; one for the centrodistal joint; and one for the tarsometatarsal joint.

There are only three metatarsal bones in the horse and the third metatarsal bears the majority of the animal's weight. The second and fourth metatarsal bones are reduced to plantar 'splint' bones that fuse to the third metatarsal. The lower hindlimb of the horse is similar to the lower forelimb.

Small mammals

The rabbit has a separate bone, known as the os acetabuli, which forms the structure of the hip joint. In addition, the femur is more flattened in the rabbit, making this bone less suitable for the intramedullary pin techniques used for fracture repair. In the majority of small mammals there are four digits in the hindlimb, with the exception of guinea pigs where there are three, and hamsters and gerbils where there are five.

Birds

The pelvis has separate pubis bones, which instead of meeting in the midline actually support the musculature of the ventral body wall. The pelvis fuses dorsally with the **synsacrum**.

The tibia in birds is fused with the proximal row of tarsal bones to form the **tibiotarsus**. The distal row of tarsal bones is fused with the metatarsal bones (which themselves are fused together into one bone) to form the **tarsometatarsus**. Thus, the avian equivalent of the hock is actually an intertarsal joint and is known as the **suffrago joint**.

The hindlimbs of most birds have four digits. In parrots, the first and fourth digits point caudally, and the second and third digits point cranially (known as a **zygodactyl limb**). In most raptors and passerines (such as canaries and finches), the first digit points caudally, and the second, third and fourth digits point cranially (known as an **anisodactyl limb**).

Reptiles

In chelonians, the pelvis is rotated so that the ilium is near vertical and the ischium and pubis point ventrally and cranially. In females, the pubic bones are not fused together, in order to allow egg laying.

Splanchnic skeleton

A splanchnic bone is one that develops within the soft tissues. In many male animals, including the dog, ferret, hamster and gerbil, a bone is present within the penis. This is known as the **os penis**. It is absent or only partially present in male cats.

Joints

A joint occurs where two or more bones join together or articulate. Different degrees of movement are present in different types of joint. Joints are classified as follows:

- **Fibrous** – little or no movement
- **Cartilaginous** – little or no movement
- **Synovial** – a wide range of movement.

Terminology

The range of movement of a joint can be described using the following terms:

- **Flexion** – bending the limb by decreasing the angle of the joint
- **Extension** – straightening the limb by increasing the angle of the joint
- **Adduction** – moving the limb distal to the joint towards the midline/body
- **Abduction** – moving the limb distal to the joint away from the midline/body
- **Gliding** – flat surfaces moving over each other (e.g. in the carpus)
- **Rotation** – movement shown by a pivot joint
- **Circumduction** – moving one end of a bone (usually the end distal to the joint) in a circular motion
- **Protraction** – lengthening the limb by moving distal limb away from the body
- **Retraction** – shortening the limb by moving the distal limb towards the body
- **Supination** – turning the lower surface of the paw downwards
- **Pronation** – turning the lower surface of the paw upwards.

Fibrous joints

Fibrous joints are present as **sutures** in the skull, or **syndesmoses** between two areas of bone.

Cartilaginous joints

Cartilaginous joints can present as **synchondroses**, which are joints between the epiphyses and diaphyses in growing animals, or as **symphyses**, which are joints between the mandible bones of the lower jaw and the pubic bones of the pelvis.

Synovial joints

Synovial joints (**diarthroses**; Figure 3.34) are characterized by

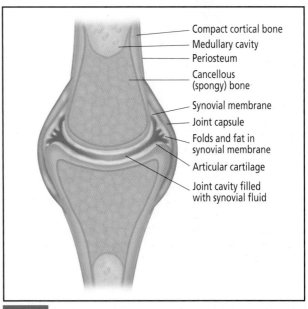

Compact cortical bone
Medullary cavity
Periosteum
Cancellous (spongy) bone
Synovial membrane
Joint capsule
Folds and fat in synovial membrane
Articular cartilage
Joint cavity filled with synovial fluid

3.34   A synovial joint.

the presence of:

- Synovial membrane
- Fibrous joint capsule
- Articular surfaces
- Synovial fluid
- Ligaments
- Meniscus/menisci.

Synovial joints can be further described according to the range of movement they allow (Figure 3.35).

Ligaments

Ligaments are thickened bands of fibrous tissue which connect bones and form the capsules of joints.

Stifle

The stifle comprises the femur, tibia, fibula and patella. These bones are held in place by four different ligaments:

- The **medial collateral ligament** joins the femur to the proximal tibia on the medial side of the stifle joint
- The **lateral collateral ligament** runs from the femur to the fibula on the lateral side of the stifle joint
- The **cranial cruciate ligament** runs from the lateral condyle of the femur to the caudal tibial plateau
- The **caudal cruciate ligament** runs at right angles to the cranial cruciate ligament, attaching the femur to the tibia.

In dogs there are also two small sesamoid bones (fabellae) caudal to the stifle joint, situated in the origin of the gastrocnemius muscle. Located between the condyles of the femur and the tibia are menisci; wedge-shaped pieces of cartilage sitting both laterally and medially. These prevent some of the lateral movement of the femur in relation to the tibial plateau. The menisci also have nerve endings, which provide information to the nervous system about the pressure within and the position of the stifle joint.

Joint	Type of movement	Examples
Condylar	Convex surface which fits on to a concave surface to allow flexion and extension	Stifle (between femur and tibia; Figure 3.36)
Ellipsoidal	Sliding	Radiocarpal joint
Hinge	In one plane	Elbow (between humerus and radius/ulna)
Pivot	Rotational	Atlanto-axial joint; radius and ulna
Plane	Sliding	Between carpal and tarsal bones
Saddle	In one plane	Phalanges
Spheroidal (ball and socket)	Rotational	Hip (between femur and acetabulum)

3.35 Classification and range of movement of synovial joints.

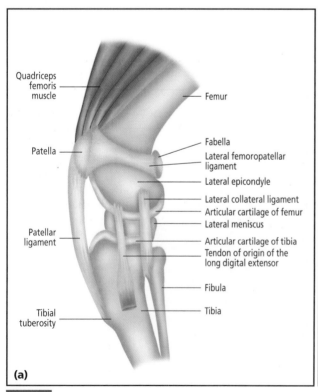

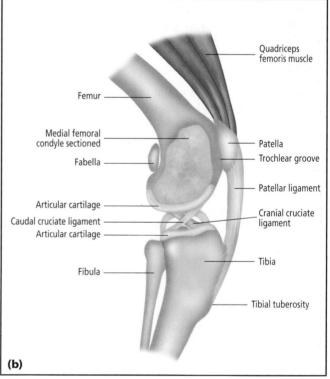

3.36 Structure of the left stifle joint. **(a)** Lateral view. **(b)** Medial view.

Muscular system

There are three basic types of muscle: skeletal, smooth and cardiac (Figure 3.37).

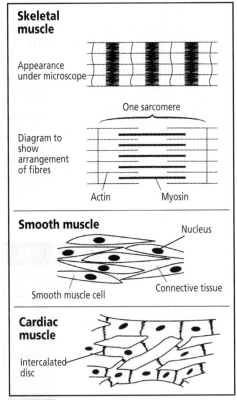

Skeletal muscle

Appearance under microscope

One sarcomere

Diagram to show arrangement of fibres

Actin   Myosin

Smooth muscle

Nucleus

Smooth muscle cell

Connective tissue

Cardiac muscle

Intercalated disc

3.37 Structure of muscle tissue.

Skeletal muscle

Skeletal (**striated** or **voluntary**) muscle is found in association with the skeleton. It consists of individual muscle cells known as **muscle fibres**, which are grouped together in bundles called **fascicles** by connective tissue called **perimysium**. Many perimysium-bound bundles are further grouped together, and the whole muscle is then surrounded by **epimysium**. Each muscle fibre contains many **myofibrils**. The basic unit of a myofibril is the **sarcomere**, which comprises **actin** and **myosin** filaments.

The structure of a skeletal muscle is shown in Figure 3.38. The muscle **origin** is the proximal attachment to the skeleton. The main part of the muscle is known as the **muscle belly**. The

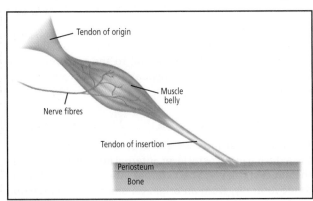

Tendon of origin

Muscle belly

Nerve fibres

Tendon of insertion

Periosteum

Bone

3.38 Muscle and tendon insertion.

distal part of the muscle then attaches to the skeleton at the point of **insertion**. Muscles are attached to bones via **tendons**, which consist of connective tissue. Where a tendon is closely related to a bone, a **bursa** may be present to act as a protective cushion between the bone and the tendon. Surrounding the tendon is a connective tissue layer (the **synovial sheath**), which allows the smooth movement of the tendon over the bone and provides nutrients to the tendon.

Skeletal muscles are stimulated to contract by an impulse from a neuron. The first stage of contraction is initiated by an increase in the intracellular calcium concentration. This allows the actin and myosin filaments to move and overlap one another, resulting in contraction of the muscle.

Forelimb muscles

The muscles of the forelimb of the dog are shown in Figure 3.39 and described in Figure 3.40.

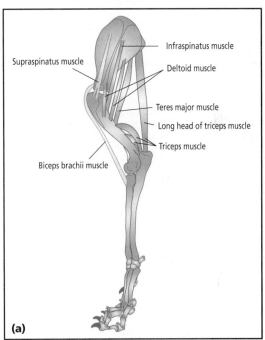

Infraspinatus muscle

Supraspinatus muscle

Deltoid muscle

Teres major muscle

Long head of triceps muscle

Triceps muscle

Biceps brachii muscle

(a)

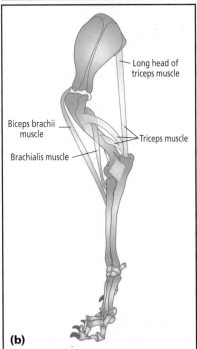

Long head of triceps muscle

Biceps brachii muscle

Triceps muscle

Brachialis muscle

(b)

3.39 Lateral views of the muscles of the forelimb of the dog. **(a)** Muscles that move the shoulder joint. **(b)** Muscles that move the elbow joint.

Muscle	Origin	Insertion	Function
Trapezius	Mid cervical and thoracic vertebrae	Spine of the scapula	Abductor of the forelimb

Brachiocephalicus:
  Cleidobrachialis
  Cleidocervicalis
  Cleidomastoideus
	Cervical region	Humerus	Advances the forelimb

Latissimus dorsi	Caudal thoracic and lumbar vertebrae	Medial humerus	Flexes the shoulder and retracts the forelimb
Supraspinatus	Supraspinous fossa	Proximal tuberosities	Stabilizes the shoulder
Infraspinatus	Infraspinous fossa	Lateral tubercle of the humerus	Stabilizes and abducts the shoulder
Triceps	Caudal border of the scapula and tricipital head of the humerus	Olecranon	Flexes the shoulder and extends the elbow
Biceps brachii	Supraglenoid tubercle	Radial tuberosity	Extends the shoulder and flexes the elbow
Brachialis	Proximal caudal aspect of the humerus	Radial tubercle	Flexes the elbow

Carpal flexors:
  Flexor carpi radialis
 	
  Flexor carpi ulnaris
 	
  Deep digital flexors
 	
  Superficial digital flexors
	
	Medial epicondyle of the humerus and medial radius
	Medial epicondyle of the humerus and caudal ulna
	Medial epicondyle of the humerus, caudal ulna and medial radius
	Medial epicondyle of the humerus
		
		Palmar side of metacarpal 2 and 3
		
		Accessory carpal bone
		
		Flexor surface of distal phalanges 1–5
		Palmar surface of phalanges 2–5
			Flex the carpus

Carpal extensors:
  Extensor carpi ulnaris
  Extensor carpi radialis
 	
  Common digital extensor
 	
  Lateral digital extensor
	
	Lateral ulna
	Lateral supracondylar crest of the radius
	Lateral epicondyle of the humerus
	
	Lateral epicondyle of the humerus
		
		5th metacarpal
		Tuberosities on 2nd and 3rd metacarpals
		Extensor processes of distal phalanges 2–5
		Proximal ends of all phalanges and distal ends of phalanges 3–5
			Extend the carpus

Digital flexors:
  Deep digital flexor
 	
  Superficial digital flexor
	
	Medial epicondyle of the humerus, distal radius (medial) and ulna (caudal)
	Medial epicondyle of the humerus
		
		Flexor surface of distal phalanges 1–5
		
		Palmar surface of phalanges 2–5
			Flex the digits

Digital extensors:
  Common digital extensor
 	
  Lateral digital extensor
	
	Lateral epicondyle of the humerus
	
	Lateral epicondyle of the humerus
		
		Extensor processes of distal phalanges 2–5
		Proximal ends of all phalanges and distal ends of phalanges 3–5
			Extend the digits

3.40 Muscles of the forelimb of the dog.

Hindlimb muscles

The muscles of the hindlimb are shown in Figure 3.41 and described in Figure 3.42. In addition, the Achilles tendon (common calcanean tendon) inserts on the point of the hock (the calcaneus; see Figure 3.33), allowing connection of the gastrocnemius muscle to the hock.

Epaxial muscles

The epaxial muscles lie dorsal to the transverse processes of the vertebrae. They are arranged in three parallel rows, which run from the neck to the lumbar area, and extend the vertebral column.

Hypoaxial muscles

The hypoaxial muscles lie ventral to the transverse processes of the vertebrae. The hypoaxial muscles cause flexion of the neck.

Intercostal muscles

The intercostal muscles are arranged in three layers: the **external intercostal** layer, **internal intercostal** layer and the **subcostal** layer. The external intercostal muscles run caudoventrally, from an origin on one rib to an insertion on another rib. Internal intercostal muscles run cranioventrally.

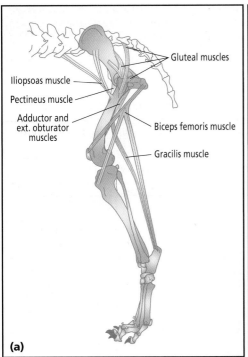

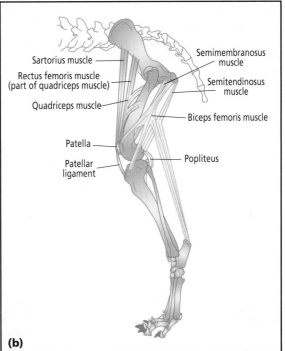

(a)

(b)

3.41

Lateral views of the muscles of the hindlimb of the dog. **(a)** Muscles that protract, retract, adduct and abduct the hindlimb. These muscles also flex and extend the hip. **(b)** Muscles that move the hip and stifle joint.

Muscle	Origin	Insertion	Function
Biceps femoris	Ischial tuberosity	Various insertions including the patella, tibial crest and calcaneus	Retracts the hip, flexes/extends the stifle and extends the hock
Semimembranosus	Ischial tuberosity	Medial distal femur and medial proximal tibia	Retracts the hip and flexes the stifle
Semitendonosus	Ischial tuberosity	Tibial crest and calcaneus	Retracts the hip and extends the stifle and hock
Quadriceps femoris: 　Vastus lateralis 　Vastus intermedius 　Vastus medialis 　Rectus femoris	 Proximal femur Proximal femur Proximal femur Ilium	Tibial tuberosity	Extends the stifle
Pectineus	Prepubic tendon and pelvis	Distal femur	Adducts the hip
Gastrocnemius	Caudolateral distal femur	Calcaneus	Flexes the stifle and extends the hock
Hock flexors: 　Long digital extensor 　Lateral digital extensor 　Cranial tibialis 　Fibularis brevis 　Fibularis longus	 Lateral epicondyle of the femur Proximal third of the fibula Proximal tibia laterally Lateral tibia and fibula distally Proximal tibia and fibula	 Dorsal surface of distal phalanges 2–5 Phalanges of 5th digit Metatarsal 1 and proximal end of metatarsal 2 Proximal end of metatarsal 5 Plantar surface of all metatarsals and 4th tarsal bone	Flex the hock
Hock extensors: 　Superficial digital flexor[a] 　Gastrocnemius 　Semitendinosis 　Biceps femoris	 Lateral supracondyle of the femur and sesamoid Medial and lateral supracondyles of the femur Lateral ischial tuberosity Sacrotuberous ligament and ischial tuberosity	 Tuber calcanei and distal metatarsophalangeal joints Via calcaneal (Achilles) tendon on tuber calcanei Medial tibia Tibial crest, tuberosity and merges into calcaneal (Achilles) tendon	Extend the hock
Deep digital flexor	Head of fibula	Bases of the distal phalanges	Flexes the digits
Digital extensors: 　Long digital extensor 　Lateral digital extensor 　Medial digital extensor	 Lateral epicondyle of the femur Proximal third of the fibula Medial aspect of the femur	 Distal phalanges 2–5 Digit 5 Digits 1 and 2	Extend the digits

3.42   Muscles of the hindlimb of the dog. [a]Also flexes the digits.

Diaphragm

The diaphragm separates the thoracic and abdominal cavities in mammals. It is dome-shaped, pointing toward the thorax, situated underneath the ribs. The central area is made of a tendon with muscle around the edge. Dorsally the diaphragm is divided into left and right **crura** (singular: **crus**). There are three openings in the diaphragm, which allow blood vessels and other organs to pass from the thorax to the abdomen. The **aortic hiatus** allows the aorta, azygous vein and thoracic duct to pass through the diaphragm. The **oesophageal hiatus** lies ventral to the aortic hiatus and allows the oesophagus and vagal trunks to pass through the diaphragm. The **caval foramen** is found in the central tendon and allows the caudal vena cava to pass through the diaphragm.

Horses

The muscles of the forelimb and hindlimb of the horse are illustrated in Figure 3.43. The important muscles, tendons and ligaments of the forelimb are described in Figure 3.44, those of the hindlimb in Figure 3.45 and those of the torso in Figure 3.46.

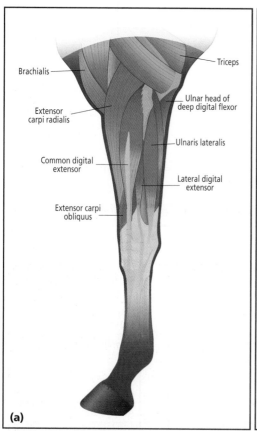

(a)

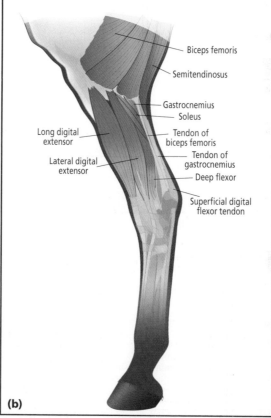

(b)

3.43 **(a)** Lateral view of the muscles of the forelimb of the horse. **(b)** Lateral view of the muscles of the hindlimb of the horse.

Structure	Origin	Insertion	Action
Muscles			
Biceps brachii	Distal scapula	Radius	Flexion of the elbow
Brachiocephalicus	Cranial cervical vertebra	Proximal: shoulder Distal: humerus	Lateral movement of the head and neck; protraction of upper limb and extension of the shoulder
Deltoid	Scapula	Proximal humerus	Flexion and abduction of the shoulder
Extensor carpi radialis	Humerus	Metacarpal bones I, II and III	Extension of the carpus and flexion of the elbow
Flexor carpi radialis	Humerus	Metacarpal bone III	Flexion of the carpus and extension of the elbow
Latissimus dorsi	Caudal thoracic and cranial lumbar vertebrae	Caudal humerus	Retraction of the limb and flexion of the shoulder
Pectoral	Sternum and first four ribs	Scapula and humerus	Adducts, protracts and retracts the forelimb
Rhomboideus	Nuchal ligament	Scapula	Extends the shoulder; pulls scapula cranially and dorsally; raises the head

3.44 Muscles, tendons and ligaments of the forelimb of the horse.

continues ▶

Structure	Origin	Insertion	Action
Muscles *continued*			
Supraspinatus	Cervical vertebrae deep to trapezius muscle	Scapula	Maintains shoulder extension
Triceps brachii	Scapula and proximal humerus	Ulna (olecranon process)	Extension of the elbow joint
Tendons			
Common digital extensor	Distal humerus and proximal radius	Phalangeal bones I, II and III	Extension of the carpus and joints between phalangeal bones I, II and III; flexion of the elbow
Deep digital flexor	Medial humerus and ulna (olecranon)	Palmar aspect of phalangeal bone III	Extension of the elbow; flexion of the carpus and phalangeal bones I, II and III
Lateral digital extensor	Lateral elbow	Phalangeal bone I	Extension of the carpus and phalangeal bones I, II and III
Superficial digital flexor	Medial humerus and caudal radius	Phalangeal bones I and II	Extension of the elbow; flexion of phalangeal bones I, II and III
Ligaments			
Carpal check	Distal carpus	Proximal deep digital flexor tendon	Extension of the elbow; flexion of the carpus and phalangeal bones I, II and III
Radial check	Distal radius	Proximal superficial flexor tendon	Extension of the elbow; flexion of phalangeal bones I, II and III
Suspensory	Proximal caudal metacarpus	Dorsal extensor tendon at the level of distal phalangeal bone II	Support the fetlock joint

3.44 *continued* Muscles, tendons and ligaments of the forelimb of the horse.

Structure	Origin	Insertion	Action
Muscles			
Gastrocnemius	Caudal distal femur	Calcanean tuber (point of the calcaneus)	Flexion of the stifle; extension of the hock
Peroneus tertius	Distal femur	Calcanean tuber, fourth tarsal bone, dorsal surface of third tarsal bone and metatarsal bone III	Ensures that the hock flexes when the stifle flexes
Semimembranosus	Tuber ischii of the pelvis and the sacrosciatic ligament	Distal femur	Extension of the hip; adduction of the hindlimb
Semitendinosus	Tuber ischii of the pelvis and the coccygeal vertebrae	Proximal tibia	Extension of the hip and hock joint
Superficial gluteal	Tuber coxae of the pelvis	Proximal femur	Flexion of the hip
Tendons			
Deep digital flexor	Proximal tibia	Plantar aspect of phalangeal bone III	Extension of the hock; flexion of the metatarso-phalangeal joint and interphalangeal joints
Lateral digital extensor	Lateral collateral ligament of the stifle and proximal tibia and fibula	Long extensor tendon and metatarsal bone III	Flexion of hock; extension of the metatarso-phalangeal joint and interphalangeal joints
Long digital extensor	Distal femur	Dorsal proximal surface of phalangeal bones I, II and III	Flexion of the hock; extension of the metatarso-phalangeal joint and interphalangeal joints
Superficial digital flexor	Distal femur	Calcanean tuber and plantar aspect of phalangeal bones I and II	Extension of the hock; flexion of the metatarso-phalangeal joint and interphalangeal joints
Ligaments			
Tarsal check	Distal tarsus	Proximal deep digital flexor tendon	Extension of the hock; flexion of the metatarso-phalangeal joint and interphalangeal joints

3.45 Muscles, tendons and ligaments of the hindlimb of the horse.

Structure	Origin	Insertion	Action
Muscles			
Abdominal oblique (external and internal)	Ribs	Pelvis	Abdominal wall support; aid respiration
Intercostal	Rib to rib	Rib to rib	Lateral and medial movement of the chest wall
Longissimus dorsi	Pelvis (ilium) and sacral and thoracic vertebrae	Cervical (4–7), lumbar and thoracic vertebrae and ribs	Extension of the head and neck; lateroflexion of the spine
Rectus abdominis	Costal cartilage (4–9) and the sternum	Pubis of pelvis	Abdominal wall support; aid to respiration
Sternocephalicus	Sternum	Mandible	Flexion of the head and neck
Transversus abdominis	Lumbar vertebrae and medial aspect of the last ribs	Linea alba	Abdominal wall support; aid to respiration
Ligaments			
Nuchal	Occipital protuberance of the skull	Cranial thoracic spinous processes	Extension of the neck and head

3.46 Muscles and ligaments of the torso of the horse.

Stay apparatus

The stay apparatus system is unique to equids and comprises a series of muscles, tendons and ligaments, which, in both the forelimbs and hindlimbs, allow the passive maintenance of the standing position with minimum muscular effort. This is achieved by locking the joints to reduce muscle contraction, enabling the bodyweight to be borne even when the horse is asleep.

In the forelimb (Figure 3.47a) the shoulder joint is prevented from flexion by the biceps tendon. The carpus is prevented from flexion by the extensor carpi radialis muscle. The fetlock is prevented from over-extension by the suspensory apparatus (interosseous and distal sesamoidean ligaments holding the proximal sesamoid bones) and supported by the tension in the accessory check ligaments and distal superficial and deep flexor tendons. The pastern joint is prevented from over-extension by the axial and abaxial palmar and straight sesamoidean ligaments, which cross its palmar/caudal aspect.

In the hindlimb (Figure 3.47b), similar ligaments hold the distal limb (below the hock) in place as those described in

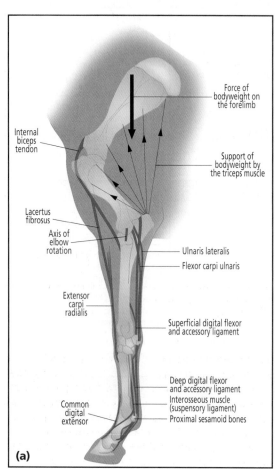

(a)

Internal biceps tendon

Lacertus fibrosus

Axis of elbow rotation

Extensor carpi radialis

Common digital extensor

Force of bodyweight on the forelimb

Support of bodyweight by the triceps muscle

Ulnaris lateralis

Flexor carpi ulnaris

Superficial digital flexor and accessory ligament

Deep digital flexor and accessory ligament

Interosseous muscle (suspensory ligament)

Proximal sesamoid bones

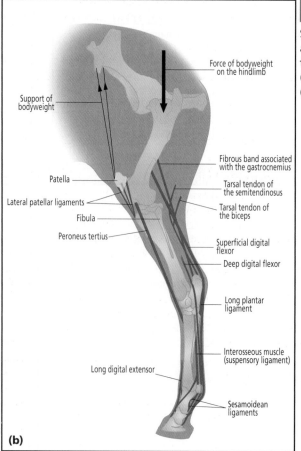

(b)

Support of bodyweight

Patella

Lateral patellar ligaments

Fibula

Peroneus tertius

Long digital extensor

Force of bodyweight on the hindlimb

Fibrous band associated with the gastrocnemius

Tarsal tendon of the semitendinosus

Tarsal tendon of the biceps

Superficial digital flexor

Deep digital flexor

Long plantar ligament

Interosseous muscle (suspensory ligament)

Sesamoidean ligaments

3.47

Stay apparatus in the horse.
(a) Forelimb.
(b) Hindlimb.

the forelimb, the only difference being that the superficial digital flexor tendon provides strong support to the lower limb. Above the hock, the peroneus tertius muscle is important as it coordinates the action of the stifle and hock, and ensures that one cannot be flexed without the other being flexed. Thus, the stifle joint may be locked into place by extending the joint. Extension of the stifle joint results in movement of the patella proximally. The patella is then rotated medially, allowing the parapatellar cartilage and medial patellar ligament to hook over the protuberance of the medial patellar ridge of the distal femur. This effectively stops the patella from moving distally, and so locks the stifle. As a result, via the peroneus tertius muscle, the hock is also locked in place.

Birds

Significant adaptations to the skeletal muscles are present in birds in order to enable flight, including:

- No diaphragm
- Large **superficial pectoral** muscles for movement of the wings downwards.
- **Deep pectoral** muscles (also known as the **supracoracoideus** muscles) beneath the superficial pectoral muscles, the tendon of which passes through the triosseal canal in the coracoids bone and attaches to the dorsal surface of the humerus, allowing upward movement of the wings.

Reptiles

Most of the body wall muscles in chelonians are reduced due to the presence of dermal bone, which forms the shell. In addition, although there is no true diaphragm in reptiles, chelonians may have partial muscular sheets which resemble this muscle.

Lizards have a similar muscular structure to mammals. Snakes have no limbs, but do have a strong segmented ventral body wall muscle used to create a wave of contraction from cranial to caudal, which raises the ventral scales propelling the snake forwards. This is enhanced by contraction of the intercostal body wall muscles, which makes the snake adopt a sinusoidal movement.

Smooth muscle

Smooth muscle is found in visceral structures such as the blood vessels, the gastrointestinal tract, the uterus and the bladder. The basic structure of the smooth muscle cell is different to that of skeletal muscle, with overlapping cells arranged in sheets or bundles. Smooth muscle lacks sarcomeres; this is obvious visually as they have no striations. However, the muscle cell still consists of **actin** and **myosin** filaments.

Contraction of smooth muscle is involuntary and controlled by the autonomic nervous system or hormones. As with skeletal muscles, contraction is initiated by an increase in the intracellular calcium concentration.

Cardiac muscle

Cardiac muscle is found in the heart and comprises branched muscle cells linked by **intercalated discs**. The basic structure is similar to that of skeletal muscle. Contraction of the heart muscle is controlled by a conduction system (see below).

Nervous system

Neurons

The main cell of the nervous system is the neuron (Figure 3.48). A nerve consists of many neurons. The neuron is a simple cell comprising:

- A **cell body** located at one end of the neuron containing the **nucleus**
- A series of thick **dendrons** or fine **dendrites** (short filaments of the cell body), which carry nerve impulses *toward* the cell body
- A single **axon**, which carries impulses *away* from the cell body toward other neurons. The axon may be a few millimetres or up to a metre in length
- **Nerve endings** at the end of the axon, which connect one neuron with another at a **synapse** or with a muscle cell at a **neuromuscular junction**.

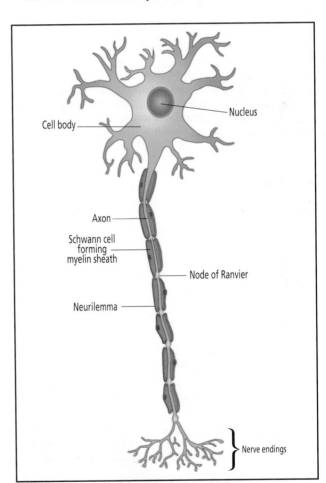

Cell body

Nucleus

Axon

Schwann cell forming myelin sheath

Node of Ranvier

Neurilemma

Nerve endings

3.48 Structure of a neuron.

The axon is often surrounded by an insulating cell, known as a **Schwann cell**. Such neurons are referred to as **myelinated,** as the Schwann cell produces a white lipoprotein sheath known as myelin around the axon, forming a neurolemmal membrane (**neurilemma**). Myelinated axons have a rapid rate of impulse transmission. The axon can still receive nutrients despite the myelin sheath as there are small gaps between adjacent Schwann cells, known as **nodes of Ranvier.**

Some axons do not have protective outer cells and are referred to as **non-myelinated** neurons. They are relatively uncommon and generally have slower rates of impulse transmission (e.g. neurons in the retina of the eye and in the grey matter of the brain and spinal cord).

Impulse conduction

At the synapse or neuromuscular junction there is a gap between the end of the axon and the next cell. In order for the electrical impulse to 'jump' across this gap, a chemical known as a **neurotransmitter** is released from the axon. The most common neurotransmitter is **acetylcholine**; however, both noradrenaline and adrenaline may be present in various neurons.

When the impulse reaches the nerve ending, voltage-sensitive calcium channels open, allowing calcium ions to enter the nerve ending from the extracellular and synaptic spaces. This influx of calcium ions causes the release of the chemical neurotransmitter into the synaptic gap or space, which then diffuses across the gap to the next neuron or muscle cell. The neurotransmitter binds to the adjacent cell, causing either more ion channels to open or further chemicals to be released, which results in continuation of the electrical impulse.

What happens in the postsynaptic neuron or muscle depends on whether the presynaptic neuron is inhibitory or excitatory. The presence of a synapse means that there is an 'all-or-nothing' phenomenon, in that either the impulse will cross the synapse or it will not; there is no gradation of response.

Structure

The nervous system is broadly divided into two parts:

- **Central nervous system** (CNS) – comprises the brain and spinal cord

- **Peripheral nervous system** (PNS) – comprises all nerves arising from the CNS.

Central nervous system

There are two components to the CNS: the brain and the spinal cord. Within the CNS, two types of tissue are found:

- **Grey matter** – peripherally located in the cortex of the cerebellum, but centrally located in the medulla of the spinal cord and cerebrum
- **White matter** – peripherally located in the cortex of the spinal cord and cerebrum, but laterally located in the medulla of the cerebellum.

The grey matter largely consists of non-myelinated neurons or those portions of the neuron that are not normally covered in myelin (e.g. the cell body). Accumulations of cell bodies are often referred to as **nuclei**. These nuclei act as relay centres for many subconscious neurological pathways from the brain to the spinal cord.

The white matter consists of myelinated neurons, or those portions of the neuron that are normally covered in myelin (e.g. the axon).

Brain

The brain (Figure 3.49) is divided into three areas:

- The **forebrain** – comprising the cerebrum (telencephalon) and the diencephalon
- The **midbrain** (mesencephalon) – comprising the tectum, tegmentum and the cerebral peduncle (crus cerebri)
- The **hindbrain** – comprising the medulla oblongata, pons and cerebellum.

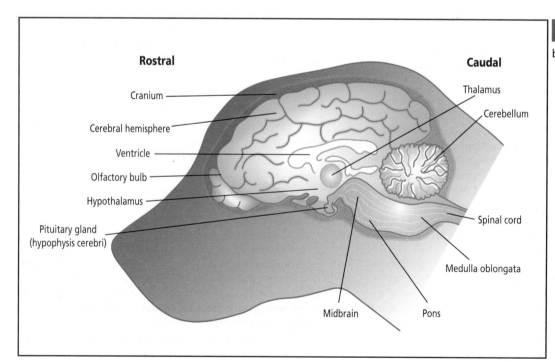

3.49 Structure of the brain in the dog.

Rostral Caudal

Cranium
Cerebral hemisphere
Ventricle
Olfactory bulb
Hypothalamus
Pituitary gland (hypophysis cerebri)
Thalamus
Cerebellum
Spinal cord
Medulla oblongata
Midbrain Pons

Cerebrum

The cerebrum (telencephalon) consists of paired lateral cerebral hemispheres (often referred to as the **neopallium**), which are the most obvious external feature of the brain, as well as the **paleopallium** (the rostroventral part of the brain connected to the olfactory lobe) and the **basal nuclei**, which have connections to the olfactory and sensory motor centres.

The surface of the cerebral hemispheres is highly folded (the tops of the folds are known as **gyri**; the bottom of the folds are known as **sulci**); this allows the brain to increase its surface area massively without increasing its overall size. The two hemispheres are separated by the **longitudinal fissure** into which the **falx cerebri** (a fold of the meninges) projects. The two hemispheres are connected by a band of white tissue known as the **corpus callosum**, which runs just beneath the dorsal surface of the cerebrum, forming the roof of the **lateral ventricles** (two fluid-filled areas, one in each hemisphere, located beneath the outer cerebral hemispheres).

The cerebrum can be further subdivided into cortical lobes, according to the overlying skull bone structure:

- Frontal lobe (rostral)
- Parietal lobe (dorsal)
- Occipital lobe (caudal)
- Temporal lobe (lateral)
- Olfactory lobe (ventrorostral; connected to the olfactory nerves via the olfactory bulb on the ventral surface).

Diencephalon

The diencephalon forms the most rostral part of the **brainstem**. Only the ventral part of this structure, known as the hypothalamus (see Figure 3.49), can be visualized. The diencephalon consists of three main parts:

- Hypothalamus
- Thalamus
- Epithalamus.

The **hypothalamus** forms the ventral and lateral walls of a cerebrospinal fluid-filled structure of the brain known as the third ventricle (Figure 3.50), which lies medially beneath the lateral ventricles. The hypothalamus contains a number of **nuclei** which are involved in hormonal regulation and connect the CNS with the autonomic nervous system (ANS). One of these connections is to the pituitary gland, which lies immediately ventral to the hypothalamus.

The **pituitary gland** (see Figure 3.49) consists of an anterior and a posterior lobe. The **posterior lobe** is an outgrowth of the hypothalamus and comprises neural tissue directly linked to the hypothalamus. It is responsible for the secretion of:

- Oxytocin
- Antidiuretic hormone (ADH).

The **anterior lobe** is adjacent to the posterior lobe and is responsible for the secretion of:

- Follicle-stimulating hormone (FSH)
- Luteinizing hormone (LH)
- Growth hormone (GH)
- Thyroid-stimulating hormone (TSH)

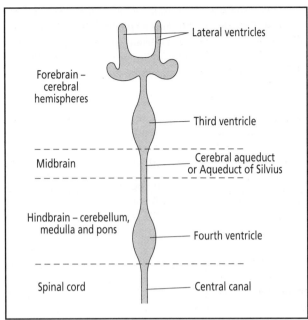

3.50 General plan (dorsal view) of the ventricular system and its position within the brain.

- Prolactin
- Adrenocorticotrophic hormone (ACTH).

These hormones are released by the anterior lobe in response to hormones secreted by the hypothalamus and posterior lobe. These hormones and their function are discussed more fully in the Endocrine system section (below).

The **thalamus** is also surrounded by the third ventricle. The thalamus comprises a large number of **nuclei**. The role of the thalamus is to relay signals between the cerebrum and the brainstem. It receives incoming (afferent) signals from most sensory systems (with the exception of the nose, whose signals enter the forebrain through the olfactory bulbs and olfactory lobe) and acts as feedback control for most motor pathways.

The **epithalamus** is the most dorsal part of the diencephalon and contains the **pineal gland**, which is responsible for the regulation of reproductive activity as influenced by day length.

Mesencephalon

The ventral surface only of the mesencephalon (midbrain) can be seen in the intact brain. It has a lumen, known as the **aqueduct of Silvius** (see Figure 3.50), which joins the larger fluid-filled third and fourth ventricles. It has three parts (dorsal to ventral):

- Tectum
- Tegmentum
- Cerebral peduncle (crus cerebri)

The **tectum** lies dorsal to the aqueduct and consists largely of paired swellings, known as **colliculi**, which are connected to the thalamus and visual pathways (involved with the blink and pupillary reflexes) and are also spatial awareness integration centres.

The **tegmentum** is the main core of the midbrain and comprises the **reticular formation**, which contains the significant **nuclei** of the cranial nerves, including the **oculomotor (III)**, **trochlear (IV)**, and **trigeminal (V)** nerves. In addition, the nuclei of the **red nucleus** (so called because of its prominent vascular supply) are found here. These nuclei are connected to the basal nuclei of the telencephalon and also control motor movement.

The **cerebral peduncle** (crus cerebri) can be seen from the ventral surface of the intact brain. This is a nerve fibre tract connecting the brainstem with the telencephalon.

Medulla oblongata and pons

The medulla oblongata and the pons, although apparently grossly separate, are in fact continuations of one another, situated ventral to the cerebellum with the fluid-filled **fourth ventricle** (see Figure 3.50) lying between them and the cerebellum.

The **pons** is the most rostral part of the hindbrain and supports the middle cerebellar peduncles, bridging the two hemispheres of the cerebellum. It has many functions, including the control of respiration.

The **medulla oblongata** is caudal to the pons and continuous with the spinal cord. It has a series of decussating nerve fibres, forming significant tracts (e.g. the 'pyramids' tracts). In addition, many of the cranial nerves emerge from the CNS at this point, including the **trigeminal (V)**, **abducens (VI)**, **facial (VII)**, **vestibulocochlear (VIII)**, **glossopharyngeal (IX)**, **vagus (X)**, **accessory (XI)** and **hypoglossal (XII)** nerves. The **olivary** and **pontine nuclei** are also located in the medulla oblongata, along with the **reticular formation**; these are all important regulators of the feedback mechanisms controlling motor function, The reticular formation is also responsible for transmitting impulses that increase the animal's awareness of its surroundings when aroused. A decrease in the activity of the reticular formation tends to result in lethargy or sleep.

Cerebellum

The cerebellum is the spherical folded structure that sits immediately caudal to the cerebral hemispheres on the dorsal aspect of the pons and medulla oblongata. It has two main lateral hemispheres and a central body known as the **vermis**. The arrangement of white and grey matter is reversed in the cerebellum compared with the cerebrum and spinal cord, as the grey matter is located in the outermost cortical areas and the white matter in the central medulla. The cerebellum is attached to the brainstem by three paired peduncles: the cranial peduncle attaches it to the midbrain, the middle peduncle attaches it to the pons, and the caudal peduncle attaches it to the medulla oblongata. The cerebellum is responsible for CNS involvement with balance and coordination of postural and locomotive activities.

Birds

The avian brain is notable for its lack of folds (there are no gyri or sulci). Birds also have a reduced olfactory bulb and significantly enlarged optic nerve and optic lobes, which sit caudoventral to the cerebral hemispheres.

Reptiles

The reptilian brain is significantly smaller in relation to the whole body mass compared with small mammals and birds; however, the basic structure of the brainstem is similar to the mammalian form. Reptiles have two cerebral hemispheres, but these are lyssencephalic (i.e. have no folds, gyri or sulci). A **dorsal ventricular ridge** (DVR) is present, arising from the lateral wall of the forebrain, which receives sensory input from the eyes, ears, nose and skin. The DVR relays the sensory information received to the cerebral hemispheres, diencephalon and efferent motor pathways. Snakes have prominent olfactory bulbs (as do some other species).

Some species have a **parietal eye**, which is a projection of the parietal part of the telencephalon connected to the pineal gland. This is well developed in species such as the green iguana and tuatara (which has a lens and a retina within the structure) and its function is to impart day length details to the brain to help regulate circadian rhythms and seasonal changes in metabolism and sexual behaviour.

Meninges

There are three membranes that protect the CNS and retain the cerebrospinal fluid:

- Dura mater
- Arachnoid mater
- Pia mater.

Dura mater

This is the outermost membrane and is largely attached to the periosteum of the inside of the cranium. In the spinal cord it is separated from the periosteum of the vertebral bodies by epidural fat deposits, creating an epidural space which is used for anaesthesia (see Chapter 23).

Arachnoid mater

This is the next membrane and consists of large blood vessels supported by tough collagen fibres. The gap between the arachnoid mater and the dura mater (known as the **subdural space**) is filled with fat.

Pia mater

This is a thin fibrous membrane, which in the cranium is closely adherent to the surface of the brain. It contains small blood vessels that supply nutrients to the nervous tissue. The gap between the pia mater and the arachnoid mater (known as the **subarachnoid space**) is filled with cerebrospinal fluid.

Reptiles

There are only two membranes in reptiles: the **pia arachnoid** and the **dura mater**. The space between the membranes is referred to as the subdural space and is filled with cerebrospinal fluid.

Cerebrospinal fluid

The function of cerebrospinal fluid is to cushion and supply some nutrients to the nervous tissue. It is produced by a series of **choroid** (vascular) **plexuses**, which lie in the lumen of the **ventricles**. There are four main ventricles (see Figure 3.50):

- Two lateral ventricles in the forebrain (one in each hemisphere), just below the corpus callosum
- The third ventricle is situated around the thalamus in the centre of the brain
- The fourth ventricle is situated in the medulla oblongata.

The ventricles are connected: the lateral ventricles communicate across the midline with one another and caudally with the third ventricle. The third and fourth ventricles communicate via the **cerebral aqueduct** (aqueduct of Silvius), which runs through the midbrain. The fourth ventricle communicates with the **central canal** of the spinal cord.

Spinal cord

The spinal cord extends from the medulla oblongata, exiting the cranium via the **foramen magnum** of the skull, through the spinal column in the vertebral canal created by the meninges lining the linked lumens of the vertebral bodies. It terminates before the end of the spinal column in a series of fine nerves known as the **cauda equina**. A pair of nerves from the spinal cord exit at each intervertebral joint. These nerves carry both afferent (sensory) and efferent (motor) neurons to the musculoskeletal and visceral organs.

The spinal cord consists of an outer cortical layer of **white matter** and a central butterfly-shaped core of **grey matter** (Figure 3.51). The white matter is formed from myelinated neurons, which ascend to and descend from the brain. The grey matter consists of non-myelinated neurons and cell bodies, which connect afferent and efferent neurons. In the midline is the **central canal**, which connects the spinal cord with the ventricles of the brain and contains cerebrospinal fluid.

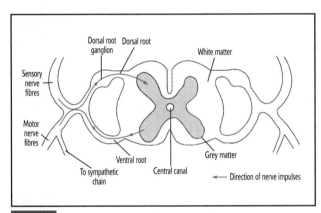

3.51 Cross-section through the spinal cord.

Nerve number	Nerve name	Function
I	Olfactory	Sensory nerve from the nasal mucosa (smell)
II	Optic	Sensory nerve connecting the eye to the sight centre of the brain
III	Oculomotor	Motor nerve supplying the muscles of the eye, eyelid and ciliary body
IV	Trochlear	Motor nerve supplying the dorsal oblique muscles of the eye
V	Trigeminal	Sensory nerve of the head/face. Very important nerve as it supplies a large number of structures within the head. Motor nerve supplying various muscles of the head/face
VI	Abducens	Motor nerve supplying the extrinsic muscles of the eye
VII	Facial	Motor nerve supplying various muscles (e.g. ears, eyelids, lips)
VIII	Vestibulocochlear	Sensory nerve for balance (from the semicircular canals of the inner ear) and hearing (from the cochlea of the inner ear)
IX	Glossopharyngeal	Sensory nerve from the taste buds of the tongue and the pharynx. Motor nerve supplying the pharynx, root of the tongue, palate and some salivary glands
X	Vagus	Sensory nerve from the pharynx and larynx. Motor nerve supplying the larynx. It also carries parasympathetic motor fibres to the heart and other visceral organs (e.g. stomach and intestines)
XI	Accessory	Motor nerve supplying various muscles (e.g. trapezius and brachiocephalic)
XII	Hypoglossal	Motor nerve supplying the tongue

3.52 Cranial nerves.

Peripheral nervous system

The PNS is the means by which the CNS communicates with the organs and tissues of the body. Peripheral nerves comprise cranial and spinal nerves and consist of:

- **Sensory** or **afferent nerve fibres**, which collect information from the environment and transmit it to the CNS
- **Motor** or **efferent fibres**, which are responsible for carrying information from the CNS to the target tissues and organs, and control their activity.

Cranial nerves

Most cranial nerves (Figure 3.52) originate in the hindbrain and exit the cranium through various foramina. Many of these foramina, which can be seen on the skull, are accumulated around the base of the middle ear. Most have either a sensory or a motor function, but some such as the trigeminal, glossopharyngeal and vagus have a mixed motor and sensory function.

Spinal nerves

The spinal nerves are paired at each intervertebral junction (one left and one right) and exit through their respective **intervertebral foramina**. Each of the paired spinal nerves has a **dorsal root** and a **ventral root** (see Figure 3.51).

- The **dorsal root** is where the sensory nerves enter the spinal cord, relaying information from the sensory bodies to the cord. There is a small swelling where the cell bodies of the sensory neurons are located; where they form synapses is known as the **dorsal root ganglion**.
- The **ventral root** comprises motor nerves exiting the spinal cord on the way to the somatic muscles and visceral organs. The **sympathetic nervous system** is supplied by these motor nerve fibres. There is no corresponding ventral root ganglion.
- As the dorsal root has a sensory function and the ventral root has a motor function, a spinal nerve is a **mixed nerve**.

In the region of the forelimbs and hindlimbs, the spinal cord is thicker than normal. This is due to the large number of nerves passing into and out of the spinal cord. In addition, the spinal nerves anastomose (join together) to form the main nerves supplying the limbs. This anastomosis of spinal nerves is referred to as a **plexus**: the **brachial plexus** supplies the forelimb; the **lumbosacral plexus** supplies the hindlimb.

- The **brachial plexus** consists of the last three cervical and first two thoracic spinal nerves. It is located deep beneath the scapula and supplies the structures of the forelimb, with the exception of the trapezius, omotransversarius, brachiocephalicus and rhomboideus muscles, and the skin over the upper shoulder region.
- The **lumbosacral plexus** consists of the fourth lumbar through to the second sacral spinal nerves. It supplies the structures of the hindlimb, with the exception of a few proximal areas of skin.

Spinal reflexes

Due to the dual sensory and motor function of the spinal nerves, they can form a **reflex arc** from sensory organ to spinal cord and then motor function, without going via the brain. Spinal reflexes (e.g. patellar reflex) can be used to ascertain whether there has been damage to the nerves at a local level. They do not indicate whether the spinal cord is intact above the reflex arc. However, if the animal vocalizes or turns to look at the site where the stimulus is being performed, this indicates that the sensation has been perceived at a higher, conscious level in the brain; therefore, the spinal cord above the reflex must be intact.

These reflex arcs are often referred to as:

- **Monosynaptic** – when there is only one synapse/connection and therefore only two nerves involved with the reflex
- **Polysynaptic** – when there is more than one synapse and therefore more than 2 nerves involved with the reflex.

Neurons in other segments of the spinal cord can also modify reflex arcs. If the modifying neurons are situated above the reflex arc, they are called **upper motor neurons**. If the modifying neurons are located below the reflex arc (rare), they are called **lower motor neurons**. When testing, if the reflex response is present but exaggerated, it may indicate that although the nerves responsible for the reflex arc are intact, the modifying nerves above or below that segment in the spinal cord may be damaged.

Reflex arcs can be overridden by the brain. For example, the local reflex may be to remove a limb from a noxious stimulus; however, the brain can override this reflex in order to keep the limb where it is. These are called **conditioned reflexes** and are learned.

Common reflex arcs

Pedal reflex

This is also known as the flexor or withdrawal reflex in response to a painful stimulus. Pain receptors present in the skin are stimulated, resulting in flexion of the muscles to move the limb away from the stimulus.
▶

Panniculus reflex

This is a twitch response of the skin over the back in response to a stimulus in that area.

Patellar reflex

Tapping the patellar ligament stretches the quadriceps muscle, which in turn results in contraction of the quadriceps muscle. This contraction causes the lower limb to be extended.

Anal reflex

This is a twitch response of the anal sphincter in response to a touch stimulus of the perianal skin.

Thoracolaryngeal reflex

This reflex is seen in the horse. A slap in the saddle region on one side of the chest produces a flickering adductor movement of the contralateral side of the larynx, as determined by endoscopy or gentle palpation of the extrinsic laryngeal muscles. This reflex is absent in some horses with recurrent laryngeal neuropathy and cases of cervical vertebral stenosis.

Autonomic nervous system

This is the unconscious visceral nervous system, which supplies motor innervation to most of the vital organs (heart, gut, bladder) as well as the endocrine and exocrine glands. There are two aspects to the ANS (Figure 3.53):

- Sympathetic nervous system
- Parasympathetic nervous system.

Sympathetic nervous system

This is the system of 'fright, flight and fight' and is responsible for a number of functions (Figure 3.54). The preganglionic nerves arise from the first thoracic through to the fourth lumbar vertebral space. They then pass into the ventral roots of the first thoracic to fourth lumbar spinal nerves, before exiting and joining the ganglia of the **sympathetic trunk**. The sympathetic trunk runs parallel to the spinal cord along the length of the neck and back, starting at the cranial cervical ganglion and ending in the diffuse splitting of nerves into the tail region (Figure 3.53). For this reason, the preganglionic nerves of the sympathetic nervous system are short, whereas the postganglionic fibres are long.

Parasympathetic nervous system

The parasympathetic nervous system generally opposes the actions of the sympathetic nervous system (Figure 3.54). The preganglionic neurons originate as discrete nuclei in the brainstem. They are often distributed within the cranial nerves (e.g. oculomotor, facial, glossopharyngeal and vagal). There is also a **sacral outflow** of the parasympathetic nervous system, which arises from S1–S2 and innervates the pelvic organs such as the bladder and genitals. The preganglionic nerves of the parasympathetic nervous system are long, whereas the postganglionic fibres are short.

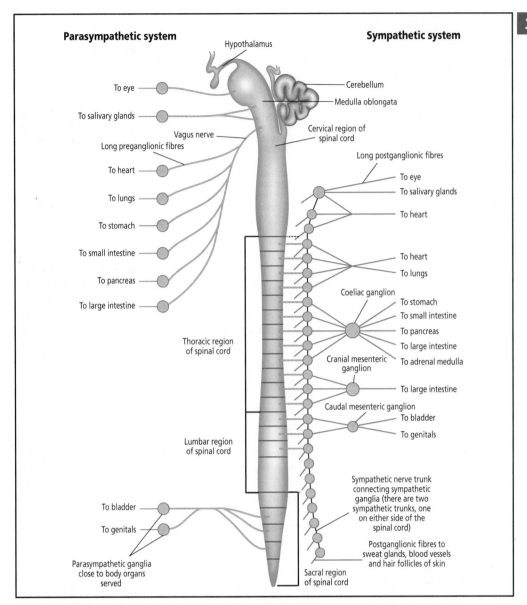

Structure innervated	Sympathetic effect	Parasympathetic effect
Bladder	Relaxes bladder muscle Increases bladder sphincter tone	Contracts bladder muscle Decreases bladder sphincter tone
Blood vessels	Vasodilatation	Vasoconstriction
Eyes	Dilates pupil Relaxes ciliary muscle (lens becomes flattened for far vision)	Constricts pupil Contracts ciliary muscle (lens becomes more convex for near vision)
Gastrointestinal tract	Reduces activity of the gut and stomach Inhibits secretions from the pancreas Dries salivary secretions	Increases activity of the gut and stomach Increases secretions from the pancreas Increases salivary secretions
Heart	Increases heart rate Increases contractility Increases conduction velocity of the atrioventricular node	Decreases heart rate Decreases contractility Decreases conduction velocity of the atrioventricular node
Lungs	Dilates bronchioles Increases respiratory rate Inhibits secretions	Constricts bronchioles Decreases respiratory rate Increases secretions
Skin	Causes piloerection Localized secretion from sweat glands (paws)	No effect on hairs Generalized secretion from sweat glands
Uterus	Gravid: contracts uterus Non-gravid: relaxes uterus	Variable response

3.54 Functions of the sympathetic and parasympathetic nervous systems.

Special senses

The special senses are smell, sight, hearing, taste and touch.

Smell

There are numerous sensory neurons (**olfactory nerves**) responsible for conducting the sensation of smell to the brain. The olfactory nerves traverse small holes in the cribriform plate of the ethmoid bone (the rostral part of the calvarium, the bone that immediately surrounds the brain) and pass directly into the olfactory lobe of the brain. The olfactory lobe is situated close to the nasal cavity. For a smell to be detected, molecules are trapped in the mucus lining the caudal nasal passages and dissolved. This creates a chemical reaction that stimulates the nerve endings.

Dogs

Dogs have some of the most tightly coiled nasal conchae of any animal, which increases the surface area of the nasal cavity and enhances the sense of smell.

Birds

Most birds have a reduced reliance on their sense of smell compared with mammals and reptiles. The nostrils are generally found at the base of the beak; however, in waterfowl they may be found more rostrally, and in birds such as the kiwi they may be found on the very distal tip of the bill.

Reptiles

Reptiles can detect smells via the sensory mucosa in the nasal passages in conjunction with the olfactory nerves. However, those reptiles (such as snakes) that particularly utilize their sense of smell for hunting also have an enlarged **vomeronasal organ** in the maxilla. The tongue darts out of the mouth and traps the scent molecules in the saliva coating its surface. The tongue is then withdrawn and the tip immediately pushed into this organ in the roof of the mouth.

Some reptiles also appear to have additional nostrils located around the maxilla. In the case of boid snakes, these pits are found around the upper lip; in the case of some vipers, there are two small pits which face cranially located between the eye and the true nares. These are **heat-sensitive** pores and not nostrils at all. In boids these pores are not very sensitive, but do allow the snake to locate prey in the dark. In pit vipers the pores are highly sensitive to heat differences and because they face forward have 'binocular' heat-sensing capabilities, allowing the snake to accurately judge how far the prey is in front of them.

Sight

Position of the eyes

In predators (e.g. cats and dogs) the eyes are to the front of the head, whereas in prey species (e.g. rabbits) the eyes are to the side of the head to give a greater field of vision. Cats, in particular, have excellent binocular vision (i.e. the field of view of each eye overlaps, allowing good depth perception). This is essential when hunting prey.

Structure of the eyes

The anatomy of the eye is shown in Figure 3.55.

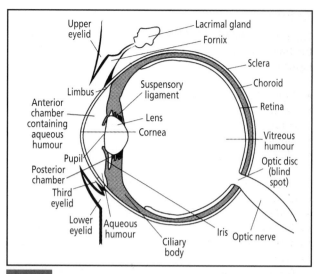

3.55 Longitudinal section through the eye.

Sclera and cornea

The **sclera** ('white' of the eye) is the opaque outer protective coating of the eye. The muscles responsible for movement of the eye (see below) originate at the sclera and attach to the periosteum.

The **cornea** is the transparent outer protective coating of the eye. The cornea does not normally contain any blood vessels; however, in some diseases blood vessels can enter the cornea, resulting in areas of opacity. Corneal cells receive their nutrition from the lacrimal fluid and aqueous humour. The cornea is very sensitive to stimuli due to the presence of numerous nerve endings (branches of the ophthalmic nerve). The closing of the eyelids in response to something touching the cornea is known as the **corneal reflex**.

The junction at which the sclera and cornea meet is known as the **limbus**.

Uvea

Beneath the outer connective tissue layer, is the vascular layer. This consists of:

- **Choroid** – found underneath the sclera, from the optic nerve to the limbus
- **Ciliary body** – found adjacent to the limbus
- **Iris** – found anterior to the ciliary body.

The **choroid** contains blood vessels. Situated in the dorsal part of the choroid is the **tapetum lucidum**, an area which reflects light and aids vision in the dark. It is this structure that makes the eyes of dogs and cats shine in the headlights of a car. The colour of the tapetum lucidum varies according to age and breed in dogs. In puppies it has a blue/violet appearance, which changes to green/yellow as the animal gets older.

The **ciliary body** suspends the lens via **zonular fibres**, which collectively are known as the **suspensory ligament**. The ciliary muscle controls the shape of the lens.

The **iris** consists of pigment cells, which give colour to the eye, and smooth muscle, which controls the amount of light entering the eye by contracting and dilating the **pupil**.

The space between the lens and the cornea is filled with **aqueous humour**. This space is divided into an **anterior chamber** (between the iris and the cornea) and a **posterior chamber** (between the iris and the lens).

Retina

The retina contains light-sensitive cells and is connected to the brain via the **optic nerve**. The retina comprises different layers of cells:

- Pigmented cells (outer layer)
- Receptor cells (**rods** are responsible for black and white vision; **cones** are responsible for colour vision)
- Bipolar ganglion cells
- Multipolar ganglion cells.

Situated where the optic nerve exits the eye is the **optic disc**. There is no retina in the area of the optic disc, so this is a **blind spot**. A series of blood vessels run across the surface of the retina, arising from the retinal artery and radiating out from the optic disc. These blood vessels supply nutrients and oxygen to the cells of the retina.

The **vitreous body** is found caudal to the lens and consists of vitreous humour and connective fibres. The vitreous body keeps the shape of the eye.

Eyelids

The upper and lower eyelids join at the medial and lateral canthi (singular: canthus) and are secured by the **palpebral ligaments**. Each eyelid consists of a thin outer layer of skin, overlying a musculofibrous layer. At the edge of the eyelid (next to the eye) is a more fibrous area known as the **tarsus**, which gives structure to the eyelid. Along the margin of the eyelid are **Meibomian glands (tarsal glands)**, which secrete an oily material. Located beside these glands are the eyelashes or **cilia**. The inner surface of the eyelid is lined by **conjunctiva**.

Located at the ventromedial aspect of the eye is the **third eyelid**. This is not a true eyelid but a T-shaped piece of cartilage, the nictitating membrane, covered by conjunctiva. The third eyelid provides protection for the eyeball and secretions from the **Harderian gland**.

Lacrimal gland

Situated dorsolaterally to the eye is the lacrimal gland. This is responsible for tear production. Lacrimal fluid is spread across the eye by blinking, and drains from the eye through the **punctum lacrimale** found at the medial aspect of the lower lid. The punctum lacrimale is connected to the **nasolacrimal duct**, which drains into the nasal cavity.

Movement of the eyes

Movement of the eyes is controlled by the muscles attached to the sclera, including:

- Retractor bulbi muscle
- Dorsal rectus muscle
- Ventral rectus muscle
- Medial rectus muscle
- Lateral rectus muscle
- Dorsal oblique muscle
- Ventral oblique muscle.

These muscles are supplied by a number of cranial nerves, including:

- Oculomotor nerve
- Trochlear nerve
- Abducens nerve

- Facial nerve
- Trigeminal nerve, which is responsible for transmitting sensory information from the eye.

Formation of an image

The formation of an image can be considered as a four step process:

1. Light rays from an object pass:
   a. Through the **cornea** and the **pupil** to hit the **lens**
      - The cornea plays a part in focusing the light on to the retina
      - The iris alters in size and controls the amount of light entering the eye
   b. Through the lens to be focused on to the **retina**
      - The curvature of the lens is altered by the ciliary muscles and focuses the light rays on to the retina
   c. Through the layers of the retina to the **photoreceptor cells**. Some light is reflected back to the retina by the **tapetum lucidum** to stimulate more receptor cells.
2. Resulting nerve impulses, generated by the photoreceptors, travel along the nerve fibres of the **optic nerve** to the **brain**.
3. On the ventral surface of the brain, a proportion of nerve fibres cross via the **optic chiasma** to opposite sides of the brain so that each cerebral hemisphere receives information from both eyes.
4. Information is carried to the **visual cortex** of the cerebral hemispheres, where it is interpreted as an image. The image formed on the retina is smaller than the original and inverted but the brain automatically modifies it.

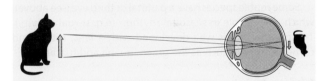

Horses

The lens in the eye of the horse does not have a great ability to change shape and, therefore, may not be the sole mechanism for focusing light on the retina. The retina is not perfectly round; it is sloped or 'ramped'. This means that horses might be able to 'find' a location on the retina where the light is in focus by simply raising or lowering their head. Horses often raise their head to 'focus' on objects close to them and lower them to focus on objects far away.

Small mammals

Most commonly kept small mammals are prey species and thus have laterally situated eyes. In the rabbit there is little binocular vision; each eye provides a separate image to the brain which has to be interpreted. This gives the rabbit a near 360 degree field of view. The third eyelid contains a large amount of lymphoid tissue, which can become reactive and swell when stimulated by antigens. The Harderian gland also enlarges in bucks during the breeding season. The single large punctum lacrimale in the lower lid is easy to cannulate for flushing the tear duct or for injecting radiopaque dye for the investigation of nasolacrimal duct disease.

Birds

Sight is the main sense in birds; therefore, they have relatively enormous eyes compared with body size. Birds have excellent colour vision. Predators (such as the raptors) tend to have more forward facing eyes, which provide binocular vision; prey species tend to have more laterally placed eyes, enabling a wider field of vision.

Ocular structures

Birds have large pear-shaped eyeballs. Small bones (**scleral ossicles**) support the anterior globe at the junction of the sclera and cornea. The surface of the retina has no obvious blood vessels; instead there is a **pecten oculi**, a vascular plexus of capillaries near the optic disc, which provides nutrients to the inside of the eye. The iris comprises both skeletal and smooth muscle; therefore, constriction and dilatation of the pupil is partially under voluntary control.

Periocular structures

Birds have an infraorbital sinus, which has only soft tissue in the lateral wall. This means sinusitis results in puffing around the eye. The lower (main) eyelid is devoid of glands. There is a nictitating membrane which lies on the medial aspect of the eye. Ocular movement is limited as the globe is so large; however, it is possible for each eye to move independently. Occasionally, there is no bony septum between the eyes and the structures are so large that they touch one another.

Reptiles

The upper and lower eyelids in snakes are fused over the corneal surface, forming the transparent 'spectacle', which is shed with the rest of the skin each time the snake sloughs.

Some reptile species have a parietal or third eye (see above), which plays a role in seasonal rhythms (e.g. sexual activity). The parietal eye is well developed with a lens, retina and cornea in species such as the green iguana and tuatara.

Hearing

The ear has two main functions: hearing and balance. The ear consists of three parts (Figure 3.56):

- Outer ear
- Middle ear
- Inner ear.

Outer ear

The outer ear consists of the **auricle** (pinna or ear flap) and the **external acoustic meatus** (ear canal). The auricle comprises cartilage (auricular cartilage) covered with skin. It is funnel-shaped, although this can vary between species and breeds, and can be moved toward the source of a sound. The ear canal is formed from cartilage and bone. It is lined with epithelium, which has a high concentration of ceruminous (secreting ear wax) and sebaceous glands. The ear canal is L-shaped, making treatment of external ear disease difficult in some cases.

Middle ear

The middle part of the ear is found within the temporal bone of the skull. Situated between the outer ear canal and the middle ear is the **tympanic membrane** (ear drum); this transmits

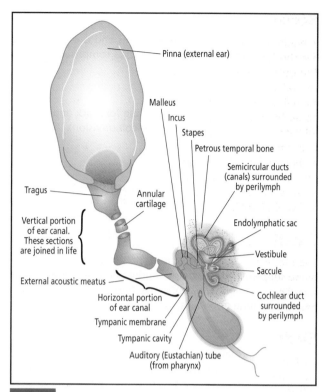

Labels: Pinna (external ear); Malleus; Incus; Stapes; Petrous temporal bone; Semicircular ducts (canals) surrounded by perilymph; Tragus; Annular cartilage; Endolymphatic sac; Vertical portion of ear canal. These sections are joined in life; Vestibule; Saccule; External acoustic meatus; Horizontal portion of ear canal; Cochlear duct surrounded by perilymph; Tympanic membrane; Tympanic cavity; Auditory (Eustachian) tube (from pharynx)

3.56 Cross-section through the ear.

sound vibrations to the middle ear. The middle ear contains the three **auditory ossicles**, known as the **malleus** (hammer; attached to the ear drum), **incus** (anvil) and **stapes** (stirrup).

The ventral part of the temporal bone expands into the tympanic bulla, which is very prominent in some species. It is thought that the tympanic bulla improves hearing ability. The **auditory (Eustachian) tube** connects the middle ear to the nasopharynx. It is responsible for ensuring equalization of air pressure between the middle ear and the atmosphere; it does this by opening slightly when the animal swallows (e.g. the sensation of ear 'popping' when you ascend in an aeroplane).

Inner ear

Located within the inner ear are the bony canals which contain **perilymph**. Within these are the delicate membranous canals which contain **endolymph**. Together, these form **semicircular ducts (canals)**, which allow the animal to maintain balance, and the **cochlea**, which is involved with hearing.

The endolymph in the semicircular canals contains hairs and crystals. The crystals move in response to movement of the head, resulting in stimulation of the hairs. These minute hairs are connected to nerves, which coalesce to form the vestibulocochlear nerve, allowing transmission of movement to the brain. The three semicircular canals are arranged at right angles to one another, thus providing a three-dimensional (3D) form, allowing the brain to determine the movement and position of the head more accurately.

The cochlea is shaped like the shell of a snail and is filled with fluid. This fluid allows the reverberation of sound to stimulate nerve endings. These impulses are transmitted via the vestibulocochlear nerve to the brain, which then interprets them as sound. Between the semicircular canals and the cochlea are the utricle and saccule, which are principally responsible for interpretation of linear acceleration and thus help control posture and balance.

Horses

In equids the auditory tube is massively dilated to produce a diverticulum (volume = 300–500 ml) called the **guttural pouch**. The guttural pouch sits between the nasopharynx and the ventral skull. Each pouch is divided caudally into a larger medial and smaller lateral compartment by the stylohyoid bone. The guttural pouch is closely related to cranial nerves VII (lateral compartment), IX, X, XI and XII, as well as to the sympathetic nerve and the cranial cervical ganglion (all within the medial compartment). The internal carotid artery runs in a fold of mucosa in the medial compartment of the guttural pouch, and the maxillary artery runs along the lateral wall of the lateral compartment.

Small mammals

The rabbit has elongated pinnae, which have an excellent blood supply. The lateral/marginal ear vein is used for blood sampling and intravenous drug administration. Chinchillas have a very prominent tympanic bulla.

Birds

Birds have no pinnae, but often have a very short external ear canal before the tympanic membrane. The outer ear is frequently covered by short feathers. There is one auditory ossicle, the columella, attached medially to the vestibular window and laterally to the extracolumella cartilage, which in turn connects with the tympanic membrane. The cochlea is only slightly curved and has a blind-ending apex, known as the lagena, the function of which is not clearly understood.

Reptiles

Chelonians and lizards posses a tympanic membrane, but have only one auditory ossicle. Snakes do not have ears; the single auditory ossicle connects with the quadrate bone of the skull, allowing vibrations to be sensed and transmitted to the brain. Reptiles do not have a cochlea but do have a well developed semicircular duct system. This suggests that the ears are mainly used for balance rather than hearing. However, it is clear that reptiles can 'hear' or detect both ground and air vibrations.

Taste

The taste buds are the primary organ for flavour detection. Dogs and cats have numerous taste buds scattered across the surface of the tongue, soft palate and epiglottis. As with the detection of smell, the chemical causing the 'taste' (gustation) dissolves in the mucus/saliva and stimulates the taste buds. Sensory signals are then sent via the facial, glossopharyngeal or vagus nerves, depending upon the location of the taste bud, to the brainstem.

Birds

Birds have a reduced number of taste buds, but can still readily discern different flavours.

Reptiles

Taste buds in a vestigial form have been found scattered across the oral mucosa and tongue in most reptiles.

Touch

Touch receptors are present in the skin (for details on the anatomy of the skin, see the Integument section below) alongside receptors for pain, heat, pressure and cold.

- Pain receptors are present in the epidermis as free nerve endings.
- Bulbous corpuscle endings are present in the dermis and are stimulated by heat or cold. These nerve endings are encapsulated.
- Lamellar corpuscles comprise concentric layers of cells in the subcutis, which respond to pressure.
- Meniscoid corpuscles end in cup-shaped discs in the dermis and epidermis and act as touch receptors. Tactile hairs (**vibrissae**) on the muzzle and eyes are also responsible for the sensation of touch.

Horses

The skin receptors sense changes in temperature, pressure and pain, encouraging the horse to yield to the pressure of a rider and to protect itself against parasites.

Small mammals

Many small mammals have tactile hairs around their muzzles and lower lips. For example, rabbits cannot see beneath the mouth and so rely on the tactile hairs to locate food.

Birds

Birds have tactile bristles around the beak and face.

Reptiles

Rudimentary corpuscles have been described in the skin of reptiles, particularly around the mouth and ventral aspect of the body (especially snakes). These corpuscles allow reptiles to interpret their surroundings. Reptiles do have heat receptors, but do not seem to respond to intense heat; therefore, they should be protected from heat lamps as severe thermal burns can result if the animal is too close to a heat source for a prolonged period of time.

Cardiovascular system

The cardiovascular system consists of the vessels and organs involved in the transport of blood around the body. The main components are the heart, arteries, veins and blood.

Heart
Anatomy

The heart (Figure 3.57) is responsible for pumping blood continuously around the body. It sits in the thorax within the mediastinum. Anterior to the heart in young animals is the thymus. The heart is surrounded by a sac known as the **pericardium**, which is attached to the base of the heart. This sac is also attached to structures surrounding the heart and keeps it in place in the thorax. The layer of pericardium in contact with the heart is known as the **visceral pericardium**; the outer layer is known as the **parietal pericardium**. The pericardium contains a small amount of **pericardial fluid**. This fluid allows the heart to contract freely within the pericardium.

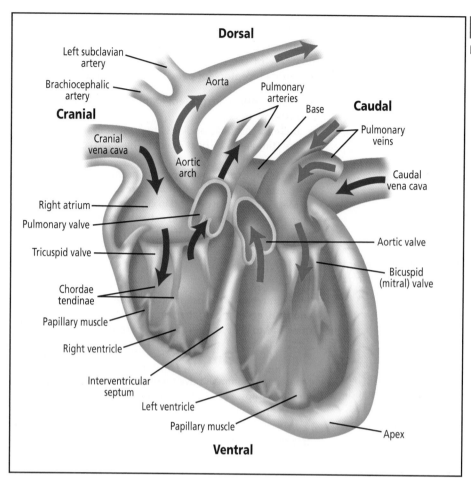

Dorsal

Left subclavian artery

Brachiocephalic artery

Cranial

Aorta

Pulmonary arteries

Base

Caudal

Cranial vena cava

Aortic arch

Pulmonary veins

Caudal vena cava

Right atrium

Pulmonary valve

Tricuspid valve

Aortic valve

Bicuspid (mitral) valve

Chordae tendinae

Papillary muscle

Right ventricle

Interventricular septum

Left ventricle

Papillary muscle

Apex

Ventral

3.57 The structure of the heart and direction of blood flow.

The heart has three layers of cardiac muscle: the **epicardium** (outer layer), the **myocardium** (thick middle layer) and the **endocardium** (thin and relatively smooth inner layer).

The heart consists of four chambers: **right atrium, left atrium, right ventricle** and **left ventricle**. The wall of the left ventricle is much thicker than that of the right ventricle; this can be appreciated on a visual examination of the heart. The right side of the heart is separated from the left side by a **septum** or wall of tissue that runs the length of the heart. Between the left and right atria this is known as the **interatrial septum**, and between the left and right ventricles it is known as the **interventricular septum**. On the outside of the heart, the atria and ventricles are separated by the **coronary groove**, which contains the major vessels of the **coronary artery**.

The atria and ventricles are also separated by **atrioventricular (AV) valves**. Valves are present in the heart to prevent blood from flowing backwards (i.e. from the ventricles into the atria). The AV valves are attached to **papillary muscles** (projections from the heart wall) via strands of tissue known as **chordae tendinae**. The chordae tendinae allow the AV valves to move, resulting in blood from the atria entering the ventricles. However, when the heart contracts the chordae tendinae prevent the AV valves from swinging back into the atria, thus ensuring that the valves remain blood-tight. The combination of AV valves and chordae tendinae has the appearance of a parachute.

The AV valve between the right atrium and right ventricle is known as the **tricuspid valve** as it has three cusps or segments. The AV valve between the left atrium and left ventricle is known as the **bicuspid** or **mitral valve** and has two cusps. In addition to the tricuspid and bicuspid valves, there are also valves present where blood leaves the right ventricle and enters the pulmonary artery (**pulmonary valve**) and where blood leaves the left ventricle and enters the aorta (**aortic valve**). The pulmonary and aortic valves are also known as **semilunar valves** because of their half-moon shape.

Contraction

- Contraction of the heart is known as **systole**.
- Relaxation of the heart is known as **diastole**.

The heart contracts due to electrical activity in the cardiac muscle cells. A conduction system (Figure 3.58) allows the transmission of electrical impulses in a controlled manner, resulting in contraction of the heart. Abnormalities in the conduction system can lead to irregularities in the rhythm of contraction, known as arrhythmias.

Within the heart there are specialized areas of cells that control the rate at which the heart contracts. These areas are called **pacemakers**, and are predominantly located in the **sinoatrial node** (SA node; Figure 3.58a). The SA node is the beginning of the conduction system and initiates a wave of contraction in the atria (Figure 3.58b). The electrical impulse then passes to a second group of specialized cells located at the top of the interventricular septum. This area is called the **atrioventricular node** (AV node). From the AV node the impulse travels down the interventricular septum in the **bundle of His** (Figure 3.58c). The electrical impulse is then distributed to the ventricles in the part of the conduction system known as the **Purkinje fibres/tissue**. These structures are not apparent to the naked eye but can be seen under a microscope. The nerve fibres directly innervate the cardiac muscle cells.

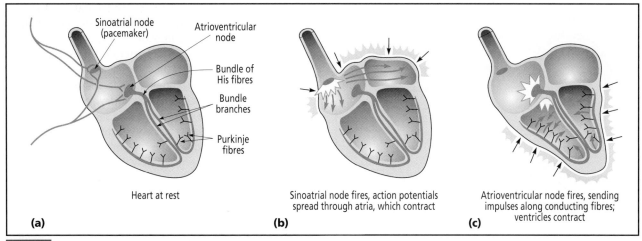

Sinoatrial node
(pacemaker)

Atrioventricular
node

Bundle of
His fibres

Bundle
branches

Purkinje
fibres

Heart at rest

Sinoatrial node fires, action potentials
spread through atria, which contract

Atrioventricular node fires, sending
impulses along conducting fibres;
ventricles contract

(a)

(b)

(c)

3.58 The conduction mechanism of the heart.

There is a potential difference across the cell membrane of a cardiac muscle cell, with the inside of the cell being more negatively charged. When the cell is stimulated, the permeability of the cell membrane to potassium and sodium is altered; sodium moves into the cell and potassium moves out. This results in an electrical impulse and contraction of the cell.

Heart sounds

Closure of the AV valves due to contraction of the ventricles results in the **first heart sound** ('lub'), which can be heard on auscultation. In most animals closure of the right and left AV valves cannot be heard separately; however, in conditions where this does arise it results in a 'split' first heart sound. Closure of the pulmonary and aortic valves (predominately the aortic valve) following contraction and emptying of blood from the ventricles results in the **second heart sound** ('dub'); this signals the end of systole.

Blood pressure

Due to contraction and relaxation of the heart, the pressure within the blood vessels is constantly changing. The pressure in the blood vessels when the heart contracts is known as the **systolic pressure**. The pressure when the heart relaxes is the **diastolic pressure**. Measurement of blood pressure using an inflatable cuff and Doppler probe on a distal limb determines only the systolic pressure.

Horses

The heart lies in the ventral section of the mediastinum. In horses, the mediastinum is incomplete allowing communication between the two sides of the chest. The size of the heart varies with breed; thoroughbreds have markedly larger hearts than draft horses. The heart lies within the second to sixth intercostal spaces. Auscultation of the mitral valve is easiest over the fifth intercostal space on the left side, just caudal to the point of the elbow. Auscultation of the tricuspid valve is ideal over the ventral third and fourth intercostal spaces on the right side.

Small mammals

In rabbits the heart is relatively small compared with overall body mass. In addition, the right AV valve has only two cusps.

Birds

In birds the heart is relatively large compared with body mass. It has a **sinus venosus**, which is formed at the confluence of the right cranial vena cava and caudal vena cava. The sinus venosus is separated from the right atrium by two muscular SA valves. The right AV valve has a single muscular flap and no chordae. The AV bundle gives off a fascicle, which encircles the AV opening and innervates the right AV valve. The pulmonary veins combine to form a single vessel before entering the left atrium. The entrance to the vein is guarded by a valve to prevent reflux.

Reptiles

In reptiles the heart has three chambers: two atria and a common ventricle. A fourth chamber is present in the form of the **sinus venosus**, which is separated from the right atrium by two valves.

The pacemaker for the heart is believed to lie within the wall of the sinus venosus. The single ventricle functionally separates oxygenated and deoxygenated blood via a series of muscular ridges.

Arteries
Anatomy

The wall of an artery consists of three layers known as tunics (Figure 3.59).

- The **internal tunic** (*tunica interna* or *tunica intima*) is thin and consists of endothelium.
- The **middle tunic** (*tunica media*) is the thickest layer and comprises elastic tissue and smooth muscle.
- The **outer tunic** (*tunica adventitia*) is made up of connective tissue. Within this layer in large arteries are small blood vessels, which supply nutrition to the artery itself. This is because it is not possible for large arteries to absorb nutrients directly from the bloodstream due to the thickness of the arterial wall.

The artery is designed to withstand the high pressure of blood from the heart. Elastic tissue is important in the arterial wall because it allows the artery to expand during systole, when blood is being forced around the body, and to recoil during diastole, when the heart relaxes. Recoil of the

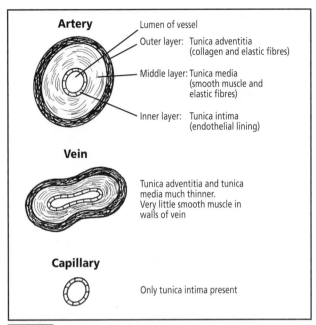

3.59 Structure of an artery, vein and capillary.

arteries also forces blood around the body. The smooth muscle controls the diameter of the artery and regulates the flow of blood to different organs. Due to the presence of elastic tissue and muscle, arteries do not need valves to control blood flow. As the arteries get smaller there is a larger proportion of smooth muscle to elastic tissue.

Arterial system

The main artery is the **aorta**, which arises from the left ventricle of the heart and travels in a caudal direction underneath the vertebrae dorsally. The aorta has many branches (Figure 3.60), which supply the major organs, including:

- The **coronary artery**, which supplies the heart muscle
- The **brachiocephalic trunk**, which divides into the common carotid and subclavian arteries
- There is a **common carotid artery** on the left and right

side of the body. These vessels arise separately and travel up either side of the neck. The common carotid artery ends by dividing at the level of the larynx into the **external** and **internal carotid arteries**. These vessels supply the structures of the head

- The **subclavian artery** supplies the forelimb, neck and cervicothoracic area. There is a subclavian artery on the left and right sides of the body. The subclavian artery becomes the **axillary artery** and continues as the **brachial artery** as it passes down the forelimb
- The **renal arteries**, which supply the kidneys and adrenal glands
- The **ovarian/testicular arteries**, which supply the gonads
- The **coeliac artery**, which supplies the stomach, spleen and liver
- The **cranial mesenteric artery**, which supplies the small intestine
- The **caudal mesenteric artery**, which supplies the large intestine
- The **external iliac artery**, which branches into the **femoral artery**. The femoral artery supplies the hindlimbs
- The **internal iliac artery**, which supplies the pelvic organs.

Arteries continuously split into smaller and smaller vessels, like branches of a tree. As arteries become smaller they are known as **arterioles**.

Birds

In birds the aorta curves to the right rather than to the left as in mammals. The common carotid artery is very short and divides rapidly in the base of the neck to form the **vertebral artery** and the internal carotid artery. The subclavian artery provides a large **pectoral trunk** to the pectoral muscles. The kidneys are supplied by a **cranial**, **middle** and **caudal** artery. The pelvic limbs are supplied by an **ischial artery**, which continues in the thigh as the femoral artery. The **ischiatic artery** (larger than the femoral artery) also supplies the leg and divides distally into the **popliteal** and **cranial tibial arteries**.

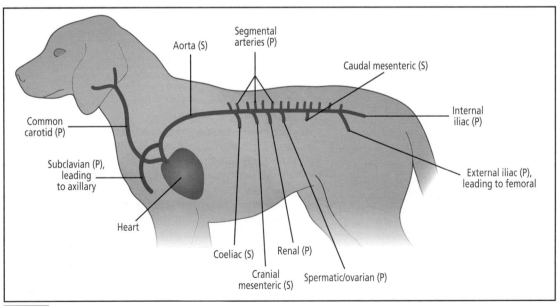

3.60 Diagrammatic representation of the major arteries of the dog. P = paired vessels; S = single vessel.

Reptiles

In reptiles two aortas exit the heart (right and left), which merge to form a single abdominal aorta halfway down the body. The common carotid artery bifurcates in the neck region and connects to the carotid duct to form the right and left internal and external carotid arteries. There is a variable number of renal arteries in reptiles: 1–2 in snakes; up to 4–5 in agamids and chameleons.

Capillaries

When arterioles branch they divide into smaller vessels until the walls are only one cell thick: these vessels are known as capillaries (see Figure 3.59). The wall of a capillary comprises only the internal tunic (see above) and thus consists of endothelium. Capillaries form an interlacing network within the vital organs, allowing the exchange of fluid, gases and nutrients to and from the surrounding tissues. For this reason, capillaries are not watertight but are in fact full of small holes which allow molecules smaller than blood proteins to move by osmosis between the capillary lumen and the body cells.

Veins

Anatomy

Although similar in construction to arteries, the walls of veins are thinner (see Figure 3.59) and have valves along their length to prevent the backflow of blood. In addition, veins collapse in on themselves rather than holding their shape like arteries.

- The **internal tunic** is thin and does not have an elastic membrane. The main function of this layer is the formation of the valves. Each valve comprises two or three cusps. These valves are present in veins exposed to intermittent pressure and are greatest in number in veins leaving muscles and in the distal limbs. These valves aid the movement of blood back to the heart and are necessary due to the much lower blood pressure found in veins compared with arteries.

- The **middle tunic** is thinner in veins than in arteries and consists of more smooth muscle than elastic tissue.
- The **outer tunic** consists of connective tissue.

Venous system

Blood returns to the right atrium of the heart via the venous system (Figure 3.61), including:

- The **coronary sinus**, which returns blood from the heart wall
- The **cranial vena cava**, which is formed by the junction of the external jugular and subclavian veins. The cranial vena cava runs through the thorax in the mediastinum
- There are two pairs of **jugular veins** within the neck: the **internal jugular vein**, which is located beside the common carotid artery; and the **external jugular vein**, which runs from the angle of the jaw, down the neck and into the thorax. The external jugular vein drains the head
- The **subclavian vein** drains the forelimbs and receives blood from the **cephalic**, **radial** and **ulnar veins**
- The **caudal vena cava**, which is a large vein that traverses the abdomen dorsally just underneath the spinal vertebrae. The right and left **internal iliac veins** from the pelvic area join together to form the caudal vena cava. The **external iliac veins** (which drain the hindlimbs) then join the caudal vena cava. As it passes through the abdomen towards the thorax, the **renal** and **hepatic veins** also join the caudal vena cava. The vessel passes through the diaphragm and into the thorax via the **caval foramen**, which is located in the ventral part of the diaphragm. The caudal vena cava then travels forward and enters the right atrium of the heart
- The **azygous vein** is formed by the union of the first **lumbar veins**, and passes into the thorax through the **aortic hiatus** in the diaphragm, where it receives blood from the **intercostal veins**. The azygous vein then travels forward and enters the right atrium. However, the anatomy of the azygous vein can vary between different species.

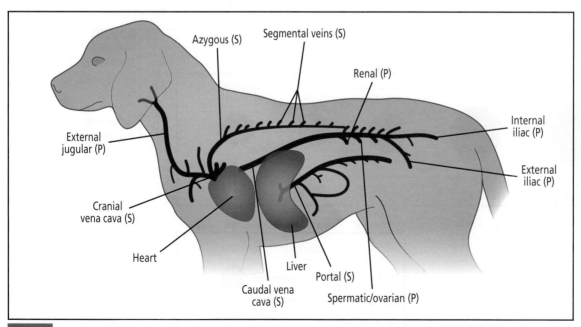

3.61 Diagrammatic representation of the major veins of the dog. P = paired vessels; S = single vessel.

Birds

There are no brachiocephalic veins in birds, instead the left and right cranial venae cavae are formed by the union of the jugular and subclavian veins. The right jugular vein is dominant and often 2–3 times the size of the left. The **brachial vein** drains the wing and can be seen running along the ventral surface. The external iliac vein (rather than the ischiatic vein) provides the main drainage for the leg. The external iliac vein is derived from the **femoral vein**, which in turn is derived from the **popliteal** and **tibial veins**.

In birds a **renal portal system** is present, whereby venous blood from the hindlimbs and caudal end of the body can travel back to the heart either by passing through the renal parenchyma or by being diverted through other vessels. This means that any nephrotoxic drug injected into the legs or caudal half of the bird's body is likely to do more damage to the kidneys than if it were injected into the cranial half of the body.

Reptiles

In many reptiles, such as lizards, a midline **ventral abdominal vein** is present. The **hepatic portal vein** joins the ventral abdominal vein. A **renal portal system** is present and is a complex anastomosis of vessels, including the **caudal** and **iliac veins**. As with birds, the significance of the renal portal system is that blood from the caudal part of the body can pass through the kidneys prior to returning to the heart.

Blood

Blood comprises a cellular component and a fluid component. The cellular component consists of red blood cells, white blood cells and platelets. The blood cells have many different functions, including the carriage of oxygen, providing immunity and blood clotting. The fluid component consists of plasma, which contains many different proteins including albumin, globulins and nutrients.

Blood cells

Haemopoiesis

This is the process by which blood cells are produced from the bone marrow in the long bones, pelvis, sternum and skull in the young animal, and in the epiphyses of the long bones, pelvis, sternum and skull in the adult animal. The spleen and liver can also take part in production when there is an increased demand for blood cells.

Erythropoiesis

This is the process by which red blood cells (erythrocytes) are produced from the bone marrow (Figure 3.62). The process is stimulated by **erythropoietin** produced by the kidney. As red blood cells develop, the nucleus condenses and is present until the developing red cell becomes a **reticulocyte**. Reticulocytes are present predominantly in the bone marrow with only a few released into the circulation in the healthy cat and dog. However, in anaemia increased numbers of nucleated red blood cells and reticulocytes can be seen in the circulation.

Red blood cells

These are the most predominant type of blood cell. Mammalian red blood cells or **erythrocytes** are circular in shape with a depression in the centre, giving them a disc-like

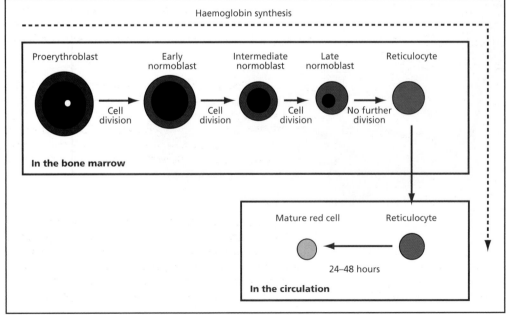

3.62

Erythropoiesis. The developing red blood cells become progressively smaller and accumulate haemoglobin. They are released into the circulation as reticulocytes. (Reproduced from the *BSAVA Manual of Canine and Feline Clinical Pathology, 2nd edition*)

appearance. The depression in the centre on either side increases the surface area of the red blood cell and allows for a greater transfer of oxygen. Red blood cells contain haemoglobin, which is required to carry oxygen and gives the cells their red colour. Red blood cells are produced in the bone marrow (see above) and after entering the circulation survive for approximately 120 days. When the cells become damaged or die they are removed from the circulation by the spleen.

White blood cells

White blood cells or leucocytes (Figure 3.63) are involved in the cellular and humoral immune response (see Chapter 5) and comprise:

- Neutrophils
- Lymphocytes
- Eosinophils
- Basophils
- Monocytes.

White blood cells are often seen as a white layer above the red blood cells when blood is centrifuged. This white layer is also known as the 'buffy coat'.

Neutrophils

In dogs and cats neutrophils (polymorphonuclear leucocytes) make up the majority of white blood cells in the circulation. Roughly 70% of the white blood cells are neutrophils and 30% are lymphocytes. The other white blood cells are present only in very small numbers.

Neutrophils are easily identified due to the large nucleus and numerous granules in the cytoplasm. The neutrophil nucleus consists of 2–5 lobes and appears segmented. Neutrophils are short-lived and usually only survive in the circulation for 1–4 days.

Neutrophils attack infectious agents; they phagocytose foreign material and release enzymes to digest any infecting organism (see Chapter 5). Neutrophils are also the predominant cells present in pus. The presence of immature neutrophils (also called band cells as the nuclei are less segmented than mature cells) and an increased number of neutrophils (neutrophilia) are suggestive of an infection.

Lymphocytes

There are two types of lymphocyte: **T lymphocytes** produced by the thymus and **B lymphocytes** produced by the bone marrow. These are very important cells in the immune response. Lymphocytes are larger than red blood cells and have a relatively large, dense, round nucleus; the cytoplasm of the cell can be stained pale blue for examination. The lifespan of lymphocytes can vary from a few days to years.

Eosinophils

These cells are much less common than neutrophils. The nucleus in eosinophils generally has two lobes and the cytoplasm contains numerous granules. Following standard staining (e.g. with Romanowsky stains) these granules appear bright red on examination, making eosinophils very distinctive. The main function of eosinophils is to fight parasitic infections. Increased numbers of eosinophils can also be seen in allergic conditions.

Basophils

In cats and dogs basophils make up only 1% of white blood cells and are difficult to locate in normal blood. The nucleus is separated into separate lobes and the cytoplasm contains numerous granules. Basophils appear similar to eosinophils, but the granules appear blue when stained with Romanowsky stains. Basophils are involved in inflammation and can contribute to allergic reactions.

Monocytes

These are the largest type of white blood cell and have an oval or horseshoe-shaped nucleus. Monocytes are produced in the bone marrow and travel in the bloodstream to the connective tissue of the skin, spleen, brain and other organs. When monocytes enter the connective tissue they are known as macrophages and are responsible for phagocytosis (see Chapter 5).

Blood cell	Appearance	Function
Neutrophil		Phagocytosis
Lymphocyte		Cellular immune response
Eosinophil		Immune response to allergens and parasites
Basophil		Immune response to allergies
Monocyte		Phagocytosis

3.63 Appearance and function of white blood cells. (May–Grunwald–Giemsa stain except basophil (Rapi-Diff); original magnification X1000) (Photographs reproduced from the *BSAVA Manual of Canine and Feline Clinical Pathology, 2nd edition*)

Platelets

These are very small cells and have no nucleus. Platelets originate from a giant cell, known as a **megakaryocyte**, located in the bone marrow. On examination, platelets are usually seen clumped together. Once in the circulation platelets have a lifespan of approximately 10 days. Platelets are involved in the clotting mechanism and are also known as thrombocytes.

Horses

Red blood cells in horses have a marked tendency to form **rouleaux** (stacks) (Figure 3.64).

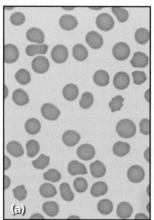
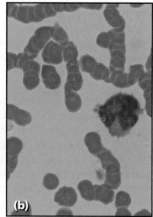

3.64   Appearance of red blood cells from a horse. **(a)** Normal. **(b)** Red blood cells in rouleaux formations; a reactive monocyte is also present. (Leishman's stain; original magnification X400) (Courtesy of T Greet)

Small mammals

There are a couple of unusual white blood cells found in small mammals:

- Rabbits – **pseudoeosinophil**, which is really a neutrophil, but when stained for examination looks more like an eosinophil
- Guinea pigs – **Kurloff cell**, which is a circulating mononuclear cell with a large inclusion (Kurloff body), commonly seen in mature female guinea pigs during gestation.

In addition, there tend to be more lymphocytes than neutrophils.

Birds

The red blood cells are nucleated and oval in shape (Figure 3.65). Neutrophils are known as **heterophils**; they have a lobed nucleus and cigar-shaped granules in the cytoplasm, which appear red when stained for examination. Heterophils are the first line of defence during an infection. The avian platelet is also nucleated.

Reptiles

The red blood cells are nucleated and oval in shape (Figure 3.66). Neutrophils are known as **heterophils**; they have a lobed nucleus and cigar-shaped granules in the cytoplasm, which appear red when stained for examination. Heterophils are

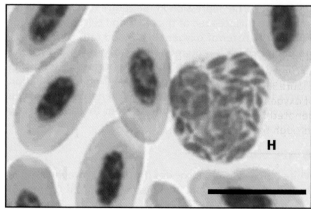

3.65   Appearance of red blood cells and heterophil (H) from a bird. (Bar = 10 μm; Hemacolor stain) (Reproduced from the *BSAVA Manual of Psittacine Birds, 2nd edition*)

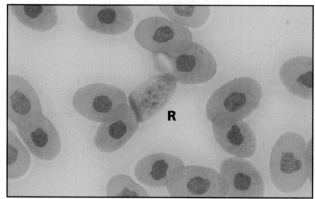

3.66   Appearance of red blood cells and a reticulocyte (R) from a reptile. (Wright–Giemsa stain; original magnification X1000) (Reproduced from the *BSAVA Manual of Reptiles, 2nd edition*)

the first line of defence during an infection. Circulating **plasma cells** may be seen in cases of immunogenic stimulation. Snakes often have a circulating mononuclear cell, known as an **azurophil**, which may be found in small numbers in healthy individuals, but which can become elevated in chronic infections. The reptilian platelet is also nucleated.

Plasma

Plasma is the fluid part of blood and contains many different substances, including:

- **Proteins** – albumin, fibrinogen and globulins are large molecules which contribute to the osmotic pressure of the plasma
- **Gases** – oxygen and carbon dioxide
- **Electrolytes** – sodium, potassium, calcium, magnesium, chloride and bicarbonate ions
- **Nutrients** – amino acids, fatty acids and glucose are transported around the body in the plasma
- **Waste products** – urea and creatinine are transported to the kidneys and liver for excretion
- **Hormones and enzymes** – transported around the body in the plasma
- **Antibodies and antitoxins** – form part of the immune system.

Circulation

Systemic

Blood returning from the body enters the heart via the cranial (left and right) and caudal venae cavae at the right atrium (Figure 3.67). This blood is venous and has a low concentration of oxygen and high concentration of carbon dioxide (deoxygenated). The blood then passes from the right atrium through the tricuspid valve and into the right ventricle.

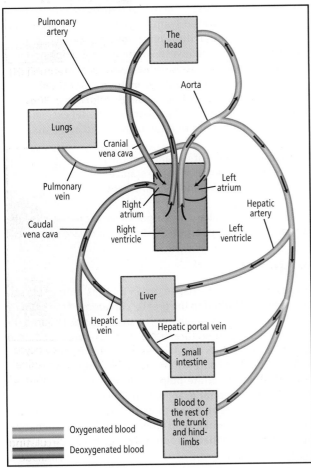

▬▬	Oxygenated blood
▬▬	Deoxygenated blood

3.67 Circulation of blood around the body.

From the right ventricle blood is pumped to the lungs in the pulmonary arteries, where it becomes oxygenated and carbon dioxide is removed. The oxygenated blood then returns to the left atrium via the pulmonary veins. The blood passes from the left atrium through the bicuspid or mitral valve and into the left ventricle. Blood leaves the left ventricle in the aorta and is pumped around the body.

Pulmonary

Deoxygenated blood leaves the right ventricle in the pulmonary trunk, which then divides into the pulmonary arteries (these are the only arteries that transport deoxygenated blood). The pulmonary arteries then branch and enter the lungs. Within the lungs the pulmonary arteries follow the bronchi and divide further into arterioles, where the blood becomes oxygenated in the alveoli. Oxygenated blood is transported to the left atrium of the heart in the pulmonary veins, which join together before leaving the lungs. Valves are absent from these veins.

Hepatic portal system

Blood from the gastrointestinal system contains the products of digestion, which need to be transported to the liver to be metabolized. The hepatic portal vein drains the spleen, abdominal digestive organs, caudal oesophagus and rectum. The three main vessels that form the portal vein are the cranial and caudal mesenteric veins (which drain the intestines) and the splenic vein. The hepatic portal system bypasses the heart.

Clotting

Blood clotting involves platelets and proteins known as clotting factors. Vitamin K is required by the liver to produce clotting factors, including II, VII, IX and X. A cascade or consecutive series of reactions occurs when blood clots.

1. **Primary aggregation** – when the endothelium (internal tunic) of blood vessels is damaged platelets are induced to clump together.
2. **Secondary aggregation** – the clumped platelets release chemicals, which induce further platelet aggregation.
3. **Blood coagulation** – factors present within the plasma, damaged blood vessels and platelets induce a cascade of reactions, resulting in the formation of **fibrin** from fibrinogen (Figure 3.68), which is found circulating in the bloodstream.
   a. **Intrinsic pathway** – the formation of fibrin is controlled by a protein present in the bloodstream known as Factor XII. The intrinsic pathway is initiated by damage to the endothelium and occurs whenever blood comes into contact with any substance other than intact epithelium.
   b. **Extrinsic pathway** – the formation of fibrin is initiated by thromboplastin, which is present on the cell membrane of most cells. The extrinsic pathway is activated when thromboplastin comes into contact with blood, following damage to the vessel walls.

   The activated factors produced by the intrinsic and extrinsic pathways join together, resulting in the formation of **thrombin**, which in turn initiates the formation of fibrin. Fibrin forms a meshwork of fibres (skeleton of the clot), which traps more platelets and cells of the immune system. The clot is present to protect the tissue whilst healing takes place.
4. **Clot dissolution** – fibrinolytic mechanisms break up the clot.
5. **Clot retraction** – the clot contracts due to a chemical reaction, closing down the defect.
6. **Clot removal** – the clot is removed by an enzyme known as a **plasmin**.

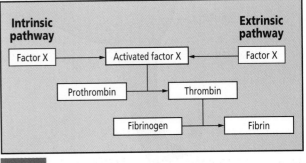

3.68 Fibrin system.

Lymphatic system

The lymphatic system is responsible for the transportation of fluid (**lymph**) from the cells to the right side of the heart. Fluid is transported to the body tissues in capillaries and forced out by the pressure from the left side of the heart to bathe the cells. However, as there is no pressure to force the fluid back into the capillaries, it has to enter the lymphatic system of vessels to be returned to the heart. In addition to the transportation of fluid, the lymphatic system is also involved with the immune system: the lymph nodes, spleen, thymus and submucosal deposits of lymphoid tissue in the intestines, tonsils and pharynx play a role in this function. Lymphoid tissue acts as the first line of defence and helps control localized infections (see Chapter 5).

Lymphatic vessels

Lymphatic vessels have thin walls and pass through all the tissues in the body (Figure 3.69). They begin as blind-ending vessels, similar to capillaries, and consist of a thin endothelial lining which is permeable to fluids and proteins. The lymphatic vessels join together and drain into two main vessels:

* **Thoracic duct** – situated in the dorsal abdomen. The initial section of the thoracic duct is dilated and called the **cysterna chyli**
* **Anterior vena cava** – the thoracic duct passes cranially through the diaphragm at the aortic hiatus and opens into the anterior vena cava.

The lymphatic system also carries fat from the intestines to the bloodstream. In the intestines there are blind-ending lymphatic ducts into which passes the fat that has been absorbed from the gut lumen. These lymphatic ducts are called **lacteals.**

Movement of fluid through the lymphatic system is aided by pulsating blood vessels situated alongside the lymphatic vessels, and by the contraction and relaxation of the surrounding muscles.

Lymph nodes

Lymph nodes are pale, bean-shaped structures situated intermittently along the length of the lymphatic vessels (Figure 3.69). Each lymph node is enclosed in a capsule made from connective tissue. This connective tissue extends into the lymph node itself as **trabeculae**, along which the blood vessels travel. Lymphoid tissue fills the space between the outer capsule and in the connective tissue trabeculae. This tissue is divided into an outer **cortex** and an inner **medulla**. Within the cortex are **follicles** or **germinal centres**, which are areas of highly concentrated lymphocytes. These areas appear darker than the rest of the lymph node when examined under a microscope. Lymphatic vessels entering the lymph node are known as **afferent vessels**; those vessels leaving the lymph node are known as **efferent vessels**.

Lymph nodes found near the surface of the animal (superficial lymph nodes) can be palpated on clinical examination. The main lymph nodes that can be palpated in the dog are:

* Submandibular – at the angle of the jaw
* Prescapular – anterior to the scapula
* Popliteal – just behind the stifle joint

The parotid, axillary and inguinal lymph nodes may also be palpated in dogs, especially if they are enlarged.

Spleen

The spleen is a strap-shaped organ that sits on the left side of the body attached to the greater curvature of the stomach by the gastrosplenic ligament. The spleen looks similar to the liver in colour and texture. It has a tough outer connective tissue capsule, parts of which extend into the body of the spleen. Follicles (concentrated areas of lymphoid cells) are found within the **white pulp** of the spleen, which appears pale when stained for examination. The more vascular areas of the spleen are referred to as the **red pulp**, and appear darker than the white pulp when stained for examination. The thick capsule that surrounds the spleen contains a large

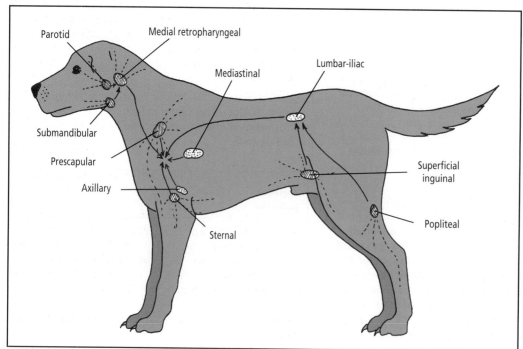

3.69 Lymph nodes and lymphatic vessels in a dog. (Reproduced from the *BSAVA Manual of Canine and Feline Oncology, 3rd edition*)

amount of smooth muscle. This allows the size of the spleen to vary greatly: as the muscle relaxes, the spleen becomes engorged with blood and so increases in size; as the muscle contracts, red blood cells are released into the circulation and the spleen becomes smaller. The functions of the spleen include: immunity, removal of damaged cells from the bloodstream and the production and storage of red blood cells.

Thymus

The thymus is located in the thoracic cavity, cranial to the heart. It is at its largest in the young animal and decreases in size as the animal gets older, disappearing completely in dogs and cats by the time they reach reproductive maturity. The thymus has an outer **cortex**, which is densely populated with lymphocytes, and an inner **medulla**. The sole function of the thymus is to contribute to the immune system by producing T lymphocytes (see Chapter 5).

Submucosal deposits of lymphoid tissue

As well as being located in the thymus, spleen and lymph nodes, discrete collections of lymphoid tissue are found throughout the body. These collections are classified according to their location:

- Peyer's patches or gut-associated lymphoid tissue (GALT) – located throughout the intestines
- Skin-associated lymphoid tissue (SALT)
- Mucosa-associated lymphoid tissue (MALT).

Lymphoid tissue is also present in the tonsils and around the pharynx.

Horses

The superficial lymph nodes normally palpable in the horse include:

- Submandibular
- Prescapular
- Subiliac
- Inguinal.

The spleen lies dorsally on the left side of the cranial abdomen, largely underneath the ribcage. It is triangular in shape with the apex pointing ventrally.

Small mammals

Small mammals have lymph nodes, a spleen and lymphatic tissue within the digestive tract (e.g. rabbits possess a so-called caecal 'tonsil'). The thymus is usually present in adult animals as it does not markedly reduce in size with age.

Birds

Most birds do not have lymph nodes, with the exception of some waterfowl which possess a single coelomic lymph node. Instead, the lymphatic tissue is often located within other organs such as the liver and kidneys. Birds do possess a spleen, but its size and shape varies with species: it is often spherical in psittacine birds and strap-like in passerine birds.

Thymic tissue is present (even in adults) as islands of cells throughout the cervical and cranial coelomic regions. In addition, birds have a unique type of lymphatic tissue located in the dorsal cloacal region, known as the **Bursa of Fabricius**. This is the site of B lymphocyte production and reduces in size with age, disappearing in the adult bird.

Reptiles

Reptiles do not have discrete lymph nodes but instead have islands of lymphatic tissue within other organs such as the liver and kidneys. Some reptiles have a separate spleen, but in many (particularly snakes) the spleen is fused with the pancreas to form a **splenopancreas**. Thymic tissue is found in the cervical region and anterior coelomic cavity, and may persist in the adult.

Respiratory system

The respiratory system comprises the nose, pharynx, larynx, trachea, bronchi and smaller airways, lungs and diaphragm. Its function is to facilitate the passage of oxygen into the body and carbon dioxide out of the body.

Anatomy

The upper respiratory tract consists of the nose, nasal cavities, pharynx, larynx and trachea (Figure 3.70). The lower respiratory tract consists of the lungs, bronchi, bronchioles and alveoli.

Nose and nasal cavities

The external part of the nose is known as the nasal plate; the central fissure of the nasal plate is called the **philtrum**. The outer part of the nose is lined with epithelium, which continues into the entrance of the nares where it is gradually replaced with mucosa. The nasal cavities are lined with **olfactory mucosa**, which is well supplied with sensory nerves and serous olfactory glands. Secretions from the olfactory glands help to keep the mucosa moist. The two nasal cavities are separated by the nasal septum, which is made of cartilage. Located alongside the nasal septum is the **vomeronasal organ** (which is highly developed in some reptiles). This is responsible for the detection of pheromones, and also plays a role in behaviour.

Situated within the nasal cavities are the **dorsal**, **ventral** and **ethmoidal conchae**.

- Dorsal and ventral conchae – these are folds of cartilage.
- Ethmoidal conchae – these are scrolls of cartilage located in the caudal part of the nasal cavities. The space between the cartilage scrolls is known as the **ethmoidal meatus**.

The dorsal, ventral and ethmoidal conchae provide a large surface area for the filtering (removal of dust and bacteria), moistening (with secretions from the olfactory glands) and warming (to near body temperature) of inspired air. Connected to the nasal cavities are the **paranasal sinuses**. In the dog there are two main paranasal sinuses:

- The **maxillary sinus** – found in the maxillary bone of the skull
- The **frontal sinus** – found in the frontal bone of the skull.

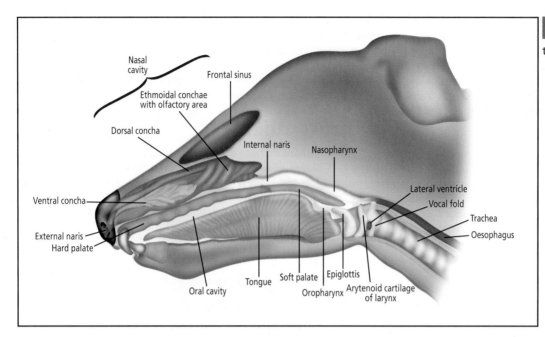

3.70 Midline section through a dog's head.

The paranasal sinuses humidify and warm inspired air, and also help to lighten the skull. In addition, they have a role in voice resonance and so are generally larger in the male.

Pharynx

The pharynx is the part of the respiratory tract that connects the nasal cavities to the larynx. It also communicates with the mouth. The pharynx is divided by the palate into:

- The **nasopharynx** – which is connected to the caudal nasal cavities
- The **oropharynx** – which is connected to the caudal oral cavity.

Larynx

The larynx is a 'box' consisting of a group of cartilages (Figure 3.71):

- **Epiglottis** – the most rostral of the cartilages. It is spade-shaped and attached to the tongue and thyroid cartilage

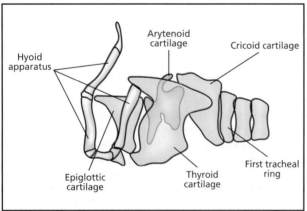

3.71 Structure of the larynx. (Reproduced from the *BSAVA Manual of Canine and Feline Head, Neck and Thoracic Surgery*)

- **Thyroid** – this is the largest of the cartilages and forms the floor of the larynx
- **Arytenoid** – this forms the inside of the larynx and supports the vocal chords
- **Cricoid** – a ring-like structure which articulates with the thyroid cartilage and trachea.

The functions of the larynx include:

- Preventing the entry of foreign material into the respiratory tract during swallowing (**deglutination**)
- Regulating the flow of gases into the respiratory tract
- Contributing to vocalization.

Trachea

The trachea consists of C-shaped rings of cartilage connected by fibrous connective tissue and smooth muscle, and lined with ciliated epithelium. Dorsally the C-shaped rings are incomplete and the free ends are connected by soft tissue. The trachea passes into the thorax at the thoracic inlet and traverses the mediastinum. The mediastinum is the space between the lungs which is bound by the pleurae (see Figure 3.9) and where the heart, thymus and blood vessels are located. The trachea splits into two bronchi at the level of the heart base. The function of the trachea is to allow airflow from the larynx to the lungs.

Bronchi, bronchioles and alveoli

The bronchi are similar in structure to the trachea, but the cartilage rings are complete. The bronchi divide further into bronchioles. As the bronchioles become smaller the amount of cartilage present decreases, finally disappearing completely. The bronchioles continue to divide to the level of the terminal bronchioles and end in the alveolar ducts (Figure 3.72). Each alveolar duct terminates in a number of alveoli, the appearance of which can be likened to a bunch of grapes attached to their stalk. The alveoli are lined with a single cell thick pulmonary membrane covered in capillaries, across which gaseous exchange takes place.

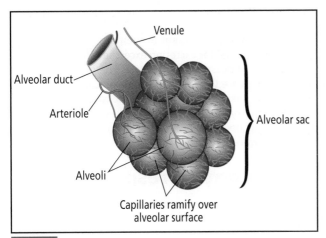

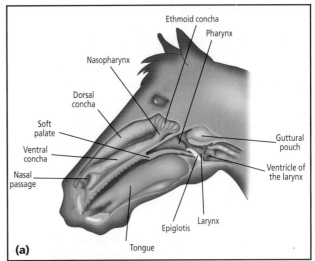

3.72 The terminal air passages.

Lungs

The lungs lie within the thoracic cavity, on either side of the mediastinum. Each lung is covered by a connective tissue layer known as the **pulmonary pleura** (visceral pleura). This is separated from the parietal pleura, which covers the inside of the thoracic cavity, by a small space known as the **pleural space** (see Figure 3.9).

The lungs consist of bronchi, bronchioles, alveoli, blood vessels and connective tissue (parenchyma). Each lung is divided into lobes (Figure 3.73): the left lung comprises the cranial, middle and caudal lobes; the right lung comprises the cranial, middle, caudal and accessory lobes.

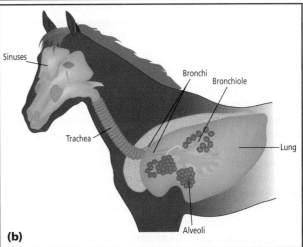

3.74 (a) Upper respiratory tract of the horse.
(b) Lower respiratory tract of the horse.

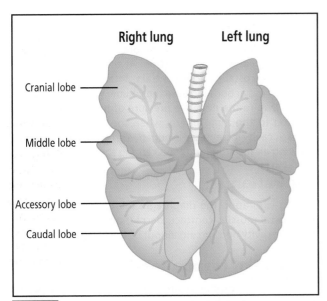

3.73 The lobes of the lungs in a dog.

Horses

Horses are obligate nasal breathers. The Eustachian tube connects the middle ear to the guttural pouch (see above section on Hearing), which lies lateral and dorsal to the pharynx (Figure 3.74a). The guttural pouch is protected by a cartilaginous flap, which opens during swallowing. This, along with the elevated soft palate, helps prevent entry of foreign material into the respiratory tract during swallowing.

The soft palate forms a continuous muscular sheet from the hard palate to the roof of the pharynx. There is a hole towards the caudal part of the soft palate called the **intra-pharyngeal ostium**, in which the rostral laryngeal cartilages fit snugly, forming an airtight and food-tight seal. The only time this junction is disrupted in normal animals is during swallowing, when for less than one second the soft palate is elevated to block off the back of the nasal cavities and the larynx moves rostrally and closes. This coincides with the propulsion of a food bolus from the back of the mouth into the oesophagus; the epiglottis tilts over the closed **rima glottidis** to prevent food material being inhaled. The structures immediately resume their respiratory position after swallowing.

The most significant feature of the equine larynx is the outpouching of the laryngeal mucosa. This occurs laterally between the vocal and vestibular folds within the thyroid cartilage to form the **laryngeal ventricles**. Laxity in the muscles that contract the ventricles results in the eversion of the ventricles into the lumen of the larynx. This laxity commonly results from a degeneration of the **recurrent laryngeal nerve**. The condition is usually seen on the left side, as a consequence of the elongated course of the left nerve around the aortic arch. The left laryngeal muscles may become paralysed (**laryngeal hemiplegia** or **recurrent laryngeal neuropathy**). The most significant muscle is the **left cricoarytenoid muscle**, which is the only abductor (dilator) of the rima glottidis (laryngeal valve), and causes laryngeal obstruction during exercise. Affected horses, in particular young males, make a 'whistling' or 'roaring' noise on inspiration.

The trachea is located ventrally and slightly to the right of the midline. The cartilages are C-shaped, with the free ends bridged by the **trachealis muscle**. The right and left lungs are more equal in size compared with many other species (Figure 3.74b). There is no external evidence of lobation, except the presence of an accessory lobe, which is attached to the base of the right lung, and the fact that the cranial lobes narrow from the main body of the lungs. The left lung has a deep cardiac notch, so the heart has considerable contact with the inside of the chest wall between the third and sixth ribs on the left-hand side.

Small mammals

Small herbivores are obligate nasal breathers. Many small rodents have a **palatal ostium** (an opening through the soft palate to access the trachea). The division of the lungs into lobes is generally less obvious. The diaphragm is more deeply domed and is the main impetus for inspiration.

Birds

Birds have one nasal concha. The main sinus is the **infraorbital sinus** (Figure 3.75), which sits below the eye and has no lateral bony wall. The glottis lacks an epiglottis, thyroid cartilage and vocal folds. The glottis is held closed at rest. The trachea has complete signet ring-shaped cartilages supporting its structure. The trachea may be coiled inside the sternum in some waterfowl. Some birds (e.g. penguins) have a midline septum dividing the trachea in two as far cranially as the glottis. Male ducks have a **diverticulum (bulla)** of the trachea just inside the body cavity. The **syrinx** (avian voice box) may be found at the caudal end of the trachea.

The lungs are semi-rigid in birds and thus do not significantly inflate or deflate during inspiration and expiration. The lungs are attached to the underside of the dorsal body wall and protected by the **notarium**. There are nine **air sacs** in most species. There is no diaphragm in birds, and the common body cavity is referred to as the **coelom**.

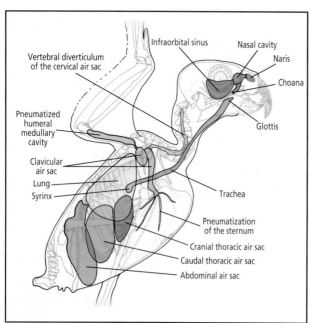

3.75   Respiratory system of the bird. (© Nigel Harcourt-Brown)

Reptiles

There are salt glands present in the nares of some reptiles (e.g. green iguana) for excreting excess salt. Non-crocodilian reptiles do not possess a hard palate. The rings of cartilage in the trachea are O-shaped in chelonians, and C-shaped in lizards and snakes. The lungs are more alveolar and elastic than those in mammals. In many snakes (such as colubrids) the left lung becomes reduced, leaving only a major right lung (see Figure 3.86). There is no true diaphragm in reptiles.

Physiology of respiration

Terminology

- **Total lung capacity** – the total volume of air in the lungs.
- **Tidal volume** – the volume of air breathed in or out in one normal breath.
- **Functional residual volume** – the volume of air left in the lungs after one normal breath.
- **Vital capacity** – the maximum volume of air that can be forced out of the lungs.
- **Residual volume** – the volume of air left in the lungs after forced expiration.
- **Anatomical dead space** – the volume of air which does not reach the alveoli. This is equal to the volume of the trachea, bronchi and bronchioles.

The application of these terms with regards to general anaesthesia is discussed in Chapter 23.

Inspiration

During inspiration the diaphragm contracts, becoming flatter and moving in a caudal direction. At the same time the external intercostal muscles contract, lifting the ribcage outwards. These actions increase the volume within the thoracic cavity. Due to the negative pressure of the pleural space in relation to the atmosphere, when the volume within the thoracic cavity increases, the negative pressure increases, thus drawing air into the lungs and causing them to inflate.

Expiration

During expiration the diaphragm relaxes and the internal intercostal muscles contract, decreasing the volume of the thoracic cavity and forcing air out of the lungs.

Control of respiration

Inspiration and expiration are controlled by a number of different systems, including:

- Neural control
- Humoral control.

Neural control

When the lungs inflate, receptors in the bronchi and bronchioles send impulses to the respiratory centre in the medulla and pons of the hindbrain, which inhibits further inspiration and stimulates expiration. This is called the **inflation reflex** or **Hering Breuer reflex**. When the lungs deflate, the respiratory centre initiates the next inspiration. This is called the **deflation reflex**.

Humoral control

Respiration is also controlled by various chemicals in the blood, including carbon dioxide, which is monitored by the medulla of the hindbrain. When carbon dioxide levels in the blood increase, ventilation increases; when carbon dioxide levels in the blood decrease, ventilation decreases. The medulla only monitors carbon dioxide levels. Oxygen levels in the bloodstream are monitored by **chemoreceptors** in the carotid arteries and the aortic arch.

Birds

During inspiration the sternum moves downwards and the ribcage outwards, thereby increasing the volume of the coelom. This increased coelomic volume allows air to be drawn through the lungs and into the series of air sacs, which act as passive bellows. The respiratory cycle is complex in birds and occurs over two inspirations and expirations.

- The **first inspiration** draws air into the lungs, much of it bypassing the areas of gaseous exchange and moving directly into the caudal air sacs (caudal thoracic and abdominal).
- During the **first expiration**, air in the caudal air sacs moves back through the neopulmonic part of the lungs and into the paleopulmonic sections (from caudal to cranial), where gaseous exchange occurs.
- The **second inspiration** allows air moving cranially from the first expiration to move into the cranial air sacs.
- The **second expiration** allows air in the cranial air sacs to be expelled through the secondary and primary bronchi.

Digestive system

Anatomy

The basic components of the digestive tract (Figure 3.76) are:

- Mouth
- Pharynx
- Oesophagus
- Stomach
- Small intestine
- Large intestine
- Liver and gallbladder
- Pancreas.

Although the general structure of the digestive system is similar, differences arise depending on whether the animal is a carnivore (meat eater), herbivore (plant eater) or omnivore (eats a mixture of meat and plants). Herbivores are of two broad types: ruminants (foregut fermenters, e.g. cattle) have highly developed stomachs; hindgut fermenters (e.g. horses) have a highly developed large intestine and caecum.

Mouth

The mouth extends from the lips to the pharynx. It is divided into a cavity between the teeth and cheeks (**buccal space** or **cavity**) and the **central cavity**. The central cavity is bound by the hard palate, teeth (see Skull section above), gums and tongue.

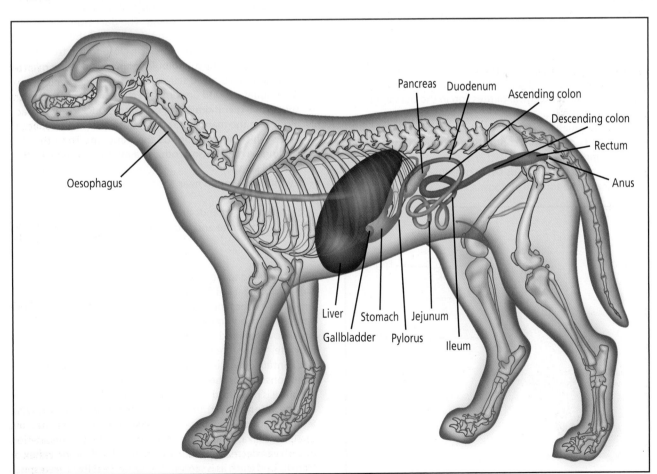

3.76 Digestive tract in the abdomen of a dog. The length of the intestines has been reduced in order to simplify the diagram.

Lips

The lips comprise a covering of skin with underlying muscles and tendons and an inner layer of mucosa. The skin of the lips is well supplied with sebaceous glands, which provide waterproofing and scent. The **facial nerve** innervates the lips and controls movement. Some larger breeds of dogs have impressive lip folds, which are prone to infection. The function of the lips is to bring food into the mouth (**prehension**). The degree to which the lips are involved in this process varies between species, being very important in herbivores such as horses and rabbits, but less important in cats and dogs.

Cheeks

The cheeks are lined with stratified squamous epithelium (**buccal mucosa**). The cheeks or **buccae** are controlled by the **buccinator muscle**. The function of the cheeks is to move the food bolus from one side of the mouth to the other (along with the tongue) during chewing; this function is highly developed in herbivores.

Palate

The **hard palate** forms the roof of the mouth and consists of the incisive bone rostrally (which holds the incisors), maxillary bone laterally and palatine bone. The bones are covered in keratinized epithelium, which protects the underlying structures. Caudally the hard palate merges into the **soft palate**, which is lined with the same epithelium but comprises soft tissue rather than bone.

Tongue

The tongue consists of a number of different parts (Figure 3.77), including:

- Apex – tip of the tongue
- Body – main part of the tongue
- Root – where the tongue attaches to the mouth
- Median groove – central depression in the dorsal surface of the tongue
- Papillae – small projections on the surface of the tongue
- Frenulum – tissue that connects the tongue to the floor of the mouth
- Lyssa – an area of fibrous tissue present on the ventral surface of the tongue in dogs.

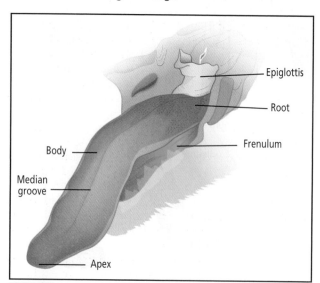

Body

Median groove

Apex

Epiglottis

Root

Frenulum

3.77 The structure of the tongue.

The tongue is attached to the hyoid bones and the mandible. It is covered in keratinized mucosa, which protects it from the trauma of **mastication** (chewing). Papillae are present to some degree on all tongues; they are well developed in cats, giving the tongue a rough appearance which can easily be seen with the naked eye. Some of the papillae contain taste buds. The tongue consists of skeletal muscle controlled by the **hypoglossal nerve**. The specific muscles present in the tongue are:

- Geniohyoideus
- Genioglossus
- Hyoglossus
- Styloglossus.

The tongue has many functions, including:

- Prehension
- Lapping
- Grooming
- Vocalization (in combination with the vocal folds)
- Heat loss through panting.

Salivary glands

Salivary glands are present in cats, dogs and other mammals. The four main salivary glands in the dog and cat are:

- **Parotid** – found at the base of the ear. The duct from the parotid gland exits rostrally and opens into the mouth opposite the upper fourth premolar tooth in the buccal space/cavity.
- **Mandibular** – found at the angle of the jaw and is smaller that the parotid gland. The duct from the mandibular gland runs along the floor of the mouth and opens on the sublingual caruncle close to the frenulum of the tongue. The mandibular gland produces a mixture of serous and mucoid saliva
- **Sublingual** – found underneath the tongue. The sublingual gland drains via one single duct located alongside the mandibular duct, but has many smaller ducts which open alongside the frenulum. The sublingual gland also produces a mixture of serous and mucoid saliva
- **Zygomatic** – found near the eye in the dog.

Small salivary glands are also present on the lips, cheeks, tongue, soft palate and pharynx.

Saliva

This is required to moisten the mouth and provide lubrication. Saliva forms part of the non-specific immune system; it continuously washes the mouth and reduces the level of bacteria. Saliva is also required for the initial mechanical and chemical breakdown of food: the saliva of dogs and herbivores contains amylase, which breaks down starch; the saliva of cats does not contain amylase as they are carnivores. In addition, saliva is responsible for the excretion of minerals found in tartar.

Saliva is produced continuously, but the rate of production can be altered by the autonomic nervous system (ANS). Stimulation of the parasympathetic branch of the ANS can increase saliva production; stimulation of the sympathetic branch can decrease production. Eating food, or the anticipation of food (such as is seen in the classical Pavlovian reaction), can stimulate production of saliva. Fear and dehydration decreases the level of saliva and leads to a dry, tacky mouth.

Pharynx

The pharynx is defined by the base of skull, the mandible and the larynx. It comprises three parts:

- The **nasopharynx** – which is connected to the caudal nasal cavities
- The **oropharynx** – which is connected to the caudal oral cavity
- The **laryngopharynx** – which is connected to the oesophagus and lies alongside the larynx.

The act of eating involves three stages:

1. Prehension – taking food into the mouth.
2. Mastication – chewing food.
3. Deglutition – swallowing food.

The **swallowing reflex** is finely controlled to ensure that food does not enter the airway. A network of nerve impulses stimulate the nasopharynx and larynx to close, and the oropharynx to open, allowing the food bolus to pass into the oesophagus.

1. The soft palate is elevated to close off the nasopharynx.
2. The laryngeal muscles close the larynx; this means that the animal cannot breathe for a short time.
3. The tongue moves the bolus of food from the back of the mouth to the cranial oesophagus.
4. Peristaltic waves begin at the cranial end of the oesophagus to move the food bolus down into the stomach.

Oesophagus

The oesophagus consists of four layers:

- Outer layer – connective tissue
- Muscle layer – mainly striated muscle, changing to smooth muscle distally. In the dog the entire oesophagus comprises striated muscle. There are two layers of muscle: an inner circular layer and outer longitudinal layer
- Submucosa layer
- Inner layer – mucosa (stratified squamous epithelium).

The oesophagus passes down the left side of the neck. It enters the thorax and traverses the **mediastinum**, passing dorsal to the heart, through the diaphragm and into the abdomen, where it enters the stomach at the **cardiac sphincter**. A sphincter is a muscular valve which controls the passage of gut contents. However, the cardiac sphincter is not a true sphincter as it opens with only the pressure of a food bolus: this allows passage of food into the stomach, and the return of food to the oesophagus when the animal regurgitates or vomits. The oesophagus is innervated by the **vagus nerve**, which controls peristalsis.

Stomach

The stomach has a curved appearance: the smaller cranial curve is known as the **lesser curvature**; the larger caudal curve is known as the **greater curvature**. The dorsal part of the stomach is the **fundus** (Figure 3.78a), which receives food from the oesophagus via the **cardiac sphincter**. The main part of the stomach is the **body**, where food is mixed with saliva and

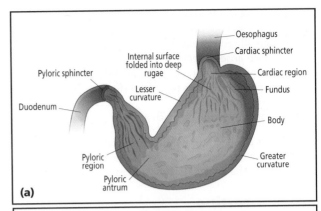

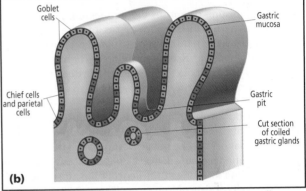

3.78   **(a)** Cross-section through the stomach wall. **(b)** Section showing the gastric pits.

gastric secretions. From the body, ingesta moves to the **antrum** before entering the **pylorus**. From the pylorus food can either enter the **duodenum** via the **pyloric sphincter**, or return to the body of the stomach for further breakdown.

The stomach wall consists of six different layers:

- Serosa – outer layer
- Smooth muscle – three layers: longitudinal (top layer), circular (middle layer) and oblique (bottom layer)
- Submucosa
- Mucosa – inner layer consisting of glandular, columnar epithelium covered with mucus.

Different parts of the mucosa contain different types of gland (Figure 3.78b). The cardiac and pyloric mucosa contain mucus-secreting glands (**goblet cells**). The glands in the mucosa of the body (**gastric glands**) produce **pepsinogen (chief cells)** and **hydrochloric acid (parietal cells)**. Pepsinogen is converted into its active form **pepsin** by hydrochloric acid in the lumen of the stomach. The hormone **gastrin** is also secreted by the stomach into the bloodstream. Gastrin stimulates the production of hydrochloric acid.

Gastric secretions (mucus, pepsinogen and hydrochloric acid) are stimulated by the sight or smell of food, the act of eating and the presence of food in the stomach. Inhibition of secretion occurs when the stomach contents reach a pH <2 or when the ingesta passes into the duodenum. The muscular layers of the stomach contract at different intervals to help break down food and move the ingesta towards the pyloric sphincter (e.g. the antrum contracts up to four times per minute, depending on the amount of food present). It should be noted that nutrients are not absorbed from the stomach.

Emptying of the stomach is carefully controlled by the nervous and endocrine systems. The speed at which the stomach empties also depends on the type of food consumed:

high fat meals result in slower gastric emptying, so that fat breakdown can take place in the jejunum without it being overloaded. Blood is supplied to the stomach via the **coeliac artery**, which arises directly from the aorta. Branches of the coeliac artery initially supply the lesser and greater curvatures and then spread out to the rest of the stomach. Venous drainage is via the **portal vein**.

The functions of the stomach are:

- To act as a collecting chamber for food
- To initiate the mechanical breakdown of food
- To initiate the enzymatic breakdown of food.

Small intestine

The small intestine comprises the duodenum, jejunum and ileum. Ingesta from the stomach passes into the **duodenum**. This is a short section of intestine situated on the right side of the abdomen and fixed in position by tight connective tissue. The pancreatic duct and common bile duct are located here, allowing pancreatic enzymes and bile to enter the gastrointestinal tract.

From the duodenum, ingesta passes into the **jejunum**. This part of the intestine is very long and coiled within the abdomen. The final part of the small intestine is the **ileum**, which can be identified by the lack of villi on the mucosa. The ileum meets the large intestine at the **ileocolic junction**. The small intestinal wall consists of four layers (Figure 3.79a):

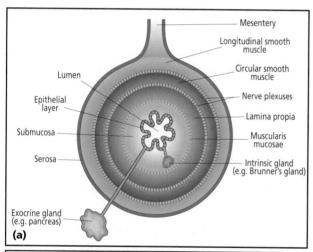

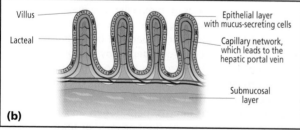

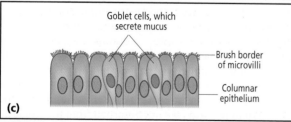

3.79   **(a)** Cross-section through the intestine wall. **(b)** Detail of the villus structure. **(c)** Detail of epithelium.

- Serosa – outer layer
- Smooth muscle
- Submucosa
- Mucosa – inner layer where the villi (finger-like projections; Figure 3.79b) are located. Along the villi are even smaller projections, known as **microvilli**, which are collectively termed the **brush border** (Figure 3.79c). The intestinal glands are also found in this layer.

Blood is supplied to part of the duodenum by the **coeliac artery**. The remainder of the duodenum along with the jejunum, ileum and the ileocolic junction is supplied by the **mesenteric artery**. Venous drainage is via the **cranial** and **caudal mesenteric veins**. Lymphatic vessels from the small intestine drain into the **cysterna chyli**, which forms part of the **thoracic duct** and returns the lymphatic fluid to the venous bloodstream.

The functions of the small intestine are:

- Enzymatic digestion of food
- Absorption of nutrients following digestion of food.

Digestion of food within the stomach and small intestine takes place through the action of various secretions (Figure 3.80). The villi increase the surface area of the small intestine that the ingesta comes into contact with. Within each villus is a capillary which absorbs nutrients and lacteals which absorb chyle (a milky liquid containing digested fat).

Large intestine

The large intestine comprises the caecum, colon and rectum. The **caecum** is a blind-ending diverticulum found at the ileocolic junction. The size of the caecum varies between species. In the rabbit the caecum is a large organ, which is required to break down fibre. In the dog and cat the caecum is **vestigial**, as vegetation only makes up a small part of the diet, or none at all.

Ingesta from the ileum passes into the colon. The **colon** consists of an **ascending** portion, a **transverse** portion (moving from right to left) and a **descending** portion (moving from the left flank to the pelvic cavity). From the colon, ingesta passes into the rectum. The **rectum** lies dorsally above the organs of the reproductive and urinary tracts. Movement of faeces out of the rectum is controlled by the **anal sphincter**. Located on either side of the anal sphincter are the **perianal sacs**, which are also known as the **anal glands**: this term is not strictly correct as they are not true glands. These sacs are lined with glandular epithelium, which secretes fluid used to scent mark territory. Each time the animal defecates, these sacs should empty.

Blood is supplied to the ascending and transverse colon by the **cranial mesenteric artery**. The descending colon and rectum are supplied by the **caudal mesenteric artery**. Venous drainage is via the cranial and caudal mesenteric veins.

The functions of the large intestine are:

- Microbial digestion:
  - Breakdown of fibre
  - Production of essential amino acids
  - Production of B vitamins and vitamin K
- Resorption of water and electrolytes.

As these functions take some time, gut transit is slower in the large intestine than in the small intestine.

Origin of secretion	Digestive juice	Contents	Action	Comments
Stomach				
Goblet cells	Gastric juices (the hormone gastrin is produced as food enters the stomach and stimulates the gastric pits to secrete gastric juices)	Mucus	No enzyme action. Lubricates food. Protects gastric mucosa from autodigestion	
Parietal cells		Hydrochloric acid (HCl)	Denatures protein. Creates a pH of 1.3–5. Converts pepsinogen to active pepsin	Protein digestion is made easier. Acid pH kills most pathogenic bacteria
Chief cells		Pepsinogen	When activated by HCl, pepsin converts protein to peptides	Peptides are small molecules
Small intestine				
Liver	Bile	Bile salts	Emulsifies fats to produce small globules. Activates lipases	As chyme enters the duodenum, the gallbladder contracts forcing bile along the bile duct
Exocrine pancreas	Pancreatic juice (produced in response to gastrin and the hormone cholecystokinin which is secreted by duodenal cells as chyme passes through the pyloric sphincter)	Bicarbonate	No enzyme action. Neutralizes the acid pH	Neutral pH stops action of pepsin and enables intestinal digestive enzymes to act
		Trypsinogen	Inactive	Converted to active trypsin by enterokinase present in succus entericus. Spontaneous conversion is prevented by a trypsin inhibitor
		Trypsin	Activates other enzyme precursors. Converts peptides and other proteins to amino acids	Amino acids are absorbed into the bloodstream
		Lipase	Converts fats to fatty acids and glycerol	Activated by bile salts
		Amylase	Converts starches to maltose	Starches are plant carbohydrates
Brunner's glands as succus entericus and crypts of Lieberkuhn	Intestinal juices (produced in response to the hormone secretin, which is secreted as chyme passes through the pyloric sphincter)	Maltase	Converts maltose to glucose	Glucose is absorbed by the blood capillaries
		Sucrase	Converts sucrose to glucose and fructose	Glucose and fructose are absorbed by the blood capillaries
		Lactase	Converts lactose to glucose and galactose	Glucose and galactose are absorbed by the blood capillaries
		Enterokinase	Converts trypsinogen to trypsin	Trypsin is activated
		Aminopeptidase	Converts peptides to amino acids	Amino acids are absorbed into the bloodstream
		Lipase	Converts fats to fatty acids and glycerol	Fatty acids and glycerol are absorbed into the lacteals

3.80   Processes involved in digestion.

Liver and gallbladder

The liver is a solid organ located between the stomach and the diaphragm. It is divided into lobes, the pattern of which varies between species. In the dog six lobes are present:

- Left lateral
- Left medial
- Right lateral
- Right medial
- Quadrate
- Caudate.

The liver consists of cells, known as **hepatocytes**, arranged in hexagonal lobules. Located between the lobules are the **bile canaliculi**; this is where bile is secreted and then transported to the gallbladder. The liver receives blood from both the hepatic artery and the portal vein. The **hepatic artery** provides oxygenated blood from the aorta to the liver cells.

The portal vein transports absorbed products of digestion from the gastrointestinal tract to the liver for metabolism. Venous drainage is via the **hepatic vein**.

The functions of the liver are:

- Metabolism of carbohydrate, protein and fat absorbed from the intestines
- Production of bile
- Neutralization and destruction of drugs and toxins
- Manufacture, breakdown and regulation of hormones
- Manufacture of enzymes and proteins (e.g. albumin)
- Removal of old red blood cells from the circulation
- Storage of iron and vitamins A, D, E and K.

The liver generates heat when carrying out these processes and is a major contributor to the maintenance of body temperature in endothermic animals.

The **gallbladder** is situated between the quadrate and right medial lobes of the liver. Its function is to store bile until it is required for digestion.

Pancreas

The pancreas is a glandular structure comprising an **endocrine** and an **exocrine** component. The endocrine section is responsible for the production of insulin and glucagon (see Endocrine system below). The exocrine section produces **bicarbonate** and **enzymes**, which are required for digestion. Bicarbonate neutralizes acid from the stomach, ensuring that the ingesta entering the small intestines is less acidic. The digestive enzymes produced by the pancreas (see Figure 3.80) include:

- Trypsin – which breaks down protein
- Lipase – which breaks down lipids
- Amylase – which breaks down starch.

Horses

The digestive system of the horse is shown in Figure 3.81.

Mouth

The hard palate is wide, prominently ridged and merges into the soft palate. The tongue is long, wider at the tip than at the base, and is covered with taste buds. The main salivary glands are paired and include the parotid (largest), mandibular, sublingual and buccal glands.

Stomach

The stomach is small in relation to body mass and is mainly situated on the left side of the cranial abdomen. Externally,

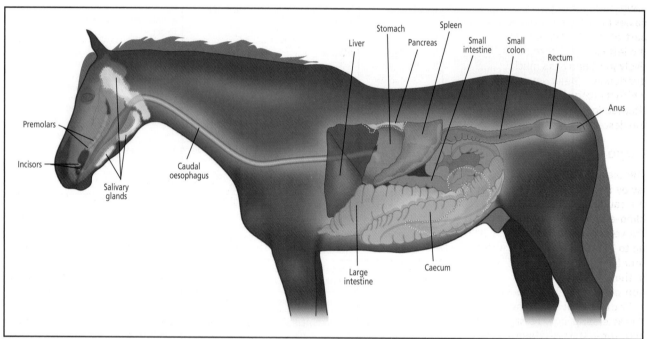

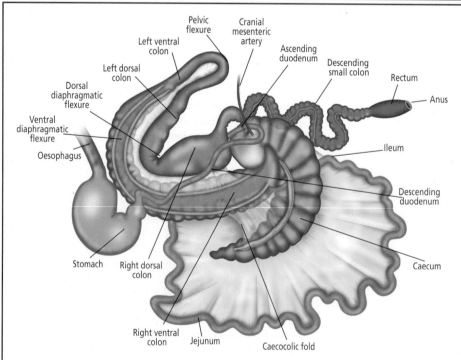

3.81 Digestive tract in the horse.

the shape of the stomach is similar to that of dogs and cats. Internally, there is a marked step in the lining of the stomach, known as the **margo plicatus**, which divides the cranial non-glandular section from the caudal glandular section. The non-glandular part of the stomach resembles the oesophagus in structure. The caudal part of the stomach has gastric and pyloric glandular zones with acid- and protease-secreting glands. The cardiac sphincter is well developed, thus vomiting is rare.

Small intestine

The small intestine is approximately 25 metres in length. The duodenum is short and commences ventral to the liver, where it forms a **sigmoid flexure**, first dorsally and then ventrally, as it moves in a caudal direction. At the first bend of the sigmoid flexure, the pancreas and bile duct empty from a single papilla into the duodenum. The duodenum then continues until it reaches the level of the right kidney, where it passes medially around the root of the mesentery. The final part of the duodenum passes cranially and ventrally below the left kidney to continue as the jejunum. The ileum is relatively short and has a much thicker wall than the jejunum and duodenum. The ileum ends in the base of the caecum, into which it protrudes on a papilla. Most of the small intestine is situated in the left dorsal part of the abdomen, along with the descending colon.

Large intestine

The caecum is shaped like a giant comma. It extends aborally (away from the mouth) from its opening on the right side of the caudal abdomen. The base is located dorsally with the blind-ending apex running ventrally and cranially, ending on the ventrum of the abdomen. The caecum has a capacity of up to 30 litres and can measure a metre in length. There are four longitudinal muscles (**taeniae**) over most of the length of the caecum. These muscles pull the caecum into a series of non-permanent folds (**haustrae**).

The colon has ascending, transverse and descending limbs. The ascending limb is U-shaped and has four parallel sections with three flexures (bends). The most important is the second, known as the **pelvic flexure**, and this is where the colon narrows most significantly. It is often the site at which obstructions occur, as it is the point where the ingesta becomes less fluid. The pelvic flexure is also where the four taeniae reduce to three. The taeniae give the colon a haustrated appearance. The transverse colon is short (moves from right to left) and located cranially to the root of the mesentery. The descending limb is much narrower than the rest of the colon and has its own separate mesentery. It has two taeniae and is haustrated.

The caecum and colon act as giant fermentation vats. They contain large numbers of bacteria and protozoa, which digest the cellulose-based diet, producing volatile fatty acids that can be absorbed. The caecum and colon also absorb the vast proportion of ingested water and can be considered equivalent to the bovine rumen. Thus, horses are known as **hindgut** herbivores.

Liver

The liver varies in form and size between breeds. It is predominantly located on the right side of the cranial abdomen. There are four main lobes: left, right, caudate and quadrate. Horses do not have a gallbladder, but there is a prominent biliary system and the bile duct opens into the cranial duodenum on the papilla shared with the main pancreatic duct.

Ruminants

Mouth

The tongue is long and fleshy and covered with taste buds. It is raised caudally to form a fleshy hump, known as the **torus**, which is separated from the rostral flatter part of the tongue by a groove known as the **lingual fossa**.

Cattle produce over 100 litres of saliva per day. The saliva is alkaline and helps to buffer the volatile fatty acids produced by fermentation of food. The three main glands are:

- Parotid – which lies ventral to the external ear canal
- Mandibular – which lies medial to the mandible and extends to the atlantal fossa caudal to the skull
- Sublingual – which is divided into two parts: one part lies lateral to the tongue on the floor of the mouth; the other part lies more rostrally.

There are other minor salivary glands scattered throughout the mucosa of the mouth and oropharynx.

Oesophagus

The oesophagus possesses striated muscle along its whole length, which is important as it allows **eructation** – the regular regurgitation of partially digested food (cud) from the rumen to the mouth, where further mastication occurs. The oesophagus traverses the neck and mediastinum before passing through the diaphragm to empty into both the reticulum and rumen at the cardia via the reticular groove.

Stomach

The first three stomachs are the **reticulum**, the **rumen** and the **omasum** (Figure 3.82), collectively known as the forestomachs. All play a role in the fermentation of fibrous food material and thus have a large symbiotic bacterial and protozoal population. Next is the 'true' acid-secreting stomach, similar to that seen in monogastric animals, known as the **abomasum**. The forestomachs are relatively poorly developed in the infant ruminant. The reticular groove is closed in young animals, meaning that suckled milk bypasses the forestomachs and enters directly into the abomasum. The groove persists in adult animals, but does not close during eating. Certain chemicals (e.g. copper) can stimulate closure.

Rumen

This is the largest of the stomachs, occupying nearly the whole of the left side of the abdomen. The rumen starts at the cardia dorsally and ruminoreticular fold ventrally, which separates it from the reticulum around the level of the eighth rib, and extends caudally to the pelvis. It moves medially and crosses the midline both ventrally and caudally. The rumen is divided incompletely by pillars into a number of chambers. The major pillars run horizontally around the rumen, dividing it into dorsal and ventral sacs. Smaller vertical pillars create a caudodorsal and a caudoventral blind sac at the caudal end of the rumen, and a craniodorsal sac (known as the **atrium ruminis**) that communicates with the reticulum. The mucosa lining the rumen is the same as the reticulum, except it is not thrown up into ridges but into papillated projections, which increase the surface area of the stomach, enhancing absorption of volatile fatty acids produced by microbial fermentation.

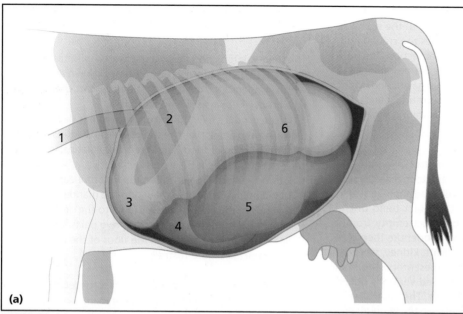
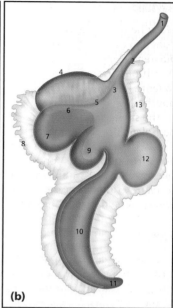

3.82 **(a)** Position of the stomachs in a ruminant. 1 = oesophagus; 2 = spleen; 3 = abomasum; 4 = reticulum; 5 = ventral sac of the rumen; 6 = dorsal sac of the rumen. **(b)** Stomachs of the ruminant and associated structures. 1 = oesophagus (cranial); 2 = cardia; 3 = atrium ruminis; 4 = dorsal sac of the rumen; 5 = part of the greater curvature corresponding to the right longitudinal groove of the rumen; 6 = part of the greater curvature corresponding to the left longitudinal groove of the rumen; 7 = ventral sac of rumen; 8 = greater omentum; 9 = reticulum; 10 = abomasum; 11 = pylorus; 12 = omasum; 13 = lesser omentum.

Reticulum

This is the smallest, most cranial stomach and is intimately related to the rumen. The reticulum is divided from the rumen by a series of internally projecting folds, known as **pillars** or **pilae**. The most prominent is the **ventral ruminoreticular fold**. The reticulum lies just caudal to the diaphragm, predominantly on the left side, between the sixth and eighth ribs. The mucosa lining the reticulum consists of harsh stratified epithelium, which is thrown up into ridges to create a reticular pattern of four-, five- and six-sided geometric shapes. The reticulum is relatively larger in sheep and goats compared with the other stomachs.

Omasum

This is a more spherical stomach that communicates with the rumen. It lies to the right of the midline, sandwiched between the rumen and reticulum on the left, and the liver and body wall on the right. The mucosa lining of the omasum is thrown into a series of deeply laminated folds, which have free edges and numerous papillae. The omasum empties into the abomasum. The omasum is relatively smaller in sheep and goats compared with the other stomachs.

Abomasum

This is typical of the monogastric stomach and lies to the right of the midline. It is loosely divided into two parts: a fundus and a body. The mucosa lining is glandular and folded longitudinally into **rugae**. There is a projection or torus of mucosa and submucosa from the lesser curvature, which narrows the exit to the outflow tract from the pylorus.

Small intestine

The abomasum empties into the duodenum. The first part of the duodenum is joined to the liver by the **lesser omentum**.

Large intestine

The caecum is the widest part of the gastrointestinal tract, but has no haustrae. It is separated from the colon by the opening to the ileum. The colon is divided into ascending, transverse and descending limbs. The ascending limb is complexly wound. The transverse section limb crosses the midline cranial to the mesenteric artery, before emptying into the descending limb.

Liver and gallbladder

The liver is situated on the right side of the cranial abdomen. It is flanked by the reticulum, rumen, omasum, duodenum, gallbladder and pancreas on the visceral surface and the diaphragm cranially. There are four main lobes: left, right, quadrate and caudate, with a couple of processes of the caudate lobe. Ruminants possess a gallbladder.

Pancreas

The pancreas has two lobes and lies adjacent to the duodenum.

Omentum

Omenta are thin but tough serosal sheets of tissue that help support the abdominal organs, principally the gastrointestinal tract. They are especially well developed in ruminants. The **greater omentum** is attached to the dorsal abdomen and supports (with two separate sheets) the distal oesophagus, rumen, reticulum, abomasum and duodenum. The greater omentum is used as a fat store. The **lesser omentum** is related to the liver. The omental sheets enclose a space, known as the **omental bursa**, which communicates with the rest of the peritoneum via the epiploic foramen located close to the liver.

Small mammals

Many herbivores have a narrow oral cavity compared with dogs and cats. They have no canine teeth, but rather have a **diastema** (gap) between the incisors and premolars (see Dentition, above). The tongue is relatively immobile in rodents. Hamsters and chipmunks have well developed cheek pouches, which are used to store food.

The stomach in hamsters is divided into a glandular and a non-glandular part. Rabbits, guinea pigs and chinchillas have a capacious intestine and caecum designed to house bacterial and protozoal populations, which digest hemicellulose and cellulose. The caecum and colon are often folded into haustrae to improve fermentation by longitudinal bands of muscle known as taeniae. Ferrets have no caecum and a short colon.

Birds

The tongue varies from muscular and mobile in psittacine birds to strap-like in passerine birds. Birds have a **crop** (Figure 3.83), a diverticulum of the oesophagus located at the base of the neck, which acts as a food storage chamber. Some species produce crop 'milk' from the crop lining, which is used to feed young animals (e.g. pigeons and doves).

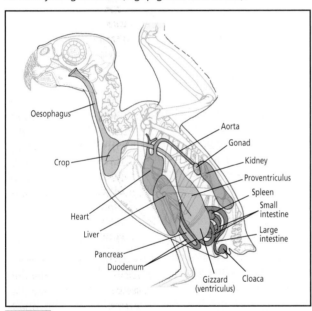

3.83 Viscera of a bird. (© Nigel Harcourt-Brown)

Birds have two stomachs: an acid-secreting stomach (**proventriculus**), followed immediately by the **ventriculus** (gizzard). The ventriculus can be sac-like (e.g. raptors) or muscular (e.g. seed-eating birds) and helps to grind food. A significant duodenal loop is found in birds. Caeca (singular: caecum) are not present in all species, and where they do occur are often paired. Birds have a short large intestine, often referred to as a rectum.

Birds possess a **cloaca**, a communal chamber into which the gastrointestinal, urinary and reproductive tracts empty before exiting the body through the vent. The cloaca is split into three chambers:

- The **coprodeum**, which receives faeces from the gastrointestinal tract
- The **urodeum** into which the ureters and reproductive tract empty. It is separated from the coprodeum by a fold
- The **proctodeum**, which is the last chamber.

A bilobed liver is present. Some species have a gallbladder; however, it is often absent in psittacine birds. Biliverdin is the main bile pigment in birds.

Reptiles

The tongue may be fleshy and immobile in chelonians; fleshy and mobile in many lizards; and strap-like and mobile in snakes. The lack of a diaphragm means that there is no division between 'abdominal' organs such as the liver and intestines, and 'thoracic' organs such as the heart and lungs. Instead there is a single coelomic cavity (Figures 3.84 to 3.86).

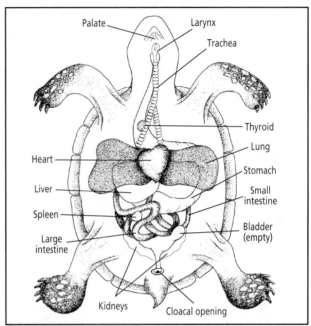

3.84 Main organs in the body cavity of a tortoise (plastron removed). (Reproduced from the *BSAVA Manual of Reptiles, 2nd edition*)

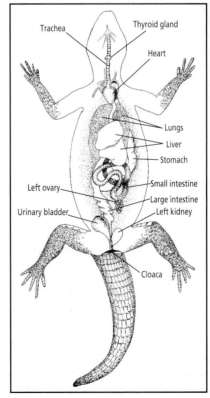

3.85 Main organs in the body cavity of a lizard. (Reproduced from the *BSAVA Manual of Reptiles, 2nd edition*)

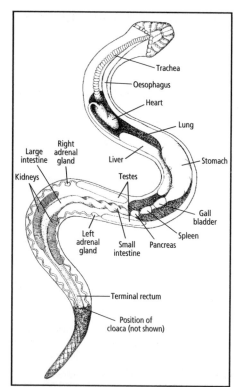

| **3.86** | Main organs in the body cavity of a snake. |

(Reproduced from the *BSAVA Manual of Reptiles, 2nd edition*)

The large intestine may be multi-chambered in hindgut fermenters such as the green iguana. Reptiles possess a cloaca, which is similar in structure to that found in birds. The liver is generally bilobed and the main bile pigment is biliverdin. The pancreas may be fused with the spleen to form a splenopancreas, particularly in snakes.

Physiology of digestion

The functions of the gastrointestinal system are to receive and digest food so that the nutritional requirements of an animal can be met, and to excrete waste products. The process of digestion involves: the movement of ingesta along the gastrointestinal tract; mechanical breakdown of food; enzymatic breakdown of food; absorption of nutrients; and the excretion of waste.

Nutritional requirements

The nutrients required by animals (see Chapter 13 for details) are:

- Water
- Proteins
- Fats
- Carbohydrates
- Minerals
- Vitamins.

Movement of ingesta

Waves of smooth muscle contractions (**peristalsis**) move ingesta along the gastrointestinal tract. Peristalsis is controlled by pacemakers situated throughout the gastrointestinal tract.

Distension of the intestine can also stimulate muscular contractions. Even in a relatively empty gastrointestinal tract there are waves of peristaltic contractions, beginning at the stomach and moving caudally, pushing waste material and bacteria out of the rectum.

Mechanical breakdown

The mechanical breakdown of food is initially carried out by chewing, and continued by contractions of the stomach.

Enzymatic breakdown

Dogs have a small amount of amylase present in saliva, which begins to break down starch in the mouth. However, the majority of enzymatic digestion occurs from the stomach onwards (for further information, see Chapter 13).

- Pepsin begins the breakdown of proteins into peptides, which are further broken down to amino acids at the level of the **brush border** in the small intestine.
- Fats (triglycerides) are emulsified in the stomach and broken down in the small intestine by the action of pancreatic lipase. Bile acids act as a detergent and emulsify the fats for digestion.
- Carbohydrates are broken down to monosaccharides by pancreatic and intestinal disaccharides.

Absorption

Absorption of nutrients from the gastrointestinal tract into the bloodstream occurs from the duodenum onwards (see Figure 3.80). No absorption takes place in the oesophagus or stomach. The highest levels of absorption occur in the duodenum and jejunum. From the jejunum to the rectum, the level of absorption decreases with mainly water and electrolytes being absorbed from the large intestine.

Excretion of waste

Defecation is the process by which animals excrete solid waste products from the colon and rectum. The anal sphincter is the muscular end of the gastrointestinal tract. It is usually in a state of constriction, thus ensuring that the opening to the large intestine remains closed. Relaxation of the anal sphincter (usually under voluntary control) allows the passage of faeces. Contraction of the abdominal muscles whilst the glottis is closed increases the abdominal pressure and results in excretion. In dogs the entire rectum is emptied, which means that softer faeces will always be seen towards the end of defecation. This is normal and not suggestive of a gastrointestinal tract problem.

Neonatal gastrointestinal tract

The small intestine in neonates allows antibodies (large molecules) to pass directly into the bloodstream for a few hours after birth, rather than being broken down and absorbed. This results in a transfer of immunity from the dam to the offspring via the maternally derived antibodies (MDA) present in the colostrum. The extent to which this transfer occurs varies between species: it is minimal in humans where most of the MDA transfer occurs via the placenta; it is predominant in dogs, cats and ruminants, where colostral antibodies are an essential part of immunity (see Chapter 5).

Ruminants

Reticuloruminal contraction cycle

This regular cycle facilitates the mixing of ruminal contents. The cycle starts with two contractions of the reticulum, which pushes the reticular contents into the atria ruminis of the rumen. This then stimulates contraction of the dorsal sac of the rumen, followed by contraction of the ventral sac of the rumen: each wave of contraction moves in a cranial–caudal direction. The force of the contractions is determined by mechanoreceptors, which detect how full/stretched the reticulum and rumen are with ingesta. These contraction waves occur approximately every 2–3 minutes.

Regurgitation

Ruminants have a highly fibrous diet and regular regurgitation of the cud for remastication helps to further break down the fibre. Contraction of the reticulum pushes ingesta to the cardiac sphincter. The ingesta is then pulled cranially into the oesophagus when the animal inspires against a closed glottis. Once the ingesta is in the distal oesophagus, a reverse peristaltic wave of striated muscle contraction occurs, propelling the cud to the mouth where it is chewed and then swallowed.

Eructation

Due to the microbial breakdown of ingesta, large amounts of gas (chiefly methane and carbon dioxide) are produced, which must be eructed to prevent the life-threatening condition bloat. The contractions occur purely within the rumen (where the gas is situated): the ventral sac of the rumen contracts first, followed by the dorsal sac: each wave of contraction moves in a caudal–cranial direction. Once at the cardiac sphincter, gas moves into the distal oesophagus and a reverse peristaltic wave propels it to the mouth: this is eructation.

Endocrine system

The endocrine system is a collection of ductless glands, which produce hormones and deliver them into the bloodstream, lymph or tissue fluid.

Terminology

- **Hormones** are chemicals that travel through the bloodstream until they reach their target organ and exert an effect.
- **Autocrine** – of or relating to a hormone that has an effect on the original cell that produced it.
- **Endocrine** – of or relating to a hormone that is transported in the bloodstream to the target organ.
- **Exocrine** – of or relating to a hormone that is released through a duct or ducts.
- **Paracrine** – of or relating to a hormone that has an effect on local cells.

The secretion of many hormones is controlled by **negative feedback**. In simple terms, negative feedback is where increased levels of a hormone are detected by a gland and result in decreased levels of hormone production by that gland. Positive feedback has the opposite effect: increased levels of a hormone are detected by a gland and result in even more hormone being produced by that gland.

Hormones can be grouped according to the type of molecules present:

- Proteins – growth hormone, insulin, adrenocorticotrophic hormone (ACTH)
- Peptides – thyroid-stimulating hormone (TSH), oxytocin
- Amines – dopamine, adrenaline
- Steroids – cortisol, progesterone.

Hypothalamus

The control centre of the endocrine system is the **hypothalamus** (see Central nervous system, above). The hypothalamus sits at the base of the brain and connects the endocrine system with the nervous system (see Figure 3.49). The hypothalamus produces **releasing hormones**, which in turn control the pituitary gland.

Pituitary gland

The **pituitary gland (hypophysis)** responds to the releasing hormones secreted by the hypothalamus by producing **stimulating hormones**, which are sent out to individual organs. The pituitary gland comprises an anterior and a posterior section, which produce different hormones.

Anterior pituitary gland

The anterior pituitary gland (**adenohypophysis**) produces the following hormones:

- **Adrenocorticotrophic hormone (ACTH)** – which targets the adrenal gland cortex and stimulates the release of corticosteroids and mineralocorticoids
- **Follicle-stimulating hormone (FSH)** – which targets the Sertoli cells in males causing spermatogenesis. In females it targets the ovaries stimulating growth of the follicles which contain the ova (eggs)
- **Growth hormone (GH)** – also known as **somatotropin**. It acts on all tissues of the body, stimulating growth by increasing the uptake of amino acids and protein production. Fat deposition is also increased by GH
- **Luteinizing hormone (LH)** – which targets the Leydig cells in males and stimulates the release of testosterone. In females it targets the ovaries causing ovulation and the development of the corpus luteum. LH has various functions. It is released spontaneously in the bitch, but is only released in response to mating in the queen
- **Prolactin** – which targets the mammary glands to stimulate development during pregnancy and milk let down following parturition
- **Thyroid-stimulating hormone (TSH)** – which targets the thyroid gland and stimulates the release of thyroxine. Thyroxine controls metabolic rate.

Posterior pituitary gland

The posterior pituitary gland (**neurohypophysis**) is connected to the hypothalamus and produces two hormones:

- Antidiuretic hormone (ADH) – also known as **vasopressin**. It is released in response to an increase in plasma osmotic pressure (as detected by baroreceptors). ADH targets the distal convoluted tubules in the kidney, increasing their permeability. This causes an increase in

the resorption of water, thus increasing plasma volume and reducing the volume of urine produced
- Oxytocin – which targets the uterus during parturition causing contraction of the smooth muscle. It also acts on the muscles lining the mammary glands, resulting in milk let down.

Pineal gland

The pineal gland is located within the brain and produces **melatonin** in response to daylight length. Melatonin is responsible for the functions of the body related to photoperiod such as reproduction, behaviour and coat changes.

Thyroid gland

The thyroid gland lies over the trachea, caudal to or at the level of the larynx. In dogs and cats the thyroid gland is divided into two lobes, which sit on either side of the larynx. The gland comprises follicles within a connective tissue capsule. Parafollicular cells (also known as C-cells) are located between the follicles. Parafollicular cells produce **calcitonin**, which is responsible for the control of blood calcium levels. Calcitonin decreases the blood calcium level by stimulating deposition of calcium in bone, decreasing calcium absorption from the gastrointestinal tract and increasing excretion of calcium in the urine.

Thyroid-stimulating hormone (TSH) targets the thyroid gland resulting in the secretion of **thyroxine** (T4) and **triiodothyronine** (T3). The secretion of these hormones is controlled by negative feedback: increased levels of thyroxine are detected by the anterior pituitary gland, resulting in a decrease in the secretion of TSH. Thyroid hormones act on virtually all cells in the body. They control metabolic rate and are essential for normal growth. Thyroid hormones have an effect on the skin, skeleton, cardiovascular system, neurological system and reproductive function.

Parathyroid glands

The parathyroid glands are found in close proximity to or sometimes embedded within the thyroid gland. There are two parathyroid glands associated with each lobe of the thyroid gland, resulting in a total of four parathyroid glands. They are much small and paler than the thyroid gland. The parathyroid glands produce **parathyroid hormone** (**PTH**), which is involved in the control of blood calcium levels. PTH has an antagonistic effect to that of calcitonin: it increases blood calcium levels by releasing calcium from bones, increasing calcium absorption from the gastrointestinal tract, accelerating vitamin D activation and decreasing excretion of calcium in urine by stimulating calcium resorption in the distal tubules of the kidneys. PTH also decreases blood phosphate concentrations by increasing phosphate deposition in bone.

Kidneys

The kidneys produce **erythropoietin**, which stimulates the bone marrow to produce red blood cells. The production and release of erythropoietin is regulated by the arterial oxygen concentration in a manner that is poorly understood.

Adrenal glands

The adrenal glands are small bean-like structures that lie in the dorsal abdomen craniomedial to the kidneys. They consist of an inner medulla and outer cortex, which is covered in a connective tissue capsule.

Cortex

The adrenal gland cortex is divided into three different zones:

- Zona glomerulosa (outermost)
- Zona fasciculata
- Zona reticularis.

Adrenocorticotrophic hormone (ACTH) from the anterior pituitary gland acts on the adrenal cortex, stimulating the production of mineralocorticoids and glucocorticoids. The adrenal gland cortex also produces sex hormones (androgens and oestrogens). However, the significance of these hormones is not clear as the majority of the sex hormones are produced by the gonads.

Mineralocorticoids

These are produced by the **zona glomerulosa** and include **aldosterone**, which controls the level of sodium and potassium in the body. Aldosterone is produced via the renin–angiotensin–aldosterone pathway (see below).

Glucocorticoids

These are produced by the **zona fasciculata** and **zona reticularis**. Glucocorticoids, such as **cortisol**, are produced in a circadian rhythm (in dogs levels of cortisol are higher in the morning and lower in the evening; in cats levels of cortisol are lower in the morning and higher in the evening). Cortisol has diverse effects in the body. Its main functions are: metabolism of carbohydrates, proteins and fats; and the promotion of gluconeogenesis. Cortisol also reduces the inflammatory process and the immune response. Levels of cortisol increase if an animal is stressed.

Medulla

The adrenal gland medulla is connected to the nervous system and is responsible for the 'flight or fight' response via the release of **adrenaline** (epinephrine) and **noradrenaline**. The release of adrenaline is stimulated by hypoglycaemia, stress, decreased blood pressure and hypothermia. The adrenal glands have a good vascular supply, which allows adrenaline to be quickly released into the circulation. Adrenaline increases glucose production by the liver, increases blood glucose concentrations, increases blood supply to the skeletal muscles and increases heart rate. It also causes relaxation of the gastrointestinal smooth muscle, urinary retention, dilatation of pupils and sweat production.

Gastrointestinal hormones

Gastrin is released from G cells in the stomach, duodenum and pancreas. Secretion of gastrin occurs in response to the presence of peptides (from food) in the stomach. Gastrin stimulates hydrochloric acid release by the stomach lining. **Cholecystokinin** is released from I cells in the lining of the duodenum. It stimulates pancreatic and bile secretions to aid digestion. **Secretin** is released from S cells in the duodenum. It helps control the pH of gastrointestinal tract contents.

Pancreas

The pancreas is located in the mesentery of the duodenum. It has both exocrine and endocrine components. The exocrine section produces digestive enzymes which are secreted into the gastrointestinal tract (see Digestive system, above). The endocrine section comprises the **Islets of Langerhans**. These islets consists of three different cells:

- Alpha cells – which produce glucagon
- Beta cells – which produce insulin
- Delta cells – which produce somatostatin.

Glucagon production is stimulated by low blood glucose concentrations or stress. It acts on the liver to break down stored glycogen into glucose (glycogenolysis) and to increase the production of glucose (gluconeogenesis). Glucagon also increases lipolysis. **Insulin** production is stimulated by high blood glucose concentrations, as well as by the gastrointestinal hormones gastrin, cholecystokinin and secretin. Insulin stimulates the uptake of glucose into the cytoplasm of cells and the production of glycogen, triglycerides and proteins. Insulin has the opposite effect to glucagon. **Somatostatin** has a regulatory role inhibiting the release of both glucagon and insulin.

Reproductive glands

Follicle-stimulating hormone (FSH) and luteinizing hormone (LH) are **gonadotrophins**. They are released from the anterior pituitary gland (see above) and stimulate the reproductive organs. More detail on their actions is given in Chapter 26.

Testosterone

Testosterone is the predominant hormone in males. It is produced by the Leydig cells in response to LH.

Oestrogen

In males oestrogen is produced by the Sertoli cells in the seminiferous tubules. In females it is produced by the developing follicles during the oestrous cycle. It is responsible for the physical and behavioural signs of oestrus.

Progesterone

Progesterone is produced by the corpus luteum and is present in both pregnant and non-pregnant females. It is responsible for the maintenance of pregnancy and the signs associated with metoestrus.

Birds

Hormones such as prolactin and thyroxine help control the cycle of feather moulting and regrowth. The principal corticosteroid produced by the adrenal glands in birds is **corticosterone** rather than cortisol.

Reptiles

Reptiles produce vasotocin rather than oxytocin during egg production. The parietal eye (situated on the top of the head in reptiles such as the green iguana) and the pineal gland are responsible for the production of melatonin in reptiles. Melatonin controls seasonal variations in reproduction and activity. The thyroid gland plays an important role in the homeostatic mechanisms of hibernation.

Urinary system

Kidneys

The kidneys in dogs and cats are often described as bean-shaped. They are found in the **retroperitoneum** close to the dorsal body wall. The right kidney is positioned slightly more cranially than the left kidney. The cranial pole of the right kidney is located in a depression of the caudate process of the liver. The left kidney can be mobile, especially in cats.

The kidney is surrounded by a tightly adherent capsule and consists of three main areas (Figure 3.87):

- The outer cortex (often dark in colour as it is more vascular)
- The inner medulla (often light in colour as it is less vascular)
- The renal pelvis.

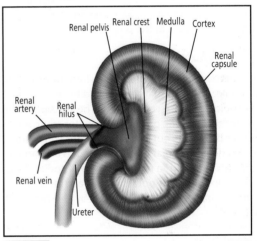

3.87 Longitudinal section through a kidney.

The **nephron** (Figure 3.88) is the functional unit of the kidney. It comprises a vascular plexus known as the **glomerulus**

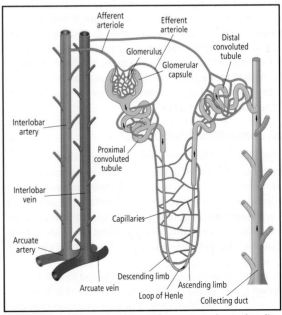

3.88 A kidney nephron. The arrows show the direction of urine flow.

surrounded by the **Bowman's capsule** (glomerular capsule), located in the cortex. An afferent arteriole supplies the glomerulus and an efferent arteriole drains it. The Bowman's capsule leads to the **proximal convoluted tubule**, which in turn leads to the **loop of Henle** located within the medulla. The loop of Henle leads to the **distal convoluted tubule** situated within the cortex. The distal convoluted tubule then leads to the collecting duct, which is located in the medulla. The renal pelvis is where the collecting ducts merge into the neck of the ureter.

Physiology of urine formation

Glomerulus

The glomerular blood vessels are tightly adhered to a basement membrane. Blood flows through the glomerulus and, due to the blood pressure, water, electrolytes and other substances are forced through the holes in the wall of the glomerulus into the **glomerular space**. The holes are large enough to allow molecules such as urea, haemoglobin and simple sugars to leave the glomerulus, but will not allow larger molecules such as albumin to pass. This process is known as ultrafiltration and results in the production of urine.

Proximal convoluted tubule

The urine produced in the glomerulus moves into the proximal convoluted tubule. It is here that sodium and the majority of the water (around 75%) are reabsorbed. The resorption of sodium provides the osmotic potential for water resorption. In order to pump sodium out of the proximal convoluted tubule and into the peritubular blood vessels, it is exchanged for potassium. Thus, there is a net resorption of sodium and water and a net excretion of potassium. In addition, many drugs (e.g. penicillin) are actively excreted by the proximal convoluted tubule.

Loop of Henle

The urine passes from the proximal convoluted tubule into the descending limb of the loop of Henle. The descending limb has a thin wall and allows water to pass out of the lumen and into the interstitial tissue by osmosis. The urine then passes into the ascending limb of the loop of Henle. The ascending loop has a thick squamous epithelium, which prevents water from leaving the lumen. Sodium, potassium and chloride are pumped out of the ascending limb and into the interstitial tissue. This creates an osmotic gradient between the interstitial tissue (high osmotic concentration) and the descending limb (low osmotic concentration), allowing water to diffuse out of the lumen.

Distal convoluted tubule

From the loop of Henle the urine passes into the distal convoluted tubule. It is here that more sodium is reabsorbed, and potassium and hydrogen are excreted. Hydrogen excretion is important as it enables the body to maintain the **acid–base** balance. **Aldosterone** regulates sodium absorption and potassium excretion in the distal convoluted tubule. Aldosterone is produced via the **renin–angiotensin–aldosterone pathway**:

1. If an animal is dehydrated or suffers blood loss, the reduced blood flow to the glomerulus results in the release of the hormone **renin** from the granular cells in the juxtaglomerular apparatus of the kidney.
2. Renin acts on the plasma protein **angiotensinogen** to convert it to **angiotensin I**.
3. Angiotensin I is converted to **angiotensin II** by **angiotensin-converting enzyme** in the lungs.
4. Angiotensin II stimulates the production of **aldosterone** from the adrenal gland cortex. Angiotensin II also causes the afferent arteriole to constrict, reducing blood flow to the glomerulus and thus increasing blood pressure.
5. Aldosterone acts on the distal convoluted tubule to increase sodium resorption and potassium excretion. Water is consequently reabsorbed by osmosis, thereby increasing plasma volume.

Collecting duct

Urine passes from the distal convoluted tubule into the collecting duct. Each collecting duct collects urine from a number of nephrons. Antidiuretic hormone (ADH), released by the posterior pituitary gland in response to an increase in osmotic pressure or low blood pressure, acts on the collecting ducts to increase resorption of water. The urine then moves through the collecting ducts and into the renal pelvis, where it drains into the ureter.

Ureters

Each kidney has a single ureter, which drains the renal pelvis and transports the urine to the urinary bladder. The ureters are retroperitoneal and suspended within a fold of visceral peritoneum known as the **mesoureter**. The ureters are lined with transitional epithelium, which allows some expansion of the lumen. The transitional epithelium is supported by a sheath of smooth muscle, which helps propel urine from the kidney to the urinary bladder by peristaltic waves of contraction.

Urinary bladder

The bladder is situated within the retroperitoneum; although, when full it projects into the caudal abdomen. The bladder receives urine from the ureters, which enter through the **trigone** on the dorsal surface. The oblique angle at which the ureters enter the trigone prevents the reflux of urine from the bladder. The base of the trigone (triangle) lies between the two ureteral entrances with the apex at the **urethral orifice**. Urine is discharged from the bladder into the urethra at the level of the **pelvic inlet**.

A **lateral ligament** connects the lateral surface of the bladder to the lateral pelvic wall. A **median ligament** connects the ventral surface of the bladder to the symphysis of the pelvis and the midline of the body wall as far cranially as the umbilicus. In addition, there is a **middle ligament** which in the foetus contains the **urachus**. This is the stalk of the **allantois**, which disappears after birth leaving a peritoneal fold.

The urinary bladder is lined with transitional epithelium. The wall of the bladder comprises three layers of smooth muscle with a muscular sphincter at the bladder neck. These muscles are innervated by the **pudendal nerve** (somatic innervation), the **hypogastric nerve** (sympathetic innervation) and the **pelvic nerve** (parasympathetic innervation).

Urethra

The urethra is a simple structure lined with transitional epithelium, which is supported by a sheath of smooth muscle and connective tissue.

In male dogs the urethra runs from the neck of the bladder to the prostate gland, where it is joined by the **deferent duct**. The section of the urethra that runs through the prostate gland is called the **prostatic urethra**. As it exits the prostate gland, the urethra runs caudally through the pelvis to the pelvic brim. This part is called the **membranous urethra**. The urethra then moves ventrally, beneath the perineal surface, before travelling cranially to run through the penis on the ventral surface of the body. This part is termed the **cavernous urethra** and is surrounded by erectile tissue (see Figure 3.89a). The external urethral orifice is found on the tip on the penis.

In tomcats, the course of the urethra diverges from that of male dogs once it has passed through the pelvis. In cats the urethra runs through the penis in the perineal region. Tomcats also have an additional urethral section: there is a short length of urethra cranial to the prostate gland, located between the opening to the bladder and the prostate gland. This is known as the **pre-prostatic urethra**. Tomcats also have a pair of **bulbourethral glands**, which open into the lumen of the urethra close to its caudal end (see Figure 3.89b). The external urethral orifice is found on the tip of the penis.

The function of the urethra in males is to transport urine, sperm and spermatic fluid from the bladder and prostate gland to the penis for excretion.

In females the urethra runs from the bladder neck, through the pelvis, to the floor of the vagina. Its only function is to transfer urine from the bladder to the vagina for excretion. The external urethral orifice is located in the vestibule caudal to the vagina.

Horses

The right kidney lies ventral to the last 2–3 ribs and the first lumbar transverse process. It is heart-shaped and sits in a depression of the liver. It is attached ventrally to the pancreas and base of the caecum. The left kidney lies ventral to the last rib and the first three lumbar processes. The kidneys have a **modified unipyramidal** structure. This means that at some point in their evolution horses had lobulated kidneys; however, the surface of the kidneys in modern horses is smooth and the only evidence of lobulation is in the arrangement of the interlobular arteries.

The ureters in horses are wide as they leave the kidneys and rapidly narrow as they move caudally. The ureters enter at the neck of the urinary bladder. The urethra in the male runs caudally from the bladder, before travelling ventrally over the rim of the caudal pelvis and finally moving cranially through the penis, which terminates cranial to the cranial edge of the pelvis on the ventral abdomen. The urethra in females is short and opens into the vestibule caudal to the vagina.

Small mammals

In small mammals that live in desert conditions, such as gerbils, the loop of Henle in the kidneys is comparatively longer than that of dogs. This means that gerbils can concentrate urine much more effectively.

Birds

Birds have long, thin trilobed kidneys (see Figure 3.83), which are attached to the ventral surface of the synsacrum. Approximately 50% of the nephrons in the kidney have no loop of Henle. The ureters empty directly into the **urodeum** section of the **cloaca**; thus, there is no urinary bladder in birds. The main waste product of protein metabolism is **uric acid** rather than urea. In addition, birds have a renal portal system (see section on Veins, above).

Reptiles

The kidneys in chelonians and lizards are compact (see Figures 3.84 and 3.85). The kidneys in snakes are long and thin (see Figure 3.86). The nephrons in the kidney have no loop of Henle. Some male reptiles have a sexual segment to the kidney, which is responsible for producing spermatic fluid. The ureters empty directly into the urodeum section of the cloaca. Many chelonians and lizards possess a urinary bladder, but snakes do not. As the ureters empty into the urodeum, urine is not sterile even when a urinary bladder is present. The main waste product of protein metabolism is uric acid rather than urea. In addition, reptiles have a renal portal system (see section on Veins, above).

Reproductive system

For more information on the physiology of reproduction see Chapter 26.

Male reproductive system
Anatomy

The reproductive system of the male dog and tomcat are shown in Figure 3.89. The male reproductive tract comprises the testicles, epididymis, deferent duct, spermatic cord, urethra, penis, prostate gland and bulbourethral gland.

Testicles

The testicles are round to oval and found outside the abdomen in the **scrotum**. The temperature in the scrotum is slightly lower than core body temperature, and this is optimal for sperm production. The testicles consist of:

- Leydig cells (interstitial cells)
- Sertoli cells
- Spermatogenic cells.

Epididymis

The epididymis is part of the testicle, but appears grossly to be adhered to its outer surface. Sperm are produced in the main part of the testicle and then transported to the epididymis in ducts. The epididymis becomes narrower and tapers into the deferent duct.

Deferent duct

The deferent duct (also known as the **vas deferens** or **ductus deferens**) transports sperm from the epididymis to enter the urethra at the neck of the bladder.

Spermatic cord

The spermatic cord travels from the epididymis up into the abdomen. The spermatic cord and testicle are surrounded by a layer of connective tissue (an outpouching of the peritoneum) known as the **vaginal tunic**.

A number of structures can be found within the spermatic cord:

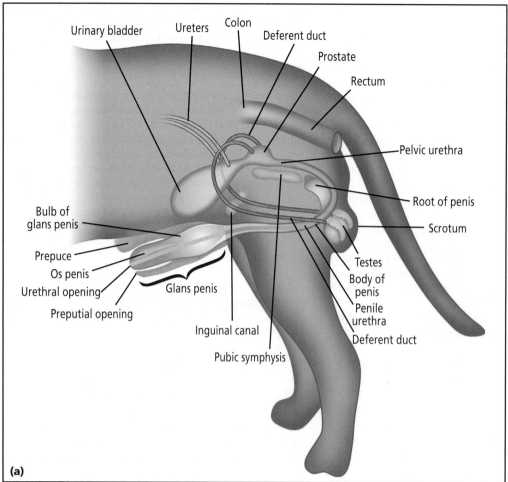

(a)

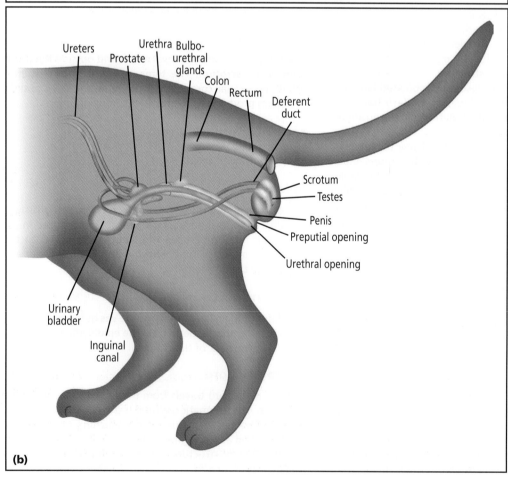

(b)

3.89

(a) Reproductive and lower urinary tract of a dog. **(b)** Reproductive and lower urinary tract of a tomcat.

- Deferent duct
- Testicular artery and vein
- Lymphatic vessels
- Nerves
- Cremaster muscle – which is responsible for raising/lowering the testicle depending on the surrounding temperature.

Penis

The penis consists of erectile tissue, which has a profuse blood supply. In dogs the penis is present on the ventral abdomen, running from the **ischial arch** of the pelvis cranioventrally along the perineum. There is a small bone, known as the **os penis**, present dorsal to the urethra. In tomcats the penis is found under the tail, ventral to the anus. It points caudally (rather than cranially) and is covered in **barbs**, which are thought to be partly responsible for the induction of ovulation in the queen during mating.

Accessory glands

The accessory glands are responsible for the production of spermatic fluid. This fluid not only transports but also provides nutrition for the sperm and contains hormones that are important in fertilization. Various accessory glands are found along the male reproductive tract, including:

- Prostate gland – a single gland found around the urethra at the neck of the bladder. It is present in both dogs and tomcats
- Bulbourethral glands – paired glands located on the dorsal aspect of the urethra near the pelvic exit. These glands are absent in dogs and vestigial in tomcats.

Sperm

Sperm comprise four main parts:

- **Acrosome** – this is a cap-like structure found on the head of the sperm. It is derived from the Golgi apparatus
- **Head** – this is where the nucleus is located
- **Mid-piece** – which contains mitochondria
- **Tail** – which provides motion.

Horses

An adult male horse is called a **stallion**. The testicles are located within the scrotum, which lies ventral to the pubic brim and between the hindlegs. The testicles usually lie with the long axis horizontal, but can be brought vertical by strong contraction of the cremaster muscles.

The penis is **musculocavernous** in conformation: it begins proximally with two crura penes attached to the ischial arch, which curve ventrally and cranially between the hindlegs and merge into a single **corpus cavernosum**. This has a ventral groove where the erectile tissue of the **corpus spongiosum** lies. The corpus spongiosum expands distally to form the terminal part of the penis (glans). The urethra also runs in the ventral groove of the corpus cavernosum, surrounded by the corpus spongiosum, and terminates at the glans on a small papilla or process.

The paired retractor muscles of the penis lie ventral to the **bulbospongiosus muscle**, which is located ventral to the **corpus spongiosus muscle**. The bulbospongiosus muscle aids voiding of urine and semen when contracted.

The penis is housed within a prepuce or sheath. This has additional internal folds, which allow enlargement of the penis when engorged. The prepuce contains many glands, which secrete a substance known as **smegma** that can build up around the terminal end of the urethra and in the sheath.

The accessory sex glands, starting at the bladder neck and moving caudally, include:

- Vesicular glands (paired) – also known as seminal vesicles. These are large (10–12 cm), smooth, bladder-like organs
- Prostate gland (singular) – which has two lateral lobes
- Bulbourethral glands (paired) – which lie dorsolateral to the urethra at the caudal pelvic outlet.

Small mammals

Ferrets

A male ferret is called a **hob**. The penis is located on the ventral abdomen. The os penis is J-shaped. Ferrets possess a prostate gland.

Rabbits

A male rabbit is called a **buck**. Mature males have obvious scrotal sacs, although it is possible for the testicles to move through the **inguinal canal** and into the abdomen. By applying pressure on either side of the urethral opening it may be possible to extrude the penis. The penis is conical and has no central slit. There is no os penis. Rabbits possess a prostate gland, vesicular glands, bulbourethral glands and coagulating glands. These accessory glands are found along the deferent duct and urethra, and produce seminal fluid.

Guinea pigs

A male guinea pig is called a **boar**. The **inguinal ring** is permanently open, through which a fat body from each testicle protrudes into the abdomen. A spicule-like os penis is present. Guinea pigs possess a prostate gland, vesicular glands and coagulating glands.

Rats and mice

Male rats have obvious testicles from approximately 5 weeks of age. However, the testicles may not always be present in the scrotum as the inguinal canal remains open throughout life. A spicule-like os penis is present. Rats possess ampullary, bulbourethral, preputial, prostate and vesicular accessory glands. Male mice have similar glands and a very pungent odour.

Hamsters and gerbils

Male hamsters and gerbils have obvious testicles and a spicule-like os penis. In addition, they have similar accessory glands to rats and mice.

Birds

A male bird is called a **cock**. Males possess two intra-abdominal testicles, located cranial to the kidneys. Most male birds do not have a penis, with the exception of some waterfowl and ratites (such as the ostrich). Instead semen is transferred from the male to the female via apposition of the cloacas. During the breeding season male birds may show up to a 10-fold increase in the size of the testicles.

Reptiles

Chelonians

Male tortoises have one penis, which lies in the ventral cloaca. Male tortoises also have a longer tail and more distal vent than females. In addition, the plastron in males may have a concave appearance.

Lizards

Male lizards have two hemipenes located in the base of the tail, similar to those seen in snakes. For this reason the base of the tail in males may appear wider than in females. Males may also have pores in the skin along the underside of the thighs (e.g. in agamids and iguanids) or in front of the vent (e.g. in geckos).

Snakes

Males possess intracoelomic testicles, located cranial to the kidneys. Male snakes have a pair of **hemipenes** (singular, **hemipenis**), which are situated at the base of the tail. The hemipenes are inverted sacs at rest and only become obvious during mating. Snakes are sexed using a blunt-ended surgical probe, which is inserted through the vent and advanced cranially. In male snakes, the probe can be inserted a length equal to 8–16 subcaudal scales.

Physiology

The main hormones associated with the male reproductive tract are:

- Follicle-stimulating hormone (FSH) – which targets the Sertoli cells causing spermatogenesis and the production of oestrogen
- Luteinizing hormone (LH) – which targets the Leydig cells causing the production of testosterone
- Testosterone – which influences spermatogenesis, development of the male reproductive tract and development of male secondary sexual characteristics.

Female reproductive system

Anatomy

The reproductive system of the bitch (Figure 3.90) and queen are similar in structure. The female reproductive tract comprises the ovaries, uterine tube, uterus, cervix, vagina and vulva.

Ovaries

The ovaries are paired and lie caudal to the kidneys. The ovary is suspended from the abdominal wall in the **mesovarium**, part of which is folded into the **ovarian bursa**. The ovarian bursa is a pouch-like structure which completely covers the ovary. The ovary is attached to the dorsal body wall by the **ovarian ligament**.

The ovaries are small and round or oval. However, the shape of the ovary changes during the oestrous cycle as follicles appear on its surface in response to follicle-stimulating hormone (FSH). Each follicle releases an ovum (egg) in response to a surge in luteinizing hormone (LH). Located close to each ovary is the **infundibulum**, which 'catches' the ovum when it is released and transports in through the **uterine tube** (also known as the **Fallopian tube**) to the uterus.

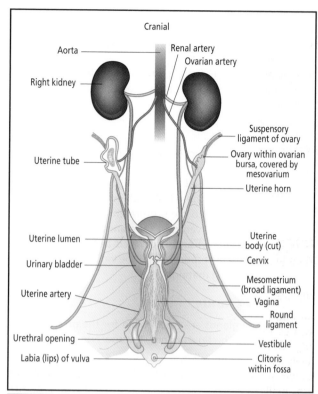

3.90 Ventrodorsal view of the urogenital system of a bitch.

Uterus

The uterus comprises two horns, which join together at the **uterine body**. The length of the **uterine horn** varies depending on the species. Animals that have a large number of offspring per pregnancy (e.g. dogs and cats) have long uterine horns. Animals that have one or two offspring per pregnancy (e.g. cows) have shorter uterine horns.

The uterus consists of an outer layer of connective tissue, a central layer of muscle (**myometrium**) and a highly vascular inner layer (**endometrium**). Blood is supplied to the uterus via the uterine artery, which runs parallel to the uterine body from caudal to cranial on either side.

Cervix, vagina and vulva

The cervix is a short thick-walled sphincter, which separates the uterus from the vagina. It is closed most of the time but opens during oestrus and for parturition. The vagina extends from the cervix to the external urethral orifice, where the urinary tract joins the reproductive tract. The vulva is the external opening to the reproductive tract.

Mammary glands

These are modified skin glands that are found on either side of the midline in pairs. The number of mammary glands varies between breeds, but in general bitches have five pairs and queens have four pairs. Each gland consists of glandular epithelium lined with secretory epithelium. Milk from the sinuses drains into teat canals, which open on the surface at teat orifices (Figure 3.91). Milk is produced in response to progesterone and prolactin. Milk let down or excretion in response to suckling is due to muscular contractions induced by oxytocin.

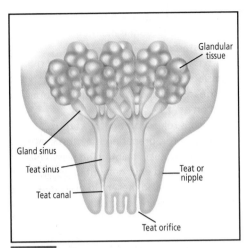

Glandular
tissue

Gland sinus

Teat sinus

Teat or
nipple

Teat canal

Teat orifice

3.91 Structure of a mammary gland.

Horses

An adult female horse is called a **mare**. The ovaries are located in the dorsal abdomen, just cranial to the cranial edge of the iliac wings of the pelvis. The ovaries are relatively large and have a prominent indentation on one side known as the **ovulation fossa**. The infundibulum is situated proximally opposite the ovulation fossa within the uterine tube, which is approximately 20 cm in length. The infundibulum continues as the **ampulla**, which narrows into the **isthmus**, before opening into the cranial end of the uterine horn. The **uterotubular junction** is able to determine whether an ovum is fertile and prevents infertile ova from entering the uterus.

The uterus has two short horns and a large uterine body. The horns lie within the abdomen and are suspended from the dorsal wall by the **broad ligaments**. The cervix is short and projects caudally into the cranial vagina, creating a space around the cervix known as the **fornix**. The vagina is a similar length to the uterine body and lies ventral to the rectum and dorsal to the bladder and urethra. It is mainly retroperitoneal, although, the cranial edge is covered with peritoneal lining. There is a transverse fold cranial to the opening of the urethra, which is the remains of the **hymen**.

The **vestibule** is located caudal to the vagina, starting at the urethral opening and sloping steeply in a ventral direction over the ischial arch of the pelvis. The vulva is found caudal to the vestibule and contains the **clitoris** in its ventral commissure. The clitoris is very prominent in mares in heat, when it can be seen between the **labia** (external folds) as the mare moves: a feature known as 'winking'. Laterally and ventrally the clitoris is separated from the labia by a **fossa glandis**, which is where the organism that causes contagious equine metritis can be found.

The udder is located on the caudal ventral abdomen in the pelvic area. There are two teats; each teat is supplied by 2–3 duct systems and generally has two draining sinuses. The surface of the udder is covered in sebaceous and sweat glands.

Small mammals

Ferrets

A female ferret is called a **jill**. The urogenital opening is located ventral to the anus. Jills are seasonally polyoestrous and induced ovulators. This can lead to problems in unmated

females as they do not ovulate, but instead remain in oestrus. This results in high levels of oestrogen, which can impair red blood cell production, leading to anaemia, which can be fatal in many cases. Normal gestation lasts 41–42 days. Pseudo-pregnancy lasts a similar length of time.

Rabbits

A female rabbit is called a **doe**. The ovaries lie caudal to the kidneys. The uterus has no uterine body: the two uterine horns each possess a cervix, which projects into the vagina. This arrangement is described as being **duplex**. The urethra also opens into the vagina. The vulva is rounded with a central slit. Does are induced ovulators and cycle every 12–16 days during the breeding season if they are not mated. The ano-genital distance in females is shorter than in males.

Guinea pigs

A female guinea pig is called a **sow**. Guinea pigs have a **bicornuate** (heart-shaped) uterus, with two uterine horns, a single uterine body and a single cervix. Guinea pigs are non-seasonally polyoestrous and spontaneous ovulators. Each oestrous cycle lasts for approximately 16 days.

Following mating a **copulatory plug** forms, which falls out of the vagina after a few hours. It is thought that this plug may prevent further matings by other males. At the end of pregnancy, the release of relaxin and progesterone stimulates relaxation of the pelvic ligaments. This allows the pubis and ischium to separate to facilitate delivery of the young. However, this is usually only fully achieved in animals mated for the first time when they are young, before complete ossification of the pelvis.

Rats and mice

Rats and mice have a duplex uterus: the two parallel uterine horns each possess a cervix and join to the cranial vagina. However, from the external surface, the uterine horns appear to fuse cranially to the cervices, so some texts still refer to the uterus in rats as being bicornuate. The urethra and vagina have separate openings. Rats and mice are non-seasonally polyoestrous with an oestrous cycle of approximately 5 days. Gestation lasts 21–23 days in rats and 19–21 days in mice.

Hamsters and gerbils

Female hamsters and gerbils are seasonally polyoestrous and spontaneous ovulators. They have a 4-day oestrous cycle and a gestation length of 15–18 days.

Birds

A female bird is called a **hen**. Egg production is the most obvious feature of avian reproduction. In most species only the left ovary is present, located cranial to the kidney. An **oocyte** is released from the ovary into the infundibulum during ovulation. The oocyte travels down the **oviduct** (a tube-like structure) towards the cloaca. It is in the oviduct that the oocyte is coated in albumen (the egg white) and that the shell membranes become thicker. It takes on average 20 hours for the oocyte to travel from the ovary to the cloaca.

Reptiles

Female reptiles have paired oviducts. The oviducts comprise: the infundibulum, the magnum, the isthmus, the shell gland/uterus and the muscular vagina. The vagina opens into the urodeum portion of the cloaca.

Chelonians

Female tortoises have paired ovaries and can produce eggs twice a year. Some female tortoises have a hinge on the caudal part of the plastron to make egg-laying easier. They may also have longer hindlimb claws than males, which are used for digging holes in preparation for egg-laying. Eggs are produced in a similar manner to those in birds, but the shell is more leathery. The temperature at which the eggs are incubated determines the sex of the offspring.

Lizards

Female lizards can be **oviparous** (egg-bearing), **viviparous** (bear live young) or **ovoviviparous** (eggs are produced internally, but when the young are 'born' they are not inside an egg). Sex determination in lizards is mainly chromosomal, with the exception of geckos where the temperature at which the eggs are incubated determines the sex of the offspring: higher incubation temperatures result in males.

Snakes

Most species of snake have paired ovaries. Eggs travel from the ovary to the uterus via the oviduct. Female snakes can be oviparous (e.g. kingsnakes and pythons) or viviparous (e.g. garter snakes and boa constrictors). Sex determination in snakes is chromosomal. Snakes are sexed using a blunt-ended surgical probe, which is inserted through the vent and advanced cranially. In female snakes, the probe can be inserted a length equal to 2–6 subcaudal scales.

Physiology

The normal activity of the ovaries is controlled by hormones (see also Chapter 26):

- Follicle-stimulating hormone (FSH) – which is produced by the anterior pituitary gland. It stimulates the ovary to develop follicles, which release oestrogen. Oestrogen has a negative feedback effect on the pituitary gland and decreases the amount of FSH released
- Luteinizing hormone (LH) – which is produced by the anterior pituitary gland. A surge of LH is released prior to ovulation and causes the release of the ovum from the follicle. Once the follicle has ruptured, scar tissue is formed. This scar tissue is known as the corpus luteum (yellow body). The corpus luteum is maintained by LH and produces progesterone
- Oestrogen – which is released from the follicles of the ovary. It is responsible for most of the physical and behavioural changes associated with the bitch or queen being 'in season' ('on heat')
- Progesterone – which is released from the corpus luteum. It is responsible for: preparing the uterus to receive fertilized ova (zygotes), maintaining pregnancy and causing mammary gland enlargement in pregnancy and pseudopregnancy. It is also present in pregnant and non-pregnant animals following oestrus.

Integument

The integument is the outer covering of the animal and comprises the skin, fur, claws and hooves.

Skin

Structure

The basic structure of the skin comprises the **epidermis**, the **dermis** (Figure 3.92) and the **subcutaneous** connective tissue. The thickness of each layer varies in different parts of the body and between species; for example, in areas prone to abrasion such as the footpads, the epidermis is thicker to protect the underlying structures. In dogs and cats, the skin is thicker dorsally and thinner ventrally. The thickness of the skin ranges from 0.5–5 mm in dogs and 0.4–2 mm in cats.

Epidermis

The epidermis consists of 4–5 layers of cells, which are constantly replaced from the basal layer:

- Stratum corneum
- Stratum lucidum
- Stratum granulosum
- Stratum spinosum
- Stratum basale.

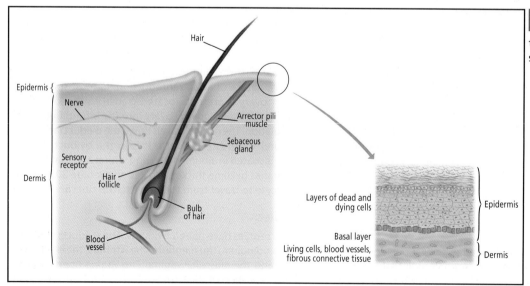

3.92 Cross-section through the skin to show its structure.

Stratum corneum

This comprises many layers of cells known as **corneocytes** (47 layers have been described in skin from the flank of a dog). Corneocytes consist of **keratin** and provide a waterproof covering to the skin. These cells are dead. The outer corneocytes are continuously sloughed and replaced by cells from lower layers. On average, it takes 22 days for cells from the basal layer to reach to stratum corneum. However, this can vary depending on trauma and disease.

Stratum lucidum

This layer is only present on the nose and footpads. It consists of dead cells that contain lipid, which give the nose and footpads a glassy appearance.

Stratum granulosum

This is the granular layer. In this layer cells begin to die and are filled with keratin, which gives them a granular appearance under a light microscope. The nuclei of the cells are shrunken. This layer can be two cells thick in areas where hair is present, and up to 8 cells thick in areas where hair is absent.

Stratum spinosum

The cells in this layer have a spiky appearance and are still alive and nucleated. This layer is 1–2 cells thick in areas where hair is present, and up to 20 cells thick in areas where hair is absent.

Stratum basale

This is the basal layer. It is the lowest layer of the epidermis and consists of a single layer of cells. The cells in this layer replicate by mitosis to replace those lost from other layers of the epidermis. **Melanocytes**, which give the skin its pigment, are present in this layer.

Dermis

This layer is where the blood vessels, lymphatic vessels, nerves, sweat glands, sebaceous glands and hair follicles are found, surrounded by a dense, elastic connective tissue. **Arrector pili muscles** (which cause hairs to stand on end) associated with hair follicles are also present in the dermis.

Hair

This is important for insulation, perception and to act as a barrier against injury. Hair comprises an inner medulla, an outer cortex and an overlying cuticle. Hairs that do not have a medulla (known as lanugo) are only found in fetal dogs and cats.

Hair follicles develop from epidermal cells. They can be single (simple follicles) or grouped (compound follicles). Hair follicles grow down into the underlying dermis to form a **hair cone**, which overlies a **hair papilla**. From the hair cone, keratinized cells grow to form a hair (Figure 3.93). The hair coat can be divided into **primary hairs** (outer coat) and **secondary hairs** (undercoat). Most hairs in dogs and cats are present as compound follicles, consisting of 2–5 primary hairs surrounded by secondary hairs. Each primary hair emerges through a separate pore and has an associated arrector pili muscle, sebaceous gland and sweat gland. Secondary hairs emerge through a common pore and only have an associated sebaceous gland.

Specialized hair cells can also be found in dogs and cats:

- **Sinus hairs** – these are also known as whiskers or vibrissae and are found on the muzzle, eyelids, lips and face. In cats they are also located on the palmar aspect

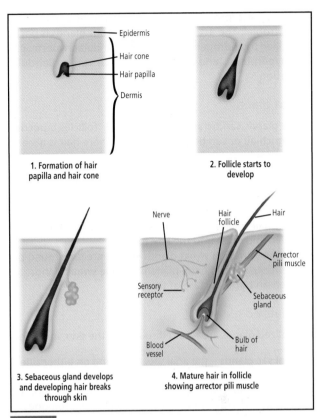

1. Formation of hair papilla and hair cone

2. Follicle starts to develop

3. Sebaceous gland develops and developing hair breaks through skin

4. Mature hair in follicle showing arrector pili muscle

3.93 The structure and formation of hairs.

of the carpus. These hairs are very thick, stiff and have a profuse blood supply. Sinus hairs act as slowly adapting mechanoreceptors

- **Tylotrich hairs** – these are found scattered throughout the skin amongst the primary and secondary hairs. Tylotrich hairs are strong and thick and present as a single hair within a large follicle. Tylotrich hairs acts as fast-acting mechanoreceptors.

The direction in which the hairs grow gives rise to **hair tracts**. Hair in different parts of the body will grow in different directions. Hair growth can be divided into three phases:

- Anagen – rapid growth phase
- Catagen – transitional phase
- Telogen – resting phase when no growth takes place.

Hair growth is affected by seasonality, breed, sex, temperature, nutrition, genetics and hormones such as thyroxine and cortisol. Hair replacement in dogs and cats is usually in a mosaic pattern. Dogs and cats may shed more hair during the spring or autumn; however, this can be affected by central heating, thus they may shed hair all year round. The final length of the hair is determined by genetics. Once this predetermined length has been reached the hair enters a resting phase.

Sebaceous glands

Sebaceous glands are associated with hair follicles. There tends to be a larger number of sebaceous glands in areas where the hair follicle density is low (e.g. mucocutaneous junctions, interdigital spaces, chin and the dorsal neck, rump and tail). Sebaceous glands are not found on the footpads or nasal planum. Sebaceous glands produce **sebum** (a waxy/oily substance), which is secreted into the hair follicles. Sebum forms an emulsion over the surface of the skin that provides waterproofing, retains moisture and acts as an antimicrobial. The activity of the sebaceous glands is partly controlled by androgens, which cause glandular hypertrophy and hyperplasia, and oestrogens, which cause glandular involution.

Sweat glands

Sweat glands can be associated with hair follicles (**apocrine** or **epitrichial**) or can be found in areas where hair is absent, such as the footpads (**eccrine** or **atrichial**).

- Apocrine (epitrichial) sweat glands – the distribution of apocrine sweat glands is similar to that of sebaceous glands in that a greater number are found in areas of poor hair follicle density. Apocrine sweat glands are coiled and open into the hair follicle.
- Eccrine (atrichial) sweat glands – these are only found on the footpads and nasal planum. Eccrine sweat glands open on to the surface of the skin.

Specialized glands

Specialized glands are found throughout the skin, including:

- **Anal sac glands** – the anal sacs are found on either side of the anus. These sacs are lined with epithelium, which consists of specialized sebaceous glands that produce a strong smelling oily substance containing pheromones. When the animal defecates, the anal sacs empty, providing a means of scent marking
- **Perianal (circumanal) glands** – which are responsible for pheromone production
- **Ceruminous glands** – the external auditory canal of the ear is lined with ceruminous glands, which produce cerumin (ear wax)
- **Tail (supracaudal** or **preen) gland** – in dogs this oval gland is located at the level of the fifth to seventh coccygeal vertebrae. The hair coat in this area comprises stiff, coarse primary hairs. The surface of the skin can be yellow and waxy, and is more obvious in older, entire male dogs. In cats the tail gland runs the length of the tail on the dorsal surface.

Eyelid skin

Cilia or eyelashes are only present on the upper eyelids of dogs and cats. **Meibomian (tarsal) glands** are a type of sebaceous gland and open at the mucocutaneous junction. **Zeis glands** are sebaceous glands associated with the cilia. **Moll's glands** are apocrine sweat glands associated with the cilia. The **Harderian gland** is an accessory lacrimal gland, which produces tears.

Footpads

These consist of thickened epidermis, covering a fatty vascular structure called the **digital cushion**. Dogs and cats have seven footpads on the forepaws and five footpads on the hindpaws. There are three types of footpad (Figure 3.94):

- Digital – these footpads protect the distal interphalangeal joints
- Metacarpal/metatarsal – these footpads protect the metacarpal–phalangeal and metatarsal–phalangeal joints
- Carpal – these footpads are also known as stopper pads and lie distal to the carpus in the forepaw

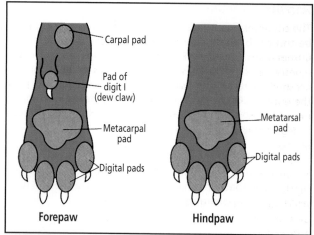

3.94 Ventral view of the forepaw and hindpaw showing the footpads in a dog.

Small mammals

Many rabbits have a **dewlap** (ruff or fold of skin on the neck). Rabbits do not have footpads, but instead the palmar/plantar aspect of the foot is covered with dense fur. The number of sweat glands in rabbits and rodents is reduced. Hamsters have lateral flank scent glands. Gerbils have a ventral scent gland located near the umbilicus. Gerbils also have **fracture planes** in the skin of the tail; this means that the skin is easily degloved if the tail is grasped firmly.

Birds

The epidermis and dermis are thinner in birds. Feather follicles, rather than hair follicles, are present and give rise to several types of feather:

- **Primary** or **flight feathers** – which are located on the manus of the wings. These are strong vaned feathers with a central rachis and interlocking barbs and barbules
- **Secondary feathers** – which attach to the ulna of the wings. These feathers are similar in form to the primary feathers
- **Down feathers** – which have a limited rachis and no interlocking barbs. These feathers are used for insulation
- **Contour feathers** – which are a smaller version of the primary feathers. They cover the down feathers and provide the overall shape and coloration of the bird
- **Filoplume feathers** – which are associated with the primary and contour feathers. They have a long thin unvaned rachis and a small tuft of barbs at the distal end. The root of these feathers is highly innervated, allowing the bird to subconsciously alter the position of the primary and contour feathers during flight
- **Bristle feathers** – which are usually found around the face. These feathers are innervated and allow sensory information to be relayed to the central nervous system.

Birds have a reduced number of sweat glands. The **uropygial** or **preen gland** is located at the base of the tail. It produces an oily substance which, when spread over the feathers, acts as a waterproofing agent. Some species, such as emus, ostriches and bustards, do not have a uropygial gland.

Reptiles

The epidermis contains a large amount of keratin, which can be thrown into folds to create scales. Chelonians have an **intradermal bone**, which forms the carapace. Lizards undergo a process known as **ecdysis**, where small patches of old skin are shed and replaced. Snakes also undergo ecdysis, but slough the entire body skin in one piece after the production of a new skin beneath the old one.

Pigment cells may be prominent in some species (e.g. chameleons) and can be controlled by mood and neural stimulation. A parietal eye may be present in reptiles such as the tuatara (see Nervous system section above). Some species of reptiles (e.g. green iguanas) have fracture planes in the tail, which allow the entire tail to be shed if it is grasped roughly by a predator. The tail often regrows in a process known as **autonomy**. Integumentary sensory organs are often found in the scales on the flanks of reptiles (e.g. crocodilians). These organs detect changes in water pressure associated with the movement of prey.

Function

The skin has many functions, including:

- Adnexa production – hairs, claws and hooves
- Antimicrobial – secretes antimicrobial agents
- Communication – alters appearance by raising the hairs if the animal is frightened
- Excretion of waste products in sweat (low levels)
- Indicator of general health (e.g. can be used to evaluate shock and jaundice)
- Motion and shape – flexible and elastic to allow movement
- Pheromone production
- Pigmentation – colour of the hair coat and skin helps prevent damage from solar radiation
- Prevents water and electrolyte loss
- Protection – provides a physical barrier, preventing chemicals and organisms from entering the body
- Sensation – heat, cold, touch, pressure, itch and pain
- Storage of fats, electrolytes, vitamins, carbohydrates and proteins

- Temperature regulation – hair coat, cutaneous blood supply (vasodilatation and constriction) and sweat glands
- Vitamin D production
- Waterproofing.

Claws

Claws are highly keratinized structures, which are continuous with the epidermis and dermis. The **distal phalanx** is located within the claw. The coronary band is found around the base of the claw, and it is from here that most nail growth occurs (Figure 3.95).

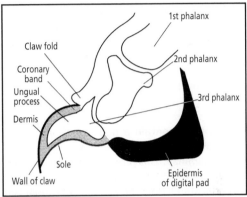

3.95 Longitudinal view of the toe in a dog, showing the claw.

Hooves

The hoof (Figure 3.96) covers the distal phalanx in horses. The forelimb hoof is generally circular; the hindlimb hoof is more oval. The keratinized **wall** of the hoof is the protective external structure. It grows from the **coronary dermis**, which runs around the proximal edge of the wall at the level of the **coronary band**. The wall is covered by a thin layer of rubbery horn, known as **periople**, which is thicker at the **coronet** and **bulbs** of the **heel**, but very thin over the distal wall. The wall

3.96 Structure of an equine hoof.

Proximal phalanx
Middle phalanx
Coronary band
Sensitive laminae
Distal phalanx
White line
Hoof wall
Sole
Digital cushion
Superficial digital flexor tendon
Deep digital flexor tendon
Navicular bone
Frog

tapers towards the bulbs of the heel, where it runs axially to form the **bars** of the hoof. The bars merge into a V-shaped structure known as the **frog**. The frog is soft and provides some cushioning to the foot. The **sole** fills the space between the wall and the frog, forming most of the palmar/plantar aspect of the hoof. The fusion of the wall and the sole is known as the **white line** and is used by farriers as a guide when placing nails.

The dermis is located deep to the capsule of the hoof. There is a coronary, frog, laminar, perioplic and solar dermis. The coronary and laminar dermis are associated with the wall and are richly innervated as well as highly vascularized. The surface of the coronary dermis contains papillae. Cells covering the papillae produce **intratubular horn**; cells located between the papillae produce **intertubular horn**. The coronary and laminar dermis form folds of tissue, called **primary** and **secondary laminae**. There are two types of primary laminae:

- Dermal (sensitive) – produced from the laminar dermis
- Epidermal (insensitive) – produced from the coronary dermis.

The primary laminae contain a number of secondary laminae. The secondary laminae interlock the dermal and epidermal primary laminae. This process is known as **interdigitation**.

The subcutis is located below the dermis and connects it to the distal phalanx, the cartilages of the hoof and the tendons. The subcutis layer is generally thin. However, beneath the coronary and frog dermis it is enlarged with fat and elastic tissue to form the **coronary cushion** and the **digital cushion**, respectively. These cushions are bound by lateral cartilages. The coronary and digital cushions provide some pliability and 'give' against the concussive forces which occur when the hoof contacts the ground.

References and further reading

Ashdown RR and Done SH (2011) *Color Atlas of Veterinary Anatomy: Volume 2: The Horse, 2nd edn.* Mosby, St Louis

Boyd JS, Paterson C and May AH (2001) *Color Atlas of Clinical Anatomy of the Dog and Cat, 2nd edn.* Mosby, St Louis

Colville TP and Bassert JM (2008) *Clinical Anatomy and Physiology for Veterinary Technicians, 2nd edn.* Mosby, St Louis

Cunningham JG and Klein BG (2007) *Textbook of Veterinary Physiology, 4th edn.* WB Saunders, Philadelphia

Dyce KM, Sack WO and Wensing CJG (2010) *Textbook of Veterinary Anatomy, 4th edn.* WB Saunders, Philadelphia

Kainer RA and McCracken TO (1998) *Horse Anatomy: a Coloring Atlas.* Alpine Publications, Loveland, CO

Kainer RA and McCracken TO (2002) *Dog Anatomy: a Coloring Atlas.* Teton New Media, Jackson Hole, WY

Raynor M (2006) *Horse Anatomy Workbook* (Allen Student). JA & Co Ltd, London

Self-assessment questions

1. Describe the positions of anatomical features on a diagram or a live animal using the following terms: cranial, caudal, medial, lateral, proximal, distal, ventral, dorsal, plantar and palmar.
2. Define diffusion and osmosis.
3. What organelles are found within a cell?
4. Name and describe the two types of cell division.
5. Name the body cavities in (a) a dog; and (b) a lizard.
6. In an immature animal how does a long bone grow?
7. What are the dental formulae for a mature dog, a kitten and a mature rabbit?
8. Tendons attach what to what?
9. List the cranial nerves (names and numbers).
10. Name the chambers and valves through which blood passes in the heart.
11. What are the names of the four stomachs of a cow?
12. The beta cells of the pancreas are responsible for the secretion of which hormone?
13. What is the function of parathyroid hormone?
14. Leydig cells are responsible for the production of which hormone?
15. What is the name of the outermost layer of the skin?

Chapter 4

Genetics

Susan E. Long

Learning objectives

After studying this chapter, students should be able to:

- **Describe the structure of DNA**
- **Define the terms:**
  - **Autosome, sex chromosome**
  - **Gene, gene locus, allele**
  - **Dominant, recessive, epistasis**
  - **Homozygous, heterozygous**
- **Describe mitosis and meiosis and explain the difference**
- **Define Mendel's first and second laws and describe their modern interpretation**
- **Describe methods for identifying animals carrying a recessive gene**
- **Describe X inactivation and show how this is demonstrated in tortoiseshell cats**
- **Define inbreeding, line breeding, outcrossing and heterosis**
- **Describe the health schemes for:**
  - **Hip dysplasia and elbow dysplasia in dogs**
  - **Inherited eye disease in dogs**
  - **Polycystic kidney disease in cats**
- **Describe the principles of DNA testing**

Introduction

In the last ten years, genetics has been one of the most exciting and fast changing of the biological sciences. However, it has taken over a century of scientific research to get to where we are today. It is generally considered that the science of genetics began in the latter part of the 19th century when Gregor Mendel, a monk who had been experimenting with peas, showed that characteristics (traits) were passed on in a predictable manner. He suggested that each trait was governed by a pair of 'factors'; these later became known as genes. Today, genes are defined as segments of DNA (deoxyribonucleic acid) that are inherited between generations.

It was not until 1953 that James Watson and Francis Crick published a paper describing the double helix structure of DNA, the molecule within the nucleus that was by then acknowledged as containing the genetic information.

In the 1960s techniques were developed for growing peripheral blood lymphocytes in culture and fixing the cells so that each chromosome from the nucleus was separated and visible under the light microscope. This technique led to the investigation of many chromosomal anomalies.

In 1984 a technique was developed by Alec Jeffreys, whereby restriction enzymes were used to cut the DNA molecule at defined sites, and the fragments obtained were separated on an agarose gel. The result was a 'bar code'-like pattern unique to that particular DNA. This technique later came to be known as 'genetic fingerprinting'. In 1987, the polymerase chain reaction (PCR) was developed, which enabled the amplification of even very small pieces of DNA so that they could be examined. In more recent years techniques for DNA sequencing have been used to map entire genomes.

Modern-day genetics is often divided into molecular genetics, cytogenetics, Mendelian genetics and population genetics.

- **Molecular genetics** deals with the molecular structure and manipulation of DNA.
- **Cytogenetics** deals with chromosomes, which are strands of coiled DNA, linked to protein molecules.
- **Mendelian genetics** deals with the inheritance in individuals of characteristics that are governed by a single gene or a very small number of genes.
- **Population genetics** deals with the inheritance of characteristics or traits within a population of individuals. These traits may be governed by many genes, which individually obey the principles of Mendelian genetics but which are also affected by environmental factors.

Genetic material

DNA

DNA has a unique structure (Figure 4.1). It consists of two chains of sugar and phosphate molecules (the 'backbone') joined together by other molecules, rather like the rungs of a ladder. The 'steps' of the ladder are formed by pairs of bases: either adenine (A) and thymine (T), or guanine (G) and cytosine (C). A always links with T, and G always links with C. For example, if on one side of the ladder there is a sequence of AGTAACGGC, then on the other side of the ladder the

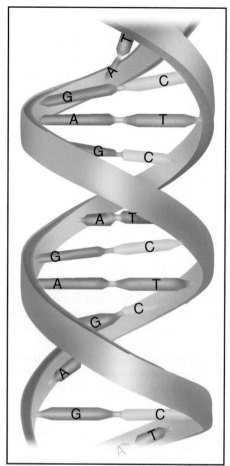

4.1 The structure of DNA. The 'steps' of the 'ladder' are a sequence of **base pairs** and their structure is such that they cause the sides of the ladder to twist, forming a double spiral, or double helix.

RNA

Ribonucleic acid (RNA) is another form of nucleic acid. It differs from DNA in that the base thymine is replaced by uracil (U). That is, adenine pairs with uracil (AU) in RNA instead of thymine (AT) as in DNA. RNA is important in the process of protein production from the genetic code.

Mitochondrial DNA

Most DNA is located in the nuclei of cells. However, a small amount of DNA is found in the mitochondria, the organelles within the cell that generate energy via respiration (see Chapter 3). The mitochondrial DNA (mtDNA) is passed on to offspring down the female line only (i.e. mtDNA is maternally inherited). This is because the mitochondria in mammalian sperm are usually destroyed by the egg after fertilization. Mitochondrial DNA can therefore be used to investigate an individual's maternal lineage.

Genes

Genes are specific sequences of nucleotides, the base pairs of which act to instruct the production of proteins. A protein is made up of a sequence of amino acids. Each amino acid is coded for by a group of three nucleotides, known as a codon. The order of codons within the gene determines the order of amino acids and hence the identity of the protein produced. There are special codons at the start and end of each gene (start and stop codons) and these identify the region of DNA to be used as the blueprint for protein production, and therefore ensure that the correct amino acid sequence (and thus the correct protein) is produced.

Protein synthesis

A gene contains the necessary information to make a protein. How the sequence of codons within the gene is read and the protein produced is the central dogma of molecular genetics.

Getting from the gene to the protein requires two steps. Firstly, in the nucleus, the double chain of DNA is 'unzipped' and the bases separated from their partners. This forms a template for the production of RNA, whereby spare bases within the nucleus attach to those of the unzipped DNA, recreating the pattern of bases; although, as previously mentioned, in RNA the thymine is replaced with uracil. The new strand of bases is known as messenger RNA (mRNA). The production of RNA from the DNA template is called **transcription.**

In the next step the mRNA moves out of the nucleus and attaches to a structure within the cytoplasm known as a ribosome. The ribosome moves along the strand of mRNA, reading the codons and matching them to their corresponding amino acid. As the ribosome travels along the mRNA strand it produces a chain of amino acids, joined together in the right sequence to form the correct protein. This second process is called **translation.**

Gene loci

Each gene has a specific location on a specific chromosome; this is called the **gene locus.** Since chromosomes within a nucleus are in pairs, it follows that genes also come in pairs.

If a gene locus occurs on a sex chromosome, this gene is said to be **sex-linked.**

sequence *must be* TCATTGCCG. Thus, the steps of the ladder are a sequence of 'base pairs'. The structure of the base pairs is such that they cause the sides of the ladder to twist, forming a double spiral, or **double helix.**

A nucleotide consists of a phosphate molecule plus a sugar molecule and a base. Genes are specific sequences of nucleotides that code for the production of proteins. In between the genes, the base pairs have a random or non-coding sequence and this is often called **junk DNA.** Over millions of years, individual variation in the non-coding part of DNA has developed because changes in this part of the DNA do not affect the viability of the animal. It is possible to detect this individual variation and so produce **genetic fingerprints.** DNA can be broken into small pieces by attacking certain base pair sequences using enzymes called restriction enzymes. These particular sequences of bases occur at different sites along the DNA molecule in different individuals. If these broken pieces are separated in an agarose gel by electrophoresis, the differently sized pieces move at different rates. When stained, this results in a pattern like a barcode that is different for different animals and this is the genetic fingerprint.

A microsatellite is a short DNA sequence that is repeated many times within the animal or organism. (It is called a microsatellite because these short sequences separate on an agarose gel at some distance from the other DNA fragments.) The number of repeats at a particular site is highly variable between individuals of the same species and is therefore characteristic for that individual.

Genes are usually expressed in the same way in either sex, but some genes control characteristics that are only expressed in one sex. Such genes are said to be **sex-limited**; they are only 'turned on' in individuals of one gender and not the other. Some genes or gene combinations are not compatible with life and these are said to be **lethal genes** or **lethal factors**. If an individual receives such a gene or genes, that individual dies.

Some definitions

Nucleotide: A phosphate molecule + a sugar molecule + a base.

Gene: The unit of inheritance; a sequence of nucleotides that codes for a protein.

Locus: The place along the chromosome at which the gene is located.

Sex-linked gene: A gene situated on a sex chromosome. The orange coat colour gene in cats and the gene for haemophilia A in dogs are both found on the X chromosome and are therefore examples of sex-linked (or X-linked) genes.

Sex-limited gene: A gene that is expressed in one sex only. The genes associated with milk quality in cats are carried by both males and females but can only be expressed in the females; therefore these genes are said to be sex-limited.

Lethal genes: A gene or gene combination that is not compatible with life. The gene that causes lack of a tail in the cat is the manx gene. When two copies of this gene are present, this is lethal and the embryo dies *in utero*.

Genotype: The genetic make-up of an organism.

Phenotype: The physical result of the interaction of gene effects and the environment.

Diploid: Applied to cells containing the normal number of chromosomes.

Haploid: Applied to cells containing half the normal number of chromosomes.

Environmental influence on gene action

Gene expression may be influenced by the environment. This 'environment' may be within the animal, for example its hormonal status. Alternatively, it may be the outside environment, such as temperature or infectious challenge. In general, these effects are seen in traits that are governed by many genes and are studied in population genetics.

Mutations

Mutations are permanent changes in the sequence of DNA. If a mutation occurs in a somatic cell (i.e. a body cell other than sperm or eggs), division of this cell will produce a new cell containing the mutation; however, this mutation will not be passed to any offspring. If a mutation occurs in a germ cell (i.e. a cell that gives rise to either sperm or eggs),this mutation can be passed on to offspring. Most mutations do not occur in parts of the DNA where genes are located, but if they do, one of two things may happen:

* The change is so great that the gene can no longer produce an instruction for its protein. In this case, the gene is destroyed and lost. If this occurs in an embryo, it may result in an abnormality or even death of the organism

OR

* The change allows coding, but a slightly different instruction is produced. The gene still exists but there has been a small change. A gene that has been changed is said to be an allele of the original gene.

Not all mutations are 'bad'; most have a neutral effect, i.e. they are neither advantageous nor disadvantageous with regards to the survival of the individual. A few mutations are advantageous and convey a competitive advantage to the individuals that carry them.

Alleles

Alleles are alternative forms of a gene that have developed as a result of mutations. A gene can have any number of alleles, depending on how often mutations have occurred at that place in the DNA. However, an individual has a maximum of two alleles per gene. This is because alleles of a single gene are found at the same locus on a chromosome, and there are only two copies of each chromosome within each cell.

* If there are two different alleles in the cell, the animal is said to be **heterozygous** for that gene.
* If there are two copies of the same allele, the animal is said to be **homozygous** for the gene.

Chromosomes

Within the cell nucleus, the DNA molecule is very tightly folded and coiled and is surrounded by protein to form the chromatin fibres of the chromosomes. The chromosomes are usually considered in pairs. One of each pair is inherited from each parent. The chromosomes in a pair are alike in morphology and the function of genes that they carry, and are therefore said to be **homologous** chromosomes (meaning 'same').

Each species has a characteristic number of chromosomes. For example, the number of chromosomes per diploid cell is 38 for cats, (Figure 4.2), 78 for dogs, and 64 for horses. If all the chromosomes from one cell in any of these species were weighed, the total weight of the genetic material would be more or less the same; in other words, they have roughly the same amount of genetic material but it is divided into a different number of pieces.

Sex chromosomes and autosomes

Two of the chromosomes are called the **sex chromosomes** and are designated X and Y. In mammals, females have two X chromosomes (XX), and males have one of each of the sex chromosomes (XY). In males the Y chromosome is inherited from the father and the X chromosome from the mother. In females one X chromosome is inherited from the mother and the other X chromosome from the father. Thus females are said to have a maternal and a paternal X chromosome.

The X chromosome carries a number of genes that are involved in the everyday function of the cell. The Y chromosome is usually quite small, has very few genes and carries the main genes responsible for determining differentiation of a male.

The chromosomes that are not the sex chromosomes are called **autosomes**.

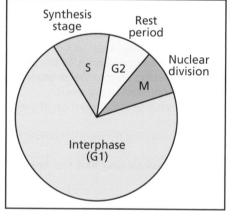

4.2 Cat chromosomes. **(a)** Karyotype showing $2n = 38$,XY. Stained by Giemsa-banding. **(b)** Fluorescence microscopy image of metaphase, following hybridization with chromosome-specific DNA paint probes, showing the X chromosome (red) and Y chromosome (bright green). *(Courtesy of Professor MA Ferguson-Smith and Dr Fentang Yang, Cambridge University Centre for Veterinary Science)*

Chromosomal abnormalities

It is possible to use an ordinary light microscope and various staining techniques to examine chromosomes and any abnormalities (see Figure 4.2). The normal chromosome number is called the **diploid** number. Half the normal number, i.e. that found in the ovum and sperm, is called the **haploid** number. Chromosome abnormalities may be numerical (i.e. too many or too few), structural or a combination of the two.

There are a number of possible structural chromosome anomalies. Bits may be missing (deletions); parts of one chromosome may be swapped with another (reciprocal translocation); or whole chromosomes may stick together (e.g. centric fusion translocation). Chromosomal abnormalities often mean that the affected chromosomes have difficulties pairing during cell division. This is most apparent during meiosis (see later) and so chromosome anomalies often result in reduced fertility or even sterility.

The cell cycle and cell division

When a cell is carrying out its normal day-to-day functions, it is said to be in **interphase (G1)**. In order to replicate itself, it first has to synthesize new genetic material – the **synthesis (S)** stage. This is followed by a resting stage, called **G2** (G stands for 'gap'). Then there is separation of the new genetic material into the two new cells; this is the nuclear division or **M phase**. The two new cells can then function normally, so they are again said to be in interphase. Thus, there is a **cell cycle** (Figure 4.3). Sometimes, there is a period at the end of G1 called G0, or G zero, where the cell exists in a quiescent state. It can be considered either as an extension of G1 or a distinct phase outside the cell cycle.

When a cell divides, the chromosomes must replicate exactly; otherwise the new cells would not be coding for the same characteristics. Many cells in the body are continually

4.3 The cell cycle.

replicating (e.g. cells from the lining of the intestine) and it is important that the new cells can carry on the functions of the old. Thus the division of the nucleus is an incredibly important process and occurs via a process known as mitosis. Mitosis refers to the replication and subsequent division of the contents of the nucleus, usually followed by cell division. Mitotic division results in two new cells with nuclei (and hence genetic material) that are exactly the same as in the original cell.

Sperm and eggs are produced using a different mechanism of cell division, known as meiosis. In this process the new cells contain only half the amount of the original DNA (i.e. they are haploid), and the genes may become slightly shuffled. Thus, when a sperm fertilizes an egg, the new embryo has the correct amount of genetic material (i.e. it is diploid) and contains a mixture of DNA from the mother and father.

Mitosis

Mitosis occurs after the S phase of the cell cycle, and so each chromosome already has an exact replica of itself (see Chapter 3). The original and replica chromosomes are joined together at the centromere. In the S phase, the two copies of the same chromosome held together at the centromere are called chromatids (Figure 4.4).

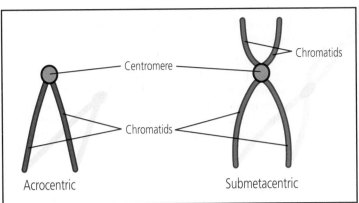

4.4 Diagrammatic representation of metaphase chromosomes. When the centromere is at the end of the chromosome it is said to be **acrocentric**. When the centromere is not in the centre of the chromosome it is said to be **submetacentric**. If it were in the centre it would be **metacentric**.

The final separation of the chromosomes and creation of two new cells is a dynamic process, but for the purposes of description it is divided into four stages:

1. **Prophase** –All chromosomes condense and become shorter and thicker.
2. **Metaphase** – The nuclear membrane breaks down and the chromosomes line up in the middle of the cell and become attached to spindle fibres.
3. **Anaphase** –The centromere divides, allowing the old and new chromosomes to separate and move to different sides ('poles') of the cell.
4. **Telophase** – The nuclear membrane forms around each group of chromosomes to create two new nuclei. The cytoplasm divides to form two new cells.

Meiosis

A different type of cell division is necessary for those cells that are going to develop into **gametes** (eggs and sperm). This is called meiotic division. It is made up of two cell divisions (**meiosis I** and **meiosis II**), during which the number of chromosomes in the daughter cells are halved. The stages are similar to those of mitotic division, i.e. prophase, metaphase, anaphase and telophase, but the first meiotic division is a longer and more complicated process (Figure 4.5).

The chromosomes must be separated into different gametes in such a way that the total number is halved and yet one copy of each pair of alleles present in the parent cell remains. In this way, when the two gametes fuse to form a zygote, the new individual has the correct number of chromosomes for

4.5 Meiosis.

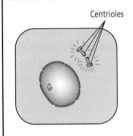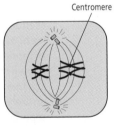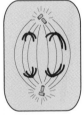

Interphase I

Prophase I
This is divided into five stages: leptotene, zygotene, pachytene, diplotene and diakinesis. During this time the chromosomes contract and crossing over takes place.

Metaphase I
Homologous pairs of chromosomes lie side by side on the cell spindle so that there are two rows of chromosomes (unlike in mitosis when there is a single row).

Anaphase I
The spindle fibres contract and homologous chromosomes separate to opposite ends of the cell. The centromeres do not divide as in mitosis.

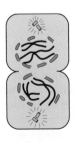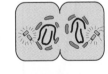

Telophase I
This is the stage of cytoplasmic division. In the female two separate cells are produced (the ovum and first polar body) but in the male cytoplasmic division is often incomplete and the cell has a dumb-bell shape with two sets of chromosomes.

Prophase II
The chromosomes remain contracted.

Metaphase II
This is like mitotic metaphase. The chromosomes line up one below the other on the equator of the spindle.

Anaphase II
Like mitotic anaphase. The spindle fibres contract, the centromere divides and the chromatids are pulled apart and move to opposite ends of the cell.

Telophase II
The cytoplasm divides. In the female this forms the ovum and second polar body and in the male the spermatids.

the species and the correct combination of genes in order that each cell can perform its function. Thus, each individual receives half its chromosomes (and so half the genes) from one parent and half from the other.

Before meiosis I, new DNA is synthesized in the S phase of the cell cycle, as with mitosis, and the new chromosomes are held together at the centromeres.

In meiosis I, prophase is much longer than in a mitotic division and so it is described as having five stages: leptotene; zygotene; pachytene; diplotene; and diakinesis. During the latter stages of meiotic prophase, crossing over takes place (Figure 4.6).

During metaphase I the chromosomes line up in the centre of the cell, with homologous chromosomes lying side by side. The homologous chromosomes then move to opposite ends of the cell, so that half the chromosomes are on one side and half on the other. This is anaphase of the first meiotic division. Telophase I initiates the division of the cytoplasm into two cells, and by Interphase II two cells are formed, each with a diploid chromosome number. The second cell division begins immediately and this process is identical to mitosis. Thus, from one original cell, four new cells are formed, each of which contains half the original number of chromosomes. The new individual inherits the genetic material from each parent but with some variation because of the crossing over.

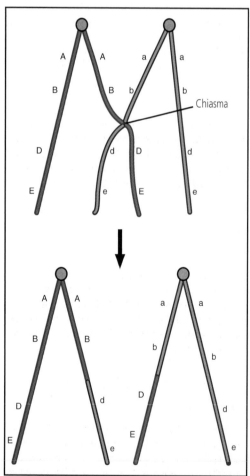

4.6 Crossing over. During prophase 1 of meiosis, homologous chromosomes, each comprising two chromatids, come to lie next to each other. At random points the chromatids break and reunite with their homologous partners. Thus, alleles that were on one chromosome cross over to the homologous chromosome.

Differences between mitosis and meiosis

- In meiotic prophase I, the homologous chromosomes lie side by side. In mitotic prophase they do not.
- In meiotic metaphase I, the homologous chromosomes line up on the metaphase plate side by side. In mitosis they line up one below the other.
- In meiotic telophase I, the nuclear membrane does not reform and a second division begins immediately.

Inheritance

Mendel's laws

Gregor Mendel (1822–1884) was the first to propose 'laws' governing inheritance. The laws were formulated so that people could calculate the expected outcome of crossing animals or plants, even though at that time the mechanism of inheritance was not understood.

Mendel's first law

Mendel's first law states that **alleles separate** to different gametes. It is now known that this is because alleles are on different homologous chromosomes and these separate to different gametes during meiosis.

Mendel's second law

Mendel's second law states that there is **independent assortment** of pairs of alleles, i.e. alleles of different genes separate at random. For the most part, this is true. However, it is now known that gene loci that are close together on a chromosome are more likely to be inherited together and so it is not an entirely random process. This is because gene loci can be separated during crossing-over. If two genes lie far apart on a chromosome, there is a greater chance of a cross-over event than if they are lying close together. Genes lying close together on a chromosome are said to be 'linked' or to show linkage. This is an advantage if both genes are desirable but a disadvantage if a breeder is trying to retain one gene and eradicate the other.

Dominant and recessive genes

If the cells of an individual contain two different alleles of a gene (**heterozygous**) it might be expected that both alleles would be 'expressed', i.e. their effects would be apparent in the organism's appearance or physiology. Although this does occur in some circumstances, when the alleles are 'co-dominant' (for example, the genes coding for blood groups), this is often not the case. **Recessive** alleles are only expressed if there are two copies of the same allele in the cell (**homozygous**). Alleles that can be expressed when only one copy is present and which can suppress the other allele are said to be **dominant**. The different types of alleles are represented by a capital letter for a dominant allele and a lower case letter for a recessive allele.

Example

The black coat-colour allele in the Labrador is dominant to the brown allele that codes for chocolate. Therefore, the black allele is designated *B* and the brown allele is designated *b*.

A black Labrador can have either *BB* or *Bb* alleles, because black is dominant to brown and the *B* allele will suppress the expression of the *b* allele. Thus *BB* and *Bb* animals have the same phenotype (i.e. the same appearance) but a different genotype (i.e. different genetic makeup).

Chocolate Labradors must all be *bb*, because brown is recessive and can only be expressed if two copies of the allele are present.

Identification of animals carrying a recessive gene

Animals homozygous for a particular gene will always breed true when bred together; however, heterozygous animals will sometimes produce offspring that are homozygous for the recessive gene. Usually (but not always), the recessive gene is unwanted and so breeders would like to be able to identify those animals that are heterozygous for a recessive gene and avoid breeding from them.

Identification of the recessive carrier can be done by test mating to a homozygous recessive animal. This test mating is known as the **back cross to the recessive**. Such a mating is useful if the recessive gene involves something like coat colour, but is not possible if the homozygous animal has an abnormality or demonstrates a disease. In that case, the mating has to be with a known heterozygous carrier.

The animals that are mated are the **parent generation** and the offspring are the **filial or F₁ generation**. If the offspring were to be mated they would produce the **F₂ generation** and so on.

Test mating with a homozygous recessive animal

If you have a black Labrador and you want to know whether its genotype is *BB* (i.e. homozygous for the dominant *B* black allele) or *Bb* (i.e. heterozygous for the recessive *b* brown allele) then you can cross it with a chocolate (*bb*) Labrador.

- If the black Labrador is *BB* then all the offspring will be black puppies (although with the genotype of Bb).
- If the black Labrador is *Bb*, it will still produce black puppies, but it may also produce chocolate (*bb*) puppies.

How this arises is demonstrated below.

Checkerboard for determining the genotype of offspring: *Bb* (father) x *bb* (mother)

	Sperm of father	
	B	b
Eggs of mother		
b	Bb	bb
		Offspring
b	Bb	bb

It can be calculated mathematically that if the black Labrador produces seven black puppies when mated to the chocolate Labrador then you can be 99% sure that its genotype is *BB*. The more black puppies that are produced, the more certain you can be that the genotype is *BB*. If just one chocolate puppy is produced, irrespective of the number of black, then you know that the black Labrador must be *Bb*. You do not have to mate the black Labrador to the same chocolate Labrador to get the offspring; it is the number of offspring that is important.

Test mating with a known heterozygous carrier

For some genes it is not possible to carry out a mating with the homozygous recessive animal and so a heterozygous carrier of the recessive has to be used. We will use the black and chocolate coat colour of the Labrador as an example again.

If a black Labrador has previously produced a chocolate puppy, then that black Labrador *must* be *Bb*, i.e. a known heterozygote. You can therefore mate your unknown black Labrador with this known heterozygote. If the unknown Labrador is really *Bb*, the checkerboard will be:

	Sperm of father	
	B	b
Eggs of mother		
B	BB	Bb
		Offspring
b	Bb	bb

This time 16 black puppies would have to be produced before you could be 99% sure that the animal was *BB* and not *Bb*. Again, these puppies do not have to be produced from a single mating and the birth of just one chocolate puppy will prove the dog to have been *Bb*.

Epistasis

The terms dominant and recessive apply to the interaction of alleles. Some genes can interact with other genes that are not their alleles, i.e. they suppress the effect of genes at a different locus. These genes are said to have epistatic effects on the other genes, or to show **epistasis**. An example is the albino gene blocking the expression of all coat-colour genes.

Sex chromosomes and X inactivation

The Y chromosome is usually quite small and carries the genes that code for maleness. Very few other genes are carried on the Y chromosome. In contrast, the X chromosome is often one of the largest chromosomes and carries a number of genes that are important in the day-to-day metabolism of the cell. Since females have two X chromosomes (XX) and males have one X chromosome and one Y chromosome (XY), it follows that females must receive twice the number of genes that are carried on the X chromosome compared with males. In order to compensate for this, only one X chromosome in each cell of a female is activated and the genes on this chromosome are functional. The other X chromosome becomes highly contracted and most of the genes are inactivated and non-functional. This is called the **Lyon hypothesis of X inactivation and gene compensation** (after the person who first put forward the hypothesis). The decision as to which X chromosome is to become inactive in a cell (i.e. the paternal or maternal X chromosome) is a random process and is settled very early on during embryogenesis. Thereafter, all the daughter cells have the same X chromosome inactivated. Thus, a female has some cells where the paternal X chromosome has activated genes and other cells where it is the maternal X chromosome that has activated genes.

The tortoiseshell coat colour and male tortoiseshell cats

The tortoiseshell coat colour in cats is a mixture of ginger and black/tabby etc., and is usually only seen in females. It is produced as a result of the epistatic effects of the sex-linked orange (O) gene on the autosomal black/tabby etc. genes. In cells with an O gene on the X chromosome, the hair colour will be ginger even if there are other coat-colour genes on the autosomes. Therefore, male cats may have an X chromosome that carries the orange gene and be X^OY. This produces the ginger coat colour. Alternatively, their X chromosome may not have the orange gene and therefore they are X^-Y and their autosomal coat colour genes will be expressed.

Females, with two X chromosomes, have three possibilities: X^-X^- cats will be black or tabby etc. depending upon which autosomal genes they have; X^OX^O cats will be ginger (it *is* possible to have ginger female cats); and X^-X^O cats will be tortoiseshell, i.e. patches of ginger and patches of black/tabby etc. There are patches of colour because in a female cell only one X chromosome is functional and the other is inactivated (Lyon hypothesis, see above). Since the inactivation takes place at random at about day 12 of gestation in the cat, there are groups of cells with a different active X chromosome and therefore groups of cells in the skin that produce the ginger coat colour or black or tabby.

In theory, male tortoiseshell cats should not occur. However, a few do appear and they are chromosomally abnormal in that they either have an extra X chromosome in each cell (e.g. XXY, called the **Klinefelter syndrome**) or have more than one cell line (i.e. they are **chimaeric**, e.g. XX/XY or XX/XXY or XY/XXY etc.). The XXY Klinefelter cats have always been infertile. Some of the chimaeric cats with a normal XY cell line are fertile but an XY cell line does not guarantee fertility.

Multifactorial inheritance and the influence of environment

Some characteristics are governed by single genes but many characteristics are controlled by the cumulative effect of many genes. Such characteristics are said to be **polygenic.**

Sometimes, when a characteristic is controlled by many genes the expression of the characteristic can vary in degree. That is, the characteristic is said to show **variable expressivity**. All animals carrying the main gene for the trait express it; however, the expression is modified by other genes to create variation in expression.

Some other polygenic characteristics show **incomplete penetrance**. That is, not all animals carrying the major genes express them, because of modification by minor genes. However, all the animals that *do* express the trait do so to the same extent.

Some characteristics are also affected by the environment. For example, the size of a dog will depend on many genes but also on the amount of food available. When the environment can influence a characteristic, as well as genes, that characteristic is said to be **multifactorial**. It is obvious that these characteristics will have great variation and be very difficult to control by selection.

The proportion of the variation of a characteristic within a population that is due to different genes (i.e. not the variation in environment) is called the **heritability** of the characteristic. For example, if only half the variation is due to variation in genes, the heritability is 50% (also written as 0.5).

Parentage analysis

The ability to identify the parentage of an individual depends upon two basic facts:

- There is genetic variation – no two individuals are *exactly* alike genetically, because regions of DNA show **polymorphism**
- An individual inherits its genes from its parents – the genotype can be traced back to the parents.

In most circumstances the dam is known and it is the sire that is in doubt. If neither parent is known, the process is more complicated but the principles are the same. Parentage analysis can be carried out in two ways:

- **By looking at the expression of genes and alleles** in the individual and possible parents. This is what is done when parents are identified using **blood typing**. Red cell surface antigens, white cell surface antigens and serum proteins can be examined and those of the individual and putative sires can be compared. If the offspring displays a characteristic that is not found in the dam, it is assumed to have been inherited from the sire. All sires without that characteristic can therefore be excluded. The more characteristics that are examined, the more sires there are that can be excluded, until only one possible candidate remains. This technique is therefore an 'exclusion' technique. It tells you very definitely which animal is *not* the father but only gives a probability of which animal *is* the father.
- **By looking at the DNA itself**. This is usually described as DNA profiling.

DNA profiling

This involves looking at DNA **microsatellites,** which are tandem repeats of base pairs found at the same site along the genome in different animals of the same species. They are highly polymorphic (i.e. there can be a different number of repeats) but related individuals inherit the same number of repeats. For the purposes of international comparability, the microsatellites are tested to ensure that there is sufficient variation in a population before it is used. The more microsatellites used, the easier it is to exclude possible parents. A trial by the American Kennel Club showed that the use of 10–15 microsatellites could provide a universal canine panel.

Microsatellites that are associated with a trait are called

markers, because they mark the presence of the gene responsible for the trait and are inherited along with that gene.

DNA profiling can be carried out using any cells that contain DNA. In practice, the most convenient source of cells is from a blood sample. Alternatively, cells from the buccal mucosa can be collected on a swab, but this does not generally provide as many cells from which to extract the DNA for analysis.

As a result of parentage analysis, possible parents can be *excluded* with 100% certainty on the basis that they could not have been able to contribute to the genome of the individual.

Those that are not excluded *could* be a parent. The aim is to use sufficient tests such that the probability of two *possible* parents having the same combination would be so small as to be negligible.

Genome sequencing

The new molecular genetic techniques have allowed sequencing of whole genomes. The dog's genome was sequenced in 2005 and the cat's in 2007. This has meant that genes can be mapped to chromosomes and this is allowing the identification of carriers of undesirable genes.

Breeding strategies

When breeders wish to ensure that animals breed true, they try to make them homozygous for the genes governing the desirable characteristics. The quickest way to increase homozygosity is to inbreed.

Inbreeding

Inbreeding is the breeding of two individuals more closely related than the population as a whole. Related individuals are more likely to have the same alleles and so more likely to produce offspring that will be homozygous for the genes. The more closely related the individuals, the more likely it is that the offspring will be homozygous at any particular gene locus. This is called the **coefficient of inbreeding,** and is defined as the probability that two alleles at any locus will be alike by descent, i.e. the alleles will be alike because they have been inherited down the maternal and paternal line through a common ancestor (Figure 4.7).

Unfortunately, inbreeding creates a higher occurrence of homozygosity, and will therefore fix the 'bad' alleles as well as the 'good' alleles. This is why inbreeding is generally considered dangerous. The chances of good or bad alleles being fixed are the same.

One way to reduce the intensity of inbreeding (and hence reduce the likelihood of producing homozygosity for a bad gene – or a good gene) is to carry out **line breeding.**

Line breeding

Line breeding is a form of inbreeding that involves mating within a certain family or line and which aims to maintain a relationship with a particular popular ancestor (e.g. show champion). Whilst the animals to be mated are related, they are not as closely related as, for example, father and daughter or brother and sister. They are more likely to be grandparents and grandchildren or cousins. The rationale is that whilst the relatives are chosen because they have the same 'good' alleles for the required trait, it is hoped that they will have

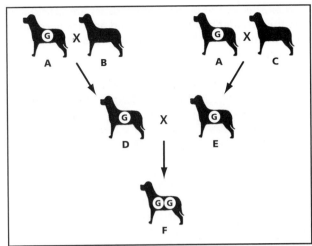

4.7 How an individual can be homozygous for a gene, by descent. The individual F will inherit genes from individual A through the paternal and maternal lines. Thus it is possible for two copies of the same allele to be inherited by F (one via the maternal line and one via the paternal line), who will therefore be homozygous by descent.

different 'bad' alleles for the other characteristics. The hope is that the offspring will be homozygous for the chosen trait but remain heterozygous for all the possible bad alleles.

Outcrossing

The best way to reduce the chances of the offspring being homozygous for any given allele is to outcross. Outcrossing (or outbreeding) is the mating of two individuals less closely related than the population as a whole. Outcrossing masks the effect of recessive alleles, because unrelated individuals are unlikely to have the same unwanted recessive alleles. The offspring of an outcross show **hybrid vigour**, or **heterosis,** i.e. they are often 'bigger and better' than their parents. The major disadvantage of outcrossing is that the F_1 generation will not breed true, because they are heterozygous and not homozygous for their alleles.

Breed variation

Cats and dogs have been kept as pets for hundreds of years and during this time humans have selected certain characteristics that were deemed either useful or attractive. This has resulted in considerable breed variation. In the past, desirable characteristics were those that made the dog suitable for a particular use, e.g. hunting or ratting. However, when animals were bred just for showing, the 'desirable' characteristics became much more subjective and less practical. In recent years there has been increasing unease as to the welfare of animals that are bred deliberately with what are, essentially, physical abnormalities, e.g. the short maxilla and enlarged soft palate of the Bulldog. Currently, veterinary professional organizations and dog breeding organizations are collaborating to develop welfare codes for dog breeding.

There are over 170 different breeds of dog, divided into seven groups: Hound; Gundog; Terrier; Utility; Working; Pastoral; and Toy (see Appendix 1). Each breed has characteristics defined by the Kennel Club.

In cats, there are 40 different breeds recognized by the Cat Fanciers' Association.

In all species the breed characteristics are artificial in that they are defined by humans and are not necessarily those characteristics that make the animal best adapted to its environment.

Hereditary diseases and health schemes

Hereditary diseases or abnormalities are caused by genes and can be passed from one generation to the next. Diseases or abnormalities that are present at birth are said to be **congenital**. Not all congenital diseases or abnormalities are hereditary, however. For example, a viral infection during gestation may result in the birth of abnormal offspring; this would be congenital but not genetic.

Conversely, not all genetic diseases manifest at birth; it may take a number of months or years for the defect to become apparent. This is true for a number of genetic eye defects.

Health schemes are designed to identify animals carrying unwanted genes. This is easy when the problems are caused by dominant genes, as every animal carrying even one copy of a dominant gene will express that gene and so can be eliminated from the breeding population. This results in a reduced frequency of the abnormal gene in the population. Reduction is more difficult when the defect is caused by recessive genes. In these cases, only homozygous individuals will express the defect and, whilst these can be removed from the breeding population, the heterozygous carriers will remain. Unfortunately, the majority of genetic abnormalities show a recessive mode of inheritance.

Traditionally, heterozygous carriers have been identified by test matings (where they are backcrossed to the recessive) but it is increasingly possible to identify carriers using molecular genetic techniques.

Polygenic conditions, such as hip and elbow dysplasia, are also difficult to control because it is the *combination* of genes that causes the problem and many animals may have some of the genes but appear completely normal.

British Veterinary Association (BVA)/Kennel Club/ International Sheep Dog Society Eye Scheme

Details of this scheme can be found at: www.thekennelclub. org.uk/item/310.

This was the first health scheme to be set up in Britain. It currently covers 11 hereditary eye conditions in 56 different breeds. The causal gene and mode of inheritance of an anomaly can be different in different breeds, but many are recessive. Although any breed can be examined for eye disease, only the results of those breeds that appear on Schedule A of the eye scheme (see below) are sent to the Kennel Club for inclusion on computer records.

Interpretation of the morphology of the eye and its structures is very complex and so all the examinations are carried out by veterinary specialists in ophthalmology. These specialists comprise the Eye Panel Working Party. Dogs are best first examined before they are a year old, and thereafter an annual examination will reveal any later developing anomalies.

The breeds and conditions are divided into Schedule A and Schedule B. Schedule A lists the known inherited eye diseases in the breeds for which inheritance of the condition has been scientifically proven, and often its mode of inheritance. For the breeds in Schedule A, a certificate is issued with results of 'affected' or 'unaffected', and these results are recorded and published by the Kennel Club. Schedule B lists those breeds in which the conditions are, at this stage, only suspected of being hereditary and are 'under investigation'. With further work, breeds and conditions in Schedule B may be confirmed as inherited and therefore moved to Schedule A.

BVA/Kennel Club Hip Dysplasia Scheme

Details of this scheme can be found at: www.thekennelclub. org.uk/item/313.

Hip dysplasia is a polygenic multifactorial condition of the hips. Clinically, there is a malformation of both the femoral head and acetabulum of the hip, which results in lameness, pain and degenerative joint changes. It is a particular problem in certain breeds of dog where the genes responsible for the condition have been concentrated, presumably during the inbreeding that produced the breed. The condition is exacerbated by increased exercise and rapid growth in the young prepubescent animal. Although hip dysplasia is more common in larger breeds, any dog of any breed can be screened.

The basis of the scheme is the radiographic examination of young adult animals in order to identify signs of malformation. For most breeds, the examination takes place after the animal is 12 months old but for giant breeds it is delayed until they are 18 months old.

The radiographs are taken by the client's own veterinary surgeon and are then interpreted by a panel of experts overseen by the British Veterinary Association (BVA). It is very important for accurate interpretation that the radiographs are taken with the animal in the correct position (see Chapter 18). A number of parameters are assessed on each hip by a member of the panel of experts and each parameter is given a score. The total for each examined point is the hip score. The lowest score, 0, indicates normality; the highest score, 106, indicates the worst possible expression of hip dysplasia.

Once the radiograph has been scored, the result is returned to the client's own veterinary surgeon and a copy sent to the Kennel Club for recording on the registration database and publication in the Breed Records Supplement. Over the years, a number of dogs have been examined from each breed and so it is possible to calculate a 'breed mean score' (BMS) for hip dysplasia. The recommendation is that only animals with a score well below the BMS should be used for breeding purposes. The BVA informs the Kennel Club of registered dogs with a score of 8 or less and no more than 6 on either hip. By following these recommendations the aim is slowly to reduce the BMS. The genes responsible for the condition will then be reduced in the breed.

BVA/Kennel Club Elbow Dysplasia Scheme

Details of this scheme can be found at: www.thekennelclub. org.uk/item/309.

Elbow dysplasia is the abnormal development of the cartilage of the elbow joint, with resultant wear leading to secondary osteoarthritic changes and, eventually, lameness.

Like hip dysplasia, the condition is polygenic and multifactorial. In the dog, there are three primary lesions: osteochondritis dissecans (OCD); fragmented or ununited coronoid process (FCP); and ununited anconeal process (UAP).

The health scheme is run in a similar manner to the hip dysplasia scheme. Two radiographic views of the elbow joint are required: extended lateral and flexed lateral. The client's own veterinary surgeon takes the radiographs when the animal is one or more years old and these are examined by a panel of experts. Each elbow is graded on a 0–3 scale, with 0 indicating normality and 3 indicating severe elbow dysplasia.

The names and scores of dogs graded under the scheme, together with the results, are sent to the Kennel Club for publication and inclusion on the relevant documents. It is recommended that only animals with a grade of 0 or 1 are used for breeding.

Feline Advisory Bureau (FAB) Polycystic Kidney Disease Screening Scheme

Details of this scheme can be found at: www.fabcats.org/breeders/infosheets/pkd/pkd_scheme.php.

Polycystic kidney disease (PKD) is a disease in which a large number of fluid-filled cysts form within the kidney. The condition is caused by a single autosomal dominant gene; this means that every animal carrying even a single copy of the gene will show clinical signs. Homozygosity for the gene causes such gross abnormal development of the kidneys that there is prenatal death. The condition is particularly common in Persian cats and exotic shorthair breeds.

There are now two ways of checking for the condition. The screening programme is based upon ultrasonographic examination of the kidney by an approved veterinary specialist. The cats should be over 10 months old in order that, when no cysts are found, there is confidence that small cysts have not been missed. A copy of the result of the scan is sent to the FAB.

A gene test is available that identifies all cats with the abnormal gene. This test can be carried out at any age and requires either a blood sample or mouth swab.

Molecular genetic screening

Molecular genetic screening (also known as DNA testing) is becoming increasingly common as our understanding of the various conditions at the molecular level improves. Molecular screening can differentiate between affected and carrier animals, as well as normal animals. New genetic tests are being developed all the time. There are a number of commercial companies offering these services. In the UK, the Animal Health Trust offers molecular genetic screening for a number of diseases in dogs, cats, horses and cattle. The tests can usually be carried out using mouth swabs, which means that breeders themselves can send in samples. A few tests require more nuclear material and hence a blood sample is required.

The Animal Health Trust currently offers tests for 15 different inherited abnormalities in the dog and for PKD in the cat. Undoubtedly, more tests will become available in time. Details of the conditions and breeds involved can be found on their website (www.aht.org.uk/genetics_tests.html).

Some diseases for which a genetic screening is offered are shown in Figure 4.8.

Condition	Mode of inheritance	Breeds affected
Centronuclear myopathy	Autosomal recessive	Labrador Retriever
Ceroid lipofuscinosis	Autosomal recessive	English Setter, Tibetan Terrier, American Bulldog
Canine leucocyte adhesion deficiency (CLAD)	Autosomal recessive	Irish Setter
Cerebellar ataxia	Autosomal recessive	Italian Spinone
Factor VII deficiency	Autosomal recessive	Airedale, Beagle, Giant Schnauzer, Scottish Deerhound
Congenital stationary night blindness	Autosomal recessive	Briards
Copper toxicosis	Autosomal recessive	Bedlington Terrier
Fucosidosis	Autosomal recessive	English Springer Spaniel
Hereditary cataract	Autosomal dominant	Australian Shepherd
	(Schedule B)	French Bulldog
	Autosomal recessive	Staffordshire Bull Terrier
Early-onset hereditary cataract	Autosomal recessive	Boston Terrier
Phosphofructokinase deficiency	Autosomal recessive	English Springer Spaniel
Progressive retinal atrophy	Autosomal recessive	English Springer Spaniel, Irish Setter, Sloughi
	Autosomal recessive	Miniature Long-haired Dachshund, Smooth-haired Dachshund
PDP1 deficiency	Autosomal recessive	Clumber and Sussex Spaniels
Urate stones /uric acid excretion (canine hyperuricosuria)	Autosomal recessive	Russian Black Terriers, Bulldogs, Dalmations and Dalmatian crosses.
von Willebrand's disease		Irish Red and White Setters

4.8 Diseases for which a genetic screening is offered.

Further reading

Long SE (2006) *Veterinary Genetics and Reproductive Physiology: A Textbook for Veterinary Nurses and Technicians*. Elsevier, Oxford (2006)

Nicholas FW (2010) *Introduction to Veterinary Genetics, 3rd edn.* Blackwell Publishing, Oxford

Robinson R (1991) *Genetics for Dog Breeders, 2nd edn.* Pergamon, Oxford

Vella CM, Shelton LM, McGonagle JJ and Stanglein TW (1999) *Robinson's Genetics for Cat Breeders and Veterinarians, 4th edn.* Butterworth-Heinemann, Oxford

Self-assessment questions

1. Describe the components of a DNA molecule.
2. Which type of cell division results in the haploid number of chromosomes?
3. What is the difference between dominance and epistasis?
4. How can you check whether a black Labrador is carrying the yellow gene?
5. What coat colour would the sire of a female tortoiseshell cat have?
6. What is meant by the term multifactorial inheritance?
7. How might you check which of two possible sires is the true father?
8. What is the procedure for hip examination under the Hip Dysplasia Scheme?
9. Why should polycystic kidney disease in cats be fairly easy to eradicate?
10. What type of tissue sample is necessary for DNA profiling?

Chapter 5

Infection and immunity

John Helps, Karen Coyne and Susan Dawson

Learning objectives

After studying this chapter, students should be able to:

- **Understand and define the common terms listed in bold type throughout the chapter**
- **Describe relationships between microorganisms and host in health and disease**
- **List factors that may influence the occurrence, onset and severity of disease**
- **List possible routes of entry of infectious agents into the host, with examples**
- **Describe how pathogens establish, spread and multiply within the host, triggering disease**
- **List ways in which infectious agents may be shed and transmitted**
- **Understand the principles involved in the control of infectious disease**
- **Describe the functional components of the immune system**
- **Understand the underlying principles of vaccines and vaccination**
- **Understand the principles of hypersensitivity and other immune disorders**

Principles of infection and infectious disease

Definitions

- **Infection** is the **colonization** of an individual (host) by a foreign microorganism. Infectious agents that cause harm are termed **pathogens**; these can live within or on the host and disrupt physiological function.
- **Disease** occurs when normal bodily functions are sufficiently impaired to reduce performance, leading to specific recognizable clinical signs. Though infection is a common cause of disease, there are many other potential causes. ▶

- Infectious diseases may be **contagious**, i.e. spread through **contagion** directly or indirectly from one individual host to another. Important examples of contagious diseases are given in Chapters 13 and 20. The ability of a pathogen to spread varies and is dependent on:
    - **Transmissibility:** the capacity to pass from one host to another, typically determined by the ability of the pathogen to survive outside the body
    - **Infectivity:** the ability to penetrate host defences.
- **Pathogenicity** is the ability of a pathogen to cause disease, and it is dependent on both its capacity to spread and its ability to harm the host, or virulence (Figure 5.1).
- **Epidemiology** is the study of the occurrence, spread and distribution of disease in populations and is of vital importance in the design and monitoring of effective control policies.
- **Endemic** refers to a disease present at a normal level in a country or region. For example, myxomatosis is now **endemic** in wild rabbits in the UK and feline calicivirus (FCV) is **endemic** in the domestic cat population
- **Epidemic** refers to a disease where a pronounced increase in incidence has been observed within a country or geographical region. The foot-and-mouth **epidemic** in the UK in 2001 led to controls on movement and widespread slaughter of infected and at-risk livestock.
- **Pandemic** refers to epidemic disease that spreads across many countries or continents, e.g. The 2009 'flu pandemic was a global outbreak of a new strain of influenza A virus, H1N1 (referred to as 'swine 'flu'). In contrast to the regular seasonal epidemics of influenza, these pandemics occur sporadically.
- **Epizootic** is sometimes used to refer to an animal disease epidemic. An example of an epizootic would be the outbreak of canine parvovirus in the 1970s, or, more recently, distemper in red foxes in Italy. Although widespread vaccination helped to control its spread, recent reports suggest that the prevalence of canine parvovirus in the UK is increasing.

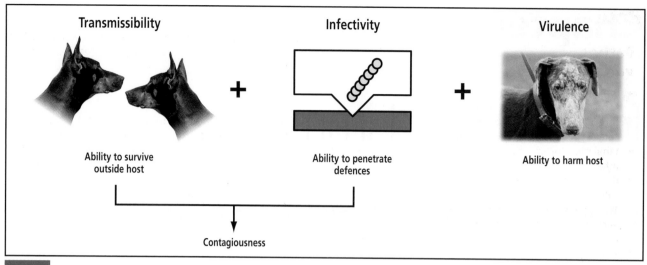

5.1   Factors influencing pathogenicity.

The resident microflora

Most microorganisms, or microbes (see Chapter 6), are useful to humans or even vital for life; relatively few are associated with ill health. The skin, oral cavity, conjunctiva, gastrointestinal tract and distal urogenital tracts all house a varied resident microflora, consisting of billions of microbes – principally bacteria. These organisms are described as commensal, because they share the body and usually do no harm; furthermore their presence may help to prevent colonization by more harmful organisms.

Non-contagious disease

Microbes that normally live benignly on or within the host or environment can cause disease. Such infections, most commonly bacterial, are less likely to lead to disease in other in-contact individuals, but gain advantage in the affected host because normal innate immunity (see below) is weakened or bypassed, or abnormal local conditions favour infection. Common examples include:

- Cat-bite abscesses
- Wound infections
- Bacterial skin infection (pyoderma)
- Bladder infection (bacterial cystitis).

Factors influencing occurrence and severity of disease

In order to trigger disease, pathogens need to:

- Penetrate host defences and establish themselves
- Multiply on or within host tissues
- Overcome the initial natural defence mechanisms inside the host
- Harm the host in some way.

The expression of disease in an individual depends on a balance between the nature of the infectious challenge and the resistance of the host. The capacity of an infection to cause disease is determined by:

- The infective dose, i.e. the number of agents, such as bacteria or viral particles
- The virulence of the agent; this may vary between different strains.

Host susceptibility may be increased by:

- Immaturity
- Stress (e.g. transport, novel environment)
- Concurrent disease
- Genetic factors (e.g. inbreeding, breed predispositions)
- Lack of or reduction in immunity (e.g. immunosuppressive illness such as feline immunodeficiency virus)
- Medication (e.g. immunosuppressive drugs such as corticosteroids)
- Malnutrition.

Based on the balance between the infectivity of an agent and host susceptibility, a number of outcomes are possible:

- The pathogen may be eliminated by the immune system without consequence to the host
- Subclinical infection may occur, i.e. an animal is infected but does not show any clinical signs of disease. There is a possible risk of transmission to other animals
- Disease may occur, associated with infection and risk of transmission to others.

The **incubation period** for an infectious disease is the time interval elapsing between exposure to the causative pathogen and the first clinical signs appearing. For many diseases this period is a few days, but it may be weeks, months or even years. Dose and virulence of the infecting pathogen, as well as host susceptibility, can affect both incubation period and the severity of disease, so that within a group of infected individuals both the severity and onset of clinical signs can vary markedly.

Routes of entry

Pathogens infect new hosts via a variety of routes:

- Ingestion (taken in via the mouth): in contaminated food or water; during hunting or mutual grooming; through coprophagia (ingestion of faeces); through contact with infected items (fomites, see below)
- Inhalation (breathing in) of infected particles (droplet infection) (e.g. kennel cough, equine influenza)
- Direct contact with saliva/nasal secretions (e.g. feline calicivirus, *Streptococcus equi* (strangles))
- Through the skin: through bite or surgical wounds; via vectors such as fleas, ticks or mosquitoes (e.g. Lyme disease (borreliosis), *Dirofilaria immitis* (heartworm))
- Via skin contact (e.g. ectoparasites, ringworm)
- Across mucous membranes: gastrointestinal and respiratory epithelia are frequent entry routes; *Leptospira* bacteria may penetrate intact mucosae as well as damaged skin
- Across the placenta or during birth (e.g. *Toxocara canis*, feline panleucopenia, feline leukaemia virus).

Spread within the host

Pathogens commonly establish and multiply at the point of entry. For many viral pathogens, this is in the epithelial cells of the gastrointestinal or respiratory tracts. From these initial entry points spread to local lymph nodes may then occur. Infection may remain localized in response to a rapid immune response and/or because of a preference (predilection, tropism) for certain cell types. Alternatively, the agent may spread into the blood circulation. The occurrence of virus within the blood is called **viraemia**. Bacterial infection may also remain localized, but serious infections can seed systemically via the bloodstream (**bacteraemia**). **Septicaemia** occurs if bacteria actively multiply in the bloodstream leading to sepsis.

How pathogens trigger disease

Harm may be caused in a variety of ways.

- The cells within tissues may be destroyed by the pathogen itself. For example, in order to reproduce and propagate, viruses 'hijack' the normal metabolic processes of the host cell, finally rupturing and destroying the cell as new virus particles leave to infect other host cells.
- Biological poisons (toxins) may disrupt normal physiological function. The presence of toxins in the circulation is called **toxaemia**. In severe sepsis, circulatory collapse caused by endotoxic shock is a potentially life-threatening consequence. (See Chapter 6 for more discussion on microbial toxins.)
- The response of the immune system to infection may cause damage. For example, in feline infectious peritonitis (FIP), damage occurs as a result of the body's immune response to attempt to eliminate the coronavirus that triggers the disease. This may damage organs, commonly including the kidneys, eyes and central nervous system ('dry' form of FIP), or may lead to exudation of large quantities of fluid into the chest or abdominal cavity ('wet' form of FIP). See also 'Allergy and hypersensitivity reactions', below.

Transmission

For pathogens to succeed and propagate they need to both infect a host and have the capacity to spread to other susceptible individuals.

Direct transmission

This involves the spread of pathogens by direct contact. Direct transmission is particularly important for fragile pathogens such as feline leukaemia virus (FeLV) and feline immunodeficiency virus (FIV), because they are unable to survive for long outside the host. Examples of direct transmission include bites, scratches and droplet spread.

Indirect transmission

This occurs if infection is acquired from a contaminated environment or via a vector.

Mechanical vectors

Also known as fomites, these may be inanimate objects such as bedding, grooming kits, feed buckets/bowls and litter trays. People may also act as vectors by transporting infection on skin, clothing or shoes. For example, canine parvovirus persists for many months or years in the environment and is susceptible to few disinfectants. Virus is excreted by infected puppies for only a few days. Because of the virus's survival ability, indirect spread via ingestion from an environment contaminated by the faeces of infected dogs is the most significant route. Direct ingestion of the faeces of an infected dog (coprophagia) would also be a possible route of transmission.

Biological vectors

These are organisms that may not cause disease in their own right but may convey infectious agents from one host to another. A number of significant canine diseases, for which dogs travelling to Europe and beyond may be at risk, are transmitted by biological vectors. Important examples of such vectors include: sandflies, which transmit leishmaniasis; ticks, which may transmit a number of serious infections including Lyme disease (borreliosis), babesiosis and ehrlichiosis; and mosquitoes, which may carry the *Dirofilaria immitis* heartworm.

Horizontal transmission

This term is sometimes applied to direct or indirect spread of infections between individuals of the same generation.

Vertical transmission

In some infections, transmission occurs from dam to offspring, either before or during birth. Possible effects of fetal infection include:

- Fetal death, resorption, mummification, abortion or stillbirth
- Birth of individuals showing clinical signs of disease
- Poor viability (e.g. fading kittens or puppies)
- Birth of infected carriers showing no disease signs (i.e. animals that are subclinically infected).

Different infective agents may be excreted or 'shed' by a variety of routes. Careful consideration of likely routes of transmission enables appropriate disease control measures to be implemented.

Routes of transmission

- In saliva, via bites (e.g. rabies, FIV).
- In nasal or ocular discharges (e.g. feline upper respiratory tract disease: feline calicivirus, feline herpesvirus; *Chlamydophila felis* conjunctivitis in cats; strangles in horses, caused by the bacterium *Streptococcus equi*).
- In urine (e.g. leptospirosis; infectious canine hepatitis).
- In faeces or vomitus (e.g. canine parvovirus; bacterial enteritis; panleucopenia; salmonellosis).
- In blood, via a biological vector (e.g. feline infectious anaemia caused by *Mycoplasma haemofelis* is transmitted by fleas; equine infectious anaemia caused by a retrovirus transmitted via biting flies).
- In milk (e.g. feline leukaemia virus; FIV; *Toxocara*).
- Across the placenta (transplacentally) to the fetus *in utero* (e.g. *Toxocara canis*; panleucopenia; equine viral arteritis).
- By aerosol, i.e. airborne (e.g. 'kennel cough'; canine distemper; equine influenza).
- By skin contact (e.g. ectoparasites; ringworm).
- During coitus or parturition (e.g. panleucopenia; FIV; contagious equine metritis (CEM)).

Carriers

In some diseases infected animals, known as carriers, may continue to shed infective agents despite showing minimal or no signs of disease.

- Cats infected with feline herpesvirus (FHV) carry infection throughout their lives and may 'shed' virus intermittently, throughout life, with or without signs of disease, following episodes of stress. Between periods of shedding, the infection remains latent (dormant) and the virus cannot be isolated on swabs.
- In contrast, cats infected with feline calicivirus (FCV) shed virus continuously, following apparent recovery from disease. Unlike FHV infection, most FCV-infected individuals eliminate the infection completely within weeks or months; however, a small proportion of some cats can remain subclinically infected for years.
- Another example of an infectious disease that can result in a carrier state is strangles in horses; following infection, horses can continue to shed the causative bacterial agent *Streptococcus equi* for prolonged periods.

Controlling infection and disease

A range of measures must be taken in order to contain the potential spread of infection between animals and to humans (see 'Zoonoses', below) and to reduce the risk of disease occurring. Hygiene measures are further discussed in Chapter 12 and include:

- Efficient cleaning and appropriate use of disinfection of accommodation, paying attention to potential fomites

- Careful cleaning and disposal of faeces, urine, body fluids and discharges; appropriate disposal of contaminated waste
- Good hygiene in all stages of storage, handling and preparation of pet food. High-quality tinned and dry diets are available and avoid the potential hazards of offering raw meat, which can potentially present a source of food-poisoning bacteria and parasites.

Animal management risks should be considered:

- Quarantine animals with suspected contagion and newly introduced animals of unknown health status (see below)
- 'Barrier nurse' cases of suspected infectious disease (see later).

To manage disease risk factors, the following actions should be considered.

- Wear suitable protective clothing whenever handling animals; change clothing if it becomes soiled.
- Observe regular hand hygiene – wash/disinfect hands between patients (Figure 5.2) and before touching any potential fomites (consider pens, clinical notes, cigarettes, door handles, food, cups, etc.).
- Ensure good draught-free ventilation and low stocking rates in multi-animal facilities, such as kennels and catteries. Avoid mixing animals in large groups and in the same airspace.
- Rest accommodation following occupation for as long as practicable, depending on the likely persistence of the infectious agent(s) of concern, to reduce the risk of residual environmental contamination.
- Minimize stress through good husbandry. Ensure optimum nutrition and prompt attention to any ancillary health issues.
- Control disease vectors, such as external parasites. Where appropriate, reduce populations of stray animals, via rescue centres and neutering programmes.
- Use appropriate vaccines in animals, both routinely and targeted where specific disease risks are identified.
- Consider animals more at risk of infection due to severity of underlying disease.

Owners should be educated regarding disease risks, hygiene and good husbandry, including parasite control and vaccination.

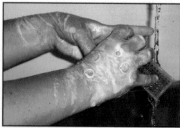
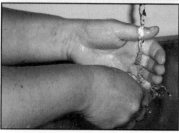

5.2 Hands should be washed thoroughly between handling each patient.

Zoonoses

Zoonoses (singular: zoonosis) are diseases that are transmissible from animals to humans. Some are potentially life-threatening (e.g. rabies, leptospirosis), while others may pass unnoticed unless an individual is particularly susceptible; toxoplasmosis, for example, is mainly a risk in pregnant or immune-suppressed individuals. Figure 5.3 lists some important examples of zoonotic infections.

Apparently healthy animals may harbour infection and it may be unclear that an animal carries a zoonosis, so care should always be exercised. In addition to the general risk-reduction measures listed above, some special precautions should be taken.

Precautions against the spread of zoonotic infections

- Do not allow animals to lick humans (particularly on the face and mouth) and especially children, as they have higher susceptibility and lower awareness of basic hygiene.
- Facilities and utensils for animal food preparation and washing up should be separate from those for human use. ▶

- Avoid unnecessary exposure to infections: reduce unnecessary animal handling and ensure that handling technique minimizes risk (e.g. from bites/scratches).
- Pregnant women and immunocompromised individuals should be especially vigilant about personal hygiene after animal contact, since infection risks are greater.
- Always seek medical advice if human infection is suspected.
- Tetanus immunization is advisable for all veterinary nurses. If working with wild animals, zoo animals or captive primates, vaccinations against rabies, tuberculosis and hepatitis should also be considered.

Nosocomial infections

Infections acquired by patients in hospital are termed nosocomial infections and are of particular concern because the patient's immunity may be compromised by underlying disease, drugs, surgery, invasive supportive care (e.g. intravenous or urinary catheters), malnutrition or stress. Poor hygiene and transfer of pathogens between patients, combined with the potential for build-up of antimicrobial resistance, lead to increased risk of exposure and of more severe consequences if infection occurs.

Disease/infection	Risk sources
Major enteric infections	
Campylobacter spp.	Contaminated food (esp. poultry meat); faeces of livestock, poultry, dogs, cats, wild birds
Salmonella spp.	Contaminated food; faeces of carrier mammals including livestock and pets, and of birds, reptiles and fish
Escherichia coli (Strain VTEC O157)	Contaminated food; faeces of healthy carrier livestock and birds
Cryptosporidiosis	Contaminated water; livestock (esp. calves, lambs)
Notifiable animal diseases in the UK	
Anthrax	Cutaneous form from contact with imported infected hide (very unlikely)
Avian influenza (fowl plague)	Airborne from infected poultry
Bovine spongiform encephalopathy (causes variant Creutzfeld–Jakob disease in humans)	Ingestion of contaminated beef
Bovine tuberculosis (TB)	Unpasteurized milk (now unlikely in the UK). Most cases due to human TB
Brucellosis	Contact with infected aborting cattle
Rabies [a]/European bat lyssavirus (EBL-2)	Mammalian hosts (esp. dogs) via bites. Risk in UK of EBL from bites from infected bats.
West Nile virus (WNV) [a]	Mosquito transmission – wild birds, horses
Other important zoonoses	
Hydatid disease [b]	Dog faeces
Leptospirosis	Water-borne; urine of infected rats, dogs, cattle
Orf	Viral skin infection of sheep
Pasteurellosis	Animal bites – cats and dogs
Psittacosis	Infected birds (esp. psittacines)
Ringworm	Contact with infected dogs, cats, livestock and wildlife (e.g. hedgehogs)
Toxocariasis	Dogs, cats (roundworms)
Toxoplasmosis	Cat faeces; uncooked meat

5.3   Some important examples of zoonoses. [a] Disease currently absent from UK; [b] _Echinococcus granulosus_ tapeworm in UK; _E. multilocularis_ currently absent from UK but present in mainland Europe.

Examples of nosocomial infections include:

- Urinary tract infection following repeated catheterization
- Wound infection following surgery (e.g. MRSA, see below)
- Diarrhoea due to overgrowth of antibiotic-tolerant microbes (e.g. clostridia).

Nosocomial infections may be minimized by:

- Effective cleaning and disinfection of kennels/housing between patients
- Good barrier nursing technique
- Reducing infection risk through:
  - Good wound management, e.g. changing soiled bandages
  - Correct management and hygiene of indwelling catheters and drains
  - Good antibacterial stewardship.

Antibacterial agents, although helpful in treating susceptible infections, may select for resistant microorganisms. An increase in antimicrobial resistance has reduced the ability to treat some formerly treatable infections in humans and animals. To reduce the build-up of resistance, antibiotics should be used only when strictly necessary and never as a substitute for good patient care and practical infection control measures.

MRSA: meticillin-resistant *Staphylococcus aureus*

Staphylococcus aureus is a commensal bacterium of the skin and nasal passages of humans. In certain situations, especially where the patients are hospitalized, the bacterium can cause disease including food poisoning, septicaemia, skin infections and post-surgical wound infections. Some *Staphylococcus* species are commensal on the skin and in the oral cavity and nasal passages of animals, although *S. aureus* is less commonly present in animals than in people. However, it has been shown that cats that have contact with people are more likely to have *S. aureus* present on their skin, and the isolation of identical isolates from a cat and human in contact suggest that interspecies transmission may occur.

Of major concern to human medicine is the development of antibacterial resistance within *S. aureus* to a wide range of antibacterial agents. These include the drug meticillin, hence MRSA (meticillin-resistant *Staphylococcus aureus*). MRSA is a major concern in hospitals and healthcare units, and can cause high morbidity and mortality during outbreaks. Although MRSA isolates are, by definition, resistant to all the groups of penicillin drugs, via the *MecA* gene, they can still be sensitive to other antibacterials. However, there is an increasing tendency for resistance to build up against other antibacterial drugs, and treatment in some cases is becoming very problematical. Healthy nasal carriers occur in the human population, making elimination of the organism difficult. There are also community-acquired infections, with MRSA isolates increasingly recognized in people.

MRSA has been isolated from several different species of animals and in some cases there has been an association with a known infected human. Some of the animals infected with MRSA have been healthy, whereas others have had systemic disease, skin infections or surgical wounds.

Isolates collected from dogs and cats in the UK have been found to be similar to the main epidemic strains. In contrast, some equine isolates of MRSA are not the same as currently recognized human strains. The majority of equine cases are related to soft tissue infections, resulting from wound and post-surgical incisions and intravenous catheter sites. To date, the actual prevalence of MRSA in animal species is unknown but overall it appears to be low. Particular strains of MRSA (e.g. ST398) are found in a high proportion of pig farms in the Netherlands and other mainland European countries and these strains can spill over into the human population, causing infections in people in contact with pigs.

Sterilization and disinfection

- **Sterilization is the complete elimination of microorganisms from equipment and surfaces.** To achieve this, surgical equipment is typically subjected to high temperatures and pressure within an autoclave (see Chapter 24).
- **Disinfection is the physical or chemical destruction of microorganisms.** A range of chemical disinfectants is available in order to achieve this (see Chapter 12).

Because pathogens vary in their structure and properties, their susceptibility to different disinfectants also varies; true sterilization may be difficult to achieve by chemical means. For optimum effect, an appropriate disinfectant needs to be selected, instructions for the correct dilution should be carefully followed and the product should be used in a physically clean environment.

Good wound management

All wounds, whether clean or contaminated (see Chapter 25), need proper care to reduce the risk of complications:

- Sterile gloves should be worn at all times
- All swabs, cotton buds or instruments entering the wound should be sterile
- Irrigation fluids used for flushing should be sterile
- Bandaging materials should also be sterile
- Dressings should always be changed regularly and whenever they become soiled or wet
- Self-trauma should be prevented if necessary by using an Elizabethan collar and providing adequate pain relief
- Careful disposal of soiled dressings, bandages, swabs, etc., is required (see Chapter 2).

Isolation and quarantine

Isolation

This is the physical segregation of an animal or group of animals suspected of having, or proven to have, a contagious disease, so as to eliminate the potential for transmission to other susceptible individuals. Isolation is also required for the exclusion of infections from 'high health status' animals, such as specific pathogen-free (SPF) animals used in research.

A self-contained isolation ward should be established with its own facilities for washing and disposal. It should hold a range of stock solely for use within the unit, including:

- Gloves, gowns, masks and overshoes – for protection of personnel and clothing from contamination
- Bedding, food bowls, litter trays
- Disinfectants
- Medications, syringes, needles
- Appropriate diagnostic/monitoring equipment.

Ideally, the ward's entrance and its ventilation should be separate from those of the main practice. A footbath at the entrance, for disinfecting footwear, and the allocation of different personnel to the isolation unit are useful precautions.

Potential routes of transmission (see above) should be carefully considered when designing procedures to avoid the spread of infection. The risk of spread of airborne pathogens can be minimized by reducing the number of animals in the same airspace and ensuring a good rate of air exchange. Within buildings, positive pressure ventilation may be used to encourage airflow from cleaner to potentially contaminated zones.

Barrier nursing

This is the term describing the precautions used in nursing an animal kept in isolation. This subject is discussed in Chapter 12.

Quarantine

This is the segregation of individuals of unknown disease status for a period prior to entry to a new premises or country, to limit the risk of disease introduction.

In the UK, quarantine is most commonly associated with preventing the entry of rabies. The UK has been free of terrestrial rabies since 1922, although endemic European bat lyssavirus (EBLV2) has been identified in Daubenton's bats and has been responsible for causing 'bat rabies' in humans. Prior to the PETS travel scheme, 6 months of compulsory quarantine for all pet dogs and cats entering the UK successfully prevented reintroduction of the disease.

Pet Travel Scheme (PETS)

The Pet Travel Scheme for dogs, cats and ferrets replaced the 6-month quarantine rule for dogs and cats entering the UK from designated countries, including EU member states, the USA, Japan, Australia, New Zealand and many rabies-free islands. The scheme operates via certain carriers and designated entry points within the UK, including Eurotunnel, major ports and airports. For animals that fail to comply with PETS rules, the 6-month quarantine rule still applies.

'Pet Passports', recognized throughout the EU, hold all the relevant certification in booklet form and double as entry documents for many EU countries, simplifying export procedures.

To qualify for entry or return to the UK, a number of criteria have to be met. For an animal new to the Scheme, these are (in chronological order):

1. Identichip implantation.
2. Rabies vaccination.
3. Blood sample (2–4 weeks after vaccination, usually at 21 days) and serological testing of this to show adequate rabies immunity. **With effect from 1 January 2012, pets travelling from EU member states and 'listed' Third countries which the EU considers do not present a high risk of rabies will no longer be required to have a blood test after vaccination against rabies.**
4. A correctly completed Pet Passport, with the relevant identification, vaccination and blood testing details. ▶

5. A waiting period after vaccination. For most countries (EU member states and 'listed' Third countries) this is 21 days. For the UK the waiting period is currently 6 months from the date of blood testing before animals can be considered for entry. **With effect from 1 January 2012, the waiting period before entering the UK after rabies vaccination will be reduced from 6 months to 21 days for pets from EU states and 'listed' Third countries, and to 4 months from 'unlisted' Third countries.**
6. A visit to a veterinary surgeon 24–48 hours prior to the return to the UK for tick and tapeworm treatment and certification to that effect. **With effect from 1 January 2012 there will be no requirement for tick treatment before embarkation to the UK. A similar approach is under consideration for tapeworm treatment.**

In order to keep 'passports' valid, rabies boosters must be repeated within the duration of immunity of the particular vaccine used.

Changes to the scheme will come into effect on 1 January 2012. The up-to-date requirements of the Department for Environment, Food and Rural Affairs should always be checked: see www.defra.gov.uk.

The immune system

This is the defence system by which the body protects against disease by detecting and resisting microbial or parasitic invasion. The immune system must distinguish invasion of these pathogens from the host's own healthy cells and tissues in order to function properly.

The immune system functions on three basic levels: physical barriers, innate immunity and acquired immunity. Throughout life, individuals are continuously exposed to a range of foreign antigens. These are delivered to the immune system, such that over time the individual can become resistant to a wide range of pathogens.

Physical barriers

Physical barriers to invasion (the skin and the surfaces of the gastrointestinal, respiratory and urogenital tracts) provide an initial obstacle. The movement of mucous secretions up the respiratory tract, coughing, sneezing, urine flow, vomiting and diarrhoea all aid in clearing pathogens.

Innate immunity

Innate immunity constitutes the next layer of defence. Components of innate immunity are either pre-existing or rapidly activated:

- **Pre-existing**: e.g. enzymes such as lysozyme in tears and saliva, and various proteins that can bind to bacteria and hasten their destruction
- **Rapidly activated**: cells such as macrophages and neutrophils can recognize molecules on the outside of invading microbes before engulfing (by phagocytosis) and destroying them (Figure 5.4). Inflammation allows blood flow to increase to areas of damaged tissue, allowing such cells to be directed to the site of injury.

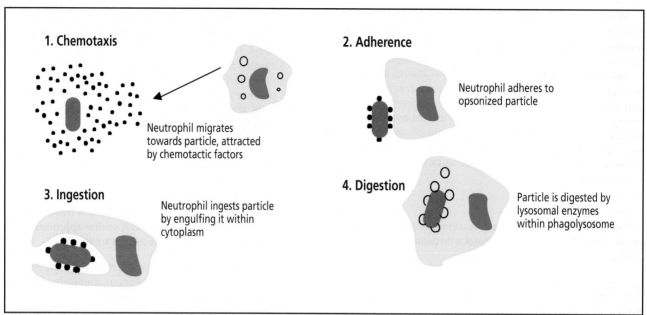

1. **Chemotaxis**

Neutrophil migrates towards particle, attracted by chemotactic factors

2. **Adherence**

Neutrophil adheres to opsonized particle

3. **Ingestion**

Neutrophil ingests particle by engulfing it within cytoplasm

4. **Digestion**

Particle is digested by lysosomal enzymes within phagolysosome

5.4   The process of phagocytosis. (1) **Chemotaxis**: neutrophils are attracted to areas of infection by chemical factors from bacteria or damaged cells. (2) **Adherence** of the neutrophil is facilitated by presence of **opsonins** such as antibodies or protein components known as **complement**. (3) **Ingestion**: The neutrophil engulfs the particle within its cytoplasm. (4) **Digestion**: the particle is digested within a phagolysosome by lysosomal enzymes.

Innate immunity is a vital and effective layer of defence, but many pathogens successfully overcome it, and more sophisticated and specific approaches are therefore required.

Acquired immunity

Acquired immunity recognizes and responds to specific foreign pathogens. Following infection, the immune system learns to produce specific cells and antibodies directed precisely against the particular pathogen involved. In contrast to the rapid response of innate immunity, this active immunity takes several days to begin to act against infections not previously encountered by the host. However, because specific memory cells are formed following initial exposure, a much more rapid response may be expected if challenged by the same pathogen again.

Active immunity is initiated when components of foreign substances and microbes that trigger immune recognition (antigens) are collected by antigen-presenting cells (e.g. dendritic cells and macrophages) and delivered to lymph nodes, where they are presented to lymphocytes. Some lymphocytes specifically recognize the antigen and become activated.

There are two major divisions of acquired immunity: humoral and cellular.

Humoral immunity

Humoral immunity (Figure 5.5) is associated with B lymphocytes (B cells), which mature within bone marrow. Activated B lymphocytes develop into plasma cells, which manufacture proteins called **antibodies** (composed of immunoglobulins). Antibodies lock on to specific foreign antigens and neutralize them, or facilitate the binding of other components of the immune system. Humoral immunity can be measured by assessing the level of specific antibodies in the blood. Such tests are commonly used as diagnostic tests for specific infections, e.g. feline leukaemia virus (FeLV) (see Chapter 19).

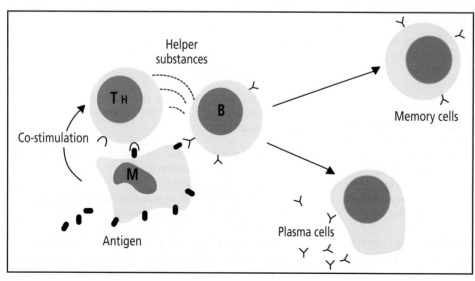

Helper substances

Co-stimulation

Antigen

Memory cells

Plasma cells

5.5   B cells differentiate into antibody-producing plasma cells and memory cells. Interaction with, and stimulation by, antigen-presenting cells such as macrophages (M) and helper T cells (T_H) is needed for this to occur.

Humoral immunity can be acquired via passive transfer of antibodies. In nature, this is by passage of **maternally derived antibodies** (MDA) across the placenta and in the first milk (colostrum) from a dam to her offspring. Whereas in humans the vast majority of MDA pass across the placenta before birth, in dogs and cats few MDA are received in this way and the vast majority are present in the colostrum. The intestine of neonatal animals is initially permeable to the passage of these antibodies, allowing an efficient transfer into their circulation. However, the efficiency of this transfer declines rapidly within hours of birth and this means that significant delays to colostral intake by young animals may lead to poor passive immunity and increased risk of infection. Whereas active immunity invokes immunological memory, passive immunity confers only *temporary* protection. Within a few weeks of birth, MDA decline to non-protective levels, whereupon young animals become more susceptible to disease.

Cellular immunity

Cellular or cell-mediated immunity does not involve antibodies, instead it is associated with the activity of T lymphocytes (T cells), which mature within the thymus. Activated T lymphocytes manufacture chemical messengers called cytokines, which help to direct immune cell functions and responses. There are a number of different types of T lymphocyte:

- **Helper T cells** recognize processed antigen and coordinate macrophages and B cells in the immune response, promoting immune function (see Figure 5.5)
- **Cytotoxic T cells** destroy cells infected with intracellular pathogens such as viruses
- **Suppressor T cells** keep the immune system in check by suppressing immune reactions within tolerable limits. Decreased activity of these cells is one mechanism by which the immune system may begin to damage the body's own tissues and organs (see 'Autoimmune disease', later).

Principles of vaccination

The purpose of a vaccine is to stimulate an active immune response in the recipient against one or more specific pathogens, such that an improvement in clinical outcome is seen following infection. Resulting immunity varies, depending on the pathogen and vaccine, from full protection of the host against clinical disease, infection and shedding (sterilizing immunity) to simply a reduction of clinical signs following infection. The contribution made by vaccination towards preventing and reducing the incidence of major infectious diseases in humans and animals is, without doubt, enormous. Many serious contagious diseases are seldom seen today, but continued widespread vaccination is essential if this is to remain so.

Immunization may be passive or active.

- **Passive immunization**: This involves administration of antisera or antitoxins containing concentrated antibodies against either a pathogen or a toxin, respectively. Used in the treatment of disease or at the time of possible exposure, passive immunization cannot give long-term protection, because the levels of antibody decline over several weeks. An important example is the preventive use of tetanus antitoxin in horses with wounds and for therapy of animals with clinical tetanus.
- **Active immunization**: Most vaccines stimulate immunity by exposing the immune system to foreign antigens associated with specific infections. Immunological memory stimulated by such exposure means that, if challenged by the same infections, acquired immunity quickly neutralizes or minimizes the threat.

Types of vaccine

There are three broad categories of vaccine product designed for active immunization (see also Chapter 8): attenuated (live) vaccines; inactivated (killed) vaccines; and subunit, recombinant and vector vaccines.

Attenuated (live) vaccines

Live vaccines usually contain weakened (attenuated) strains of the pathogen, i.e. strains that cannot cause disease in the host. The immune response following vaccination with such products mimics what occurs following natural infection. Good cellular and humoral immunity is usually stimulated, and a protective immune response can often be expected rapidly after one dose. A potential concern when using live vaccines is reversion of the vaccine strain to virulence, although stringent trials required for licensing make this an unlikely scenario.

Inactivated (killed) vaccines

Inactivated vaccines remove the potential for reversion to virulence by containing pathogens that have been inactivated or killed. Many inactivated vaccines contain an **adjuvant**. An adjuvant is an agent that stimulates (irritates) the immune system to find and react to the vaccine agent. Killed vaccines often also require two or more doses to stimulate an effective response (Figure 5.6) and are usually better at stimulating humoral than cell-mediated responses. In some cases, the immunity acquired from a killed vaccine may not be as durable or complete as that from a live equivalent.

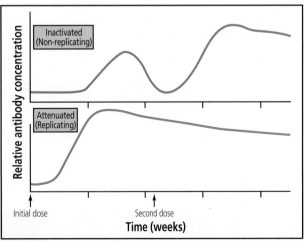

5.6 Comparison of antibody responses following inoculation with an inactivated vaccine (top) and a live attenuated vaccine (bottom). In this example, one dose of live vaccine is adequate to stimulate active immunity whereas a second dose of the inactivated product is required to stimulate a protective 'anamnestic' response.

Inactivated toxins used as vaccines are known as toxoids. Most commonly used in horses, tetanus toxoid stimulates active immunity to give longer-term protection in contrast to antitoxins, which are for short-term treatment and prophylaxis only.

Subunit, recombinant and vector vaccines

Subunit vaccines contain a small fragment or fragments of pathogen that contain the necessary antigens. Some are termed **recombinant vaccines** because they are manufactured using genetic engineering techniques. One advantage of recombinant vaccine technology is that there is virtually no chance of the host becoming ill from the agent, since it is just a single protein, not the organism itself. Traditional vaccine risks come from the organism not being totally weakened (attenuated), or a reversion to a virulent (disease-causing) form. Adjuvants may be one vaccine component responsible for some expected adverse effects such as local swelling at the injection site, malaise and fever.

Vector vaccines try to combine the potential advantages of live vaccines with some of the advantages of using an inactivated subunit vaccine. In vector vaccines the useful subunits are incorporated into a different non-pathogenic live virus. One feline leukaemia vaccine currently available in the UK uses a canarypox virus, genetically modified to contain important feline leukaemia virus (FeLV) antigens, to stimulate immunity. An advantage of vector vaccine technology is that an adjuvant may not be needed to stimulate the immune response adequately.

Administering vaccines

Vaccine antigens available for use in dogs, cats and rabbits in the UK at the time of writing are listed in Figure 5.7.

For dogs

• Canine distemper.
• Infectious canine hepatitis.
• Canine parvovirus.
• Leptospirosis (*Leptospira canicola* and *L. icterohaemorrhagiae*). Rabies.
• Kennel cough:
  – Canine parainfluenza virus [a]
  – *Bordetella bronchiseptica* [b]
• Canine herpesvirus.
• Tetanus toxoid.

For cats

• Feline panleucopenia.
• Cat 'flu:
  – Feline calicivirus
  – Feline herpesvirus
  – *Bordetella bronchiseptica* [b]
• *Chlamydophila felis*.
• Feline leukaemia virus.
• Tetanus toxoid.

For rabbits
Myxomatosis. Viral haemorrhagic disease.

5.7   Disease antigens currently available as vaccines for small animals in the UK. [a] Parenteral or intranasal combined vaccines available. [b] Intranasal vaccine available.

Some vaccines contain single components (e.g. parvovirus alone) but, for convenience, a number of different components are often packaged together as a **multivalent** vaccine, conferring activity against more than one pathogen. Recommendations for use of different vaccines vary and are detailed within product data sheets. Live vaccines are often freeze-dried, requiring reconstitution with a diluent prior to use (Figure 5.8).

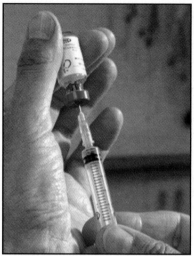

5.8   Preparing a vaccine for use.

Not all vaccines are administered by injection. Figure 5.9 shows a *Bordetella* vaccine being administered intranasally to a cat. Intranasal administration stimulates the rapid formation of specific antibodies on the lining of the respiratory tract, which neutralize infection at the point of entry. Intranasal vaccines typically work within a few days and can be effective in the face of MDA, allowing some such products to be used to protect even very young animals.

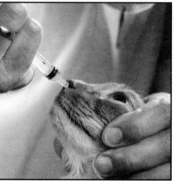

5.9   Intranasal vaccination in a cat.

Primary vaccination

Primary vaccination describes the initial administration or course of administrations that establishes immunity. Significant levels of passive antibodies (e.g. MDA) can interfere with the immune response to the vaccine. The recommendations for timing of primary vaccine course doses are based on an understanding of when MDA will decline to levels that will not interfere with the immune response (Figure 5.10).

• Canine vaccines currently in use in the UK have recommendations for the final dose of the primary course to be given at 10 or 12 weeks of age; for cats, 12 weeks is most commonly the age at which the final dose of the primary course is given. Some vaccine guidelines now recommend a later finish, especially in puppies in areas where canine parvovirus is common. The WSAVA

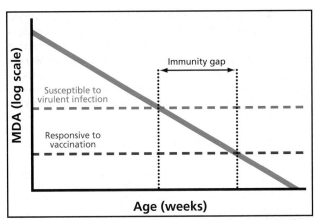

5.10 The fall in maternally derived antibodies (MDA) is depicted by the solid line. As MDA interferes with response to vaccination, the final vaccination is timed to coincide with the expected decline in MDA to a point where a response is possible. The period between the decline in MDA to non-protective levels and vaccinal immunity developing is known as the **immunity gap**. Animals exposed to infection during this period will not be protected.

Vaccination Guidelines Group (VGG) established in 2006 published key opinion recommendations on best practice for the vaccination of dogs and cats and is available on the WSAVA website www.wsava.org.

- The greatest immunity is passed on to a foal from a mare if she is vaccinated 1–3 months before foaling. The foal can then begin the primary course of vaccinations at 5–6 months. If the mare has not been vaccinated, the mare and foal should receive a tetanus antitoxin injection within 24 hours of foaling. The foal can then begin its tetanus vaccine course at 6 weeks of age and its 'flu course from 3 months.

A **turnout period** (often around 7–14 days) should be carefully observed following final vaccination before protective immunity is established and individuals can be exposed to risk; during this time animals should not be allowed outside or in contact with others that may pose a disease risk.

Booster vaccinations

Booster vaccinations are required in those individuals where immunity may decline to non-protective levels. For some UK canine vaccines against distemper, hepatitis and parvovirus, the recommended licensed intervals have changed

to every 3 or 4 years (though recommendations vary with manufacturer). Available evidence shows that annual boosters against other diseases, such as leptospirosis, are still essential to maintain optimal immunity. A similar approach is taken with cats and it is therefore important to check manufacturer's guidelines.

Immune-mediated disorders

Allergy and hypersensitivity reactions

Allergy is a state of exaggerated immune sensitivity induced by exposure to a particular, usually otherwise harmless, antigen (or allergen), resulting in harmful immunological reactions on subsequent exposures. Allergies may be localized problems in one organ (e.g. skin, intestinal tract, respiratory tract) or can result in systemic and potentially life-threatening reactions.

Hypersensitivity reactions are the inappropriate immune responses that result from exposure to a foreign antigen, and are the underlying mechanisms for allergies as well as a number of other important autoimmune diseases (see below) and rare drug and vaccine reactions. Different forms occur. A type I (immediate-type) hypersensitivity reaction is perhaps the most familiar and is the classical underlying mechanism for allergic reactions such as hay fever in humans, urticaria (wheals) and atopic dermatitis. Clinical signs vary from mild and localized (hay fever) through to systemic and life-threatening (anaphylactic shock).

Other hypersensitivity reactions are underlying mechanisms for a number of diseases, including autoimmune disease. Figure 5.11 summarizes the different types of hypersensitivity reactions seen in animals and gives examples of diseases where such reactions are noted.

Autoimmune disease

Autoimmunity occurs if the immune system reacts to one or more of the body's own tissues as foreign. Although rare, such conditions can prove life-threatening and difficult to manage. Examples include: pemphigus complex, where the immune system specifically attacks the skin and/or

Hypersensitivity reaction	Type	Components	Disease examples
I	Immediate-type	Antigen binds to IgE antibodies on mast cells, which release histamine and other inflammatory mediators	Atopy; hay fever; urticaria; anaphylactic shock
II	Antibody-dependent or cytotoxic	Antibodies attach to antigens on the body's own cells (e.g. red blood cells), triggering their destruction	Immune-mediated haemolytic anaemia; transfusion reactions; pemphigus complex; babesiosis
III	Immune complex	Immune complexes of antibody and antigen form in tissues (e.g. joints, kidneys, blood vessels), precipitating damage	Immune-mediated polyarthritis; glomerulonephritis; vasculitis
IV	Delayed-type	A cell-mediated reaction involving cytotoxic T cells, helper T cells and macrophages	Tuberculosis; allergic contact dermatitis; feline infectious peritonitis (FIP)

5.11 Hypersensitivity reaction types.

mucocutaneous junctions; rheumatoid arthritis; and immune-mediated haemolytic anaemia (IMHA), which is characterized by the breakdown of red blood cells, resulting in anaemia. Some types of endocrine disease, such as diabetes and hypothyroidism in dogs, may also arise as a result of an immune-mediated destruction of glandular tissues.

Graft rejection

Transplanting organs and tissues is a regular occurrence in human surgery and there is now some interest in the veterinary field. A potential problem is rejection of the graft or implant because the recipient's immune system may recognize transplanted tissue as foreign and attack it. Careful tissue matching reduces such risks; nevertheless, lifelong use of immunosuppressive drugs by the recipient is usually necessary.

Acknowledgement

The authors would like to thank Intervet/Schering-Plough Animal Health for their assistance with the preparation of the charts and images used in this chapter.

Further reading

Day MJ (1999) *Clinical Immunology of the Dog and Cat*. Manson Publishing, London

Day MJ, Horzinek MC and Schultz RD (2010) WSAVA Guidelines for the Vaccination of Dogs and Cats. *Journal of Small Animal Practice* **51**, 338–356. The full version of the Guidelines is available online at www.wileyonlinelibrary.com/journal/JSAP – see Volume 51, Issue 6 (DOI: 10.1111/j.1748–5827.2010.00959a.x)

Greene (2006) *Infectious Diseases of the Dog and Cat, 3rd edition*. WB Saunders, Philadelphia

NOAH *Compendium of Data Sheets for Veterinary Products*

Thrusfield N (2005) *Veterinary Epidemiology, 3rd edition*. Wiley Blackwell, Oxford

Tizard IR (2004) *Veterinary Immunology – An Introduction, 7th edn*. Elsevier, Philadelphia

Useful websites

MRSA:
www.thebellamossfoundation.com

Pet Travel Scheme:
www.defra.gov.uk/wildlife-pets/pets/travel/index.htm

WSAVA vaccine guidelines:
www.wsava.org

Self-assessment questions

1. Using specific examples, describe the main routes of entry for pathogens into hosts.
2. Using specific examples, describe how pathogens can be transmitted between hosts.
3. What three levels does the immune system function on?
4. How do physical barriers provide obstacles to pathogen invasion?
5. What is the difference between innate immunity and acquired immunity?
6. Define a zoonotic infection and list five zoonotic pathogens that can infect cats.
7. Describe three different types of vaccines available.
8. Which types of patients are at the highest risk of nosocomial infections?
9. Describe the precautions required whilst nursing a patient with MRSA infection.
10. Why is the timing of puppy, kitten and foal vaccinations important?

Chapter 6

Elementary microbiology

Maggie Fisher and Helen Moreton

Learning objectives

After studying this chapter, students should be able to:

- **Understand the different types of microbes encountered in animals**
- **Describe the important bacterial, viral and fungal infections of companion animals**
- **Describe the theoretical and practical skills necessary to identify microbial infection in animals**
- **Describe the measures used to control and treat infectious diseases**

6.1 Relative sizes of microorganisms. A white blood cell (lymphocyte) is shown for comparison.

Introduction

The microorganisms described in this chapter represent a very small proportion of all microorganisms and are those that interrelate with animal hosts in some way. They vary in size from the relatively large ringworm fungi to viruses that can only be seen with an electron microscope (Figure 6.1). The major similarities and differences between the different types of microorganism are shown in Figure 6.2.

There are several ways in which microorganisms can relate to hosts (Figure 6.3). Some microorganisms may be beneficial or neutral in effect; however, the focus of this chapter will be upon those that have the potential to harm their hosts by causing infection or disease in dogs, cats, exotic pets and horses. A few important organisms that are carried by cats and dogs without clinical signs but are capable of causing disease in humans (i.e. are zoonotic) are included.

Characteristic	Bacteria	Viruses	Fungi	Protozoa	Algae
Size	0.5–5 μm	20–300 nm	3–8 μm (yeasts)	10–200 μm	Approximately 20 μm
Cell arrangement	Unicellular	Non-cellular	Unicellular or multicellular	Unicellular	Unicellular or multicellular
Cell wall	Present; mainly peptidoglycan	Absent	Present; mainly chitin	Absent	Present; mainly cellulose
Nucleus	No true membrane-bound nucleus	Absent	Membrane-bound nucleus	Membrane-bound nucleus	Membrane-bound nucleus
Nucleic acids	DNA and RNA	DNA or RNA	DNA and RNA	DNA and RNA	DNA and RNA
Reproduction	Asexual by binary fission	Replicate only within another living cell	Asexual and sexual by spores, budding in yeast	Asexual and sexual	Asexual and sexual

6.2 Major similarities and differences between different types of microorganism.

continues ▶

Characteristic	Bacteria	Viruses	Fungi	Protozoa	Algae
Nutrition	Mainly heterotrophic – can be saprophytic or parasitic; a few are autotrophic	Obligate parasites	Heterotrophic – can be saprophytic or parasitic	Heterotrophic – can be saprophytic or parasitic	Autotrophic
Motility	Some are motile	Non-motile	Non-motile except for certain spore forms	Motile	Some are motile
Toxin production	Some form toxins	None	Some form toxins	Some form toxins	Some form toxins

6.2 *continued* Major similarities and differences between different types of microorganism.

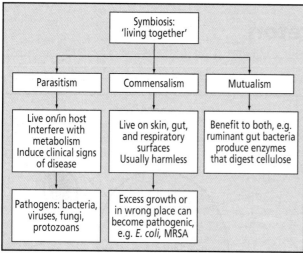

6.3 Relationships between microorganisms and animal hosts.

Microorganisms obtain their nutrition from a variety of sources and some have more specific nutritional requirements than others (see Figure 6.2).

- **Heterotrophic organisms** utilize carbon in the form of organic carbon from other organisms for growth.
- **Autotropic organisms** produce their own food from simple inorganic molecules.
- **Saprophytic organisms** live off dead or decaying matter.
- **Parasitic organisms** live in or on a living organism at the expense of the other organism – the host.

Viruses

Structure and naming

Viruses are extremely small and are sometimes not classified as living organisms, as they are incapable of reproduction without a host cell. A virus particle, or **virion**, is little more than a package containing instructions for the recreation of further virus particles. Each virus particle is composed of two parts (Figure 6.4):

- *Nucleic acid* – RNA or DNA (never both) forming a **central core**
- *A protein coat* – the **capsid**.

Together, these two parts form the **nucleocapsid**. For some viruses, this is all that an individual virus particle will comprise.

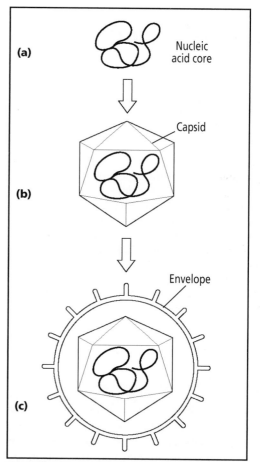

6.4 General virus components: **(a)** central core of nucleic acid; **(b)** capsid surrounding the nucleic acid to form a nucleocapsid (with icosahedral symmetry); **(c)** in addition, some viruses possess an outer envelope.

Various shapes of virus nucleocapsid have been identified:

- Helical
- Icosahedral
- Complex (poxvirus)
- Composite (some bacteriophages).

Some viruses have an additional envelope around the outside, often formed of the host cell membrane (Figure 6.4c). Each of the helical or icosahedral shapes of the nucleocapsid can be enveloped or non-enveloped (Figure 6.5), giving four possible basic shapes for viruses. In fact, there are no animal viruses (only plant viruses) that are helical and non-enveloped, so viruses of dogs and cats can be grouped by and large into the other three types. Viruses have been classified together on the basis of structural similarities. For example, the group of viruses causing true 'flu are the influenza viruses.

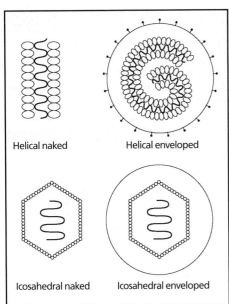

6.5 Helical and icosahedral viruses may be enveloped or non-enveloped (naked).

Helical naked · Helical enveloped

Icosahedral naked · Icosahedral enveloped

Viral replication

A virus is only able to attach to cells that carry a compatible receptor. For example, influenza viruses can only attach to ciliated epithelial cells in the respiratory tract. This specificity of viruses for specific tissues is known as tissue tropism. Viruses normally have only one or two host species that they are able to infect, e.g. parvovirus in dogs does not infect cats, and measles virus will only infect humans and apes. Once attached, virus particles are taken into the host cell (Figure 6.6) by fusing the virus envelope with the host cell membrane or, in the case of non-enveloped viruses, by causing the host cell to engulf the virus particle into the cell. Once inside the cell, the virus is able to switch the cell's normal metabolism to obey the instructions of the virus. The virus may cause this to happen immediately, so that the cell begins to produce the constituents of new virus particles within hours of infection. Alternatively, as in the case of feline leukaemia virus (FeLV), the virus may join to the host cell's own nucleic acid for an extended period before making any changes to cell metabolism. New virus particles are then assembled and released from the cell. Depending on the virus, this may leave the host cell intact or may cause its rupture and destruction.

Transmission

Viruses are transmitted from host to host either directly (e.g. by a cat licking feline calicivirus in nasal secretions from the face of another cat) or indirectly (e.g. a dog licking the floor of a kennel that had been occupied by a dog with parvovirus infection and had not been adequately cleaned). Different viruses have adapted their means of transmission according to their structure (which affects their ability to survive in the environment) and their location in the host. For example, a respiratory tract virus is often transmitted by virus particles being sneezed from one host into the air breathed in by another host. This is ideal for influenza virus, as these enveloped viruses are not very robust and do not survive for extended periods in the environment. An ability to survive in the environment for longer periods is beneficial for canine parvovirus. The virus must be licked up and ingested by another dog for infection of the gastrointestinal tract to occur.

Incubation

Once a host animal has been infected with a small number of virus particles, there is a time lag before the symptoms that are associated with the infection are seen; this is the **incubation period**. During this time, the virus reaches the cells that it can invade and initially infects a small number of cells in order to increase the number of virus particles. Clinical signs are seen once large numbers of virus particles infect a large number of cells.

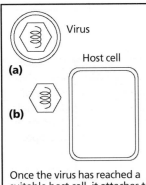

Once the virus has reached a suitable host cell, it attaches to receptor sites on the host cell membrane. **(a)** Enveloped virus **(b)** Naked virus

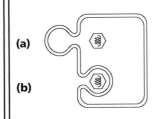

(a) The envelope of the virus may fuse with the cell wall and release the nucleocapsid into the cell or **(b)** the virus may be taken into the cell by endocytosis.

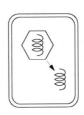

The virus enters the host cell and the protein coat (capsid) breaks down to release the viral nucleic acid.

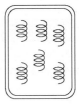

The viral nucleic acid replicates (either in the host cell cytoplasm or nucleus) and directs the host cell metabolism to make new virus material.

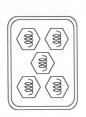

The new viruses are assembled.

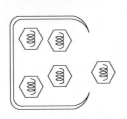

They leave the host cell either by rupture of the cell membrane (naked viruses); or

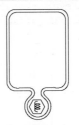

through the cell membrane (enveloped viruses).

6.6 Replication of animal viruses.

Viral diseases

Some infections in dogs and cats that are caused by viruses are shown in Figures 6.7 and 6.8. Some examples of viral infections of horses and exotic pets are shown in Figures 6.9 and 6.10. More medical details of viral diseases in small animals can be found in Chapter 20.

Diagnosis of viral infections

Viral infections may be diagnosed on the basis of clinical signs and the animal's history. Often there are several infections that may cause similar signs and it may be important to be able to confirm the particular virus present. This may be carried out in a number of ways, including the following:

Name of virus	Disease caused	Nucleic acid type	Shape of nucleocapsid	Enveloped
Parvovirus	Parvovirus	DNA	Icosahedral	No
Canine adenovirus 1 (CAV-1)	Infectious canine hepatitis	DNA	Icosahedral	No
Canine adenovirus 2 (CAV-2)	Infectious canine tracheobronchitis	DNA	Icosahedral	No
Canine distemper virus	Distemper	RNA	Helical	Yes
Canine parainfluenza virus	Part of kennel cough syndrome	RNA	Helical	Yes
Rabies virus	Rabies	RNA	Helical	Yes
Canine herpesvirus	Disease and death in very young pups	DNA	Icosahedral	Yes
Canine coronavirus	Vomiting and diarrhoea	RNA	Helical	Yes

6.7   Some viral diseases of dogs.

Name of virus	Disease caused	Nucleic acid type	Shape of nucleocapsid	Enveloped
Feline parvovirus (panleucopenia)	Feline infectious enteritis	DNA	Icosahedral	No
Feline herpesvirus	Feline rhinotracheitis; cat flu	DNA	Icosahedral	Yes
Feline calicivirus	Cat flu	RNA	Icosahedral	No
Feline coronavirus	Feline infectious peritonitis (FIP)	RNA	Helical	Yes
Feline leukaemia virus	Feline leukaemia	RNA	Icosahedral	Yes
Feline immunodeficiency virus	FIV infection	RNA	Icosahedral	Yes
Rabies virus	Rabies, although cats are less susceptible to infection than dogs	RNA	Helical	Yes

6.8   Some viral diseases of cats.

Name of virus	Disease caused	Nucleic acid type	Shape of nucleocapsid	Enveloped
Influenza virus	Equine influenza or 'flu	RNA	Helical	Yes
Equine herpes virus (EHV) 1	Equine herpesvirus infection	DNA	Icosahedral	Yes
Equine arteritis virus (EAV)	Equine viral arteritis (EVA)	RNA	Icosahedral	Yes
African horse sickness virus (AHSV)	African horse sickness (AHS)	RNA	Icosahedral	No
Equine rotavirus	Diarrhoea	RNA	Icosahedral	No

6.9   Examples of viral infections of horses.

Name of virus	Disease caused	Nucleic acid type	Shape of nucleocapsid	Enveloped	Host species
Canine distemper virus	Canine distemper	RNA	Helical	Yes	Ferret
Hamster polyomavirus	HaPV infection	DNA	Icosahedral	No	Hamster
Herpesvirus	Herpes virus infection	DNA	Icosahedral	Yes	Tortoise
Myxoma (a poxvirus)	Myxomatosis	DNA	Brick-shaped, slightly pleomorphic	Yes	Rabbit
RHV virus	Haemorrhagic fever	RNA	Icosahedral	No	Rabbit

6.10   Examples of viral infections of exotic pets.

- Virus particles are too small to be seen with the light microscope but they may be seen with an electron microscope
- Large numbers of virus particles may clump together in cells; the clump may then be seen with the light microscope. Large groups of rabies virus are seen in cells of animals infected with rabies; these are known as Negri bodies. An animal can only be examined for these and a number of other virus-related changes at post-mortem
- Serology may be carried out to detect the specific antibody produced by the host in response to infection (e.g. FIV). In some cases the virus protein (antigen) can be detected directly in serum (e.g. FeLV)
- Polymerase chain reaction (PCR) can be used to amplify and detect the nucleic acid of the virus (e.g. canine distemper).

Treatment of viral infections

Viral infections can be combatted in a number of ways. Treatment of viral infections in animals normally involves supportive nursing, for example:

- Fluids (oral and intravenous) (see Chapter 22) to prevent dehydration in the case of canine parvovirus infection
- Tempting foods for cats with cat 'flu
- Antibacterials to limit secondary bacterial infection.

Animals may also be vaccinated in order to stimulate an immune response (see Chapters 5 and 8).

There are now some specialized treatments for a few viral infections. These are mainly used in humans for HIV (human immunodeficiency virus), the shingles form of chickenpox and for herpes simplex (the cause of cold sores).

Some antiviral treatments are also used in companion animals, though this is mainly confined to ophthalmic treatment and to treatment of cats infected with feline leukaemia or feline immunodeficiency virus (e.g. zidovudine for FIV). Some interferon-containing treatments are commercially available, indicated for example to combat parvovirus infection in dogs.

Prevention of viral infection

As viral infections are difficult to treat once the animal is infected, control has been aimed at preventing infection, particularly of severe viral diseases. This can be done at a number of levels:

- A country can have a border policy to prevent entry of diseases that are not present in that country, e.g. countries seek to prevent entry of rabies by quarantine or vaccination policies (see Chapter 5)
- Accommodation can be designed to avoid or limit the spread of infection, e.g. catteries may be designed so that airborne viruses are not readily transmitted from cat to cat (see Chapter 12)
- Suitable disinfectants can be used to kill viruses that may be present in animal cages between occupants (see Chapter 12), e.g. to prevent the transmission of parvovirus between dogs
- Individual animals may be protected by vaccination, e.g. canine distemper, canine parvovirus, feline leukaemia. More details about vaccination may be found in Chapters 5 and 8.

Prions

Prions are very small protein particles that cause infections within the central nervous system, leading eventually to the death of the animal. The incubation period is usually long; it takes from 2 months to 20 years before signs of disease become apparent. Until relatively recently, the study of prion diseases was highly specialized work carried out by only a few people. Researchers had investigated scrapie, which is a transmissable spongiform encephalopathy of sheep, caused by a prion, and has been recorded in Europe for the last 200 years. Interest and research in prion infections increased greatly following the outbreak of bovine spongiform encephalopathy (BSE), which was first identified in the UK in the mid 1980s. It appears that BSE may be transmissible to humans as a result of eating infected beef. Over 150 deaths have been attributed to such infection resulting in variant CJD (vCJD) a form of the human encephalopathy, Creutzfeldt–Jacob disease (CJD). Around 20 cases of a similar disease, feline spongiform encephalopathy (FSE), in cats and other felids have been recorded since 1990. Affected cats exhibit nervous signs and incoordination. Much research effort is now aimed at being able to confirm disease in the live animal. At present, diagnosis is normally based on the appearance of brain tissue at post-mortem examination.

Bacteria

Size and shape

Bacteria (singular: bacterium) are single-celled organisms and most range in size from 0.5 μm (micrometres or microns; 10^{-6} m) to 5 μm in length, though there are some exceptions. The shape and physiology of bacteria present in infections are used to identify their species and thus assess prognosis and suitable treatments.

Three basic shapes are generally recognized and these are sometimes used as a means of classification and naming of bacteria:

- Cylindrical or rod-shaped cells (Figure 6.11a) are called **bacilli** (singular: bacillus). Some bacilli are curved (Figure 6.11b) and these are known as **vibrios**
- Spherical cells are called **cocci** (singular: coccus). Some cocci exist singly while others remain together in pairs after cell division and are called **diplococci**. Those that remain attached to form chains are called **streptococci** (Figure 6.11c) and if they divide randomly and form irregular grape-like clusters they are called **staphylococci** (Figure 6.11d)
- Spiral or helical cells are called **spirochaetes**.

Structure

Some of the structures shown in the generalized bacterial cell depicted in Figure 6.12 are common to all cells; others are only present in certain species or under certain environmental conditions.

Bacteria are commonly stained with the Gram stain, which differentially stains many bacteria either purple (Gram-positive) or pink (Gram-negative) depending on the structure of their cell wall.

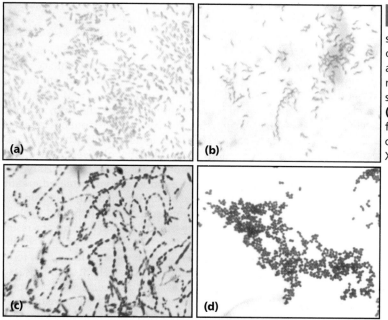

6.11 Classification of bacteria by shape. These preparations have all been stained with Gram stain: Gram-negative organisms appear pink; Gram-positive organisms appear purple. **(a)** Rods. **(b)** *Campylobacter* sp. rods appear bent; single rods appear banana-shaped and pairs resemble flying seagulls. **(c)** *Streptococcus* sp. cocci showing chain formation. **(d)** *Staphylococcus* sp. cocci showing characteristic clumping. (Original magnification X500) (© Andrew Rycroft)

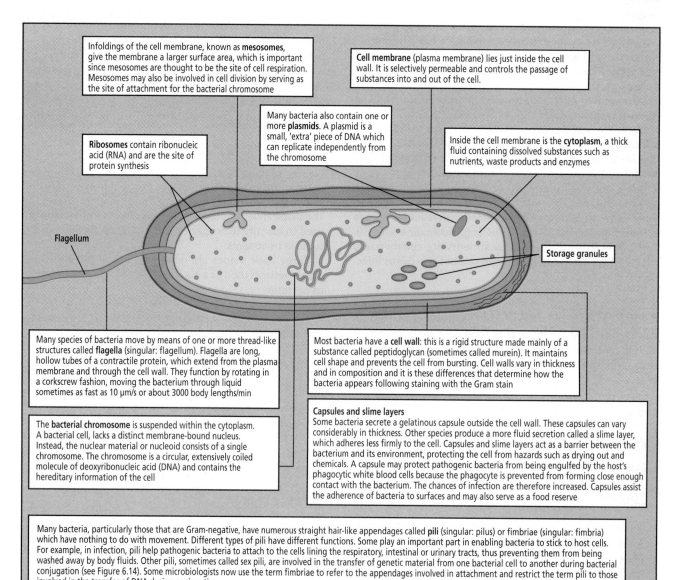

Infoldings of the cell membrane, known as **mesosomes**, give the membrane a larger surface area, which is important since mesosomes are thought to be the site of cell respiration. Mesosomes may also be involved in cell division by serving as the site of attachment for the bacterial chromosome

Cell membrane (plasma membrane) lies just inside the cell wall. It is selectively permeable and controls the passage of substances into and out of the cell.

Many bacteria also contain one or more **plasmids**. A plasmid is a small, 'extra' piece of DNA which can replicate independently from the chromosome

Ribosomes contain ribonucleic acid (RNA) and are the site of protein synthesis

Inside the cell membrane is the **cytoplasm**, a thick fluid containing dissolved substances such as nutrients, waste products and enzymes

Flagellum

Storage granules

Many species of bacteria move by means of one or more thread-like structures called **flagella** (singular: flagellum). Flagella are long, hollow tubes of a contractile protein, which extend from the plasma membrane and through the cell wall. They function by rotating in a corkscrew fashion, moving the bacterium through liquid sometimes as fast as 10 μm/s or about 3000 body lengths/min

Most bacteria have a **cell wall**: this is a rigid structure made mainly of a substance called peptidoglycan (sometimes called murein). It maintains cell shape and prevents the cell from bursting. Cell walls vary in thickness and in composition and it is these differences that determine how the bacteria appears following staining with the Gram stain

Capsules and slime layers
Some bacteria secrete a gelatinous capsule outside the cell wall. These capsules can vary considerably in thickness. Other species produce a more fluid secretion called a slime layer, which adheres less firmly to the cell. Capsules and slime layers act as a barrier between the bacterium and its environment, protecting the cell from hazards such as drying out and chemicals. A capsule may protect pathogenic bacteria from being engulfed by the host's phagocytic white blood cells because the phagocyte is prevented from forming close enough contact with the bacterium. The chances of infection are therefore increased. Capsules assist the adherence of bacteria to surfaces and may also serve as a food reserve

The **bacterial chromosome** is suspended within the cytoplasm. A bacterial cell, lacks a distinct membrane-bound nucleus. Instead, the nuclear material or nucleoid consists of a single chromosome. The chromosome is a circular, extensively coiled molecule of deoxyribonucleic acid (DNA) and contains the hereditary information of the cell

Many bacteria, particularly those that are Gram-negative, have numerous straight hair-like appendages called **pili** (singular: pilus) or fimbriae (singular: fimbria) which have nothing to do with movement. Different types of pili have different functions. Some play an important part in enabling bacteria to stick to host cells. For example, in infection, pili help pathogenic bacteria to attach to the cells lining the respiratory, intestinal or urinary tracts, thus preventing them from being washed away by body fluids. Other pili, sometimes called sex pili, are involved in the transfer of genetic material from one bacterial cell to another during bacterial conjugation (see Figure 6.14). Some microbiologists now use the term fimbriae to refer to the appendages involved in attachment and restrict the term pili to those involved in the transfer of DNA during conjugation

6.12 Components of a generalized bacterial cell and their functions.

Naming bacteria

All bacteria, in common with plants and animals, are named according to the binomial system. The first word starts with a capital letter and indicates the genus (plural: genera) to which they belong (e.g. *Escherichia*). This is followed by the species name all written in lower case (e.g. *coli*). Thus *Escherichia coli* is one of the species of the genus *Escherichia*, just as *Homo sapiens* (modern humans) is one of the species of the genus *Homo*. The generic name is frequently shortened to an initial letter, e.g. *Escherichia coli* becomes *E. coli*; *Staphylococcus aureus* may be seen written as *Staph. aureus*. Both generic and specific names are written *in italics*.

Endospores

Some species of bacteria produce dormant forms called endospores (or simply **spores**), which can survive in unfavourable conditions. They are formed when the vegetative (growing) cells are deprived of some factor, e.g. when the supply of nutrients is inadequate. It is important to note that endospore formation (or **sporulation**) is not a method of reproduction: one vegetative cell produces a single spore which, after germination, is again just one vegetative cell. Spore formation is most common in the genera *Bacillus* and *Clostridium*. These genera contain the causative agents of tetanus, anthrax and botulism. These diseases are zoonoses, affecting domestic pets, farm animals and humans. Species susceptibility to each disease varies; for example, dogs only infrequently suffer from tetanus, whilst horses are very susceptible and require routine vaccination, as do humans.

Many endospore-forming bacteria are inhabitants of the soil, but spores can exist almost everywhere, including in dust. They are extremely resistant structures that can remain viable for many years. They can survive extremes of heat, pH, desiccation, ultraviolet radiation and exposure to toxic chemicals, such as some disinfectants. The reason why endospores are so resistant is not completely understood, but heat resistance is thought to be due to the fact that a dehydration process occurs during spore formation, which expels most of the water from the spore. The spore develops within the bacterial cell, and under the microscope it appears as a bright, round or oval structure.

The fact that spores are so hard to destroy is the principal reason for the various sterilization procedures that are carried out in veterinary practice. Common techniques employed to kill spores include:

- Autoclaving (moist heat, 121°C under pressure 6.9 kPa for more than 15 minutes)
- Tyndallization (repeated steaming)
- Dry heat (160°C for at least 2 hours).

Conditions necessary for bacterial growth

Bacteria can grow and reproduce only when environmental conditions are suitable. The essential requirements for growth include:

- A supply of suitable nutrients
- The correct temperature (the temperature at which a species of bacterium grows most rapidly is the optimum growth temperature; most mammalian pathogens grow best at normal body temperature)
- The correct pH (the majority of mammalian pathogens grow best at pH 7–7.4)

- Water
- The correct gaseous environment (many species of bacterium can grow only when oxygen is present).

Bacteria that must have oxygen for growth are called strict or **obligate aerobes**. Some, known as **obligate anaerobes**, can only grow in the *absence* of oxygen, while others, the **facultative anaerobes**, grow aerobically when oxygen is present but can also function in the absence of oxygen. A few species, the **microaerophiles**, grow best when the concentration of oxygen is lower than in atmospheric air, e.g. *Campylobacter* spp.

Reproduction of bacteria

If their environment is suitable, bacteria can grow and reproduce rapidly. The time interval between successive divisions is called the **generation time**. In some bacteria the generation time is very short; for others it is quite long. For example, under optimum conditions the generation time of *E. coli* is 20 minutes, whereas for the tuberculosis bacterium *Mycobacterium tuberculosis* it is approximately 18 hours. Given appropriate conditions, growth is exponential, i.e. one bacterium produces two, then two produce four, and so on.

Bacteria reproduce asexually by simply dividing into two identical daughter cells, a process called **binary fission** (Figure 6.13). Prior to cell division, the cell grows; once it has reached a certain size, the circular chromosome or nucleoid replicates to form two identical chromosomes. As the parent cell enlarges, the chromosomes are separated and the cell membrane grows inwards at the centre of the cell. At the same time, new cell wall material grows inwards to form the septum and this divides the cell into two daughter cells. These may separate completely, but in some species (e.g. streptococci, staphylococci) they remain attached to form the characteristic chains or clusters. Replication of pathogenic bacteria usually takes place outside the host's cells – unlike pathogenic viruses, where reproduction is intracellular.

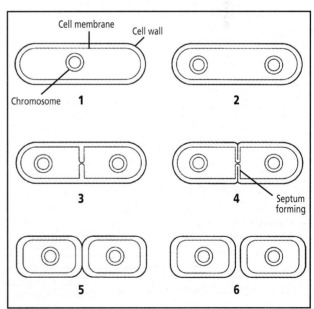

6.13 Replication of bacteria by binary fission. **1,2.** The cell grows and the chromosome replicates to form two identical chromosomes. **3.** As the cell enlarges, the chromosomes are separated and the cell membrane grows inwards at the centre of the cell. **4.** At the same time, new cell wall material grows inwards to form the septum. **5,6.** The cell divides into two daughter cells.

Conjugation

The process of conjugation (Figure 6.14) involves the passage of DNA from one bacterial cell (the donor) to another (the recipient) while the two cells are in physical contact. The cells are pulled together by an appendage called the **sex pilus**, which is formed by the donor cell. Once contact has been made, the pilus retracts so that the surfaces of the donor and recipient are very close to each other. The cell membranes fuse, forming a channel between the two cells, and DNA then passes from the donor to the recipient.

Frequently, a plasmid (see Figure 6.12) is transferred from the donor to the recipient but sometimes part of the donor

cell chromosome, or even the whole chromosome, is transferred. Conjugation is important because the recipient acquires new characteristics. For example, one plasmid, the R plasmid, carries genes for resistance to antibiotics.

Conjugation is rare among Gram-positive bacteria but common among those that are Gram-negative. It is sometimes regarded as a primitive type of sexual reproduction but this is misleading because, unlike sexual reproduction in other organisms, it does not involve the fusion of two gametes to form a single cell.

Identification of bacteria

It can be important to identify the bacteria causing an infection, for example so that appropriate antibacterials can be selected for treatment. The simplest and quickest way to identify bacteria is to make a smear and stain it with Gram stain, which involves a sequence of steps. As well as indicating whether the bacterium is Gram-positive or Gram-negative, this also allows the structure of the bacterial cell to be observed.

There are often several bacteria that look alike at this stage and so it may be necessary to culture the bacterium so that the identity can be determined more precisely. Figure 6.15 shows how this process might occur for the investigation of an infection causing otitis externa in a dog's ear.

Practically, samples are often cultured initially in order to obtain quantities of a pure growth of the bacterium responsible for the infection. The characteristics of the colony can then be observed and there is enough bacterial material to carry out any further tests that are necessary. Culture also allows an experienced microbiologist to differentiate important colonies from those of bacteria that are normally present or otherwise insignificant in the infection.

Bacterial cultivation in the laboratory

The cultivation of bacteria in the laboratory requires an appropriate nutrient material or culture medium (see Chapter 19). The culture medium must contain a balanced mixture of the essential growth requirements – carbon, nitrogen and water. Culture can also be used as a method of bacterial identification, as many bacteria have specific individual requirements for optimal growth.

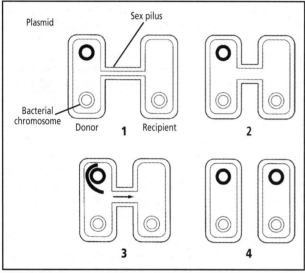

6.14 Sequence of events in conjugation. **1.** Donor and recipient cells are pulled together by the sex pilus, which is formed by the donor cell. **2.** The pilus retracts, bringing the two cells very close to each other, and the cell membranes fuse to form a channel between the two cells. **3.** The plasmid replicates and one strand passes through the channel to the recipient. **4.** The two cells separate. The recipient becomes a potential donor, because it now has the plasmid.

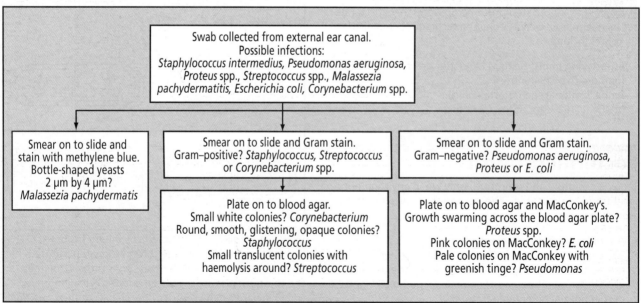

6.15 Flow chart for the identification of bacteria or *Malassezia pachydermatis* from a dog with chronic otitis externa. Further identification and sensitivity tesing is carried out as required.

Respiratory requirements

The different oxygen requirements of bacteria, described above, can be used in helping to identify bacterial pathogens, as can the detailed biochemical pathways that they use to provide energy. Bacteria that will grow in the amount of oxygen in the air may be cultured in an incubator. For anaerobes and microaerophiles (including most *Campylobacter* species), Petri dishes containing appropriate culture medium can be placed in an anaerobic jar to minimize atmospheric oxygen and encourage the growth of the bacteria. If the appropriate conditions for a particular organism are not provided, its presence may not be recognized as it will not grow in the laboratory. Respiratory mechanisms of any particular bacterium can be identified by testing for the presence of enzymes that are involved in oxidative processes, such as catalase and cytochrome oxidase.

Diseases caused by bacteria

A variety of bacteria are capable of infecting dogs and cats; some can cause signs of infection in the dog or cat. Examples of some important disease-causing bacteria have been given in Figures 6.16, 6.17 and 6.18. Sometimes the same bacterium is responsible for causing disease in a number of species; other infections are more species-specific.

Name of bacterium	Disease caused	Susceptible species	Gram staining	Shape	Aerobic
Salmonella spp.	Diarrhoea	Dog	Negative	Rods	Yes
Campylobacter spp.	Diarrhoea	Dog	Negative	Curved rods (see Figure 6.11b)	Yes (but prefer less oxygen than in air)
Bordetella bronchiseptica	Kennel cough	Dog	Negative	Short rods	Yes
Leptospira spp.	Leptospirosis	Dog	Negative	Helically coiled (spirochaete)	Yes
Borrelia burgdorferi	Lyme disease	Dog	Negative	Helically coiled (spirochaete)	Yes
Streptococcus spp.	Infection, particularly in puppies, occasionally otitis externa, metritis	Dog	Positive	Cocci (arranged in chains) (see Figure 6.11c)	Yes
Staphylococcus spp.	Pyoderma or wound infection	Dog	Positive	Cocci (arranged as bunches of grapes) (see Figure 6.11d)	Yes
Clostridium tetani	Tetanus (rare)	Dog	Positive	Long rods	No
Mycoplasma felis	Mycoplasmal conjunctivitis	Cat	Negative	Pleomorphic as there is no rigid cell wall	Yes
Pasteurella spp.	Cat-bite abscess (other organisms may also be involved)	Cat	Negative	Rods or coccobacilli	Yes

6.16 Some bacterial diseases of dogs and cats.

Name of bacterium	Disease caused	Gram staining	Shape
Rhodococcus equi	Summer pneumonia	Positive	Coccobacilli
Salmonella spp.	Diarrhoea, zoonotic	Negative	Rods
Streptococcus equi equi	Strangles	Positive	Cocci, often in chains
Taylorella equigenitalis	Contagious equine metritis	Negative	Short rods

6.17 Examples of bacterial disease of horses.

Name of bacterium	Disease caused	Susceptible species	Gram staining	Shape
Chlamydophila psittaci	Psittacosis	Birds, zoonotic	Negative (require specialized stains)	Cocci
Mycobacterium avium	Avian tuberculosis	Birds	Positive (but stain very poorly so alternative 'acid-fast' stains used)	Rods
Pasteurella multocida	Pasteurellosis (including respiratory disease)	Rabbits ('snuffles') and other species	Negative	Rods or coccobacilli
Salmonella spp.	Salmonellosis	Range of reptiles, zoonotic	Negative	Rods
Staphylococcus aureus	Pyoderma and ulcerative dermatitis	Ferrets, hamsters, mice, rats	Positive	Cocci

6.18 Examples of bacterial infections of exotic pets.

The clinical signs of infection may be: directly associated with the presence of the bacterium; or related to damage caused to local tissue by the presence of the infection, the inflammatory reaction stimulated by the infection or due to toxins produced by bacteria.

Rickettsias and chlamydias

Both rickettsias and chlamydias possess a cell wall like other Gram-negative bacteria but both need to live inside other cells, i.e. they are **obligate intracellular organisms**. These bacteria are responsible for a number of diseases in animals.

Rickettsias

- These are transmitted by vectors such as ticks, lice, fleas and mites.
- A particularly pathogenic species is the tick-transmitted infection *Ehrlichia canis*, which is endemic in France and the Mediterranean basin.
- Rickettsias are often seen on cytological examination of blood smears during clinical pathology examinations.

Chlamydias

- Various strains of *Chlamydophila* (formerly *Chlamydia*) *psittaci* are the cause of psittacosis in psittacine birds (parrots, parakeets) and mammals. Psittacosis is a zoonotic infection that humans can acquire by inhaling the organism in the airborne dust or from cage contents of infected birds.
- Feline pneumonitis is caused by *Chlamydophila felis*, which may also cause conjunctivitis in the cat. The bacteria are transmitted by inhalation of infectious dust and droplets and by ingestion. There is also evidence to suggest that vector-borne infection may occur.

Identification

Generally, the identification of rickettsias and chlamydias is more difficult and thus more specialized than that of most bacteria. Diagnosis of infection may be based on demonstration of the organisms themselves or on the demonstration of increased antibody titres in paired serum samples. Rickettsias are smaller than most bacteria and are barely visible using a light microscope. They can only be cultivated in tissue culture or in the yolk sac of embryonated eggs. Typically, they are rod-shaped and measure about 0.8–2.0 μm.

Mycoplasmas

Mycoplasmas are tiny bacteria-like organisms but they do not possess a cell wall. Examples include: *Mycoplasma felis*, a cause of chronic conjunctivitis in cats; *Mycoplasma hyopneumoniae*, the cause of enzootic pneumonia in pigs; and *M. cynos* in dogs. Damage caused by *Mycoplasma* spp. infection of the respiratory tract may predispose the animal to secondary bacterial infection.

Mycoplasmas will grow on agar-based media (Figure 6.19) but, as they are so fragile, isolation and identification are specialized skills.

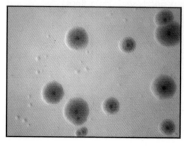

6.19 *Mycoplasma* spp. growing on specialized culture medium.
(© Andrew Rycroft)

Toxins

Toxins are poisonous substances that have a damaging effect on the cells of the host. The effects of the toxin are felt not only in the affected cells and tissues but also elsewhere in the body as the toxin is transported through the tissues. Two types of toxin are recognized.

Exotoxins

Exotoxins are proteins produced mainly by Gram-positive bacteria during their metabolism. They are released into the surrounding environment as they are produced. This can be into the circulatory system and tissues of the host or, as in food poisoning, into food that is then ingested. Microbial toxins include many of the most potent poisons known and may prove lethal even in small quantities. The body responds to the presence of exotoxins by producing antibodies called **antitoxins**, which neutralize the toxins, rendering them harmless.

As proteins, exotoxins are destroyed by heat and by some chemicals. Chemicals such as formaldehyde are used to treat toxins so that they lose their toxicity but not their ability to elicit an immune response. These treated toxins are called **toxoids** and will stimulate the production of antitoxins if injected into the body. For example, tetanus toxoid is used widely as the vaccine to induce immunity to tetanus.

Endotoxins

Endotoxins are a part of the cell envelope of Gram-negative bacteria (lipopolysaccharide) and are released mainly when the cells die and disintegrate. Compared with exotoxins, they are less toxic, cannot be used to form toxoids and are able to withstand heat. Blood-borne endotoxins are responsible for a range of non-specific reactions in the body, such as fever. At higher levels they can sometimes result in a serious drop in blood pressure (a condition commonly called **endotoxic shock**.

Aflatoxin

Toxins are not made exclusively by bacteria. The saprophytic fungus *Aspergillus flavus* produces a toxin called aflatoxin. The fungus grows in warm, humid conditions and contaminates a variety of agricultural products such as peanuts, cereals, rice and beans. Aflatoxin has been implicated in the deaths of many farm animals that have been fed on mouldy hay, corn or on peanut meal.

Effects of toxins

The effects of toxins are usually very specific. For example, when spores of the anaerobic tetanus bacillus *Clostridium tetani* get into a wound that provides favourable conditions, they may germinate and grow in the tissues. The bacteria do not spread through the tissues but secrete an exotoxin that travels along peripheral nerves to the central nervous system, where it interferes with the regulation of neurotransmitters that control the relaxation of muscle. This leads to uncontrollable muscle spasms and paralysis. Tetanus toxin is called a **neurotoxin** because of its activity in the nervous system.

Unlike tetanus, which is caused by exotoxins produced while the organism is growing within the host, botulism, caused by the saprophytic bacterium *Clostridium botulinum*, is the result of ingestion of food containing the toxins. In botulism, the exotoxin affects the nervous system, leading to paralysis; it too is therefore a neurotoxin.

Other exotoxins formed outside the body include those produced by *Staphylococcus aureus*, the bacterium that causes staphylococcal food poisoning. This is an **enterotoxin** because it functions in the gastrointestinal tract, causing vomiting and diarrhoea.

Commensal bacteria carried by cats and dogs

There are a number of bacteria (known as commensals) that are normally carried by cats and dogs without causing any clinical signs. However, in certain circumstances, disease can result from infection. Both of these examples are potential zoonoses:

- *Bartonella henselae* is a small Gram-negative bacterium present in a proportion of the cat population and is not normally pathogenic to cats. It may be transmitted to a human in the course of a cat scratch and may result in a local or more general infection in the person, so-called cat-scratch disease.
- Some *Staphylococcus aureus* developed resistance to meticillin (meticillin-resistant *Staphylococcus aureus*, or MRSA) in the 1960s. Since then some strains have developed resistance to many antibacterials. These resistant bacteria can live on the skin or in the nasal passages of dogs, cats or humans without clinical signs. However, if infection establishes in a wound or other organ, severe damage can be caused. As the organism is resistant not only to meticillin but also to other antibacterials, the infection can be very difficult to treat. The presence of infection in a veterinary hospital ward may necessitate the closure of the ward and thorough cleaning until the infection is eliminated (see Chapter 5).

Treatment of bacterial infections

Bacterial infections can occur in many different locations within an animal and so the treatment will depend on the location and the type of bacteria present (see also Chapter 5).

Choice of antibacterial agent

- A surface infection or a cat-bite abscess might be treated with local cleaning with an antibacterial wash (e.g. chlorhexidine).
- Other infections can be treated with systemic antibacterials or antibiotics. Depending on the infection, treatment may be administered by mouth or by injection. Some antibacterials can be administered intravenously when speed of activity is essential. Some antibacterials are termed broad-spectrum and are effective against a range of Gram-positive and Gram-negative organisms. Others are effective against a more narrow range of organisms, and so it is necessary to have an idea of the infection present in order to choose an appropriate antibacterial agent. See Bacterial sensitivity testing, below.
- Choice of an antibacterial also requires an understanding of where the drug will reach in the body. For example, if treatment of cystitis is required, an antibacterial that is not broken down before it reaches the urinary tract should be selected.
- Some antibacterials can destroy the microflora necessary for normal functioning. This is a particularly important consideration when choosing a treatment for small mammals such as rabbits, gerbils and hamsters.

Bacterial sensitivity testing

It is important to identify the antibacterials to which the bacteria causing an infection will respond. A bacterial sensitivity test can be conducted where, for example, the bacteria are spread on an agar plate and discs containing different antibacterials are placed on top. After incubation, the patterns of growth around the discs are examined:

- If the growth occurs right up to a disc, that antibacterial will not be effective
- If there is a wide zone of inhibition of bacterial growth around a disc, the antibacterial contained in that disc is likely to be effective (see Chapter 19).

Fungi

There are many different fungi (as can be seen by looking at a mouldy slice of bread) but only a few are able to infect animals. Fungi grow aerobically (using oxygen) and gain their energy from the organic substances on which they grow. They can be divided into two categories and the fungal pathogens seen in small animal veterinary practice include both types.

- Moulds (Figure 6.20) are multicellular. Example: the 'ringworm' dermatophytes
- Yeasts (Figure 6.20) are unicellular. Examples: *Malassezia pachydermatis* and *Candida albicans*.

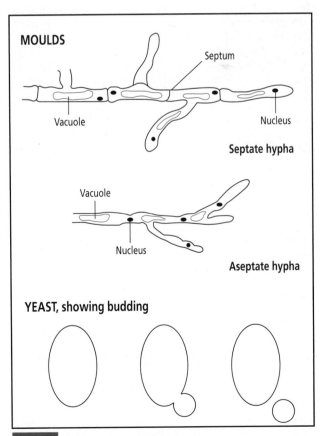

6.20 Different forms of fungi.

Dermatophytes

Fungal infections of keratin (the horny tissue that forms nail, hair and skin) can affect horses, cats, dogs, rabbits and guinea pigs. The condition broadly known as ringworm is caused by dermatophytes such as the species *Trichophyton mentagrophytes* (in dog, cat, rabbit and guinea pig), *Microsporum canis* (in dog and cat) and *Trichophyton equinum* (in horses) amongst others.

In its most obvious form, ringworm appears as circular areas of hair loss with active fungal infection around the edge of the lesion (Figure 6.21). The lesions may be small and discrete or large and coalescing, with an irregular outline. Some are not very inflamed and cause little irritation, whilst others may show severe inflammation. A more marked reaction is common in dogs.

Transmission may be directly from affected animal to animal, or to humans (many dermatophytes are zoonotic). Long-haired cats, in particular, may appear normal but may be carriers of infection. There may also be indirect transmission via bedding, cages, rugs, grooming tools, etc. Ringworm spores can remain viable in the environment for prolonged periods.

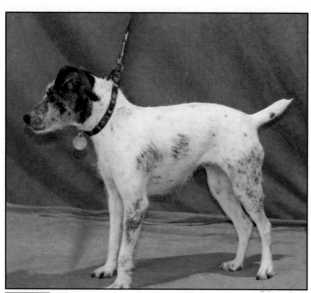

6.21 Ringworm lesions on a Jack Russell Terrier. (Courtesy of David Duclos)

Diagnosis

This can be performed by staining hair pluck or skin scrape samples, by examining for fluorescence with a Wood's lamp (for species that fluoresce) and/or by culture on specialist media (see Chapter 19).

Treatment

Topical

Treatments include a fungicidal wash (such as enilconazole) or painting the affected area with povidone–iodine. Topical treatment is usually repeated after an interval to effect a full cure. It may be possible to treat the area of a discrete lesion only, or it may be necessary to wash the whole animal. In severe or non-responsive cases, e.g. some long-haired cats, it will be necessary to clip the affected part or even the entire animal to facilitate treatment.

Systemic

Itraconazole or ketoconazole can be administered orally for the treatment of dermatophytes. Griseofulvin is administered in tablet or granule form and has to be given for a prolonged period as the levels build up gradually in the skin; it is now rarely used in small animals but is still occasionally used in horses. Care, including the wearing of gloves, should be taken when handling griseofulvin, as it is teratogenic (i.e. it can cause malformation of a fetus in a pregnant woman).

Candida albicans

The yeast *Candida albicans* is often present in the intestinal tract of animals without causing disease but it can become pathogenic in certain circumstances. *Candida* infections are usually opportunistic, i.e. they take advantage of a young, debilitated or immunocompromised animal and cause disease. Infection may also be seen after prolonged antibacterial treatment or following skin damage such as that incurred in a burn. The infection is known as 'thrush' and is commonly seen on mucous membranes, e.g. in the mouths of foals, puppies or kittens. Rarely, it can occur at mucocutaneous junctions, or systemically when it can very rarely cause septic arthritis in foals. Humans can acquire the infection but transfer of infection would be highly unlikely unless the person were immunocompromised in some way (for example, a person with HIV).

- Infection of the skin of a dog may appear as an ulcer that does not respond to antibacterial therapy.
- Infection of the mouth may appear as a white growth and ulceration of the affected area in a puppy or kitten and may be associated with unwillingness to suck.
- In birds, *C. albicans* can infect the crop, particularly after prolonged antibacterial treatment.

Treatments for candidiasis include clotrimazole or miconazole (topically), or fluconazole (systemically).

Malassezia pachydermatis

Malassezia pachydermatis is a yeast that may be found on normal skin. In some situations, particularly seborrhoeic conditions, overgrowth may cause pruritic dermatitis (localized or generalized) or otitis externa, usually in dogs, but cats are sometimes infected. Infection occurs most commonly in warm summer months. Lesions may appear greasy and may have a distinct odour.

Suspected lesions can be sampled by pressing adhesive tape to the area (see Chapter 19). The strip is stained with methylene blue, attached to a microscope slide and examined microscopically. *Malassezia* appear as small, blue, bottle-shaped yeasts (see Chapter 19). As they are present on normal skin in low numbers, significant infection is indicated by an increase in numbers, perhaps when multiple organisms are seen in each high-power field of view under the microscope. Infection can be treated with a shampoo containing chlorhexidine and miconazole.

Other fungal infections

Occasionally, dogs, cats and other companion animals develop internal fungal infections. A number of different fungi can be responsible. For example, *Aspergillus fumigatus* can infect the nasal passages of the dog, the guttural pouches of horses and the respiratory system of birds. Fungi such as *Saprolegnia* spp. can infect fish and may cause severe disease and death.

Acknowledgements

Andrew Rycroft is acknowledged and thanked for his constructive comments on this chapter.

Further reading

Gillespie S and Bamford K (2000) *Medical Microbiology and Infection at a Glance*. Blackwell Science, Oxford

Heritage J, Evans EGV and Killington RA (1996) *Introductory Microbiology*. Cambridge University Press, Cambridge

Quinn PJ, Markey BK, Carter ME, Donnolly WJ and Leonard FC (2002) *Veterinary Microbiology and Microbial Disease*. Blackwell Publishing, Oxford

Trees A and Shaw S (1999) Imported diseases in small animals. *In Practice* **21**, 482–491

Self-assessment questions

1. Define the terms 'parasitic', 'commensal' and 'symbiotic'.
2. What distinguishes a virus from other organisms?
3. Give examples of viral infections in dogs, cats, horses and exotic pets.
4. Describe the structure of a bacterial cell.
5. How do bacteria replicate?
6. Give examples of bacterial infections in dogs, cats, horses and exotic pets.
7. What does MRSA stand for and why is it an important infection?
8. What are the considerations in choosing a suitable antimicrobial drug?
9. What are bacterial toxins?
10. How is ringworm identified?

Chapter 7

Elementary parasitology

Maggie Fisher, Vicky Walsh and John McGarry

Learning objectives

After studying this chapter, students should be able to:

- **Describe the ectoparasites and endoparasites that affect dogs, cats, horses and common exotic pets**
- **Describe the geographical distribution and zoonotic potential of parasites**
- **Identify parasites on the basis of their location on or in the host and their morphology**
- **Describe how the life cycle of a parasite determines the possible routes of infection**
- **Discuss options for prophylaxis to prevent parasite infection**
- **Discuss treatment options for parasite control**

Definitions

- **Parasite:** One eukaryotic organism living off another (the host) to the advantage of the parasite.
  - **Ectoparasites** live on the outside of the host.
  - **Endoparasites** live inside the host.
- **Eukaryote:** Organism in which the chromosomes are enclosed in a nucleus (this includes animals, plants and fungi).
- **Direct life cycle:** The parasite passes directly from one host to the next without having to infect an alternative or intermediate host.
- **Indirect life cycle:** The parasite requires one or more intermediate hosts to complete its life cycle.
- **Definitive host:** The primary host in which the parasite reaches maturity and, if applicable, reproduces sexually.
- **Intermediate host:** The secondary host in which the parasite undergoes some stage(s) of its development, but without sexual reproduction.
- **Paratenic host:** An organism in which the parasite can survive but does not develop further.
- **Vector:** An organism that can physically transmit a parasite from one host to another.

Ectoparasites

Ectoparasites belong to the Phylum Arthropoda in the animal kingdom and have a chitinous outer shell or **exoskeleton**. They include:

- **Insects**, where the adult has three pairs of legs and the body is divided into three parts: head, thorax and abdomen (e.g. lice, fleas)
- **Arachnids**, where the adult has four pairs of legs and the body is divided into two parts only: cephalothorax and abdomen (e.g. mites, ticks).

Usually it is the adult stage, often together with the immature stages, that is parasitic, although there are cases where it is only the immature form that is parasitic.

Ectoparasite morphology is illustrated below and diagnostic features are described in Chapter 19.

Insects

The diagnosis and control of insect ectoparasites are described in Figure 7.1.

Lice

Infection with lice is also known as **pediculosis** and it can be seen in a range of animals including cats, dogs, horses, rabbits, rodents and birds. Lice are subdivided into biting/chewing lice (Figures 7.2 and 7.3) and sucking lice (Figure 7.4), reflecting their manner of feeding. Infection is transmitted by close contact, as the louse spends its entire life cycle on the host, or via fomites, e.g. if eggs are collected on grooming equipment. Individual louse species are, however, highly host-specific and will not survive if transferred to a different host.

Large numbers of lice cause intense irritation and concomitant self-inflicted injury. In addition, the sucking lice may cause anaemia if they are present in large enough numbers. Young or debilitated animals are often the worst affected. Biting/chewing lice can transmit the tapeworm *Dipylidium caninum* to dogs.

Life cycle

Adult female lice lay their eggs individually and cement them to hairs. The eggs ('nits') are just visible to the naked eye (Figure 7.5). When these hatch, immature lice that are identical to the adult emerge and, after several moults, become adults. The whole life cycle takes about 2–3 weeks.

Parasite	Diagnosis	Control
Lice	Demonstration of the eggs attached to hairs. Visualization of the adult louse. The adult lice may be seen with the naked eye on close examination of an animal's haircoat or may be seen in a skin scrape/brush	Thorough cleaning of environment and grooming equipment, etc. Topical surface treatment with an insecticidal wash, spray or spot-on
Fleas	Demonstration of an adult flea or their faeces in the coat of a dog or cat by combing the coat thoroughly, preferably with a very fine-toothed comb (e.g. a human louse comb). The animal may be brushed over a sheet of damp white paper. Flea faeces will be seen on the paper as small black dots. Since they contain a large amount of undigested blood, a ring of red is seen around the black spot when moistened. There is also a skin test for allergy to fleas	Control of the environment at stages: – Vacuuming, particularly around where the pet sleeps – Applying an environmental insecticide and/or an insect growth regulator such as methoprene or pyriproxyfen, for example, to kill the immature stages. Depending on the formulation, these products may be applied to the animal or directly to the environment. The chitin synthesis inhibitor (lufenuron) is given orally to the dog or cat or by injection to the cat. It prevents eggs hatching and/or larval development
		Control of adult fleas on the animal: – Thorough grooming, e.g. using a human louse comb – Applying an insecticide in the form of, for example, a spray, impregnated collar, powder, shampoo or spot-on. The active ingredient in insecticides is often a synthetic pyrethroid, phenylpyrazole (fipronil), neonicotinoid (nitenpyram, imidacloprid), avermectin (selamectin) or metaflumizone
Fly larvae	An affected animal will often stop eating and appear restless and later depressed. The animal should be thoroughly examined to find the larvae and thus diagnose the problem	In order to treat the infestation, the first step is to remove the larvae: – Wash the affected area with a mild antiseptic solution, ensuring that the larvae are removed in the process – Lightly towel-dry the area. Apply antiseptic ointment. Any underlying problem (e.g. diarrhoea) that may have predisposed the animal to becoming 'fly blown' should be investigated and treated, and an antiparasitic agent such as cyromazine applied

7.1   Diagnosis and control of insect ectoparasites.

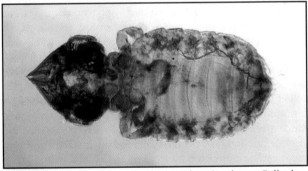

7.2   Dorsal view of the biting/chewing louse *Felicola subrostratus*. Found on cats, it is approximately 2 mm long. If viewed from the side, the louse would appear dorsoventrally flattened.

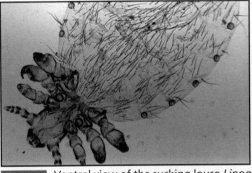

7.4   Ventral view of the sucking louse *Linognathus setosus*. Found on dogs, it is approximately 2 mm long. Sucking lice tend to have elongated, narrow heads.

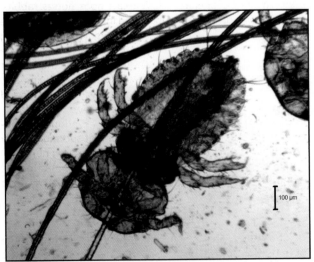

7.3   The species of biting/chewing louse found in dogs is *Trichodectes canis*. Biting lice tend to have shorter, broader heads than sucking lice.

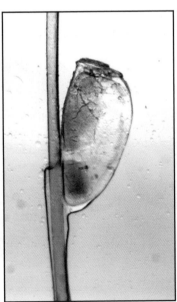

7.5   Louse egg ('nit') attached with 'cement' to the shaft of hair.

Fleas

Adult fleas bite the host in order to take a blood meal. The area that has been bitten shows something of an inflammatory reaction and causes some irritation. A heavy flea infestation may cause anaemia. Fleas can also transmit other pathogens, including *Dipylidium caninum* (a tapeworm, see later) and the agents that cause feline leukaemia (FeLV) and feline infectious anaemia. Fleas are also implicated in the spread from cat to cat of *Bartonella henselae*, the bacterium responsible for cat scratch disease in humans (see Chapter 6). It is believed that a cat's claws may be coated in the bacteria, probably derived from the cat grooming infected flea faeces out of its coat.

Some animals become sensitized to **allergens** (particular, usually otherwise harmless, antigens that induce an exaggerated immune sensitivity, resulting in harmful immunological reactions on subsequent exposures) in flea saliva, and develop severe lesions after just a few bites. This is known as flea allergic dermatitis (FAD).

The species of flea may be identified by the appearance of the head. Most fleas on cats and dogs are the 'cat flea' *Ctenocephalides felis felis* (Figure 7.6) (often abbreviated to *C. felis*) but dogs in a dog-only situation (e.g. Greyhound kennels) may be infected with the 'dog flea' *Ctenocephalides canis*. Infrequently other fleas, e.g. hedgehog fleas (*Archaeopsylla erinacei*), are found on cats or dogs.

Rabbits can be infested with *C. felis,* particularly if they are living in a household with dogs or cats. Wild rabbits are often infested with *Spillopsyllus cuniculi*, a species of flea that tends to stay attached in one place. Rats, mice and ferrets can also be infested with fleas. Birds have their own species of flea, the immature stages of which live in the bird's nest.

Life cycle of the cat flea

The life cycle of the cat flea is shown in Figure 7.7. The adult is laterally compressed, which allows it to move readily between the host's hairs. The female flea feeds, then mates on the host and lays eggs. These are smooth and fall off into the environment, particularly in the area around where the animal usually lies. After 2–14 days the eggs hatch out into larvae that look like small maggots. These feed on skin debris, the faeces of adult fleas and other organic matter in the environment. After about a week, each mature larva spins a cocoon and pupates. The outside of the cocoon is sticky and so bits of debris from the environment stick to it. After a further 10 days (though this can be considerably longer in cold or dry conditions) the adult flea is fully developed inside the pupa. Before it emerges, it waits for signs of a host being available, e.g. pressure on carpets (this is one explanation for the stories that occur of occupants going into an empty house and being bitten by fleas within hours). Once emerged from the pupal case, the flea will locate a host and jump on to it. Treatment of fleas should ideally be aimed at all stages of the life cycle (see Figure 7.1)

Dipteran flies

Larvae

Myiasis ('fly strike') is the invasion of living tissue by the larvae of dipteran flies (usually green or blue bottles). The life cycle is shown in Figure 7.8. The flies lay their eggs on a suitable site, which might be, though is not necessarily, on an animal, such as in the fleece of a sheep or around the anus of a rabbit. Flies are particularly attracted to a smelly animal, e.g. one that is soiled by diarrhoea, and so attraction can be minimized by ensuring that animals are kept clean. The larvae (maggots) hatch after as little as 12 hours and begin to traumatize the skin surface and feed off the damaged tissue. Larval development can be prevented by treating the animal with a larval growth inhibitor such as cyromazine. After two moults the mature larvae drop to the ground. Here they may overwinter as larvae before pupating or they may pupate immediately. Eventually the adult fly emerges from the pupal case.

7.6 Lateral view of the head of the cat flea, showing the characteristic combs (arrowed).

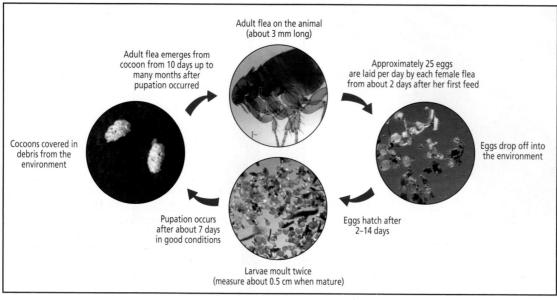

7.7

Life cycle of the cat flea.

Adult flea on the animal
(about 3 mm long)

Adult flea emerges from cocoon from 10 days up to many months after pupation occurred

Approximately 25 eggs are laid per day by each female flea from about 2 days after her first feed

Cocoons covered in debris from the environment

Eggs drop off into the environment

Pupation occurs after about 7 days in good conditions

Eggs hatch after 2–14 days

Larvae moult twice
(measure about 0.5 cm when mature)

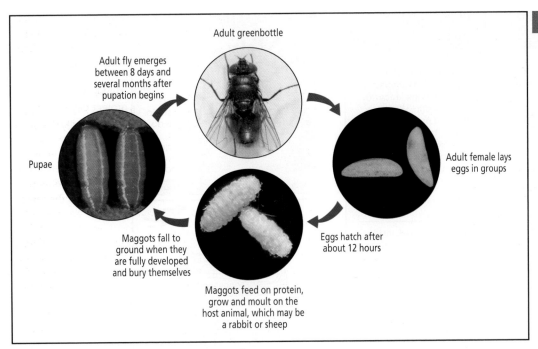

Adult greenbottle

Adult fly emerges between 8 days and several months after pupation begins

Pupae

Adult female lays eggs in groups

Maggots fall to ground when they are fully developed and bury themselves

Eggs hatch after about 12 hours

Maggots feed on protein, grow and moult on the host animal, which may be a rabbit or sheep

Bot flies (*Gasterophilus* spp.) lay their eggs on horses' hairs in late summer; they can be seen as small off-white specks attached to hairs (Figure 7.9). Once hatched from the eggs, the larvae burrow into the mouth, or are licked by the horse as it grooms. Later on in development the larvae attach themselves to the intestinal mucosa of the horse (Figure 7.9c), most commonly in the stomach or proximal small intestine, depending on bot species. Hence this is another form of myiasis. Once fully mature, the larvae detach and are passed in faeces, whereupon they pupate before developing into adult flies in the summer months. Bots can be controlled by regular removal of the eggs from the hairs of the horse or by anthelmintic treatment in the autumn using a product that is effective against bot larvae.

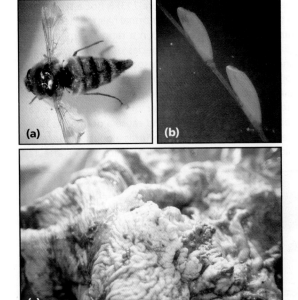

7.9 *Gasterophilus intestinalis.* **(a)** 'Bot' fly. Note the bee-like appearance. The adult flies hover close to horses, which often react to their presence. **(b)** Bot eggs attached to hair. **(c)** Bot larvae attached to the mucosa of a horse's stomach.

Adults

A number of species of biting and nuisance flies feed off horses in the summer and can cause restlessness and irritation in horses. Horse owners utilize a variety of methods, including fringes and fly repellents, to prevent flies affecting horses during the summer months.

Some horses develop an allergic response to the bites of small *Culicoides* spp. (midges). Affected horses typically show self-inflicted trauma from rubbing the tail, head and mane. The condition is known as 'sweet itch' and, once developed, individuals normally show clinical signs each summer. It can be difficult to control, with various methods including repellents used in an attempt to prevent the condition.

Flies may also act as vectors in the transmission of infections (see Chapter 6). *Culicoides* spp., for example, transmit the virus responsible for African Horse Sickness, and flies are responsible for the transfer of *Thelazia* spp. larvae, a worm that occurs on the surface of the eye of horses. In small animals, sandflies can transmit leishmaniasis and mosquitoes may carry the heartworm, *Dirofilaria immitis*.

Arachnids

The arachnids of veterinary importance are the ticks and the mites. The immature larvae that emerge from the eggs of these ectoparasites look like smaller versions of the adult, except that they have only three pairs of legs, whereas the nymph and adult stages each have four pairs of legs.

Mites

Most parasitic mites are permanent ectoparasites (they spend their entire life cycle on the host); exceptions include *Dermanyssus gallinae* (red mite of poultry) and *Trombicula autumnalis* (the 'harvest mite', where it is only the larva that is parasitic). Mites may be subdivided into the burrowing and the surface mites. Both types cause dermatitis, which may or may not be pruritic (itchy), depending on the species of mite present. Diagnosis is usually by inspection of coat brushings under a low power stereomicroscope or by examination (at higher power) of skin scrapes or hair plucks (see also Chapter 19). Specific guidance on diagnosis and treatment of each mite is given in Figure 7.10.

Parasitic	Diagnostic samples	Treatment
Sarcoptes scabiei	Skin scrapes or blood test	Mite infections may be treated with a suitable acaricide such as amitraz, selamectin or imidacloprid and moxidectin. Where no authorized product is available, treat with e.g. fipronil. Also treat the environment in *Cheyletiella* infection.
Notoedres	Skin scrapes	
Cnemidocoptes	Skin scrapes	
Demodex	Skin scrapes or hair plucks	
Cheyletiella	Coat brushings or sellotape strips (adult mite and/ or eggs)	
Otodectes cynotis	Ear wax	Clean the ear canal; instil ointment containing suitable acaricide, often in combination with antibiotic. Also treat in-contact animals to clear potential reservoirs of infection. Alternatively, selamectin or moxidectin spot-on may be used: these are typically applied to the back of the neck or behind the shoulder blades

7.10 Diagnosis and treatment of mites.

Burrowing mites

Burrowing mites create small tunnels within the surface layers of the skin. They lay their eggs within small nests within these tunnels. There are four burrowing mites seen in domestic pets: *Sarcoptes scabiei* var. *canis*; *Notoedres* spp.; *Cnemidocoptes* spp.; and *Trixacarus caviae* (a burrowing mite found on guinea pigs).

Sarcoptes scabiei var. canis

This mite (Figure 7.11) affects dogs and, very rarely, cats and horses. *S. scabiei* causes mange in rodents and scabies in humans. Animals become infected by close contact with infected animals or by acquiring mites or eggs that are present in bedding or the environment. *S. scabiei* is a permanent ectoparasite; however, mites may be shed by heavily infected individuals and in good conditions can survive in the environment for several days. Often the tips of the ears, elbows and then the face are the first areas affected, but large areas of the body may be infected in severe cases. Affected areas become hairless, thickened and inflamed. This is partly due to the effect of the mites themselves and partly due to the trauma that the animal causes by rubbing and scratching the affected area – the condition is very pruritic. Sarcoptic mites from dogs will attack humans but normally the lesions are small and self-limiting.

Notoedres spp.

The burrowing mite of the cat (Figure 7.12) is very rarely seen in the UK but it causes similar signs to *Sarcoptes scabiei* in the dog. *Notoedres* infestation also occurs in rats.

Cnemidocoptes spp.

These mites are the cause of 'scaly leg' and 'scaly face' in birds, particularly budgerigars.

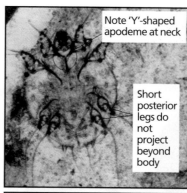
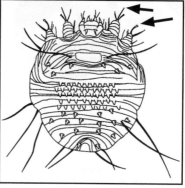

7.11 Adult *Sarcoptes* mite (0.4 mm long). The drawing (dorsal view) shows the short, stubby legs that barely project beyond the body, spines and pegs, terminal anus, and pedicles with suckers (arrowed) at the ends of the legs. (Courtesy of Donald Mactaggart)

Note 'Y'-shaped apodeme at neck

Short posterior legs do not project beyond body

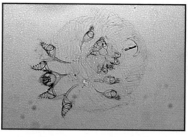

7.12 Dorsal view of adult female *Notoedres* mite (0.36 mm long) showing concentric circles on body and the dorsal anus.

Demodex spp.

This small cigar-shaped mite (Figure 7.13) is not a typical burrowing type and may be found in normal hair follicles without necessarily causing any problem, in a range of mammalian hosts. Each host has a specific species of *Demodex* mite. In companion animals, clinical signs associated with infection are most commonly seen in dogs and hamsters. In young dogs with an apparent genetic predisposition and in older dogs with immunosuppression, the number of *Demodex* mites can, however, increase dramatically and cause a dermatitis that is characteristically an area of non-pruritic alopecia. In localized demodicosis, where lesions are small, the face is often affected,

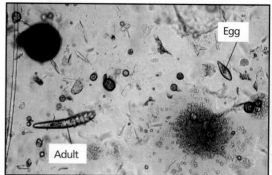
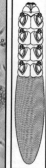

Egg

Adult

7.13 *Demodex* mite, showing cigar-shaped body (0.2 mm long) plus an egg. (Courtesy of Donald Mactaggart)

particularly around the eyes or mouth. Affected animals may appear to be wearing spectacles. Generalized demodicosis can affect any area, with involvement of the feet being especially painful and problematic. *Demodex* can be trickier to find than the other burrowing mites as it is smaller and dwells deep within the hair follicle; hair plucks are often useful.

Surface-feeding mites

Otodectes cynotis

These are the ear mites of the dog, cat and ferret (Figure 7.14). They live within the ear canal, often stimulating a dark brown waxy discharge, particularly in cats. The mites may be seen on the surface as small white moving dots, and secondary bacterial infection may result in a pus-like discharge. Some dogs, and particularly cats, are infected without showing clinical signs. Some cats and most dogs will shake their heads and rub their ears when infection is present. This may result in trauma to the ears and haematoma formation in the ear flap.

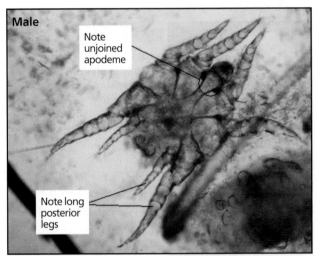

Male

Note unjoined apodeme

Note long posterior legs

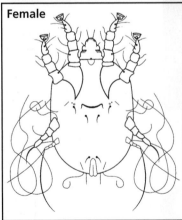

Female

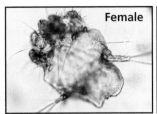 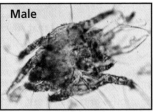

Female   Male

7.15 *Chorioptes* mites.

7.14 Dorsal view of *Otodectes* mite (0.4 mm long). Note the longer legs protruding from the body and unjoined pedicles (stalks) with suckers on the ends. (Courtesy of Donald Mactaggart)

Psoroptes spp.

Ear 'canker' in rabbits is caused by *Psoroptes cuniculi*. The mites cause crusting on the inside of the pinnae of affected rabbits. Occasionally horses are infected with *Psoroptes* spp. mites, causing an itchy mange.

Chorioptes spp.

Infection with *Chorioptes* mites (Figure 7.15) causes chorioptic mange in horses. This typically affects the caudal aspect of the lower limbs, especially in heavy horses with feathered fetlocks and in the winter time. Some horses tolerate infestation; in others the condition can be extremely pruritic.

Affected horses commonly stamp their hindfeet, chew their forelimbs and rub their legs on their companions or on the stable or fenceposts. Badly affected horses often have thickened skin and scabs, particularly around the pasterns. Some horses develop bleeding sores, and secondary bacterial infection can cause lameness and swollen legs. Treatment includes clipping the feathers and washing legs with antibacterial scrub in addition to antiparasitic drugs.

Cheyletiella spp.

Dogs, cats or rabbits affected with this fur mite may be described as having 'walking dandruff', since infection often leads to the production of excess scale and the mites (Figure 7.16) are large enough to be just visible with the naked eye. Infection does not usually cause any marked loss of hair. Often the mites will move on to humans handling animals; although the mites will not survive for long periods, they may bite, resulting in small raised red spots and pruritus.

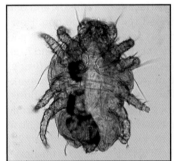 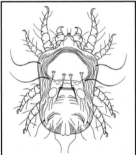

7.16 Dorsal view of *Cheyletiella* mite (0.4 mm). Note the 'comb' on the end of each leg and the large palps on either side of the head, each with a large claw.

Trombicula autumnalis

This mite, as its name suggests, normally becomes a problem in late summer and autumn, and is often associated with specific geographical areas such as the Cotswolds and Edinburgh. The larval mites (Figure 7.17) attach themselves to the legs of passing animals, including dogs or cats, and feed, causing intense irritation to the host.

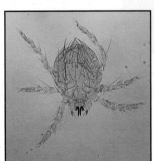

7.17 *Trombicula autumnalis* (harvest mite) larva (1 mm long, orange-brown in colour). Note that there are only three pairs of legs.

Dermanyssus spp.

This is the 'red mite' that sucks the blood of chickens and occasionally other animals. All stages live off the host, e.g. in the eaves of poultry houses. The mites visit chickens to feed, particularly at night. Infection causes irritation and debility, with anaemia in heavy infections. Control is by cleaning the henhouse and treatment with an acaricide.

Ticks

In small animal practice it is usual to encounter just one or two ticks on a cat or dog, with an owner who is concerned about how to get rid of them. A heavy tick burden may cause anaemia; however, the main health problem associated with ticks is their ability, even in low numbers, to transmit infections, such as the Lyme disease agent *Borrelia burgdorferi*. Horses can also be infested with ticks and, depending on the circumstance, may have a few ticks or a considerable burden. Ticks on livestock are also important in many parts of the world as carriers or 'vectors' of disease (see Chapter 5).

Since the advent of the Pet Travel Scheme there has been an increased opportunity for some of the tick-transmitted diseases present in mainland Europe to be introduced into the UK. In order to prevent infected ticks entering the UK, it is currently mandatory for dogs or cats to be treated with an approved acaricide (a substance that is toxic to ticks and mites) before their return to the UK. Details of the latest requirements may be found on the Defra website (www.defra.gov.uk); see also Chapters 5 and 16.

Several species of tick may affect dogs in the UK and one of these (*Ixodes canisuga*) is host-specific to the dog. However, by far the most common ticks seen on small animals and horses are the sheep tick (*Ixodes ricinus*) (Figures 7.18 and 7.19), particularly in country dwellers, and the hedgehog tick (*Ixodes hexagonus*), especially in urban areas. These ticks are remarkably cosmopolitan and will attach to many different hosts. Initially all that is visible is a small greyish swelling, firmly attached to the animal. Inspection reveals pairs of legs close to the attachment with the host; the mouthparts (Figure 7.20) are buried into the animal's flesh. As the tick ingests the host's blood it increases in size and may turn a red-brown colour. Once the tick has fed fully it will drop off its host. Diagnosis is based on finding the ticks. The identification of the species of tick is a specialized skill.

Individual ticks may be removed by dabbing them with a cotton-wool bud that has been treated with an acaricide. Once dead, the tick can be gently removed. A number of tick removal devices are also available. At times of tick challenge it may be worthwhile carrying out prophylactic treatment to ensure that any ticks are repelled from the dog or cat and that any that do attach are killed soon afterwards. There are a number of products available to achieve this, some of which will protect against flea infestation at the same time (see Chapter 8).

WARNING

- Never try to pull off a live tick unless using an effective 'tick remover', as its mouthparts may be left embedded in the animal and may become a focus for infection.
- Avoid local application of a spot-on acaricide to remove a tick close to an animal's mouth.

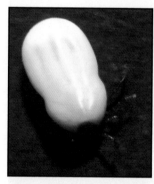

7.19 Engorged adult female sheep tick *Ixodes ricinus*, measuring approximately 7 mm. Note the small dark brown scutum or plate near to the head.

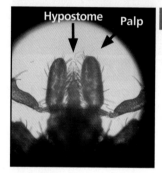

7.20 Mouthparts of a tick.

7.18 Life cycle of the sheep tick.

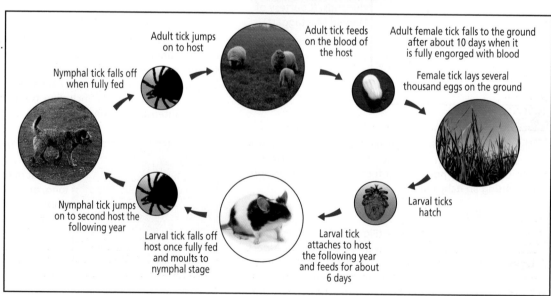

Adult tick jumps on to host

Adult tick feeds on the blood of the host

Adult female tick falls to the ground after about 10 days when it is fully engorged with blood

Female tick lays several thousand eggs on the ground

Nymphal tick falls off when fully fed

Larval ticks hatch

Nymphal tick jumps on to second host the following year

Larval tick falls off host once fully fed and moults to nymphal stage

Larval tick attaches to host the following year and feeds for about 6 days

Endoparasites

Endoparasites may be divided into **helminths** and **Protozoa**.

- **Helminths** are the 'worms' and are subdivided into three types:
  - Flukes (found in the liver of sheep, cattle and, rarely, horses but do not normally affect dogs or cats in the UK)
  - Tapeworms (cestodes)
  - Roundworms (nematodes).
- **Protozoal parasites** are small unicellular organisms.

Figure 7.21 lists the species in each category seen in equine and small animal veterinary practice.

Helminths
Cestodes (tapeworms)

A cestode is tape-like and has no alimentary tract. It is composed of three parts: the head or scolex; an area behind this where segments or proglottids form; and finally the maturing segments (Figure 7.22). Tapeworms are hermaphrodites, with a set of male and female reproductive organs in each segment. As the segment matures, reproduction takes place and eggs then develop within the segment, so that when fully mature it is simply an egg-containing structure. Each tapeworm has an immature stage (the metacestode) that develops in an **intermediate host**; the exact structure varies according to the species of tapeworm.

Tapeworms found in cats and dogs in the UK are *Echinococcus granulosus* (dogs), *Dipylidium caninum* (dogs and cats)

Parasite group	Species	Host
Helminths		
Cestodes (tapeworms)	*Echinococcus granulosus granulosus* (sheep strain) *Echinococcus equinus* *Echinococcus multilocularis* [a] *Dipylidium caninum* *Taenia* spp. *Anoplocephala perfoliata*	Dogs Dogs Dogs and cats Dogs and cats Dogs and cats Horses
Nematodes (roundworms):		
Ascarids	*Toxocara canis* *Toxascaris leonina* *Toxocara cati* *Parascaris equorum*	Dogs Dogs and cats Cats Horses
Hookworms	*Uncinaria stenocephala* *Ancylostoma tubaeforme* [b] *Ancylostoma caninum*	Dogs Cats Dogs
Whipworm	*Trichuris vulpis*	Dogs
Heartworm	*Dirofilaria immitis* [c]	Dogs and cats
Capillaria	*Capillaria plica* *Capillaria hepatica*	Dogs Dogs
Pinworms	*Oxyuris equi*	Horses
Lungworms	*Aelurostrongylus abstrusus* *Angiostrongylus vasorum* *Oslerus osleri* (formerly *Filaroides osleri*) *Dictyocaulus arnfieldi*	Cats Dogs Dogs Horses and donkeys
Strongyles	*Strongyloides westeri* Cyathostomins Large strongyles	Horses Horses Horses
Eyeworm	*Thelazia* spp.	Horses
Habronema	*Habronema* spp.	Horses
Protozoa		
Coccidia	*Isospora* sp. *Cryptosporidium parvum* *Sarcocystis* spp. *Toxoplasma gondii* *Neospora caninum* *Hammondia* sp.	Dogs and cats Dogs and cats Dogs and cats Cats Dogs Cats
Flagellates	*Giardia* sp.	Dogs and cats
Piroplasm	*Babesia* sp. [d]	Dogs

7.21 Species of endoparasite commonly found in dogs, cats and horses. [a] Mainland Europe only; [b] Hookworm infection occurs rarely in cats in the UK; [c] Not UK – endemic in the Mediterranean area; [d] Not in the UK, though infected dogs may be imported from the southern part of mainland Europe.

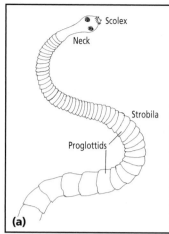

7.22 **(a)** A typical adult cestode. **(b)** A mature proglottid. (Reproduced from Urquhart *et al.*, 1996, with the permission of Blackwell Publishing.)

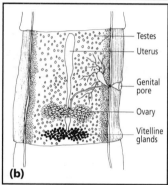

and the *Taenia* species (one species in cats and several species in dogs). Their presence is not normally a problem to the final host, though the sight of tapeworm segments is repugnant to owners. There is more often a problem with infection of the intermediate host (see Figure 7.26), either because the tapeworm cysts cause disease or because affected meat is condemned as unfit for human consumption. There is just one tapeworm, *Anoplocephala perfoliata,* found in horses: when present in large numbers it can cause colic. Most importantly, it does not respond to ivermectin anthelmintic and an appropriate drug must be used (see below).

Tapeworm definitions

Adult tapeworm:

- **Scolex**: Head of a tapeworm – used for attachment to the host's intestine using suckers and the rostellum (where present) for attachment
- **Rostellum**: The anterior part of the scolex, present in most tapeworms; it is a protrusible cone and is armed with hooks in some species
- **Strobila**: The chain of individual segments
- **Proglottid**: Name for each individual segment that makes up the strobila.

Immature tapeworms (metacestodes):

- **Cysticercus**: Fluid-filled cyst containing a single invaginated scolex attached to the cyst wall
- **Cysticercoid**: Single evaginated scolex (this is the form found in invertebrate intermediate hosts)
- **Hydatid cyst**: Large cyst containing many scolices, some loose in the fluid inside and some contained within 'brood capsules'
- **Coenurus**: A cyst with many invaginated scolices attached to the cyst wall.

Dipylidium caninum

This is probably the most common tapeworm of cats and dogs in the UK. The intermediate host is the flea, and also the biting louse *Trichodectes canis* in the case of the dog. Infection is normally diagnosed by the presence of motile segments (shaped like rice grains) containing 'egg packets' (Figure 7.23) in the faeces or around the anus. The life cycle is shown in Figure 7.24. Control depends on treating the existing infection and eliminating any flea or louse problem to break the transmission cycle. *Dipylidium caninum* occasionally infects humans.

7.23 A *Dipylidium caninum* 'egg packet'.

Adult *Dipylidium caninum* in the small intestine of a dog or cat

Motile segments passed in the faeces

Prepatent period (time from infection to egg-laying) about 3 weeks

Scolex attaches to the intestinal wall

Cysticercoid released in the small intestine

Eggs or onchospheres in egg packets are released from the segment into the environment

Eggs eaten by the larval flea

Flea groomed off readily by host and ingested

Cysticercoid (the metacestode or larval form) develops as the flea develops. Infected flea moves slowly and clumsily

7.24 Life cycle of *Dipylidium caninum*.

Taenia spp.

Dogs and cats may be infected with taeniid tapeworms when they eat raw meat, either in the form of uncooked meat or offal or through catching and eating prey containing the intermediate stages. The life cycle of *Taenia hydatigena* is shown in Figure 7.25, and the final and intermediate hosts of a range of *Taenia* species are shown in Figure 7.26. Diagnosis is based on seeing segments passed by the animal. More rarely, eggs liberated from the segments are seen during microscopic examination of a faecal sample. *Taenia* eggs (Figure 7.27) are smaller than those of *Toxocara* (see Figure 7.33), measuring about 40 μm in diameter. Control is based on treating the current infection and then preventing the animal having access to uncooked flesh, which is something that is easy to do where the animal is fed by the owner but more difficult if the infection is derived from wild prey.

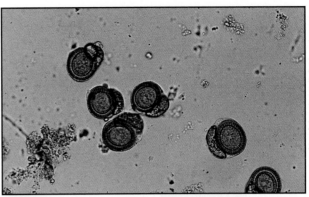

7.27 *Taenia* spp. eggs, each approximately 40 μm in diameter.

Rabbits are the intermediate hosts of *Taenia serialis*. Infection may occur as a result of grass eaten by rabbits being contaminated with eggs passed by dogs or foxes. Cysts (*Coenurus serialis*) are normally located in connective tissue and can appear similar to a subcutaneous abscess. Affected animals may show other clinical signs including decreased appetite. Treatment involves the surgical removal of cysts.

Echinococcus granulosus granulosus

This organism has a dog-to-sheep life cycle (Figure 7.28). It is an important zoonotic pathogen that occurs in the UK but is fortunately fairly rare. It is endemic in two areas of the UK (Wales and the Hebrides), where dogs have the opportunity to feed on sheep carcasses on the hills. Following accidental ingestion of eggs, hydatid cysts can develop in humans, particularly in the liver or lungs.

The adult parasite is very small, only about 6 mm long, and several thousand may be present in the intestine of a single dog. Dogs in affected areas should be regularly treated with an effective anthelmintic and denied access to sheep carcasses. If a human ingests a proglottid or individual eggs, then a hydatid cyst may develop in the liver or lungs in the same way as it will develop in the sheep. This forms a space-occupying lesion that may grow to some considerable size. Treatment of affected people is based on anthelmintics followed by draining the cyst and then surgically removing the wall of the cyst. This is quite a hazardous procedure for the patient.

Echinococcus multilocularis

This is a related tapeworm found in continental Europe, where it was particularly recognized in Switzerland but has now spread to include a wide area of central Europe, including Germany and eastern France. The intermediate stage, a multilocular invasive cyst, is normally found in rodents but humans can also be infected. Dogs, foxes and cats can act as final hosts, though cats are considered to be a poorer host. This parasite is the reason for the necessity to treat animals returning to the UK with praziquantel. Up-to-date information about this and other requirements of the pet travel scheme may be found on the Defra website.

Echinococcus granulosus equinus

This species of tapeworm has a dog-to-horse life cycle. It occurs particularly where hounds are fed on horse offal. Horses are infected when they graze pasture contaminated with eggs. It is not believed to pose a zoonotic risk.

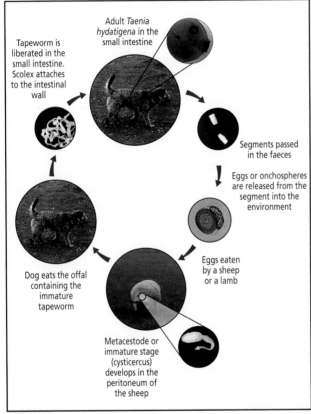

Adult *Taenia hydatigena* in the small intestine

Tapeworm is liberated in the small intestine. Scolex attaches to the intestinal wall

Segments passed in the faeces

Eggs or onchospheres are released from the segment into the environment

Eggs eaten by a sheep or a lamb

Dog eats the offal containing the immature tapeworm

Metacestode or immature stage (cysticercus) develops in the peritoneum of the sheep

7.25 Life cycle of *Taenia hydatigena*.

Taenia species	Final host	Intermediate host
T. taeniaeformis	Cat	Rat or mouse (*Cysticercus fasciolaris* in the liver)
T. serialis	Dog	Rabbit (*Coenurus serialis* in connective tissue)
T. pisiformis	Dog	Rabbit (*Cysticercus pisiformis* in the peritoneum)
T. ovis	Dog	Sheep (*Cysticercus ovis* in muscle)
T. hydatigena	Dog	Sheep/cattle/pig (*Cysticercus tenuicollis* in the peritoneum)
T. multiceps	Dog	Sheep/cattle (*Coenurus cerebralis* in the central nervous system)

7.26 Hosts of *Taenia* tapeworms.

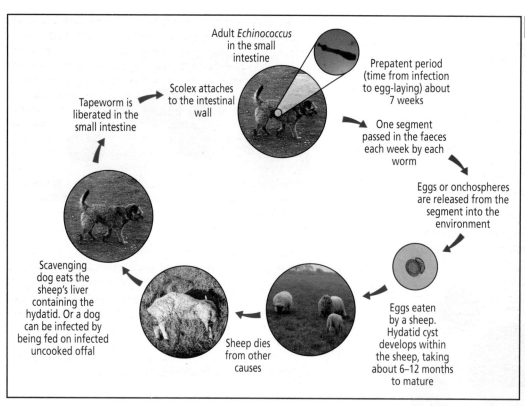

Adult *Echinococcus* in the small intestine

Scolex attaches to the intestinal wall

Tapeworm is liberated in the small intestine

Prepatent period (time from infection to egg-laying) about 7 weeks

One segment passed in the faeces each week by each worm

Eggs or onchospheres are released from the segment into the environment

Scavenging dog eats the sheep's liver containing the hydatid. Or a dog can be infected by being fed on infected uncooked offal

Sheep dies from other causes

Eggs eaten by a sheep. Hydatid cyst develops within the sheep, taking about 6–12 months to mature

Anoplocephala perfoliata

The equine tapeworm *Anoplocephala perfoliata* attaches to the intestinal mucosa in the area of the ileocaecal junction. When present in large numbers it can cause colic associated with ileocaecal intussusception and ileal impaction. Unlike the tapeworms found in cats and dogs, it is short and stout in appearance, with segments broader than they are long (Figure 7.29). The eggs cannot be reliably detected by faecal examination; a blood test to detect antibodies is more reliable. The intermediate hosts are small free-living oribatid mites, which live in pasture; horses become infected as they ingest infected mites whilst grazing.

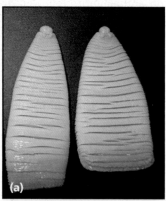

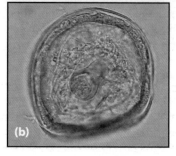

7.29 *Anoplocephala perfoliata.* **(a)** Adult, typically attached to the intestine close to the ileocaecal junction. **(b)** Egg.

Cestode infections in exotic pets

Birds and other animals, such as rabbits, mice, rats and hamsters, may all be infected with adult tapeworms specific to the host species. In most cases infection has no effect on the host. Occasionally a heavy tapeworm burden in hamsters may be associated with weight loss and perhaps intestinal blockage. In each case the intermediate host is an invertebrate such as a beetle or mite.

Treatment of cestode infections

Adult tapeworms can be killed by a number of anthelmintics. These may be products that have activity only against tapeworms, in which case they are known as **cestocides**. Alternatively, the preparation may have activity against other helminths, particularly nematodes, as well as tapeworms; these are known as **broad-spectrum anthelmintics** (see Chapter 8). It is much more difficult to kill the immature tapeworm infections in the intermediate hosts and this is not usually carried out; hence surgical removal is the treatment of choice in affected sheep and rabbits. Unfortunately there are no specific prophylactic treatments available for treatment of dogs; however, where *Echinococcus* spp. are endemic, regular treatment at 4- or 6-weekly intervals (depending on species) will remove adult worms before they begin egg laying, and hence will reduce environmental contamination with eggs and the zoonotic risk. There are a number of anthelmintics containing praziquantel or pyrantel at an elevated dose rate that are effective against tapeworms in horses.

Nematodes (roundworms)

Nematode worms are round in cross-section and have a digestive tract. Most have a direct life cycle but some (e.g. lungworms) have a slug or snail as an intermediate host. Others may be carried by a paratenic host.

Ascarids

An important nematode group seen in small animal veterinary practice are the ascarids (especially *Toxocara canis*, *Toxascaris leonina* and *Toxocara cati* in dogs and cats). These large fleshy worms (Figure 7.30) are most numerous and frequent in young animals.

Ascarids also occur commonly in exotic pets, including reptiles (e.g. tortoises) and birds (especially parakeets). In horses, particularly foals, there is one species, *Parascaris equorum* (Figure 7.31). In each case, the ascarid species is host-specific and heavy burdens may be associated with poor growth or intestinal impactions.

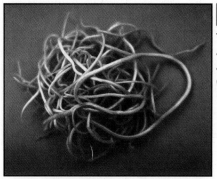

7.30

Typical appearance of adult ascarids (approximately 10 cm long).

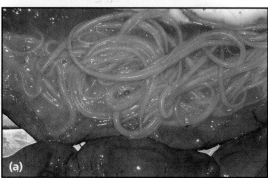

(a)

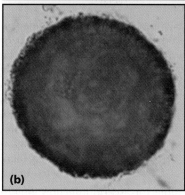

(b)

7.31

(a) *Parascaris equorum* adult worms in the intestine of a foal.
(b) Egg.

Toxocara canis

This is a very important worm, as it is a zoonotic pathogen and can also cause disease in young puppies. Its life cycle is shown in Figure 7.32.

Puppies are first infected before birth by larvae that pass from the bitch's muscles to her uterus after about the 42nd day of pregnancy. These larvae migrate through the liver and lungs of the young puppies and are then coughed up and swallowed. They remain in the small intestine, where they develop to adult worms by the time the puppies are 3 weeks old. Puppies can receive further infection from infective eggs

in the environment and by infective larvae that pass in the mother's milk, but the majority of the infection will usually have occurred across the placenta. Puppies that have a heavy *Toxocara* burden will typically be stunted, with distended bellies; they may vomit and/or have diarrhoea, and severe infections may lead to a total blockage of the intestine. As immunity develops following exposure, and possibly related to an increase in age, puppies begin to expel their *Toxocara* infection spontaneously from about 7 weeks of age. Most have expelled all of their adult worms by 6–7 months of age. Normally, further larvae that are ingested pass from the intestine to muscle, where they enter a resting state.

Adult worms pass large numbers of eggs; as many as several thousand eggs per gram of faeces in a 3-week-old puppy. Each egg is surrounded by a thick wall (Figure 7.33), which is very resistant to physical and chemical damage. The eggs are not immediately infective but require time for a larva to develop inside. In ideal conditions this will take about 14 days, but it may take much longer in low temperatures. Since the larva remains in the shell until eaten by an animal, the eggs may remain infective in the environment for at least 2 years. If the animal that ingests the eggs happens to be a bitch, the larvae remain in this resting state until she becomes pregnant; some of the larvae will migrate to infect her puppies; and others will remain to infect her subsequent litters.

Control of *Toxocara canis*

The aims are:

- Control of infection in the dog, to prevent disease in puppies and to prevent eggs being put into the environment
- Prevention of infection in children.

Control in dogs is based on the following:

- Prenatal infection in puppies may be controlled by treating the bitch, prior to whelping, with a product that will kill the migrating larvae, e.g. fenbendazole, from the 40th day of pregnancy to 2 days post whelping
- Alternatively, puppies may be treated at regular intervals with a suitable anthelmintic, starting from 2 weeks of age. The bitch should be treated at the same time
- Reducing the number of eggs in the environment is very difficult once the eggs are present. Scorching with a flame-thrower has been found to be the most effective method, but education of the dog-owning public is the best way to reduce egg output in the future.

The most important methods of preventing children from becoming infected are to ensure that:

- Dogs defecate in specified areas in parks
- 'Pooper scoopers' or other means of appropriate faecal disposal are used
- Children wash their hands before eating
- Children are discouraged from handling young puppies unless the animals have been thoroughly wormed.

Larvae that are accidentally eaten by other animals (including humans) migrate from the intestine and enter a resting state in other tissues. If a human ingests a large number of infective eggs and these all migrate together through the body, a condition known as **visceral larva migrans** may

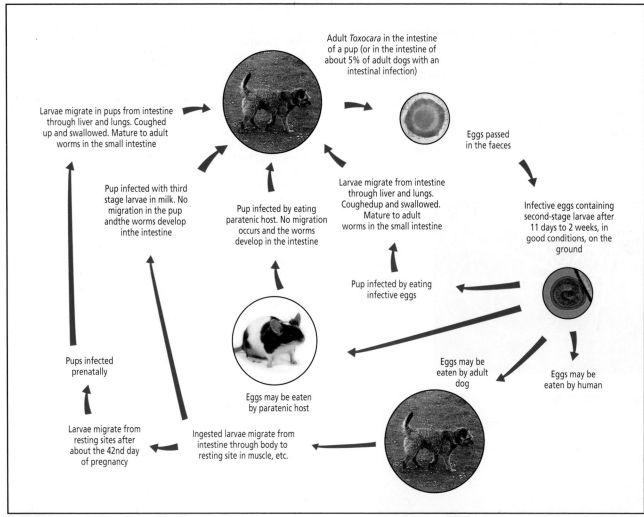

7.32 Life cycle of *Toxocara canis*.

The following labels appear around the diagram:

Adult *Toxocara* in the intestine of a pup (or in the intestine of about 5% of adult dogs with an intestinal infection)

Larvae migrate in pups from intestine through liver and lungs. Coughed up and swallowed. Mature to adult worms in the small intestine

Eggs passed in the faeces

Pup infected with third stage larvae in milk. No migration in the pup and the worms develop in the intestine

Pup infected by eating paratenic host. No migration occurs and the worms develop in the intestine

Larvae migrate from intestine through liver and lungs. Coughed up and swallowed. Mature to adult worms in the small intestine

Infective eggs containing second-stage larvae after 11 days to 2 weeks, in good conditions, on the ground

Pup infected by eating infective eggs

Pups infected prenatally

Eggs may be eaten by paratenic host

Eggs may be eaten by adult dog

Eggs may be eaten by human

Larvae migrate from resting sites after about the 42nd day of pregnancy

Ingested larvae migrate from intestine through body to resting site in muscle, etc.

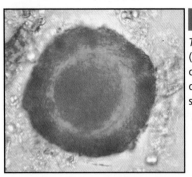

7.33

Toxocara canis egg (approximately 80 μm diameter). Note the dark contents and dark shell with pitted edge.

develop, associated with signs of damage to the organs through which the larvae are migrating. If only a few larvae are ingested, they will usually migrate through the human body without any signs of illness. However, in the rare case where they come to rest in the eye, sight dysfunction or even blindness may result. Infection is usually seen in children, as they are the most likely to have unhygienic habits.

To perpetuate their life cycle, dormant larvae in the tissues of birds or animals other than dogs depend upon their paratenic host being eaten by a dog.

In some adult dogs, for one reason or another, including a low level of challenge, adult worms will develop in the small intestine. Lactating bitches are particularly likely to have a patent infection, probably due to the change in their hormonal status. Their infection may come from a number of sources, including young worms passed by the pups that the bitch ingests as she cleans up around the nest. Usually the bitch expels her remaining infection shortly after the pups are weaned.

Single-sample surveys showed 5–10% of dogs are infected; in a recent Swiss survey, with monthly sampling over 12 months, 30% of dogs were infected at least once during the year.

Toxocara cati

This organism is responsible for ascarid infection in cats, particularly kittens. It is transmitted to kittens by their mothers' milk; infection also occurs through infective eggs in the environment and ingestion of paratenic hosts (Figure 7.34). Unlike *T. canis,* it is NOT transmitted via the placenta. A heavy infection may cause stunting of growth in kittens and a pot-bellied appearance.

The adult worm can be distinguished by the appearance of the alae or 'wings' either side of the head end (Figure 7.35) but the egg is grossly indistinguishable from that of *T. canis*.

Control is by regular treatment of kittens from about 3 weeks of age until they are several months of age. Kittens are infected via the milk and so will be about 6 weeks of age before the first infection becomes patent.

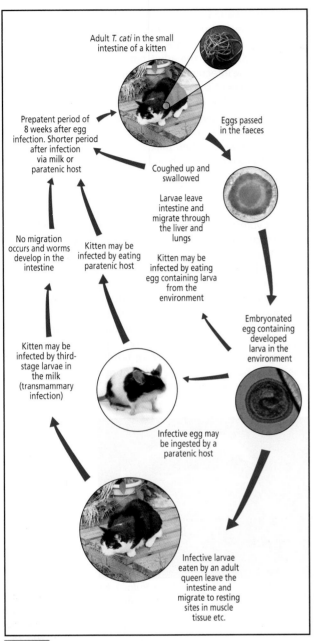

7.34 Life cycle of *Toxocara cati*.

Toxascaris leonina

Toxascaris leonina will infect both cats and dogs. Its life cycle is shown in Figure 7.36. It has rarely been implicated as a zoonosis. There is no prenatal infection; infection is therefore usually first seen in adolescent animals. The worm is not normally associated with clinical signs, since large burdens are reasonably well tolerated. The egg (Figure 7.37) can be distinguished by the smooth outer wall to its shell.

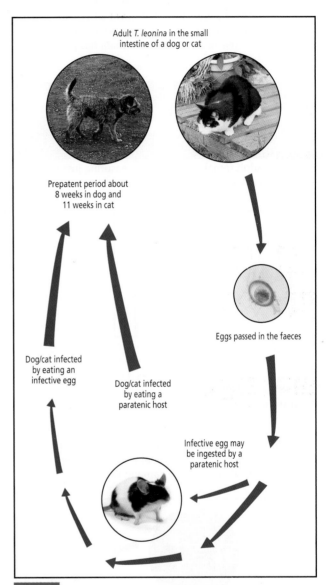

7.36 Life cycle of *Toxascaris leonina*.

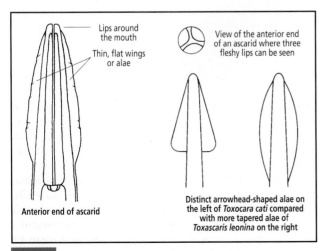

7.35 Anterior end and alae of adult ascarids.

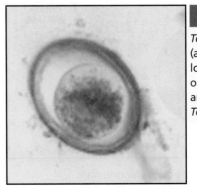

7.37

Toxascaris leonina egg (approximately 85 μm long). Note the smooth outer wall. Contents are paler than those of *Toxocara* species.

Hookworms

Hookworms are short stout worms with hooked heads (Figure 7.38). *Uncinaria stenocephala* and *Ancylostoma caninum* occur in the small intestine of the dog. Of the two species, *U. stenocephala* is the more common in the UK and is known as the northern hookworm; it is particularly seen in Greyhounds or in hunt kennels. *Ancylostoma braziliensis* infects the skin and intestinal tract of dogs and cats in tropical and subtropical regions; its larvae may also be zoonotic. The species may be distinguished by the appearance of the head: *A. caninum* has three pairs of large teeth; *A. braziliensis* (Figure 7.39) has two pairs of similar teeth; and *U. stenocephala* has plates in the mouth cavity.

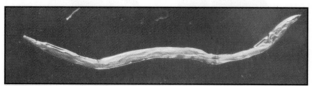

7.38 Adult female hookworm measuring just over 1 cm in length.

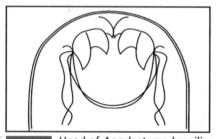

7.39 Head of *Ancylostoma braziliensis*, showing two pairs of teeth at the entrance to the buccal capsule. *Uncinaria stenocephala* has a similarly sized buccal capsule but with cutting plates instead of teeth. *A. caninum* has three pairs of teeth.

The life cycle of *U. stenocephala* is shown in Figure 7.40. The worms attach to the intestinal mucosa by their mouthparts. They use their teeth to damage the surface and then

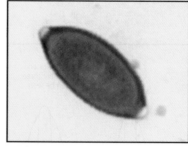

Eaten by dog. Prepatent period about 3 weeks

Eggs passed in the faeces

Larvae develop within egg

First-stage larvae liberated from the egg shells

Develop to infective third stage larvae in the environment

7.40 Life cycle of *Uncinaria stenocephala*.

feed off the tissue fluids, particularly blood in the case of *A. caninum*. A heavy burden of *Uncinaria* spp. may cause a dog to be thin and *Ancylostoma* spp. may cause anaemia.

Eggs produced by the adult female worms are passed in the faeces. The infective larvae of both worms may penetrate the skin. Larvae of *Uncinaria* spp. simply cause dermatitis, as they are incapable of travelling further, whereas those of *Ancylostoma* spp. may travel to the intestine and develop into adults. Bitches may also infect their puppies with *Ancylostoma* spp. larvae via their milk.

Cats can be infected with hookworm but infection appears to be rare in the UK.

Whipworm

Trichuris vulpis, the whipworm of the dog, has a whip-like appearance (Figure 7.41). The worms burrow into the mucosa of the large intestine, leaving the thicker caudal end in the intestinal lumen. A low burden is well tolerated but a heavy infection may be associated with bloody mucus-filled diarrhoea. The eggs in which the larvae develop are characteristic (Figure 7.42) and are covered in a thick shell, which makes them resistant to damage in the environment. Eggs containing infective first-stage larvae may survive for several years in the ground. *T. vulpis* therefore tends to cause problems when dogs have access to permanent grass runs, but clinical signs are rarely seen in the UK.

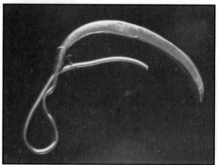

7.41 Whipworm (*Trichuris vulpis*). Note the wide posterior end and the narrow anterior end normally buried in the mucosa of the large intestine (1–3 cm).

7.42 *Trichuris vulpis* egg (approximately 70 μm long). Note plugs at both ends.

Equine intestinal nematodes

Strongyloides westeri is a slender worm that inhabits the small intestine of foals, which acquire infection through ingestion of larvae within the mare's milk. These larvae will have activated and moved from their resting place in the mare's abdominal wall and into the mammary gland. A heavy infection can cause diarrhoea and weight loss. The condition can be diagnosed by identification of the thin-walled eggs (Figure 7.43), each containing a larva, in a faecal sample.

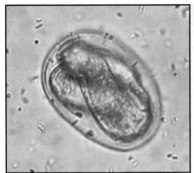

Strongyloides westeri egg.

Cyathostomins

The most common nematodes found in horses are a large group of species commonly known as the cyathostomins, or small strongyles; their life cycle is illustrated in Figure 7.44. Horses are infected when they ingest third-stage infective larvae from pasture, and the larvae develop initially within the wall of the large intestine. Some larvae undergo a state of arrested development or hypobiosis, continuing their development the following spring. As they mature, the developing worms leave the intestinal mucosa to inhabit the lumen of the large intestine. Where large numbers emerge simultaneously they can cause severe diarrhoea, a condition known as larval cyathostomosis, most commonly seen in the spring. It is therefore important to control cyathostomins to prevent disease. This can be achieved by management measures such as regular removal of dung from pasture and monitoring the worm egg count in the horse's dung and with anthelmintic treatment. As resistance of the cyathostomins to anthelmintics is becoming more widespread, a move away from regular anthelmintic treatment towards monitoring and treatment based on the presence of a low but significant worm count is being encouraged.

The large strongyles to be considered the most pathogenic worms in horses; however, each of the three species, *Strongylus vulgaris, S. edentatus* and *S. equinus,* have long developmental periods in the horse before reaching maturity, and they are very susceptible to ivermectin and related anthelmintics. The life cycle of *S. vulgaris* is shown in Figure 7.45 and a typical egg in Figure 7.46.

The larvae of *S. edentatus* and *S. vulgaris* migrate outside the intestine before they return to the large intestine to mature into adult worms. It is believed that the use of these

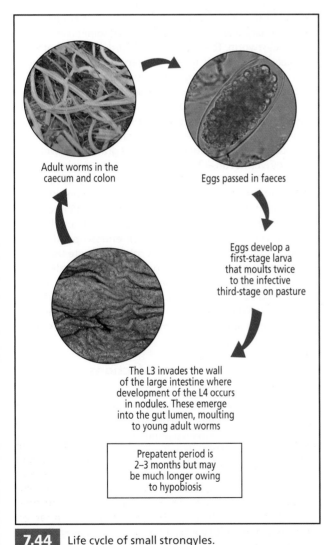

Adult worms in the caecum and colon

Eggs passed in faeces

Eggs develop a first-stage larva that moults twice to the infective third-stage on pasture

The L3 invades the wall of the large intestine where development of the L4 occurs in nodules. These emerge into the gut lumen, moulting to young adult worms

Prepatent period is 2–3 months but may be much longer owing to hypobiosis

7.44 Life cycle of small strongyles.

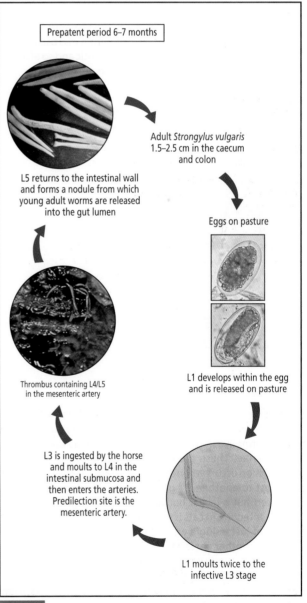

Prepatent period 6–7 months

Adult *Strongylus vulgaris* 1.5–2.5 cm in the caecum and colon

L5 returns to the intestinal wall and forms a nodule from which young adult worms are released into the gut lumen

Eggs on pasture

L1 develops within the egg and is released on pasture

Thrombus containing L4/L5 in the mesenteric artery

L3 is ingested by the horse and moults to L4 in the intestinal submucosa and then enters the arteries. Predilection site is the mesenteric artery.

L1 moults twice to the infective L3 stage

7.45 Life cycle of *Strongylus vulgaris*.

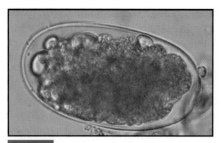

7.46   A typical cyathostomin/large strongyle egg.

anthelmintics has hugely reduced the prevalence of large strongyle parasites. The irony is that using ivermectin to remove these troublesome parasites has arguably allowed the tapeworms and small strongyles (previously considered essentially benign) to become more common.

Oxyuris equi

The pinworm *Oxyuris equi* inhabits the large intestine, and the female worms crawl out of the anus to lay their eggs around it. Therefore, eggs (Figure 7.47) cannot be reliably detected in faecal samples; instead a piece of transparent adhesive tape should be pressed on to the skin around the anus and then placed on a glass slide and examined with a microscope. The presence of female worms can be very pruritic and so affected horses may rub their tails against, for example, fences.

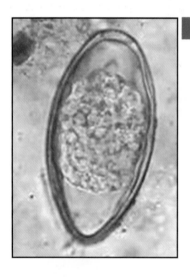

7.47   *Oxyuris equi* egg.

Heartworm

Dirofilaria immitis does not occur in the UK but may be seen in dogs that have been imported from warmer countries. The adult worms live in the heart; immature larvae are known as microfilariae. These are dispersed in the host's blood and transmission occurs when a mosquito transfers the larvae from one host to another. A light infection in a dog may be well tolerated but a larger burden can lead to right-sided heart failure. Infection in cats is somewhat less common but clinical effects of just a single worm can be severe.

This is another parasite to consider when owners are planning to take their pet to mainland Europe, as heartworm is endemic from the Mediterranean area of France southwards. Prophylactic treatment should be carried out by owners, using one of the treatments now authorized in the UK and following datasheet instructions.

Bladder and liver worms (*Capillaria* spp.)

Adult worms of *Capillaria plica* live in the bladder and so the eggs are passed in the urine of affected dogs. The eggs appear very like *Trichuris* eggs, but are smaller and have less distinct plugs. Infection is rarely seen in the UK.

Capillaria hepatica is a parasite of rats, particularly wild rats. The adult worm lives in the liver of the host, where it lays its eggs. These are only released when the rat dies or is eaten by another animal. Cats, dogs and humans may be infected, but this occurs very rarely.

Other *Capillaria* species that are specific to birds may cause diarrhoea in pigeons.

Lungworms

Cats become infected with *Aelurostrongylus abstrusus* (cat lungworm) by eating a slug or snail containing the infective larvae. The adult worm lives within the lung tissue of the cat. Infection with many worms may cause coughing, but a few worms often go unnoticed. Adult female worms produce larvae (rather than eggs) that are coughed up and swallowed. Diagnosis is confirmed by finding larvae in the faeces, using the Baermann technique (see Chapter 19).

Dogs acquire *Angiostrongylus vasorum* infection through eating a snail containing the infective larvae, or ingesting larvae once they have developed within a slug or snail. Transmission of this infection in England was confined to Cornwall and South Wales before 1990 but it is now being seen in most of the country. The slender adult worms live in the pulmonary artery of the dog, hence it is sometimes referred to as a heartworm. The adult females produce eggs that travel to the alveoli and hatch; the larvae then penetrate the alveolar walls. The larvae are coughed up, swallowed and passed in the faeces. Clinical signs include coughing and dyspnoea.

In the horse and pony *Dictyocaulus arnfieldi* has had historical importance. Its natural host is the donkey, in which many infestations are subclinical. It was an important differential diagnosis for coughing horses at grass but is well controlled by ivermectin anthelmintics and is now a relatively rare condition. The life cycle of *Dictyocaulus* spp. is direct and a mollusc intermediate host is not required for transmission.

The adult worms of *Oslerus osleri* live in small nodules at the bifurcation of the trachea (in dogs, particularly Greyhounds). The nodules can be seen on endoscopy; they may cause coughing in some dogs, but others tolerate their presence without showing clinical signs. The adult female worms produce larvae that are coughed up and swallowed. The life cycle is direct (i.e. the parasite passes directly from one host to the next without having to infect an alternative or intermediate host) and the bitch may infect her puppies as she grooms them.

Diagnosis of nematode infections

It is important that faecal samples are fresh and are quickly picked up from the ground; otherwise the sample can become contaminated with free-living nematodes and their eggs from the environment. The main diagnostic methods are modified McMaster techniques to detect nematode eggs in faeces and the Baermann technique (see Chapter 19) to detect larvae.

Treatment of nematode infections in dogs and cats

Treatment of nematode infections is carried out in three main situations.

Regular or routine treatment

A broad-spectrum anthelmintic with additional cestocidal activity is often used to remove any infections that may have accumulated since the animal was last wormed. Adult dogs and cats will usually be treated at intervals ranging from 1 (in high-risk situations) to 3 months depending on the likelihood of infection. There is now an option to control nematodes and fleas at the same time by using either selamectin or imidacloprid plus moxidectin (Advocate, Bayer Animal Health) in cats and dogs, or lufenuron plus milbemycin (Program Plus, Novartis Animal Health) in dogs; all of which are administered at monthly intervals (see Chapter 8). Like cestodes, there is no prophylactic treatment available, although some treatments are effective against immature treatments and thus will prevent maturation of infections.

Toxocara infections in puppies and kittens

Since these infections occur in the vast majority of litters, it is normal to control them by treating all puppies and kittens regularly, at 2-weekly intervals from 2 weeks of age in puppies and 3 weeks in kittens until weaning.

Diagnosed nematode infection

Where the presence of a nematode infection has been diagnosed as the cause of a clinical problem, the product with the best activity against that infection will usually be chosen for treatment of the animal. Where regular treatment is not conducted, regular faecal examinations are an alternative.

Treatment of nematode infections in horses

Wherever possible, anthelmintic treatment of horses should be combined with an appropriate mix of pasture management and faecal worm egg counting. Ideally, a strategy should be customized to the individual horse, taking into account factors such as age, management and whether it lives alone or with others.

In recent years, primarily because of increased concerns about the development of anthelmintic resistance, there has been a move away from regular repeated anthelmintic treatment and this has been replaced with two main approaches:

- **Strategic dosing:** Treatments are targetted at key times of year, e.g. larvicidal treatment of encysted cyathostomins in the late autumn and winter. The rigid application of such an approach can mean that problems can arise if, for example, there are early or late peaks in larval numbers on pasture
- **Targeted strategic treatment:** This adapts strategic dosing to incorporate additional management information such as that derived from worm egg counts.

Protozoal parasites
Coccidia

Coccidia may cause marked diarrhoea in young animals, particularly lambs, birds and rabbits. A typical coccidian life cycle is shown in Figure 7.48.

7.48

Life cycle of *Eimeria* spp. (Redrawn from Urquhart *et al.*, 1996, with the permission of Blackwell Publishing.)

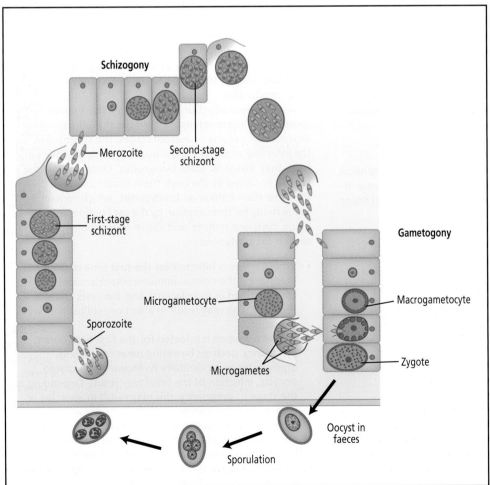

Isospora

Two species infect cats and another two infect dogs. The animals are infected when they ingest either sporulated oocysts (oocysts are not sporulated until a few days after they have been passed in the faeces) or infected intermediate hosts. Reproduction occurs in the cells lining the small intestine. Infection is usually associated with few clinical signs, but there may be transient diarrhoea. Heavy infection may cause severe diarrhoea in puppies and kittens.

Eimeria

Rabbits may be infected with any of three *Eimeria* species:

- *Eimeria intestinalis* and *E. flavescens* infect the caecum, causing diarrhoea and emaciation.
- *E. stiedae* infects the bile ducts in the liver, causing wasting, diarrhoea and excess urine production.

Diagnosis is based on finding oocysts in the faeces (Figure 7.49). It should be noted, however, that the small rod-like organisms often found in the faeces of sick rabbits are not Coccidia and are not believed to be significant. Treatment such as sulphonamide may be given in rabbits' drinking water, or to pet rabbits on an individual basis. Control is based on making sure that the rabbits have clean bedding and that droppings or diarrhoea are not allowed to build up in the feeding area.

Chickens, in common with other species of bird, are susceptible to several species of coccidian and in commercial flocks they may be the reason for significant losses. The most common species affecting poultry are:

- **Eimeria tenella:** Pathogenic coccidian located in the caecum. Young chicks are most commonly affected, with high morbidity and mortality. Faeces from affected birds may contain visible blood
- **E. necatrix:** Develops in the small intestine and caecum and may be associated with morbidity and mortality
- **E. acervulina** and **E. maxima:** Both develop in the upper part of the small intestine. Infection is typically associated with weight loss.

Prevention of disease can be achieved by careful attention to hygiene, although this can be difficult (e.g. with frequently used runs, wooden chicken houses), and anticoccidial drugs may be required.

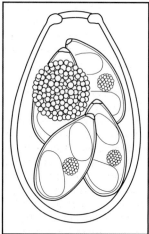

7.49 Sporulated oocyst of *Eimeria* spp. (Reproduced from Urquhart *et al.*, 1996, with the permission of Blackwell Publishing.)

Cryptosporidium parvum

This small protozoan parasitizes epithelial cells in the small intestine. Both asexual and sexual reproduction occur in the intestine; and small oocysts, the result of sexual reproduction, are passed in the faeces. Infection occurs by ingesting sporulated oocysts; this has been associated with diarrhoea in young puppies and kittens and the young of other domestic animals including foals. Humans may be infected, usually only causing a transient diarrhoea, though severe diarrhoea may be associated with infection in immunocompromised individuals. Diagnosis is based on finding the oocysts (4.5–5 μm diameter) in the faeces. Identification may be assisted by staining with Ziehl–Neelsen, as the oocysts are acid-fast, or by immuno-fluorescence techniques. There is currently no authorized treatment for the infection in small animals or horses.

Sarcocystis

This organism has a more complex life cycle. The intermediate hosts are ruminants, pigs or horses. Large unsightly cysts are formed in muscle and so infected meat is condemned. In addition, infection may result in marked illness in the infected animal. The final host for each species is the dog or the cat. For example, *Sarcocystis tenella* (also known as *S. ovicanis*) is a parasite of sheep and dogs. Reproduction occurs in the small intestine without clinical signs. The oocysts, measuring approximately 10–15 μm, are already sporulated when passed.

Sarcocystis neurona is the cause of equine protozoal myeloencephalitis, a disease affecting the central nervous system of horses in the USA and potentially in those imported from there.

Toxoplasma gondii

The final host for *T. gondii* is the cat (Figure 7.50). Sexual reproduction occurs in the epithelial cells of the small intestine. Oocysts are produced that are passed in the faeces. The cat usually shows no sign of infection and normally, after excreting oocysts for about 10 days, becomes immune and stops production.

Asexual reproduction can occur in the extra-intestinal (outside the intestine) tissue of almost any animal. Following ingestion of oocysts or asexual stages, the sporozoites leave the intestine and travel to tissue, particularly muscle or brain. Here they divide to form tachyzoites. Once an immune response is started by the host, these undergo slower division; they are then known as bradyzoites, which remain in the tissue ready for consumption by the cat (definitive host). The tissue cysts are minute and cause few problems except in certain circumstances:

- Where a ewe is infected for the first time during pregnancy, the normal immune responses are compromised in the placenta and the cysts are able to replicate. This may result in abortion, stillbirth or weak lambs
- Where a woman is infected for the first time during pregnancy, perhaps by eating meat containing bradyzoites or accidentally swallowing sporulated oocysts, infection of the fetus may result. Depending on the stage of pregnancy, this may result in abortion or severe abnormalities or in no clinical signs at all. Fortunately, infections during human pregnancy are not common. Further information and leaflets can be obtained from Tommy's, The Baby Charity (www.tommys.org), who have taken over the work of the Toxoplasmosis Trust in the UK

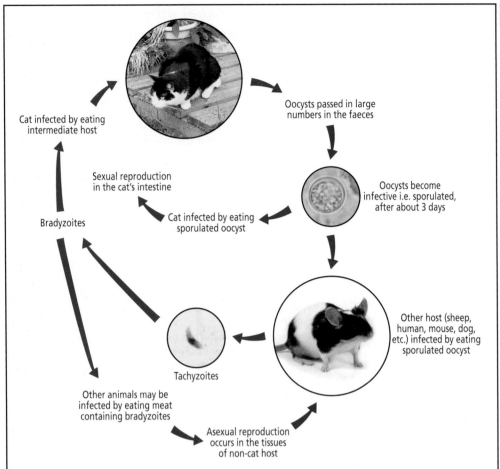

Cat infected by eating intermediate host

Oocysts passed in large numbers in the faeces

Sexual reproduction in the cat's intestine

Cat infected by eating sporulated oocyst

Oocysts become infective i.e. sporulated, after about 3 days

Bradyzoites

Other host (sheep, human, mouse, dog, etc.) infected by eating sporulated oocyst

Tachyzoites

Other animals may be infected by eating meat containing bradyzoites

Asexual reproduction occurs in the tissues of non-cat host

- Infection in humans may be associated with malaise and 'flu-like symptoms that vary in severity from individual to individual
- Cysts in immunosuppressed individuals may begin to undergo rapid division and cause severe tissue lesions.

In order to try to prevent these infections occurring:

- Farmers are advised to prevent cats, particularly young cats, from getting into food stores intended for sheep
- Sheep can be vaccinated against *Toxoplasma gondii*
- Pregnant women are advised to take precautionary measures. For example, they should not clean out cat litter trays, they should wear gloves when gardening, they *should not assist with lambing ewes,* and they should ensure that all meat is thoroughly cooked before eating it.

There is no effective treatment to prevent cats shedding the oocysts. Children who have been infected prenatally are treated with antiprotozoals to prevent any long-term effects.

Neospora caninum

This parasite causes incoordination in young dogs and abortion in cattle. In the past, infection was normally ascribed to *Toxoplasma gondii*. It is believed that the dog is the final host for this parasite. Treatment of affected puppies may be necessary. Breeding bitches can be screened serologically for signs of infection.

Hammondia

This is another protozoan parasite where the cat is the final host. Infection is not normally associated with clinical signs. Sexual reproduction occurs in the intestine of the cat and oocysts are produced that appear similar to those of *Toxoplasma*. The intermediate hosts for *Hammondia* are rodents and so the presence of these oocysts does not present a human health risk.

Giardia spp.

This flagellate protozoan may parasitize the small intestine of humans and domestic animals. The species in mammals is *Giardia intestinalis,* also known as *G. duodenalis* and *G. lamblia.* It is still unknown how important *Giardia* infection in pet animals is as a source of human infection, although some strains of *G. intestinalis* have been identified as potential zoonoses, whilst others are not. The species in mice and other small rodents is *G. muris.* Infection may cause death in cagebirds such as cockatiels and budgerigars.

Infection may be asymptomatic or may be associated with transient or chronic diarrhoea. Puppies are at greatest risk. Occasionally infections occur in foals. Diagnosis is based on demonstration of the cysts (Figure 7.51), which are small (approximately 10 μm) and may be passed intermittently in the faeces. Even when a sample is positive, cysts may be present in low numbers, so a sensitive detection technique is used, such as centrifugal flotation using saturated zinc sulphate solution. The cysts can then be stained with Lugol's iodine to increase visibility. It is suggested that collecting samples for 3 days and pooling the sample may increase the chance of

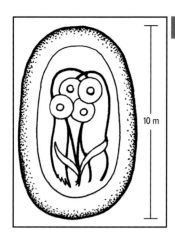

7.51 Cyst of *Giardia* spp.

10 m

detecting the cysts, which are excreted intermittently. Other methods of diagnosis include ELISA and PCR. Treatment can be carried out with repeat doses of benzimidazoles, such as fenbendazole, or metronidazole. Cleaning and hygiene, to eliminate cysts and hence prevent re-infection, are important parts of controlling an outbreak.

Encephalitozoon cuniculi

E. cuniculi is a microsporidian parasite of rabbits that can also affect humans and a variety of other animals. Microsporidia were classified as Protozoa but their classification is currently under review. Rabbits are infected by ingestion of spores from the environment or from infected rabbit urine. Between 7.5% and 68.1% of rabbits have seroconverted, i.e. have antibodies in the blood, which is indicative of exposure to infection. However, disease only develops in a proportion of these animals. Signs of disease are varied, and include head tilt, ill-thrift (failure to grow, gain weight or maintain weight in the presence of apparently adequate food supplies), weight loss and renal failure, as infection localizes in a number of organs, particularly the nervous system and kidneys. Treatment consists of symptomatic treatment and administration of fenbendazole to eliminate the infection. There is also evidence that treatment with fenbendazole may be useful to eliminate the parasite in infected but asymptomatic animals.

Other protozoal infections

Some protozoal infections are not endemic in the UK but clinical disease may be seen in animals that are imported from, for example, parts of Europe, where the disease is endemic. These include *Babesia*, a parasite that infects the red blood cells of dogs, thereby causing anaemia. This is a tick-transmitted infection endemic in central and southern Europe. Infection can result in acute disease with fever, jaundice and even death if the infection is particularly severe or is not treated rapidly.

Leishmaniosis is caused by a flagellate protozoan (*Leishmania* spp.) and is transmitted by sandflies. It occurs in many warmer parts of the world, including the Mediterranean area. Incubation can be particularly long and it is often extremely difficult to clear the infection completely with drug treatment. Dogs, particularly rescued animals, infected with *Leishmania* are not infrequently imported into the UK and may be increasingly seen in veterinary practices. Signs of infection are various and can include dermatological signs, such as localized alopecia, and systemic signs including weight loss.

These infections often pose treatment challenges as the appropriate medicines are often not readily available. More information on imported diseases may be found in the vector-borne disease guidelines at www.esccap.org.

Additional information on exotic pets

Examples of parasites in exotic pets have been included throughout the main text and are further summarized in Figure 7.52. The range of parasites in these species is large, however, and BSAVA Manuals and other books should be consulted for more complete details.

Host	Parasite group							
	Ectoparasites					*Endoparasites*		
	Lice	Fleas	Flies	Mites	Ticks	Cestodes	Nematodes	Protozoa
Rabbits	D Haemodipsus ventricosus	D Spillopsyllus cuniculi Ctenocephalides felis	D Lucilia spp.	D Psoroptes cuniculi Cheyletiella parasitivorax Listrophorus gibbus	D Various	D Cysticercus pisiformis Coenurus serialis	d	D Eimeria intestinalis E. flavescens E. stiedae
Mice	D Polyplax serrata	D Ctenocephalides felis		D Myobia musculi Myocoptes musculinus		d	d	d
Rats	D Polyplax spinulosa	d		D Radfordia ensifera Notoedres muris		d	d	d

7.52 Summary of parasites found in exotic pets. D: can be the cause of disease; d: may be present but rarely causes disease. Data compiled from Harcourt-Brown (2007); Harcourt-Brown and Chitty (2005); Keeble and Meredith (2009); Klingenberg (2004); Meredith and Johnson-Delaney (2009) and Paterson (2006).

continues ▶

Host	Parasite group							
	Ectoparasites					**Endoparasites**		
	Lice	Fleas	Flies	Mites	Ticks	Cestodes	Nematodes	Protozoa
Hamsters		D *Ctenocephalides felis*		D *Demodex* spp.				
Guinea pigs	D *Gliricola porcelli*			D *Trixacarus caviae*		d		D *Eimeria caviae*
Ferrets		D *Ctenocephalides felis*		D *Otodectes cynotis* *Sarcoptes scabiei*	D *Ixodes* spp.			
Parrots	d	d		D *Dermanyssus gallinae*	d	d	D *Ascaridia* spp.	D *Giardia* spp. *Eimeria* spp.
Budgerigars	d	d		D *Cnemidocoptes* spp. *Dermanyssus gallinae*			d	D *Ascaridia* spp.	D *Giardia* spp. *Eimeria* spp.
Tortoises			D Various		D Various		D Ascarids	D *Hexamita* spp.
Bearded dragons				D *Ophionyssus natricis*	D Various		D Ascarids	D *Isospora* spp.

7.52 *continued*   Summary of parasites found in exotic pets. D: can be the cause of disease; d: may be present but rarely causes disease. Data compiled from Harcourt-Brown (2007); Harcourt-Brown and Chitty (2005); Keeble and Meredith (2009); Klingenberg (2004); Meredith and Johnson-Delaney (2009) and Paterson (2006).

Further reading

Harcourt-Brown F (2007) *Textbook of Rabbit Medicine.* Butterworth Heinemann, London

Harcourt-Brown N and Chitty J (2005) *BSAVA Manual of Psittacine Birds, 2nd edn.* BSAVA, Gloucester

Keeble E and Meredith A (2009) *BSAVA Manual of Rodents and Ferrets.* BSAVA, Gloucester

Klingenberg RJ (2004) Parasitology. In: *BSAVA Manual of Reptiles, 2nd edn,* ed. SJ Girling and P Raiti, pp.319–329. BSAVA Publications, Gloucester

Meredith A and Flecknell P (2006) *BSAVA Manual of Rabbit Medicine and Surgery, 2nd edn.* BSAVA Publications, Gloucester

Meredith A and Johnson-Delaney C (2009) *BSAVA Manual of Exotic Pets, 5th edn.* BSAVA, Gloucester

Overgaauw PAM (1997) Aspects of *Toxocara* epidemiology: toxocarosis in dogs and cats. *Critical Reviews in Microbiology,* **23**, 233–251

Paterson S (2006) *Skin diseases of Exotic Pets.* Blackwell Publishing, Oxford

Taylor MA, Coop RL and Wall RL (2007) *Veterinary Parasitology, 3rd edn.* Blackwell Publishing, Oxford.

Trees A and Shaw S (1999) Imported diseases in small animals. *In Practice* **21**, 482–489

Useful websites

ESCCAP: provides guidelines for parasite control in dogs and cats: www.esccap.org

BSAVA review of worm control in cats; **BSAVA** review of worm control in dogs: www.bsava.com

Self-assessment questions

1. Define the terms 'ectoparasite' and 'endoparasite'.
2. Describe how you could differentiate between an insect and an arachnid.
3. Describe how you could differentiate between a burrowing and a surface mite.
4. List the zoonotic ectoparasites and zoonotic endoparasites found in dogs and cats.
5. Define the terms 'permanent' ectoparasite and 'direct life cycle'.
6. State the four ways in which dogs can become infected with *Toxocara canis.*
7. Compare and contrast the above transmission routes with those of *Toxocara cati.*
8. Based on the above transmission routes, identify prevention and treatment options for both *T. canis* and *T. cati.*
9. State the most common cestode of the dog and cat and describe how this tapeworm is transmitted.
10. Identify the cestode that has to be treated for under the Pet Passport Scheme.
11. Give examples of pathogens that ticks are responsible for transmitting.

Chapter 8

Medicines: pharmacology, therapeutics and dispensing

Sally Argyle, Debra Kennedy and Tim Greet

Learning objectives

After studying this chapter, students should be able to:

- **Understand basic pharmacological terminology and principles**
- **Name the main routes of administration of drugs including any equipment required and particular precautions that should be taken**
- **List the main classes of drug used in veterinary practice**
- **Apply the legislation governing veterinary medicines in the United Kingdom; this will include:**
  - **The legal categories of veterinary medicines**
  - **Legislation concerning the requisition, storage, dispensing, prescribing, record keeping requirements and disposal of these medicines**
- **Describe COSHH regulations and Health and Safety requirements specifically in relation to the storage, handling and administration of drugs in the practice and practice pharmacy**
- **Calculate drug doses accurately when presented with typical drug formulations**
- **Recognize adverse drug reactions and be familiar with the suspected adverse reactions surveillance scheme (SARSS)**

Introduction

Terms used in pharmacology

- **Pharmacology** is the science of drugs and their effects on living organisms.
- **Pharmacodynamics** refers to the effects of the drug on the organism; i.e. what the drug does to the body.
- **Pharmacokinetics** refers to the effects of the body on the drug; i.e. how the body handles the drug in terms of its absorption, distribution around the body, metabolism and, finally, excretion from the body (Figure 8.1).

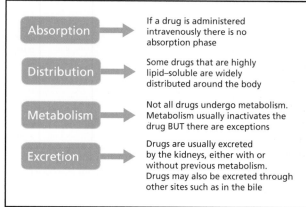

8.1 Phases associated with the pharmacokinetics of drugs within the body.

- Most drug metabolism occurs in the liver. Usually metabolism inactivates the drug, but on occasion a drug may require hepatic metabolism to become active. An example of a class of drug requiring activation would be the angiotensin converting enzyme (ACE) inhibitors, which include benazepril. Importantly, a number of drugs are capable of interfering with the liver's ability for drug metabolism. If enzyme levels are increased this will decrease the efficacy of drugs that are metabolized by those reactions. However, if enzymes are inhibited this increases the risk of toxicity from drugs relying on them for their metabolism. If an animal has liver disease, this may similarly affect its ability to handle drugs that require hepatic metabolism.
- Most drugs are excreted from the body through the kidneys, although excretion through the bile into the gastrointestinal tract is significant for quite a few. Animals with renal disease may have a decreased ability to eliminate these drugs from the body and they may need to be given at a reduced dose or avoided altogether. Drug datasheets are the most appropriate source of information for specific drug concerns and these should be used to provide information on use of drugs in animals with pre-existing renal or liver disease and on any potential drug interactions.

continues ▶

continued

- **Bioavailability** can be defined as the percentage of an administered drug that reaches the systemic circulation.
- **Clinical pharmacology:** The pharmacology of most drugs is determined in young healthy animals. Drugs may not behave in precisely the same way in individual patients, perhaps due to concurrent disease or other medications. Clinical pharmacology refers to the study of drugs in individual patients.
- **Therapeutics** refers to the use of drugs to treat diseases or conditions.

The **therapeutic index** of a drug gives an idea of its safety *versus* toxicity. It is based on a population of animals and is defined as the ratio of the maximum dose that is non-toxic to the minimum dose that is effective:

$$\frac{\text{Maximum 'safe' dose}}{\text{Minimum effective dose}}$$

Drugs that have a low therapeutic index, such as the cardiac glycosides, have very little margin between the doses required to obtain the desired effect and those doses that are associated with adverse effects. Modifying the dose of drugs with a low therapeutic index would be most critical, for example, if there were evidence of liver or renal disease that might decrease an animal's ability to metabolize or eliminate the drug, since even relatively small changes in plasma levels may be associated with toxicity.

- **Dispensing** is the physical act of giving out drugs. Pharmacists and veterinary practices are permitted to dispense drugs.
- **Prescribing** refers to 'prescription-only medicines'. Prescribing may involve a written instruction (a prescription), which may then be taken to a pharmacist or another veterinary practice, or may be the physical act of dispensing or administering the prescription medicine by an appropriate person.

Medicines and nomenclature

Drugs are referred to by both **trade names** and **generic names**. The generic name is the non-proprietary name for the drug and is recognized internationally. Generic names will be used in this chapter. The **recommended International Non-proprietary Name (rINN)** must be used under European law. The **British Approved Names (BANs)** for certain drugs have been recently modified so that all BANs are in line with the rINNs. Examples include changing frusemide to furosemide, and lignocaine to lidocaine.

The veterinary pharmaceutical industry manufactures and distributes veterinary medicines under a strict Code of Practice. The **Veterinary Medicines Directorate (VMD)**, or **European Medicines Agency (EMEA)**, must be satisfied that all regulations concerning efficacy, quality and safety have been adhered to before a drug can be authorized ('licensed'). All authorized veterinary medicines have a marketing authorization number and distribution category (see later).

Medicine formulations
Oral formulations

Drugs that are absorbed through the gastrointestinal tract into the blood circulation are said to have a **systemic effect**, as they are transported around the body. Some oral medications are designed to have a **local effect** within the gastrointestinal tract and are not absorbed into the circulation. Examples of those having a local effect include laxatives, activated charcoal, and cytoprotectants such as sucralfate.

Tablets and caplets

In tablets and caplets the active ingredient is combined with an **excipient** (an inert substance used as a diluent or vehicle) and compressed.

- Tablets/caplets may be scored to allow easy splitting to reduce the risk of fragmenting. Figure 8.2 shows a variety of scored and unscored tablets and caplets.
- Some preparations are enteric-coated, enabling the drug to pass through the stomach without causing irritation, while others need to be protected from the acids produced by the stomach.
- Other forms of coating are used to control the rate of dissolution and absorption. They can also make tablets more palatable.

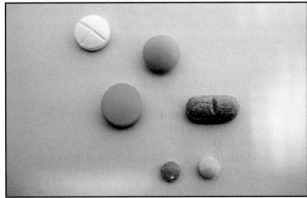

8.2 A selection of tablets and a caplet (brown) used for oral medication.

> **WARNING**
>
> It is important not to split or crush sustained-release preparations as this will destroy their sustained-release characteristics. Once a drug has been crushed or split it is exposed to air and moisture; this can cause some drugs to degenerate very quickly. Enteric-coated tablets should not be crushed or split without consulting the manufacturer.

Capsules

Capsules are a useful way of administering drugs that are very bitter and irritate the oral mucosa. The outer case of the capsule is made of gelatine or glycerine; some comprise two halves that contain powder or granules. Granulated preparations enable a sustained release of drug. Liquids are enclosed in sealed cases. Empty gelatine capsules are available in various sizes, enabling some capsules to be made up with smaller/larger doses if required (Figure 8.3).

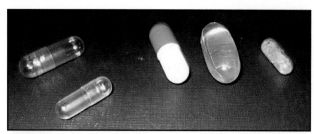

8.3 Capsules. From left to right: empty capsules; capsules containing powder, liquid, and granules.

Granules, pastes and powders

These oral formulations can have a local or systemic effect depending on their action.

- Anthelmintics, laxatives and probiotics can be found in granule and paste formulations. In horses, a paste format can be an especially useful way of administering oral medications.
- Powdered preparations are used to administer nutritional supplements, as they can be sprinkled on food or made into pastes for oral administration.

Mixtures

The main components are the solvent (the liquid base) and the solute (the drug). A wide range of drugs are available in this form as an alternative to the solid formulation. Mixtures are useful for medicating exotic pets and young animals, when accurate dosing in small volumes is required.

- **Solution**: The solute is completely dissolved in the solvent, forming a homogeneous mixture.
- **Suspension**: The solute does not dissolve in the solvent due to the large particles, forming a heterogeneous mixture. A suspension should be mixed by shaking gently before use.
- **Syrup/linctus**: A concentrated solution of refined sugar dissolved in distilled water to produce a thick viscous liquid.
- **Emulsion**: A mixture of two or more immiscible liquids that tends to have a cloudy appearance. An emulsifier is required to stabilize the emulsion.

Other formulations available include **boluses**, which are administered orally, and **suppositories**, which are inserted into the vagina or rectum. These types of formulations are more commonly used in large animal species.

Topical formulations

Topical formulations are used directly on the skin, eyes, ears and mucous membranes. They are generally used to treat local conditions but there are preparations that are well absorbed through the skin and into the systemic circulation. Examples of the latter include emodepside, a topically applied anthelmintic used to treat gastrointestinal roundworms in the cat, and glyceryl trinitrate, which may be used in the treatment of acute heart failure.

- **Cream**: Used to apply drugs to the skin, the base is a mixture of oil and water. As most drugs in creams are hydrophobic, they are released from the water after evaporation.

- **Ointment**: Used to apply drugs to the skin or mucous membranes, it is a semi-solid preparation of oil/water. The base will depend on the action of the drug and the site of application; bases include hard or soft paraffin, wax and wool fat.
- **Lotions**: Applied to unbroken skin and often have a cooling/calming effect. They are a mixture of oil and water and contain an emulgent to prevent separation.
- **Shampoos/wipes**: Preparations can be medicated or non-medicated and are specially formulated for animal skin. They may contain pesticides or other medications for the treatment of parasites or skin conditions.
- **Spot-on/pour-on**: Liquid preparations applied to the skin that have a slow-release effect. They are used to deliver pesticides and anthelmintics. Some formulations are species-specific. Care must be taken not to overdose. If used on food-producing animals (meat or eggs) there is a withdrawal period and owners must be informed.
- **Aerosols**: Release liquid droplets or suspensions under pressure. They are used to deliver pesticides and antiseptics to the skin.
- **Patches**: Transdermal patches are applied to the skin and are used to deliver a controlled release of drug that has a systemic effect. Fentanyl patches are used for their analgesic properties in the care of cancer patients and perioperatively in small animals and horses.
- **Nebulizers/inhalers**: The drug is mixed with air or gas to produce a fine mist or aerosol that can be inhaled to treat respiratory diseases; e.g. steroids and bronchodilators.

Parenteral formulations

Parenteral administration refers to any route other than the gastrointestinal route, but the term is generally used to refer to medicines administered by **injection**.

> ### WARNING
>
> All preparations and equipment necessary to administer injections must be sterile.
>
> Manufacturer's datasheets should be consulted to determine specific routes appropriate for administration, as serious complications can occur if a preparation is not administered via the correct route.

- **Single- and multi-dose vials or bottles**: These bottles are sealed with a rubber diaphragm. If it is stipulated that a medicine must be used within a given time (see manufacturer's datasheet) it must be labelled with the date the vial or bottle was broached. Single-dose vials must be used immediately once opened and any remaining product discarded in accordance with current regulations. A selection of multi-dose vials is shown in Figure 8.4.
- **Ampoules**: Used for single-dose administration, these are made of glass with a thin neck that can be snapped off (Figure 8.5). It is advisable to cover the neck with a swab or tissue to prevent cuts from glass splinters. Sometimes the preparation can sit in the neck of the ampoule and needs to be moved down by gently tapping, before the neck is broken.
- **Collapsible bags**: Made from plastic and available in many volumes and preparations, these are generally used for administering intravenous infusions, as they

collapse during administration to prevent air leaking into the infusion set (Figure 8.6).

- **Implants**: Compressed sterile pellets that are implanted subcutaneously; these serve as a depot, releasing the drug over a period of time. Hormone preparations are most commonly delivered in this type of formulation.

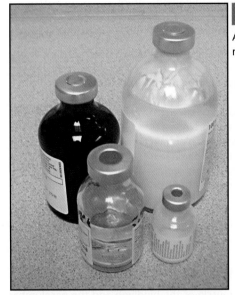

8.4

A selection of multi-dose vials.

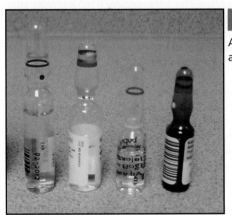

8.5

A selection of ampoules.

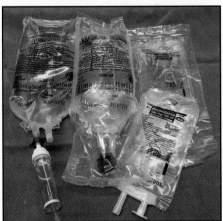

8.6   Collapsible infusion bags are usually packaged in an outer wrapping enabling them to be used in a sterile manner. Left to right: Hartmann's solution, unwrapped, part used and attached to a giving set; Ringer's solution, wrapped; metronidazole infusion, unwrapped and wrapped.

Procedure for loading a syringe with a drug prior to injection

1. Select the drug prescribed, ensuring it is the correct preparation.
2. Choose the most appropriate syringe and needle.
3. Remove the syringe from the sealed packaging without contaminating the tip.
4. Break the seal on the needle and remove it.
5. Push the hub of the needle on to the tip of the syringe firmly.
6. Shake the bottle/vial gently to mix, if required, and swab the rubber diaphragm with an alcohol swab. Invert the bottle/vial.
7. Remove the needle cap and insert the needle through the rubber diaphragm in the top of the bottle/vial.
8. Pull the plunger back slowly to the required dose Keep the needle below the level of liquid, as this will prevent air entering the syringe.
9. Remove the needle and carefully replace the needle cap.
10. Check for air bubbles. Gently tap the barrel to dislodge any bubbles that are in the liquid and push the plunger to expel any air into the needle cap.

Practical tips

- To aid loading the syringe, especially if dispensing a suspension, inject the same volume of air into the vial prior to loading. It is important not to inject excessive amounts of air into the vial as this may cause the needle and syringe to separate, contaminating the operator with leakage or spray.
- When reconstituting a powder, inject the water or diluent into the vial keeping the needle above the level of liquid. To relieve the pressure inside the vial, release the pressure on the plunger to allow air into the syringe.

Routes of medicine administration

There are a number of important factors to consider when deciding the route of administration:

- The disease and how it affects the body
- The drug being prescribed and how it is formulated
- The condition and temperament of the animal
- The owner's ability to administer the drug.

The administration of medicines by veterinary nurses is regulated under the **Veterinary Surgeons Act 1966 (Schedule 3 Amendment) Order 2002**. This states that only listed veterinary nurses (either RVN or VN) who are registered with the RCVS can administer medicines under the **direction** of a veterinary surgeon. Student veterinary nurses enrolled with the RCVS for training can administer medicines under the **direct supervision** of a veterinary surgeon or listed veterinary nurse.

Oral administration

Oral medications travel through the digestive tract. Once absorbed from the intestine, they pass through the liver before reaching the circulation and then the site of action. Some medicines are not absorbed from the gut and act locally. This may have an effect on the bioavailability of the drug.

Advantages of oral administration:

- Convenient and easy for the owner to medicate, especially when the animal is on long-term medication.

Disadvantages of oral administration:

- The absorption and distribution of the drug is relatively slow when compared to parenteral administration
- It is not a suitable route if the patient is unconscious, vomiting or difficult to dose
- Food in the stomach can affect the absorption of some drugs, e.g. erythromycin and pimobendan, and so must be given on an empty stomach
- Some drugs cause irritation to the stomach and intestine, causing vomiting and diarrhoea
- Gastric acid in the stomach can destroy (denature) drugs, e.g. insulin
- Liver enzymes may break down a drug before it is able to reach the systemic circulation, e.g. glyceryl trinitrate.

Equipment and techniques are described later in the chapter.

Parenteral administration

Routes of parenteral administration include:

- Intravenous
- Intramuscular
- Subcutaneous
- Intraosseous
- Epidural
- Intrathecal
- Intradermal
- Intra-articular
- Intraperitoneal
- Intra-arterial
- Subconjunctival.

Intravenous administration

Intravenous (i.v.) administration involves direct delivery of medicine into the venous blood. Commonly used sites for venepuncture include the cephalic vein, the lateral saphenous vein (or the medial saphenous vein in cats), the external jugular vein and the auricular vein (this is especially used in rabbits). Other sites may be used when medicating exotic pets and these will depend on the species.

When administering long-term medication, i.e. fluid infusions, over-the-needle cannulae are used in peripheral veins and can remain in place for 72 hours, or longer with careful maintenance. Leaving a cannula *in situ* for >72 hours should be considered on a case-by-case basis. Through-the-needle cannulae are longer and are used for jugular veins; they are the only cannulae suitable for monitoring central venous pressure. This type of cannula has a long-term use, but strict aseptic techniques must be followed.

Advantages of i.v. administration:

- Drugs are administered directly into the systemic circulation and thus have 100% bioavailability
- The drug action at the site is achieved quickly with predictable blood plasma levels
- Drugs that are irritant to tissues are given by this route, e.g. cancer chemotherapeutic drugs.

Disadvantages of i.v. administration:

- Aseptic technique is essential to avoid introducing infection
- The drug must be in solution, as particles in suspension may obstruct small blood vessels and cause death
- Injections should be given *slowly* to avoid serious effects on the heart and brain
- Accidental extravascular injection of irritant drugs can cause severe tissue damage
- Intravenous catheters require regular maintenance to prevent blockage or the catheter dislodging (see Chapter 17).

Equipment and techniques are described later in the chapter.

Intramuscular administration

The quadriceps muscle of the hindlimb and the paralumbar area are commonly used for intramuscular (i.m.) administration in the dog and cat. It is important to avoid damaging major blood vessels and nerves around the site of injection, e.g. the sciatic nerve in the hindlimb. The sites used when medicating exotic pets vary according to species.

In the horse, intramuscular injections are often administered into the mid-cervical musculature. This is best avoided in smaller horses and in very young foals, as it has been associated with accidental spinal injection. Similarly, the brisket has been used but this area is prone to oedematous swelling so is also best avoided. The most satisfactory intramuscular site is the gluteal region. If a large volume of viscous drug is to be injected into a small pony or foal, it may be better to divide the dose and use different sites; however, this may depend on the temperament and ease of handling of the patient. If there are reasons not to inject at these sites, it is probably better to use the intravenous route with an appropriate preparation. It is possible to use other intramuscular sites, e.g. quadriceps, but the risk of complications is greater.

Repeated use of one particular site will make the muscle group very sore and can upset the patient. Alternating sides, and even sites, is therefore good practice, especially if administering twice-daily injections of a large volume or for a long period.

Advantages of i.m. administration:

- Drugs in suspension can be given intramuscularly
- Drugs are absorbed more quickly than by the subcutaneous route.

Disadvantages of i.m. administration:

- Only small volumes can be administered at one site up to 2 ml in cats and up to 5 ml in dogs
- Injections may be painful and cause localized reactions
- Accidental intravenous injection can occur unless the syringe is drawn back after insertion to check that it is not in a blood vessel.

Subcutaneous administration

Subcutaneous (s.c.) administration involves injecting medicine into areas of loose skin. This is usually at the scruff of the neck, where skin is loose, has a poor nerve supply and lacks large blood vessels. Fluids injected into this site must be non-irritant to prevent irritation or necrosis of tissue. This route is seldom used in horses.

Advantages of s.c. administration:

- Larger volumes of fluid can be injected into the scruff of the neck, although it is preferable to use smaller volumes over several sites to reduce discomfort
- This route is generally pain-free, although this depends on the drugs being injected.

Disadvantages of s.c. administration:

- Absorption can take at least 30 minutes, due to the lack of large blood vessels. This is therefore not the route of choice for the administration of fluids to patients in shock where there is peripheral vasoconstriction
- It is possible to damage small blood vessels
- Local reactions to drugs can occur, causing swelling and irritation.

Intraosseous administration

This is the administration of a medicine directly into the **bone marrow** in the medulla of a long bone. This route may be used when intravenous access is compromised or in very small mammals, birds and chelonians. The needle can be placed into the intertrochanteric fossa of the femur, the tibial crest, the greater tubercle of the humerus, or the ilium. The route is seldom used for hydration in horses but has been used to administer local antibiotics in foals with osteomyelitis or a septic physis.

Advantages of intraosseous administration:

- Large volumes of fluid and blood transfusions can be given via this route
- No special equipment is necessary; intraosseous needles are available but spinal needles or hypodermic needles can be used.

Disadvantages of intraosseous administration:

- Strict aseptic technique must be used
- It is difficult to maintain access once the animal is mobile.

Epidural administration

Strict aseptic technique is used for epidural administration. Injections are given into the **vertebral canal** outside the dura mater. This route is used to administer preoperative, long-acting local anaesthesia and analgesia to animals undergoing orthopaedic surgery (see Chapter 23). It can provide analgesia for up to 8 hours.

Epidural administration is used in horses to provide analgesia for surgery of the perineum and genital tract in mares, occasionally as an obstetrical aid, and to reduce straining in some cases of rectal prolapse. It can also be used to provide analgesia for severe orthopaedic pain affecting the hindlimbs.

Intrathecal administration

Intrathecal administration requires strict aseptic technique. Injections are given into the **subarachnoid space**, which contains cerebrospinal fluid. This route is used for the injection of contrast media for myelography in small animals and horses under general anaesthesia. Careful monitoring of the animal is essential during this technique, as it can be associated with respiratory depression. This route is also used occasionally in the treatment of medical conditions, e.g. for the administration of tetanus anti-toxin in cases of tetanus.

Intradermal administration

This route is used for skin allergy testing in small animals and horses; very small volumes of allergens are injected into the **dermis**. It is also used for administering vaccines, e.g. myxomatosis vaccine in rabbits.

Intra-articular administration

This route is used for administering drugs, e.g. corticosteroids, directly into a **joint cavity**. It is also used for lavage of infected joints and to instil antibiotic preparations. Aseptic technique is essential. The procedure is usually carried out under sedation and analgesia. This technique is commonly used in the treatment of joint disease in horses and is frequently used to instil a local anaesthetic into the joint for the diagnosis of lameness.

Intraperitoneal administration

This route may be considered for administering large volumes of fluid when intravenous access is compromised or in small mammals (not birds or reptiles). It is not used routinely, as absorption of drugs through the peritoneum is variable and there is a risk of puncturing an abdominal organ. Strict aseptic technique is required.

Intracardiac administration

This is where drugs are administered directly into the muscle or ventricle of the heart during cardiopulmonary resuscitation, e.g. adrenaline. This route is seldom used in horses.

Intratracheal administration

For intratracheal administration, drugs are injected directly into the trachea or given through an endotracheal tube. This route is used during cardiopulmonary resuscitation, e.g. for the administration of adrenaline.

Intra-arterial administration

This route is not routinely used for administering drugs; it is more commonly used to monitor blood gases and blood pressure during surgery and in intensive care patients (see Chapters 21 and 23).

Subconjunctival administration

Subconjunctival administration involves giving an injection into the **conjunctival membranes** of the eye. This route is not commonly used in small animal veterinary medicine.

This route is occasionally used in horses with ocular infections, for the injection of anti-inflammatory preparations. It is sometimes also used to conduct the 'Mallein' test for glanders in equine species, although the antigen is more usually injected topically into the conjunctival sac rather than subconjunctivally, as the animal is more tolerant of this.

Topical administration

Administration to the skin

It is important to consult the manufacturer's instructions regarding application and frequency of use. Gloves should always be worn when applying skin preparations to prevent exposure to the drug and to the condition being treated. Advice to owners, and demonstrations, may be necessary concerning the amount of preparation needed and sites to be used.

> **WARNING**
>
> Observe animals for local or systemic reactions caused by absorption from the skin or by oral ingestion (as a result of the patient licking the treated area).

Administration to the eye

Some eye injuries can be very painful, and this must be considered when applying medication to the eyes, in order to prevent the animal from undergoing unnecessary stress and potentially biting. It may be necessary to have a second person present to hold the animal.

As the eyes are normally continuously bathed with tears, medication must be applied frequently. When applying any preparation, care must be taken not to touch or damage the surface of the eye with the nozzle or fingers.

Topical ocular preparations are commonly used in equine patients. In some horses this is achieved more effectively after the insertion of a subpalpebral catheter. As with small animals, good restraint is necessary.

> **WARNING**
>
> - Some ophthalmic preparations require gloves to be worn during administration. Always check the manufacturer's instructions.
> - Excessive tear production, swelling around the eye and pawing at the face are signs of local irritation.
> - Blepharospasm, corneal ulceration, delayed epithelial healing and miosis are contraindicators to most ophthalmic preparations.

How to apply ointment to the eye

1. Tilt the head back slightly.
2. Using your fingers, gently pull down the lower eyelid and administer the ointment along the inner canthus.
3. Release the eyelid.
4. When the animal blinks the ointment will coat the surface of the eye.

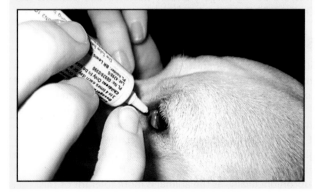

How to apply liquid eyedrops

1. Tilt the head back slightly.
2. Using your fingers, gently pull open the upper and lower eyelids to expose the eye, if possible.
3. Administer the appropriate amount of drops on to the eye, as directed, and release the eyelids.

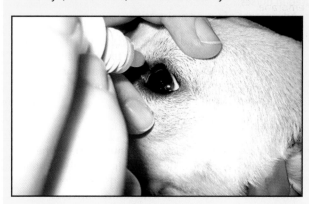

Administration to the ear

It may be necessary first to clean the external ear canal of wax, debris or hair, as this may prevent penetration of the drug that is being administered. Avoid using anything that can be pushed deep into the canal, to prevent rupture of the tympanic membrane. The ear should be examined first, to ensure that the tympanic membrane is intact, as most ear medications and cleaners are contraindicated if this is ruptured. It is advisable to wear gloves when treating or administering preparations. It may be necessary for a second person to hold the animal, depending on the severity of the condition and temperament of the animal being treated.

How to administer aural preparations

1. Hold the pinna gently to stretch out the ear canal. This is especially important with long-eared dogs, to allow the preparation to drain down the canal.
2. Administer the drops into the ear as directed.
3. Before releasing the pinna, massage the external ear canal to ensure adequate distribution.

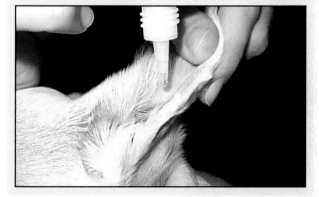

> **WARNING**
>
> Head shaking or tilting, ataxia, and problems with hearing are all clinical signs of ototoxicity contraindicating the use of aural preparations.

Methods of administration using other routes

Nebulization/inhalation

Drugs are mixed with air or gas to pass via the nose or mouth into the lungs, where they are absorbed through the mucous membrane.

- **Nebulization**: Small, portable machines are available for treating small animals and birds. The animals need to be in an enclosed space, e.g. an incubator or small cage. The vaporizer is placed as close to the patient as possible, for maximum effect. The duration of exposure depends on the species and drug being administered. In horses, drugs may be nebulized using a proprietary nebulizer and mask for the treatment of small airway disease (Figure 8.7).
- **Inhalation**: A vaporizer is used to mix volatile anaesthetics with oxygen or an oxygen/nitrous oxide mix, before they are administered into the lungs via an endotracheal tube. Inhalers, used for treating asthma in cats, are attached to a mask that covers the cat's mouth and nose; this allows the cat to inhale the vapour (Figure 8.8a). Hand-held inhalers are available for horses for daily administration of treatment by owners for the management of chronic small airway disease (Figure 8.8b).

Nasal lining/conjunctival administration

Drugs that would be broken down by enzymes in the gastrointestinal tract are administered through the mucous membranes of the nose and eye, e.g. desmopressin in the management of diabetes insipidus. The drug can be sprayed into the nose or applied as drops into the eye (see above).

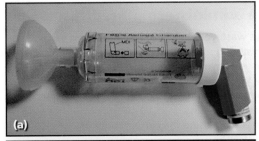

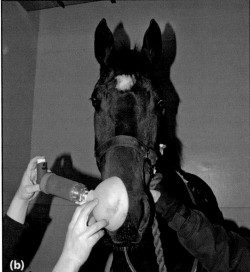

8.8 Inhalers. **(a)** A dosing chamber attached to an inhaler, suitable for an asthmatic cat. **(b)** A hand-held inhaler being used on a horse. (b, courtesy of Emily Haggett)

Rectal administration

This route can be considered if administering fluid therapy, although fluid must be instilled into the colon for absorption to take place, not the rectum. Rectal administration is not suitable for animals with diarrhoea or severe dehydration. The rectal route is also used to give enemas: a Higginson syringe is used to flush liquid into the rectum and colon to expel the faecal contents (see Chapter 17). Administration of fluid per rectum is very much a route of last resort in horses, but enemas are commonly administered to foals to aid the passage of meconium and in the treatment of meconial impaction.

Equipment and techniques used to administer medicines

Legislation and patient safety

- All drugs must be prescribed by the veterinary surgeon in charge of the case.
- Listed veterinary nurses must ensure all drugs administered to animals in their care are recorded in their notes or on inpatient sheets, in accordance with the practice protocols.
- Any changes in an animal's condition during or after the administration of a drug must be reported to the veterinary surgeon immediately.

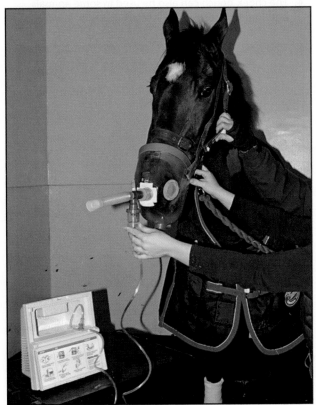

8.7 An equine nebulizer in use. (Courtesy of Emily Haggett)

Before administering medicines:

- **Always wash your hands before preparing or administering medication**
- Ensure you have the correct patient
- Ensure you have the correct medication
- Ensure you are administering the correct dose and frequency
- Ensure you are using the correct route of administration

Oral medications

Equipment is available to aid the administration of tablets (Figure 8.9):

- **Pill guns** are useful for dosing animals, particularly cats
- **Pill crushers** enable tablets to be crushed into a fine powder; this is then either mixed with food or made into a paste for administration through feeding tubes
- **Pill splitters** allow accurate dosing of tablets/caplets that are not already scored; the manufacturer's data sheet must be checked to ensure the preparation can be split.

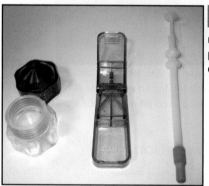

8.9 From left to right: pill crusher; pill splitter; pill doser.

Oral administration of tablets or caplets

1. Hold the top of the muzzle with one hand.
2. Use your second hand to hold the tablet and also to pull the lower jaw down gently.
3. Place the tablet on the tongue and push it to the back of the mouth.
4. Close the patient's mouth and gently stroke its throat to encourage swallowing.

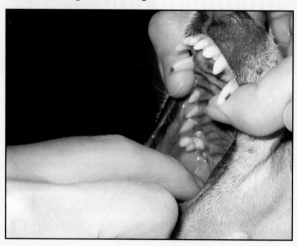

> **WARNING**
>
> Some tablets are associated with irritation of the oesophagus and should therefore be followed by a food or water bolus to prevent the preparation from residing in the oesophagus. Examples include doxycycline and clindamycin.

Oral administration of liquid preparations

1. Dispense the liquid preparation into an appropriately sized syringe.
2. Hold the patient's head gently, but securely, with one hand.
3. Using your other hand, place the syringe into the side of the mouth behind the canine teeth and administer the liquid slowly into the mouth.

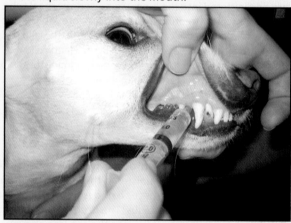

4. The cheek pouch can also be used in some animals but liquid must be administered slowly or it will run out of the animal's mouth.

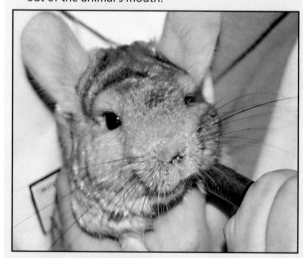

5. Support the animal's head and stroke its throat to encourage swallowing.

> **WARNING**
>
> Animals having difficulty swallowing (because of trauma, disease or surgery) must not be forced to take food or medication, as this could lead to aspiration pneumonia.

Feeding tubes and **crop feeders** are available in a range of gauges and lengths (Figure 8.10); tubes can be cut down to appropriate length for dosing small and exotic pets.

Although oral administration of medication is commonly employed in horses, it is equally common and in some ways more reliable to administer fluids or medication via nasogastric intubation, particularly in sick or inappetent patients.

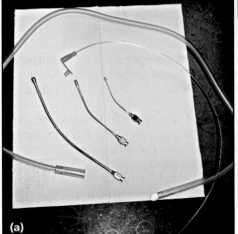

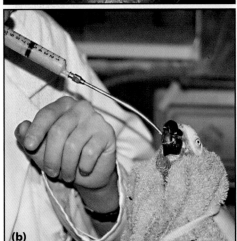

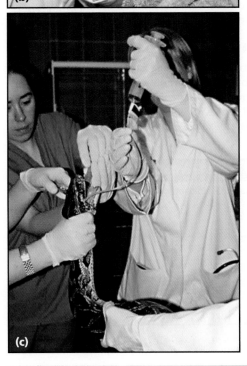

8.10

(a) A selection of crop and feeding tubes.
(b) Dosing of a bird using a crop feeder.
(c) Oral dosing of a snake.

(a)

(b)

(c)

Inserting a nasogastric tube into a horse

1. With the patient adequately restrained, the tube is passed via the ventral nasal meatus into the oesophagus, timing the push into the oesophagus as the horse swallows.
2. It is possible to visualize the tube sliding down the left side of the trachea or to palpate it in the cervical region at this site.
3. Confirmation of the presence of the tube in the stomach, by the smell of gastric contents, is important.
4. Air felt on exhalation, even though the horse may not be coughing (the horse has a relatively insensitive cough reflex), should alert the operator to the fact that the tube has inadvertently been passed into the trachea and must be withdrawn.

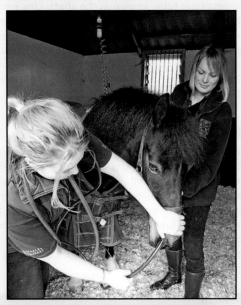

WARNING

The administration of fluids and liquid paraffin into the lower airway may have potentially fatal consequences.

Parenteral administration

Before administering a parenteral preparation:

- Consider the volume to be administered. Use a syringe appropriate to the volume to ensure accurate dosing, e.g. a 0.6 ml injection will require a 1 ml syringe
- Consider the viscosity of the preparation; it is difficult to draw a thick suspension through a 23G needle!
- Consider the species and injection site; 26G to 21G needles are generally used in dogs and cats to ensure the injection is as pain-free and atraumatic as possible.

Needles

There are many different types of needle available (Figure 8.11). The needle of choice is dictated by the procedure to be performed and site of administration.

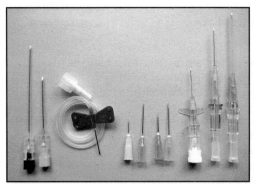

8.11 Some needle/cannula types: (left to right) spinal needles; butterfly needle; hypodermic needles; intravenous cannulae.

The **hypodermic needle** is used to administer most parenteral preparations. A hypodermic needle consists of a hollow stainless steel tube, known as the **shaft**. One end of the shaft is cut at an angle, to make a sharp point, or **bevel**, to assist penetration of the skin. Attached to the syringe is the **hub**; this has a universal colour code to reflect the **gauge** (G) of the needle. The gauge refers to the diameter of the shaft, a 6G being the largest and a 31G the smallest. All gauges are available in different lengths.

Syringes

The **hypodermic syringe** is used to administer parenteral preparations. Hypodermic syringes consist of a transparent plastic **barrel** that is graduated, indicating the volume size. The **plunger** is pushed or pulled within the barrel and is tipped with a rubber seal to prevent liquid escaping. The tip of the barrel is open, with a **luer fitting**, enabling the attachment of hypodermic needles or luer connectors.

Syringes are available with different tips depending on their function (Figure 8.12).

WARNING

- Ensure all air bubbles are removed before administering insulin as they can reduce the dose significantly. Ensure you use the correct syringe for the insulin being administered, as formulations are available in 40 IU/ml and 100 IU/ml.
- Some drugs can be absorbed into the plastic, or react with chemicals in the plastic of syringes. Consult *the manufacturer's data sheet if a preparation is not intended for immediate use.*

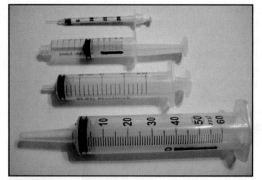

8.12 Some syringe types. From top to bottom: insulin syringe; luer-lock tip syringe; hypodermic luer-tip syringe; catheter-tip syringe.

- Luer-lock tip syringes are used when administering cytotoxic drugs.
- Catheter-tip syringes can be attached directly on to catheters and feeding tubes.
- Bulb syringes are used to flush and lavage wounds.
- Insulin syringes are for the administration of insulin only. They are graduated in units, not millilitres, and have a 25G needle attached; to reduce the amount of dead space, the needle does not have a hub.

Cannulae

There are many different cannulae available and it will depend on the function and site of use as to which is most suitable. The **intravenous cannula** (see Figure 8.11) is made of flexible nylon. This prevents damage to the lumen of the vessel and surrounding tissue. A **trochar** allows puncture of the skin into the lumen of the vein; the cannula is threaded into the vein and the trochar removed. The cannula has a luer fitting, allowing attachment of ports, adapters, infusion sets and syringes. Each practice will have its own protocols with regard to equipment, techniques and maintenance procedures (see Chapter 22).

Infusion pumps/syringe pumps

These are used to deliver accurate rates of fluids and doses of medication (see Chapter 22).

Injection sites and techniques

Figure 8.13 provides a summary of parenteral routes of administration of drugs to a variety of exotic species. Comprehensive information on administering medicines to exotic pets can be found in the *BSAVA Manual of Exotic Pets* and the *BSAVA Manual of Exotic Pet and Wildlife Nursing*.

Patient type	Intravenous	Subcutaneous	Intramuscular	Intraperitoneal	Intraosseous
Small mammals (ferrets, rabbits, rodents)	Jugular vein; marginal ear vein; cephalic vein; lateral tail vein	Dorsal body; 'scruff'	Quadriceps; lumbar	Off midline, caudal to umbilicus	Proximal femur; proximal tibia; proximal humerus
Birds	Jugular vein; brachial vein; medial metatarsal vein	Precrural fold	Pectoral (breast)	Not applicable	Distal ulna; proximal tibiotarsus
Snakes	Ventral coccygeal vein	Dorsal lateral third, over ribs	Intercostal	Cranial to vent on lateral body wall (intracoelomic)	Not applicable

8.13 Sites for the parenteral administration of drugs to exotic pets.

continues ▶

Patient type	Intravenous	Subcutaneous	Intramuscular	Intraperitoneal	Intraosseous
Lizards	Ventral tail vein; jugular vein	Loose lateral skin, over ribs	Quadriceps; triceps	Ventral, off midline, caudal to ribs	Proximal/distal femur; proximal tibia
Chelonians	Jugular, dorsal tail	Loose skin on limbs	Quadriceps, triceps, pectoral	Ventral, cranial to hindlimb in fossa	Bridge between plastron and carapace; femur
Amphibians	Femoral vein; midline abdominal vein	Dorsal area over shoulders	Triceps	Ventrolateral quadrant (intracoelomic)	Not applicable
Fish	Caudal vein	Not applicable	Dorsal lateral epaxial musculature	Rostral to ventral on lateral surface (intracoelomic)	Not applicable

8.13   *continued* Sites for the parenteral administration of drugs to exotic pets.

Intravenous injection

In small animals, administration of drugs through the **jugular vein** usually requires a catheter ('central line') to be placed. This is used in dogs or cats when animals require intensive care or long-term therapy.

Injection into the cephalic vein of a dog or cat

1. Prepare the injection as prescribed.
2. Soak swabs with an alcohol-based solution. A dry swab and microporous tape will also be required.
3. An assistant will need to restrain the animal gently by holding its head with one hand, while extending its forelimb from behind the elbow, with the other hand. The animal can be in sternal recumbency or in a sitting position.
4. Clip the area of the intended venepuncture.
5. Prepare the area using the alcohol swabs.
6. The assistant will need to 'raise' the vein by using the thumb to restrict blood flow.
7. Remove the needle cap and insert the needle through the skin into the vein. If the needle is in the vein, when the plunger is pulled back slightly, blood will appear in the syringe.
8. When the needle is in the correct position the assistant must lift their thumb to release pressure on the vein.
9. Push the plunger to administer injection slowly directly into the vein.
10. Remove the needle from the vein and immediately apply direct pressure to the site, using a dry swab to prevent haemorrhage.
11. Securely position the swab over the injection site.

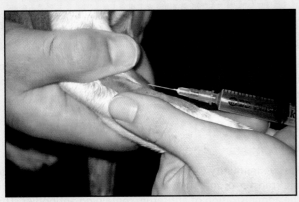

Starvation prior to a contrast study in the foal should be limited in order to maintain fluid and electrolyte balance. A neonate foal should have fluids withdrawn for no more than 2 hours. For a foal on a solid diet, solids may be withdrawn for up to 8 hours, but fluids for 4 hours at most.

In horses, the jugular vein is the usual site for intravenous injection. The vein is large in all equine species and usually easy to penetrate with a needle. It is preferable to clip the area in animals with a long or thick hair coat, and aseptic skin preparation is advised. If the jugular vein is not prominent it is usually possible to raise it by pressing a thumb on the downstream side.

If there is any doubt about injecting into a vein that has previously been used, and possibly already compromised, an alternative site should be used. In this regard, it is valuable to practise using lateral thoracic, cephalic and saphenous veins. It is essential to avoid bilateral jugular thrombosis, which usually results in venous and lymphatic stasis of the head and significant respiratory obstruction.

A variety of needle diameters may be used in horses but they should all have a minimum length of 40 mm (1½ inches). It is preferable to use a wider bore for viscous or irritant drugs to avoid perivascular injection. Caution should be observed when inserting the needle to avoid inserting it too deeply or at too steep an angle. Inadvertent injection into the carotid artery can have catastrophic consequences, as can injection of irritant chemicals around the neurovascular bundle; this may result in damage to the recurrent laryngeal or sympathetic nerves, with consequent development of iatrogenic laryngeal hemiplegia or Horner's syndrome.

Subcutaneous injection

An assistant may be required, depending on the temperament of the animal. Normally this injection is well tolerated and causes little or no stress.

> **WARNING**
>
> Manufacturers of vaccines advise against using any sterilizing solutions on the skin prior to injection, in order to prevent contamination of the vaccine.

Subcutaneous injection

1. Prepare injection as prescribed.
2. Select an area at the back of the patient's neck (the 'scruff').

continues ▶

continued

3. Remove the cap from the needle and with your other hand gently raise the skin slightly.
4. Insert the needle at a slight angle below the skin; pull back on the plunger to ensure no blood vessels have been damaged.
5. If no blood appears in the hub, administer the injection by pushing the plunger. If blood appears, remove the needle from the site; replace the needle and select another site.

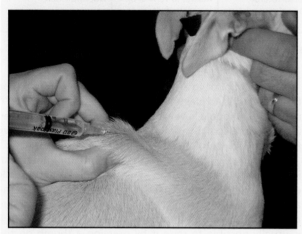

Intramuscular injection

An assistant will need to restrain the animal firmly, as this is generally a painful injection.

Intramuscular injection

1. Prepare injection as prescribed.
2. Isolate the area for injection (for example, the lumbar muscles in a dog).
3. Insert the needle into the muscle and pull back on the plunger slightly. If no blood appears, administer the injection.
4. Remove the needle and rub the site gently to aid distribution and reduce the stinging sensation.

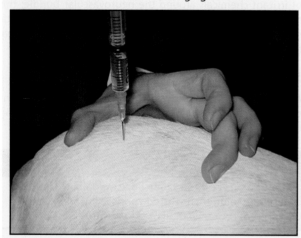

The technique for intramuscular injection in horses is the same as for cats and dogs. The injector must be aware that some horses find the procedure sufficiently uncomfortable to the point where they will resist it forcibly, and so appropriate restraint is important.

Safe handling and disposal of equipment

- All syringes and equipment contaminated with medicinal preparations must be classed as hazardous and treated accordingly (see Chapter 2).
- All 'sharps' must be disposed of immediately after use. This includes needles, syringes with attached needles, part-used syringes, broken glass, scalpels, blades and sharp sections of infusion sets. Sharps bins must be of an approved design (Figure 8.14). All sharps contaminated with animal blood or pharmaceuticals must be put into yellow sharps containers for high temperature incineration. The lid is colour coded to reflect the type of waste. The bin must have a handle and be sealed once full. **Contaminated sharps** are disposed of in a **yellow** bin with a yellow or orange lid.
- Sharps and consumables contaminated with **cytotoxic** pharmaceuticals must be used with great care and disposal of contaminated equipment requires special handling. These must be disposed of in **yellow and purple** containers. A yellow bin with a purple lid for contaminated sharps and yellow and purple disposal bags for clinical items and bedding must be used.

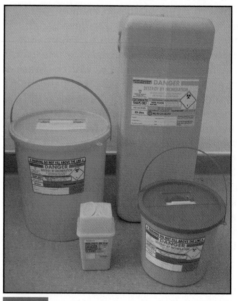

8.14 Approved containers for the disposal of 'sharps'.

Classes of drugs used in veterinary medicine

When discussing drugs, they tend to be divided into groups or classes either by the body system that they act on, or by the specific effect that they have.

Immunological agents

Vaccines

Passive immunity (see also Chapter 5) can be due either to the transfer of maternal antibodies to offspring or due to the administration of antiserum containing antibodies. This type of immunity is short-lived (1–3 months). Maternal immunity may interfere with vaccination and this is why vaccination programmes are not initiated until maternal immunity is considered to have waned (e.g. 12 weeks for canine distemper virus).

Active immunity develops when the immune system is challenged, either by a naturally occurring infection or by the administration of a vaccine. This stimulates the individual's own immune response. This type of immunity is generally much longer lasting than passive immunity.

- **A vaccine** comprises antigenic material that is given to an animal in order to induce an immune response, usually against bacteria, viruses or parasites. The vaccine may contain **live** organisms that are still capable of

replication, or **inactivated** organisms that cannot replicate. Inactivated vaccines usually require more than one dose.
- **An adjuvant** is an agent which, when added to a vaccine, enhances the immune response. Examples are aluminium hydroxide and aluminium phosphate.
- **Toxoids** are toxins obtained from microorganisms that have been modified so that they will still induce an immune response but are no longer deleterious. Tetanus toxoid is the main example.
- **A multivalent vaccine** provides protection against more than one infectious disease.

Figure 8.15 provides a summary of the main vaccines currently in use for companion animals and horses in the UK.

Disease or agent	Type of vaccine	Species	Additional information
Bordetella bronchiseptica	Live	Dogs and cats	Intranasal administration
Canine adenovirus 2	Live	Dogs	Two doses 2–4 weeks apart. Immunity has been demonstrated for 3 years
Canine distemper	Live	Dogs and ferrets	Two doses 2–4 weeks apart. Immunity has been demonstrated for 3 years. In ferrets adverse reactions have been reported. Observe the ferret for at least 30 minutes following vaccination
Canine parainfluenza	Live	Dogs	Two doses 2–4 weeks apart. Annual revaccination is recommended
Canine parvovirus	Live	Dogs	Two doses 2–4 weeks apart. Immunity has been demonstrated for 3 years
Leptospirosis	Inactivated bacterial	Dogs	Two doses 2–4 weeks apart followed by annual revaccination
Rabies	Inactivated	Dogs and cats	Single dose every 2–3 years, depending on brand
Tetanus antitoxin	Antiserum derived from horses	Dogs	Protective effect of 2–3 weeks' duration
Chlamydophila psittaci	Inactivated	Cats	Two doses 3–4 weeks apart, then annually
Feline calicivirus	Live attenuated	Cats	Two doses 3–4 weeks apart, then annually
Feline leukaemia virus	Inactivated	Cats	Two doses 3–4 weeks apart, then annually
Feline panleucopenia	Live attenuated	Cats	Two doses 3–4 weeks apart, then annually
Feline rhinotracheitis virus	Live attenuated	Cats	Two doses 3–4 weeks apart, then annually
Myxomatosis	Live Shope fibroma virus	Rabbits	Single vaccine immunity lasts about 6 months
Viral haemorrhagic disease	Inactivated	Rabbits	Single dose from 3 months of age. Annual revaccination is recommended
Combined equine influenza and tetanus	Inactivated	Equine	First dose from 5 months of age; 2nd dose 21–92 days later; 3rd dose 150–215 days after 2nd dose; then every 2 years. (Notes: FEI regulations require 6-monthly vaccinations for influenza)
Equine herpesvirus 1 and 4	Inactivated	Equine	1st, 2nd doses at 4–6 weeks of age then every 6 months. Also given to pregnant mares at 5th, 7th and 9th months of gestation
Equine influenza	Inactivated	Equine	First dose from 5 months of age; 2nd dose 21–90 days later; 3rd dose 150–215 after 2nd dose; then annually. (Notes: may be alternated with the combined influenza/tetanus vaccine; FEI regulations require 6-monthly vaccinations for influenza)
	Iscom	Equine	First dose from 5 months of age; 2nd dose 21–90 days later; 3rd dose 150–215 after 2nd dose; then annually. (Notes: may be alternated with the combined influenza/tetanus vaccine; FEI regulations require 6-monthly vaccinations for influenza)

8.15 Examples of the main types of vaccines available in the UK for small mammals and horses. It should be noted that several companies may manufacture a vaccine for a particular disease, and the type of vaccine (i.e. live or inactivated) and the recommended dosing protocol may vary depending on the manufacturer.   *continues* ▶

Disease or agent	Type of vaccine	Species	Additional information
Equine viral arteritis	Inactivated	Equine	First dose from 9 months of age; 2nd dose 3–6 weeks later; then every 6 months. Used only in breeding stallions and must have a negative EVA blood test prior to vaccination
Rotavirus	Inactivated	Equine	Given to pregnant mares at 8th, 9th and 10th months of gestation.
Streptococcus equi equi ('strangles')	Live	Equine	Submucosal injection. First dose from 4 months of age; 2nd dose 4 weeks later. High-risk horses: booster every 3 months. Do not give during pregnancy or lactation
Tetanus	Inactivated	Equine	First dose from 5 months of age; 2nd dose 4–6 weeks later; then every 2 years (Note: combined vaccine may be used instead)
Tetanus antitoxin	Antiserum	Equine	Foal: 3 ml s.c. or i.m. Adult: 7.5–10 ml s.c. or i.m. Given i.v. for therapy

8.15 *continued* Examples of the main types of vaccines available in the UK for small mammals and horses. It should be noted that several companies may manufacture a vaccine for a particular disease, and the type of vaccine (i.e. live or inactivated) and the recommended dosing protocol may vary depending on the manufacturer.

Chemotherapeutic agents

Antimicrobials

Definitions

- An **antimicrobial** agent is a substance that has the effect of killing or inhibiting the growth of microorganisms, including bacteria, viruses, fungi and protozoa. Antimicrobials may be naturally occurring, semi-synthetic or synthetic.
- An **antibacterial** is a substance that has an inhibitory or lethal effect specifically against bacterial organisms. Again, it may be naturally occurring, semi-synthetic or synthetic.
- An **antibiotic** is a substance produced by a microorganism that has the effect of killing or inhibiting the growth of other microorganisms.

However, although the definitions are clear, these three terms are often used interchangeably.

Antivirals

Antiviral compounds tend to be of limited usefulness, and treatment of viral disease is generally supportive.

- Aciclovir only has efficacy against herpes viruses. It is not authorized for veterinary use but has been used in the management of feline herpes virus 1 infection and in reptilian herpes virus infections. Aciclovir cannot eradicate latent viral infections and is applied topically.
- Zidovudine is not authorized for veterinary use but may be of benefit in the management of feline immunodeficiency virus (FIV) infection.
- Omega interferon is marketed specifically for the management of infections with canine parvovirus, FIV and feline leukaemia virus (FeLV).

Antibacterials

Definitions

- **Bactericidal** antibacterial agents kill the bacterial organism.
- **Bacteriostatic** antibacterial agents inhibit the growth of the bacteria and hence rely on the host's own immune system to deal with the inhibited bacterial population.

General principles of antibacterial use are as follows:

- The **spectrum of activity** of the drug must be known. Antibacterials vary in their ability to have an effect on anaerobic organisms, Gram-positive organisms and Gram-negative organisms.
- The **site of infection** must be considered, with regard to whether the drug can achieve sufficient concentrations at this site. Not all antibacterials are handled by the body in the same way, and certain locations are harder to penetrate than others.
- **Host factors** will play a role. Certain species are particularly intolerant of certain antibiotics. If the animal is very young or very old, or is suffering from a condition such as renal or hepatic disease, this may make it necessary to exclude certain drugs or modify dosing regimens.
- The **side effects** of the antibacterial must be considered, as well as **potential drug interactions** if the animal is on other medication.
- Antibacterials should be used prudently, and only where absolutely necessary, in order to minimize the development of **bacterial resistance**. Narrow-spectrum antibacterials are preferable. The correct dose and dosing regimen should be followed, and treatment given for an appropriate duration. The use of classes such as the fluoroquinolones and third-generation cephalosporins should be minimized; these should be reserved for situations where other antibacterials are not effective.

Figure 8.16 summarizes the main classes of antibacterials used in veterinary medicine.

Antifungals

The different types of fungal infection that require treatment (see Chapter 6) vary from systemic, which are often severe and life-threatening, to superficial, which are more common and not as serious. Often, systemic mycoses occur in immunocompromised patients. Fungal infections require prolonged treatment. In the case of topical management, adequate exposure to the agent is essential; clipping of hair or nails is an important part of treatment. Figure 8.17 summarizes the main classes and examples of antifungal agents.

Class	Mechanism of action	Subdivision	Spectrum of activity	Class examples
Beta-lactams	Interfere with the synthesis of the bacterial cell wall. Bactericidal. Most are sensitive to beta-lactamase, which is produced by some organisms. Clavulanic acid can be added to inhibit this enzyme	Narrow-spectrum penicillins	Mainly Gram-positives and anaerobes	Penicillin G, penicillin V
		Aminopenicillins	Increased activity towards Gram-negative organisms	Ampicillin, amoxicillin
		Beta-lactamase-resistant penicillins	Specifically beta-lactamase-producing Gram-positive organisms	Meticillin, cloxacillin
		Antipseudomonal penicillins	*Pseudomonas* spp.	Ticarcillin, piperacillin
		Cephalosporins: Divided into generations 1 to 4	1st generation is broad-spectrum: Gram-positives, Gram-negatives and anaerobes. Going from 1st to 4th, oral bioavailability decreases and Gram-negative spectrum increases	1st: Cefalexin 2nd: Cefuroxime 3rd: Ceftiofur, cefovecin 4th: Cefquinome
Aminoglycosides	Interfere with protein synthesis. Bactericidal		Primarily Gram-negative aerobes	Gentamicin, neomycin, amikacin
Tetracyclines	Interfere with protein synthesis. Bacteriostatic		Broad-spectrum: Gram-positive, Gram-negative, *Chlamydophila*, *Rickettsia*	Oxytetracycline, doxycycline
Potentiated sulphonamides	Inhibit the metabolic pathway involved in folic acid synthesis. Combination generally bactericidal	Combination of two classes of agent: a diaminopyrimidine and a sulphonamide	Broad-spectrum: Gram-positive, Gram-negative and some protozoal organisms	Trimethoprim/sulfadiazine
Lincosamides	Inhibit bacterial protein synthesis. Bacteriostatic or bactericidal.		Gram-positives and anaerobes	Clindamycin, lincomycin
Macrolides	Inhibit bacterial protein synthesis. Bacteriostatic or bactericidal.		Gram-positives and anaerobes	Erythromycin, tylosin, azithromycin, clarithromycin
Nitroimidazoles	Damage bacterial DNA. Bactericidal		Anaerobes	Metronidazole
Fluoroquinolones	Damage bacterial DNA. Bactericidal		Broad-spectrum, especially Gram-negatives and Gram-positives	Enrofloxacin, marbofloxacin
Chloramphenicols	Inhibit bacterial protein synthesis. Bacteriostatic		Broad-spectrum	Chloramphenicol, florfenicol

8.16 Summary of the main classes of antibacterial drugs.

Class	Examples	Mode of action	Spectrum of activity	Additional information
Griseofulvin	Griseofulvin	Disrupt the mitotic spindle. Fungistatic	Dermatophytes (ringworm)	Given orally. Avoid in cats
Azoles	Ketoconazole, miconazole, itraconazole	Inhibit the formation of the fungal cell membrane. Fungistatic	Broad-spectrum	Some suitable for systemic use (itraconazole, ketoconazole); others only suitable for topical use (miconazole)
Polyenes	Nystatin, natamycin, amphotericin B	Interfere with the fungal cell membrane. Fungicidal	Broad-spectrum	Amphotericin B is highly toxic for systemic use. Natamycin and nystatin are primarily used in topical preparations
Miscellaneous	Iodine preparations	Mechanism of action unclear		

8.17 Summary of the main classes of antifungal drugs.

Drugs used in the treatment of parasitic infections

Antiprotozoals

Protozoal organisms may affect a wide variety of animal species. Examples include *Giardia duodenalis, Toxoplasma gondii, Leishmania infantum, Babesia canis* and *Babesia equi*. Some antibacterial agents have antiprotozoal activity; these include the potentiated sulphonamides, clindamycin and metronidazole. There are also drugs with specific antiprotozoal activity.

Anthelmintics

Anthelmintics are drugs used to treat internal helminth parasites (see Chapter 7). Figures 8.18 to 8.20 summarize the main anthelmintic classes used in veterinary medicine and their activities against tapeworms and nematodes.

A number of parasites of equine species have developed resistance to commonly used anthelmintics and it is important to consider other management aids (e.g. regular paddock dropping collection or cross grazing) when considering parasite management (see Chapter 7).

Class	Examples	Mode of action	Spectrum of activity	Additional information
Benzimidazoles	Fenbendazole (D,C,H), mebendazole (H), febantel (D)	Bind to tubulin in the parasite	Mainly roundworms, some activity against tapeworms	Duration of exposure to the anthelmintic is important
Avermectins and milbemycins	Ivermectin (H), selamectin (D,C), milbemycin oxime (D,C), moxidectin (D,C,H)	Interfere with nerve transmission in the parasite	Termed endectocides; have activity against some external parasites as well as nematodes	Toxicity seen with ivermectin in collies and related breeds (e.g. Old English Sheepdog, Shetland Sheepdog, Australian Shepherd Dog)
Tetrahydropyrimidines	Pyrantel (D,C,H)	Interfere with nerve transmission in the parasite	Nematodes	
Cyclodepsipeptides	Emodepside (C)	Binds to the latrophilin receptor in the parasite and interferes with nerve transmission	Gastrointestinal nematodes	Authorized for use in cats and can be applied topically
Praziquantel	Praziquantel (D,C,H)	Interferes with calcium handling by the parasite	Specifically effective against tapeworms	Can be administered topically, orally or by injection
Miscellaneous	Piperazine (D,C)	Causes flaccid paralysis	Nematodes	Very safe, even in very young animals
	Nitroscanate (D)	Interferes with energy production	Nematodes and some tapeworms	Quite irritant if tablets are broken

8.18 Summary of the main classes of anthelmintic drugs. C = cats; D = dogs; H = horses

Anthelmintic	Effective against		
	Dipylidium	Taenia	Echinococcus
Praziquantel	✓✓	✓✓	✓✓
Nitroscanate	✓✓	✓✓	✓
Fenbendazole		✓✓	

8.19 The activity of selected anthelmintic agents against common tapeworms of dogs and cats. ✓ denotes good activity; ✓✓ denotes excellent activity.

Anthelmintic	Effective against					
	Toxocara / Toxascaris		Whipworm (Trichuris)		Hookworm (Uncinaria)	
	Adult	Immature	Adult	Immature	Adult	Immature
Selamectin	✓				✓	
Moxidectin	✓	✓	✓	✓	✓	✓
Milbemycin	✓	✓	✓	✓		
Fenbendazole	✓	✓	✓	✓	✓	✓
Febantel	✓	✓	✓	✓	✓	✓
Nitroscanate	✓	✓			✓	✓
Piperazine	✓				✓ (high dose)	
Emodepside	✓	✓				

8.20 A summary of the effectiveness of selected anthelmintics against hookworms, whipworm and gastrointestinal roundworms of dogs and cats. ✓ indicates effectiveness.

Ectoparasiticides

Ectoparasitides are drugs used to treat or prevent external parasite infestations, such as with fleas, lice, ticks and mites (see Chapter 7). There is a large range of drugs and drug classes and many preparations contain combinations of drugs, either to increase the spectrum against ectoparasites or to include activity against both internal and external parasites.

- **Endectocides** are antiparasitic drugs that control both internal and external parasites. They comprise two closely related classes of drugs, the avermectins and the milbemycins. Examples include moxidectin (a milbemycin) and selamectin (an avermectin). Selamectin is effective against fleas, lice and sarcoptic mites; moxidectin is effective against fleas, lice, and sarcoptic and *Demodex* mites.
- **Fipronil** is a widely used topical preparation that rapidly kills adult fleas by interfering with nerve transmission. It is also effective against ticks. A single application gives continued activity for up to 4 weeks.
- **Imidacloprid** is licensed for flea control in dogs, cats and rabbits. It kills the adult fleas by interfering with nerve transmission and is also applied as a spot-on preparation.
- **Environmental control agents** interfere with either egg production or larval development. Examples:
  - Lufenuron interferes with larval chitin production, preventing the production of eggs. It is administered to the host animal orally or by injection
  - Methoprene and pyriproxyfen are juvenile hormone analogues that inhibit normal larval development. They are usually applied to the environment, although methoprene exists in a combination preparation with fipronil that is applied directly to the host animal.
- **Pyrethroids** work by interfering with nerve transmission in the parasite. Examples include permethrin, preparations of which are widely used in dogs to prevent bites from fleas, ticks and sandflies. **Cats are very sensitive to the toxic effects of pyrethroids. Canine formulations must never be used in cats, and toxicity may even arise from cats grooming dogs that have been treated with these preparations. Aquatic animals and ferrets are also susceptible.**

Cancer chemotherapeutic agents

Drugs are frequently used in the treatment of neoplastic diseases in small animals. They are of particular importance in neoplastic diseases that are not amenable to surgical management, e.g. lymphosarcoma, leukaemia. Drugs may also be used as an adjunct to surgery, for example to reduce tumour size prior to surgery. Drugs used to destroy tumour cells are termed **cytotoxic** drugs; these target cell growth and cell division. Chemotherapeutic drugs may be divided into a number of categories, each of which work by different mechanisms and at different stages in the cell growth cycle.

Types of anti-cancer drugs

- **Alkylating agents**: Cause cross-linking and breaking of DNA molecules, interfering with DNA replication and RNA transcription. Examples include cyclophosphamide, ifosfamide and chlorambucil. Cisplatin also behaves in many respects like an alkylating agent.
- **Mitotic spindle inhibitors:** Bind to cytoplasmic microtubular proteins and arrest mitosis in metaphase. Examples include vincristine and vinblastine. ▶

- **Antimetabolites:** Mimic normal substrates needed for nucleic acid synthesis. They inhibit cellular enzymes or lead to the production of non-functional molecules. Examples include methotrexate and cytarabine.
- **Antitumour antibiotics:** Bind to DNA and inhibit DNA and RNA synthesis. An example is doxorubicin.
- **Glucocorticoids:** Cytolytic for lymphoid tissues and therefore useful in the treatment of some lymphoid malignancies. Their mechanism of anti-tumour action is unclear.
- **Miscellaneous**: Other agents with a variety of mechanisms of action are used in chemotherapy (e.g. platinum compounds).

WARNING

Many of these agents are highly toxic. Safety precautions should be strictly adhered to regarding the handling, dispensing, administration and disposal of these drugs (see below and the *BSAVA Small Animal Formulary, 7th edn*).

Many cytotoxic drugs are also immunosuppressant, and drugs such as prednisolone and cyclophosphamide are used in the treatment of conditions such as immune-mediated haemolytic anaemia and thrombocytopenia.

Anti-inflammatory drugs

The two main categories of anti-inflammatory drugs are the corticosteroids and the non-steroidal anti-inflammatory drugs (NSAIDs). They decrease the production of certain inflammatory mediators and have analgesic, antipyretic and anti-inflammatory effects.

Corticosteroids

These have been mentioned above in the context of cancer chemotherapy. Corticosteroids (Figure 8.21), such as prednisolone, suppress a wide range of inflammatory mediators and processes. They may be used in the management of certain inflammatory processes. Particularly at high doses, they will also suppress the immune response.

Side effects of corticosteroids

Corticosteroid use, especially if prolonged, may be associated with a variety of significant side effects. These may be seen in any species, but dogs, for example, appear to be particularly susceptible. Side effects may include:

- Increased susceptibility to infections
- Hyperglycaemia and diabetes mellitus
- Loss of muscle mass
- Osteoporosis
- Atrophy of the skin
- Decreased ability to heal
- Gastric ulceration
- Polyuria and polydipsia
- Behavioural changes
- Iatrogenic Cushing's syndrome
- Water and sodium retention and potassium loss
- Corneal ulceration
- Laminitis in the horse
- Suppression of the hypothalamic–pituitary–adrenal axis.

Drug	Glucocorticoid activity	Mineralocorticoid activity	Duration of activity
Hydrocortisone (naturally occurring endogenous)	1	1	8–12 hours
Prednisolone	4	0.8	12–36 hours
Dexamethasone, betamethasone	30	Minimal	24–48 hours
Fludrocortisone	15	150	8–12 hours

8.21 A comparison of a selection of corticosteroids. The numbers represent relative activity in relation to the endogenously produced corticosteroids (hydrocortisone); hence, hydrocorticosterone is given the designation 1. Mineralocorticoid activity controls sodium/potassium and water balance. Aldosterone is the main mineralocorticoid produced by the body. Glucocorticoid activity is more associated with the effects on metabolism, inflammatory and immune responses. However, most drugs have some degree of both mineralocorticoid and glucocorticoid activity.

Corticosteroids are commonly used in horses. There is always a slight concern when using them because of the risk of inducing laminitis; it is therefore important to ascertain whether a horse or pony is prone to laminitis before administering a corticosteroid preparation. It is recommended that all clients are warned about the risk of this occurrence, although in practice the incidence is low. Prednisolone administered orally is safe and is well tolerated in the horse. It is commonly used for the treatment of chronic conditions. Intrasynovial medication with corticosteroids (usually triamcinalone or methylprednisolone) is a commonly employed therapy for lame horses when the pain is associated with the synovium.

NSAIDs

Non-steroidal anti-inflammatory drugs specifically inhibit the enzyme cyclooxygenase, which is responsible for the production of eicosanoids important in the inflammatory process. Side effects can include gastrointestinal ulceration, renal toxicity and hepatotoxicity. Examples of NSAIDs include ketoprofen, meloxicam, carprofen and firocoxib. NSAIDs may be used either short term (e.g. in the management of postoperative pain) or long term (e.g. in the management of osteoarthritis). Figure 8.22 illustrates NSAIDs authorized for use in the UK. Some of the newer NSAIDs are defined as being

Drug name	COX-2-selective?	Species	Routes of administration	Treatment duration
Carprofen	No	Dogs, cats, horses	i.v., s.c. (not horse), oral (dog, horse)	Cats: single dose. Dogs: up to 5 days. Horses: up to 10 days
Firocoxib	Yes	Dogs, horses	Oral, i.v. (horse only)	Dogs: long term, with care. Horses: treat up to 14 days
Flunixin	No	Horses	Oral, i.v.	Horses: up to 5 days
Ketoprofen	No	Dogs, cats, horses	s.c., i.m. (not cat), i.v. (not cat), oral (not horse)	Cats: up to 5 days. Dogs: up to 30 days if low dose rate used. Horses: up to 5 days
Mavacoxib	Yes	Dog	Oral	Dogs: initial dose followed by second dose 2 weeks later, then monthly for up to 6 months
Meloxicam	No	Dogs, cats, horses	s.c. (dog and cat), i.v. (horse), oral	Cats, horses: up to 14 days. Dogs: long term, with monitoring
Phenylbutazone	No	Dogs, horses	Slow i.v. (horse), oral	Dogs: initial 2-wk course with reduced dose in week 2; may be extended at lower dose if required. Horses: can be used long term, with care
Robenacoxib	Yes	Dogs, cats	Oral, s.c.	Cats: up to 6 days. Dogs: long term, with monitoring
Suxibuzane	No	Horses	Oral	Horses: long term, with care
Tepoxalin	No	Dogs	Oral	Dogs: initially up to 7–10 days, then re-evaluate
Tolfenamic acid	No	Dogs, cats	Oral, s.c., i.m. (dog only)	Cats, dogs: up to 3 days
Vedaprofen	No	Dogs, horses	Oral (gel)	Horses: up to 14 days

8.22 NSAIDs authorized in the UK for use in dogs, cats and horses.

COX-2-selective. This means that they are less likely to inhibit the enzyme COX-1, which is the main enzyme associated with normal physiological functions. In other words, there should be a decreased risk of side effects such as gastric ulceration if a COX-2 selective agent is used.

WARNING

- Cats are particularly susceptible to the toxic effects of paracetamol (and other non-licensed NSAIDs), due to a reduced ability to metabolize the drug. Its use should therefore be avoided in this species.
- Aspirin can also cause toxicity in cats, since the excretion of the drug is slow. Aspirin can still be used in cats (for prevention of thromboembolism) provided that dosing frequency is decreased and aspirin is usually administered only three times per week.
- The use of corticosteroids and NSAIDs in conjunction should be avoided. Using both increases the risk of gastric ulceration, which is a serious side effect of both drug categories.

NSAIDs are the most commonly used anti-inflammatory medications in equine practice. A very effective and inexpensive drug is phenylbutazone, which is well tolerated even for long-term therapy at the correct dose rate. However, increased doses are associated with ulceration of the gastrointestinal tract, renal disease and death in extreme cases. It is used extensively in treating orthopaedic conditions, colic and as a general anti-inflammatory agent. Suxibuzone is a related drug and has a lower ulcerogenic effect than phenylbutazone.

Flunixin meglumine is also commonly used in horses and is an effective anti-inflammatory drug with strong action against the cardiovascular effects of endotoxaemia. This has particular clinical significance when used indiscriminately for treating horses with abdominal pain as it masks the early signs of endotoxaemia that might indicate a surgical problem, thus potentially delaying corrective surgery. Ketoprofen also appears to have a masking effect on endotoxaemia in colic patients. Meloxicam is an increasingly commonly used NSAID with a lower risk of gastrointestinal ulceration. It seems, however, to have a less profound clinical analgesic effect, but is used commonly in foals, which are at greater risk of severe gastric ulceration.

Drugs acting on the respiratory system

A variety of drug classes have specific effects on the respiratory system. These are summarized in Figure 8.23. Antimicrobials may also be used to manage infections involving the respiratory tract.

Drugs may be administered systemically but nebulization for certain drugs is also a possibility. This can allow high concentrations to be delivered directly to the location desired and may minimize systemic side effects.

Drugs acting on the cardiovascular system

Drugs used in the management of cardiovascular disease target the heart, blood vessels or kidney (Figure 8.24). Some drugs have an effect on more than one of these. The main drugs used are summarized in Figure 8.25.

Drug class	Examples	Effect on the respiratory tract
Bronchodilators	Theophylline, terbutaline, salbutamol	Dilate the airways
Mucolytics and expectorants	Bromhexine, acetylcysteine	Make mucus less viscous and therefore easier to expectorate (cough up)
Antitussives	Codeine, butorphanol	Act on the coughing centre in the brain to suppress coughing
Respiratory stimulants	Doxapram	Act on the respiratory centre in the brain to stimulate respiration
Anti-inflammatories	Antihistamines, e.g. diphenhydramine; NSAIDs, e.g. meloxicam; corticosteroids, e.g. prednisolone	Reduce inflammation produced by the release of inflammatory mediators

8.23 The main drug classes used in the management of respiratory disease.

Drugs acting on the heart
- Cardiac glycosides
- Phosphodiesterase inhibitors
- ACE inhibitors
- Calcium channel blockers
- Antiarrhythmics

Drugs acting on blood vessels
- ACE inhibitors
- Calcium channel blockers
- Nitric oxide donors

Drugs acting on the kidney
- Diuretics
- ACE inhibitors

8.24 Drugs used in the management of cardiovascular disease may act on the heart, vasculature and/or kidneys. ACE = angiotensin converting enzyme.

Drug class	Examples	Effects
Cardiac glycosides	Digoxin	Slow the ventricular heart rate; mild positive inotropic effect
Phosphodiesterase inhibitors	Pimobendan	Positive inotropes; sensitize the heart to calcium
ACE inhibitors	Ramipril	Dilate blood vessels; diuretic effect; reduce adverse changes in heart structure
Calcium channel blockers	Amlodipine, diltiazem	Dilate blood vessels; slow heart rate
Nitric oxide donors	Glyceryl trinitrate	Dilate blood vessels
Antiarrhythmics	Lidocaine	Help to control or abolish abnormal heart rhythms
Diuretics	Loop diuretics: furosemide; thiazide diuretics: hydrochlorothiazide; potassium-sparing diuretics: spironolactone	Increase urine production by the kidney. Different classes act on different regions of the nephron

8.25 The main drug classes used in the management of cardiovascular disease. A positive inotrope increases the force of the contraction of the heart. ACE = angiotensin converting enzyme.

Drugs acting on the urinary and reproductive systems

Urinary tract

The process of urination is controlled by both the parasympathetic and the sympathetic nervous systems (see Chapter 3). The large detrusor muscle is involved in contraction and emptying of the bladder and is controlled by the parasympathetic nervous system. A drug that acts like the parasympathetic nervous system is called a **parasympathomimetic**. By contrast, the sympathetic nervous system is responsible for maintaining the tone in the urinary sphincter. A drug that acts like the sympathetic nervous system is called a **sympathomimetic**. Clinical problems associated with the urinary

tract, together with the drugs used to treat or manage these conditions, are summarized in Figure 8.26.

Reproductive system

The majority of drugs acting on the reproductive system are hormones. The main ones used, along with their effects and indications, are shown in Figures 8.27 and 8.28. Further information on their use is given in Chapter 26.

Drugs acting on the digestive system

These drug classes, together with examples and effects, are summarized in Figure 8.29.

Condition	Class of drug used	Example
Urinary incontinence associated with weakness of the urethral sphincter	Sympathomimetics	Phenylpropanolamine, ephedrine hydrochloride
	Synthetic oestrogens	Estriol
Atony of the bladder	Parasympathomimetics	Bethanecol
Spasm of the urethra	Sympathetic antagonists (block action of sympathetic nervous system)	Prazosin
Urolithiasis (prescription diets more commonly used)	Urinary acidifiers for struvite calculi	Ethylenediamine
	Urinary alkalinizers for urate calculi	Sodium bicarbonate
Cystitis	Antimicrobials	Ampicillin, amoxicillin ± clavulanate, cefalexin, trimethoprim/sulphonamides

8.26 The main conditions associated with the urinary tract and the types of drugs used in their management.

Class of drug	Examples	Indications and effects
Oestrogens	Estriol	Urinary incontinence in the bitch
	Estradiol benzoate	Misalliance in dogs
Progestogens	Proligestone, megestrol acetate, medroxyprogesterone acetate, delmadinone	Used to postpone or suppress oestrus in cats, dogs and ferrets. Management of male behavioural problems
Androgens	Testosterone	Management of feminization associated with oestrogen-producing testicular tumours. Suppression of oestrus and false pregnancy in the bitch. Testosterone-responsive alopecia and incontinence in male dogs
Progesterone receptor antagonists	Aglepristone	Termination of pregnancy in the bitch up to day 45
Prolactin inhibitors	Cabergoline	Prevention of lactation and control of false pregnancy. May help chronic egg laying in birds
GnRH agonists	Deslorelin	Induction of temporary infertility in entire healthy male dogs. Prevents oestrus in ferrets

8.27 The main drug classes used to control reproductive function in small animals, including exotic pets.

Class of drug	Examples	Indications and effects
Progestogens	Altrenogest	Prevention of oestrus. Maintaining pregnancy
GnRH analogues	Goserelin, buserelin	Ovarian stimulation. Induction of ovulation
Alpha-hypophamines	Oxytocin	Induction of parturition. Encouraging placental removal after birth. Treatment of endometritis
	Carbotocin	Treatment of endometritis (longer action than oxytocin)
Antidopaminergics	Domperidone	Encouraging milk production in lactating mares
Prostaglandin analogues	Luprostenol, cloprostenol	Luteolysis and induction of oestrus

8.28 The main classes of drugs used to control reproductive function in equine species.

Class of drug	Examples	Effects
Emetics	Apomorphine (an opioid), xylazine (an alpha-2 agonist)	Induce vomiting
Antiemetics	Maropitant, metoclopramide, ondansetron	Suppress vomiting
Anti-ulcer drugs	Ranitidine and cimetidine (H2-antagonists), omeprazole (proton pump inhibitor)	Decrease gastric acid production
Cytoprotectants	Sucralfate	Protect and encourage healing of gastrointestinal erosions and ulcers
Prokinetics	Metoclopramide, cisapride	Increase intestinal contractions and promote forward movement of ingesta
Antidiarrhoeals	Loperamide, diphenoxylate	Increase segmental contractions and decrease peristaltic contractions
Laxatives	Liquid paraffin (emollient laxative), ispaghula, sterculia (bulk laxatives), magnesium sulphate (osmotic laxative)	Promote faecal evacuation
Appetite stimulants	Benzodiazepines (e.g. diazepam), cyproheptadine	Act on the satiety centre in the central nervous system
Adsorbents	Activated charcoal, bismuth salts	Adsorb toxins and drugs from the gastrointestinal tract
Drugs used in hepatic disease	Ursodeoxycholic acid, S-adenosylmethionine (SAMe), silybin	Mechanism of action not entirely clear. Used as part of a supportive therapy. May have protective and antioxidant effects

8.29 The main drug classes affecting the digestive system.

Drugs acting on the nervous system

Drugs acting on the nervous system can be categorized as:

- Sedatives
- Local anaesthetics
- General anaesthetics
- Muscle relaxants
- Anti-epileptics
- Behaviour-modifying agents.

Sedatives, local and general anaesthetics and muscle relaxants are discussed in Chapter 23.

Anti-epileptics

True or primary epilepsy is characterized by recurrent seizures, with no active underlying disease process in the brain. Ideally, drug treatment aims to prevent seizure activity while avoiding adverse effects. In reality this can be a difficult balance to strike, and a reduction in seizure frequency and or seizure severity may be a more realistic goal.

The most common drug used in chronic management of epilepsy in small animals is **phenobarbital**, which works by potentiating the effect of the inhibitory neurotransmitter gamma-aminobutyric acid (GABA) in the central nervous system. Since phenobarbital can affect liver enzymes, increasing its own metabolism and that of other drugs, therapeutic drug monitoring (TDM) is important. Potassium bromide works in a similar way to phenobarbital and may be used in combination or on its own.

Therapeutic drug monitoring

TDM refers to monitoring plasma levels of certain drugs and using this as a guide, in conjunction with clinical response, to inform dosing regimes. It is often used for drugs that have a low therapeutic index, e.g. digoxin.

The benzodiazepine **diazepam** is the treatment of choice for animals presented with status epilepticus (persistent seizure). Status epilepticus is life-threatening and therefore requires treatment that can be administered intravenously and reaches the central nervous system rapidly. Diazepam also works through enhancing the transmission of GABA at its receptors in the brain. If the seizuring is refractory to diazepam, then anaesthesia may be induced with an agent such as propofol or a barbiturate such as phenobarbital. A disadvantage of the barbiturates is that there is often a lag time before sufficient levels reach the central nervous system.

Benzodiazepines (mainly diazepam and midazolam) are commonly used in the treatment of status epilepticus in foals.

Behaviour-modifying agents

A number of drugs used in human medicine for the management of behavioural or depressive disorders are used in veterinary medicine. They are indicated for a variety of disorders, including compulsive behaviours, urine spraying, separation-related behaviours, excessive grooming and feather plucking. Examples include:

- **Clomipramine**: authorized for veterinary use; acts to block the re-uptake of both noradrenaline and serotonin in the brain; has been used in dogs, cats and birds
- **Selegeline**: authorized for veterinary use; inhibits the metabolism and therefore increases levels of the neurotransmitter dopamine in the brain; used in both dogs and cats
- **Sertraline**: not authorized for veterinary use but has been used in dogs; acts to block the reuptake of serotonin within the brain.

WARNING

All these drugs lower the seizure threshold and so should ideally be avoided in animals with epilepsy.

Drugs acting on the musculoskeletal system

The anti-inflammatory drugs (both NSAIDs and corticosteroids, see above) form an important part of both the acute and chronic medical management of musculoskeletal disorders.

Pentosan polysulphate, polysulphated glycosaminoglycans and hyaluronic acid are examples of **chondroprotective agents**. They are used to try and minimize degenerative changes in cartilage and synovial fluid and may be administered directly into the joint or given parenterally.

Drugs acting on the endocrine system

Endocrine disease usually results from either an overproduction or an underproduction of the endogenous hormones; therefore drugs designed to treat or manage endocrine disease either are hormone replacements or act to inhibit or reduce production of the endogenous hormone. Figure 8.30 summarizes the main endocrine diseases and the drugs used in the management of these conditions. Figure 8.31 gives more detail on specific insulin preparations available.

Drugs acting on the eye

Figure 8.32 shows the main types of drugs that may be used on the eye. Systemically administered drugs may also reach therapeutic concentrations in the eye provided they are well distributed around the body and are lipid-soluble. The main method of drug administration to the eye is topical administration of drops or ointment (see earlier).

Drugs acting on the ear

Drugs administered to the ear include:

- Antimicrobials, e.g. neomycin and gentamicin. Some antimicrobials such as the aminoglycosides are ototoxic and can cause deafness (irreversible) or vestibular signs (reversible)
- Antifungals, e.g. clotrimazole
- Anti-inflammatories, e.g. betamethasone
- Acaricides, e.g. tiabendazole.

Gland affected	Condition	Drugs used in management
Adrenal gland	Hyperadrenocorticism (Cushing's disease): overproduction of endogenous glucocorticoid	Trilostane: inhibits the enzyme important for corticosteroid synthesis and is the drug of choice. Mitotane and ketoconazole have also been used
	Hypoadrenocorticism (Addison's disease): underproduction of mineralocorticoid and glucocorticoid	Fludrocortisone, which has mineralocorticoid activity. Prednisolone may be used as an adjunct
	Equine Cushing's disease	Pergolide, trilostane
Endocrine pancreas	Diabetes mellitus: underproduction of endogenous insulin, leading to hyperglycaemia	Insulin (see Figure 8.31 for additional information)
	Hyperinsulinaemia: overproduction of insulin, leading to hypoglycaemia	Dextrose, glucocorticoids
	Equine metabolic syndrome (insulin resistance)	Metformin
Pituitary	Diabetes insipidus: deficiency of antidiuretic hormone (ADH)	Desmopressin, an ADH analogue without vasoconstrictor properties
Thyroid	Hypothyroidism: lack of thyroid hormone – mainly in dogs	Levothyroxine (T4)
	Hyperthyroidism: overproduction of thyroid hormone – mainly in cats	Carbimazole, methimazole. Both act by inhibiting the enzyme important in the synthesis of thyroid hormone

8.30 A summary of the main endocrine diseases and the drugs used in their management.

Type of insulin	Formulation	Properties	Products available
Short acting	Soluble (neutral) insulin	Ideal for management of ketoacidosis, as can be given i.v. Onset: 0–30 min Peak effect: 0.5–5 h Duration: 1–8 h	Human licensed product of bovine origin
Intermediate acting	Insulin zinc suspension (IZS)	Onset 30–60 min Peak effect 1–10 h Duration 4–24 h	Veterinary licensed products of porcine origin
Long acting	Protamine zinc insulin (PZI)	Onset 1–4 h Peak effect 4–14 h Duration 6–28 h	Human licensed products of bovine origin

8.31 Veterinary licensed insulin formulations. The properties given refer specifically to the dog; the duration of activity in the cat is significantly shorter. All times are approximate averages and doses need to be adjusted for individual patients.

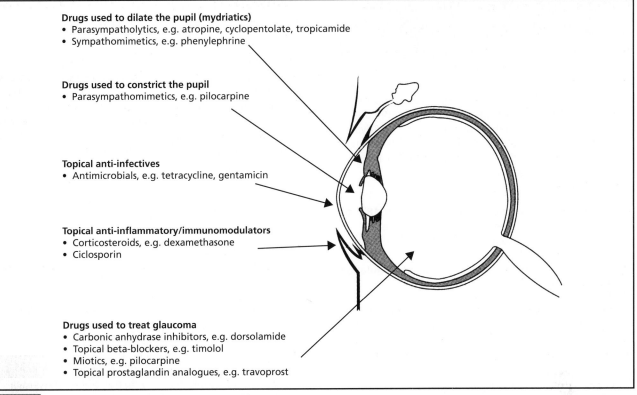

Drugs used to dilate the pupil (mydriatics)
- Parasympatholytics, e.g. atropine, cyclopentolate, tropicamide
- Sympathomimetics, e.g. phenylephrine

Drugs used to constrict the pupil
- Parasympathomimetics, e.g. pilocarpine

Topical anti-infectives
- Antimicrobials, e.g. tetracycline, gentamicin

Topical anti-inflammatory/immunomodulators
- Corticosteroids, e.g. dexamethasone
- Ciclosporin

Drugs used to treat glaucoma
- Carbonic anhydrase inhibitors, e.g. dorsolamide
- Topical beta-blockers, e.g. timolol
- Miotics, e.g. pilocarpine
- Topical prostaglandin analogues, e.g. travoprost

8.32 Drugs used on the eye.

Drugs acting on the skin

Treatment may be achieved by systemic or topical administration of drugs. Topical treatments may be formulated as shampoos, sprays, powders, ointments, lotions, gels or creams. The formulation is important, as it may aid in the penetration of the active ingredient to the skin. If the condition is affecting deeper layers of the skin or if the disease is widespread, a systemic approach may be more appropriate. Treatment should aim to:

- Alleviate symptoms
- Tackle the underlying cause.

While the symptomatic approach is quite straightforward, the aetiology of the skin disease may often be difficult to ascertain; even if the cause is identified it may not be possible to prevent exposure of the animal. For example, many dogs suffer from allergic skin disease associated with allergens such as house dust mites and fleas. Flea control may be relatively straightforward to implement but house dust mite exposure is unavoidable, although vacuuming may reduce levels of the mite. Figure 8.33 summarizes the types of agents used in the treatment and control of skin disease.

> **WARNING**
>
> Many of the agents used topically can penetrate the skin of the operator as well as the animal. In particular, care should be taken with the application of topical corticosteriods, and disposable gloves should always be worn when applying these agents (gloves should be dispensed to owners along with the drug).

Condition	Class of drug	Route of administration	Examples
Lozalized or generalized pyoderma	Antimicrobials	Systemic	Clindamycin
		Topical	Neomycin
Control of fleas	Ectoparasiticides	Systemic	Lufenuron
		Topical	Fipronil
Inflammatory and immune-mediated disorders	Corticosteroids	Systemic	Prednisolone
		Topical	Dexamethasone
Dermatophytosis	Antifungals	Systemic	Griseofulvin
		Topical	Miconazole
Seborrhoea	Keratolytics	Topical	Selenium sulphide

8.33 Examples of drug classes used to treat some skin conditions.

Legal aspects of medicines

Introduction

Legislation exists that governs the manufacture, importation, storage, handling, dispensing, prescribing, supply and disposal of medicines. In addition, bodies such as the Royal College of Veterinary Surgeons (RCVS), the British Veterinary Association (BVA) and the BSAVA provide additional guidelines and recommendations.

The legislation includes:

- **The Veterinary Medicines Regulations 2005 (VMR)** – this is reviewed and updated in October of each year
- **The Misuse of Drugs Regulations 2001**
- **Health and Safety at Work etc. Act 1974**
- **Control of Substances Hazardous to Health Regulations 1999 (COSHH).**

The purpose of the VMR legislation is to ensure the **safety, quality** and **efficacy** of veterinary medicines. The **Veterinary Medicines Directorate (VMD)** is the executive agency of Defra that is responsible for ensuring that these criteria are met.

Legal categories of veterinary medicines

In the UK authorized veterinary medicines are divided into several legal categories. These determine who may supply and prescribe these medicines.

POM-V: Prescription-Only Medicine – Veterinarian

- A POM-V may only be dispensed once it has been prescribed by a veterinary surgeon.
- A POM-V may only be dispensed following a clinical assessment of the animal (s) under his/her care by the prescribing veterinary surgeon.
- If the prescribing veterinary surgeon is also supplying the drug then no written prescription is required.
- Before prescribing the product, the veterinary surgeon must be satisfied that the person who will use the product is competent to do so.
- A current list of POM-V medicines is available on the VMD website, www.vmd.gov.uk.

Veterinary medicinal products (VMPs) are generally included in this category as a result of one or more of the following:

- The preparation contains a new active ingredient
- There are safety issues or concerns
- It is deemed that specialized veterinary knowledge is required for its use
- The drug has a narrow safety margin
- Government policy.

Medicated feedstuffs previously classified as MFS are now also in the POM-V category.

Each practice must advise clients, by means of a prominently displayed sign, of the top 10 most commonly prescribed or supplied POM-Vs and their prices. In addition clients must be advised that prescriptions are available.

POM-VPS: Prescription Only Medicine – Veterinarian, Pharmacist, Suitably Qualified Person (SQP)

- A POM-VPS may only be supplied once it has been prescribed (in writing or orally) by a registered qualified person (RQP), namely:
  - A veterinary surgeon
  - A pharmacist
  - A Suitably Qualified Person (SQP).
- A prior clinical assessment is not a prerequisite.

A VMP is generally included in this category when:

- It is used to reduce or prevent endemic disease in herds or flocks or individual animals
- There is deemed to be some risk for the user, consumer, animal or environment, but users can be made aware of this by verbal or written advice
- Adequate training can be given for regular use.

Medicated feedstuffs previously classed as MFSX are now POM-VPS.

Prescribers and dispensers

- For both POM-V and POM-VPS, a client may request a written prescription if they do not wish to purchase the VMP from the prescriber.
- For POM-V, only a vet may write the prescription but it may be supplied by another vet or a pharmacist on that vet's prescription.
- For POM-VPS, any RQP may prescribe it and it may be supplied by any other RQP on that prescription.

NFA-VPS: Non-Food Animal Medicine – Veterinarian, Pharmacist, Suitably Qualified Person

- May be supplied by an RQP, namely:
  - A veterinary surgeon
  - A registered pharmacist
  - A registered SQP.
- No prior clinical assessment or examination is necessary.
- Must be for non-food animals.

AVM-GSL: Authorized Veterinary Medicine–General Sales List

- May be supplied by any retailer; there are no restrictions on their supply.
- VMPs are placed in this category when:
  - There is a wide safety margin
  - They are used for common ailments
  - Special advice on their use is not required.

Suitably Qualified Persons

An SQP is an individual who is registered as an SQP with the Animal Medicines Training Regulatory Authority (AMTRA). To be eligible, they must have passed the required examinations. They are then able to supply medicines that are classified as NFA-VPS or POM-VPS. The SQP must have registration appropriate for the product range supplied:

continues ▶

continued

SQP type	Permissible medicines	Card colour
R-SQP	all VPS medicines	Red
G-SQP	Farm animal and equine	Orange
K-SQP	Farm and companion animal	Pink
E-SQP	Equine and companion animal	Yellow
L-SQP	Farm animal	White
J-SQP	Equine	Blue
C-SQP	Companion animal	Green

Compendia are produced for each category, detailing the drugs that may be supplied by an individual holding the appropriate SQP registration.

Controlled Drugs

These are regulated by the Misuse of Drugs Regulations 2001 and are a division of human POM medicines. They are divided into five Schedules; these determine the requirements for their requisition, storage, record keeping, prescribing, supply and disposal. Controlled Drugs (CDs) for use in animals may only be prescribed by a veterinary surgeon and supplied by a veterinary surgeon or pharmacist in accordance with that prescription.

Classification of Controlled Drugs

Schedule 1

- Includes LSD and cannabis. Veterinary surgeons have no authority to possess or prescribe these.

Schedule 2

- Special requirements for requisition, prescribing, record keeping, storage and disposal.
- Examples include etorphine, morphine, pethidine, fentanyl and secobarbital.
- Requisition must be made in writing to the supplier, signed by the veterinary surgeon; it is now permissible to produce a typed requisition, but this must still be signed by the veterinary surgeon.
- Must be stored in a locked and permanently secured cabinet (except secobarbital), which can be opened by a veterinary surgeon or person authorized by him/her (Figure 8.34). It is not acceptable to have a communal key or one that is kept in a drawer.
- A Controlled Drugs Register must be maintained, recording all purchases and each individual supply within 24 hours.
- Destruction must take place in the presence of a person authorized by the Secretary of State.
- All invoices must be kept for a period of 2 years.

Schedule 3

- Subject to the same prescription and requisition requirements as Schedule 2.
- Do not need to keep a record in a register, unlike Schedule 2.
- Examples include pentobarbital, phenobarbital, buprenorphine, pentazocine, diethylpropion and temazepam. ▶

- Buprenorphine, diethylpropion and temazepam must be kept under safe custody (locked secure cabinet). It is advisable that all Schedule 3 drugs are locked away.
- Invoices must be kept for a period of 2 years.

Schedule 4

- Exempt from most of the restrictions of controlled drugs.
- Includes most benzodiazepines plus ketamine and anabolic steroids.
- Invoices must be kept for a period of 2 years. **Ketamine may be subject to misuse; the RCVS therefore states that it should be stored in the Controlled Drugs cabinet and its use recorded in an informal register.**

Schedule 5

- Certain preparations containing codeine and morphine in less than specified amounts.
- Exempt from all of the requirements other than invoices need to be kept for 2 years.

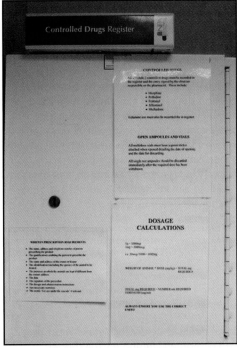

8.34

Secure and locked Controlled Drug cabinet.

Controlled Drugs Register

- Records must be kept for all Schedule 2 drugs with a separate part of the Register for each drug.
- It must be in a bound book.
- An indelible entry must be made within 24 hours of each use or supply.
- Entries must be in chronological order.
- The Register for each drug should include a running total.
- Entries must be signed by the veterinary surgeon.
- Records must be kept for 2 years from the date of the last entry.

Figure 8.35 illustrates the entries required.

Entries made when a Controlled Drug is received				
Date received	Name and address of supplier	Amount received	Form in which received	Running total
Entries made when a Controlled Drug is supplied				
Date supplied	Name and address of person supplied	Name and signature of veterinary surgeon	Amount supplied	Form in which supplied	Running total

8.35 Entries required for Controlled Drugs, both on receipt and when supplying/prescribing/administering.

The prescribing cascade

The legislation requires that when administering a medicine to an animal or a group of animals, a product that is authorized ('licensed') in that species for that condition or indication should be used.

If such a product is not available, and in order to avoid unacceptable suffering, a veterinary surgeon responsible for the animal may exercise his/her professional judgement according to the 'cascade'. The options are available in the following order:

1. A veterinary medicinal product authorized in the UK for another condition in the same species or for use in another animal species for the same condition ('off-label use').
2. If no such product is available, then either a medicinal product authorized in the UK for human use, or a veterinary medicinal product not authorized in the UK but authorized in an EU member state for use in any animal species* (in the case of a medicine for a food-producing animal it must be for a food-producing species – a Special Import Certificate will be required.)
3. Finally, if (and only if) there is no product that is suitable, a veterinary medicinal product may be prepared extemporaneously by a veterinary surgeon, a pharmacist or a person holding a manufacturer's authorization, as prescribed by the veterinary surgeon.

If a veterinary surgeon considers there is not a suitable product authorized in the UK or other EU member state, an application for a Special Treatment Certificate (STC) may be made to import a product from outside the EU.

If the animal being treated is a **food-producing animal**, additional requirements must be fulfilled:

- A withdrawal period (see below for details) must be specified. If no withdrawal period for the species concerned is indicated, a standard minimum withdrawal period of **not less** than the following must be specified:
  - 7 days for eggs and milk
  - 28 days for meat from mammals and poultry
  - 500 degree days for meat from fish (where degree days is the cumulative sum of mean daily water temperature in degrees Celsius following the last treatment)
- Specific records must be kept for 5 years, including the date the animal(s) were examined, name and address of the owner, identification and number of animals treated, diagnosis, product details including batch number, doses administered or supplied, duration of treatment and withdrawal period recommended.

When the cascade is employed, it is recommended that the veterinary surgeon:

- Keeps records of all unauthorized and off-label use of drugs
- Informs the client
- Ideally obtains the client's written consent.

Any product prescribed under the cascade must be administered by a veterinary surgeon or by an individual acting under the direction of a veterinary surgeon.

Withdrawal periods

Withdrawal periods relate to medicines used in food-producing animals (see above). This includes clients with 'backyard' chickens kept for eggs or meat. The horse is considered to be a food-producing animal unless it specifically states otherwise in the animal's passport. **Horses that are never to be used for human consumption must be clearly identified on their passport.** These animals should be treated with veterinary medicinal products with a UK market authorization for use in horses as a first choice. If there is no suitable authorized product available, the cascade (see above) may be used to select a suitable alternative.

If it is unclear from the passport whether or not a horse is intended for human consumption, it should be presumed that the horse **is** to enter the human food chain, and these cases should therefore be treated the same as horses that are **not** specifically designated (as per passport) as **not for human consumption**. Administration of the following drugs is prohibited in these animals:

- *Aristolochia* spp.
- Chloramphenicol
- Chloroform
- Colchicine
- Dapsone
- Dimetridazole
- Metronidazole
- Phenylbutazone.

This list is updated on the Veterinary Medicines Directorate website. Other veterinary medicinal products may be used with a withdrawal period of 6 months or as defined by its maximum residue level (see below), whichever is the shorter.

Regulations about horses with or without passports are detailed in the VMD website (www.vmd.gov.uk).

A **maximum residue level** (MRL) is the residue of an administered drug that is permitted in food of animal origin under EU law. This therefore relates to meat, milk, eggs and honey. The withdrawal period is the time required from administration of a particular drug until the levels in animal tissues have fallen below the MRL. The responsibility for ensuring that withdrawal periods are observed lies with the animal keeper and the veterinary surgeon. The purpose of the withdrawal period is to ensure consumer safety. Drugs authorized for food-producing animals state the withdrawal periods that must be observed on their datasheets for the species in which they are licensed.

Many competition horses are bound by the rules of their respective governing bodies concerning use of therapeutic substances and those involved in a particular sport must be aware of the current regulations.

The Small Animal Exemption Scheme (SAES)

Certain veterinary medicines may be imported, marketed and supplied in the UK without a marketing authorization. The pets covered include aquarium fish, cagebirds, homing pigeons, terrarium animals, small rodents, ferrets and rabbits. Products containing antibiotics, narcotics or psychotropic agents are not included in the scheme. Products intended for parenteral, ophthalmic or aural administration may not be included in the scheme. The product must be clearly labelled, stating that it is being marketed under this scheme and these products do not have to prove safety quality and efficacy. However, they must be manufactured under the same stringent conditions as authorized medicines. Products included in the scheme include some antiparasitic drugs and some anthelmintics.

Prescriptions

Prescriptions are required for POM-V and POM-VPS drugs. A prescription is a means of defining the product, its dose and other relevant instructions. It must be issued in writing unless it is being supplied by the person issuing the prescription.

Certain information is legally required on a written prescription:

- Name and address of prescriber
- Credentials of the prescriber, e.g. MRCVS
- Name and address of the person receiving the prescription
- A description of animal(s)
- Where the animals are kept, if not at owner's address
- Drug, dose and instructions (including withdrawal period if required)
- Note if prescribing under the cascade
- The date of supply
- The signature of the person issuing the prescription
- A statement saying 'For animals under my care'
- Any repeat instructions.

'For animals under my care'

For the purpose of prescription medicines, the RCVS defines this term as follows:

- The vet has responsibility for the animal(s)
- This is real and not nominal
- The animal(s) has been seen at prescribing or recently or often enough
- The vet must keep the clinical records of this animal or group of animals.

Other points should be considered when writing a prescription:

- The prescription must be written in indelible format
- The prescription is valid for 6 months from the date of writing
- Prescriptions for Controlled Drugs are valid for 28 days
- Use of decimal places should be avoided, for example, 500 mg rather than 0.5 g. If decimal places must be used, a 0 should be placed before (i.e. 0.5 g, not .5g)
- Micrograms, nanograms or other units must not be abbreviated
- Only the minimum amount required for treatment should be prescribed
- Certain abbreviations may be used for dosing instructions:
  - Once daily: uid or sid (avoid od)
  - Twice daily: bid or bd
  - Three times daily: tid or tds
  - Four times daily: qid or qds.

Figure 8.36 illustrates a standard form of prescription.

Record keeping

There are a number of requirements for keeping records. These apply to records of all prescription drugs, records for drugs used in food-producing species and records of Controlled Drugs, which have already discussed above.

Prescription drugs

This includes drugs classified as POM-V and POM-VPS. Records of all incoming and outgoing transactions must be made. These records should include:

From: *Address of practice*
Telephone No.   *Date*
 	
Animal's name   *Owner's name*
                                                Owner's address
 	
Rx   *Print name, strength and formulation of drug*
        Total quantity to be supplied
        Amount to be administered
        Frequency of administration
        Duration of treatment
 	
        For animal treatment only
        For an animal under my care
 	
Non-repeat/repeat X *1, 2 or 3*
                        Name and Signature of veterinary surgeon

8.36 An example of a written prescription, illustrating the information required.

- The date and nature of transaction
- The identity of the drug, including **batch numbers** (for non-food animal medicines the batch number need only be recorded when first received or used, not at every subsequent transaction)
- The quantity received or supplied
- The name and address of the supplier or recipient
- A copy of any prescriptions and the name and address of the person who wrote the prescriptions
- Whether the cascade was used.

Records must be kept for 5 years.

Food-producing species

For food-producing species, there are requirements for both the veterinary surgeon and the owner of the animal.
On purchase of a product, the owner must record:

- The name of drug
- The date of purchase
- The quantity
- The withdrawal period (see above)
- The name and address of supplier.

At the time of administration, the owner must record:

- Their name
- The date of administration
- The quantity administered
- The identity of the treated animal
- The name of the veterinary surgeon (if the product is administered by a veterinary surgeon).

The veterinary surgeon must also keep a record of prescription drugs, as above, including details of any drugs prescribed under the cascade and withdrawal periods recommended.

Audits

A detailed audit must be carried out annually, reconciling records of all incoming and outgoing transactions, any damaged or out-of-date stock and any discrepancies recorded. Computerized records must be adequately backed up. These records can be checked by the Veterinary Medicines Directorate during practice inspections.

Labelling

All medicines supplied by the practice, other than POM-Vs (see below), must be labelled in accordance with the Veterinary Medicines Regulations (VMR). Generally, such medicines must be supplied in a container (with labelling) specified by the marketing authorization for the medicine. Any additional labelling must not obscure any of the pre-existing information. If the manufacturer's data sheet contains directions for the species and condition then there is no legal requirement for any additional labelling. It is advised that, in addition, such medicines are labelled with the name and address of the practice supplying the medicine.

For POM-V medicines

All POM-V medicines supplied by the practice **must** be labelled with the following information:

- The name and address of animal owner
- The name and address of the approved premises supplying the medicine

- The date of supply
- The words 'Keep out of reach of children'
- The words 'For animal treatment only' unless the package or container is too small for it to be practicable to do so
- The words 'For external use only' for topical preparations
- The name and quantity of the product, its strength and directions for use.

For medicines supplied under the cascade

There are **additional requirements** for medicines supplied under the cascade:

- Identification of the animal or group of animals
- The name of the veterinary surgeon who has prescribed the product.

And, unless specified on the manufacturer's packaging:

- Any special precautions
- The expiry date
- Any necessary warnings for the user, target species, administration or disposal of the product.

The purpose of appropriate labelling is to ensure that the drug can be used safely and effectively. The label should ideally be computer-generated but if handwritten must be legible and written in indelible ink.

Suspected Adverse Reactions Surveillance Scheme (SARSS)

The VMD administers the SARSS scheme. This is a method whereby unwanted or adverse effects associated with drug administration are reported. Veterinary surgeons, pharmacists and veterinary nurses are not, at present, legally required to report adverse reactions; however, this process is vitally important for ensuring drug safety and efficacy.

Anyone can report an adverse reaction. Reports can be made online via the VMD website (www.vmd.gov.uk) or forms can be downloaded and posted in. The company manufacturing the drug should also be informed.

Pharmacy management

Registration

As of 1 April 2009, all premises from which veterinary medicinal products are to be supplied must be registered with the Royal College of Veterinary Surgeons (RCVS).

Stock control

The medicines in a pharmacy will reflect the type of work undertaken in the practice. The stock of a referral practice specializing in orthopaedic surgery will differ from that of a busy first-opinion small animal practice. Efficient stock control ensures that capital is not tied up unnecessarily.

It is good practice to have a named person responsible for stock control. Managing stock levels to ensure efficient running of a practice is essential.

Factors to consider:

- The frequency of ordering stock, i.e. daily or weekly
- The availability of stock required, e.g. a special order may take 2 weeks to arrive
- The frequency with which a medicine is used. Identify those medicines that are required out of necessity but are rarely used and are likely to expire before use, e.g. adrenaline and atropine
- The viability of the drug, i.e. long or short expiry date
- The facilities available for storage
- Seasonal variations – there may be a high demand for vaccines or medicines to treat allergies in the summer months.

When managing stock, it is sensible to:

- Dispense medicines with the shortest expiry date first
- Store medicines with the same batch number together.

After considering these factors a maximum/minimum level of stock should be set for each product.

It is prudent and good practice to take advantage of special deals and bulk orders with manufacturers and wholesalers, although the consequences should be considered, i.e. stock needs to be sold before expiry.

Issuing prescriptions to clients for medicinal preparations that are not normally kept in stock will prevent supplies of unused stock being stored.

Ordering stock

All practices should have a protocol for ordering veterinary medicinal products and equipment to ensure accurate records are kept for future reference. It is a legal requirement to keep records concerning all veterinary medicinal products for a minimum of 5 years. As previously mentioned, an audit of all stock should be carried out at least once a year.

Many practices have a direct computer link to a veterinary wholesaler. This enables access to product information, current prices and a scanning system for ordering products. It is possible to have an automated ordering system that monitors stock levels and replaces stock as and when necessary.

The date of delivery from the wholesaler or manufacturer should be recorded unless it is on the delivery note or invoice, which is retained. The date of first use of each batch should be recorded. This enables a product recall to be carried out if required.

A requisition to supply a veterinary surgeon with a Controlled Drug must be made in writing by the registered veterinary surgeon and be received by the supplier (e.g. an authorized veterinary wholesaler) before the delivery of a Schedule 2 or 3 Controlled Drug can be made. The requisition must be signed by the veterinary surgeon and must include the veterinary surgeon's name, professional qualifications and address.

Storage

Upon delivery of stock, all items must be checked to ensure the correct products have been delivered, the products are in date and there is no damage to the products or packaging.

Stock that requires refrigeration should be stored immediately to prevent deterioration. Stock should be stored out of direct sunlight.

Stock rotation is essential when new stock is received to ensure older stock is used first.

All products that are hazardous or inflammable must be stored at ground level in secure cabinets if required, in accordance with current safety regulations. Schedule 2 Controlled Drugs must be kept in a secure, lockable and immovable cabinet that can only be opened by a veterinary surgeon or person authorized by him or her (see Figure 8.34). Each individual supply must be recorded within 24 hours, as detailed above. Subject to certain exemptions, Schedule 3 drugs must also be kept in a locked secure cabinet; although it is advised that *all* Schedule 3 drugs are kept in a locked secure cabinet. Ketamine may be subject to misuse and should therefore be stored in the Controlled Drugs cabinet and its use recorded in an informal register.

Medicinal products should be stored in accordance with the manufacturer's recommendations *whether in a practice or a vehicle*. In order to maintain their stability and viability consideration must be given to the following factors:

- **Temperature control**: Some products must be stored in a refrigerator to prevent instability, e.g. insulin and vaccines. The temperature should be maintained between 2°C and 8°C. Cytotoxic drugs must be stored in a separate lockable fridge (Figure 8.37). Products stored on the shelf are stored at an ideal temperature range of 8–15°C, and should not exceed 25°C. There must be proper monitoring and recording of maximum and minimum temperatures in the refrigerator, pharmacy and storage rooms. Temperature records may be subject to inspection
- **Light**: All preparations should be stored out of direct sunlight, as this can cause chemical reactions. Drugs that are particularly light-sensitive are stored in dark bottles or packaging
- **Hydrolysis**: Humidity and dampness can cause chemical changes. Antibiotics are particularly sensitive to this.
- **Oxidation**: Damage to packaging or ill-fitting lids can cause excessive exposure to oxygen in the air, causing colour changes and deterioration of fat- or wax-based preparations.

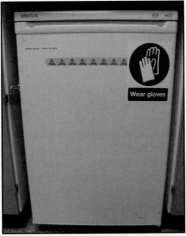

8.37

Locked refrigerator used for the storage of cytotoxic drugs.

> **WARNING**
>
> Biological samples and food must not be stored in refrigerators used to store medicines.

Packaging

Many different types of material are used, such as plastic, glass, aluminium foil, tin, and cardboard (Figure 8.38).

- **Glass** is used to store a range of preparations as it generally does not cause chemical reactions and can be sterilized. Liquid preparations that are for external use must be dispensed into fluted bottles that are recognizable by touch. Plain glass bottles are used for oral liquid preparations.
- **Plastics** are light and convenient to use for most products.
- **Metals** are used in foil strips, tubes and aerosol cans.
- **Paper/cardboard** – No medicinal preparation can be dispensed into paper envelopes alone. It can be used for sachets, as an outer container for additional protection and for labelling.
- **Closures** are generally made of plastic with a child-resistant lock. They must provide protection and be leak-proof.
- **Bulk containers** – Preparations must be repackaged into containers most appropriate to the formulation, i.e. if it is light-sensitive the packaging must reflect this.
- **Unit packaging** is available in the form of blister packs for tablets and capsules, and strip packs for liquid preparations.

- A pharmacy manual detailing standard operating procedures and Control of Substances Hazardous to Health (COSSH) assessments should be read by all those dispensing medicines.
- Contamination should be prevented by the use of measuring containers, gloves and pill counters (Figure 8.39) to ensure minimum exposure to the drug. Spills and breakages should be dealt with immediately and any packaging/drugs disposed of according to current legislation.
- Good hygiene practices should be in place. Hands should be washed between each preparation. All equipment used should be washed to prevent cross-contamination. It is important to keep the pharmacy clean and free from dust, and it is vital that work benches are cleaned regularly. No food or drink should be stored or consumed in a pharmacy.
- Liquid preparations should be dispensed in amber bottles.
- Bottles containing topical preparations should be fluted in order that they may be recognized by touch. This does not apply to prepackaged eyedrops or eardrops.
- All stock should be kept in order, ensuring lids are closed and bottles are clean. Damaged and expired stock should be checked for regularly.
- Returned medicines *must not be re-used*, as the required storage and viability cannot be guaranteed.

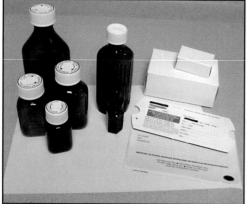

8.38 Examples of packaging available for dispensing medicines.

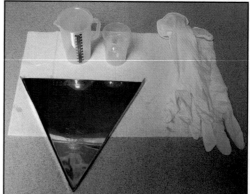

8.39 Equipment used for dispensing tablets.

Packaging regulations

- Child-resistant containers must be used unless otherwise requested.
- Paper or plastic envelopes are unacceptable as the sole containers for the dispensing of medicinal products.
- Tablets and capsules must be dispensed in crush-proof and moisture-proof containers.
- Sachets and manufacturer's strip or blister pack medicines should be dispensed in paper board cartons or wallets or paper envelopes.

WARNING

Particular care should be taken when dispensing and administering cytotoxic drugs (Figures 8.40).

Dispensing medicines

- The pharmacy must be a designated area within the practice, with no access available to members of the general public.
- All those dispensing medicines should be suitably trained.

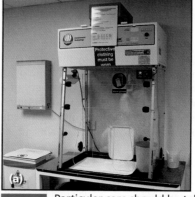

8.40 Particular care should be taken with cytotoxic drugs. **(a)** Hood and associated equipment used for dispensing.

continues ▶

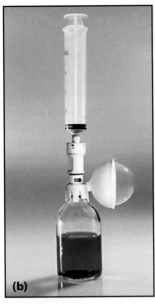

8.40 *continued* Particular care should be taken with cytotoxic drugs. **(b)** The closed Phaseal system for administration of cytotoxic drugs. (Courtesy of Cave Veterinary Specialists)

It is important to have knowledge and understanding of the classifications of drugs and their indications. Information on drugs can be found in manufacturers' datasheets, the National Office of Animal Health (NOAH) Compendium of Datasheets for Animal Medicines and the *BSAVA Small Animal Formulary*. These provide information on drug uses, formulations, dose according to species, any adverse effects and contraindications and any possible drug interactions.

It is a legal requirement that only the minimum amount of drug is prescribed to treat the animal, except when the packaging of the product prohibits this. It is an offence to break up bulk packaging to supply smaller amounts unless the marketing authorization allows it.

Advice to owners

A veterinary surgeon prescribing a POM-V or POM-VPS medicine must be satisfied that the person who will administer the product will do so safely and will use it for the purpose for which it is authorized. If the veterinary surgeon is not present when the medicine is handed over, he/she must authorize the transaction and be satisfied that the person handing it over is competent to do so.

Information for clients

- Clients must be made to understand why the drugs have been prescribed. The methods of administration and the techniques required to administer the drug must be discussed.
  - It may be necessary to demonstrate techniques such as the use of pill guns, filling syringes with medication and tube feeding, to ensure the client is confident and understands what is required.
  - Shaving the hair over the site of injection to aid the administration of insulin can prove beneficial to those clients that are hesitant, until they become more proficient and confident.
  - Some exotic pets, particularly chelonians, may have feeding tubes placed to aid administration of food and drugs. ▶

- Any special instructions on the label (e.g. 'To be given before food', 'Shake well before use', 'Keep refrigerated', 'Wear gloves') should be highlighted.
- The client should be alerted to any potentially harmful medications. They must be instructed as to the necessary precautions needed when administering these drugs, and gloves should be provided with the medication if necessary. Potential side effects and contraindications should be discussed and the client instructed to contact the practice immediately should any occur.
- It is also important to ask clients about their own sensitivity to medicinal products, e.g. penicillin, as it may be necessary to dispense an alternative medication.
- The client should be told whether the course of treatment should be stopped after a required number of days or continued until the medication is finished. Clients may be encouraged to return any unused medication and containers for safe disposal.

WARNING

Be aware of client confidentiality when discussing any details concerning their animal's history and treatment.

Disposal of medicines: unused, expired and damaged stock

All practices have a duty to ensure that:

- All waste is stored and disposed of responsibly
- Waste is only handled or dealt with by those authorized to do so
- Appropriate records are kept of all waste that is transferred or received.

The **Hazardous Waste (England and Wales) Regulations 2005** implement the European **Waste Framework Directive WFD (2006/12/EC)**, which controls the disposal of all forms of hazardous waste. Classification of waste has been replaced by **European Waste Catalogue (EWC) codes**. All pharmaceutical waste is classified under Healthcare Waste. The British Veterinary Association has produced guidelines (see Chapter 2).

Medicinal waste
Whole pharmaceuticals

This includes returned, out of date and damaged pharmaceutical products. Damaged stock includes spillages and breakages. Spilled drugs should be contained with a 'spill kit' (sand, sawdust or cat litter) and the content and amount recorded. The container should be disposed of in the pharmaceutical waste bin. The medicines should be collected into a leak-proof container. *Liquids and solids must be kept separate and should not be mixed.* Contents must be recorded and the records made available to the disposal contractor.

Controlled Drugs

The disposal of Controlled Drugs has additional requirements. All Schedule 2 drugs must be denatured before disposal. Denaturing kits may be purchased from veterinary wholesalers. The waste may then be disposed of in the standard pharmaceutical waste bin. This bin must be re-coded as denatured controlled drug. The process must be witnessed by an individual authorized by the Home Office. It must also be recorded in the Controlled Drugs Register and signed by the witness. Residual amounts of drug in used vials needles or syringes do not need to be denatured before disposal. Schedule 3, 4 and 5 Controlled Drugs must also be denatured, but their destruction does not need to be witnessed by an authorized person.

Cytotoxic and cytostatic drugs

Cytotoxic and cytostatic drugs are classed as hazardous waste. They fall into the European Waste Catalogue (EWC) code 18 02 07, which dictates that they must be separated from other pharmaceutical waste and disposed of by specialist contractors, who must destroy them by incineration. Waste must be put into yellow and purple containers and purple-lidded sharps bins (see Chapter 2). Items for disposal include unused medicines, residue, contaminated syringes, needles, cannulae and protective clothing.

Medicines must be defined by their hazardous properties:

H6	Toxic teratogenic
H7	Carcinogenic
H9	Infectious
H10	Toxic for reproduction
H11	Mutagenic.

The following medicines are included in these categories: cancer chemotherapeutic drugs, antiviral medication including aciclovir ophthalmic ointment, ciclosporins, some hormone preparations including prostaglandins, e.g. delmadinone, aglepristone, estradiol.

The EWC code and the H code must be clearly visible on the waste container. Transporting this type of waste by unlicensed vehicles is illegal.

Residue pharmaceuticals

Used vials or bottles of injectable medicines

This waste includes empty multi-dose bottles, vaccine bottles and empty tablet containers and syringes (discharged of contents). Snap-top vials should be placed in the sharps bin.

Needles

The Environment Agency states that all sharps are Hazardous Waste. Clear advice is given in the BVA 'Good Practice Guide to Handling Veterinary Waste'. The Environment Agency also advises that needles should not be separated from the syringe body but that they must be disposed of together in a yellow-topped sharps bin. Provided a practice has carried out training and a risk assessment, separation of syringe and needle may be considered. The syringe may then be disposed of in the pharmaceutical waste container. The needles are disposed of in the yellow-topped bin.

Management of health and safety at work

The **Health and Safety Executive** (HSE) requires that practices assess risks in the workplace, take precautions to avoid risk, and review and revise the risk assessments as necessary. If there are more than five people employed, all risk assessments must record any significant findings. The areas that need to be addressed concerning the handling and dispensing of drugs are:

- The handling of medicines, including cytotoxic drugs
- The spillage of medicines
- Waste disposal.

As a result of the risk assessment, **standard operating procedures (SOPs)** should be drawn up.

Control of Substances Hazardous to Health Regulations 2002

The COSHH Regulations 2002 require that employers assess the risks to health and safety posed by exposure to veterinary medicines and other substances used in the practice and then take necessary measures to protect their employees. Exposure to veterinary medicines tends to take place during dispensing and administering; careful consideration should therefore be made concerning drug formulations and the methods of administration required.

Exposure may be caused by any of the following:

- **Absorption through the skin and mucous membranes**: Some drugs require the use of protective clothing or wearing gloves. Needles and syringes should be firmly attached to prevent the drug leaking or it being sprayed as the plunger is pressed
- **Ingestion**: Food or drink must not be consumed or stored in a pharmacy. Strict hygiene policies should be in place including regular washing of hands, especially after preparing and administering medications
- **Accidental injection**: Loaded syringes should never be carried in a pocket and needle caps should be replaced with care. Accidental injection of oil-based vaccines should be dealt with immediately to prevent serious reactions
- **Inhalation**: The use of masks will help reduce the risk of irritation of the respiratory tract from powders and aerosols. Scavenging of anaesthetics removes toxic and hazardous gases from operating theatres.

Drugs and other substances are classified into low, medium or high risk.

Low- and medium-risk substances

These can be grouped according to therapeutic group, type or route of administration. Standard measures to control exposure can be used for the whole group. Examples of groups include:

continues ▶

continued
- Antibiotics
- Vaccines
- Injectable anaesthetics
- Inhalation anaesthetics
- Steroids
- Disinfectants.

Any specific risks must be identified, e.g. penicillin allergy.

High-risk substances

High-risk substances must have detailed individual assessment. These substances include:

- Oil-based vaccines
- Cytotoxic drugs
- Glutaraldehyde disinfectant
- Hormones
- Tilmicosin.

Measures to control risk to these substances must be explained to employees.

Safety datasheets

Safety datasheets must be provided for all medicines stocked. They can be in either hard copy or electronic format, but access to data in an emergency is essential.

Report of Injuries, Disease and Dangerous Occurrences Regulations 1995 (RIDDOR)

An employer must report any death, certain injuries or disease and dangerous occurrences (see Chapter 2).

Calculation of drug doses

EXAMPLE 1

A 15 kg dog has acute vomiting. The drug of choice is the antiemetic maropitant at a dose rate of 1.0 mg/kg. The preparation is available at a strength of 20 mg/2 ml. What volume should be injected?

The total dose required in mg is
15 kg × 1.0 mg/kg = 15 mg
The preparation contains
20 mg/2 ml = 10 mg/ml
The volume to be injected is the total required dose divided by the concentration:
15 mg (dose) divided by 10 mg/ml = 1.5 ml

EXAMPLE 2

An acaricidal preparation used to treat demodicosis in dogs is available as a 5% w/v concentrated solution. This has to be applied to the dog at a concentration of 25 mg/100 ml. What volume of water needs to be added to 1 ml of the concentrated solution to achieve this? ▶

A 5% solution is equivalent to
5 g in 100 ml = 5000 mg/100 ml = 50 mg/ml
Required strength
= 25 mg/100 ml = 0.25 mg/ml
The concentrated solution is 50/0.25 = 200 times more concentrated than the required solution. Therefore take 1 ml of the concentrated solution and add water to make it up to 200 ml.

EXAMPLE 3

A 500 ml bag of fluids contains a drug at a concentration of 0.1% w/v. How many ml/h will you need to administer to a 35 kg animal in order to achieve a dose rate of 8 mg/kg/h?

A 1% solution would contain 10 mg/ml, so a 0.1% solution would contain 1 mg/ml of drug

The required dose per hour for a 35 kg animal would be
35 × 8 = 280 mg
Therefore, in order to receive 280 mg/h from a solution that has 1 mg/ml of drug, the animal would have to receive 280 ml of fluid per hour.

EXAMPLE 4

A 34 kg dog presents with ventricular tachycardia. A bolus of lidocaine i.v. at a dose rate of 2 mg/kg must be administered. The preparation available is a 2% w/v solution. What volume of lidocaine should be given?

The dose required by the dog is
2 mg/kg (dose rate) × 34 kg (bodyweight) = 68 mg

A 1% solution contains 1 g/100 ml or 10 mg/ml. A 2% solution contains 20 mg/ml.
The volume to be administered is the total required dose divided by the concentration:
68 mg (dose) divided by 20 mg/ml (concentration)
= 3.4 ml of the 2% solution.

EXAMPLE 5

A lovebird needs to be treated with the antibacterial enrofloxacin. The bird weighs 50 g and requires an oral dose of 15 mg/kg. The enrofloxacin preparation available contains 25 mg/ml. What volume needs to be administered to the bird?

The bird weighs 50 g = 0.05 kg
The dose required by the lovebird is
15 × 0.05 = 0.75 mg
The volume required
= 0.75 divided by 25 = 0.03 ml
However, it is recommended that any volume less than 0.1 ml should be diluted to ensure accurate dosing. Therefore 0.1 ml of enrofloxacin is diluted with water to a total volume of 1.0 ml, providing a 2.5 mg/ml solution rather than a 25 mg/ml solution.
The volume now required is
0.75 divided by 2.5 = 0.3 ml.

Further reading

BSAVA Guide to the Use of Veterinary Medicines, available at www.bsava.com

Ramsey I (2011) *BSAVA Small Animal Formulary, 7th Edition.* BSAVA Publications, Gloucester

Saunders R and Whitlock E (in preparation) Nursing of hospitalized patients. In: *BSAVA Manual of Exotic Pet and Wildlife Nursing,* ed. M Varga *et al.* BSAVA Publications, Gloucester

Wanamaker BP and Lockett-Massey K (2004) *Applied Pharmacology for the Veterinary Technician, 3rd Edition.* Elsevier, St. Louis

Useful websites:

Veterinary Medicines Directorate (Executive Agency of the Department for Environment, Food and Rural Affairs): www.vmd.gov.uk

National Office of Animal Health (NOAH): www.noah.co.uk

Animal Medicines Training Regulatory Authority (AMTRA): www.amtra.gov.org.uk

www.feicleansport.org for information on equine anti-doping and controlled medication regulations

---

Self-assessment questions

1. List all topical preparations available in your practice, including sites of administration and any special indications required.
2. What are the routes most commonly used for administering medicines?
3. List the types of packaging used for veterinary medicines. When dispensing veterinary medicines, what are the legal requirements for packaging and labelling preparations?
4. What are the storage, prescribing and record-keeping requirements for a Schedule 2 controlled drug?
5. What do you understand by the term 'pharmacokinetics' of a drug?
6. What are the main classes of drugs that might be used in the management of respiratory disease?
7. Name two classes of drug commonly used in the treatment of heart disease.
8. What action should you take if you suspect that an animal has experienced an unexpected adverse effect to a drug that it has recently been given?
9. List the four legal categories of veterinary medicinal products.
10. Identify three examples of drugs used for cancer chemotherapy. Discuss the precautions that are required in the handling, administration and disposal and of these drugs.
11. What is a diuretic and when would such a drug be used?
12. Why is it important that horses never to be used for human consumption are clearly identified on their passport?

Chapter 9

Client communication and practice organization

Carol Gray and Carole Clarke

Learning objectives

After studying this chapter, students should be able to:

- **Describe the basic skills involved in verbal and non-verbal communication**
- **Recognize the structure of a consultation using a common consultation model**
- **Consider the components of informed consent**
- **Incorporate good communication in admission and discharge procedures**
- **Describe communication techniques for dealing with difficult situations**
- **Describe the aims and basic organization of common nursing clinics**
- **Describe the principles of good record-keeping and organization**
- **Describe the principles of handling appointments and reception duties, including processing payments and debt control**
- **Describe the range of materials and equipment necessary to support a veterinary practice**
- **Consider all the relevant issues when controlling stock and ordering supplies**

Principles of communication

- True communication is a **two-way process** – one person sends a message and another receives it.
- In fact, communication is based on a helical model: feedback from the receiver will strongly influence the sender of the message, and cause the sender to adapt the message or to reinforce it, to add further information or to stop transmission.

It is accepted that 93% of the meaning of a message is transmitted non-verbally: 55% of meaning is transmitted by facial expression or body language, with 38% by vocal tone; only 7% of the meaning of a message is transmitted by the actual words spoken.

Non-verbal communication consists of:

- Facial expression
- Posture
- Hand gestures
- Proxemics (personal space)
- Haptics (touch)
- Appearance
- Paralanguage.

Facial expression can give away how we are feeling before we even realize that it has happened (see later explanation regarding affective and cognitive responses), so it is very important that we consciously monitor what our faces are communicating.

Posture can influence communication – compare the response if you speak to another person with your arms folded, or with your arms held by your side. Seated posture is even more telling – the best posture when speaking to someone else in a seated position is to have feet together, hands lying palm upwards on knees, neither arms nor legs crossed, and leaning forward towards the other person. Similarly, positioning yourself on the opposite side of the consulting table puts up a barrier between you and the client. Try positioning yourself on the short side of the table (around the corner from the client) or even standing on the same side of the table, and see what difference that makes!

Some people use their **hands** continuously to embellish their verbal communication. This is a very personal style, but can be quite distracting to the client. If hand gestures are saved for important points, they can help to emphasize vital information.

Proxemics concerns the space between people. What is desirable varies between different cultures and individuals, so be aware that your idea of a friendly chat may make the client feel uncomfortable – if you are picking up signals of unease from the client, try moving a little further away.

Haptics concerns touch. Many people are uncomfortable about touching clients, and touch can be misinterpreted by emotionally distressed clients. It is said that the safest form of touch is a hand placed on the upper arm. However, touch depends very much on personal communication style and empathy. If you are a natural user of touch, it will happen without even thinking about it. If you ever find yourself wondering, 'Should I touch this client?' then the answer will inevitably be 'No'.

Appearance is important, as most people will make a decision about how they feel about you within the first few seconds of meeting you. It is important to look professional, with a clean and tidy uniform. Research from human health sciences suggests that people have no particular preference between a dress-style uniform or a smart polo shirt and trouser combination.

Paralanguage includes the little add-ons that we use to enhance the meaning of our words or to facilitate a conversation, e.g. 'hmmm' or 'uh-huh' to encourage someone to keep talking. It also includes the rate and tone of our speech, and any inflections used (e.g. the Australian inflection, where the pitch of the voice is raised at the end of each sentence, to make it sound like a question even when it's not).

One-way communication

The ultimate vehicle for one-way communication is the written word. Brochures, flyers, websites, advertisements – they all rely on the meaning of the words used being unambiguous. They have to say exactly what they want the reader to understand. There is no margin for error. This is why proofreading – for spelling, grammar and meaning – is essential for all written material that is prepared for public scrutiny. The content should be tested on members of the target audience. If producing literature for clients, make sure that you have not used veterinary jargon. You may know what 'perioperative complications' are, but will your clients?

Public information about a veterinary practice must be accurate. Information about the practice is also likely to be transmitted by interpersonal communication ('word of mouth'), and disgruntled clients will probably tell more people about their experiences than satisfied clients will.

Two-way communication

Telephone calls are a more severe test of communication skills:

- Why is the person on the other end reacting like this?
- Have we missed an important cue (it is more difficult to pick up verbal cues than non-verbal ones)?
- Does the receiver of the telephone call understand the sender correctly?

Telephone communication can be practised by sitting with your back to another person and talking, with a third person observing and giving feedback. If you recreate usual topics for telephone calls, this can feel quite realistic. Some ideas for telephone scenarios are available from NUVACS (the National Unit for the Advancement of Veterinary Communication Skills) at www.nuvacs.co.uk.

Telephone communication at least allows us to use pitch and tone of voice, and rate of speech, to convey extra meaning. That is, unfortunately, not the case with email. The increasing use of email as a message medium can create communication problems. Rapid replies to emails can be misconstrued, and lead to difficulties. Email etiquette is an important factor to consider. Email communication is like a slow-motion version of the telephone call. It takes longer to rectify an incorrect interpretation by the receiver, and you have to wait until the end of the message to question any difficult points.

Email etiquette

- For business emails, always start with a greeting and end with a farewell statement.
- Should you always use correct capitalization, punctuation and grammar? It is probably worth doing this, as it slows down the response and forces you to check the meaning and tone of what has been written BEFORE hitting 'send'.

Recently, video conferencing has become available and can add to the communication experience by adding observation of body language (albeit with a slight time delay). Video conferences can involve two people or larger groups. The more people involved, the more difficult it is to run the meeting or watch body language.

Communicating with clients

It is useful to have a structure for client interviews, whether as part of a consultation in a nurse clinic, when discharging an animal, or when dealing with an emergency patient that has been rushed into the practice.

The veterinary consultation model has been adapted from the Calgary–Cambridge Observation Guide for medical interviews (Figure 9.1). It provides a framework for good practice, but can also be used to evaluate communication skills.

Preparation

Preparation is an integral part of the process. This involves ensuring that both the environment (e.g. the consulting room) and the person involved (i.e. the nurse) are ready.

Preparation of the room

- **Privacy:** No interruptions; no phone calls put through; no-one using the room as a thoroughfare. This is particularly important for euthanasia consultations. Some practices use a 'code' system such as hanging an agreed symbol on the door to signify that a euthanasia consultation is in progress.
- **Safety and comfort:** Windows and doors closed to ensure safety of patient; chairs available if necessary for clients; clean and tidy environment.

Personal preparation

- **Knowledge of patient's history:** Patient's medical records available and read; any extra information to hand, e.g. test results, radiographs.
- **Mental preparation:** Brain 'in neutral', especially if previous work was emotionally demanding.
- **Appearance:** Professional; clean and tidy uniform; appropriate facial expression.

Opening the interview

It is essential that the first few seconds of the encounter go well; this is when the client decides whether they like you and can trust you.

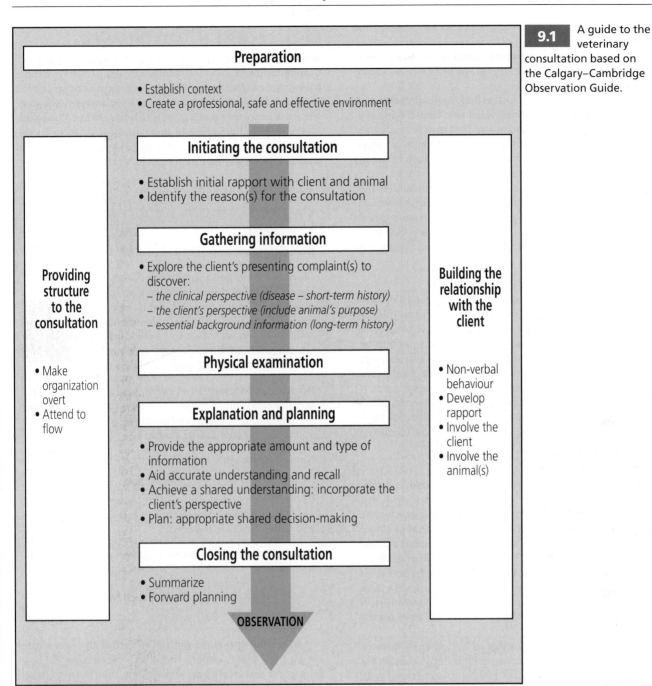

9.1 A guide to the veterinary consultation based on the Calgary–Cambridge Observation Guide.

Preparation

- Establish context
- Create a professional, safe and effective environment

Initiating the consultation

- Establish initial rapport with client and animal
- Identify the reason(s) for the consultation

Gathering information

- Explore the client's presenting complaint(s) to discover:
  - *the clinical perspective (disease – short-term history)*
  - *the client's perspective (include animal's purpose)*
  - *essential background information (long-term history)*

Physical examination

Explanation and planning

- Provide the appropriate amount and type of information
- Aid accurate understanding and recall
- Achieve a shared understanding: incorporate the client's perspective
- Plan: appropriate shared decision-making

Closing the consultation

- Summarize
- Forward planning

OBSERVATION

Providing structure to the consultation

- Make organization overt
- Attend to flow

Building the relationship with the client

- Non-verbal behaviour
- Develop rapport
- Involve the client
- Involve the animal(s)

How can you make a difference to their opinion? It is useful to open the interview by introducing yourself if you have not met the client before and explaining your role in the practice, then continuing with some general conversation. This is important because it puts the client at ease. Many people forget that taking an animal to a veterinary practice is actually quite stressful, and this can affect a client's behaviour and response. Some comments about the weather, or how hard it is to park near the surgery, or about the pet, can go a long way to easing the stress at the start. Of course, there are some cases where it is inappropriate to spend time chatting about other topics, e.g. with an emergency case or a planned euthanasia.

In nearly all cases, the first question that should be asked is an open question, i.e. a question with multiple possible answers, such as 'What has been happening with Scamp?' or 'How has he been since the last time we saw him?' The client should be allowed to reply without interruption.

The human–animal relationship

When meeting a new client and patient, it can be useful to find out what type of relationship exists between them. For example, owners may regard the same type of animal in different ways in different situations, e.g. a working horse *versus* a pet pony. Similarly, a racing Greyhound in training and a retired Greyhound living in a family home will have different value and status for their respective owners.

Culture and religion

Religion is the basis for an ethical code for many people. Judaism and Christianity have promoted kindness to animals from a standpoint of the negative effect of cruelty to animals on the perpetrator and on the animal owner. Animals are regarded as possessions in the UK

continues ▶

continued

and in most Christian nations. Damage to someone else's property is not allowed, either in law or from a religious standpoint.

Some eastern religions, such as Buddhism, Hinduism and Jainism, may give an intrinsic value to animals' lives, and their belief in reincarnation means that cruelty to animals (or ending their lives) could be interfering with a fellow human in one of their other incarnations. Such religions will not allow euthanasia under any circumstances.

The Islamic faith has identified certain animals, i.e. the pig and the dog, as 'unclean' and some Muslims would never keep a dog in the house. They may have a guard dog, which is kept outside, and it is important that their religious beliefs are acknowledged when discussing the care of their animal.

Socioeconomic status

People may attempt to use animal ownership to elevate their status socially (e.g. ownership of large aggressive dogs) or to prove that they have a certain level of wealth (e.g. ownership of very rare breeds). Clients need to be allowed to decide for themselves how they wish to spend their money and have all the options for healthcare presented without any preconceptions about wealth. It is said that we should never make judgements about what a client might be willing, or able, to spend on their pet, and this is essential when we move on to discuss decision-making.

Health status of the owner

Assistance animals include guide dogs for blind people, hearing dogs for deaf people, assistance dogs for disabled people, dogs that alert epileptic owners to imminent fits, and even companion dogs that can help people with mental health problems to lead as normal an existence as possible. The effect on the client of illness or planned surgery on such dogs is enormous and must be borne in mind when communicating risk and aftercare. If the dog is unable to work for a while, it is important to remember the effect this will have on the client's life.

Animals can have a positive effect on their owners' health just by providing companionship. Pet ownership has been associated with better health outcomes and with increased social opportunities. Many animals will have deeper associations for their owners, with memories of loved ones, for example, and this can have a massive effect on decision-making.

It should also be remembered that animals can have a negative effect on human health. For example, people with asthma may refuse to rehome their pets and continue to live with a chronic disease rather than without them. Pets may potentially cause illness or injury to people on long-term medication, such as those on warfarin or immunosuppressants. Also, the risks of zoonotic diseases, such as ringworm, toxocariasis and toxoplasmosis, should be conveyed to pet owners.

It is useful at the start of the consultation to investigate the client–patient relationship, i.e. what does *this* animal mean to *this* owner? An open question such as 'Can you tell me all about Sparky?', followed by active listening, will hopefully elicit useful information about the relationship.

Gathering information

The process of gathering information involves tactical use of summarizing and screening, and making use of open questions (those that can have a number of possible answers) and closed questions (those that have a more defined answer). However, the most important skill is LISTENING. The client will give you lots of information, much of it very useful, but how do you remember it and, more importantly, let the client know that you have been paying attention?

Example: A client with a diabetic dog has come in for a regular check-up

Nurse: How's Scamp been since we last saw him?

Client: *Well, I've been quite pleased with him, but he didn't eat his breakfast one day last week, so I didn't give him his injection. He was a bit quiet that day, but the next day he was eating really well again so we went back to his normal routine. He doesn't seem to be drinking as much, and he has definitely got more energy. I worry about hurting him when I inject him, but I suppose he's quite used to it now.*

Nurse (summarizing): So, in general things are going well, but you had a problem when he didn't eat his breakfast. He seems to be better in himself, but you are concerned about the injections hurting him.

Nurse (screening): Is there anything else we need to discuss?

Client: *We go on holiday in 2 months time. I'm not sure if we can put him in kennels or if I need to teach someone else in the family to inject him.*

Use of closed questions can investigate this new information further:

Nurse: Is there someone else in the family who could look after him?

Notice that the nurse did not interrupt the client after asking the initial question. This is very important. The basic principle is to start with open questions, then move to closed questions for specific bits of information. Other types of question may be useful, such as multiple choice, if the client does not seem to understand what is being asked. For example, 'What is Scamp's reaction to the injection – does he squeal, or turn round, or just flinch slightly?'

It is important *not* to use leading questions, such as 'He's not drinking nearly so much now, is he?' where the phrasing of the question suggests the correct answer, or the answer that the questioner wants to hear. The use of 'we' in the question can help to engender a feeling of the client and the nurse being part of a healthcare team, and will enhance the relationship. Active listening (appropriate eye contact, nodding, using verbal encouragers such as 'Yes' or 'OK') also helps to build the relationship with the client.

Giving information

The aim of giving information is to allow the client to make an informed decision, and to increase client concordance with treatment plans. In order for this to happen, information must be given in a format and style that maximizes the client's understanding, and it is important to check that understanding on a regular basis.

Information is best given in small pieces, regularly making sure that it is understood ('chunking and checking'). It is better to ask the client if they have any questions about the information given, rather than asking whether they understand what they have been told. Retention of information is increased if the verbal information is supplemented with written or visual aids. It is important to determine the client's level of knowledge before embarking on an explanation, e.g. by asking 'Have you any experience of this condition?', and to pitch language appropriately. In most cases, it is best to avoid the use of scientific or medical terminology, unless the client has indicated that they have specialized knowledge. Similarly, if the client's first language is not English, then explanations have to be carefully worded to avoid ambiguity. It is especially important to avoid the use of colloquial terms if language difficulties exist, as the meaning can be totally misconstrued (e.g. 'put him down', 'knock him out', 'put him to sleep').

Helping the client to make a decision means presenting the information so that they can make a decision. It does not mean making the decision for them. If the client asks 'What would you do if it was your pet?', how would you respond? The best way to handle this one is to acknowledge that it would be a difficult decision for you too, and then to go back over the options with pros and cons of each, perhaps sharing your thoughts on how you would try to reach a decision.

Closing the interview

It is important that the end of the interview is structured to provide a clear way forward and to delineate responsibilities. This is the time for a final summary, a final screen ('Is there anything else you wanted to discuss?') and a structure for what happens next. The client should feel adequately supported by the practice and should have a named person to contact with any queries. If a return visit is needed, the client should be asked to return on a specific day and to make sure they see the same nurse. If you have agreed to telephone the client, or have asked the client to telephone you, decide on a day and a time and enter this in the diary so that you are available at that time.

Picking up cues

Clients will often signal when they are feeling a particular emotion. This signal may be verbal or non-verbal. Most people will ignore the signal. With training, nurses can learn to pick up on cues (signals) and respond appropriately to them. It is not difficult to learn this technique, and it can avoid escalation to extreme displays of emotion (where the signals become more obvious until you *have* to react to them).

It is perhaps easiest to start with non-verbal cues. The client may look worried when the nurse gives them a particular piece of information, or when they are telling them what has been happening with their animal. Going back to the diabetic dog, the client gave a cue that she was worried about giving injections. This could be picked up and acknowledged at the time: 'You said that you are worried about the injections hurting Scamp. Perhaps we can go through your injection technique again?' This could prevent the problem escalating to eventual non-compliance where the client is so worried about the injections that they stop giving them.

Other causes of non-compliance can be identified and dealt with. For example, if a client has financial concerns about continuing treatment for a chronic condition, a discussion with the veterinary surgeon regarding choice of treatment and cheaper alternatives can be arranged. If a client cannot give the medication to the patient, offering supervision for the first few occasions or, in some cases, giving the treatment at the practice can alleviate this concern. Perhaps the client is not convinced that the treatment will help. Again, picking this up at an early stage and describing other similar, successful cases may deal with this concern. In each of these cases, it is vital to pick up cues from the client at an early stage, to ensure that the patient receives the treatment.

Most responses to cues will be empathic responses. For example, the client looks very concerned when the nurse is describing aftercare following surgery. This can be picked up on by saying, 'I can see that you are concerned about this. Is there anything in particular that is worrying you?'

Dealing with bereavement or breaking bad news

Empathy is a key communication skill in many situations, but is particularly useful for dealing with a bereaved client, or when breaking bad news to a client. Empathy means identifying the emotion being felt by the client, and acknowledging that emotion (e.g. 'I can see how upsetting this news is for you', 'I realize this makes you very angry'). Showing higher levels of empathy is positively associated with greater client satisfaction with consultations.

In cases of bereavement, the classical processes of grief (shock/denial, guilt/anger, bargaining, and acceptance) do not happen in every case, nor in that particular order. Identifying the client's emotional response correctly allows the nurse to use empathy in an appropriate way.

For example, if a client has just been told that their cat has feline leukaemia virus (FeLV), their response may be to question whether these are the correct results for their cat (denial). If the nurse can spot why this is happening, he/she can use empathy to try and help the client to move forward: 'I can see that this news is a great shock to you, and with Sparky being so young, it's difficult to take it in. I'm so sorry this has happened.'

Appropriate use of silence is very important when breaking bad news. If the client is very upset, it is pointless to carry on talking, as they will not hear a word that you say. It is something that can be practised. Silences always seem awkward to the person who is breaking the bad news, but not to the client.

The nurse should always be prepared to deal with tears. A box of tissues, handed to the client at the right moment, signifies that 'it's all right to cry' and conveys empathy. Silence is, again, an important part of dealing with a distressed client.

It is always difficult to decide whether touch can be used in this situation. If you have to think about it, don't do it. It is said that a light touch on the upper arm is the safest form, but with a client that the nurse knows well, a hug may be appropriate.

You should bear in mind the possibility of touch being misinterpreted by an emotionally distressed person, particularly if they are of the opposite sex.

Euthanasia

Clients require the most sensitive communication skills from professionals when they have decided to opt for euthanasia of their animal. This may be due to incurable disease, lack of finance to pay for treatment, because it is a kinder option for the patient, or for some other reason. The first point to remember is how the client is feeling. If they are unable to afford treatment, they may be feeling guilty, or angry that they have been put in this position. In most cases, however, the predominant feeling is grief and overwhelming sadness. It is important that the nurse learns to deal with this, as he/she will meet it frequently. Skills that can be used include:

* Giving the client time to think, speak and show emotion
* Showing empathy
* Making sure that the procedure itself goes smoothly.

It is very distressing for clients to see their pet struggle, or for the procedure to go wrong. This possibility needs to be minimized. If you can see that the animal is distressed, it may be sedated first. Some veterinary surgeons will insert an intravenous catheter to minimize the chance of failure and this also allows the client to hold the animal while the injection is given. A full description of what will happen should be explained prior to the injection being given as well as the possibility of untoward events (e.g. urination, reflex gasps).

Dealing with the financial aspect at the time of euthanasia is always difficult. The nurse should be guided by the practice policy. If the client is unknown to the practice, they should be asked to settle the payment beforehand. Whilst some clients do prefer to settle their bill at the time, for many others dealing with the money at a later date is preferable and allows them to be left with the animal afterwards, with time to say goodbye. At this stage you could also offer the clients the opportunity to keep a memento (e.g. a clipped piece of fur). **Sending the request for payment should never be combined with sending a sympathy card.**

Euthanasia should always be adequately planned for, with a double appointment booked, or at the end of surgery. It also helps if there is a dedicated room in the practice, or at least a separate exit, to avoid the client having to go back through the waiting room.

Clients vary in their responses to grief. If a client seems to be severely affected, it may be advisable to contact friends or relatives, and, if possible, the client should not be sent home on their own. Bereavement counsellors are available in most areas and their numbers should be available at the reception in each practice. Cards detailing the contact number and website address of the Pet Bereavement Support Service (PBSS) may be given to every bereaved client. Remember that you are not a trained counsellor and should not take on areas beyond your expertise. It is, however, a thoughtful act to telephone a bereaved client a few days later to see how they are coping and to offer any further support.

Dealing with anger

It is important to realize the reasons for a client's anger, to acknowledge these reasons, and to let the client know that you have acknowledged them. The main skill used in dealing with anger is empathy. This can be a very difficult response to find when faced with an angry client. It is easy to respond empathically to a bereaved client, as our instinctive response is to show the same emotion (**affective empathy**). However,

we cannot allow this instinctive response with anger. We need to use higher brain centres to employ a considered response (**cognitive empathy**). This involves remaining calm, remaining seated if possible, keeping your tone of voice low and pace of speech slow. Don't react to personal insults. An angry person needs a reaction to fuel the anger.

A checklist for dealing with anger may look like this:

* Remain outwardly calm
* Keep your voice low and even
* Try to slow things down – pause before answering, or before asking another question
* Don't interrupt the client – allow them to vent their anger
* Try to stay at a lower level than the client (but see section on personal safety below)
* Use empathy ('I can see that you are very angry, and you have had an upsetting experience')
* Try to move things forward ('I am sorry that this has happened. How can we try to put it right?').

Report any concerns you may have to your employer; it is not acceptable for you to feel bullied by a client (Equality Act 2010).

Personal safety

When dealing with anger, personal safety may be compromised. In this case, there should be some method of raising the alarm (e.g. panic buttons in consulting rooms) and an escape route (for example, avoid being trapped behind a consulting table). If a client has a history of anger, it would be sensible practice policy to ensure that no-one is left alone with them, or they should be asked to send another member of the family with the patient. It is essential to have a practice protocol on personal safety. Remember that a client with a grudge may pose a risk to every member of staff. If there are genuine concerns about the safety of practice staff, the local police should be informed.

Communicating with clients who have special needs

When clients have difficulty in communicating due to either disability or lack of English as a first language, the onus falls on the veterinary professional to make sure that the client is given the information in a way that they can understand. This may involve:

* Writing information down
* Drawing diagrams
* Repeating information
* Using an interpreter
* Using models.

In some instances a person may accompany the client to help with understanding (e.g. by translating for them), but it is important that the client makes the decision regarding their animal (especially if this decision is to give consent for surgery or in-patient treatment). In rare cases the client may have given the accompanying person the right to make the decision for them (as an agent or proxy), but this needs to be verified carefully, especially with regard to payment for treatment.

Dealing with assertive clients

Being assertive is the skill of saying what we need or want, or protecting ourselves from what we do not want, whilst respecting the needs and rights of others. It is being able to communicate appropriately in a direct, open and honest way. Assertiveness may sometimes be seen as the mid-point between passive and aggressive ways of being. This seems to be the type of client who strikes fear into everyone's hearts, but dealing with assertive clients can be less intimidating if a few golden rules are followed.

- **Acknowledge their expertise.** Most assertive clients feel that they have specialist knowledge about their animal and its condition. Treat them as if they know more than the average client. If they bring in pages printed out from the internet, acknowledge their research and share good websites with them.
- **Involve them in the decision-making process.** All clients appreciate being part of a team involved in healthcare delivery, but assertive clients will react particularly positively to this strategy.
- **Do not dismiss their ideas for treatment.** Acknowledge that they could be right, although current research may suggest an alternative method is better. Perhaps you could try the method they suggested if the first method fails? You will have to put up with 'I told you so!' but you can admit that they had a good idea.
- **Do not be afraid to admit that you do not know.** It can be difficult if a client is demanding a particular method of care, but if you have no experience of this method then say so. Refer the client to the veterinary surgeon in charge of the case.

How to improve your communication skills

- Set up a suitable encounter – this could be an actual conversation with a client (you must get consent from the client if you do this), or a role play with a colleague or with a professional actor.
- Video this encounter.
- Analyse the encounter, describe what happened, the effect this had on the communication, and evaluate your skills (this can be done either on your own or with a few colleagues).
- Reflect on the exercise – what have you learned and how will you use this?
- Start again – changes in behaviour are effected by rehearsal.

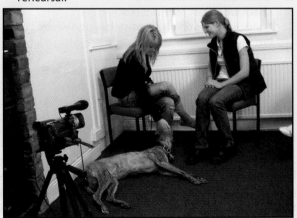

Communicating with colleagues

A team works well when each member knows exactly where he/she fits into the team, what is expected of him/her, and how to raise concerns or suggest improvements. A line management system that delineates responsibility, but also values and rewards initiative, will help to keep the team together and lead to greater employee satisfaction. Job descriptions and line management structure should be set out in contracts of employment. However, this ethos still requires effective communication between members of the team for it to work.

Providing support for colleagues

It is essential for the effective working of a team that individual members should be able to identify when one of their colleagues is stressed and requires support. This may be provided in a simple form, e.g. a chat over coffee, giving the stressed colleague a chance to talk about what is stressing them or, if the problem is more serious, providing more structured support such as telephone numbers of helplines. As with bereavement counselling, it is important to realize when the support required is outside your own area of expertise.

Regular formal communication is best achieved by holding team meetings. It can be difficult to arrange a time when everyone can attend, but it is important that meetings are not repeatedly cancelled or rescheduled. Meetings should be held at a fixed frequency and time, so that all members of the team know when they can next air their views. Some practices have a suggestion box that allows team members to post their concerns or comments anonymously. This can be a good idea, though it is better for the person with the concern to maintain responsibility for it until it is resolved. For large practices, team meetings for each group of employees (e.g. vets, nurses, receptionists) may be held, but it is important that outcomes are circulated to the whole practice to maintain communication.

- All meetings should have an agenda, with a suggested time limit for each agenda item. This prevents some items dragging on for hours and preventing discussion of other topics.
- Minutes should be taken and circulated as soon as possible after the meeting, particularly for those who were unable to attend.
- Action points should be allocated to individuals, and followed up at subsequent meetings.

Reflective practice: appraisal

Most practices will monitor the performance of individual team members via the appraisal system, and this can be a worthwhile learning experience for both the appraiser and the appraised. However, the appraisal system only works if it is regarded as important enough to warrant protected time for meetings, and if the appraisal is seen as a reflective tool. Appraisals can involve one other person, or can involve several members of the team (e.g. a veterinary surgeon, veterinary nurse and receptionist could be involved in an appraisal, although each would meet individually with the person being appraised; this is known as a 360-degree appraisal).

Preparation for the appraisal involves distribution of appraisal forms, listing the areas to be discussed, to both parties in advance of the meeting. During the meeting, the person being appraised should be asked to evaluate their own performance first, and to suggest areas for improvement or training required. The appraiser then goes through a similar list and discusses any points of contention. Eventually both should reach consensus. Discussions and action plans should be documented for future reference, with copies given to both parties. It is a useful opportunity to review and ensure that the job description still reflects the role carried out by an individual.

Key points for successful appraisals:

- Pre-arrange the meeting time
- Protect the time, and ensure it is adequate
- Use a private room with no opportunity for interruptions
- Start with positive aspects (both parties)
- Move on to areas where improvement could be made (both parties)
- Summarize and record agreed actions. Update job description if necessary
- Make sure both parties receive copies
- Arrange follow-up meeting.

Not all appraisals go well or are seen as positive experiences. However, reflection is a vital aspect of professional life. Veterinary nurses must have the ability to take responsibility for their actions, be honest with themselves, work out a plan for remedying any deficiencies, and also maximize the chance to use any specific knowledge or skills. If reflection becomes part of the team ethos, with everyone willing to assess and evaluate what they do continually, then appraisals become a formal part of that cycle. A key professional skill is practising self-appraisal and being aware of personal strengths and weaknesses. For many people, this requires practice.

One way to do this is to look at 'critical incident analysis': choose one major event in which you are involved each day; reflect on it from the perspective of all people involved (including yourself). Soon this will become a natural strategy for reflecting on your own practice.

Reflective practice: clinical audit

Practice teams can take the reflective ethos a stage further and investigate all areas of veterinary care on a regular basis. This requires someone to take responsibility for an area of practice, to investigate how this works in the practice and to compare the results with the evidence available on 'best practice'. This is known as **clinical audit**. Veterinary nurses can play an important part in this cycle by developing and investigating particular areas of interest.

Practices should implement a system of clinical governance, where important areas of the practice are subject to regular clinical audit. The areas selected will vary from one practice to another, depending on the type of work carried out, but should include both surgical and medical examples. The example below gives a rough idea of what is involved in a clinical audit.

Example: Clinical audit to review mortality rates associated with the perioperative nursing care of 'small pets'

1. Arrange team meeting to choose area for audit and get everyone on board.
2. Decide upon which species will be included (e.g. rabbits, rodents).
3. Consider what the practice does to care for small pets, i.e. what is the normal protocol (a) preoperatively, (b) during the operation, and (c) postoperatively.
4. Calculate the mortality rate for small pets undergoing surgery in the practice over the past year. This will require access to case records and operating lists. There will be variable factors, such as different types and duration of anaesthesia, and these should be taken into account.
5. Consider how this compares with reported studies (research the literature).
6. Ask whether there is anything that the practice could change to improve its mortality rates (search the literature for 'best practice').
7. Implement changes.
8. Monitor results over the next year.
9. Repeat the exercise.

Admission and discharge procedures

Surgical and medical admissions

Responsibility for admitting animals for surgical or medical interventions is likely to be delegated to the veterinary nurse. It is important to realize that this is an area where misunderstandings can develop. The veterinary nurse should be able to refer any difficult clients or situations back to a veterinary surgeon.

Admission procedure

1. Check patient identification.
2. Check client identification.
3. Check when last fed/watered.
4. Check whether on any medication, and when last given.
5. Complete patient ID tag/collar.
6. Complete inpatient cards.
7. Perform a health check.
8. Gain client consent.
9. Label possessions.
10. Advise on time to phone or time to collect.

Identification

Firstly, correct identification of the animal must be considered. There have been many horror stories of mix-ups; for example, the champion stud dog booked in for dental treatment that was mistakenly castrated in place of another dog of the same breed in the neighbouring kennel.

If an animal is microchipped or tattooed, mistakes are less likely to happen (provided that the chip or tattoo is read immediately before the operation). However, most animals will be brought in with only a collar for identification purposes (or often, in the case of cats, no means of identification at all). A more foolproof method of identification is to use disposable lightweight collars (tab band collars) for every inpatient (see Chapters 12 and 16). The collar should be marked with the patient's name and the procedure for which it has been admitted, written clearly. The name and telephone number of the practice must also be included (these can be pre-printed) in case of escape. These collars can be used for dogs, cats and rabbits. Mane tags and labelled head collars should be used for horses (see Chapter 16).

Inpatient cards

An inpatient card for every surgical patient is common practice. Two cards are best: one card can accompany the patient into theatre, to be used for intraoperative checks and monitoring; while the other is left on the kennel or stable to ensure that each animal is returned to the same place. The inpatient card should contain the following information:

- Identity of patient
- Procedure
- Description
- Temperament
- Any special requirements (e.g. medication, fluids)
- Observation records
- Accommodation in use.

Admission health check

The admission procedure should also include a full health check (see Chapter 15). This allows assessment of temperament (useful before the patient is put into a kennel), investigation of feeding regime (when last fed and watered) and detection of any clinical abnormalities. At the very least, the patient should have a physical health check that includes TPR (temperature, pulse and respiration) observations. Some practices will offer pre-anaesthetic blood tests to surgical patients, e.g. to check hepatic and renal function. This may be offered to all surgical patients, or only to those undergoing non-elective procedures. It is important to conform to **practice protocol** in this area.

Isolation

Isolation cages should be available for both dogs and cats (see Chapter 12). Any animal showing signs of an infectious disease, whether likely to be contagious or not, should be isolated, with special guidelines for nursing. If the animal is booked for an elective procedure, it should be checked by a veterinary surgeon, as the surgery may need to be postponed and the animal sent home. Particular care must be taken with potential zoonotic diseases, such as ringworm. All staff must be made aware of the risks to their health if such animals are admitted and must take suitable precautions (see Chapter 5).

Possessions

Many practices refuse to take in clients' possessions when admitting animals but it is sometimes necessary to accept them (e.g. collars and leads, cat baskets). These should be clearly labelled with the names of the client and the patient. Similarly, any other possessions taken in must be clearly labelled, with a note on the inpatient card of what has been left. When discharging the patient, the person responsible should sign to indicate that the possessions have been returned to the client.

Informed consent

When animals are admitted for any diagnostic, medical or surgical treatment, **informed consent** for any diagnostic or surgical procedure on an animal (including admission for blood sampling and radiography) must be obtained from the owner or their representative (Figure 9.2). Under English law, animals are regarded as property and owners have the ultimate sanction over what happens to their animals. Note, however, that animal welfare legislation overrides this sanction in relevant cases.

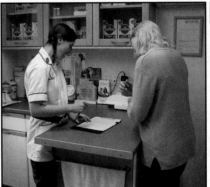

9.2 Obtaining client consent.

Informed consent requires:

- **A detailed description** of exactly what is going to be done to the animal, in language that the owner can understand. It is the veterinary professional's duty to ensure client understanding. In cases where there is a problem, such as language, disability or if the owner is not available, it would be better to postpone the procedure until this requirement can be met
- A discussion of **any side effects or risks** associated with the procedure. All material risks must be discussed with the owner, even if the chances of their happening are small. A material risk is a risk with severe consequences, e.g. death or serious injury of the animal during general anaesthesia
- A discussion of **any alternative treatments** or diagnostic options available. The client must be allowed to make a decision that is suitable for their needs, both financial and emotional
- A discussion of **who** will perform the surgery – this is especially important if a veterinary nurse is undertaking a surgical procedure under Schedule 3 of the Veterinary Surgeons Act, or if a veterinary student will be involved under supervision
- A discussion of **where** the surgery will take place, if this involves transport to another branch of the practice
- A discussion/explanation of **costs** (see below).

The person seeking to obtain the owner's consent should be appropriately trained (and qualified) to give a full explanation of the procedure. Reliance on consent forms should be minimal; the detail of the form should be explained verbally, with any scientific jargon simplified. Consent is usually confirmed via a written signature, which makes it easier for any subsequent complaints to be investigated. It is good practice, and now recommended by the RCVS, that the owner is given a copy of the consent form. There are exceptions, such as telephone consent for euthanasia while an animal is anaesthetized. In this case, two people should obtain verbal consent from the owner and this should be written in the case notes as soon as possible. Many veterinary surgeons do not ask owners of terminally ill animals to sign consent forms if they have been involved in the treatment along the way. However, it is sensible practice to get written consent for euthanasia in most instances.

Financial estimates

Consent to treatment also brings in the law of contract. That is why it is important to give financial estimates for the treatment. **Estimates** are a rough guide to cost. If they are going to be exceeded, the owner must be kept informed of this. Some elective procedures will have fixed costs; these are then **quotes** rather than estimates, and must be adhered to if the surgery proceeds normally.

Should financial information be included on a consent form? It can prevent the client from considering the other aspects of consent. It would be better practice to use two forms: one for consent to the procedure; and one for consent to financial obligations (contract).

Legal age of consent

In order to be party to a financial contract (which is what is essentially being described here), in England and Wales the person signing the form must be at least 18 years old (16 in Scotland). However, the age for legal medical consent is 16. It would be possible for a 16-year-old to give consent for the surgical procedure, but there would be no guarantee that the bill would be paid. That is why most practices insist on a minimum age of 18 for signing consent forms. This applies to both parties in the contract, so **a veterinary nurse who is 17 years of age should not be involved in the consent process.**

Discharging inpatients

If given responsibility for returning an animal to a client, it is important to know the full facts about the case or procedure, so that any client questions can be answered. It is often advisable to go through this information before returning the patient to the client, otherwise the client may be too distracted by the reunion with their animal to take in the information.

- Remember the 'chunking and checking' technique for giving information, and allow the client time to think about questions they may want to ask.
  - Avoid jargon. Make sure that the client understands what has happened, and what they need to do in terms of home care.
  - Acknowledge any concerns the client may have about aftercare.
  - Use written information, diagrams or models to enhance explanations.
  - Always end the conversation with 'Is there anything else that you would like to discuss?'
  - Finish with a final summary of your discussion and what happens next.
- Make sure that both you and the client know what happens next, and reassure them that there is a 24-hour service available for emergencies. It is useful to give them a business card with contact telephone numbers on it.

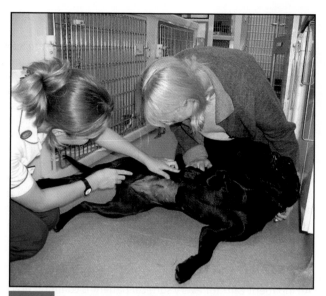

9.3   Explaining postoperative care to a client.

Discharge procedure

1. Check patient identification.
2. Check client identification.
3. Prepare discharge sheet (these may be pre-printed for common procedures).
4. Prepare medication.
5. Explain procedure/aftercare to client (Figure 9.3).
6. Collect/check possessions left with patient.
7. Bring patient through from ward.
8. Arrange next visit.
9. Collect payment if this has not already been done.

Nurse clinics

Running nurse clinics in specific delegated areas can be very rewarding, can benefit the practice financially, and offers clients a service they really appreciate.

Popular areas for nurse clinics

- Puppy and kitten advice.
- Flea and worm control.
- Dental home care.
- Support for pets that need to lose weight.
- Help and advice for senior pets.
- Advice on some behavioural problems.
- Puppy classes.

Nurses can also offer support for owners of pets with chronic conditions, such as diabetes mellitus, arthritis, urinary tract problems and allergic skin disease. Ensuring compliance with chronic treatment regimes can improve a pet's quality of life and help to reduce stress for an owner who may find giving medication difficult. Nurses can train owners to administer medications correctly and help them to gain in confidence, e.g. with insulin injections. Clients also often ask the nurse questions that they would not 'bother the vet with' but which are nonetheless important for the pet's health.

Deciding when to see clients can be problematical, particularly in a busy practice with limited consulting room space. Ideally, clients should be seen in a consulting room, or dedicated 'nurses room', but areas of reception are used in some practices. Clients can be seen by appointment at particular times, but it is a good idea for the nurse to be available at the request of the consulting veterinary surgeon so that clients identified as needing a nurse consultation can be referred immediately.

Protocols should be agreed for each type of consultation, so that veterinary surgeons and nurses know exactly which areas will be discussed and can avoid duplication of effort. Checklists are helpful. The veterinary nurse should have received adequate training and be confident to cover the areas expected. All consultations and advice should be recorded in the clinical notes. For more details on running nurse clinics, see the *BSAVA Manual of Canine and Feline Advanced Veterinary Nursing*.

Examples of protocols for nursing consultations

Dental home care

- Discuss current home care.
- Examine the mouth, use disclosing solution to show plaque.
- Discuss diet.
- Demonstrate and discuss tooth brushing and other preventive measures.
- Make recommendations for dental home care.
- Make appointment for follow-up visit.

Obesity clinic

- Weigh pet.
- Work out ideal weight and target weight.
- Discuss current feeding, exercise, treats, etc.
- Make sure pet is healthy (veterinary surgeon to check if unsure).
- Agree action plan and proposed dietary and exercise changes; issue weight chart.
- Arrange next appointment to check progress.

It is helpful to have information supporting your advice, for the client to take away. This can be produced in-house, or you can make use of the literature provided by the suppliers of products you are recommending or by BSAVA in the case of behavioural advice, and personalize it with your own and your practice details.

Puppy parties

Puppy parties can be run as single sessions or as a course and can include general care issues, nutrition, parasite control, early puppy training and, most importantly, socialization (see Chapter 11). Approximately six puppies and their families are regarded as the optimum number, though some practices run larger groups quite successfully. Nurses should seek further training in this area, particularly in behaviour management, before running groups themselves.

Location may be a problem, as many reception areas are not suitable. Good hygiene is essential, particularly if puppies are coming before completing their primary vaccination. A dedicated room is ideal, but just a dream for many nurses.

Customer service and the value of clients

The success of any practice is related to its ability to attract and retain customers (its clients). The total number of clients at any time will be determined by the rate at which new clients are joining the practice, and the rate at which they are leaving. The most common reasons for people to leave are the death of their pet or because they move away, but a surprising number of clients may leave the practice because of a perceived indifference to them or because their experience just did not match their expectations. Most will not take the trouble to complain. For most practices, more than half their new clients will come by direct recommendation from existing clients, and many new patients will be new pets acquired by the existing client base. Advertising, good practice presentation and maintaining a presence in the local news all help in attracting new clients, but retaining them after the first visit, and keeping the clients you already have is vital for the economic success of the business. It is a useful exercise to calculate how much an average client will spend with the practice over the lifetime of one pet. The figure may be surprising.

Offering the best customer service will give practices a good advantage in client retention. This is a complex area but some key points can be considered.

Key points of customer service

- Listen to the client, and ask questions to understand their need.
- Be honest at all times.
- Talk to and engage with their pet.
- Give clients your undivided attention, and respond to their concerns.
- Make sure that you are consistent in your service, so clients know what to expect (agreed protocols may help).
- Check or follow up with the client to make sure they are happy and understand everything.
- Try to add value to your service by doing a little more than expected (this can be something small, such as carrying a bag of food to the car, following up with a phone call the next day, or writing down recommendations).
- Encourage feedback on your service, particularly complaints, and act on them.
- Encourage clients to return by using reminder systems, and encouraging compliance with recommendations.
- Thank clients for recommending the practice.

Reception duties

Every client will make contact with the practice initially by telephoning or dropping into reception, and the welcome and response they receive may make or break the practice–client relationship. If possible, the nurse or receptionist on the front desk should not be distracted by other duties. Every client should be greeted immediately and given full attention. It is the receptionist's job to find out why the client has made contact and to ascertain their needs and priorities, and then to ensure that these needs are met, that the client's questions are answered and that any action required is followed up efficiently. Expectations should not just be met, but exceeded.

The nurse in reception must:

- Feel confident and in control
- Have a well organized and tidy area to work in
- Understand all the relevant practice processes and protocols
- Know how to make and record appointments
- Know which personnel are available and when
- Know how to prioritize appointments so that urgent cases are seen quickly, and be able to offer interim advice to the client
- Know how much time to allow for each appointment or visit so that the clinical staff do not 'run behind'
- Have a good rapport with the clients and a professional and friendly manner that puts clients at their ease
- Know when and where to ask for assistance
- Be able to handle sales transactions and process payments.

Working on reception can be more stressful than working behind the scenes, for two main reasons. First, the nurse is 'on show' and may be worried about how much he/she knows and how he/she comes across to others. Secondly, on reception it is more difficult to control the flow of work, and there will be busy and slack periods. Clients with difficult queries or complaints never seem to come into an empty reception area. If you are a student nurse, it may help to explain that you are learning and ask people to bear with you if you are not working as quickly as your colleagues. Clients are usually supportive if they know that someone is new to the job, particularly if they ask for help appropriately. Always have a pen and paper (or a day book) ready to note messages and call details, and a local area map may be useful for place names and large animal call planning. In quieter periods, the nurse can chat to the clients and patients and get to know them – this helps the nurse to relax and can build relationships that may last a whole career. Filing and tidying can be done along the way.

Confidence on reception and on the telephone comes with experience and practice. The more confident the nurse becomes, the more he/she will enjoy interacting with the clients and their pets (Figure 9.4).

Most practices have a sales area in reception and the nurse must be familiar with all the products and how they are used,

so that he/she can recommend them to clients. It is important to understand the practice's protocols for selling and approving prescription-only medicines (see Chapter 8).

Keeping reception and the waiting area clean and neat means walking around regularly, removing out-of-date notices and other clutter, making sure that children's toys are clean and tidy and that magazines are current and look inviting. Plants or flowers should be fresh and healthy.

Confidence and respect will be gained from having appropriate, neat and clean uniform or clothes, polished shoes and tidy hair. If you have just been working in the clinical areas, check that you have no splashes of blood or clumps of hair on your clothing.

Handling appointments

Although many veterinary practices still hold open surgeries, where clients are seen in the order they arrive, most now have at least some appointment-only surgeries. Depending on the practice's policy, appointments may be made just for a specific time, or also to see a specific veterinary surgeon or nurse. Diaries may be in book or loose-leaf form, or may be on computer. The advantage of a computerized diary is that it can be linked to the records themselves; it is also easier to amend and can often be accessed anywhere in the building, or even remotely.

Appointments may be for a set time (e.g. 10 minutes) or may be run on a flexible basis. For example, 5-minute slots may be used, with puppy vaccinations being allowed 20 minutes, suture removals 5 minutes, repeat prescription checks 10 minutes, and so on. For equine or farm calls, record clear details of call requests to help the veterinary surgeon plan the visit and take along appropriate equipment and medication.

Most people telephone for an appointment or make one on the previous visit. It is vital to ensure that the owner and animal's names have been recorded accurately. If the appointment is for a new client, a telephone number should be taken so that they can be contacted if necessary.

Priorities

Often the practice will have quiet and busy periods. The quieter times should be offered first, leaving the popular times for those who have no option but to come in then. When prioritizing appointments, consideration should be given to:

- The urgency of the case
- The preference of the owner
- Available staff
- The possibility that the client may be able to book elsewhere.

Clients may be looking for a particular time or day rather than a particular veterinary surgeon, and losing the appointment to a neighbouring practice may mean losing the lifetime value of that pet to the practice – a substantial sum of money.

Emergencies and delays

Recognition of emergencies is covered in Chapter 21. Emergency cases should be seen as soon as possible and may have to take priority over existing appointments. The situation should be explained to those waiting – most will be happy to wait. If possible, clients due for an appointment should be

9.4   A busy reception area. Confidence comes with experience.

telephoned and asked to rebook, or warned that there will be a wait. The veterinary nurse should never say, 'We are running behind' or 'The vet is busy', but should always give as much information as permitted about the nature of the emergency or difficult case without identifying animal or owner (clients are always interested in what is going on behind the scenes). For long waits, clients should be updated on the situation at least every 10 minutes or given an option to return later or rebook. The veterinary surgeons and nurses should be consulted on difficult days to decide how to handle the list. As clients with appointments arrive, they should be seen in the order of appointment rather than order of arrival, unless someone is late. Veterinary surgeons on farm or equine rounds should leave a note of the order of visits and remain in contact so that the nearest available clinician can be diverted to an emergency. Regular check-ins or mobile phone contact are also good practice for security and personal safety.

Second opinions and supersession

New clients should always be asked whether the animal is currently under treatment. It is not unusual for clients to seek a second opinion or to try a new veterinary surgeon during a course of treatment. In these situations, all veterinary surgeons must follow the guidelines in the *RCVS Guide to Professional Conduct* (currently under review). The client is free to choose whichever veterinary practice they wish, and veterinary surgeons should not obstruct a client from changing to another veterinary practice, nor should they discourage a client from seeking a second opinion. If a veterinary surgeon sees an animal that has been treated elsewhere for its current problem, the previous veterinary surgeon should be contacted as soon as possible to obtain details of the case and medications prescribed. This guidance is given in the interests of the patient, but informing a colleague of a consultation with their former client is also professional courtesy and helps them to know what has happened with the case.

The taking over of a patient in this way is termed supersession. Occasionally, a client will be embarrassed about changing practices and may attempt to withhold details of their previous veterinary surgeon. A gentle explanation that the history is important for the health of their pet usually helps them to understand why it is necessary to talk to the previous veterinary surgeon. In an emergency it is acceptable to make an initial assessment and administer any essential treatment before contacting the original veterinary surgeon.

Veterinary surgeons may also advise clients to seek a second opinion, particularly where there may be doubt about the diagnosis. In this situation, the veterinary surgeon will arrange for the second practitioner to see the case and will expect to take back responsibility for the case after the consultation.

Referral

Where further expertise or equipment is required to make a diagnosis or treat an animal, referral to another veterinary surgeon may be considered. The referral veterinary surgeon usually holds further qualifications or RCVS Specialist status in a particular field of activity. A referral letter is written, outlining the progress of the case so far and the reasons for referral, and the results of diagnostic tests may be sent, such as radiographs or laboratory reports. Following the referral consultation, a referral report is sent to the referring

veterinary surgeon, who may take over responsibility of the case again. Owners should be made aware of the level of expertise of the referring veterinary surgeon, and the probable costs. Referrals may also be made to behaviourists and alternative therapy practitioners.

Complaints

Always regard complaints as an opportunity to put things right. Many unhappy clients will just go elsewhere and never mention a problem with your service, so those who do take the time to complain often want to continue to do business with you and may actually become very loyal clients if their complaint is handled well. Complaints may be formal, for example a letter or email, or may just be a moan at reception – each needs to be handled carefully and promptly. Practices should have a complaints procedure indicating who will handle complaints, and a time frame for response. It is helpful to communicate this to a complainant. A complaint procedure should be agreed with the practice team and should include initial acknowledgement of the complaint, recording and investigating the issues, acting on the complaint and informing the client, with appropriate timescales. Follow-up action to prevent recurrence of the issues is advised.

For informal and verbal complaints particularly, always acknowledge the complaint and allow the client time and privacy to explain the issues. Listen carefully and summarize the main points if possible to check that you understand and have not missed anything. If appropriate, express regret that the client is not satisfied, and then agree a way forward. This may be to hand the complaint to the appropriate person, for example the veterinary surgeon involved or a practice manager if the complaint is not about a clinical issue. Explain what you intend to do and give a time frame for response. Always thank the client for bringing the issues to your attention.

For minor service issues, if possible, resolve the complaint on the spot by putting things right if you can, for example replacing a faulty item, or explaining a misunderstanding. Always record the complaint and the outcome for future reference and ensure that, if you are passing the issue on to someone else, they have all the information they need, including the current contact details of the complainant. Formal complaints on behalf of a client from a solicitor or from a professional body, for example the RCVS, should be acknowledged immediately and professional advice may be required. Further advice is available from the *RCVS Guide to Professional Conduct* and The Veterinary Defence Society Ltd.

Processing payments

When a practice provides a service for a client, it usually makes a charge, which may be explained orally to the client. An itemized invoice should always be produced. This may be broken down item by item, or split into categories, e.g. surgery, consultations, medication, food. Nurses sometimes find themselves feeling uncomfortable asking for payment, perhaps because an owner is emotional, or because the fee seems excessive to them. A full understanding of the case and the costs to the practice of the services given is very helpful in learning to ask for payment confidently. Ask for explanations from senior staff if you are struggling with asking for money, and try to deal with distressed owners away from the busy reception area. Never apologize for a fee or a bill, and refer difficult queries to senior staff or the veterinary surgeon in charge of the case.

VAT

Value added tax (VAT) is payable on veterinary services and on most medications, except for those that are 'zero rated' for VAT. This should be indicated on the invoice, with the net amount (fees without VAT), the VAT and the total listed. VAT is usually paid quarterly to HM Revenue and Customs (HMRC), and the practice can reclaim VAT it has spent on overheads and purchases for resale.

When quoting fees in companion animal practice, the inclusive price should normally be given. Many farm and equine practices, who deal with other businesses, may state their fees exclusive of VAT and then add the VAT to the invoice. Invoices and receipts should include the practice's VAT registration number.

Checking and recording payments

When taking payments, it is important to ensure that the bill has been properly calculated, that all charges are included, and that if treatment has been given to more than one animal, these are also included in the total. It may be difficult to collect payment later for money that was not asked for at the time the client paid.

Payments may be recorded in a day book, a receipt book, or, as in most practices, through a till or computer system. Electronic systems will produce a receipt automatically. All clients should receive a receipt for money paid.

Cash and electronic payment slips must be kept secure and it is important that clients' personal card details are not easily stolen – these may be printed in full on the payment slip.

Methods of payment

Payment may be made by cash, cheque, credit card or debit card. Practices will have their own policies regarding accepted methods of payment, each of which costs different amounts to administer. Many banks charge to deposit cash and cheques, and most charge for change. Card-handling services charge a set fee for each debit card transaction and a percentage of the payment for a credit card transaction. Cash and electronic payments are credited to the practice account immediately they are banked; cheques may take a few days to clear. Practices may have policies regarding minimum payments accepted on cards or by cheque. Taking payments is a serious responsibility and should never be rushed.

Cash

When taking cash, the amount tendered should be confirmed to the client, particularly if the practice's till does not have a 'sum tendered' key. Clients may occasionally claim to have tendered a higher sum, and mistakes are less likely if cash changing hands is counted out loud. Nurses unused to handling cash and giving change should practise before taking money in a busy reception area.

Cheques

Cheques are no longer guaranteed with a cheque guarantee card, and electronic card or BACS (Bankers' Automated Clearing Service) payment maybe more secure.

Credit and debit cards

Credit and debit card payments may require authorization and it is important to know the procedure for this and what to do if a payment is refused. Some practices allow credit or debit card payment over the telephone and may allow payment direct into bank accounts using the BACS system. In the latter case, the practice's bank details may be included on the invoice and clients can make payments direct from their bank accounts.

Reconciliation

Reconciliation is the process of balancing up the total payments taken in a period with the amounts recorded as due. By reconciling the totals, errors can be spotted early on, e.g. payments not recorded against the client's records. Proper reconciliation is vital to protect the practice against fraud, and to spot errors straight away so that clients' accounts are accurate.

Insurance

Clients with pet insurance may pay as they go and claim fees back, but some practices will accept direct payment terms with certain insurance companies, sending their accounts for payment direct to the company. In these cases, clients will still be required to pay an 'excess' (a minimum amount towards the cost of each course of treatment).

Many practices have leaflets about insurance, and these can be displayed and handed out. General insurance is regulated by the Financial Services Authority (FSA), which stipulates that, unless a person or organization is regulated by the FSA, they cannot carry out certain activities. These include:

- Giving advice on insurance, except in very general terms, or recommending particular policies or offering inducements for people to take out a particular insurance
- Assisting clients to complete proposal forms
- Collecting insurance payments.

A practice that is an Appointed Representative or Introducer Appointed Representative may specifically recommend an insurer, and staff members may be suitably trained to do this. For more information, see www.fsa.gov.uk or contact the relevant veterinary fee insurers.

Practice organization

The veterinary practice team

Veterinary practices are run in many different ways, but all rely on the skills of professional staff (veterinary surgeons and listed or registered veterinary nurses) and lay or support staff (nursing assistants, receptionists, administrators, managers, cleaners, etc.) working together as a team day to day. Roles must be agreed, and appropriate training is vital for each team member to be effective in their role. Honesty, transparency and mutual support are key attributes for a successful team, and open communication is essential for the effective delivery of clinical care.

Receptionists and managers play an important role in facilitating communications with clients and smoothing work flow through efficient handling of appointments and telephone calls as well as other resources. Assistant staff can free a nurse's time to be with patients and clients by carrying out some of the support roles such as kennel and facility cleaning, organizing supplies and maintaining routine patient care.

Legal aspects

When dealing with patients, all members of the practice team should be aware of the law governing acts of veterinary surgery. It is important that nurses and assistant staff do not undertake procedures with inadequate supervision or where they do not feel competent.

The **Veterinary Surgeons Act 1966** provides for the regulation of the veterinary profession and the registration of veterinary surgeons. It also provides for the regulation of professional education and professional conduct and for action in cases of misconduct. Under the Act, the practice of veterinary surgery is restricted to qualified veterinary surgeons registered with the Royal College of Veterinary Surgeons (RCVS).

Under the **Schedule 3 Amendment Order 2002**, listed and registered veterinary nurses and enrolled veterinary nurse students are permitted to carry out medical treatment and minor surgery (not involving entry into a body cavity), under the direction of a veterinary surgeon employer, to animals under that veterinary surgeon's care. Nurses who are not currently on the register or list are not permitted to carry out these procedures, whether or not they have passed professional examinations in the past.

There are also a number of other exemptions allowing certain minor treatment, tests or operations (e.g. artificial insemination of cattle and horses) which may be carried out by suitably trained and competent non-veterinary surgeons. The carrying out of first aid for the purpose of saving life or relieving pain is also exempted.

Enrolled student nurses carrying out treatment under the Schedule 3 exemption must do so in the course of their training, and under the supervision of a veterinary surgeon or registered veterinary nurse. In the case of minor surgery, this supervision must be direct, continuous and personal. For current advice and clarification, visit www.rcvs.org.uk. **It is a criminal offence to practise veterinary surgery outside these regulations.**

It is helpful to differentiate enrolled student nurses and registered or listed nurses clearly from other trainee and assistant nursing staff who are not permitted to perform acts of veterinary surgery. This may be by job title and uniform style and colour.

Financial control

Veterinary practices are businesses, and attracting and keeping clients is essential for the practice to survive, as is adequate cash flow. Money earned by the business is used to pay the costs of running it (premises, salaries, overheads, loan interest, etc.) and to purchase stock for sale. Money remaining is the profit, and a proportion of this will be used to improve the practice, to purchase equipment and vehicles, to pay off any loans, and to give the practice owners an adequate return for their investment.

Good financial control and effective budgeting are very important for the financial health of a practice and the job security of its staff. This area is usually the responsibility of the practice owner(s) and a practice manager or administrator. Fees should be set at levels that provide a sufficient return for the work done, and stock and drugs should be priced competitively but so that income covers the costs of purchase, storage and handling. Regular reviews and close monitoring of costs and stock invoices is essential.

As well as ensuring that the fees and prices are appropriate, it is important to ensure that clients are charged the correct fees, and that charges are not missed or forgotten, or stock given away. The veterinary nurse can monitor and audit records to ensure that clients are charged correctly for everything they have received, but this is often neglected in practice. Consumables, inpatient medications, hospitalization fees and extra treatments dispensed on visits may all be missed from time to time, and a simple method of writing up cases as they progress or whilst on farm or at stables will help to reduce missed fees.

Debt control

Speed of payment can have a huge impact on the financial health of the practice, for two reasons. First, prompt payment is essential for healthy cash flow; and with many practices running a bank overdraft or with substantial loans, cash in the bank will reduce interest charges and can be used for the business. Secondly, the longer a debt is outstanding, the less likely it is that it will be paid.

Most small animal practices work on a pay-as-you-go basis: the client is invoiced and pays at the time of treatment. Referral, mixed and equine practices may have a high level of account clients, who may be sent a regular invoice for payment within a specified period of time, generally 30 days. Discounts may be given for prompt payment, to encourage clients to pay early. Offering payment by credit or debit card, or by BACS, as well as by cash or cheque is helpful in encouraging prompt payment. There will, however, always be some who are slow to pay or who do not pay at all.

Successful debt collection depends on prompt reminders and requests for payment, prompt follow-up of any queries or complaints, and positive action if the debt is not paid. An outline of the procedure should be included in the practice's terms and conditions of business. Methods that may be used include debt collection agencies, court proceedings (usually through the small claims court) and writing to the client after a predetermined time to inform them that they must seek treatment for their animals elsewhere in future if the account is not settled. Some clients will pay when they receive this last letter, having ignored all other requests.

Avoiding a debt building up in the first place is always the best option. Good estimating, noting estimates on consent forms, clear terms and conditions of business issued to all clients, and making it clear that you expect to be paid, all help to avoid debts occurring.

If a debt is impossible to collect, it can be written off after 6 months for VAT. This means that the practice can reclaim the VAT due on the debt if it is using the accrual basis of accounting, and include the fee as a cost in the practice overheads.

Keeping and organizing records

Efficient record-keeping is essential for maintaining good communication within the practice. Accurate records aid patient care, protect the practice from legal challenges and are vital for proper stock and financial control. Records may be paper-based and electronic or include other media.

Types of records a practice might keep

- Client records with contact information.
- Supplier records.
- Medical records, including ward or hospitalization notes, anaesthetic charts, laboratory results, slides, radiographs, digital images and recordings.
- Personnel records, including salary records, recruitment records, application forms and staff reviews or appraisals.
- Financial records, bank statements and invoices.
- Payment records, electronic payment slips.
- Health and Safety records, accident records, risk assessments and local rules.
- Training records, student college reports, centre correspondence, Nursing Progress Logs (electronic and printed out), tutorial records.
- Monitoring, e.g. closed circuit television (CCTV) tapes, or recordings of telephone conversations.
- Correspondence.

Practices that keep personal records of staff or clients must comply with the **Data Protection Act 1998** (DPA). This requires that anyone holding information about living individuals in electronic format, and in some cases on paper, must follow the eight data protection principles of good information handling.

Personal information must be:

- Fairly and lawfully processed
- Processed for specific purposes
- Adequate, relevant and not excessive
- Accurate and, where necessary, kept up to date
- Not kept for longer than is necessary
- Processed in line with the rights of the individual
- Kept secure
- Not transferred to countries outside the European Economic Area, unless there is adequate protection for the information.

The DPA requires that data users, including some veterinary practices, must notify the Information Commissioner if they wish to use records for particular purposes. Practices can complete a simple checklist at www.informationcommissioner.gov.uk, where full guidance on the Act and need for notification is easy to access. Notification is straightforward with a standard fee in 2011 of £35. The DPA also gives all individuals certain rights, including the right to see information that is held about them and to have it corrected if it is wrong. Clients may request access to their records under the Act.

Clarity and accuracy

Accurate record-keeping will increase the confidence that clients have in the practice. Clarity, legibility and accuracy are vital; poorly spelt names, untidy writing or an inability to read a colleague's notes do not present a good impression.

Records should be easy to understand by anyone required to access them (Figure 9.5), such as referral clinicians, practice staff, clients, or a new practice if the client moves house. Only commonly understood abbreviations should be used, and

developing a standard list for the practice will help with this and in training junior staff. Records should be kept of every clinical examination and should include: presenting signs, history, results of the physical examination, clinical findings, differential diagnoses and treatment plan. It is good practice to outline any conversations with the client, including notes on decision-making and whether a client declines a recommended treatment.

Financial information (e.g. fees, drugs and consumables costs, payments and balance outstanding) may be kept on the clinical record. This facilitates auditing of charging, but long lines of detail regarding insurance claims and payment negotiations can make accessing the clinical lines more difficult. A separate part of the record for non-clinical notes can be helpful and makes it simpler to pass clinical notes on to another practice or veterinary surgeon.

Both financial and clinical records should be written up at the time or as soon as possible afterwards. Laptop or tablet computers and electronic notepads can be useful on visits away from the practice. Contemporaneous notes (those made at the time) are particularly valuable in solving any disputes about what was said, and are generally more accurate than notes written up later.

Medical and financial records should never be altered. If editing is necessary, a note should be included explaining why, and the alteration should be clear. Computer systems should either forbid editing or should maintain an audit trail of any editing that has taken place.

Records should be objective – based on observation and factual information, with subjective opinions included only where they are relevant, perhaps where a risk assessment has influenced decision-making or where a diagnosis is unclear. **Never should anything personal be written about a client, particularly disparaging comments or tongue-in-cheek notes.** Even the placement of exclamation marks can be misinterpreted! At any time, the records could end up in a court of law and the practice needs to be happy with their quality. Particular care should be taken not to write any false or defamatory statements about a person (libel), or make any malicious, false or injurious spoken statements about anyone (slander). Information about a person's character or financial situation should never be taken outside the practice, and it is good practice never to talk disparagingly about a client or another member of staff within the practice either.

If records are computerized, there should be a supply of temporary paper record sheets, price and data guides for use if there is a loss of power. Records can be input later when power is restored.

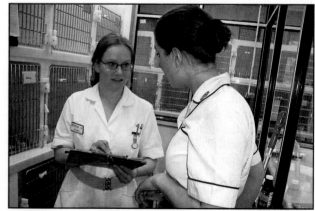

9.5 Clear and comprehensive records are essential when handing over cases to colleagues.

Filing

Records should be stored conveniently near where they are needed, using an appropriate filing system. Rarely used files can be stored away from the clinical areas, with commonly used ones in reception or close to where they are needed.

Alphabetical filing

Clients' paper or card records are generally filed alphabetically. In veterinary practice, where different members of the family may bring pets in at different times, a system based on surname and house number or pet name may be preferable to surname and initials. Computerized records can search on a number of parameters, including pet name, owner name and address, and reduce the drudgery and error of manual filing.

Chronological filing

Other records, such as dental charts, radiographs, ECGs and laboratory reports, can be filed in date order and cross-referenced on the client record. This chronological filing is much quicker to maintain than alphabetical filing, as each new record can be filed on top of the last one. Archiving old records is also simpler with this system and saves the continual file expansion required in an alphabetical system.

Electronic storage

It is now possible for laboratory results to be emailed into the practice and attached directly to client computer records, for ECG tracings and radiographs to be stored digitally, and for records to be shared between veterinary surgeons via the internet. This saves storage space and makes retrieval much faster. As electronic storage increases, however, practices will need to review their back-up systems to include the increasing number and size of files.

Labelling

All files should have a standard labelling system, whether in hard copy or electronic format. This will generally include the owner and animal name plus a reference number and date. Radiographs should be permanently identified at the time of exposure.

File markers

Non-electronic files should always be returned to their files after use – a marker can be inserted into the space as the file is removed to aid replacement (Figure 9.6). The marker can be useful if a file remains missing: staff can be alerted to chase up its return.

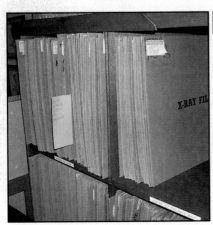

9.6 Marking where an X-ray file has been removed makes correct replacement simpler and also alerts staff that the file is missing in the meantime.

Security

Records should be recorded on permanent material, such as good quality paper or other media. Paper records should be stored securely, under lock and key if necessary.

Computers

Magnetic media such as back-up tapes or floppy discs should be stored in a clean dry place away from possible sources of radiation or magnetism. Compact discs and DVDs should be kept in protective cases and clearly identified. Computer records should be regularly backed up on to storage media, and these back-ups should be verified so that the data are reliable for restoring on to the system should the need arise. A minimum of daily backing up is recommended for medical records and financial information, and weekly for less sensitive records. Back-up files should be stored off-site or in secure fireproof safes. Many computer networks now include automatic back-up, with duplicate hard drives to take over if one fails, and some are web-based with central holding of data. Practices should verify the integrity and security of data if stored remotely by a third party.

Computers should be protected by using uninterruptible power supplies to allow controlled shut-down in the event of power loss, and by using surge protectors. It is best not to install computers in dirty areas, such as where animals are clipped or where there are high moisture levels. If this is unavoidable, regular vacuum cleaning around them will prevent dust and hair from building up, and keyboard covers should be used to protect against spills and contamination.

Records may be stolen, and so hard copies should not be left out on reception desks or in other public areas. Computers, particularly laptops, are very attractive to casual thieves; locking devices to fix them down, and alarms, are recommended. Computers should never be left in vehicles, and care should be taken if staff take laptops home with practice data on them. **Protection of data with secure passwords is essential so that unauthorized personnel cannot gain access.**

Purging, archiving and disposal

To reduce size and to comply with the DPA, old or unused files should be archived or discarded regularly. There are no legal limits on document storage times, but in general:

- **Financial, tax and PAYE records** should be kept for 6 years after the financial year end
- **Medical records, radiographs, etc.** should be kept for at least 6 years in case of legal claims, and longer if deemed necessary by the clinician
- **Practice insurance records** for employer liability should be kept indefinitely, and it may be prudent to keep Health and Safety records and staff appraisal records of current staff as long as practicable
- **Recruitment records**, such as application forms and references from unsuccessful candidates, should not be kept longer than 6 months.

Archived records should be stored securely until destroyed. Garden sheds and outhouses are not suitable; secure storage should be available. Computers should be disposed of only after permanently erasing any sensitive data and according to local waste regulations. Paper records should be destroyed by shredding or burning, or by using a professional confidential waste contractor.

Access and ownership of records

RCVS guidance recognizes that clients who now have access to their own medical records are likely to seek similar access to their pets' records. In such cases it may be helpful, on the direction of a veterinary surgeon, for a client to be offered sight of the records at the surgery by appointment at a mutually convenient time.

Case records, including radiographs and similar documents, are the property of, and should be retained by, veterinary surgeons in the interests of animal welfare and for their own protection. Copies with a summary of the history should be passed on request to a colleague taking over the case. Where a client has been specifically charged and has paid for radiographs or other reports, the client is legally entitled to them. However, the practice may choose to make it clear that they are charging not for the radiographs but for diagnosis or advice only. In appropriate circumstances they may be prepared also to provide copies of the radiographs. Practices should consider clarifying their position on ownership of and access to diagnostic material in their standard terms of business document.

Disclosure of records may be ordered in disciplinary or court hearings, and the RCVS may request copies of case records routinely in the course of investigating a complaint.

Confidentiality

The veterinary nurse must maintain the confidentiality of client and practice information at all times, and should not discuss professional or privileged information outside the practice.

*RCVS Guide to Professional Conduct** guidance on confidentiality

- The veterinary surgeon–client relationship is founded on trust and, in normal circumstances, a veterinary surgeon must not disclose to any third party any information about a client or their animal either given by the client or revealed by clinical examination or by postmortem examination. This duty also extends to associated support staff.
- In circumstances where the client has not given permission for disclosure but the veterinary surgeon believes that animal welfare or public interest are compromised, the RCVS may be consulted before any information is divulged.
- Permission to pass on confidential information may be express or implied. Express permission may be either verbal or in writing, usually in response to a request. Permission may also be implied from circumstances, for example in the making of a claim under a pet insurance policy, when the insurance company becomes entitled to receive all information relevant to the claim and to seek clarification if required.
- Registration of a dog with the Kennel Club requires a veterinary surgeon who carries out surgery to alter the natural conformation of a dog (including caesarian section) to report this to the Kennel Club.

* The guide is currently under review

If there is any doubt about the disclosure of any information, confirmation should be sought from a practice veterinary surgeon or from the RCVS. In particular, giving out details over the telephone to any third party is not recommended, due to the difficulty in identifying the parties involved. People may not be who they say they are. Where it is considered that client information should be divulged on animal welfare or public interest grounds, the severity and urgency of the issues should be considered carefully, as should the options to resolve the issue without disclosure. Involving a third party may destroy the veterinary surgeon/client relationship and make resolution of the problem more difficult.

Equipment

Every practice relies on a range of clinical and non-clinical equipment, which must be maintained and checked on a regular basis.

Practice equipment will include:

- Personal protective equipment (PPE), e.g. gloves, masks, safety goggles
- Diagnostic equipment, e.g. stethoscopes, auriscope, ophthalmoscope, glucometers
- Mechanical equipment, e.g. anaesthetic machines, mechanical ventilators, hydraulic operating tables, stocks (equine)
- Instruments and restraint equipment, e.g. large animal gags
- Electrical equipment, e.g. X-ray and ultrasound machines, endoscopes, electronic ventilators, ECG machines, anaesthetic monitors, laboratory diagnostic equipment.

More details on equipment care are given in relevant chapters but, in general, the following issues must be considered:

- Correct storage of the equipment and how it is made ready for use
- Cleaning and hygiene measures needed routinely and before and after each use
- Checks to perform before using each piece of equipment
- Regular in-house maintenance required and its frequency
- External maintenance and servicing required and its frequency
- Any legal requirements, e.g. for portable electrical equipment or gas appliances
- Who to call in the event of malfunction.

Stock

Practice stock will include:

- Drugs used within the practice, such as anaesthetics, sedatives, antibiotics, intravenous fluids, topical treatments, injectable drugs, vaccines
- Consumables used in the course of treatments, such as cotton wool, syringes and needles, disposable gloves, gowns and drapes
- Suture materials, bandages and dressings
- Drugs dispensed in the course of treatment, such as tablets, oral pastes and drenches and topical treatments (e.g. ear drops, shampoos, parasiticides)
- Food and disposable bedding for hospitalized patients
- X-ray film and processing chemicals

continues ▶

continued

- Dispensing items such as child-proof tablet bottles, boxes, dispensing bags and carriers
- Items for general sale such as pet carriers, grooming equipment, leads, toys, pet foods and supplements
- Stationery, such as headed paper, computer paper, envelopes, business cards, toner, printer cartridges
- Cleaning materials, disinfectants, washing powder
- Tea, coffee and milk.

Practices use their own systems to ensure adequate supplies, but maintaining stocks of medicines and items for sale will be the particular concern of the veterinary nurse.

Most practices buy their main supplies from one source, generally a veterinary wholesaler. Different manufacturers supply the wholesaler, who fills the practice's order, often breaking down bulk boxes ('outers') into individual units. Other items may be purchased locally or from mail order suppliers. A list of suppliers' details and the items ordered should be kept accessible.

Practices are required to audit their purchases, sales and stocks of prescription-only medicines at least annually and to record any discrepancies. Practices are also required to record the batch numbers and expiry dates of all medicines received and when each batch was first used. The aim is that, should a batch need to be recalled, practices should be able to determine to whom that batch has been dispensed. For food animals, batch numbers of all medicines used must be recorded on the clinical record; this is good practice for small animal work too.

Ordering stock

Methods will vary from practice to practice, but the principles are the same. The aim is to keep adequate stock levels for the day-to-day and emergency needs of the practice without tying up excessive resources. The value of stock on the shelf and in vehicles can be substantial, and losses can be considerable if items go out of date or are not stored correctly. If stock levels fall too low the practice may run out of items, possibly jeopardizing an animal's treatment or forcing a client to buy elsewhere.

Manual ordering

Stock is ordered when it is felt that it is needed. Either a note of ideal stock levels is made on the shelf, or an experienced staff member checks daily and 'has a feel' for when to reorder items. This can work well in small practices where stock is kept in one place and the experienced member never goes on holiday, but it is time-consuming and not particularly accurate. Alternatively, staff may note on an order pad when they sell a certain quantity of an item, so that it is reordered. This is not a reliable system and only works well for large items – not items where many small transactions are made through the day.

Computerized stock control

Hand-held computers are popular and may be supplied by the wholesaler. They hold a database of the drugs and items used and may hold stock level information. The list can often be set so that products are listed in the order in which they are stored on the shelf. The nurse can enter the product code, or scan a bar code from the product or a shelf label, to bring up that item and set either the quantity in stock (from which the computer calculates the number to order) or the quantity to

order. The complete order can then be sent electronically to the supplier. Some systems can incorporate seasonal stock requirements and automatically adjust stock levels to usage. Stock stored in multiple locations, e.g. in vehicles, may not be counted, so allowances must be made for this.

The most sophisticated systems are those that use the practice's main computer records system. Set up properly, this can be an extremely effective method of stock control, as each time a product is used it is taken from the stock quantity and when the stock level reaches the pre-set reorder level it is added to the order. The system may take time to set up and must be used accurately without being over-ridden to be successful. Orders are generated electronically and minimum stock levels can be automatically calculated according to usage, increasing as an item is used more. The system can generally handle part quantities such as individual tablets and volumes of injectable drugs, and can be extremely accurate if used properly. It is, however, only as good as the data that are input: if products are not charged for or de-stocked, there will be no reorder.

Computerized systems help greatly with stock auditing and reconciliation, as well as with batch number recording. Tracking stock discrepancies will show where stock is short, which may be due to stocking-on or de-stocking errors, pilfering, undercharging and unnoticed errors in deliveries, so is well worthwhile.

Placing the order

How a stock order is placed will depend on the system used by the veterinary wholesaler or supplier. Small suppliers may be happy taking a phone order, but written or faxed confirmation is ideal. Individual orders can be written in an order book; supplier details and contact numbers can be kept at the front, and orders checked off when they arrive. Suppliers often ask for an order number. Use your name or initials and the date if you do not have a purchase order system. Wholesalers may accept faxed orders but most prefer electronic orders, either from their own computer systems or directly from a practice management system. Many web-based ordering systems are now in use. Price lists, price updates and details of stock delivered can all be transmitted back to the practice computer.

The timing of ordering can be crucial for reliable delivery. Wholesalers have a cut-off time after which orders cannot be accepted and so it is vital to be in good time, as there are always interruptions and distractions during a busy day to take you past the deadline! Daily ordering is now commonplace and useful for keeping stock levels low and for last-minute items. Less frequent ordering, though, can be more efficient as larger quantities are handled at once, saving staff time. Interim orders can be used to top up in between.

Receiving stock

Practices should ensure that delivered goods only arrive during opening hours where possible, so that goods remain secure and can be dealt with as soon as possible.

Delivery notes

When products arrive they are generally accompanied by a delivery note (not to be thrown away with the packaging). This will detail the items supplied and may also show the price. The goods delivered should always be carefully checked, both against the delivery note and against the original order, and it is a good idea to initial the delivery note so that if there is a query everyone knows who unpacked and checked the order (Figure 9.7).

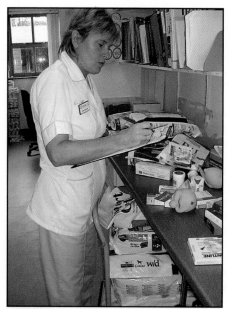

9.7   Receiving a delivery. Goods should be checked carefully against the delivery note and any discrepancies noted.

The condition of the goods and their packaging should be examined to ensure that there are no breakages or damage to the product that may make it unusable or difficult to sell. Any problems or shortages must be notified to the supplier as soon as possible; a specific time period may be stated in their terms and conditions.

For parcels delivered by courier and requiring signature, it should always be stated that the item is 'unexamined' if it is not possible to unpack and check it immediately (which would not be popular with the waiting delivery driver). If someone in the practice has signed that the goods were in good condition on receipt, it may be difficult to complain about damage later.

'Stocking-on'

If automatic computerized stock control is in operation, the items will need to be 'stocked on', i.e. added to the quantity held in stock on the computer. This can be done manually, direct to the practice computer by the supplier or by scanning in a bar code on the delivery note. Stock should only be 'stocked on' if it has actually arrived.

Unpacking

Great care should be taken not to cut hands or damage the contents when opening boxes with a sharp blade or scissors, and to be aware of the hazards of metal staples, sharp wrapping tape and sharp paper edges. Special cutting tools for boxes are available and are recommended.

Unpacking and storing

- Perishable items or those requiring special storage conditions should be unpacked and dealt with first.
  - Vaccines, some laboratory diagnostics and insulin all need to be kept refrigerated and should arrive in insulated packaging, often with cold packs. They should be checked and placed in the appropriate refrigerator immediately. If there has been a delay in delivery, prolonged storage at too high a temperature will make them unusable and they ▶

should be rejected. The rest of the order should be put away as soon as possible, using good stock rotation practice (see below) and ensuring that the delivery and any packaging do not obstruct fire exits and access ways in the practice nor present a trip hazard.
- Particular care should be taken in handling heavy items. Trolleys should be used where possible to move large items such as food bags, and heavy boxes should not be lifted on to high worktops.
- Many wholesalers use reusable packing cases that can be collected on the next delivery. Other packaging should be disposed of responsibly, recycling where possible.

Returns

Goods to be returned should be stored safely for collection or packed securely for return. Suppliers will have their own systems for returns and the practice should ensure that the return is expected and use the correct documentation, a copy of which should be kept for reconciling to a credit note later.

Organizing and maintaining stock

Poor stock organization and handling, and human error, will limit the effectiveness of any ordering system. Stock levels should be altered according to seasonal changes (generally, more flea and tick treatments are sold during summer and autumn in small animal practice), introduction of new products, and changes in prescribing habits in the practice. Involving the clinical team in controlling stock is essential.

Stock organization

- Medicines may be stored according to therapeutic category (antibiotics; steroids; non-steroidal anti-inflammatories) or product group (topicals; injectables; oral fluids; tablets) and alphabetically. It is always easiest to store medicines in one central place but this may be impractical for many practices.
- Stock should not be duplicated in several places, as this makes ordering difficult and more items are likely to go past their expiry date.
- If items are needed at point of use, a central stock area with smaller stock levels at point of use (e.g. anaesthetic agents in prep areas and injectables in consulting rooms) is a good compromise.
- Stock in vehicles should be regularly checked and rotated and kept out of sight and secure.
- In ward areas, sufficient medication for each patient should be dispensed either daily or as a course of medication and can be kept in labelled drawers or attached safely close to the kennels.
- **Make sure patients cannot access medication, particularly if it is palatable.**

Quality control

Stock must be easy to find and access and should be stored so that **older stock is used first**. Newly delivered items must be put behind or under older items, expiry dates of products should be checked so that the oldest are used first, and items that are short-dated (will expire shortly) should be rejected on delivery or used up first.

Gravity-fed sloping shelving can be useful in rotating stock. Dispensary shelving should be clearly labelled and designed so that stock fits well and can be stored with labelling clearly visible and the right way up.

Drug stock in the practice and in cars should be checked regularly for expiry dates and for general condition. Multi-dose injection bottles should be marked with the date of broaching (when the first dose was extracted) and discarded after the time period indicated in the data sheet.

Environmental control

Refrigerated products should generally be kept at 2–8°C and provision must be made for products that need to be kept away from light. Drug storage areas, including cars, should have maximum and minimum temperature recording to ensure that the temperature stays within the required range stated on the drug packaging or in its data sheet. If drugs are taken on visits, insulated cool boxes with temperature recording should be used and minimal stock carried. Cars become very cold in winter and very hot in summer, and drugs should not be left in them overnight or on non-working days. Protection from dust and extremes of humidity is also important.

Drug storage and preparation areas should be kept clean, dry and free of vermin. They should have impermeable work surfaces, and facilities for hand washing and disinfection. Food and drink should not be permitted where drugs are stored or dispensed.

Security is paramount, particularly when away from the practice. The public should not have access to the practice pharmacy or any area where drugs are stored. Where drugs are used in consulting rooms, it is vital that children and animals cannot access them or access any syringes or sharps.

Further reading

Bower J, Gripper J, Gripper P and Gunn D (2001) *Veterinary Practice Management, 3rd edn*. Blackwell Science, Oxford

BSAVA Guide to the Use of Veterinary Medicines at www.bsava.com

Hibbert SC (2008) Practice administration. In: *BSAVA Manual of Canine and Feline Advanced Veterinary Nursing*, ed. A Hotston Moore and S Rudd, pp.286–301. BSAVA Publications, Gloucester

Kurtz SM, Silverman JD and Draper J (2004) *Teaching and Learning Communication Skills in Medicine, 2nd edn*. Radcliffe Medical Press, Oxford

McLeod HL (2008) Practice administration. In: *BSAVA Manual of Canine and Feline Advanced Veterinary Nursing*, ed. A Hotston Moore and S Rudd, pp.302–312. BSAVA Publications, Gloucester

Pullen S and Gray C (2006) *Ethics, Law and the Veterinary Nurse*. Elsevier Science, Oxford

Radford AD, Stockley P, Silverman J *et al.* (2006) Development, teaching and evaluation of a consultation structure model for use in veterinary education. *Journal of Veterinary Medical Education* **33**, 38–44

RCVS (2010) *Guide to Professional Conduct*. RCVS, London (also available online at www.rcvs.org.uk) [under review]

RCVS (2008) *Guide to Professional Conduct for Veterinary Nurses*. RCVS, London (also available at www.rcvs.org.uk) [under review]

Shilcock M (2007) Organization and communication skills. In: *BSAVA Manual of Practical Animal Care*, ed. P Hotston Moore and A Hughes, pp.164–175. BSAVA Publications, Gloucester

Shilcock M and Stutchfield G (2008) *Veterinary Practice Management, A Practical Guide*. WB Saunders, Philadelphia

Silverman JD, Kurtz SM and Draper J (2004) *Skills for Communicating with Patients, 2nd edn*. Radcliffe Medical Press, Oxford

Self-assessment questions

1. What are the main components of non-verbal communication that convey to clients that you are listening to them?
2. What is the best way to give information to a client about neutering their male kitten? Think particularly about the information required to ensure informed consent is obtained.
3. A client is creating a scene in reception, complaining to the receptionist about their bill, which is more than they thought it would be. You are asked to sort it out. How would you approach this client/situation?
4. How and what would you prepare for an annual appraisal with your practice manager/line manager?
5. Describe the eight data protection principles of good information handling.
6. How can you ensure your clinical records are accurate and clear?
7. What factors should you consider when setting up an effective stock control system?

Chapter 10

Animal handling, restraint and transport

Trudi Atkinson, Jane Devaney and Simon Girling

Learning objectives

After studying this chapter, students should be able to:

- **Describe how to handle and restrain dogs, cats, horses and exotic pets correctly for examination, transportation and treatment**
- **Understand basic animal 'body language', including signals indicating fear and potential aggression**
- **Explain how to minimize fear and stress in veterinary patients during approach, handling and restraint**
- **Understand the techniques used when handling aggressive or potentially aggressive animals, and the use of any equipment that may be required**
- **Apply the principles of handling and restraint to use in everyday veterinary practice**

Introduction

A frequent task for the veterinary nurse in practice is the handling and restraint of animals requiring treatment or examination. How an animal is handled can greatly affect the ease and efficiency with which procedures are carried out. Inefficient or inappropriate handling can subject the patient to unnecessary stress and discomfort, which is not only damaging to patient welfare but may also result in the development of, or an increase in, defensive aggression towards veterinary staff. Proficiency in handling and control is one of the most essential and valuable skills for a veterinary nurse to acquire.

The aims of the nurse when restraining an animal should be as follows:

- To enable an examination or procedure, such as the application of dressings or the administration of medication, to be carried out as efficiently as possible
- To avoid injury or further injury to the patient. For example, if sharp instruments such as scissors are used to cut the animal's hair or a scalpel blade is used to take a

skin scrape for examination, injury may result if the animal moves excessively or unexpectedly. Likewise, excessive or sudden movement may result in further injury while attempts are made to examine or treat a fracture or open wound
- To prevent the animal injuring handlers, veterinary staff or other persons
- To achieve the above without causing additional or unnecessary pain or distress to the animal.

In order to handle dogs, cats, horses and exotic pets successfully it is important first to understand a little about how these species behave and are likely to respond to attempts to handle and restrain them.

Canine and feline communication

Pain and fear may cause an animal to behave very differently in the veterinary surgery from how it might do under other circumstances. An elementary knowledge of canine and feline communication can help the veterinary nurse assess the possible reactions of an individual animal in its current situation and adapt the means of handling and restraint accordingly.

Canine 'body language' and facial expressions

Figure 10.1 illustrates the typical range of canine body postures and facial expressions (changes in body posture will also occur depending on the dog's current activity).

Tail wagging

A wagging tail can have several meanings, including a willingness to interact (possibly aggressively) by an assertive dog, or a sign of appeasement by a nervous and potentially defensively aggressive dog. The veterinary nurse should always consider other aspects of the dog's body language and never assume that a dog with a wagging tail is friendly and will not bite.

Dominance, aggression and fear

'Dominance' is a commonly misunderstood concept. It is purely the ability of an individual at a given point in time to gain or maintain preferential access to a desired resource. *It is incorrect and potentially damaging to equate 'dominance' with aggression or other undesirable behaviour.* Fear is the underlying cause of almost all episodes of aggression, especially in a veterinary situation.

A fearful dog may appear confident and assertive if it has previously had the opportunity to learn that aggression can be effective in making a potential threat 'back off' or keep its distance, even if only momentarily. It is important to realize that attempts to reprimand a fearful animal will only result in an increase in fear and consequently an increase in defensive aggression (see also Chapter 11).

Feline communication

Figure 10.2 shows the typical body language of a cat.

Relaxed

- *Body*: If resting, cat may be on its back with belly exposed, or curled up. Feet may not be in contact with the ground.
- *Tail*: Extended or loosely wrapped if cat is resting. If standing or if in motion, tail may be held down in 'U' shape away from body, or upright, sometimes with curl at the end as friendly greeting.
- *Ears*: Normal 'relaxed'.
- *Eyes*: May be half closed if cat is relaxed; pupil size dependent on available light. A 'slow eye blink' may be directed towards other animals, including people, as a signal of 'non-confrontation'.
- *Vocalization*: May purr while relaxed, or chirrup or meow as friendly greeting.

Tense

- *Body:* May explore area looking for ways of escape or rest in 'ready' position with feet in contact with the ground so cat can move quickly if necessary.

Relaxed, neutral

Alert, aroused

Greeting

Fearful

Fearful, pacifying

Fearful, defensively aggressive

Overt, defensive agressive attack

10.1 Canine body language and facial expressions. (Illustrations by Priscilla Barrett; redrawn after Fox and Bekoff, 1975)

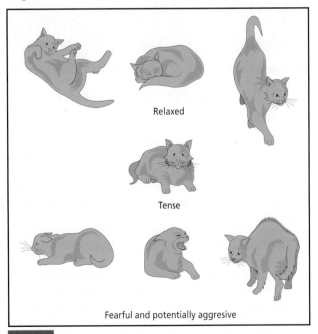

Relaxed

Tense

Fearful and potentially aggressive

10.2 Feline communication.

- *Tail*: Usually wrapped around body.
- *Ears*: Slightly flattened sideways.
- *Eyes*: Open, pupils dilated.

Fearful

- *Body*: May be held low and away from source of fear with all four feet on the ground, or may attempt to hide.
- *Tail*: Very tight to body.
- *Ears*: Flattened sideways.
- *Eyes*: Wide, with dilated pupils.

Fearful/defensively aggressive

- *Body*: Flattened and backed away from source of fear. If approached, may 'lash out' with front feet, but with body held back.
- *Tail*: Tightly wrapped or 'lashing'.
- *Ears*: Fear and submission signalled by holding ears down and to the side; however, to protect them from injury, ears are held back and down if an aggressive encounter becomes more likely.
- *Eyes*: Wide, pupils fully dilated, and focused on the source of fear.
- *Vocalization*: May growl, hiss or spit.

A cat confronted by a sudden, unexpected danger, such as an unknown or unfriendly dog, may arch its back and fluff out the hairs along its back and tail in an attempt to appear much larger than it really is.

Purring

Cats often purr when relaxed or as a way of soliciting food or attention, but they may also purr when in extreme pain or distress. This may be one way that the cat tries to reduce its level of stress, in the same way that people may whistle or hum if anxious or frightened.

Initial approach and handling of dogs and cats

Handling with the owner present

When handling any species of animal in front of its owner the veterinary nurse should always remember that how the owner witnesses their pet being handled will reflect upon the type and standard of care that they expect from the veterinary practice in general; if the pet is handled roughly or inefficiently they may choose to take their pet and their custom elsewhere. The way in which the animal is handled whilst with the owner may also affect the way that the pet behaves; this is especially the case for dogs.

It may be tempting to ask an owner to help with handling or restraining their pet, particularly if it is nervous; however, practice staff should be aware of the possibility of litigation should an owner be injured, even if the owner volunteered their services. Owners might usefully administer treats or distractions to their pet to ease examinations, etc. but

generally should be dissuaded from putting themselves in any position of potential risk. A second member of staff should be asked to help if two people are needed to restrain and examine the pet. For more information on staff and client safety see Chapter 2.

Some owners may unintentionally reinforce their pet's fear and aggression, and if an animal is difficult to handle it may be easier to deal with away from the owner. When separating dog and owner it is often more successful to ask the owner to leave the room first and then lead the dog away.

Handling dogs

It is helpful to spend a little time 'chatting' with the owner before attempting to handle or approach a dog. This time can be spent watching the dog and making a general assessment of its temperament. The dog will take cues from its owner as to whether or not something or someone is a potential threat. A minute or so talking with the owner in a 'friendly' manner can often help to convey the message to the dog that you are not a threat.

A dog may, however, still regard you as a threat, either due to a previous negative experience in a veterinary context or because of a generalized fear of strangers, and may react in a defensive and aggressive manner, not only if approached directly but also if an approach is made towards the owner. Therefore, until you are certain of the pet's temperament and its perception of you as 'friend or foe', it is advisable not to attempt to shake the owner by the hand or perform other similar actions.

- Whenever possible, a dog should be encouraged to approach the vet or nurse, rather than the vet or nurse directly approaching the dog.
- Cornering a dog, leaning over it or prolonged direct eye contact, all of which the dog may consider threatening, should be avoided.
- Crouching down to the dog's level can help with nervous individuals, but not so close that your face could be within 'biting' distance.
- **Grabbing a dog by the collar or scruff should be avoided, as this could frighten the dog and cause it to turn and bite.**

Nervous animals that are normally obedient may be reassured by giving them a few easy commands to help them relax, especially if the owner has previously associated these responses with rewards. However, veterinary staff must also be aware that if a dog has been subjected to punitive training methods, the use of commands could have the opposite effect of increasing fear and associative defensive behaviour.

Occasionally, dogs are reluctant to leave the safety of a hospital kennel and may become defensively aggressive if confronted or if attempts are made to enter the kennel in order to remove them. If a lightweight lead is left on the dog, the end can be extracted using a broom handle or cat catcher, allowing the handler to take hold of the lead safely without needing to confront the dog. In most instances, once the handler has hold of the lead the dog will leave the kennel and walk willingly with the handler.

> **WARNING**
>
> To avoid injury if leaving a lead on a dog in a kennelled situation, the lead must **never** be attached to a choke chain or slip lead and the dog must be regularly supervised.

Handling cats

Examination or procedures should be carried out on cats as soon as possible. Cats often have a limited 'tolerance period', i.e. they will put up with so much for so long and then suddenly decide that they have had enough and try to escape or become defensively aggressive. Cats often feel very vulnerable in hospital kennels. Providing a box or similar in which they can hide (Figure 10.3) can help a cat feel more secure and therefore easier to approach and handle.

Extracting a cat from a carrier

Top-opening carriers

1. Lift the lid slowly. Most cats will prefer to stay in the carrier but some may try to jump out as soon as the lid is lifted, so be prepared.
2. Stroke the cat to settle it and assess its temperament.
3. Make sure the cat is well supported underneath (see Lifting and carrying) and lift it out and on to the examination table.

Front-opening carriers

1. Open the front and try to encourage the cat out without putting a hand inside the carrier, which the cat may find threatening, making it less willing to leave the safety of the carrier.
2. If the carrier can be separated into two halves, remove the top half and lift the cat out as you would with a top-opening carrier. Some front-opening carriers have a tray in the base in which the cat sits. If so, this can be gently pulled out, bringing the cat out with it.
3. If none of the above is possible, gently tilt the carrier, which may help to encourage the cat out.

A cat should only be forcibly extracted from its carrier as a last resort; if this is necessary try to do so gently and be aware that the cat may become defensive. ***Do not pull the cat out by its scruff unless it is absolutely necessary and all other methods have been tried.*** Doing so can be frightening and potentially painful for the cat, thereby increasing the likelihood that the cat may become progressively more difficult to handle.

Once the cat is out, the carrier should be placed on the ground or otherwise out of the cat's sight. If the cat can see the carrier it may repeatedly try to get back in and may become fractious when prevented from doing so.

Moving, transporting and lifting dogs and cats

Dogs must always be on a lead attached to a well fitting collar if they are to be walked from one area of the surgery to another.

- Always check that the collar is not too tight, or so loose that the dog could slip out of it.
- For added security, use a lightweight slip lead as well.

If cats or other small animals are to be transported from one area to another, they must be securely contained in an appropriate carrier.

Lifting and carrying

Handlers should be aware of any possible medical conditions or injuries that could be causing an animal pain or discomfort before attempting to lift or carry it. Points of pain should be kept away from the handler's body as the animal is carried, to reduce the risk of causing further discomfort.

It is important to ensure that the animal is aware of the handler's approach and intent before an attempt to lift it is made.

- Small to medium-sized dogs may be lifted by one person (Figure 10.4). Assistance may be required to carry drips or open doors, etc.
- Large, heavy (>20 kg) or injured dogs should be lifted and carried by two people of similar height (Figure 10.5).
- Large, immobile or severely injured dogs are best carried by two or more people in a blanket (Figure 10.6) or on a stretcher (Figure 10.7).
- Cats should be tucked in under the arm with the forearm supporting the underneath of the cat and with the hand gently holding its front legs (Figure 10.8). The other hand can be used to stroke the cat over the head and neck, ready to take hold of its scruff if necessary.

Always follow the health and safety guidelines when lifting (see Chapter 2):

- Keep the back straight, legs slightly apart and bend at the knees
- Always get assistance before attempting to lift a heavy or awkward weight
- Keep the load close to the body.

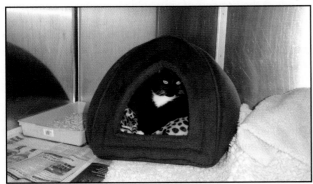

10.3   Providing a place to hide can make a cat feel more secure.

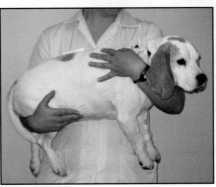

10.4

Lifting a small dog. (Courtesy of E Mullineaux)

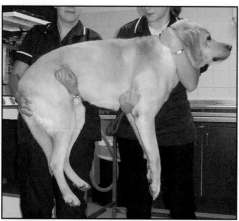

| 10.5 | Lifting a large dog requires two people. (Courtesy of J Niehoegen) |

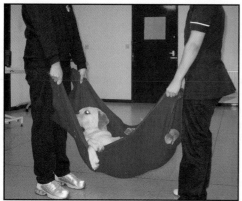

| 10.6 | Lifting a dog with a blanket. (Courtesy of J Niehoegen) |

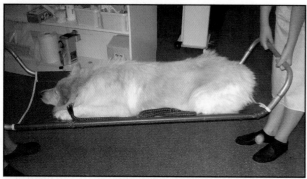

| 10.7 | Carrying a dog on a stretcher. (Courtesy of E Mullineaux) |

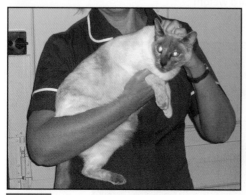

| 10.8 | Lifting a cat. |

Transport of anaesthetized or unconscious animals

Anaesthetized or unconscious animals should be transported on a wheeled trolley, or similar, and monitored at all times. To maintain the animal's airway the neck should be pulled slightly forward and the tongue extended. Placing the tongue under the patient's lower jaw will prevent the tongue falling back into the mouth and blocking the airway if the animal is not intubated.

International transport of small animals: the Pet Travel Scheme

The Pet Travel Scheme (PETS) relates to the movement of pets (dogs, cats and ferrets) into the UK. While allowing ease of movement without quarantine, there are control measures (vaccination) to prevent rabies from entering the UK. Animals travelling from 'unlisted' countries may also travel but require more stringent controls, including a 4-month waiting period and blood tests after rabies vaccination (see Chapter 5 for details). More recently, the European Parliament and Council have advised that numbers of dogs, cats and ferrets entering from one EU member state into another will be limited to five per person. This limit is applicable to all pets entering the UK and also those leaving the UK for EU destinations. A limit of five pets is already enforced for entries of animals from listed non-EU countries.

A Pet Passport may be obtained from a veterinary surgeon; in the UK this is a local veterinary inspector for Defra.

Export and import licences are required for the transport of other mammalian species and for birds, as well as for dogs, cats and ferrets to or from countries outside the Pet Travel Scheme.

For further details and current information see the Defra website.

Restraint of dogs and cats for examination or treatment

Restraint of pet animals should be firm but gentle, using no more than the minimum amount of restraint necessary. Care must be taken not to cause undue pain or discomfort by applying any more pressure than is required. It may be necessary to adjust the firmness of your hold momentarily, depending on the animal's reactions to the procedure being performed.

The means of restraint used is dependent on both the procedure to be performed and the reactions of the individual animal.

Restraint of dogs

Figure 10.9 shows two methods of steadying a dog's head. The rolled-up towel method is particularly useful with small brachycephalic breeds and can be used to prevent a dog from turning round to bite when it is not possible to use a muzzle.

Figure 10.10 shows a dog being held for cephalic venepuncture. It is often useful to have an additional person available to steady the back end of the dog if it starts to struggle.

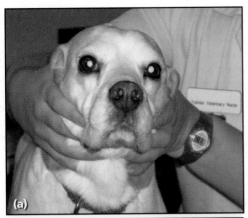

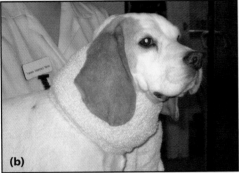

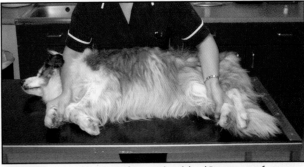

10.11	Restraining a dog on its side. (Courtesy of J Niehoegen)

10.9 Restraining a dog's head. **(a)** The hands are placed either side of the neck and the head is gently pushed forwards with the fingers. **(b)** A rolled-up towel is held firmly but gently around the dog's neck. (Courtesy of E Mullineaux)

Restraint of cats

Figure 10.12 shows general restraint for examination or treatment of the head area. The cat's body should be held close to the handler to prevent the cat from backing away. A firm but gentle hold around the front legs prevents the cat using its front claws.

Figure 10.13 shows raising of the cephalic vein or restraint for examination or treatment of the foreleg. One hand is used to steady the head the other to raise the vein or present the forelimb to the other person.

Figure 10.14 shows two methods of restraint for jugular venepuncture. In Figure 10.14a, one hand is used to restrain the forelimbs and the second to raise the cat's chin in order to present the jugular area to the person taking the blood sample. The sampler raises the vein. In Figure 10.14b one hand is used to hold the forelimbs and the other to raise the vein.

It may occasionally be necessary to hold a cat by the scruff of the neck if firmer restraint is required. However, this should be considered as a last resort, as being held by the scruff can be frightening and potentially painful and many otherwise calm and tolerant cats can become fractious and difficult to handle as soon as attempts are made to handle them by the scruff.

Distraction

Gentle distractions can often help to calm an animal and allow procedures to be carried out more efficiently.

- Talking to the animal in a calm and friendly manner, especially if the animal's name is used, can often help to distract and calm a patient.
- Fingers can be used to gently stroke, scratch or massage the animal.
- A short whistle can often 'still' a struggling dog, allowing a few moments to get a needle into a vein, take a radiograph or perform any other procedure that requires the animal to be still and distracted for a second or two.

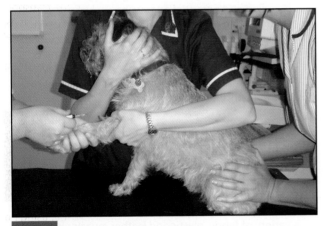

10.10 Holding a dog for cephalic venepuncture.

Figure 10.11 shows a dog being restrained on its side. It may be possible to manoeuvre a dog into this position by first getting the dog to lie down, on command if possible, or by drawing the dog's legs forward whilst it is in a sitting position and then gently rolling the dog over using the forearm to push the dog's head down whilst also holding on to the dog's legs. If the position cannot be achieved by the above method, the dog's legs that are closest to the handler are grasped and pulled away, causing the dog to fall towards the handler. The dog is then gently lowered down against the handler's chest and on to the surface. However, it is necessary to be aware that this manoeuvre and being held in this position can be frightening and may cause the dog to panic and attempt to bite. Gentle reassurance is essential and muzzling the dog beforehand may be advisable.

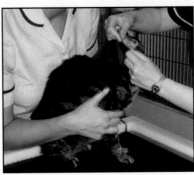

10.12	Restraint of a cat to allow treatment or examination of the head.

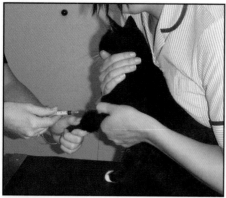

10.13 Raising a cat's cephalic vein or restraint for examination of foreleg.

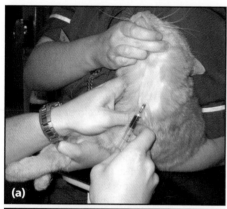

(a)

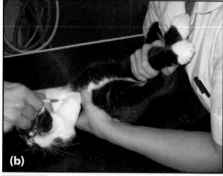

(b)

10.14 Alternative methods of holding a cat for jugular venepuncture. (**a**, Courtesy of D Mactaggart; **b**, Courtesy of E Mullineaux)

Handling difficult or aggressive dogs and cats

Many animals are scared by the veterinary clinic and what happens there. It is a strange place where potentially unpleasant things can happen. Good sensitive handling will obviously help to minimize this problem. The use of dog and cat pheromone diffusers and sprays in the clinic may also help to reduce an animal's anxiety. Remember that a frightened animal may use aggression as a defence. Any unnecessary actions that may increase an animal's fear or cause it to be fearful should therefore be avoided.

Dogs

Raising of the paw, lip-smacking, yawning and looking away are all signs of possible stress and anxiety. The handler should look for these signs and intervene before the animal shows more overt signs. Giving the animal something to do, which it knows how to do and for which it is normally rewarded (such as giving a 'sit' command), can be a good way of switching the animal into a more positive mood. However, it is important that such actions are taken before the animal gets too agitated.

Growling

If a dog growls:

- **Do** *not* attempt to punish the dog: A confrontation will only teach the dog that it has good reason to be defensive.
- **Do** *not* attempt to comfort or reassure the dog as this may be misinterpreted by the dog and so increase its fear and defensive behaviour.

Instead:

- *Do* muzzle the dog: A growl may not cause you to back off but a set of sharp teeth heading in your direction will. If this happens the dog will learn that direct aggression is effective even if a warning growl is not. Dogs that have already learnt this can be some of the most dangerous and unpredictable to handle.
- *Do* try to appear unconcerned by the growl: Backing away or appearing fearful or angry may reinforce the growling and potential aggression.
- *Do* try to understand why the dog is growling. Is the dog in pain? Is it the way in which it is being handled? Is it the procedure that is being carried out? Unless the procedure is almost finished, or is one that will only take a few seconds, it is best to stop and then continue once the dog is muzzled.

Muzzles

Whenever possible, a dog should be muzzled *before* it tries to bite. It can be far more difficult to put a muzzle on a dog that has already decided that you are a threat and has discovered that trying to bite is effective in making you back off.

A variety of fabric, plastic and leather muzzles is available (Figure 10.15). A good selection of different types and sizes should always be to hand. Note that open-ended muzzles may still allow a dog to 'nip' with its front teeth.

If a dog is to be muzzled for longer than a few minutes, it is important always to use a basket-type muzzle that allows the dog to open its mouth, enabling it to pant or vomit. A dog must never be left unattended for any length of time whilst muzzled.

If a dog is a regular patient and frequently needs to be muzzled, it is a good idea to provide the owner with a suitable muzzle to take home. The owner should be advised to put the muzzle on the dog frequently for short periods and reward the dog with food treats, play, affection, and even walks whilst wearing the muzzle. The dog will then make pleasant associations with wearing the muzzle, making it easier for the owner to put the muzzle on the dog before bringing it into the surgery.

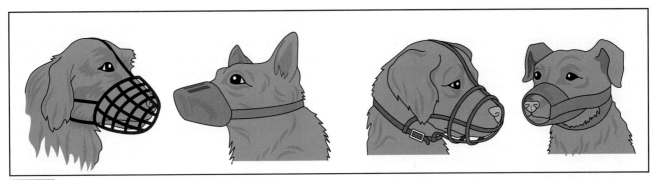

10.15 Examples of muzzles, from left to right: closed basket type; closed plastic; semi-closed leather; open-ended fabric.

Applying a tape muzzle

Figure 10.16 shows the steps in applying a tape muzzle. The tape must be pulled tight in order for the muzzle to be effective, but this can be uncomfortable for the dog and may even cause some slight injury. Therefore this muzzle should only be used in an emergency or if it is not possible to get close enough to the dog to use any other type of muzzle. Often a commercial muzzle can be placed over the tape muzzle and once securely in place the tape muzzle can be allowed to come loose.

Using a 'dog-catcher'

The noose of the dog-catcher (Figure 10.17) is dropped over the animal's head and then tightened, thereby reducing the risk of injury to the handler when taking hold of a severely aggressive dog. The use of a dog-catcher can be highly traumatic for a dog, so it should only ever be used as a last resort.

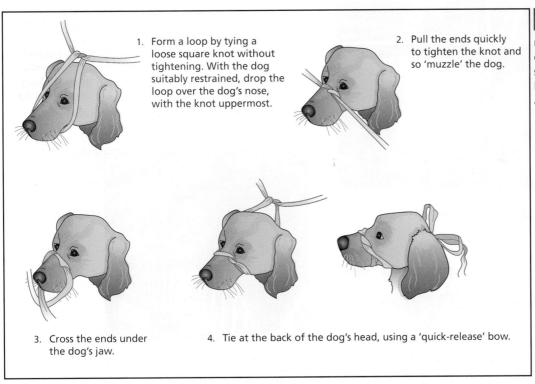

1. Form a loop by tying a loose square knot without tightening. With the dog suitably restrained, drop the loop over the dog's nose, with the knot uppermost.

2. Pull the ends quickly to tighten the knot and so 'muzzle' the dog.

3. Cross the ends under the dog's jaw.

4. Tie at the back of the dog's head, using a 'quick-release' bow.

10.16 Applying a tape muzzle. Use a length of tape or non-stretch bandage at least 100 cm long for a medium-sized dog.

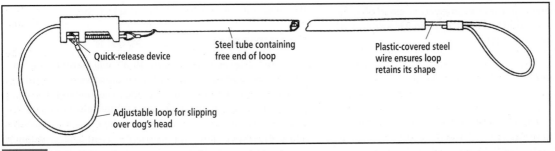

Quick-release device

Steel tube containing free end of loop

Plastic-covered steel wire ensures loop retains its shape

Adjustable loop for slipping over dog's head

10.17 A dog-catcher.

Cats

Fractious cats can often be adequately restrained by wrapping them in a large towel. An alternative is a 'cat restraining bag'. Cat muzzles may also be of use. Both cat muzzles and restraining bags can also help to calm a fractious cat (Figure 10.18).

Use of a 'crush cage' may be necessary with cats that cannot be handled. This is similar to a wire cat carrier but with a movable partition that is used to press the cat against one side of the cage, allowing an injection to be given through the mesh of the cage. If a crush cage is not available, or if the cat cannot be moved from its carrier, the lid or door of the carrier can be opened just enough to allow thick towels to be pushed into the carrier but not enough to allow the cat to escape. The towels are then used to press the cat against the side of the cage, allowing an injection to be given.

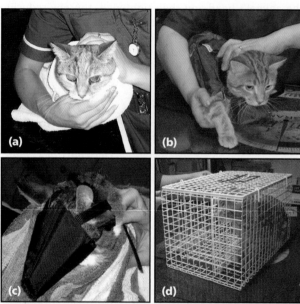

10.18 Ways of restraining fractious cats. **(a)** Wrapping in a towel. **(b)** Cat restraining bag. **(c)** Cat muzzle. **(d)** Crush cage.

Handling and restraint of horses

The principles of handling other equine species are similar to those described here for horses and ponies. Donkeys in particular can become very stressed if not used to handling or transportation. It is usual practice with donkeys to provide a companion if possible during travel and also to hospitalize them with a companion, as they become very stressed on their own. The reader is referred to *The Professional Handbook of the Donkey* for more information.

Understanding equine behaviour

Normal equine behaviour can be understood if they are observed in their natural state in a herd setting. Horses are prey animals, which affects their behaviour when placed in stressful situations. Horses are, however, also naturally inquisitive animals that will investigate things in the first instance and then escape if danger is presented. When handling a horse it is important to be aware of signals that may indicate a change in its behaviour (e.g. if it becomes fearful or aggresive), that indicate potential danger if actions are not taken.

Aggression

Horses may demonstrate aggression for a number of reasons.

- Aggression may be used as a protective mechanism; for example, a mare that is 'foal-proud' may be difficult to approach, so restraining the mare must be a priority before approaching the foal.
- Horses may become aggressive if stabled for a protracted period of time and boredom sets in, causing anxiety and/or stable guarding.
- Horses may also demonstrate aggression toward each other as normal dominance behaviour in a herd. Animals that are at the top of the 'pecking order' in their herd will want to continue this behaviour in any setting when mixed with other horses. Care must be taken not to place yourself in the area of danger from kicks or bites.

Horses displaying aggression will normally exhibit some outward signs, including tail swishing and obvious baring of teeth (Figure 10.19); the ears will lay flat against the head and some horses will strike out with the front legs or swing the quarters round to kick out with the hindlimbs.

Some stallions, in particular, are very difficult to handle, especially if used for breeding purposes. Any stallion admitted for clinical reasons into a hospital setting should be treated with caution. They should be separated, if possible, from mares and sometimes they are more cooperative when handled by male personnel.

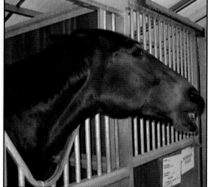

10.19 A horse showing aggression: ears flat to head and teeth bared.

Fear

Horses that display fear may also display signs of aggression. They may retreat to the back of the stable or move away in the field but, when pressed, can also kick out.

Content/normal behaviour

A 'happy', relaxed horse (Figure 10.20) will stand to the front of its stable and approach with an inquisitive mind, with the ears forward or slightly to the side. The relaxed horse will often sleep if contented in the stable/field environment. Horses are able to lock the joints of their limbs so that they can sleep whilst standing (see Chapter 3). In a herd situation, one horse may be left standing whilst the remainder are able to lie completely recumbent.

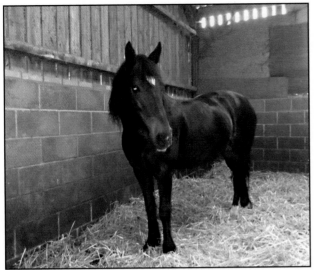

10.20 A horse showing a normal relaxed resting stance. (Courtesy of B. Cooper)

Approach

Before performing a task with the horse, everything required should be to hand so that the procedure runs smoothly without interruption. **Personal protective equipment (Figure 10.21) should include suitable footwear (preferably with steel toe caps), leather gloves, long-sleeved top and a skull cap if lungeing or trotting up.** Horses can be unpredictable and even the most placid horse can become excitable or stressed in unfamiliar surroundings.

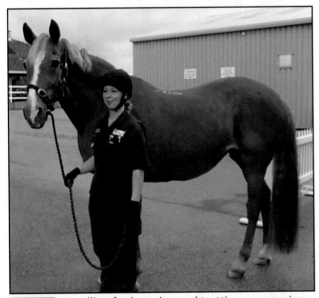

10.21 Handling for lungeing and trotting up, wearing gloves and skull cap.

Horses should be approached in the same manner whether in the field or stable. Common to many prey animals, their eyes are situated on the side of the head, enabling them to see the area to either side in a panoramic fashion. However, vision directly in front of and behind the horse is inhibited and the horse should not be approached from those angles. Traditionally, horses are taught to be led from the **near side** (the horse's left shoulder), although most horses should be able to be led from either side when necessary.

Putting on a head collar

The horse should be approached towards the shoulder and verbal communication used. At this point it may be advisable to slip the lead-rope over the neck to prevent the horse from wandering off, although most horses will happily place their nose into the head collar. The horse should never be forced into the corner of the stable. If the horse turns away and displays its hindquarters this is an indication that it is not happy, and it is important not to try and squeeze between the horse and the wall. It is far better to tempt the horse with a reward to entice it to face towards you.

How to put on a head collar

1. Ensure that you have a large enough head collar and rope to be able to secure the horse.
2. Get the horse's attention so that it knows that you are going to enter the stable.
3. Stand next to the horse's near side (left) shoulder, facing forward, and place the noseband over the nose, slowly inserting the nose through the large hole (nosepiece).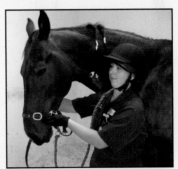
4. Take the long strap up and over behind the ears and secure the buckle fastener on the left side of the cheek.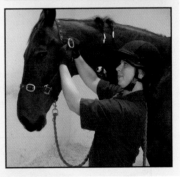
5. Make sure you can fit a hand's width under the chin; this ensures the head collar is not too tight.

Considerations when putting a head collar on a horse

- **Do not** allow the lead-rope to dangle on to the floor; this is a tripping hazard to both handler and horse

- **Do** keep the lead-rope over your shoulder to prevent tripping.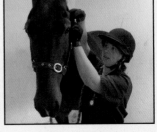

Putting on a bridle with a bit

Most horses can be led by a simple bridle or headpiece with a head collar over the top. However, more difficult or young animals may require the use of a Chifney (anti-rearing bit) (Figure 10.22). The bit is designed for in-hand use only. The Chifney attaches to a headpiece and has a single loose ring for the lead-rope to attach to at the back of the horse's chin. The thin V-shaped bit will dig into the horse's tongue if it tries to rear or pull. A Chifney must be used in experienced hands only, as it can cause injury and discomfort with insensitive use.

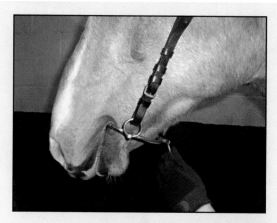

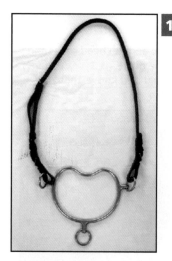

10.22 Simple headpiece with Chifney.

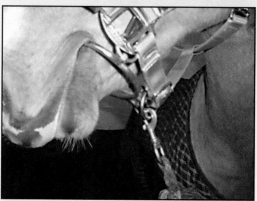

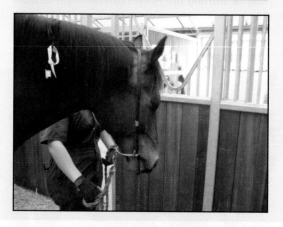

Using a Chifney bit

1. Place the bit with the top edge between the horse's lips and with a thumb behind the incisors. The bottom edge with the ring should be below the horse's jaw.
2. Secure the bridle over the ears.

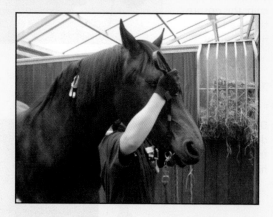

3. Check that any forelock is pulled from beneath the bridle and that the Chifney is sitting in a comfortable position in the gap between the incisors and cheek teeth.
4. Once the head collar is on, attach the lead-rope to the ring on the head collar as well as to the ring on the Chifney – this prevents undue pressure and potential injury to the horse when pulling against the Chifney, as the loop cannot travel any further away from the jaw than the head collar will allow.

▶

A bridle with a simple bit, such as a simple loose ring snaffle (Figure 10.23), may also be used for handling.

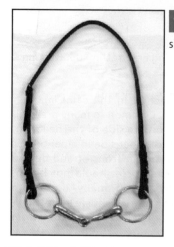

10.23 Simple headpiece with loose ring snaffle.

How to put on a bridle with a bit

1. Approach the horse from the left shoulder and place your hand around its head to secure the horse in a comfortable position; note the bridle cannot be placed with the head in an elevated position.

2. Hold the headpiece up against the head, apply gentle pressure with the bit and place your thumb in behind the incisors at the same time.

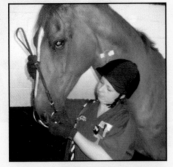

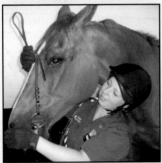

3. Once the bit has been accepted by the horse, place the headpiece over its ears.

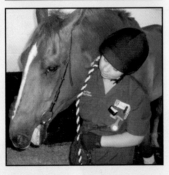

4. Once in position, adjust the headpiece to fit, so that there are no more than two creases in the edge of the lip and the bit is not dangling on the incisors.
5. Place the head collar over the headpiece to prevent the headpiece from being pulled over the head if the horse runs backwards sharply.

To remove the bridle, take hold of it from behind the ears and allow the bit to gentle drop between the incisors; a hand should be held under the nose to catch the bit to prevent it banging on the teeth.

Leading a horse

Once the head collar is on, the horse should be walked at its shoulder (Figure 10.24). The horse should not be allowed to get too far ahead as it may run off. The remaining lead-rope should never be wrapped around the handler's hand, as injury may occur if the horse rears or pulls back. The rope should be held with the right hand approximately 20 cm from the jaw and the remaining rope loosely held in the left hand. Hands should never be placed through the head collar. In a hospital environment where the animal is unknown to the nurse, it may be wise to use a simple snaffle bit and headpiece in

conjunction with the head collar to facilitate more control, especially if 'trotting up' or exercising on a lunge is to be performed. When leading a horse for dynamic evaluation a suitable level area should be sought, where the horse can be walked or trotted for 20 m in a straight line. When turning the horse (turning should be done in walk only) the handler should turn the animal away from them in a fairly wide circle to prevent the horse from treading on human toes. It is only common sense to try to ensure that this is carried out in an area from which the horse cannot escape. Potentially severe consequences can result from horses escaping on to public roads.

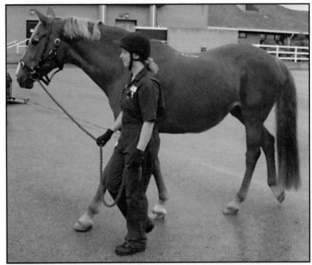

10.24 Walking the horse from the shoulder with bridle and head collar.

Tying up a horse

Horses should always be tied up using a 'quick-release' knot, allowing them to be quickly untied in case of emergency. The horse should always be tied to a bale twine or commercial rubber loop; it should never be tied to something that will not break if the horse should panic.

How to tie a quick-release knot

1. Thread the lead-rope through the bale twine and keep a small loop.

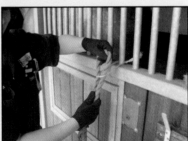

2. Thread the lead-rope through the first loop to produce a second loop.

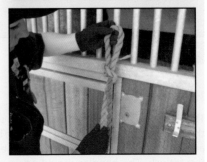

continues ▶

continued

3. Pull the knot to secure it, and thread the remaining end through the second loop made to prevent the horse from pulling on the end and untying itself.

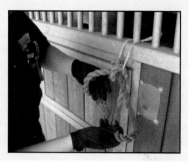

Picking up a foot

The horse should be restrained by a handler or tied to a suitable tie ring with a quick-release knot before it is approached to pick up a foot. The horse should be allowed to stand evenly, weight bearing on all four limbs, before the command to lift a foot is given.

Forefoot

The handler should stand facing the tail at all times. To lift the forefoot, the handler's hand should be placed on the shoulder of the horse and run down the caudal and then palmar aspect of the limb until the fetlock is reached. Gentle pressure should then be applied to the area and the horse commanded to lift the limb (the command would usually be 'up'). As the horse lifts the limb, the area from the dorso-medial aspect of the foot should be supported and held gently (Figure 10.25). Keeping in close contact with the horse's shoulder will allow the handler to detect any movement from the horse and anticipate the horse snatching the foot down; the handler should stay ahead of the horse to prevent injury from the horse striking out with its limb. Examining and cleaning of the hoof (see Chapter 16) should be carried out twice a day, especially in a hospital environment where the horse is standing in the stable and fungal infection can occur as a result of poor foot care.

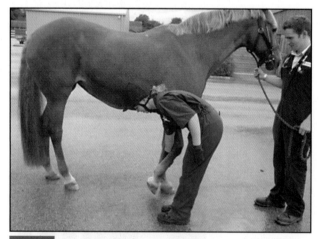

10.25 Picking up a forefoot.

Hindfoot

The hindfoot should be approached in a similar manner, with the approach from the front of the horse back to the quarters and down the caudal then plantar aspect with pressure to the fetlock. The handler should again remain close to the

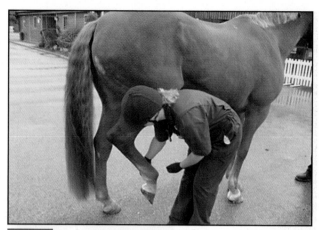

10.26 Picking up a hindfoot.

horse to minimize the risk of being kicked. The foot should not be restrained, but instead the limb should be supported, as a pressured horse will kick out (Figure 10.26).

Examination of the mouth

Some medications, such as worming, anti-inflammatory and antibiotic pastes (see Chapter 8), can be given straight into the mouth. With the horse restrained using a head collar, the syringe nozzle is inserted into the corner of the mouth so it is as near the back of the tongue as possible (Figure 10.27).

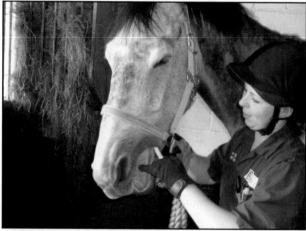

10.27 Giving oral medication to a horse. The syringe is placed in the corner of the mouth and directed towards the back of the tongue.

A cursory examination of the equine mouth can be made by gently holding the tongue in one hand through the side of the mouth between the canine and premolar teeth (Figure 10.28). To examine a horse's mouth properly, and to carry out any dental work, a gag is needed (typically a Hausmann's gag).

Apart from rasping teeth with a hand rasp, all other procedures (including any tooth extractions and use of motorized dental instruments) must be carried out by a veterinary surgeon or a BEVA-accredited equine dental technician. Removal of teeth with significant periodontal attachment is an act of veterinary surgery and may only be carried out by a veterinary surgeon. In the case of a fractious horse that needs sedation to perform an oral examination, a veterinary surgeon must be present to administer sedation or supervise the nurse. This does not prevent nurses from assisting with the preparation of the equipment and patient.

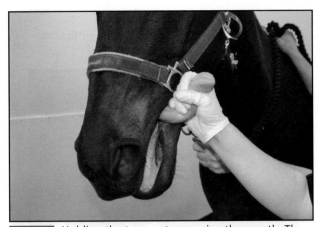

10.28 Holding the tongue to examine the mouth. The tongue is gently withdrawn into the space between the canine and premolar teeth allowing the teeth on the opposite side of the mouth to be examined.

Mouth examination procedure

A set of stocks may be used to prevent the horse from moving about during examination. The area should be well lit, to facilitate the oral examination, and quiet to prevent interruption.

1. Once the patient is *in situ,* a Hausmann's gag can be placed in its mouth. It is very important that the size of the gag fits the patient; one size will not fit all. The gag should be carefully placed on the horse. The strap must sit behind the ears in a normal headpiece position and then be tightened until the plates fit neatly between the teeth; there should be no gap between the front of the bite plate and the incisor teeth. A loose strap will allow the gag to slip and the horse's mouth to close on the vet.

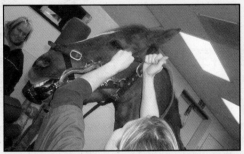

2. Once the gag is safely in place the plates can be widened one click at a time, going from one side of the gag to the other, giving the horse time to adjust each time the gag is widened. Once the gag is wide enough to allow the vet to palpate the teeth safely, examination can begin.

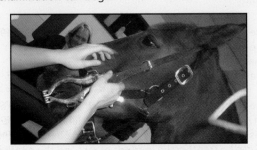

▶

3. The mouth is first washed to remove any food material.

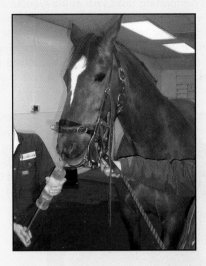

4. The dental examination can then begin, followed by any necessary dental work. Note that one hand should be placed on the gag whilst the other is in the mouth to control the horse's head. The horse may be rested several times during the procedure to prevent temporomandibular joint pain. Oral extractions may take several hours, so patience is required.

Mouth being palpated for abnormalities.

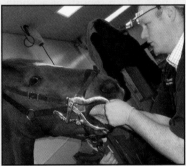

Oral examination with a head-torch.

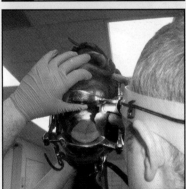

Teeth being rasped.

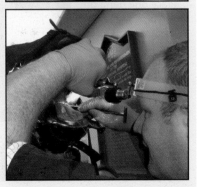

Restraint for procedures

When performing tasks such as intravenous catheterization or nerve blocks, additional restraint may be required; this may be as simple as holding the tail to keep the horse weight bearing (Figure 10.29), or lifting and holding a foreleg in order to examine a hindleg. More involved restraint techniques, such as the application of a twitch or chemical restraint, may be required in some cases.

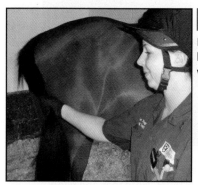

10.29

Holding the tail to keep the horse weight bearing.

Application of a 'twitch'

Applying a skin twitch to the neck or shoulder may encourage the horse to remain still for a procedure. This can be done by holding a small amount of skin firmly in the hand (Figure 10.30).

A nose twitch consists of a length of wood (or metal or rubber, which are usually much safer) with a rope attached at one end in a loop. Commercial twitches are also available. It must be placed carefully to prevent injury to the horse and the handler, and must not be left in place for more than 5 minutes.

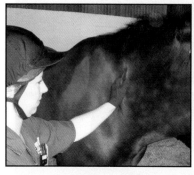

10.30 Skin twitch.

How to apply a nose twitch

A handler is required to stand at the side of the horse, and on the same side as the person applying the twitch in order to prevent the horse from jumping on to them.

1. Place one hand on the pole and your second hand through the rope, which should then be placed on the horse's upper lip.

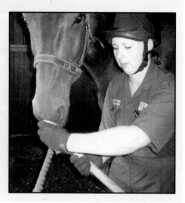

2. Slide the rope over the hand on to the lip and then twist it until it grips a firm amount of skin.

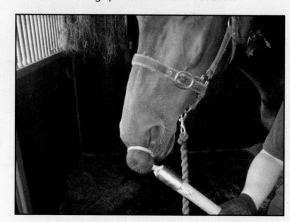

3. Twist the lead-rope over the handle of the twitch so that, should the horse throw its head upwards, the twitch will not swing and collide with the horse's head or the handler.

> **WARNING**
>
> **A twitch should never be used on an ear**, as this can cause permanent damage and may also cause the animal to become head shy.

It is essential to monitor a horse's behaviour very carefully when it is 'twitched', as of all the restraint techniques employed it is the one most commonly associated with injury to personnel. Some horses will suddenly react or strike out when 'twitched', but usually they will give signs such as closing their eyes before this happens. Under such circumstances, the twitch should be removed immediately.

Transporting horses

Legislation

Defra has specific guidelines on the transport of horses, which state that within the United Kingdom transporting a horse in a way that is detrimental to its welfare would be a breach of the Animal Welfare Act 2006. The Act states that a person commits an offence if they are responsible for an animal, either permanently or temporarily, and either cause the animal to suffer or fail to ensure its need are met.

Other legislation controlling the transport of horses includes:

- The Horses (Sea Transport) Order 1952 – amended 1958
- The Transit of Animals (Road and Rail) Order 1975 – amended 1979 and 1988
- The Welfare of Animals (Transit) Order 1997.

The Horserace Betting Levy Board also provides additional guidelines on the transport of racehorses. These give details of the size of carrier transport, the length of time a horse can be transported, periods of rest and the prevention of transporting horses that may be unfit for transport due to ill health, or transportation of mares in early pregnancy. For all horses, rest periods should be applied every 8 hours and for horses travelling over 24 hours, a 24-hour break should be given.

Equine passports

Horse owners are responsible for making sure that they have an up-to-date horse passport, so that their horse can be identified. Passport legislation covers all horses, ponies, donkeys and zebras. Foals must be registered with a suitable passport agency recognized by Defra before the foal is 6 months old or before 31 December in the year of birth, whichever is later. Owners can be fined up to £5000 for not having a passport. An equine animal cannot be moved/transported without a valid passport. The passport must be available for inspection by trading standards officers or Animal Health Officers. If a passport has been applied for, this information must be given so that the officer may check for the application with the relevant body. Passports are available from several issuing bodies, including equine breed societies.

Horse passports are important because they help to:

- Ensure horses that have been treated with certain medicines do not make it into food intended for humans (see Chapter 8)
- Prevent the sale of stolen horses.

The passport will contain details about the horse, including its appearance, which is illustrated in a diagram, microchip details (Chapter 16), age, breed/type and all the medications it has been given (if it has been declared 'intended for human consumption'). Passports require a signed statement by the owner that it is NOT intended for human consumption, otherwise it is presumed that it is intended for human consumption; this is important for the administration of medication (see Chapter 8).

Practical considerations

Transporting a horse can be stressful to the animal and this must always be taken into consideration. Horses can become dehydrated, even over a short journey, and regular water should be offered at rest breaks.

Horses should be allowed to spend at least some of the journey with their head in a lowered position, with good ventilation as this will help to decrease the risk of respiratory complications. Any horse with a pre-existing respiratory problem should preferably not be transported. If transport is necessary, then careful monitoring for further exacerbation of the disease, which could lead to pleurisy/pneumonia, is necessary.

Correct travel clothing should be used for all horses that are travelling. This should include padded bandages that cover the limb from the hoof to above the carpus and tarsus to prevent rubbing and knocks, or commercial travelling boots (Figure 10.31). Poll guards to protect the top of the head in the event of rearing in a confined space (Figure 10.32), and a tail bandage and guard to protect against rubs, are also available. A rug may be necessary, but care should be taken when transporting several horses in a small area, as overheating can worsen dehydration. A sweat rug may be applied at the end of the journey.

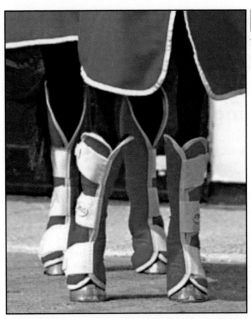

10.31
Travelling boots.

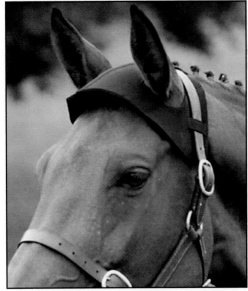

10.32
Poll guard.

Transport to the veterinary practice

Not all horses travel regularly and care should be taken not to hurry such patients when travelling to or from the surgery; owners should be advised to give themselves plenty of time to load and unload. Injured or sick horses must travel only on the authorization of a veterinary surgeon. Each case should be given special consideration; horses in splints for suspected fractures should be loaded on a flat surface if possible, with the ramp elevated to help protraction of the leg in the case of a forelimb. Horses with a forelimb fracture should travel facing backwards, whereas those with hindlimb fractures should face forwards. This will allow them to cope if the horse box has to brake suddenly. Any horse with an injury or rhabdomyolysis (tying up) should not be moved more than necessary and the transport should be for as short a distance as possible. Foals should be allowed to travel with the mare without a partition if possible. Personnel should not travel in the back with an animal, unless it is in a specially adapted ambulance.

Handling and restraint of exotic pets

Removing patients from travelling boxes

Removing exotic pets from their travelling boxes for examination can be a challenge in itself and depends to a certain extent on the type of carrying box the animal has arrived in and the species. Examples of dealing with different types of pets in differing boxes are given below; however, these should be considered in conjunction with the species-specific advice that follows. Exotic pets should be fully assessed before any attempt is made to remove them from their cages or boxes. In all cases, it is easier to remove the patient when the handler is at roughly the same level; therefore, picking the box up and placing it on to a table with a non-slip mat is preferred. In some cases with larger rabbits, it may be preferable to kneel down and remove the patient from its box on the floor.

Top-loading boxes

In most cases it is best to consider sliding a towel in underneath the lid before the lid is fully opened to ensure that the patient does not suddenly leap out, in the case of a rabbit or ferret, or fly out, in the case of a parrot. The towel may then be allowed to cover the animal whilst the lid is carefully opened and the animal scooped out of the carrying box. In the case of ferrets and rabbits that are fractious or nervous it may be advisable to grasp the scruff of the neck with one hand through the towel, whilst reaching underneath and restraining the hindlegs around the hocks. The rabbit or ferret may then be carefully lifted out and placed on to a non-slip surface.

Side-front-loading boxes

For rabbits and other small mammals in this type of box it is preferable to remove the door where possible, as this increases the opening available for removal of the patient. A towel may then be introduced and the scruff of the neck grasped, to allow the patient to be moved forward enough

to allow the hindlegs to be grasped and the animal removed as described above.

In the case of a parrot or other larger cagebird, a towel should be carefully introduced to prevent escape of the bird past the towel. This should then be draped over the head and body, and the head grasped from behind, transferring the thumb and fingers underneath the lower mandible to control the beak. The rest of the towel is then used to drape over the wings and body and the other hand is used to wrap the bird in the towel to prevent it flapping and hurting itself. The bird may then be removed from the box.

Bird cages

Many smaller cagebirds are transported to the practice in their everyday cage. This can be useful to assess the local environment and the type of droppings the bird has been passing recently, assuming it has not been cleaned out prior to the visit. However, such cages may present a problem in removing the bird safely from the cage as many small cagebirds have plentiful perches, toys (e.g. mirrors, bells) and food items that provide cover to hide behind and that could potentially cause damage. The first aim is therefore to remove the majority of these obstructions carefully from the cage.

In the case of highly nervous and flighty individuals, it may be sensible to transfer the cage into a darkened room as diurnal (day-active) birds do not see well in red light; this makes catching the patient easier. Once the cage has been depopulated of toys, etc., a small hand towel or paper towel may be introduced through the largest opening to aid the catching of the bird. This presents a larger surface area than the hand alone, and so tends to make the bird less likely to dodge around the towel and escape. It also provides something for the patient to bite on whilst trying to control the head and beak, and allows some passive restraint of the wings as well (Figure 10.33).

Rodent cages

As with bird cages there may be a lot of cage furniture inside these enclosures and the majority should be removed to allow free access. Hamsters in modular housing should be encouraged to move into their sleeping quarters, which may then be detached from the maze of tunnels.

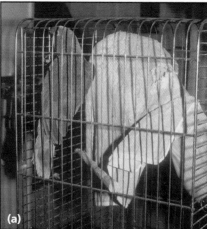 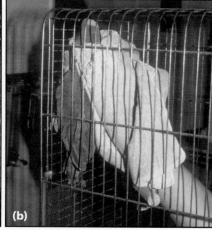 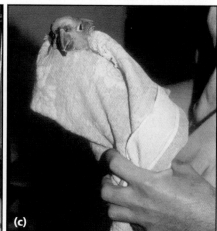

10.33 Removing a parrot from its cage. **(a)** The towel and hand are introduced into the cage. **(b)** The bird is firmly but gently grasped from the back. The head must be located first, to allow the thumb and forefingers to be positioned underneath the lower beak, in order that it can be pushed upwards thus preventing the bird from biting. The rest of the towel is then used to wrap around the bird to gently restrain its wing movement. This will avoid excessive struggling and wing trauma. **(c)** The patient may then be cocooned in the towel with the head still held extended from behind through the towel and the rest loosely wrapped around the bird's body.

Once the cage is cleared of excess furniture, a light hand towel or paper towel may be introduced and draped over the rodent to initially restrain it. The scruff of the neck may then be firmly grasped, as described below for more active and aggressive animals such as hamsters. Alternatively, the thumb and forefingers may be slid under the forelimbs and the other hand introduced to support the rear end of more docile rodents such as chinchillas and rats.

Handling and restraint of small mammals

Pet mammals come in many different shapes and sizes, and from many different backgrounds – from those more adapted to human co-habitation such as mice and rats, through to the animals more recently adopted as pets, such as chipmunks, which are still semi-wild in nature.

Assessment before handling

1. **Is the patient severely debilitated and/or in respiratory distress?**
   Examples include the pneumonic rabbit, with obvious oculonasal discharge and dyspnoea, or older rats with chronic lung disease. Excessive or rough handling of these patients is contraindicated and the journey into the veterinary practice may already have caused further stress.
2. **Is the species a tame one?**
   Examples of the more unusual small mammals that may be kept include chipmunks, marmosets and other small primates, opossums and raccoons. All of these are potentially hazardous to handlers and themselves, as they will often bolt for freedom when frightened, or turn and fight. Even the more routinely kept small mammals may be aggressive, e.g. hamsters.
3. **Is the small mammal suffering from a metabolic bone disease?**
   This is often seen in small primates, young rabbits and guinea pigs. The diet may have been inadequate with regard to calcium and vitamin D3, and exposure to natural sunlight may be absent. Hence long-bone mineralization during growth will be poor, leading to spontaneous or easily fractured bones.
4. **Does the small mammal patient require medication/physical examination?**
   If so, handling is often essential.

Rabbits

The majority of domestic rabbits are docile, but the odd aggressive doe or buck, usually those not used to being handled, does exist. The potential dangers to the veterinary nurse arise from the claws, which can inflict deep scratches rivalling those inflicted by cats, and the incisors, which can produce deep bites. Aggression is frequently worse at the start of the breeding season in March/April. In addition to the damage they may cause the handler, a struggling rabbit may lash out with its powerful hindlimbs and fracture or dislocate its spine. Severe stress can even induce cardiac arrest in some individuals. Rapid and safe restraint is therefore essential.

To this end, if aggressive, the rabbit may be grasped by the scruff with one hand whilst the other hand supports underneath the rear legs. If the rabbit is not aggressive then one hand may be placed under the thorax, with the thumb and first two fingers encircling the front limbs, whilst the other is placed under the rear legs to support the back.

When transferring the rabbit from one room to another it must be held close to the handler's chest. Non-fractious individuals may also be supported with their heads pushed into the crook of one arm, with that forearm supporting the length of the rabbit's body; the other hand is then used to place pressure/grasp the scruff region (Figure 10.34).

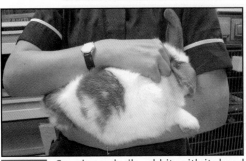

10.34 Carrying a docile rabbit, with its head in the crook of the elbow. Most rabbits find this method of restraint settling. (Reproduced from the *BSAVA Manual of Rabbit Medicine and Surgery, 2nd edition*)

Once caught, the rabbit may be calmed further by wrapping it in a towel, similar to the method used for cats, so that just the head protrudes in a 'bunny burrito' (Figure 10.35). There are also available specific rabbit 'papooses' that zip up along the rabbit's dorsum, leaving the head/ears free for blood sampling, but confining the limbs to prevent escape or self-harm. It is important not to allow rabbits to overheat in this position, as they, like a lot of small mammals, do not have significant sweat glands and do not actively pant. They can therefore quickly overheat if their environmental temperature exceeds 23–25°C, with fatal results.

Covering a rabbit's eyes will often help to calm it (Figure 10.36).

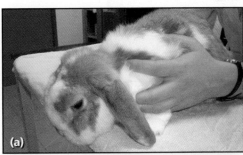

(a)

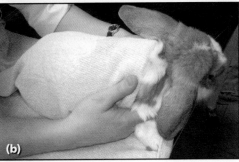

(b)

10.35 The 'bunny burrito': restraining a rabbit by wrapping it in a towel. **(a)** The rabbit is placed on a towel, facing away from the handler. **(b)** One side of the towel is wrapped firmly across the dorsum, covering the forefeet but leaving the head exposed. *continues* ▶

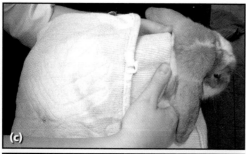

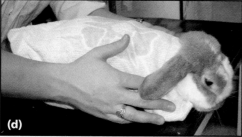

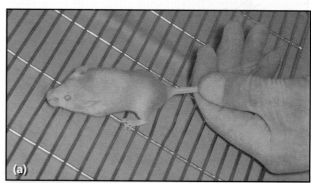

10.35 *continued* The 'bunny burrito': restraining a rabbit by wrapping it in a towel. **(c)** The back of the towel is folded up over the lumbar region. **(d)** The remaining side of the towel is wrapped across the dorsum and tucked in ventrally on the opposing side to complete the wrap. (Reproduced from the *BSAVA Manual of Rabbit Medicine and Surgery, 2nd edition*)

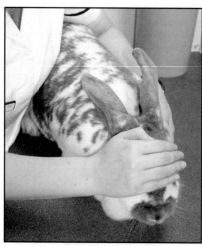

10.36 A hand over the rabbit's eyes helps to keep the animal calm. (Courtesy of C Clarke)

Trancing and turning

The method of restraint commonly known as 'trancing' (more accurately, creating a state of tonic immobility), whereby a rabbit is induced to become immobile after lowering it into a dorsal recumbency, is not recommended. Contrary to popular belief, rabbits in a state of tonic immobility are not relaxed, hypnotized or insensitive to pain. Scientists believe that this is a defence mechanism employed once a rabbit has already been 'caught' by a potential predator. By remaining very still the rabbit may appear already dead, thereby causing the attacker to release its grip momentarily and allow the rabbit to escape. Research has shown that in this state rabbits show increased heart and respiratory rates plus elevated plasma corticosterone levels, indicative of fear-induced stress. The stress caused by this procedure may prove fatal, especially for rabbits suffering from respiratory or cardiovascular disease, and the sudden transition from the passive state to one of very active escape can be instantaneous and unpredictable and may result in significant injury to the patient.

Enlisting the help of an assistant, to raise the rabbit's forelimbs off the ground, whilst keeping the rabbit's hindlimbs in contact with a solid surface, allows for ventral examination of rabbits.

Rodents
Mice and rats

Mice will frequently bite an unfamiliar handler, especially in strange surroundings. It is first useful to grasp the tail near to the base and then place the mouse on a non-slip surface (Figure 10.37a). Whilst still holding the tail, the scruff may now be grasped firmly between the thumb and forefinger of the other hand (Figure 10.37b), allowing the mouse to be turned and examined as necessary (Figure 10.37c).

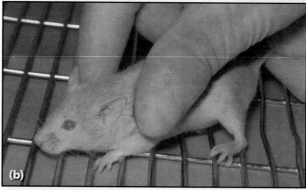

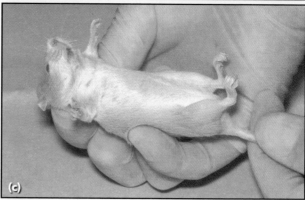

10.37 Handling techniques for mice. (Reproduced from *BSAVA Manual of Exotic Pets, 4th edition*)

Rats will rarely bite unless roughly handled (Figure 10.38). They are best picked up by encircling the pectoral girdle, immediately behind the front limbs, with the thumb and fingers of one hand whilst bringing the other hand underneath the rear limbs to support the rat's weight (Figure 10.39). The more fractious rat may be temporarily restrained by grasping the base of the tail before scruffing it with thumb and forefinger.

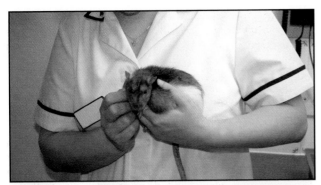

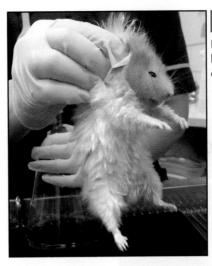

10.40

Handling a hamster. (Courtesy of Aiden Raftery)

`10.38` Holding a tame rat. (Courtesy of C Clarke)

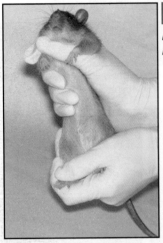

`10.39` Restraining a rat. (Reproduced from *BSAVA Manual of Exotic Pets, 4th edition*)

handler's hands mimic the swooping action of a bird of prey, startling the rodent.

For more rigorous restraint, the gerbil may be grasped by the scruff between thumb and forefinger of one hand after placing it on to a flat level surface. It is vitally important not to grasp a gerbil by the tail as this will lead to stripping of the tail's skin leaving denuded coccygeal vertebrae. This will never regrow and the denuded vertebrae will themselves undergo avascular necrosis and drop off later. Jirds and jerboas are related species, and handling techniques are the same.

Guinea pigs, chinchillas and degus

Guinea pigs are rarely aggressive, but they become highly stressed when separated from their companions and normal surroundings. This makes them difficult to catch, as they will move at high speed in their cage. To aid restraint, dimmed lighting can be used and environmental noise restricted to reduce stress levels. Restraint is also easier if the guinea pig is already in a small box or cage, as there is less room for it to escape.

To restrain a guinea pig, it should be grasped behind the front limbs from the dorsal aspect with one hand, whilst the other is placed beneath the rear limbs to support the weight (Figure 10.41). This is particularly important as the guinea pig has a large abdomen, but slender bones and spine that may be easily damaged.

Chinchillas are equally timorous and rarely if ever bite. They too can be easily stressed, and dimming room lighting and reducing noise can be useful during capture.

Some chinchillas when particularly stressed will rear up on their hindlegs and urinate at the handler, with surprising accuracy. It is therefore essential to pick up the chinchilla calmly and quickly with minimal restraint, placing one hand around the pectoral girdle from the dorsal aspect just behind the front legs, with the other hand cupping the hindlegs and supporting the chinchilla's weight.

Degus may be handled in a similar way to chinchillas.

> **WARNING**
>
> Under no circumstances should mice or rats be restrained by the tips of their tails, as de-gloving injuries to the skin in this area will easily occur.

Hamsters and gerbils

Hamsters can be relatively difficult to handle as, being nocturnal, they are never pleased at being awoken and picked up during daylight hours. If the hamster is relatively tame and used to being handled, simply cupping the hands underneath the animal is sufficient to transfer it from one cage to another.

Some breeds of hamster are more aggressive than others, with Russian, Djungarian or hairy-footed hamsters being notorious for their short temper. In these cases, the hamster should be placed on to a firm flat surface and gentle but firm pressure placed on to the scruff region with finger and thumb of one hand. As much of the scruff as possible should then be grasped, with the direction of pull in a cranial manner to ensure that the skin is not drawn tight around the eyes (Figure 10.40); hamsters have a tendency for ocular proptosis if roughly scruffed. If a very aggressive animal is encountered, the use of a small glass/perspex container with a lid for examination and transport purposes is useful.

Gerbils are relatively docile but can jump extremely well when frightened and may bite if roughly handled. For simple transport they may be moved from one place to another by cupping the hands underneath the gerbil. Small mammals should always be approached from the side and at low levels, as when they are descended upon from a great height, the

> **WARNING**
>
> Chinchillas must not be scruffed under any circumstances, as this will result in the loss of fur at the site held. Chinchillas may actually lose some fur due to the stress of the restraint, even if no physical gripping of the skin occurs. This 'fur slip' as it is known, will leave a bare patch, which will take many weeks to regrow.

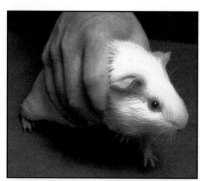

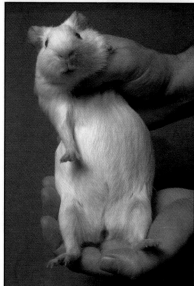

10.41 Restraining a guinea pig. The animal is first grasped around its shoulders. It can then be lifted, with the hindquarters supported.

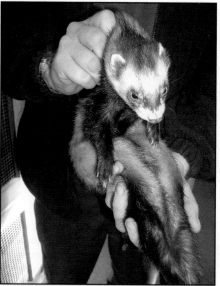

10.42 Holding a potentially aggressive ferret, using the scruff. (Courtesy of S Redrobe)

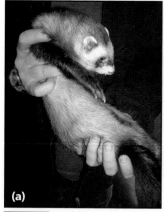

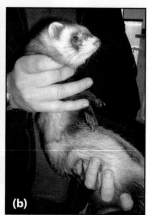

(a)   (b)

10.43 Holding a less aggressive ferret. (Courtesy of S Redrobe)

Chipmunks

There are more than 24 species of chipmunk, with the commonest seen in the UK currently being the Siberian species, although North American smaller species are also kept. Chipmunks are extremely highly strung and the avoidance of stress is essential to avoid fatalities. Generally, they are very difficult to handle without being bitten, unless hand-reared when they may be scruffed quickly, or cupped in both hands. To catch them in their aviary-style enclosures the easiest method is to use a fine-meshed aviary/butterfly net, preferably made of a dark material. The chipmunk may then be safely netted and quickly transferred to a towel for manual restraint, examination or injection/induction of chemical restraint.

Ferrets

Ferrets can make excellent house pets and many are friendly and hand-tame. Some ferrets kept as working animals, to hunt rabbits, may be less frequently handled and more aggressive.

For excitable or aggressive animals, a firm grasp of the scruff, high up at the back of the neck should be made. The ferret may be suspended from this whilst stabilizing the lower body with the other hand around the pelvis (Figure 10.42). In the case of more hand-tame animals, they may be suspended with one hand behind the front legs, cupped between thumb and fingers from the dorsal aspect, with the other hand supporting the rear limbs (Figure 10.43a). This may be varied somewhat in the more lively individuals by placing the thumb of one hand underneath the chin, so pushing the jaw upwards, and the rest of the fingers grasping the other side of the neck (Figure 10.43b). The other hand is then brought under the rear limbs as support.

Handling and restraint of birds

As with small mammals, the veterinary nurse needs to make a decision on whether the bird in question is safe to restrain. This is not only because of the danger to the nurse's welfare (in the case of an aggressive or potentially dangerous bird of prey) but also because of the medical aspects of the patient's health.

Assessment before handling

1. Is the bird in respiratory distress, and is the stress of handling therefore going to exacerbate this?
2. Is the bird easily accessible, allowing quick stress-free and safe capture?
3. Does the bird require medication via the oral or injectable route, or can it be medicated via nebulization or food or drinking water?
4. Does the bird require an in-depth physical examination at close quarters, or is cage observation enough?

It is not always necessary to restrain the bird. It is important to remember that many avian patients are highly stressed individuals, so any restraint that is performed should involve minimal periods of handling and capture.

Initial approach

The majority of avian patients seen in practice (with the obvious exception of the owl family) are diurnal (that is active during the daylight hours) and so reduced or dimmed lighting in general has an extremely calming effect. This can be used to the veterinary nurse's advantage when catching a flighty or stressed bird. In the case of Passeriformes (perching birds such as canaries and finches) and Psittaciformes (members of the parrot family, which includes budgerigars and cockatiels as well as the larger parrots), turning down the room lights or drawing the curtains or blinds is enough. For birds of prey there may well be access to the practice's or the bird's own 'hoods'; these are leather caps that slot over the head, leaving the beak free but completely covering the eyes (Figure 10.44). They are used to calm the bird when on the wrist or during handling or transporting.

It is also advisable to keep the noise levels to a minimum when handling avian patients, as the acuity of their hearing is second only to the acuity of their vision. With these two initial approaches, stress and time for capture can be greatly reduced.

Prior to capture, all obstructing items should be removed from the cage or box – e.g. toys, water bowls, food bowls. This helps to avoid self-induced trauma by the bird and reduces the time needed to capture the patient. Once these initial arrangements have been made, the avian patient can be approached.

Birds of prey

There are two main categories of birds of prey commonly seen in practice: Falconiformes (includes falcons, hawks and eagles) and Strigiformes (the owl family). Falconiformes are mainly diurnal (daylight active) and they make up the most commonly seen group of birds of prey in practice. Strigiformes are generally nocturnal (active during the hours of darkness) and so use of hoods and darkening the room will not quieten these birds. However, they generally tend to be relatively docile.

Several pieces of specific handling equipment are often used for birds of prey. Hoods (Figure 10.44) are used to calm many falcons and hawks, and many of these birds will also have **jesses** on their legs. These are the leather straps attached to their 'ankles' (lower tarsometatarsal area) and they allow the falcon to be restrained whilst on the owner's fist.

Leather gauntlets (Figure 10.44) should be worn by all handlers for all birds of prey, as their talons and the power of grasp of each foot can be extremely strong. The feet of birds of prey represent the major danger to the handler and not the beak. It is important to note that when the bird of prey is positioned on the gauntleted hand, the wrist of this hand (traditionally the left hand in European falconers) is kept above the height of the elbow. If not, the bird has a tendency to walk up the arm of the handler, with serious and painful results. The type of gauntlet should be either a specific falconer's gauntlet or one of the heavier duty leather pruning gauntlets available from garden centres.

1. Place the gauntleted hand into the cage or box or beside the bird's perch.
2. Grasp the jesses with the thumb and forefinger of the gauntleted hand and encourage the bird to step up on to the glove.
3. Once on the hand, retain hold of the jesses and slip the hood over the bird's head.

The bird of prey may then be safely examined 'on the hand' and is frequently docile enough to allow manipulation of wings and beak and for small injections to be administered or for oral dosing to occur.

If the bird of prey does not have jesses on but is trained to perch on the hand it may well step up on to the gauntlet of its own accord. If not, then you need to reduce the room lighting for Falconiformes. A blue or red light source could also be used, allowing the handler to see the bird but preventing the bird of prey from seeing normally. There are then two possible approaches:

- The bird may be grasped from behind in a thick towel, ensuring that you are aware of where the bird's head is (this is known as **casting** the bird; Figure 10.45). The bird is restrained across the shoulder area with the thumbs pushing forward underneath the beak to extend the head away from the hands. The hood can then be placed over the bird's head and the bird placed on to a gauntleted hand. The majority of birds are happier and struggle less when their feet are actually grasping something, rather than being held in a towel with their feet freely hanging.

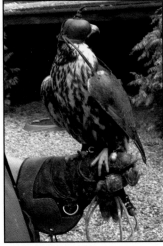

10.44 A hood keeps a raptor calm. (Courtesy of J Chitty)

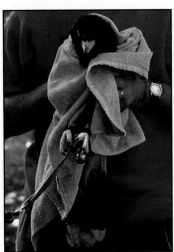

10.45 Casting a Harris' hawk. (Reproduced from *BSAVA Manual of Exotic Pets, 4th edition*)

- Alternatively, the hooded bird may be held from behind with the middle and fourth finger of each hand grasping the leg on the same side and directing the feet away from the handler. This method of holding the legs prevents the raptor from grasping one foot with the other which will cause severe puncturing of the skin, leading to secondary infections known as 'bumblefoot'.

For the majority of raptors, if they are loose in their aviary it is best to catch them at night. Owls should be caught during the day. The use of nets and towels is often required.

Finally, it is important to remember that the majority of birds of prey are regularly flown, so it is vital to preserve the integrity of their flight and tail feathers. Unfortunately, few falconers will thank you for saving their bird's life if they then cannot fly that bird until after the feathers have been replaced at the next moult; moulting usually occurs in the autumn.

Parrots and other cagebirds

Parrots are often trained to step up on to the hand. If the owner does not have the bird already trained to do this, he/she should be encouraged to do so. A tasty treat can be held in front of the bird, with the other hand just in front and above the internal perch. The treat should be at such a distance that the bird must step on to the hand to get the treat. It is important to be aware that nervous birds especially may reach down to the hand, as it is normal for many parrot species to use the beak as a third limb to help balance. The novice handler may mistake this for an attempt to bite and pull away, making matters worse as the bird is now even less sure about stepping on to the hand and may grab at the hand in a desperate attempt to pull itself on to the hand, biting in the process. All of these birds will also benefit from subdued or blue or red light to calm the bird and to allow restraint with minimal fuss.

- In psittacine birds (e.g. African grey parrots, macaws, Amazon parrots and cockatoos) the main weapon is the beak and a powerful bite is possible.
- In passerine birds (e.g. mynah birds, starlings and orioles) the main weapon may again be the beak. Although this is less damaging as a biting weapon, it may still be a sharp stabbing weapon.

Wearing heavy gauntlets is not recommended for restraint of either family group as it will not allow easy judgement of the strength of the handler's grip on the patient. Instead it is better to use dish or bath towels for the larger species and paper towels for the smaller ones as these provide some protection from being bitten without masking the true strength of the grip. The towel technique is also more beneficial than gloves alone because it presents a larger surface area for the bird to try and evade. The bird is then less likely to try and bolt for freedom, whereas a single hand can be a much smaller target and encourages escape attempts. After removal of the bird from its cage (see Figure 10.33), the limbs may then be removed from the towelling one at a time for examination or medication.

> **WARNING**
>
> Birds do not have a diaphragm and so rely solely on the outward movement of their ribcage and keel bone for inspiration. Restriction of this movement with too tight a grip can be fatal.

For smaller cagebirds:

1. A piece of paper towel may be used and then the bird transferred to the hand. Latex gloves may be worn.
2. The neck of the bird should be held between the index and middle fingers (Figure 10.46).
3. The thumb and forefinger can then be used to manipulate legs or wings.
4. The rest of the hand should gently cup the bird's body to resist struggling.
5. Care should be taken not to over-constrain as this could cause physical harm.

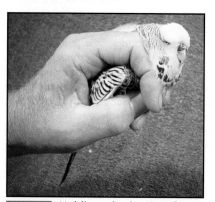

10.46   Holding a budgerigar for examination. (Reproduced from *BSAVA Manual of Psittacine Birds, 2nd edition*)

In the case of particularly aggressive parrots that are very difficult to handle, leather gauntlets may be employed. Remember that too strong a grasp around the bird's body can prove fatal.

Young and hand-tame parrots

In the case of hand-reared and very tame young parrots, these may be removed from their containers by scooping them up between the palms of both hands before being placed into a towel-lined cardboard box or shallow dish. They should never be left unattended as they could still jump out of the container and injure themselves; however, this technique may allow sufficient restraint to allow a clinical examination.

For fully feathered immature parrots it may still be necessary to towel restrain the bird to examine the vent, feet and other sensitive areas without the bird biting or flapping its wings and escaping.

Waterfowl

Ducks, geese and swans are often kept in farm situations, but are also kept by smallholders and so may well be brought in for treatment.

Restraint of these species is relatively straightforward but may become hazardous with the larger swan and goose family.

1. The first priority is to concentrate on capturing the head. This can be done manually, by grasping the waterfowl around the upper neck from behind.
2. Make sure that your fingers curl around the neck and under the bill whilst the thumb supports the back of the neck and the potentially weak area of the atlanto-occipital joint. Failing this, a swan or shepherd's crook or other such adapted smooth metal or wooden pole attached hook can be used to catch the neck – again high up under the bill.

3. Next, it is essential that the often powerful wings are controlled before the bird has a chance to damage itself or you. This can be most easily achieved by using a towel, thrown or draped over the avian patient's back and loosely wrapped under the sternum. Some practices may have access to more specialized goose or swan cradle bags, which wrap around the body, containing the wings but allowing the feet and head and neck to remain free.

4. The bird may now be safely carried or restrained by tucking its body (contained within the towel or restraint bag) under one arm and holding this close to the torso. With your other hand, the neck can be loosely held from behind just below the bill.

Toucans and hornbills

Another group of birds increasingly kept in private collections are the toucans and hornbills. These have an extremely impressive beak, with a serrated edge to the upper bill. Provided the head is initially controlled using the towel technique described above for parrots, an elastic band or tape may be applied around the bill, preventing biting. The handler still needs to be careful of stabbing manoeuvres and it may be a good idea to work with a second handler. Otherwise, restraint is the same as for Passeriformes.

Escaped birds

Where a bird is loose in a room or in an aviary flight cage, a number of methods can be applied. Again, darkening the room and reducing its area if possible are both very helpful to calm and confine the bird.

- In the case of larger parrots, throwing a heavy bath towel over the bird can confine them for long enough to allow the handler to restrain the head from behind and then wrap the patient in the towel.
- For very small birds, the investment in a fine aviary or butterfly net (preferably made of dark very fine mesh) is extremely useful to catch the bird safely, either in mid-flight or against the side of the cage or room. Larger nets are available from specialist retailers for catching the larger species of birds.

Handling and restraint of reptiles

Reptiles tend to be less easily stressed than birds and so restraint of the debilitated animal may be performed according to the degree of risk. It is still worthwhile considering one or two aspects that may make restraint dangerous to animal and veterinary nurse alike.

Assessment before handling

1. **Is the patient in respiratory distress?**
   Examples include pneumonic cases, where mouth breathing and excessive oral mucus may be present and where excessive manual manipulation can exacerbate the condition.

2. **Is the species of reptile a fragile one?**
   The small day geckos (*Phelsuma* spp.) for example are extremely delicate and very prone to shedding their tails when handled. Similarly, some species such as green iguanas (*Iguana iguana*) are prone to conditions such as metabolic bone disease whereby their skeleton becomes fragile and spontaneous fractures are common.

3. **Is the species an aggressive one?**
   Some are naturally so, for example, alligator snapping turtles (*Macroclemys temminckii*), Tokay geckos (*Gekko gecko*), and rock pythons (*Python sebae*).

4. **Does the reptile patient require medication/physical examination?**
   In these cases, restraint is essential.

Reptiles are ectothermic and so rely on their environmental temperature to maintain their body temperature. Handling periods should therefore be minimized as much as possible to prevent undue cooling of the reptile. Most reptiles commonly seen in veterinary practices require an optimum temperature range of 22–32°C.

> ### WARNING
>
> It should be borne in mind that many species of reptile have a bacterial flora in their digestive systems that frequently includes *Salmonella* spp. Personal hygiene is therefore very important when handling these patients, to prevent zoonotic diseases. Disposable gloves may be worn. Hands must always be washed thoroughly after handling.

Chelonians

This group includes all land tortoises, terrapins and aquatic turtles. Size differences in this order are not as great as for the other two reptile families, but it is still possible to see chelonians varying from the small Egyptian tortoises (*Testudo kleinmanni*) weighing a few hundred grams all the way up to adult leopard tortoises (*Geochelone pardalis*) at 40 kg, and the Galapagos tortoises, which can weigh several hundred kilograms. The majority of chelonians are harmless, although surprisingly strong. The exceptions include the snapping turtle (*Chelydra serpentina*) and the alligator snapping turtle (*Macrochelys temminckii*), both of which can give a serious bite. Most of the soft-shelled terrapins have mobile necks and can also bite; even red-eared terrapins (*Trachemys scripta elegans*) may give a nasty nip.

For the mild tempered chelonians such as the Mediterranean *Testudo* species, the tortoise may be held with both hands, one on either side of the main part of the shell behind the front legs (Figure 10.47a). For examination, to keep the tortoise still it may be placed on top of a cylinder or stack of tins. This ensures that the legs are raised clear of the table and the tortoise is balancing on the centre of the underside of the shell (plastron).

For aggressive species it is essential that the shell is held on both sides behind and above the rear legs to avoid being bitten (Figure 10.47b). In order to examine the head region in these species it is necessary to chemically restrain them.

For the soft-shelled and aquatic species, soft cloths and latex gloves (non-powdered) should be used in order not to mark the shell.

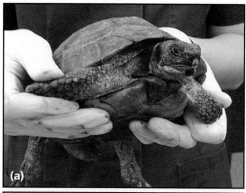

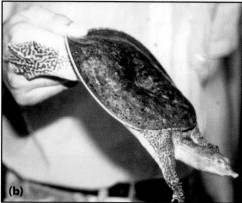

10.47 Handling chelonians. **(a)** Lifting a docile species. **(b)** Handling an aggressive species by grasping the caudal part of the carapace. (Reproduced from *BSAVA Manual of Reptiles, 2nd edition*)

Lizards

Lizards come in many different shapes and sizes from the 1.2 m long adult green iguana to the 10–12 cm long green anole (*Anolis carolinensis*). They all have roughly the same structural format, with four limbs (although these may become vestigial in the case of the slowworm for example) and a tail. The potential danger to the veterinary nurse includes their claws and teeth, and in some species such as iguanas, their tails, which can lash out in a whip-like fashion.

Geckos other than Tokay geckos are generally docile, as are lizards such as bearded dragons (*Pogona* spp.). Iguanas may be extremely aggressive, particularly sexually mature males. They may also be more aggressive towards female owners and handlers as they are sensitive to human, as well as reptile, pheromones.

Restraint

Restraint is best performed by grasping the pectoral girdle with one hand from the dorsal aspect, so controlling one forelimb with forefinger and thumb and controlling the other forelimb between middle and fourth finger. The other hand is used to grasp the pelvic girdle from the dorsal aspect (Figure 10.48), controlling one limb with the thumb and forefinger, and the other limb between middle and fourth finger. The lizard may then be held in a vertical manner with the head uppermost and the tail out of harm's way underneath the handler's arm. When holding a lizard in this manner, the handler should allow some flexibility as the lizard may wriggle, and if the restraint is overly rigid the spine can be damaged. It is then possible to present the head and feet of the lizard away from the handler to avoid injury.

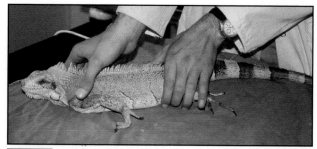

10.48 Holding the forelimbs and hindlimbs against the thorax and tailbase, respectively, restrains medium to large lizards such as this iguana. (Courtesy of S Redrobe)

Some of the more aggressive iguanas may need to be pinned down, prior to this method of handling. Here, as with avian patients, the use of a thick towel to control the tail and claws is often very useful. In some instances gauntlets are necessary for particularly aggressive large lizards, and for those which may have a poisonous bite, such as the Gila monster (*Heloderma suspectum*) and the beaded lizard (*H. horribilis*). It is important not to use too much force when restraining the lizard, as those with skeletal problems such as metabolic bone disease, may be seriously injured. In addition, lizards, like other reptiles, do not have a diaphragm and so over-zealous restraint will lead to the digestive system pushing on to the lungs and compromising respiration.

Geckos can be extremely fragile and the day geckos for example are best examined in a clear plastic container rather than physically restraining them. Other gecko species have skin that is easily damaged and so latex gloves and soft cloths should be used and the gecko cupped in the hand rather than restraining it physically.

Small lizards may have their heads controlled between the index finger and thumb to prevent biting.

> **WARNING**
>
> **It is important that lizards are never restrained by their tails.** Many will shed their tails at this time, but not all of them will regrow (show autotomy). Green iguanas, for example, will only regrow their tails as juveniles (under 2.5–3 years of age); once they are older than this, they will be left tail-less.

Vago-vagal reflex

There is a procedure that may be used to place members of the lizard family into a trance-like state. It involves closing the eyelids and placing firm but gentle digital pressure on both eyeballs. This stimulates the parasympathetic autonomic nervous system, which results in a reduction in heart rate, blood pressure and respiration rate (the vago-vagal reflex). To maintain pressure on the eyeballs, a cotton-wool ball may be placed over each closed eye and a bandage wrapped around the head, holding these in place. Provided there are no loud noises or environmental stimuli, after 1–2 minutes the lizard may be placed on its side, front, back, etc., allowing radiography to be performed without using physical or chemical restraint. Loud noises or physical stimulation, however, will immediately bring the lizard back to its normal wakeful state.

The 'trancing' of rabbits (see above) has recently been reviewed on welfare grounds, based upon recent scientific research. Such scientific evidence is not currently available for lizards. It is not yet known whether the physiological response of the lizard differs from that of a tranced rabbit or if the same welfare concerns arise. The procedure in lizards should therefore currently be viewed with an open mind.

Snakes

There is a wide range of sizes, from the enormous anacondas (*Eunectes murinus*) and Burmese pythons (*Python molurus bivittatus*) (Figure 10.49), which may achieve lengths of up to 10 m or more, down to the thread snake family (*Leptotyphylid*), which may be a few tens of centimetres long. They are all characterized by their elongated form with an absence of limbs. The potential danger to the veterinary nurse is from the teeth (and in the case of the more poisonous species, such as the viper family, the fang teeth) or, in the case of the constrictor and python family, the ability to asphyxiate the prey by winding themselves around the victim's chest or neck. With this in mind, the following restraint techniques may be employed.

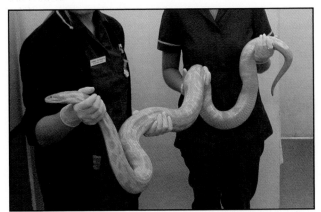

10.49 Carrying a large snake requires support from more than one handler. (Reproduced from *BSAVA Manual of Reptiles, 2nd edition*)

Non-venomous snakes

Non-venomous snakes can be restrained initially by controlling the head. This is done by placing the thumb over the occiput and curling the fingers under the chin. Reptiles, like birds, have only one occipital condyle and so the importance of stabilizing the atlanto-occipital joint cannot be overstated. It is also important to support the rest of the snake's body, so that not all of the weight of the snake is suspended from the head. With smaller species, this is best achieved by allowing the snake to coil around the handler's arm, so that it is supporting itself.

In the larger species (those longer than 3 m) it is necessary to support the body length at regular intervals (see Figure 10.49). Indeed, it is vital to adopt a safe operating practice with the larger constricting species of snake. For this reason a 'buddy system', as with scuba diving, should be operated whereby any snake longer than 2.5–3 m in length should only be handled by two or more people. This is to ensure that if the snake were to enwrap the handler, the 'buddy' could disentangle them by unwinding from the tail end first. Above all, it is important not to grip the snake too hard as this will cause bruising and the release of myoglobin from muscle cells that will lodge in the kidneys, causing damage to the filtration membranes.

Venomous and aggressive snakes

Venomous snakes (such as vipers and rattlesnakes) and very aggressive species (such as the green anaconda (*Eunectes*

murinus), reticulated python (*Python reticulatus*) and rock python (*P. sebae*)) may be restrained initially using snake hooks. These are 0.5–0.75 m steel rods with a blunt shepherd's hook at one end. They are used to loop under the body of a snake, to move it at arm's length into a container. The hook may also be used to trap the head flat to the floor before grasping it with the hand. Once the head is controlled safely the snake is rendered harmless – unless it is a member of the spitting cobra family. Fortunately it is rare to come across these in general practice, but staff who do handle them must wear plastic goggles or a plastic face visor as they may spit poison into the handler's eyes and mucous membranes, causing blindness and paralysis.

Handling and restraint of amphibians

Examination of the amphibian patient should be performed at the species' optimum body temperature. A rough guide is between 21 and 24°C, which is lower than the more usual 22–32°C reptile housing conditions.

The examination table should be covered with paper towels (unbleached) soaked in dechlorinated, preferably purified, water. Additional purified water should be on standby to be applied to the amphibian patient to prevent dehydration during the examination.

Initially it is useful not to restrain the patient until the extent of any problem is assessed, as many have severe skin lesions that are extremely fragile.

Once an initial assessment has been made, the patient may be restrained manually. It is advisable to use a pair of non-powdered hypoallergenic latex gloves. This minimizes irritation to the amphibian's skin caused by the normally acidic human skin, and prevents irritation caused by the powder in many prepacked latex gloves. The wearing of gloves is also essential for handling members of the toad family or the arrow tree frogs, which can secrete irritant or even potentially deadly toxins from their skin. These toxins can be absorbed through unprotected human skin. It may be necessary to wear goggles when handling some species of toad. The giant toad (*Bufo marinus*) can squirt a toxin from its parotid glands over a distance of several feet.

When handling the amphibian patient, the method of restraint will obviously depend on the animal's body shape.

- The elongated form of **salamanders** and **newts** will require similar restraint to that of a lizard: one hand grasps the pectoral girdle from the dorsal aspect, with the index finger and thumb encircling one forelimb and the second and third fingers the other, while the opposite hand grasps the pelvic girdle, again from the dorsal aspect in a similar manner. Some salamanders will shed their tails if roughly handled and so care should be taken with these species.
- **Large anurans** (members of the frog and toad family) can be restrained by cupping one hand around the pectoral girdle immediately behind the front limbs, with the other hand positioned beneath the hindlimbs (Figure 10.50). Care should be taken with some species that have poison glands in their skin as mentioned above. Care should also be taken with species such as the Argentinian horned frog (*Ceratophrys ornata*) as these can bite.

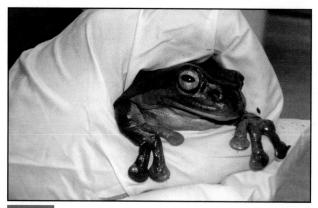

10.50 Handling a frog. (Courtesy of Gidona Goodman)

- **Aquatic urodeles** should be examined only in water, as removal from the water results in skin damage. Some of the larger urodeles, such as the hellbender species (*Cryptobranchus* spp.), can also inflict unpleasant bite wounds on handlers.

Smaller species and aquatic species may be best examined in small plastic or glass jars.

Handling and restraint of invertebrates

The species involved will naturally determine the methods by which the patient can be safely, for handler and invertebrate alike, restrained.

Many invertebrates present no direct threat to the handler. Examples include giant land snails, stick insects and cockroaches. These may be gently picked up and cupped in the hand, or allowed to walk on to a towel or similar non-slip surface.

Other species, such as those in the **mygalomorph spider family,** may present multiple hazards. These may flick setae (the small hairs that cover their abdomens) at the handler if stressed or if they feel threatened. These setae are highly irritant on the skin and are particularly dangerous if they come into contact with the conjunctiva. In addition, many of these spiders have a nasty bite. The bites are rarely fatal but still cause pain and potential harm, similar to the pain associated with a bee or wasp sting. These species should be transferred into a Perspex, glass or plastic container (Figure 10.51), and only ever handled with latex gloves. If it is necessary to pick up such a spider, it may be either cupped in paired hands or grasped with atraumatic forceps or fingers, immediately behind the cephalothorax, around its 'waist'. Protective goggles should be worn if the spider is to be removed from its container.

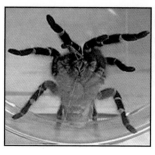

10.51 Placing a spider in a transparent container allows it to be examined easily. (Courtesy of E Morgan)

Scorpions present a similar problem, with the tail sting being the most obvious danger. The majority of scorpions kept in captivity such as the imperial scorpion, are not seriously dangerous, although the sting may be likened to a wasp or bee sting. To restrain these species safely, they may be transferred into a Perspex, plastic or glass container, or alternatively a sheet of clear plastic may be gently but firmly laid over the top of the scorpion to confine it for examination or to allow a better grasp. They may also be lifted gently by the tip of the tail using atraumatic forceps, with a sheet of card or plastic supporting the body from underneath.

Aquatic invertebrates should be examined and moved in water, using either their own tank or a clean plastic, Perspex or glass container.

Acknowledgements

Jane Devaney would like to acknowledge the assistance of the following people for the equine content of the chapter: Derek Knottenbelt; Claire Magee; and Rosie Owen. Thanks also go to the family of Max Hoare, for the use of their photographs.

References and further reading

Atkinson T and Riccomini F (2008) Behaviour. In: *BSAVA Manual of Canine and Feline Advanced Veterinary Nursing, 2nd edn,* ed. A Hotston-Moore and S Rudd, pp. 313–328. BSAVA Publications, Gloucester

Bradshaw JWS (1992) *The Behaviour of the Domestic Cat.* CAB International, Wallingford

Fowler ME and Ames L (1995) *Restraint and Handling of Wild and Domestic Animals, 2nd edn.* Iowa State Press, Ames

Fraser M and Girling S (2009) *Rabbit Medicine and Surgery for Veterinary Nurses.* Wiley-Blackwell, Oxford

Girling SJ (2003) *Veterinary Nursing of Exotic Pets.* Blackwell Publishing, Oxford

Horwitz D (2009) An update on canine human-directed aggression. *Proceedings of the American Animal Hospital Association Conference 2009*, pp. 33–37

Horwitz D and Mills D (2009) *BSAVA Manual of Canine and Feline Behavioural Medicine, 2nd edn.* BSAVA Publications, Gloucester

McBride A, Day S, McAdie T et al. (2007) Hypnosis: a state of fear or pleasure? *Proceedings of CABTSG Study Day 2007 'Emotional Homoeostasis, Stress, the Environment and Behaviour',* pp.38–40

McClean A and McClean M (2008) Academic horse training. *Equitation Science in Practice.* AEBC, Victoria

Meredith A and Johnson-Delaney C (2010) *BSAVA Manual of Exotic Pets, 5th edn.* BSAVA Publications, Gloucester

Meredith A, Redrobe S and Mullineaux E (2007) General care and management of other pets and wildlife. In: *BSAVA Manual of Practical Animal Care,* ed. P Hotston Moore and A Hughes, pp. 53–87. BSAVA Publications, Gloucester

Svendsen E (2008) *The Professional Handbook of the Donkey, 4th edn.* The Donkey Sanctuary, Sidmouth

Useful websites

http://www.defra.gov.uk/wildlife-pets/pets/travel/pets/ regulation/eu-reg.htm

Self-assessment questions

1. What are the four main aims of the veterinary nurse when restraining an animal?
2. What are the signs that could indicate that a dog or cat may be fearful and/or potentially aggressive?
3. What actions should and should not be taken when initially approaching and handling a dog or cat?
4. What are the important DOs and DON'Ts when a dog growls?
5. How is a tape muzzle applied and when should one be used?
6. What are the typical signs displayed by an aggressive horse?
7. Which position should a horse not be approached from?
8. Which direction should you face to pick up a horse's foot?
9. How often should a horse's feet be checked for problems?
10. What is the maximum length of time for a twitch to be in place on a horse?
11. What is the maximum length of time that a horse should travel without water/food?
12. How is it best to handle an aggressive male rabbit?
13. Which species of rodent should not be routinely grasped by the scruff of the neck to restrain them?
14. What type of bird will not be quietened by moving it into a darkened room?
15. When restraining a bird, what should the handler be careful not to do too firmly?
16. What important zoonotic bacteria may be carried by reptiles?
17. What defence mechanism might mygalomorph spiders employ to avoid being handled?

Chapter 11

Small animal behaviour and training

Kendal Shepherd

Learning objectives

After studying this chapter, students should be able to:

- **Understand the external factors that influence an animal's behaviour, whether deliberately applied or not**
- **Understand the principal theoretical modes of learning**
- **Translate theory into practice in order to guide behaviour appropriately**
- **Understand that aggression is a response to perceived threat and not an expression of dominance**
- **Better interpret canine body language**
- **Identify high-risk situations in the clinic and propose strategies to improve patient behaviour, particularly in minimizing the animal's need for an aggressive response**
- **Prepare clients for the requirements of behaviour therapy, including giving appropriate behavioural first aid**
- **Direct clients to receive qualified behavioural help in the same way as any other referral service**

Introduction

Unwanted behaviour, particularly if dangerous, remains a common reason for relinquishment and euthanasia, especially in the dog, and veterinary nurses may feel under pressure to help clients in what are often distressing situations. It is important that whatever the circumstances, they should not attempt to give advice or to handle an animal beyond their competence as this can have disastrous consequences for the individual and the patient, as well as the client and the practice as a whole. It is essential that any knowledge of behaviour gained during training is supplemented with further reading and education. This is to ensure that the enormous potential of veterinary nurses in caring for the mental as well as the physical well-being of the animals in their care can be fulfilled.

Whether viewed by human companions as acceptable or not, all animals are continually responding behaviourally to the environment around them and their expectations of it. This is always in a way that they perceive as likely to achieve the most advantageous results.

An animal's decision as to how to behave is based upon an amalgam of genetic factors and life experiences. The principles guiding the learning process are exactly the same, whether an animal is being trained by random environmental events (e.g. the apparent success of driving away a postman by barking), or by a human 'trainer' when teaching a dog to sit, lie down or retrieve.

Cats are almost entirely trained by non-controlled environmental events, including the inadvertent actions of their owners, whereas dogs generally spend at least some time in their lives being deliberately 'trained'. However, for the vast majority of dogs, this training tends to be very specific in nature, namely: when they are young; for a very small proportion of their lives; and in specific contexts only, such as in a training class. Deliberate training of dogs rarely extends into every area of real life, and most pertinently for veterinary staff, in the consulting room, hospitalization kennels or preparation room. The surgery can become another context in which an individual animal may be left entirely without human guidance, and therefore behaves appropriately or not entirely by accident, depending upon what history and experience has taught it.

There are several areas in which the veterinary nurse can and should be involved in dealing with behavioural issues. Answering direct questions from clients, mainly regarding what to do about perceived behavioural problems, has increased in importance owing to public awareness and demand, in addition to the delegation of responsibility to nurses by their employers. Running puppy parties and classes is advocated as the way forward in educating dogs for their future lives, not least in how to behave in a convenient way, to all-round benefit, at the surgery. What is less immediately obvious is the need to recognize the impact of what subsequently happens to an animal at the surgery upon its behaviour, whether or not an owner is present, and how all that a young dog learnt at puppy class may be undermined during veterinary treatment.

It is also impossible to treat physical ailments thoroughly without considering an animal's total environment and its behavioural responses to it. To be most effective, it is essential that the same message is delivered to both client and patient by all veterinary staff from reception through to the kennels, consulting room and operating theatre. Whether treating behaviour problems or trying to prevent them, the impact of any environment upon behaviour and the principles underlying how an animal learns must inform everything that veterinary staff do.

Influences on behaviour

An animal's behaviour at any given moment is a response to certain immediate influences. These can be divided into external and internal factors.

- **External factors** include how the animal is managed and specific features of the environment at the time the behaviour is shown.
- **Internal factors** include the animal's physiological and emotional state.

The two are linked, however, as the external environment brings about changes in both internal physiology and emotion. In simplest terms, there is an intimate three-way relationship between the environment of an animal, including its owner; how it 'feels' in terms of physiology and emotion; and the behaviour it subsequently employs (Figure 11.1).

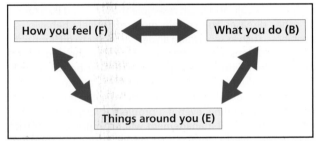

11.1 The intimate three-way relationship between the environment of an animal (E), how it 'feels' in terms of physiology and emotion (F) and the behaviour it subsequently employs (B) can be expressed as a 'universal triangle'. It is essential to take into consideration that one element of this triangle cannot be changed without immediately affecting the other two. © Kendal Shepherd.

The action an animal takes is always intended to create or restore emotional and physiological stability. Perceived problem behaviour arises when the means by which a normal animal attempts to do this are at odds with human requirements. This is of exceptional importance when trying to understand and treat canine aggression, which may well be normal behaviour from the dog's perspective, but completely unacceptable from that of the dog's owner. If an animal has become incapable of fulfilling its emotional needs through behavioural means, simply because nothing seems to work, a true behavioural problem with concurrent emotional distress can arise. The majority of cases treated, however, fall into the first category, i.e. normal animals using normal behaviour yet deemed unacceptable by their owners.

Physiology and perception not only bring about changes in the immediate behaviour of an animal but can also shape future development and behavioural tendencies in a more permanent way. For example, aggression seen during pregnancy (or false pregnancy) is intimately associated with concurrent hormonal changes in the bitch, making it more important for her to defend herself and her offspring.

Learning at this time may result in the display of future defensive aggression when a bitch is in possession of anything viewed as valuable by her, even though neither the puppies themselves (whether real or imagined), nor the hormones involved, are still present. Disease, with resulting alteration of perception and associated pain, may both contribute to and cause behaviour problems. Examples of this are aggression in hyperthyroid cats and in dogs with the chronic low-grade pain associated with bilateral hip dysplasia. Although pain may be subsequently relieved and a clinical condition treated, the learning that has inevitably occurred in the patient during the disease process, and the associations made with both companions and the environment, must not be forgotten.

In summary, to understand behaviour fully it is necessary to draw on knowledge not only from veterinary medicine but also from branches of zoology and psychology as well as animal management and nutrition. Consideration must be given not only to what an animal has actually done, but also to where, when, with and to whom and, most importantly, why.

Assessment of behaviour

As with clinical disease, in addition to their own observations, veterinary staff are reliant upon information given by the owner of a pet when gathering essential history regarding an animal's behaviour. Some owners will hold back information, either because they think it is not important or because they feel guilty about some aspect of it. It is essential to establish a bond of trust with the client when trying to extract information about their pet's behaviour and to be completely non-judgemental in attitude. There is a tendency to consider behaviour as being largely influenced either by the animal's genes (**nature**) or by the environment in which the animal lives (**nurture**). This is particularly pertinent when a dog's *breed* or *type*, as judged by conformation, is used to determine how dangerous a dog might be, rather than its upbringing, management, experience and demonstrable behavioural propensities. However, as in all animals, it must be recognized that both influences come together in any given animal to make it an individual, with individual behavioural characteristics. These two elements are considered below.

Genetics – the influence of nature

Genes provide the blueprint for the behaviour of the individual (see Chapter 4). Genetic factors not only determine what is normal but may also set certain limits. This can be seen at three levels: species-typical behaviour; breed characteristics; and individual characteristics.

Species-typical behaviour

This describes those behaviours that define a dog as a dog and a cat as a cat or an African Grey parrot as an African Grey parrot. Many popular texts will make analogies to wild relatives, such as the wolf in the case of the dog. But dogs are certainly not wolves. Their behaviour is quite different, as domestic dogs have evolved to survive in very different environments as well as to need and value human companionship and guidance. So the value of such analogies is limited and can lead to inaccurate advice. One needs to be well versed in the normal behaviours of a species in order to appreciate if something is genuinely abnormal and therefore be able to advise an owner correctly. For example, an owner may think that the behaviour of their female cat in oestrus, when rolling on the floor and 'calling', is abnormal or indicative that the animal is in pain. The jumping up of a dog is often misinterpreted as an aggressive or 'dominant' act, requiring punishment, when in fact this behaviour is simply part of the normal appeasing greeting repertoire of any dog. In the case of pet birds, there are enormous differences in the natural biology of the different species and generalizations are rarely valid.

Breed characteristics

Just as a dog is not a wolf, so all breeds of dog or cat are not alike. Thus breed characteristics also determine what is normal for an individual of that breed. Excessive vocalization might be a cause for concern in the domestic shorthaired cat but is normal in the Siamese. Similarly, the Border Collie is expected to herd and stare obsessively at sheep or tennis balls; the retriever enjoys water and having objects in its mouth; and the Greyhound, running and the chase. But expectations that a Greyhound should retrieve or want to swim are likely to be in vain and the Poodle or Bichon Frise, for example, may decline to do any of these things, despite human training efforts. At the very least, training for a task to which a breed is not already predisposed is very much harder work. The young German Shepherd Dog appears to become wary rather than inquisitive far earlier in the socialization phase than other breeds (see later). So such breed-related behavioural tendencies also predict what problems may be more prevalent in a given breed and explain why object-guarding retrievers, stranger-wary German Shepherd Dogs and jogger and bicycle-chasing Border Collies are over-represented in behaviour problem statistics. An understanding of the breed, and its associated behavioural tendencies, is of course also important when trying to advise a potential owner about a new pet.

Individual characteristics

Within any breed, there are behavioural differences and some of these have been shown to have a genetic basis. Within certain breeds, some animals are predisposed to being more fearful than others and nervousness, for example, has been reported to have a relatively high heritability. Recent studies suggest that there is an association between aggression and low serotonin levels in the Cocker Spaniel as a breed, which may in the future also help to explain certain impulsive and aggressive behaviour in individuals of other breeds. More emphasis is now being placed upon the study of personality, particularly in dogs – how such traits can be measured, and how compatible, or otherwise, they are with human requirements. Such information is particularly important when considering the prevention of behaviour problems through selective breeding as well as appreciating the limits of what training and behavioural modification can achieve.

Certain differences in behaviour are based upon the sex of an animal (genetically determined). As the effect of physiology on behaviour is very complex, however, care must be taken in assuming that behaviour is solely governed by sex hormones. For example, although urine spraying in cats is more common in males, neutering usually helps in the prevention and treatment of the problem in both sexes by altering their physiological state. Similarly, although aggression both towards other dogs and people is more common in male dogs, it is

neither a male-typical nor hormone (testosterone)-dependent behaviour, but is rather influenced by numerous physiological and social factors. Castration may indeed make matters worse in some cases, and simple generalizations about the management of behaviour by surgical means should be avoided.

Age-related changes

Sexual maturity is a time when relatively sudden changes may be seen in an animal's behaviour owing to an alteration in sensitivity to certain stimuli. At maturity, the opposite sex suddenly becomes more interesting and potentially valuable. The attention of entire animals inevitably becomes biased towards this biological need and away from other lesser essentials, such as the requirements of an owner for a dog to sit or come to call. Apparent loss of obedience control at sexual maturity in dogs is therefore a very common complaint. Such internal physiological changes also underpin other phases when certain types of behavioural change may be more or less likely. These include sensitive phases in early development (see next section), but also changes associated with ageing.

As an animal gets older, not only are there pathological changes, such as the loss of sight and hearing or pain related to arthritis, which can influence behaviour, but also specific age-related changes in the brain. This can result in a condition known as cognitive dysfunction, akin to Alzheimer's disease in humans. The presenting signs, such as house-soiling and increased vocalization, can resemble those caused by a range of other diseases and certain more exclusively behavioural problems, such as separation anxiety. In order to differentiate these conditions and protect the welfare of the dog or cat, any problem with a late age of onset must be particularly carefully evaluated by a veterinary surgeon to determine possible medical causes, before a behavioural plan is implemented. At the same time, even if a problem is largely medical in origin, behavioural management will be important in order to counter adverse learned associations during the course of ill health. If a clinic wishes to demonstrate concern for the all-round welfare of its patients, any distinction between behavioural and medical management should be avoided.

The environment – the influence of nurture

In early life, dogs and cats have 'sensitive phases' when they learn more rapidly and can therefore form impressions that affect their behaviour and temperament in a fundamental and lasting way. At this stage in life, temperament is shaped for better or worse and any damage done is much harder to undo later. Many behaviour problems arise because the animal has not been properly socialized or trained when young. It is far easier to teach appropriate behaviour from the outset, even though it may not appear to be necessary in an animal so young, than it is to correct problems later on.

Animals reared in impoverished environments often do not develop well intellectually and may have difficulty in regulating their emotions, particularly in the face of any novel feature of their environment. Such animals are not only predisposed to a variety of behaviour problems but, as the ability to learn may be impaired, these problems may also carry a worse prognosis for treatment. The socialization phase is particularly important, as it has a large impact on the way the animal will tend to respond to both physical and social features of its environment later in life. This period appears to be between the fourth and tenth week of age in the puppy and between the second and seventh week in the kitten. It is vital that pets receive pleasant experiences at this time associated with all things that human society expects them to accept later. They should be handled gently by people of both sexes, both old and young, to avoid a fear of strangers. Controlled exposure to an urban environment with all the sights, sounds and smells of traffic and various people may be one of the most important factors in building confidence at this age, which prevents fearful avoidance later in life. On the other hand, over-stressing the animal, e.g. by excessive exposure or early weaning, should be avoided, as this also interferes with the animal's learning ability. Early weaning has been implicated in fundamental emotional changes and a reduced ability to cope with stress in a range of species.

Drug therapy also affects an animal's physiological state as it alters the balance of nerve transmitters in the brain. Whilst there are some drugs, such as anti-depressants and anxiolytics, which are specifically designed for this purpose, other drugs may produce behaviour changes as a secondary affect. Phenylpropanolamine, for example, used to control urinary incontinence in dogs may also cause aggression in some cases.

Diet can also influence behaviour through its physiological effects. This ranges from simple hunger, which may also be disease-induced, to the ingestion of stimulants which result in over-activity and hence associated problems, to the manipulation of diet to maximise the availability of precursors of neurotransmitters. It is being increasingly recognized that dietary reactions may also play an important role in some behaviour problems. These are not the same as allergies, but may respond to similar dietary changes. There is also some anecdotal evidence of the benefits on both physical and mental condition of raw food feeding for both cats and dogs which is yet to be statistically tested.

Behaviour does not just happen. Whatever form it takes, it is an essential response to the situation in which an animal finds itself based upon its perception at the time. This is why so much of the management of behaviour, whether it is the immediate manner of handling the nervous dog or treating its fear in the longer term, focuses on environmental changes. Behavioural improvement must include both procedures that change the immediate response of an animal, e.g. environmental enrichment by the provision of a stuffed chew-toy, as well as procedures that are designed to bring about long-term learned changes in behaviour and underlying emotion, in other words, owner-based training. Of all the environmental influences to which an individual animal can be subjected, the actions of the owner, for better or worse are of ultimate importance.

Principles of animal learning

There is a common assumption that behaviour modification and training are in some way different. The reason for this is that a **modified behaviour** tends to imply a *reduction* in the expression of a behaviour an owner does not want, such as trying to bite passers-by or urinating in the wrong place. A **trained behaviour** assumes an *increase* in a more desirable performance, such as sitting rather than lunging at a passer-by, or urinating in the garden rather than in the sitting room. Both processes are dependent upon the alteration of an

animal's conditioned (learned) response to environmental information, most importantly that which is provided by the owner. They are both practical manifestations of the behavioural effects of an animal's learning. It is important to realize that, in practice rather than in theory, one process cannot happen without the other.

Conditioned, or learned, responses involve memories, associated emotions and their behavioural expression, and are evoked by changes in the environment. The manner in which environmental information is presented can however change (or modify) behaviour immediately, sometimes giving a false impression that a particular task has been learned. Only by consistent presentation of information in all contexts in which an animal 'behaves', will resultant behaviour be sufficiently rehearsed and learned to be able to say that 'training' has occurred (Figure 11.2).

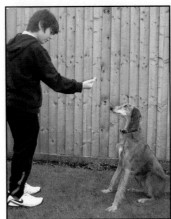

11.2 A raised hand predicting food will generate a sit response, but only if this has consistently occurred in every context of the dog's life.
© Kendal Shepherd.

Associative learning (or conditioning) occurs in one of two ways:

- **Pavlovian (or classical) conditioning** occurs when physiological and behavioural responses change as a response to previously unconnected environmental events
- **Operant (or instrumental) conditioning** occurs when an individual animal uses its behaviour to alter the response of the environment.

Classical conditioning

Classical conditioning is named after Pavlov's classical finding that once a stimulus, the ringing of a bell, which previously had no significance to dogs, was closely associated with the presentation of food, salivation (an unconditioned response that did not need to be learned) occurred equally to the sound of the bell alone as to the presentation of food. The sound of the bell had become a conditioned (or learned) stimulus predicting the arrival of food and subsequently elicited similar physiological, emotional and behavioural response as the unconditioned (unlearned) stimulus of food.

Examples of classical conditioning abound in an average dog's life: the sight of a lead predicting the excitement of a walk; the sound of a particular car engine predicting an owner's imminent arrival home; the sound of a tin-opener, rustle of a crisp packet or clicker (see later) predicting food (Figure 11.3); or the sight of a syringe in a vet's hand predicting restraint and pain (Figure 11.4). All these stimuli have no intrinsic meaning to a dog until they are reliably paired with an emotionally significant outcome.

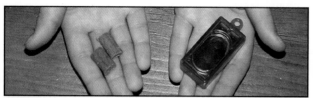

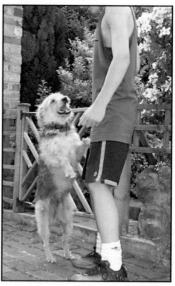

11.5 Instructing a dog to get down when jumping up in greeting will have no effect if the dog is looked at, touched, and randomly petted at the same time. © Kendal Shepherd.

11.3 A clicker becomes meaningful to a dog once reliably paired with an emotionally significant outcome, such as a food titbit. It can be used to reward both obedience (response to command) and good behaviour (e.g. tolerance of veterinary handling). © Kendal Shepherd.

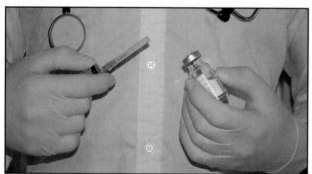

11.4 By the process of classical conditioning, the sight of a syringe in a vet's hand may come to signify impending restraint and pain. © Kendal Shepherd.

Operant conditioning

Operant conditioning is the learned effect that consequences of behaviour have upon an individual animal deciding whether the same behaviour should be performed again (operated) or not. All trained behaviour is led by its consequences, in other words what happens *after* a particular behaviour is performed. A common misconception is that a dog will sit, for example, on hearing the command word 'sit', because it has 'been told what to do'. In reality, the dog sits because the sound of the word, the appearance of the owner or trainer and the action of sitting, have all become usefully paired with a desirable consequence from the dog's perspective. This rewarding consequence may either be the gaining of something the dog wants, such as food, or the avoidance of something the dog does not want, such as a reprimand or physical coercion (positive and negative reinforcement respectively – see later). This consequence is predicted to the dog by environmental information of all kinds, verbal information being only one category upon which a dog will depend.

There is now considerable experimental evidence that visual cues are more powerful and will over-ride verbal ones, if they are not giving the same information. The simple reason why words fail in so many situations, frustrating both clients and their pets alike, is that what a person says and what their body does, or looks like, are in conflict from the perspective of their dog. Instructing a dog to 'Get down!' when jumping up in greeting will be to no avail if the dog at the same time is looked at, touched and randomly petted (Figure 11.5). In the same way, an owner may be saying 'Come ' or 'Sit', but their tone of voice, expression and posture may lead a dog to consider it would be a far better idea to run away rather than to approach and sit, if nothing in the owner's appearance predicts reward.

In all real life situations, however, the processes of **classical** and **operant conditioning** are inextricably linked. The sound of a crisp packet may herald food (*classical conditioning*) but unless a dog then uses a previously successful behaviour (*operant learning*), the food reward itself will not materialize. This is irrespective of whether the learned behaviour is convenient to us, to come and sit for example, or inconvenient, such as to jump up and grab. Some dogs may very usefully be taught that staying in their bed is a more likely way of getting the food to arrive, whereas others learn to steal when no-one is looking. Likewise, the sight of a syringe and needle may signify the association of pain, but it is the behaviour that seems to make such unpleasantness go away that will be operantly conditioned. Some dogs learn that sitting calmly does indeed eventually work in getting a veterinary surgeon to retreat, whereas others rely upon wriggling, growling and attempting to bite.

Reward and punishment

Whether a behaviour is repeated or not depends upon the reliability or predictability of consequence and this phenomenon is used in both training and behaviour modification. It is important to realize that although we tend to assume that rewards are 'nice' and punishments are 'nasty', the terms must be defined only by their results upon an animal's behaviour, therefore by the animal's own view of them, not by our human view of desirability or unpleasantness. If attempted punishments by pet owners, such as shouting or smacking, merely exacerbate problem behaviours rather than reducing them, they cannot be called punishments. In the same vein, a 'reward' in the form of a titbit of food offered for sitting is not reinforcing if, at that particular moment, a dog's preferred option is to chase ducks or escape a veterinary surgeon's clutches. This is one of the most difficult concepts for owners to grasp – that what *they* view as pleasant and rewarding, e.g. a pat on the head or a cuddle, or punishing, e.g. an angry tone of voice, a smack, or being sent to bed, is not viewed in the same way by their pet.

It is useful to remember the following rules and definitions and to visualize a practical application of each, in order to advise clients correctly:

- **Reinforcement** is defined as an environmental event that *increases* the likelihood of a behaviour being performed

- **Punishment** is defined as an environmental event that *decreases* the likelihood of a behaviour being performed.
- Both reinforcement and punishment can be **positive** or **negative**.

The **arrival** of both reinforcing and punishing events induces behavioural change as follows:

- **Positive reinforcement** is the arrival of an event, as a direct consequence of a behaviour that *increases* the likelihood of that behaviour being performed, e.g. the presentation of food as a result of sitting. If the arrival of food does indeed increase the likelihood of a dog sitting, then the food can be termed a **positive reinforcer**
- **Positive punishment** is the arrival of an event, as a direct consequence of a behaviour, that *decreases* the likelihood of that behaviour being performed, e.g. jerking on a choke chain as a result of a dog pulling ahead (Figure 11.6). But only if the application of a tight choke chain reduces the likelihood of a dog pulling in future, can it be called a **positive punishment.**

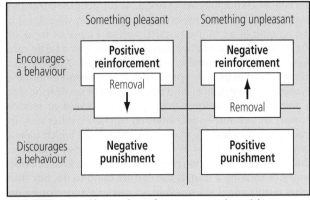

	Something pleasant	Something unpleasant
Encourages a behaviour	**Positive reinforcement** Removal ↓	**Negative reinforcement** ↑ Removal
Discourages a behaviour	**Negative punishment**	**Positive punishment**

11.7   The effects of reinforcement and punishment, both positive and negative, from the animal's perspective.

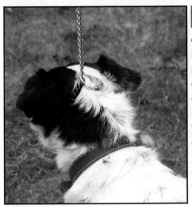

11.6   The application of a tight choke chain is an example of positive punishment only if the behaviour of pulling on the lead is reduced in the future. If behaviour does not change, it runs the risk of damage and abuse. © Kendal Shepherd.

The **removal** of both reinforcing and punishing events induces behavioural change as follows:

- **Negative reinforcement** is the removal of an event, as a direct consequence of a behaviour, that *increases* the likelihood of that behaviour being performed, e.g. the slackening (i.e. removal of tightness) of a choke chain as a result of walking to heel. Only if a slack choke chain increases the likelihood of a dog walking to heel, can it be called a **negative reinforcer**
- **Negative punishment** is the removal of an event, as a direct consequence of a behaviour, that *decreases* the likelihood of that behaviour being performed, e.g. denying a dog attention or a food reward if it jumps up. Only if the removal of the food reward decreases the likelihood of a dog jumping up, can it be called a **negative punishment.**

These rewarding or punishing consequences of behaviour are summarized in Figure 11.7. Any of them can be practically applied during training and behaviour modification to channel behaviour in a desired direction.

Many everyday items and events can be used to **reinforce** desired behaviour other than food, including toys, human attention and play. Conversely, withdrawal or denial of any

of these will constitute **negative punishment** of the behaviour that produced it. A dog that jumps up wanting attention will thus be punished by absolute denial of attention in any form. Further examples of potential **positive punishments** are: a water spray, rattle can, shouting and smacking. Withdrawal of any of these punishments will constitute **negative reinforcement** of the behaviour that produced it, so that a dog that avoids being shouted at by going to its bed, for example, will be rewarded by cessation, or lack, of shouting.

A note of caution

Explaining the principles of learning and the pressures that may be applied in order to achieve it does not imply that the end, that of a 'trained' and obedient animal, automatically justifies the means. One must be very aware of the dangers of using any punishing technique that increases threat to, or inflicts fear and pain upon, an animal in attempts to train it. While choke chains are deemed unnecessary for effective management, examples that refer to their use are given in this chapter but only to show how their application is often misunderstood. Not only should it be considered ethically unsound and contrary to principles of animal welfare to induce pain and fear in order to train any animal, but there is also a very real risk of inducing a defensively aggressive response towards any coincidental feature of the animal's environment while training is taking place. This includes innocent bystanders, human or otherwise, as well as the trainer themselves. **It is always safer, more fruitful, expedient and humane to demonstrate to an animal what is required by means of reward *before* it makes a mistake, than to punish it, by whatever means, after the event.**

Balancing reward and punishment

Underlying the use of these principles must be the understanding that negative punishment (e.g. absence of food) cannot operate without the contrast of positive reinforcement (presence of food), just as negative reinforcement (e.g. absence of choking) cannot operate without the contrast of experienced positive punishment (presence of choking). Some training classes claim that 'only reward-based methods are used'; similarly the manufacturers of punishing devices that only 'negative reinforcement' comes into play. Both these assertions imply that the essential balance between reward and punishment is not fully understood. *All* correctly used training methods must have a rewarding consequence, whether it is the gaining of a positive reward, such as a piece of food, or the avoidance of a positive punishment, such as a rattle can, water spray or the choking effect of a sliplead. The emotion of relief is an extremely potent one. It may be more relevant in certain circumstances (and therefore more reinforcing) for a dog to use behaviours that successfully avoid or reduce human threat and anger, whether applied deliberately in training or accidentally in real life, than those which gain a tasty piece of food. **As already stated, this does not mean that deliberately applying positive punishment, such as being angry or choking a dog, is the correct thing to do, nor that what a dog might do to avoid an owner's anger or being choked, is desirable or appropriate.**

Owners appear to have a natural tendency to resort by default to reprimand and attempted punishment when their dogs misbehave, implying that, for anyone involved in improving the relationship between people and their pets, a thorough grounding in the nature of punishments and how they do or do not work, and whether they are safe or advisable, is absolutely essential. A useful exercise to develop awareness of the relationship between behaviour and events is simply to observe dogs wherever they may be while asking the question, 'What is that dog doing and why?' Everyday observations will include: a dog sitting at the kerbside; a dog pulling on lead; a dog not pulling on lead; a dog chasing a ball; a dog not coming when called; a dog jumping up in greeting; a dog trying to jump off the consulting room table; and a dog sitting still.

All too often in considering behaviour, those behaviours that obviously are happening are noticed rather than those that are not happening. For example, the question 'Why did this particular dog bite?' is asked more often than the question 'Why did that particular dog not bite?'. Or, for one dog, why did it bite today when it did not bite in similar circumstances yesterday? Both questions and their answers are equally valid and are crucial to understanding fully and improving an animal's behaviour. Understanding motivation to behave 'well' and using this knowledge consistently to create more of the same behaviour, treats behaviour problems just as effectively as preventing them.

Habituation

Habituation is a form of non-associative learning, in other words, it is not connected with any particular event or feature of the environment. It is the process whereby an animal becomes used to, and learns to ignore, environmental events that have no consequence to it. In effect, environmental stimuli have neither positive nor negative significance but become emotionally neutral. Habituation is part of the socialization process in young puppies and allows the older dog to encounter new experiences without viewing them as dangerous and therefore becoming fearful. The more real-life experiences a puppy has, the less novel the world and its contents will seem later in life and the less likely fearful responses become.

Latent inhibition

Latent inhibition allows previous experiences and associations made within certain contexts to block future associations. In this way, previous good experiences and memories may protect an animal against later, less favourable, experiences in the same situation. If a dog is given tasty food in the presence of a potentially alarming stranger, once this memory and learning is in place the animal is less likely to react fearfully

or aggressively later, even if the experience is not pleasant. Awareness of the protective effect of latent inhibition is of particular importance during an animal's first contact with the veterinary practice, e.g. at puppy vaccination. It is essential that this experience is as pleasant and educational as possible if the animal is to remain tolerant and forgiving of handling and potential discomfort during later visits to the practice. Regardless of age, a dog's ability to behave well should never be taken for granted in any new situation but guided using relevant rewards as a valuable investment for the future.

Desensitization and counter-conditioning
Desensitization

Desensitization is a similar process to habituation but tends to be used in behaviour management to describe the loss of already existing negative emotions and their behavioural results that have become associated with environmental information and events. It is therefore used in treating problem behaviour rather than preventing it. Once an animal is already afraid of a particular stimulus, e.g. the sight and sound of fireworks, the stimulus must initially be presented at a low enough intensity to induce no emotional and behavioural reaction. If a dog is able to hear recorded sound, a recording of sufficient quality of various noises, including those of fireworks, may be used to gradually increase the intensity of sound to ensure continued lack of response. Success of desensitization, similar to the success of habituation, is seeing nothing, in other words, no undesirable behavioural response.

Counter-conditioning

Counter-conditioning involves the creation of new, more positive, emotional associations linked to a previously fear-inducing event. This may be achieved by presenting the animal with something that it enjoys, e.g. food or a game, in the presence of an event it would normally try to avoid, such as the appearance of the vacuum cleaner, wheelie bins, hot air balloons or noises of various descriptions. It is imperative that the animal remains calm throughout as once aroused, any attempted reward will become immaterial. The stimulus, whether real or recorded, must therefore be presented at a low enough intensity for the dog to still be able to enjoy the offered reward.

In practical terms it is not possible to create new associations with an event without operant conditioning (*how* an animal gains an emotionally significant reward) coming into play. Specifically, if a dog is asked successfully to sit in exchange for a food reward while a thunderstorm recording is played at low volume, food will both create pleasant associations with the sound as well as reward the behaviour itself. It can be difficult to convince people that the success of both desensitization and counter-conditioning exercises, as well as simple obedience training, is to see no evidence of the previously undesired behaviour. The temptation of all impatient trainers and owners is to test out success by risking failure. The ability of a dog to eat, play and respond to simple commands should therefore be used practically as a rough gauge of emotional state and as a warning of going 'too far, too fast' in training. Continuing to be able to eat and play while the intensity of stimulus increases can be taken as a measure of success of a desensitization and counter-conditioning programme. On the other hand, if negative emotions prevail and prevent a dog from eating, the exercise should be abandoned immediately as no fruitful learning can occur.

Response substitution

In behaviour management, response substitution usually refers to the specific *replacement* of a behaviour, something inconvenient to humans, with another more 'appropriate' one. For example, a dog that habitually lunges and barks at other dogs when on the lead can be taught to look to his owner instead for an expected game with a tennis ball; and jumping up in greeting can be replaced with 'sit to greet'. To achieve this, an accurate assessment must be made of *why* a dog lunges at other dogs or jumps up, in other words, its motivation, before attempting to compete with this during training. There is no point in enticing a dog with food if its over-riding desire is to play or fight. It may be necessary to combine reinforcers (e.g. tasty food + tennis ball + owner's attention) to create more behavioural leverage, as well as present a stimulus at very low intensity, for example, the sight of a dog 100 yards away, before an alternative behaviour can begin to be learned and trained.

Extinction

The process of extinction refers to a behaviour becoming gradually redundant, owing to a lack of reinforcement (negative punishment), and therefore its elimination from an animal's behavioural repertoire. This is only achieved if an expected reward is never forthcoming and it is therefore essential that this lack of reward and reinforcement is absolute and consistent. A dog that jumps up in greeting is inevitably used to being petted and cuddled in certain convenient situations but being reprimanded in others. In both cases attention given continues to reinforce the behaviour and maintain it as a result. The sudden withdrawal of attention, by folding arms and turning away, as a result of the same behaviour, is a dog's first signal that jumping up is not working as it used to. Clients must be warned of the **extinction burst**, whereby a dog may initially try harder to gain his accustomed reward. Giving in to a dog's increased demands at this time, as behaviour may seem to get worse before it gets better, is a very common reason for failure of otherwise sound advice.

Definitions and real life

Although habituation, desensitization, counter-conditioning (including response substitution) and extinction are all described as separate processes, in practical terms they generally must happen all at the same time when treating behaviour problems. There is no point in attempting to provide motivation for alternative, more convenient, behaviours (*response substitution*), if accidental or deliberate reinforcement is still continuing for what is not wanted (failure of *extinction*). However much a family may want to say hello to their dog on their return to the house, they will not be doing their visitors, or passers-by on the street, any favours by continuing to reward jumping up. The most humane way to alter emotions (*desensitization and counterconditioning*) is to train alternative behaviours (*response substitution*) using positive reward-based training methods, by which a dog will look forward (*positive emotional change*) to doing exactly as humans require, with implied loss (*extinction*) of undesirable behaviour. In this way, both emotions and behaviour are changed for the better at the same time.

Conditioned reinforcers and punishments

All potential reinforcers and punishments can be divided into:

- **Primary** – those events that do not need to be learned and are inherently rewarding (e.g. food, water, rest and play) or inherently punishing (e.g. pain and danger) to an animal
- **Secondary** – those events whose significance has to be learned, such as the sound of a whistle, the sound of a word, the sight of a raised hand or the sound of training discs or a clicker. Such stimuli, once associated with primary rewards or punishments, are termed **secondary** (or **conditioned**) **reinforcers** and **punishers**. Secondary reinforcers and punishers are used deliberately in dog training, but also occur inadvertently in every aspect of day-to-day life.

Although assumed to be intrinsically rewarding (i.e. a primary reinforcer), human praise or pleasure works most efficiently when contrasted with human displeasure or sternness. Therefore, rather than being a true positive reinforcer, it may be that praise is effective mainly via negative reinforcement; in other words, a dog learns to perform behaviours that stop humans being angry rather than those that make them pleased. Praise is also frequently linked to, and therefore predicts, more tangible rewards in the form of food and cuddles, and as such is effective also as a secondary reinforcer. A sternly issued command or pointed finger, both threatening in themselves, may be predictors of worse to come if disobedience continues. In predicting punishment, but not actually administering it, such human gestures are secondary punishers. Both secondary reinforcers and secondary punishers, as long as they are consistently followed by a primary reinforcer or punishment, come to induce the same emotional and behavioural change as the primary reinforcer or punisher that they predict.

Clicker training

Clicker training makes use of both classical and operant conditioning. Once paired with the reliable and imminent arrival of a food reward (by classical conditioning), the click becomes a 'good news' sound, inducing the same emotional change as the primary reinforcer, the food itself. It therefore becomes a sound that a dog (or other animal) wants to hear and is now a *secondary reinforcer*. Behaviours are therefore performed ('offered') by the dog in order to make the click happen and are thereby operantly conditioned. No verbal cue (later to become a 'command') is given until a certain behaviour is consistently being performed. The choice of what behaviour to perform is entirely up to the dog. The consequences of a dog's choice of behaviour are marked either with a 'click and treat' signifying success, or no click, indicating not only failure but 'try again in a different way'.

Clicker training allows for **successive approximations** – in other words, stages in progress towards a completed task, to be marked and rewarded. For example, in training an assistance dog to retrieve or pick up a set of keys, the first point at which the dog is to be 'clicked and treated' is when it is sniffing at the object on the ground. Once this is consistently being performed, the anticipated click is withheld in order to frustrate the dog into trying harder to gain a click ('raising the criteria'). Among behaviours a dog will reliably try next is to begin to mouth or pick up the object, which then earns the expected 'click and treat' for progress in the desired direction.

Failure of clicker training results from:

- Insufficient preparation in creating the close association between the sound and a food reward so that the click sound does not develop the significance that it should
- The use of the clicker as a distraction or form of 'remote control' in order to alter a dog's behaviour – if so used, the click will mark 'wrong' behaviours rather than 'right' ones
- Lack of patience in waiting for a dog to make the 'right' choice without speaking to it.

Good clicker training candidates are those dogs considered to be the most inquisitive and mischievous and who are always 'getting themselves into trouble'. Clicker training does not create behaviours – it merely selects from a dog's existing repertoire, those behaviours of which humans approve. These behaviours may then be linked together, or *chained*, to create complex sequences of behaviour, such as those required of assistance dogs. The more extensive the repertoire is to start with (the definition of a 'mischievous' dog for some people!), the more there is to select from.

Training discs

Training discs are a set of brass discs making a distinctive sound if pressed together (Figure 11.8) used correctly should signify the exact opposite of the sound of the clicker. They indicate failure or 'non-reward' and the sound of them becomes therefore a *secondary punishment*. Rather than the click predicting the arrival of a food reward, the sound of the discs is deliberately associated with removal, or loss, of food (*negative punishment*). Once trained to the significance of the sound, an animal should therefore decide for itself to desist from whichever behaviour seemed to induce the 'bad news' sound. As with the clicker, training discs are frequently misused as distractions or a means of startling a dog into behaving differently rather than truly communicating a specific educational message. Even if used correctly, training discs do not direct the animal towards 'good' behaviour but simply punish the 'bad'.

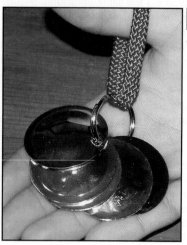

11.8 Training discs.
© Kendal Shepherd.

Vocal communication

The word, 'Yes!', if used consistently, can replace the sound of a click to mark a successful behaviour just as, by contrast, the word, 'No!' can, and should, signify simple failure and 'Try again!'. Almost universally however, the word 'No!' is used in a 'Stop it or else!' fashion in conjunction with threatening human body gestures and, as such, becomes a predictor of positive, rather than negative, punishment. The practical consequence is the considerable number of dogs presented for behaviour therapy that growl and bite when reprimanded, or in situations when historically a physical reprimand has been proved very likely. All too often a dog does not know how to pre-empt the threat of punishment: in other words, a human-approved or 'correct' behaviour has never been reinforced in the first place and punishment has been applied inconsistently to all other behavioural alternatives. If this is the case, then anxiety and subsequent aggression is a common consequence. If, however, an approved-of behaviour has already been firmly established by means of reward, a dog will know exactly how to avoid a threatened punishment. It can therefore remain in control of a situation, without the generation of uncertainty and anxiety or any need for aggression.

Advice on dog training and communication pitfalls

What is obedience?

When asked to define what constitutes an obedient dog an owner will invariably answer, 'One who does what he is told'. This implies not only a knowledge of the meaning of words on the part of their dog but also that a dog should have no other reason for behaving other than to please its owner and prevent them becoming angry. While this may well succeed in certain circumstances, this is definitely on the basis of 'more by luck than judgement'.

When beginning any discussion regarding behaviour modification or training, one should always ensure that an owner is aware that obedience training is simply the means of encouraging their dog's *own choice* of behaviour to coincide with the owner's choice. Intrinsic to successful obedience training is therefore the transfer of explicit and reliable information from owner to dog. For this to be successful, the owner must have clearly decided what it is their pet should do and they must give information to their dog equally clearly, if it is to understand what is required. Of utmost importance is that the means of giving information must also predict to the dog *why* it should comply, regardless of context. Both the words and the appearance of the owner must always predict where the reward is coming from and what form it will take. There is no point in a raised closed hand predicting food (regardless of whether food is in the hand) and smiling encouragement from a standing position being the cue for a 'sit' when a dog is young and in puppy class, for this to be converted to a downward pointed finger and a frown from a seated position on the settee when the dog is older and standing in front of the television. Similarly, if a sit has been taught with an upward yank of a choke chain and downward push of the hindquarters, this will be of no use if the dog is off lead and free in the park.

The need for an ultimate behavioural goal

One of the reasons for the success of an experienced trainer over a typical pet dog owner, whether using positive or negative reinforcement to direct behaviour, is the ability to recognize an **ultimate behavioural goal**. Experienced trainers have a specific end in sight for which they not only select the most suitable dog but also have the ability to train the dog they have already selected. A dog that shows inappropriate behaviours and traits for a given task is not likely to be selected in the first place. Successful trainers will also work towards a specific goal and appreciate that they are training their dog whenever and wherever they are with it, resulting in reliable behavioural results and expectations in their dog. These goals are clearly communicated to the dog through consistent and unambiguous signals, giving the dog information that persists across all real-life contexts.

Pet dog owners, on the other hand, frequently 'fall in love' with the most unpromising material and this often means the least suitable dogs fall into the least experienced and able hands. In general, the average pet dog owner has no idea of what they need or how to educate a dog to perform to requirements. They are not aware of the need for the giving of consistent information in all situations, alternately cuddling and reprimanding as they see fit to ultimate canine confusion. This must be taken into account in any advice given to pet dog clients but without implying fault for any ill-informed judgement or choices. However, for the majority of the time, the dog–human relationship is successful, regardless of inconsistency and such ill-informed choices, without any deliberate professional intervention. Any advice given must therefore take into account the historical and emotional needs of each party, while at the same time giving practical and educational advice.

Positive training for real life

Just as a client's primary concern regarding physical illness and injury is that the clinical sign (e.g. limping, vomiting, scratching) should go away, the ubiquitous requirement when help is needed for behaviour problems is that the dog **stops doing** whatever behaviour it is that has become irritating, dangerous or expensive, or a combination of all three. In order to try to stop a dog biting, chewing the contents of the house or urinating in the kitchen at night, for example, various means of punishment will have inevitably been tried already with little or no success.

Trying to stop behaviour using punishment, with or without forethought and planning, implies a human belief that a dog must already have 'misbehaved' in order to justify the action. Animals have no concept of 'right' or 'wrong' and punishment gives an animal no clue as to what it should be doing instead. The means whereby punishment is avoided, in other words, which behaviour is negatively reinforced, is largely left to chance and may or may not result in behavioural improvement. Human anger as a punishment all too frequently simply triggers potentially dangerous aggression.

Rarely is enough time spent deciding **how a dog should behave** in all real-life contexts, let alone training it to perform as required. The assumption is made that early training lasts for life and that a dog will continue to sit because 'we said so' rather than for anything more tangible. In addition, in situations for which a dog has not been trained and where it may find the 'right' decision impossible to make, it will often be viewed as 'disobedient' and 'stubborn' and not deserving of reward. In practical terms, however, the greatest reward must be on offer at the very times when a dog may be about to be the worst behaved, if it is to be encouraged to make the right choice. For example, the most desirable food or toy may be needed to reward tolerance and to pre-empt snapping on veterinary handling or at a passing stranger.

Using positive reward-based training methods not only ensures that behaviour is channelled consistently in the right direction but also reduces the number of decisions a dog has to make on a 'threat/no threat' (i.e. the threat of punishment versus successful avoidance) basis. Any communication with dogs that does not involve threatening them will significantly reduce, if not actually eliminate, their need for an aggressive response.

Figure 11.9 illustrates a simple means whereby dog owners can be encouraged to think ahead in preparing their pets thoroughly for when life becomes challenging. An analogy is made with teaching a child to swim. No-one needs to know how to swim in the shallow end, for there they are able to stand. But, with forethought, parents know that being able to swim will become essential once a child is out of its depth. Very few dogs are prepared in the same way.

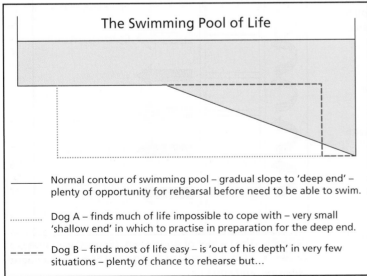

The Swimming Pool of Life

———— Normal contour of swimming pool – gradual slope to 'deep end' – plenty of opportunity for rehearsal before need to be able to swim.

············ Dog A – finds much of life impossible to cope with – very small 'shallow end' in which to practise in preparation for the deep end.

– – – – Dog B – finds most of life easy – is 'out of his depth' in very few situations – plenty of chance to rehearse but...

11.9 Dog A finds much of life hard to cope with and consequently rarely behaves well. Dog B behaves well most of the time, only rarely finding himself 'out of his depth'. But both dogs are viewed as being 'good' and behaving well when unchallenged – the equivalent of the 'shallow end'. At such times neither is deemed to need training or reward, as they are both already 'being good'. They are therefore completely unprepared for what to do in the 'deep end', when both will be considered to be behaving badly. Any attempt to alter 'bad' behaviour is then far too late, in exactly the same way as would be attempting to teach a child to swim in the deep end of the pool. To help all dogs, good behaviour must be appreciated and rewarded at all times and a slope created gradual enough for them to learn calmly and accurately in preparation for potential problem situations ahead. © Kendal Shepherd.

Obedience and 'good behaviour'

Owners are generally unaware of the difference between an **obedient** dog and a **well behaved** one. It is however perfectly possible for a dog to be obedient and not well behaved at all, or to be exceptionally well behaved without knowing the meaning of a single obedience command. Well trained obedient dogs appear to be presented as frequently for counselling, owing to their unacceptable behaviour, as are completely uneducated ones.

Often, dogs are well behaved only by chance: they are making their own choices as to what to do but their behaviour happens to be convenient and pleasurable to their owners. In effect, information from the environment is sufficient for the dog to make an appropriate decision: e.g., the television is turned on and the dog lies down at its owner's feet, or a visitor arrives and the dog lies down in its bed. Such ideal dogs may be the result of evolutionary selection for an ability to read human behaviour rather than the training skill of the owner. Commands and rewards therefore appear to be unnecessary as the dog is already doing as its owner wishes for the vast majority of the time.

The result is that the very words that are needed to give a dog successful guidance when life gets difficult, distracting or threatening are never thoroughly rehearsed when the dog is calm and amenable enough for teaching and learning. In real life, as opposed to training class, owners often try to change a dog's mind only when it has already made an inconvenient, dangerous, damaging or painful decision. They do not practise achieving a truly obedient dog, one whose choice of behaviour can be altered to coincide with theirs by means of a cue word or signal, until the situation is so distracting, exciting or threatening that the dog will find it impossible to comply.

Considerable progress may be made with many problem animals simply by making an owner aware of 'good behaviour', in other words, lack of bad behaviour, and encouraging them to notice and appreciate it in a manner meaningful to their pet rather than ignore it. Rather than expecting the dog to perform a task to earn a 'click and treat', the clicker can be used to mark and reward any behaviour that *isn't* 'bad', particularly in situations where 'bad' behaviour might have been expected. In the absence of a clicker, the spontaneously performed good behaviour should be labelled, e.g. 'Good sit' or 'Good lie down', and followed with the delivery of a food reward. Owners are thereby taught to concentrate on encouraging good behaviour from their pet, rather than waiting for the dog to misbehave and then being forced to intervene.

Top tips for real life training

- Remember that an obedience command is simply a means of giving information in order to change a dog's mind and must be continually rehearsed.
- Keep body gestures consistent in all contexts and with or without food in hand.
- Praise the behaviour, e.g. 'Good sit', not the dog – praise should maintain behaviour, not end it.
- Reward difficulty of task not quality – the puppy or adult finding it the hardest, deserves the most reward.
- Never take any 'good' behaviour for granted – reward it as often as obedience.
- Do not get angry!

Canine appeasement behaviour and body language

The appearance of appeasing (or calming) and threat-averting behaviour is, for the most part, enormously appealing to humans and is likely to have formed at least part of the basis upon which selection and rejection has been made since the domestication process began. In other words, people love dogs who look like they love them. Recognizing what appeasement behaviour looks like, understanding its purpose and responding appropriately to it are therefore all of crucial importance in preventing dogs from needing to bite. On the other hand, misunderstanding and misinterpreting the nature and purpose of appeasement behaviour frequently results in inappropriate human responses which ultimately damage a dog's trust in people with potentially disastrous results.

The Ladder of Aggression (Figure 11.10) is a sequence of calming and threat-averting gestures that dogs give with the intention of achieving an immediate reduction in the threat perceived. These gestures are nothing to do with supposed dominant or submissive states of mind. If responded to appropriately, escalation to overt and potentially damaging aggression is pre-empted and avoided. The more intense the gesture (higher up the ladder), the more important it is that a dog's expression of unease and discomfort is understood. If it is not understood, then the risk of a dog being forced to retaliate and bite as a response increases significantly.

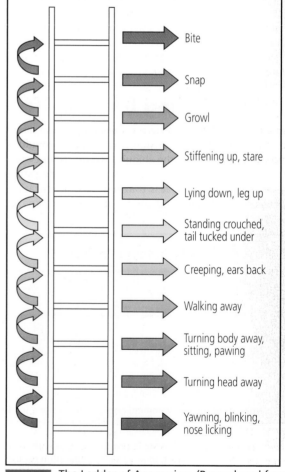

Bite

Snap

Growl

Stiffening up, stare

Lying down, leg up

Standing crouched, tail tucked under

Creeping, ears back

Walking away

Turning body away, sitting, pawing

Turning head away

Yawning, blinking, nose licking

11.10 The Ladder of Aggression. (Reproduced from *BSAVA Manual of Canine and Feline Behavioural Medicine, 2nd edn.*)

The apparently guilty dog (see middle rungs of ladder) who 'knows he has done wrong' is in reality giving threat-averting gestures designed to calm and appease. Such body language has a genetic basis and will be displayed at the instant uncertainty and threat are perceived. Once an association has been made by the dog between specific environmental information, (e.g. urine in the kitchen, a chewed sofa, raided rubbish) and an unpleasant and threatening event (e.g. human anger and punishment) then a learned attempt to pre-empt and avert a predicted threat will be made. The dog does not know that such behaviours are inherently 'wrong', nor can it make such a retrospective connection between its own previous behaviour and punishment; nonetheless, an almost universal human assumption is made that such body language indicates an acknowledgement of guilt and an apology. This in turn seems to justify the use of punishment on the premise that the dog knew it should not do it and will thereby 'learn not to do it again' (Figures 11.11 and 11.12).

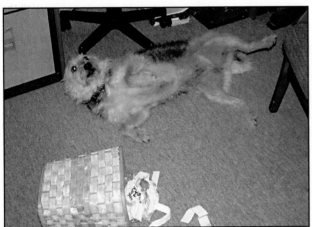

11.11   The 'lying down, leg up' gesture (see Ladder of Aggression, Figure 11.10) signifying 'You're threatening me – please stop it now' is almost universally misinterpreted as an expression of guilt. Continuing to reprimand and attempt to punish carries the risk of inducing aggression rather than improving 'bad' behaviour. © Kendal Shepherd.

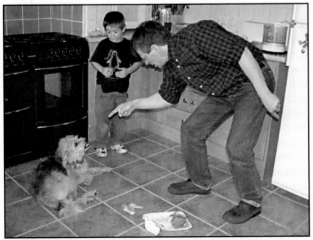

11.12   This dog has already growled in response to reprimand and is also at risk of associating the punishment with the presence of a child and its own need for an aggressive response. So-called 'unpredictable' aggression towards children may therefore emerge in the future. © Kendal Shepherd.

Such a human response merely increases the threat to an already threatened dog and is perceived as unjustified aggression, thereby warranting an aggressive response. If a dog learns that the more subtle calming and 'negotiating' stages of the Ladder of Aggression, such as turning the head away, walking away or even growling are ineffective, they may be dispensed with and a bite selected immediately as the only strategy humans seem to understand. By punishing the 'guilty' look, the very behaviours for which dogs have been selected are devalued. Many so-called 'unpredictably' aggressive dogs result from the very predictable misinterpretation by humans of the Ladder of Aggression. From a dog's perspective, much of what humans do, particularly when coercive and threatening training methods are used, is simply intrusive, unpredictable and incomprehensible.

The fallacy of dominance

Another universal area of misunderstanding for owners is the concept of dominance. Based upon historical study of captive wolves it has been wrongly assumed that the wolf pack is structured in a hierarchical manner, with aggressive behaviour being an essential feature in maintaining an individual's position within this hierarchy. It has also been assumed that so-called 'dominance' is a desirable state and that the wolf, and its relative the domestic dog, will fight to obtain it. Recent studies of free-living wolves reveal a society far more akin to that of humans, which avoids aggression whenever possible. Rather than in packs, wolves live in family units with parents guiding, teaching and only sometimes chastising their offspring. Once reaching adolescence, young wolves may leave the family group and set up a family of their own. As in human society, each individual within a family group develops an expectation of its relationship with others and the outcomes of interactions between them. The avoidance of aggression by readily understood social gestures and the use of aggression only when absolutely necessary, is a particular feature of wolves, as it is of dogs.

There is no evidence that dogs use the concept of social dominance, in other words, a desire to be in overall control, to motivate their behaviour. In fact it is very doubtful that they are capable of such a concept. Current thinking therefore measures and assesses dog behaviour in terms of what an individual has learned to expect from its companions and environment, and which of its repertoire of behaviours, including aggression, are rewarded and reinforced, rather than by any false notion of dominance or submission. Apparent 'dominance', or the appearance of controlling others, is therefore created purely by behavioural outcomes. It may become the expectation of a dog but it is never the intention. The term 'dominance aggression' is therefore a contradiction in terms and anyone referring to such a supposed diagnosis should be considered suspect in terms of their true understanding of the social nature and behaviour of dogs.

In managing behaviour, whether deliberately or accidentally, it does not matter whether the owner believes he is training his dog to sit by giving food or a dog believes it is training its owner to give food by sitting. The behaviour of both human and dog is reinforced at the same time and this is the basis of the ideal dog–human relationship. For many dogs, the balance of this relationship is accidentally skewed in their favour in many day-to-day circumstances that may lead, not to a dog thinking of itself as 'dominant' or 'in control', but to where humans seem to 'do as they are told' most of the time. For example: a dog scratches at the back door and is let out to relieve itself; a dog presents a ball at its owner's feet or lap and is obediently played with; or a dog barks and the postman leaves or the dog is taken for a walk or fed. These are not seen as significant events by humans, and indeed may be convenient and pleasurable, but have a continual and cumulative effect upon the dog's perception of the consequences of its interactions with its human companions.

This would not of itself cause a problem, if it were not for the commandeering of so-called states of 'dominance' and 'submission' into coercive management and training techniques. These dictate that if a dog is assumed to be 'dominant' or 'in control', an owner should then assume control by physical and threatening means. Threatening behaviour on the part of an owner will, in turn, elicit threat-averting behaviour on the part of their dog, which can be wrongly interpreted as 'submission' or even 'obedience' (see Ladder of Aggression). However, threatening behaviour, particularly if unexpected and unjustified, will be seen by the dog as a reason to escalate overt aggression in response.

Commonly recommended exercises, such as rolling a dog on to its back to assert 'dominance' are a *test* of canine tolerance and human control in a given context only and do nothing to create a perception of a human's supposed superiority. If applied forcefully enough, they may convince a dog that a certain person is dangerous and is to be obeyed at all costs. However, if a dog is fearful of human handling, these techniques are extremely ill-advised as they can be very dangerous. Supposed attempts at asserting dominance by humans can only be seen by the dog as acts of aggression. They are particularly risky if attempted by individuals who do not normally take control and may not be physically able to appear dangerous enough, generally women and children. Such exercises should **never** be recommended as part of either treatment or a preventive behaviour management programme when there are much more humane, informed and less risky ways of altering a dog's choice of how to behave. Rather than physically taking control of a dog's body, the humane and safe alternative is to take control of the consequences of a dog's actions in order to alter its decisions and long-term behaviour.

Prevention of behaviour problems

Pet selection and breeder responsibility

Problem prevention begins with the breeder in choosing which animals to breed from and how their offspring are reared before they are sold. If working with breeders, it is essential to emphasize the importance of their role in prevention of behaviour problem. Despite the breeder's aim to create an animal that conforms to a breed standard, an over-riding concern must be that the animal behaves in a socially acceptable way. To achieve this, the breeder of any puppy, pure or cross-bred, has a responsibility to ensure that from the start that puppy is gently but routinely exposed to the range of environmental stimuli that it will be expected to cope with in later life including, most importantly, human handling.

Owners of 'rescued' dogs will often interpret fear and aggression as the result of previous 'deliberate cruelty and abuse', but it is far more likely to be the result of a lack of appropriate environmental experience in the first 3 months of life, for which, more often than not, the breeder is responsible. The age at which caution begins to over-ride the desire to explore, and therefore the age at which the ability to learn good things about the environment begins to be inhibited by fear, is for most breeds between 7 and 8 weeks. Certain breeds, such as the German Shepherd Dog, may become fearful as early as 5 weeks of age, explaining why they have become so useful as 'guard' and 'attack' breeds. However much breeder clients may give the impression that they already 'know it all', it is a duty of the veterinary practice team to inform them of the essential nature of the socialization process and how routine exposure to real life should not be left to chance. It should be deliberately arranged by the breeder and continued in the puppy's or kitten's new home.

In selecting a new pet, in terms of both nature and nurture, it is not only important that owners appreciate the behaviour and needs of the species and breed of pet they are choosing, but also that they are honest about their own lifestyle, needs and capabilities. The criteria for purchasing only from a reputable breeder should not simply include a good pedigree, optimal diet and spotless living conditions. Particularly for dogs and cats, a highly sociable early environment may be far more behaviourally beneficial than one where hygiene and cleanliness is paramount.

Settling in a new home

Some time should be spent preparing the home for the new arrival in order that the environment provided is set up to encourage appropriate behaviour from the outset. Although an animal from the wrong environment will be stressed and may be more likely to develop problems, of over-riding importance is the early relationship with humans, which should be immediately established on sound behavioural principles. The puppy should be imagined as a much larger animal and socially acceptable behaviour encouraged by reward from the start. Owners may need advice on suitably educational toys for their pet and in the case of small mammals, reptiles and birds, standard housing is often not the same as appropriate housing if normal behaviour is to be considered (see Chapter 12).

It is essential to explain to owners of a new puppy that their new canine acquisition is much more advanced in developmental terms than they may realise. A 10-week-old puppy is the equivalent of a 5-year-old child (Figure 11.13) and is equally capable of learning to 'say please'. Treating puppies as babies, whose every demand has to be met immediately, leads the puppy to believe that demanding behaviour is what owners want. Inappropriate, inconvenient and sometimes dangerous behaviours are thus maintained into adolescence and adulthood.

Often, owners are told that a puppy must be kept indoors until at least a week after the second vaccination, resulting in a puppy's first contact with the world being as late as 14 weeks of age. An appropriate balance must be struck between the risk of infection and the risk of under-socialization and habituation, with consequent development of equally life-threatening anti-social and fear-related problems. Carrying a dog out into a town where it can see and experience the sights, sounds and smells of the city is a simple way to habituate a dog to many stimuli at minimal risk.

The reasons for neutering and its benefits are routinely discussed during puppy vaccination. Whether considering

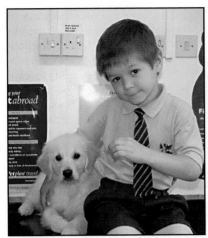

11.13 This 10-week-old puppy and 5-year-old child are developmental equivalents but will be treated very differently by average parents and dog owners. © Kendal Shepherd. (Reproduced from *BSAVA Manual of Canine and Feline Behavioural Medicine, 2nd edn.*)

spaying or castration, emphasis should be placed upon physical benefits and the prevention of conditions associated with the entire dog, such as pyometra or prostatic disease, rather than any future behavioural effects. In terms of behaviour, castration should be considered purely as a means of preventing unwanted puppies and testosterone-related behaviours such as territorial marking, rather than reliably preventing or treating other behavioural complaints, such as disobedience, poor recall, boisterousness or aggression.

Puppy parties and classes

The assumed aim of puppy parties and classes is to create a sociable animal that will be able to cope with all life events without becoming fearful or aggressive. Although the terms 'party' and 'class' are frequently used interchangeably, **puppy parties** refers to pleasantly habituating the puppy to the practice, the consulting room table, other puppies and human handling, whereas the term **puppy classes** infers specific obedience training and learning for real life as well. It may be that most veterinary premises are more suitable for the running of parties, to habituate the puppy to that particular practice and its staff, than to the more ambitious and essential role of the puppy class.

However and wherever they are conducted, for classes or parties to contribute to behavioural success, owners must be realistic as to what will be achieved by attendance. Over-optimistic expectations on the part of both dog and owner may be more damaging than not attending at all. Most owners have the frequently unrealistic requirement that their dogs should either ignore all other dogs when out walking, or 'play nicely' with them should the opportunity arise and it be convenient for the owner. But an animal cannot learn to 'play nicely' unless it has the chance to practise, nor will a dog ignore other dogs upon request unless its owner makes deliberate, concerted and continual efforts to remain the most important feature in the dog's life whatever else is happening. If such effort is not made, ignoring the owner completely in favour of the highly self-rewarding behaviour of play may be all that is learned instead.

The essential lessons of puppy class are that the dog's owner must be instructed in how to retain mental control of their dogs at all times and in all situations, and that practising

such control must continue throughout a dog's life. A common finding in treating behaviour problems later is the false assumption that puppy class lessons last for life without rehearsal and without considering it necessary to continue to reward a dog for a job well done. Puppies are given food rewards, but adults are expected to obey and tolerate anything life presents to them for human pleasure alone.

Studies have shown that puppies under the influence of pheromone treatment are calmer, less fearful, less noisy and have more successful interactions with both dogs and people during puppy class. Use of pheromones in the diffuser form in this context may therefore enhance effective learning by increasing an individual dog's social awareness and subsequent social skills.

Veterinary practices should consider running their own puppy classes, but only if the expertise exists to manage them correctly and sufficient space is available. An ill-informed, badly run and cramped puppy class may cause more problems than it alleviates. Alternatively, one of a growing number of professional puppy trainers may be used to deliver a structured programme at the practice. It is crucial to check the qualifications and experience of anyone invited to deliver classes or training in the name of the practice, as the standard of service can vary enormously. These classes should combine basic obedience training with socialization, plenty of non-threatening handling, and lots of novel stimuli provided in a controlled and pleasant environment. Puppies are taught what is acceptable and what is not (e.g. jumping up and mouthing). All vaccinated puppies can be invited to the classes and given the opportunity to mix with puppies of their own age and new people. This is not only an important service, but an excellent public relations exercise for the practice, and a lot of fun for all involved.

Minimizing behavioural damage during veterinary intervention
Reading a dog's body language

It should be remembered that:

- The purpose of appeasement behaviour is to deflect threat and restore harmony
- Devaluing appeasement behaviour forces a dog towards aggressive behaviour.

Unfortunately, appeasement behaviour is consistently ignored, misunderstood and devalued in the veterinary consulting room and surgery, to the detriment of staff, owners and the pet.

An animal's preferred option when faced with a threat is to retreat from it. The minute such retreat is unavailable, the conversion of 'flight' to 'fight' becomes more likely, if not inevitable. Raising a paw, tucking the tail under or putting the ears back are all evidence of a dog's desire for a perceived threat to diminish (see Ladder of Aggression, Figure 11.10). In cats, hunching the body or laying the ears back are similar signs of avoidance. Whenever veterinary attention and interference continues in spite of such signalling, the animal is slightly less likely to use such signals next time and more likely to opt for overt aggression. Every effort must therefore be made to understand what the animal in the clinic is trying to convey and to avoid forcing it to learn that aggression is necessary in this situation.

Vaccination

A pet's vaccination is likely to be its first experience of the practice and must be viewed as an opportunity to predict the same message as is conveyed in puppy or kitten parties/ classes. If an animal has already attended a class then there is a chance to reinforce overtly what has already been learned. If a concerted effort is not made to make the practice appear 'nice', but things are left to chance, there is the very real possibility that the animal's perception will be converted to one of 'nasty', with the risk of consequently fearful and aggressive responses. It is a sad indictment of a consistent lack of veterinary attention to the nurturing of a positive attitude among their patients, that so many clients assume that their pets 'hate coming to the vets'. By contrast, what is demonstrated at this time should not only create animals that are convenient and safe for veterinary staff to handle, but should also provide a model for humane and educational owner interactions with the pet for the rest of its life.

Whatever time is available for a vaccination consultation, the majority of it should be spent feeding or playing with the puppy or kitten, and using ample and tasty food rewards to demonstrate the principles of both associative and operant conditioning (Figure 11.14). At this stage in their lives, there are very few puppies that will not want to eat – but only if nothing nasty has happened to them first. There is little point in trying to 'make friends' after the event. Asking the owner to feed the puppy or kitten while its ears, teeth, skin and nails are examined creates pleasant associations with handling. Waiting until a puppy or kitten sits on the table before food is given, rather than pestering at the hand containing the food, demonstrates operant conditioning. If these very simple lessons are taken into every aspect of a pet's life, fewer behaviour problems will occur later.

Whether these exercises are carried out by the veterinary surgeon or the veterinary nurse, it is essential that both deliver the same message to the patient. At the point of giving the injection, owners should be asked to release the animal and tease it instead with a particularly tasty treat or toy. The owner should be instructed to present the food at the exact time of the injection (Figure 11.15). Such an approach produces animals who very rarely even notice the procedure, and who may indeed look forward positively to the next one, and prevents the apparent need to grab the animal suddenly and restrain it to prevent escape. The stimulus of restraint itself, once associated with pain, is at great risk of triggering a fearful and aggressive response during subsequent visits.

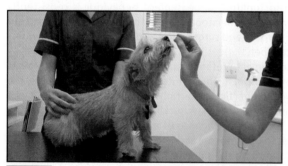

11.14 Presenting food to a puppy in the consulting room will make pleasant associations with handling through classical conditioning, as well as deliberately rewarding appropriate behaviour, such as to sit, through operant conditioning. © Kendal Shepherd. (Reproduced from *BSAVA Manual of Canine and Feline Behavioural Medicine, 2nd edn.*)

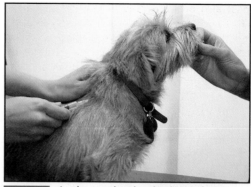

11.15 As the vaccination is given, the puppy should be played with and given food, preferably without restraint, to prevent the stimulus of restraint itself triggering painful memories and potential aggression. © Kendal Shepherd. (Reproduced from *BSAVA Manual of Canine and Feline Behavioural Medicine, 2nd edn.*)

Use of classical and operant conditioning at the surgery

Positive reinforcement of good behaviour and obedience

One of the biggest mistakes to make is to take good behaviour for granted, wherever the animal might be. This is of particular importance at the veterinary practice where the most commonly made observation by owners is that 'he used to be fine'. The simple reason a dog is no longer 'fine' in the practice is that its previous tolerance was unappreciated and unrewarded. For all dogs that are able to eat in the surgery, tasty food should be available for all staff to give routinely both to maintain pleasant associations with the premises and to reinforce good behaviour and obedience (Figure 11.16).

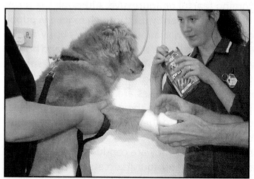

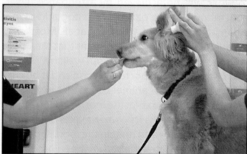

11.16 Whether a patient appears to need it or not, food should continue to be used to maintain pleasant associations and to reward tolerance of all veterinary handling procedures. © Kendal Shepherd. (Reproduced from *BSAVA Manual of Canine and Feline Behavioural Medicine, 2nd edn.*)

Owners must also be instructed in how to give clear information to their dogs and not to alter the way they give commands because they are now at the practice. A dog will not behave consistently if the verbal and visual signals given by the owner vary from one situation to another, or depending on whether they have food rewards in their hand or not. Training classes are very rarely conducted with a handbag in one hand and a baby buggy in the other, but owners must act as if they are in training class or in their kitchen at home if dogs are to be expected to behave in the same way. If a dog has been clicker-trained then this device should not be left at home at the very times when a dog might need the information it gives the most.

Even if an owner has attended training classes, when stressed and worried they frequently revert to meaningless instructions such as 'Come on, behave yourself!' that their dog has never heard before. If owners can simply be reminded to give a clear 'sit' and 'stay' command to their dog, preceded by the dog's name only, many will achieve remarkably instant results.

Veterinary staff should consider which specific behaviour will be of use, if not essential, for the future so that owners can be advised about the behaviours to rehearse at home in preparation for the visit to the practice. Conditioning positive emotional expectations and associated behaviour to commands will ensure that both behaviour and underlying emotions will remain stable if not actually improve with subsequent visits (Figure 11.17).

Commands of particular use for veterinary visits

- 'Sit!'
- 'Stand!'
- 'Lie down!'
- 'Stay!' (remain in previous position)
- 'Roll-over!'
- 'Watch me!' (watch owner rather than anything else)
- 'This way!' (follow as handler turns away)

Food should also be used to demonstrate to owners how to create pleasant associations with items or events that a dog or cat may already associate with pain or discomfort and now be afraid of. Common culprits are nail clippers, bottles of ear drops (Figure 11.18) and grooming tools. The clicker is ideal for rewarding, not obedience in this situation, but tolerance and lack of reaction.

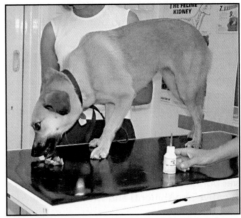

11.18 If items, such as a bottle of ear drops, are already associated with pain and discomfort, food should be used to help reverse these associations and encourage tolerance. © Kendal Shepherd. (Reproduced from *BSAVA Manual of Canine and Feline Behavioural Medicine, 2nd edn.*)

Negative reinforcement of good behaviour and obedience

Food is not the only reward that can be offered to animals, as relief from unwelcome attention or danger is also an extremely potent motivator. Although nearly all puppies are happy to eat in the consulting room, unfortunately a proportion of adult dogs simply turn and back away as a result of previous bad experiences. A typical owner response is either that, 'he won't take food from strangers', which should be interpreted as 'he's worried by strangers,' or, 'he remembers

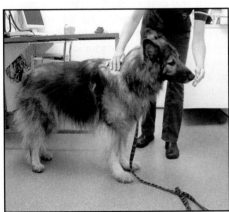
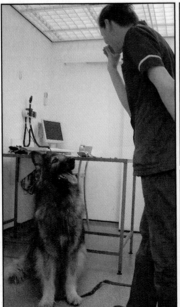
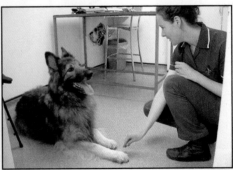
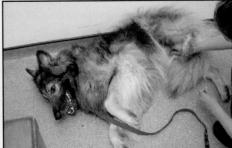

11.17 Thoroughly rehearsing simple obedience tasks *in situ* will not only train behaviours to facilitate veterinary handling, but also help keep the patient's emotions stable. © Kendal Shepherd. (Reproduced from *BSAVA Manual of Canine and Feline Behavioural Medicine, 2nd edn.*)

what happened last time' and is therefore worried by specific strangers, such as veterinary surgeons and veterinary nurses. Use can still be made of desirable events in order to try to maintain behaviour that allows a veterinary surgeon or veterinary nurse to do their job.

Most clinical tasks can be performed with a dog that reliably sits and stays sitting for a prerequisite time. The reward offered to the dog in order to maintain a 'sit' as a useful behaviour in the consulting room, is the opportunity to leave the room. This can be trained using the following procedure.

1. With the dog on the lead, approach the closed consulting room door as if to leave, putting a hand on the door as if to open it, and ask the dog to sit.
2. Open the door only if the dog obeys the request straight away (Figure 11.19)
3. If the dog does not comply immediately, in addition to not opening the door ask the owner to turn away from their dog, keeping the lead slack, thereby demonstrating how to deliver punishment effectively by withdrawal of attention (negative punishment) and without the need for threat.

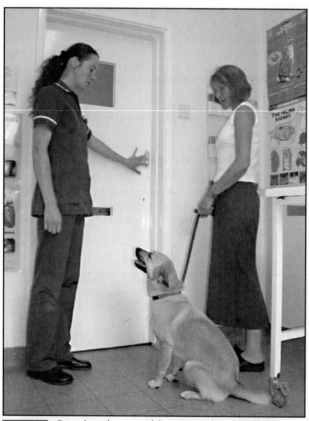

11.19 Opening the consulting room door to allow a dog to leave only if the patient sits first, can be used to reward appropriate behaviour. © Kendal Shepherd.

Most dogs will quickly learn to sit and wait for the double rewards of regaining their owner's attention and being able to leave the room. Sitting thus becomes a valuable behaviour both for veterinary staff and patient. This request can then be used to give even an anxious dog guidance in the clinic and elsewhere. A little patience is all that is required.

Using conditioned emotional responses

Although a dog may not take food if offered from the hand of a veterinary surgeon or veterinary nurse, the same food item may be readily accepted from the hand of the owner, the explanation simply being that one hand is less threatening than the other. For a certain number of dogs, however, they are simply too worried by the environment of the clinic to take food even from the hand of the owner. If the same dog is asked to sit by the owner, at the same time ensuring that the owner's body language looks as if they are relaxed and happy rather than stressed by being in the practice, a considerable proportion of dogs will not only comply with the command, but will then also accept the food item. In this situation, the previous experience of the 'sit' word and body language of the owner is being used to produce a **conditioned emotional response** (Figure 11.20).

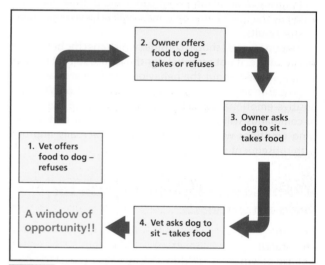

11.20 Previously existing positive emotional responses to command words and gestures, such as to sit, will induce positive emotional change in anxious or fearful dogs. © Kendal Shepherd.

Such emotional change for the better, induced when a familiar word is heard and gesture seen, allows the dog to relax sufficiently to eat. In other words, the 'sit' command results in eating rather than a dog sitting in order to gain food. It is then highly likely that a sit command issued by the veterinary surgeon or veterinary nurse will also be obeyed and food eaten as a result. Once this breakthrough in communication is made, a window of opportunity is created whereby a dog's view of the practice and consulting room can be improved.

Minimizing stress on admission

Pheromone products appear to have a calming effect on both dogs and cats in the clinic, by helping to reduce the perceived novelty of the environment. But there are also many other simple measures that can help shift the balance away from fearful or anxious expectations. The more that the same commands the dog is familiar with at home can be used at the clinic, the less novel the environment will seem. Conditioned emotional responses to standard obedience commands are invaluable in buffering the dog against potentially fear-provoking novelty. In order to minimize the impact of the hospital, it is therefore worth asking a few basic questions as part of the admission procedure. The following questions are equally relevant to day patients as to hospitalized ones, the only difference being that dogs staying overnight or longer have more opportunity for learning.

- How has your dog been trained?
  (*What emotional responses have been conditioned and why?*)
- What words does he/she know?
  (*Use the same ones!*)
- Any concerns regarding reactivity to noises?
  (*Protect dog in hospital/early intervention for treatment*)
- Where does the dog usually eliminate? On command or 'asks' to go out?
  (*Gravel, grass, earth, concrete*)
- What is the dog's reaction to other dogs?
  (*May govern kennelling choice*)
- What is usual lead restraint? How does he/she behave on the lead?
  (*Pre-prepare with Halti or Gentle leader*)
- How does the dog react to grooming, both at home and at groomer's?
  (*If better at groomer's, possibly consider owner-absent examination/basket muzzle training*)

'First aid' for common behaviour problems

The following should not be considered a comprehensive guide to the treatment of commonly encountered behaviour problems but a means of informing the client of the sort of measures that may be recommended during behaviour therapy, whether supplied in-practice or by referral elsewhere.

It is important to emphasize that there is rarely a 'quick fix' for behaviour problems, but that commitment, both in terms of time and money, is required. It is essential to determine all the causes of a problem, including any contribution that medical conditions may make, and any behaviourist the practice uses must have the recognized expertise to achieve this. At the same time, the behaviour of a considerable number of dogs will be improved, regardless of the nature of the problem behaviour, by imparting information on general principles and how to resolve commonly made mistakes as already discussed.

Aggression

Any dog bite reported to the veterinary practice should be dealt with as a matter of urgency. Although it may be the thought uppermost in an owner's mind, it is not always the case that a dog that has bitten needs to be euthanased. However, the following steps should be taken immediately to ensure that human safety and compliance with the law, as well as the welfare of the patient, are taken into account.

- Book an appointment with a veterinary surgeon, at which the history of the circumstances surrounding the bite and the damage inflicted should be taken. The

patient should be thoroughly examined to eliminate any concurrent physical malaise which may have contributed to the dog's unease. How the dog tolerates veterinary handling and examination should also be taken into account in diagnosis. Dogs with stranger-directed aggression may also dislike their attending veterinary surgeon, whereas those in conflict with their families may be perfectly tolerant of those humans of whom they have no experience or expectations. Veterinary consultation is also necessary to highlight to the owner the importance the practice attaches to all behavioural issues.

- If the bite occurred outside the house, muzzling in public places must be advised as a precaution prior to seeking further behavioural advice. This should always be by means of an open basket-style muzzle in which the dog can pant and drink and with which pleasant associations are made by the use of food titbits (Figure 11.21). If the bite has been reported to the police, and there is therefore the possibility that an interview will be conducted in the future regarding the incident, the client should be advised of their right to have a solicitor present during their interview.

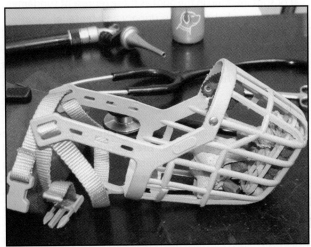

11.21 If a muzzle is to be used as a precaution, pleasant associations should first be made with it by the use of food, in routine as well as trigger situations. © Kendal Shepherd.

- Nearly all family-directed aggression within the home is the result of perceived threat on the part of the dog. Often this threat is in the form of reprimand for some misdemeanour or conflict over resources, such as who owns the sofa, rubbish bin or TV remote control. Advice to reduce confrontation with the dog immediately is therefore absolutely essential. Dogs bite because they anticipate having to defend themselves, not through any notion of 'dominance'. Human perception of right and wrong and of a 'naughty' and 'subordinate' dog fully deserving of punishment, must be set aside in favour of a more enlightened view of canine social behaviour and education.
- If the bite was directed towards children, both parties must be closely supervised when in each other's company. This must be achieved without creating tension and thereby alerting the dog to child-related

unpleasantness. Instructing children to leave the dog alone completely and, at the same time, occupying the dog with reward-based training exercises does much to improve a dog's view of children. If this is not possible, then the dog should be confined until a diagnosis is reached and treatment implemented, particularly away from visiting children.

- Refer the owners to a suitably qualified behaviourist, part of whose remit ought to be to create an accurate prognosis for the patient as with any medical condition. If the prognosis is poor, then counselling owners in their acceptance of the necessity for euthanasia is a valuable and humane service to offer. If good, then a full report on behavioural recommendations for the client and veterinary surgeon should be expected, allowing the veterinary surgeon to remain involved in treatment and in monitoring compliance and progress.

House-soiling

When asked about a house-soiling problem it is important to establish what form of elimination is involved and, if it involves urine, whether the animal is scent marking (spraying in the cat or spot marking in the dog) as these represent fundamentally different behaviours to urinary and faecal elimination. In all cases of inappropriate urination, possible medical causes should first be investigated and ruled out by a veterinary surgeon. The next step is to establish that the animal has been properly house-trained.

Cats

Feline urine spraying, where it is not due to cystitis, may be treated with a commercial preparation of feline facial pheromone and may not require any additional retraining advice. Marked areas should be cleaned with a solution of biological washing powder followed by surgical spirit. The area should then be rinsed with water and wiped dry with paper towels.

Cats that have been urine marking for some time may also stop using the litter tray. Other reasons for indiscriminate elimination include lower urinary tract disease, aversions to litter tray and/or litter, and substrate preferences, as well as anxiety and social dysfunction. It should be checked that the litter tray is positioned away from the cat's food and bed in a quiet, secluded area where the cat cannot be disturbed, that the tray is cleaned regularly and completely and that there have been no changes to the normal routine, such as a change of litter type. Bleach, ammonia-based disinfectants or strongly smelling cleaners are not recommended as the cat may be averse to the smell. If the cause is not readily identifiable and the animal is healthy, then expert behavioural advice should be sought.

Dogs

In the dog, house-soiling is most commonly a result of faulty housetraining, where the dog has not learned to distinguish adequately between substrates indoors and outdoors. It is often the case that all a dog has inadvertently been taught is that it is safer to eliminate when no-one is looking, rather than specifically where and on what.

Loss of previously well established housetraining, scent marking, disease, fear and separation distress may all result in house-soiling. Any disease must be recognized promptly, but in all cases the pet will also need retraining. This is most effectively achieved by ensuring that the dog is taken out regularly to a particular toileting area and returned indoors without comment if it does not eliminate. If it does, the behaviour should be praised ('good wee-wee!') and a reward given. This might be in the form of a titbit (the clicker being ideal to mark elimination at a distance) a game or a longer walk. It is essential that the fun does not stop as soon as the dog has eliminated or he may delay further next time. Instead, a reason to eliminate as soon as possible must be given. Neutering (surgical or chemical) can often be an effective treatment for scent marking.

Dogs may urinate during greeting and when they feel threatened, as this is a normal appeasement gesture. Owners often get upset and angry at this reaction and so may make matters worse by reprimanding their dog. Eye contact alone may be sufficient to trigger this appeasement behaviour in some dogs. Owners and visitors should be encouraged not to appear threatening in any way towards a dog particularly on entering the house, by avoiding petting and eye contact.

Dogs also eliminate when they are frightened, e.g. during thunderstorms, or distressed in some other way, e.g. by the departure of the owner.

Owner-absent behaviour

The term 'separation anxiety' is often wrongly used to describe any problem that arises in the owner's absence. Such owner complaints are more accurately described as 'separation-related behaviour' and are purely descriptive of what happens rather than assigning or identifying any specific cause.

It is frequently necessary to advise video recording the behaviour of the pet when left, in order to identify both the cause and emotional state of the pet accurately. There are many reasons why an animal may not be able to cope with the absence of its owner. These may include being overly dependent upon an owner for emotional support, in which case therapy must concentrate on creating a more emotionally stable and independent dog. Possibly, more commonly, the dog may have experienced a fear-provoking event, such as a thunderstorm, that initially occurred when the owner was out of the house. Owner departure and subsequent isolation then come to predict further thunderstorms, regardless of whether they actually occur, with consequent anticipatory anxiety.

In this case, it may be necessary to avoid leaving the animal alone at all when beginning treatment in order to avoid the inevitable set-backs caused by further anxiety and panic. Using the car as a temporary secure den or providing a companion may help, while the dog is trained gradually to cope with steadily increasing periods of isolation. Gradual and patient desensitization and counter-conditioning to the initial fear-provoking trigger will also be necessary.

A third factor may relate to the stress of confinement or barrier frustration and results in primary attempts to escape rather than to regain an owner's company. Judicious test absences and video recording while giving a dog more freedom at home may reveal a much more relaxed animal. In other cases, the owner may simply be expecting too much from a young or ageing dog. Whatever the cause, behaviour modification advice is generally essential for the long-term resolution of the problem, but this should be tailored to address the factors underlying the behaviour for maximum success. Drugs such as clomipramine or commercial preparations of dog pheromones may help speed up the rate of response in certain cases.

These problems may also occur in cats, with soiling in these cases usually associated with the owner's bed or some other personal area.

All dogs should be provided with stimulating chew toys when left alone for long periods of time. These can be made attractive at the time of leaving, by smearing them with food paste or filling them with food. The toy should be taken away when the owner returns so that access is limited and its value to the dog increased.

Dogs should also be trained to chew on appropriate items at all times, not just when left alone. Praise and rewarding attention should be given whenever a dog is chewing appropriately, rather than attention being reserved only for the stolen remote control, sock or tea towel.

Fear of noises

It is suspected that sensitivity to sounds resulting in varying degrees of fear-related behaviour is under-diagnosed among companion animals and, as already discussed, frequently underlies apparent separation anxiety and separation-related destruction and house-soiling.

The following tips may be given to an owner to help alleviate the impact of sound upon their dog but should not replace expert behavioural diagnosis and advice.

- Ask the owner to revise all basic obedience commands in exchange for food routinely throughout the day, regardless of whether the dog seems to need rewards. It is particularly important to reward a 'lie down' at a distance from the owner and for the dog to follow 'this way' when asked.
- Rather than any attempts at comforting a dog, the owner should turn and walk away (as a negative punishment) at the first sign of unease in their pet. If the dog then complies with a simple obedience request, such as to come and sit, it should be praised and rewarded.
- If the dog is not afraid of the sound of the clicker, this training tool is ideal to help a dog listen out for a rewarding sound in the environment rather than other potentially fear-provoking sounds.
- Provide a soundproof den, preferably in a position to which the dog retreats when worried. The dog should be asked to lie in it frequently throughout the day and rewarded for this rather than following the owner. The aim must be that the dog deliberately seeks out this den as a protection from sound.
- If a known noise onslaught is predicted, such as a neighbouring firework party, the giving of a starch-rich meal earlier in the day may help. Taking the dog out in the car while the party is going on may be necessary to avoid further behavioural deterioration.
- If behavioural therapy is deemed necessary, including medication, this must be instigated at the very time when it appears not to be necessary – well before the winter months when noise fears are typically worse.

A warning regarding crate training

Although the correct use of indoor crates can be very helpful, animals should not simply be caged when left alone without planning and forethought. Shutting the door may alleviate owner distress by restricting damage and soiling when getting up in the morning or on their return to the house but will do nothing to improve the animal's emotional state. It is essential to train the animal to the cage first so that going into it and remaining there with the door shut becomes a positively desirable experience. It must however also be realized that, if the door continues to need to be shut, the problem for which the crate was used in the first place, is not solved.

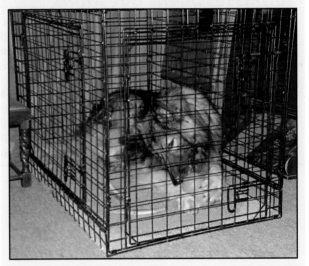

© Kendal Shepherd

Summary

In summary, behaviour should be considered in all dealings with any veterinary patient and their owner in order to achieve the following:

- To present veterinary surgeons and veterinary nurses to the public as role models
- To fulfil welfare obligations – the Animal Welfare Act 2006 Section 9 imposes a duty of care to avoid mental as well as physical suffering.
- To prevent iatrogenic behavioural damage and deterioration
- To educate the public by demonstrating learning principles and animals' choices in a humane manner
- To take the whole of any animal's life and management system into account when treating disease
- To facilitate best practice in terms of clinical care
- To improve the relationship between the clinic and client.

Acknowledgement

The author would like to thank Daniel Mills for his input to the chapter, adapted from previous editions.

Further reading

Heath S and Mills D (2005). *Client Information Handouts: Behaviour*. Lifelearn, Newmarket

Horwitz D and Mills DS (2009) *BSAVA Manual of Canine and Feline Behavioural Medicine, 2nd edn*. BSAVA Publications, Gloucester. Client handouts on behaviour available to members of BSAVA: www.bsava.com

Shepherd K (2007) *The Canine Commandments*. Broadcast Books, Bristol

Useful websites:

Animal Behaviour Training Council: www.abtcouncil.org.uk
Association of Pet Behaviour Counsellors: www.apbc.org.uk
Association for the Study of Animal Behaviour Accreditation Scheme: http://asab.nottingham.ac.uk/accred/index.php
Companion Animal Behaviour Therapy Study Group: www.cabtsg.org
Puppy School: www.puppyschool.co.uk
The APBC/CABTSG Manual of Behavioural First Aid: www.apbc.org.uk/books1.htm

Self-assessment questions

1. What is the most common reason for a dog to become aggressive?
2. How is behaviour (or what a dog decides to do) determined?
3. What information does a dog need in order to behave well?
4. Define positive reinforcement, negative punishment, positive punishment, and negative reinforcement.
5. How does an obedient dog differ from a well-behaved one?
6. Why are the terms 'dominance' and 'submission' considered to be outmoded in relation to the domestic dog?
7. What are the potentially damaging consequences of coercive training techniques?
8. Why and how should the veterinary clinic become involved in routine behaviour management?

Chapter 12

Maintaining animal accommodation

Louise Monsey and Jane Devaney

Learning objectives

After studying this chapter, students should be able to:

- **Outline optimal environmental conditions for different types of domestic animal accommodation**
- **State the advantages and disadvantages of different construction and bedding materials in relation to animal accommodation**
- **Explain the general principles and considerations of kennel, cattery and stable management in relation to an animal's needs**
- **Describe different types of specialized animal housing, including housing for exotic pets**
- **Outline the principles of cleaning and disinfection of kennel, stable and hospital environments**
- **State the principles of isolation and barrier nursing**

Animal housing

Anyone responsible for animal care should be aware of, and always bear in mind, the animal's basic needs.

The Five Freedoms

- **Freedom from Hunger and Thirst**
  By ready access to food and fresh water in order to maintain full health and vigour.
- **Freedom from Discomfort**
  By providing an appropriate environment including shelter and a comfortable resting area.
- **Freedom from Pain, Injury or Disease**
  By prevention and/or rapid diagnosis and treatment.
- **Freedom to Express Normal Behaviour**
  By providing sufficient space, proper facilities and, where necessary, company of the animal's own kind.
- **Freedom from Fear and Distress**
  By ensuring conditions and treatment that avoid mental suffering.

The Animal Welfare Act 2006 states that anyone responsible for an animal, including owners and temporary or permanent keepers, must ensure the welfare needs of an animal are met. These needs closely follow the Five Freedoms and are stated in the Act as follows:

- The need for a suitable environment
- The need for a suitable diet
- The need to be able to exhibit normal behaviour patterns
- Any need the animal has to be housed with, or apart from, other animals
- The need to be protected from pain, suffering, injury and disease.

Environmental requirements

All animal accommodation must be soundly constructed to ensure security and provide conditions that will ensure suitable temperature, humidity and ventilation. All animals should be clean, dry (unless aquatic) and comfortable at all times. Species-specific requirements will be discussed in more detail later in the chapter; however, general principles apply to all species.

Temperature

Animals must be protected from extremes of temperature. Very old and very young animals, which are more sensitive to changes in temperature, may require provision of heating or cooling. The temperature of accommodation for dogs and cats should not be allowed to drop below 7°C and the temperature in the sleeping area should not be allowed to drop below 10°C (Figure 12.1). It is often high temperatures that are more difficult to control, but the temperature of the accommodation should not exceed 26°C unless there is access to a shaded area where the animal can seek cooler temperatures.

The ambient temperature for hospitalized animals, especially for those recovering from general anaesthesia or sedation, should generally be higher, as their ability to thermoregulate may be compromised. Additional heat sources, such as warm-water beds and warm-air blankets or insulation in the form of additional blankets and bubble-wrap, may be required to treat or prevent hypothermia.

Species or area	Recommended ambient temperature
Adult dogs	7–26°C Should not drop below 7°C Sleeping area should be at least 10°C
Adult cats	10–26°C
Hospital and isolation kennels	18–23°C
Whelping/kittening and neonate accommodation	Parturition area: 18–21°C Neonates: • First week: 26–29°C • Second week: 21–26°C • Until weaning: 20°C

12.1   Environmental temperatures for housing dogs and cats.

Hyperthermic animals will usually require active cooling. Air-conditioning units can rapidly lower the environmental temperature and portable fans are useful to direct at the patient. Brachycephalic breeds may struggle with high hospital temperatures, so should be monitored carefully and cooling provided as required.

Horses will tolerate a wide range of temperatures. Most horse stables use natural rather than mechanical heating and ventilation to control temperature (Figure 12.2). Stables should therefore not be positioned near dust sources such as hay or grain sheds. Boxes facing just east of south will get the benefit of the morning sun, especially in the winter. Trees may provide a useful wind break in exposed areas but care must be taken to ensure that falling leaves do not block drains.

Small pets are particularly susceptible to hypothermia due to their high surface area to bodyweight ratio; measures should therefore be taken to prevent heat loss. The preferred ambient temperature for small mammals will vary with species (see later) but, in general, extremes of temperature should be avoided. Small mammals are particularly susceptible to damp and drafts. Careful attention should be given to the environmental temperatures provided for poikilothermic animals; they often require a temperature gradient, to allow self-regulation of their body temperature. Reptiles and fish have very specific temperature, humidity and ventilation requirements (see later).

Lighting

Lighting should be as similar to the duration and intensity of natural conditions for the species as possible. Sunlight is preferred for birds and mammals, provided shaded areas are available. Artificial lighting is usually necessary to allow animal housing to be thoroughly cleaned and animals to be checked and treated. Daylight-simulating fluorescent bulbs are available and provide a more naturally lit environment than incandescent bulbs, which emit a yellow rather than a white light. Birds and reptiles benefit from daily exposure to natural or artificial ultraviolet (UV) light. Small mammals should be provided with shelter from direct sunlight and nocturnal species will require a dark nest box to retreat to during the day.

Ventilation

Ventilation should be adequate to keep animal housing areas free from damp, noxious odours and draughts. Fans should not be placed near windows, as this would limit air movement to a small circle rather than redistributing it around the rest of the room. Under normal conditions, four to eight air changes should take place per hour, but the rate can be increased according to weather conditions, occupancy levels, presence of disease, use in isolation units or other factors. More information is given on ventilation systems later in this chapter.

Adequate ventilation is important for all species to prevent respiratory disease. Aquarium-style accommodation for small mammals is often difficult to ventilate and most small mammals are poorly tolerant of high humidity.

Beds and bedding

Beds and bedding offer warmth, comfort, security, protection and absorbency and represent the animal's own territory whilst in the kennel, stable or hospital environment. The bedding area should be large enough to enable the animal to stretch out but small enough to ensure that it feels secure. Bedding from home may comfort the animal whilst in a kennelled environment but may possibly introduce infective agents into a hospital environment. Small pets usually appreciate somewhere to hide, such as a box or plentiful bedding material. Sawdust and wood-shavings should not be used for postsurgical patients as the material may stick to wounds. Cats also often appreciate a box, igloo type bed or additional litter tray with bedding to sit in (Figure 12.3).

12.2   Stable block with natural ventilation from the central ridged roof and natural light from skylights. (Courtesy of E. Mullineaux)

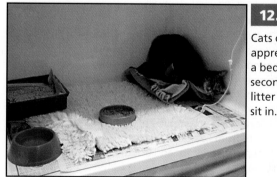

12.3

Cats often appreciate a bedded second litter tray to sit in.

Recumbent animals require a foam mattress (Figure 12.4) or an orthopaedic bed to prevent the formation of decubitus ulcers. Foam mattresses will also provide additional comfort for animals with osteoarthritis. Acrylic veterinary bedding is warm, supportive and durable and absorbs body fluids into the bottom layer leaving the top layer dry for the animal to lie on, should it not be changed immediately. Blankets are easily saturated with urine and are not as supportive. They also take longer to launder and dry. Newspaper is often used to line hospital kennels as it is usually in plentiful supply and is very absorbent (Figure 12.4). Incontinence pads are useful for recumbent or incontinent patients and may be used on top of acrylic bedding to allow easier cleaning. It is important to change the pads as soon as they become soiled.

Properties of a good bedding material include:

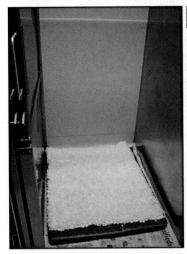

12.4 Kennel with a foam mattress (useful for recumbent and arthritic patients) covered with veterinary fleece. The kennel is first lined with newspaper.

- Good insulator
- Soft and comfortable
- Absorbs body fluids to keep the animal dry
- Non-irritant and presents no harm to the animal
- Easy to launder and disinfect
- Easy to store
- Does not damage or soil the animal's coat
- Economical – durable, long-lasting, reusable, inexpensive and difficult to chew or tear.

The advantages and disadvantages of different bedding materials for domestic animals are considered in Figure 12.5.

Type of bed/bedding	Use	Advantages	Disadvantages
Acrylic veterinary bedding	Small animal veterinary surgeries, kennels, domestic	Easy to launder. Absorbs body fluids into bottom layer, leaving top layer dry for the animal to lie on. Supportive. Does not harbour parasites. Long-lasting and durable	Expensive. May be chewed
Blankets	Kennels, domestic	Warm	Difficult to launder and dry. May be chewed. May harbour dust mites. Expensive unless donated. Several layers needed for comfort. Easily saturated with urine
Bean bags, acrylic-filled beds	Domestic	Comfortable. Supportive. Good insulators	Easy to chew. Expensive. Difficult to launder. Easily saturated with urine
Igloo-type beds	Veterinary surgeries, catteries, domestic	Allows cats to retreat and feel more secure. May reduce stress in hospitalized cats	Difficult to launder and dry. Expensive. May harbour dust mites. Easily saturated with urine
Covered foam pads and orthopaedic pet beds	Equine recovery boxes, small animal veterinary surgeries for recumbent animals	Comfortable. Warm. Supportive – excellent for recumbent animals	May be chewed or torn. Difficult to clean unless cover is durable
Shredded paper	Horses, small mammals	Comfortable. Allows nesting behaviour. Absorbent. Does not harbour parasites. Low in dust so suitable for horses with respiratory problems. Relatively cheap	Not very warm. Large amounts needed for horses. May contain ink, which may stain coat. May blow around in the wind and become heavy when wet
Straw, hay (may be barley, wheat or oat; barley most commonly used)	Horses, small mammals	Comfortable. Warm. Allows nesting behaviour. Least expensive bedding material for horses	Not very absorbent. Price fluctuates according to year and climate. May be dusty (especially wheat straw). May harbour parasites and *Aspergillus* spores (may cause or aggravate respiratory problems). Relatively expensive for small mammals. Readily eaten (especially barley straw) by some horses, resulting in impaction colic
Acrylic/nylon wadding	Small mammals	Comfortable. Warm. Does not harbour parasites	Not very absorbent. Expensive. May constrict around limbs
Newspaper	Lining of kennels/cages for small animals	Very absorbent. Usually free of charge	Not comfortable unless shredded. Urine may be drawn across paper. Animals may eat or rip. May dirty pale coats
Incontinence pads	Small animals in isolation; those with vomiting and diarrhoea or incontinence	Easy to replace. Saves continuous laundering. Useful when laid on top of other bedding	Not comfortable. May be expensive if several are used. Animals may eat or rip

12.5 Types of bedding for animal accommodation.

continues ▶

Type of bed/bedding	Use	Advantages	Disadvantages
Sawdust/shavings	Horses, base of small mammal cages	Comfortable. Allows tunnelling and nesting behaviour. Warm. Absorbent. Relatively dust-free	More expensive than straw. May harbour parasites. Not suitable for foals as ingestion may lead to colic and tends to stick to nose and eyes. Takes more time than straw to compost down. Not for hospitalized small animals as impractical to observe. May stick to wounds. May emit terpenes, which irritate mucous membranes
Presterilized peat	Horses, base of small mammal cages	Comfortable. Warm. Allows tunnelling and nesting behaviour. Does not harbour parasites. Very absorbent. Reduces odours	Expensive compared with straw. Can be heavy to muck out. Not renewable, considered to be environmentally unfriendly. Not for hospitalized small animals as impractical to change and observe animal. May stick to wounds
Hemp	Horses	Absorbent. Dust-free	Relatively expensive. May be eaten
Rubber matting	Horses	Can reduce other bedding amounts. Protective to hooves	Not recommended for use on its own as it provides little warmth. May create problems with urine scalding. Exceptional hygiene must be employed and it must be sealed at joins or should be lifted for regular cleaning as ammonia build-up can be a problem

12.5   *continued*   Types of bedding for animal accommodation.

General principles of kennel and cattery management

Although the information below applies to kennel and catteries used to board healthy dogs and cats, many of the principles of the management of such facilities can and should be applied to boarding facilities used for other species (exotic pets and horses) and veterinary facilities used to board hospitalized pets.

Managers of animal boarding establishments are responsible for:

- Providing accommodation and facilities to suit the physical and behavioural requirements of the animals held
- Providing protection for the animals in their care from adverse natural or artificial environmental conditions, other animals and interference from the general public
- Providing sufficient space for animals to stand, move around freely, stretch fully and rest
- Providing sufficient and appropriate exercise for the requirements of the animal
- Providing sufficient quantities of appropriate feed and water to maintain good health
- Protecting animals as far as possible from disease, distress or injury
- Providing prompt veterinary or other appropriate treatment in cases of disease or injury
- Maintaining the hygienic status of the premises and the health of the animals
- Directly or indirectly supervising daily feeding and watering, and inspecting the animals to ensure their welfare
- Providing adequate training and supervision of staff
- Collating and maintaining relevant records.

Licensing

The location and construction of animal boarding establishments must comply with local government requirements. Boarding kennels are licensed by local councils on an annual basis as required by the Animal Boarding Establishments Act 1963. A licence will be granted at the discretion of the local authority and will only be granted if:

- Animals will, at all times, be kept in accommodation suitable in terms of construction, size of quarters, number of occupants, exercising facilities, temperature, lighting, ventilation and cleanliness
- Animals will be adequately supplied with suitable food, water and bedding material, adequately exercised and (as far as necessary) visited at suitable intervals
- All available precautions will be taken to prevent and control the spread of infectious or contagious diseases among animals, including the provision of adequate isolation facilities
- Appropriate steps will be taken for the protection of the animals in case of fire or other emergency
- A register will be kept containing a description of any animals received into the establishment, date of arrival and departure, and the name and address of the owner. The register must be available for inspection at all times by an officer of the local authority or veterinary surgeon.

Veterinary staff are advised not to recommend boarding establishments to clients without having knowledge of or having visited the premises themselves. Clients should be advised to inspect premises and ask questions of the owner or manager of the kennels or cattery to ensure that they feel confident about the establishment before leaving their pet in its care.

Location

Animal boarding establishments (and veterinary facilities) should be located in an area that is not subject to flooding or accessible to members of the public. They must be away from sources of noise and pollution that are likely to cause injury or stress to the animals and must be far enough away from residential areas to minimize complaints regarding the noise from barking dogs. When new boarding or veterinary establishments are erected, sound-proofing should be considered. Double-brick walls, double-glazing and tree belts around the premises are all methods used in sound-proofing.

Sharing of facilities

Generally there should be no sharing of facilities, except where animals are from the same household and this has been agreed (preferably in writing) with the owner. No more than three cats from the same household should be housed together. Strays should only be boarded following licensing approval and then kept separately from other boarded animals.

Animals from the same household hospitalized in veterinary kennels may share accommodation prior to any surgery but should be separated whilst recovering from anaesthesia to avoid injuring one another. Stray animals are generally only boarded in veterinary environments if they require medical attention and then should ideally be isolated (see later) as their health status will be unknown. Veterinary surgeons have a legal obligation to provide first aid treatment to prevent pain and suffering for all animals whether they are owned, stray or wildlife. The RSPCA/BVA Memorandum of Understanding is an agreement that aims to ensure that appropriate professional treatment is available for all injured or sick animals. Adherence to this memorandum should result in a rapid and humane response to any emergency situation.

Animal identification

All animals must be clearly identified. Records that must be kept for each animal admitted for boarding include:

- The animal's name
- The owner's name, address and telephone number
- The emergency/contact telephone number of the owner/ the owner's nominee
- A description of the animal, including:
  - Sex
  - Breed or type
  - Colour
  - Age
  - Distinguishing features
  - Date of admission
  - Expected date of collection
  - Details of medical, dietary, bathing and grooming requirements
  - The animal's condition and, when possible, its weight on arrival
  - Any collar, leads or belongings brought in with the animal
  - Vaccination status
  - Name and contact number of the veterinary surgeon who normally attends to the animal.

Veterinary patients should be clearly identified on admittance to the veterinary practice to ensure that the correct animal receives the correct course of treatment. This may be through the use of name tags or consent forms attached to the front of the kennel or using a plan of the kennels which is filled in. As animals may be moved from the kennels, a disposable collar with a name label (Figure 12.6) is the most effective method of identification. Informed consent must

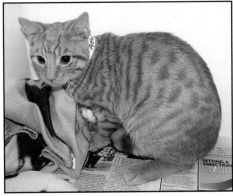

12.6 Disposable identification collar on a cat.

be obtained for all procedures carried out in a veterinary practice, usually through the use of a signed consent form. In a veterinary facility these records are likely to form part of the animal's clinical records (see also Chapters 9 and 16).

Hygiene and safety
Disease control

Disease control involves the consideration of many issues in kennel design and operation, including:

- Construction of buildings, flooring and surfaces
- Cleaning and disinfection (see later)
- Vaccination (see Chapter 5)
- Cleanliness of communal areas such as exercise areas
- Hygienic use of feeding bowls, muzzles and other equipment
- Provision and use of isolation facilities (see later)
- Efficient ventilation
- Pest and parasite control
- Veterinary care.

Cleaning and disinfection

Animal housing and exercise areas must be cleaned and disinfected so that the comfort of animals can be maintained and disease risk can be controlled. Excreta must be removed as necessary. Kennels should be cleaned out and disinfected at least once daily (Figure 12.7) and more frequently if required in hospitalized patients. Cleaning and disinfecting agents

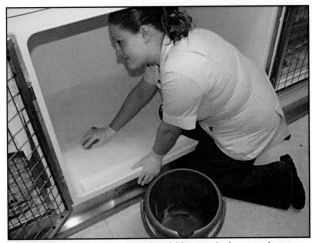

12.7 Kennel cleaning should be carried out at least once daily. NB Additional protective clothing such as an apron and facemask will be required with some disinfectant agents.

should be chosen on the basis of their suitability, safety and effectiveness (see later). Manufacturer's instructions for the use of these agents should be followed. After cleaning, animal housing areas should not be allowed to remain wet. Poor ventilation and humidity increases the spread of disease.

Pest control

Efforts must be made to control pests effectively, including insects (flies, fleas, etc.) and wild rodents, as many are disease vectors. Some pesticides and rodenticides are toxic to domestic animals and should be used with extreme care. If chemicals are used, they must only be used according to the manufacturer's instructions. All patients must be completely excluded from that part of the facility until the poisoning programme is complete.

Waste disposal

Waste disposal must be in accordance with the requirements of the local authority. Solid waste must be collected from all parts of the facility and be disposed of in a suitable fashion. The British Veterinary Association (BVA) provides general guidance on disposal of waste in a veterinary environment although the protocols set by the waste carrier used by the individual veterinary practice should be adhered to (see Chapter 2). The waste carrier and the facility where it is disposed of must be licensed with the Environment Agency. Veterinary practices should keep a record of waste for 2 years following its disposal under The Environmental Protection (Duty of Care) Regulations 1991. The practice should have a facility for storage and suitable arrangements with a registered contractor for the disposal of cadavers.

Emergencies/fire

An adequate plan must be provided to cover emergency measures. All staff should be aware of the plan. A sign should be displayed referring anyone to an emergency contact if nobody is present at the facility. Fire extinguishers should be placed at easily accessible places and fire exits should be clearly marked.

Veterinary practices should appoint (in writing) a Fire Officer, draw up a list of the Fire Officer's duties and carry out a Fire Risk Assessment (including procedures for raising the alarm and evacuation). Smoking should not be permitted in the building. Fire extinguishers and alarms should be serviced regularly (see Chapter 2).

Welfare

Vaccination

Dogs and cats should be vaccinated prior to admission to kennels and catteries (see Chapters 5 and 8). A current vaccination certificate (i.e. certifying that the vaccination was done within the preceding 12 months) must be produced. Some vaccinations (usually initial vaccination courses and kennel cough vaccinations) may take 5–14 days to produce the full immune response. Datasheet recommendations should be followed. Dogs and cats under 4 months old should not be admitted for boarding other than in exceptional circumstances, and then preferably held in isolation. All risks must be explained to the owner prior to admittance. Unvaccinated animals admitted to veterinary practices should ideally be housed in an isolation facility.

Dogs and cats should also be treated for internal and external parasites prior to admission.

Observation of animals

Each animal should be checked at least once daily to monitor its health and comfort. Any change in health status should be reported promptly to the animal boarding establishment manager.

Inpatients in a veterinary practice are routinely checked much more frequently than those in boarding establishments (see Chapter 15). The frequency of the checks will depend upon the animal's condition but typically varies from constant monitoring (for a critical patient) to every 2–4 hours. All inpatients should be examined at least daily by a veterinary surgeon.

Veterinary services

The boarding establishment manager should establish liaison with a veterinary surgeon to attend the premises whenever required. Veterinary attention must be sought for any animal showing signs of injury or disease. The animal's insurance cover should be known.

Isolation

Animals known or suspected to have a contagious disease should not be admitted for boarding, other than in exceptional circumstances. They must then be held in isolation facilities. An infected animal should never be admitted into a boarding facility where no separate, specific isolation facilities exist. The usual reason for providing these facilities is to enable the isolation of animals that have developed suspicious clinical signs after they have been admitted, since by then this will be the only course of action to protect the other animals housed.

It is recommended that there is at least one isolation kennel per 50 dogs and one per 30 cats. Isolation kennels must be separate from the main kennels and are usually physically separated by at least 5 m (this distance is based upon the distance that infectious droplets from a dog's sneeze may travel). In existing catteries there must be a minimum of 3 m physical separation from the main cat accommodation units. Cat isolation cages should have solid rather than wire mesh doors to act as sneeze barriers. Where new kennels and catteries are being built it is recommended that isolation facilities are built 10 m from the main accommodation units.

Animals that have been in contact with a contagious case should be isolated from both the contagious patient and from healthy animals. Veterinary advice should be sought in the management of specific outbreaks of disease. Facilities should be designed in such a way as to prevent cross-infection and to be easily cleaned and disinfected, e.g. non-porous kennel surfaces, minimal equipment kept within the facility, washing facilities available at the entrance to the facility, protective clothing available. Further practical details are given in 'Isolation and barrier nursing' later in this chapter.

Animals receiving medication

The boarding establishment must follow all written medication protocols they are given, unless they receive advice from a veterinary surgeon to change them. The type of drug (name, amount and description) should be noted on the animal's reception card along with details of the veterinary surgeon who prescribed the medication. The staff member administering the medication must record that each treatment has been administered (what and when) and a permanent record of this must be kept for reference purposes.

Veterinary practices must provide facilities and adequate nursing staff for the care of inpatients, with suitable arrangements for their overnight care. All hospitalized animals should have inpatient care sheets.

Nutrition

Sufficient food of adequate nutritional value must be supplied daily to every animal and fresh water should always be available. The manufacturer's instructions should be adhered to for the feeding of commercial food. Details of any special feeding requirements should be obtained from owners on admission of the animal. Owners can be encouraged to bring the pet's usual food if the kennel/cattery does not stock it.

Food should be prepared hygienically in a separate kitchen area (Figure 12.8) and should be stored appropriately (e.g. dry food should be kept in a rodent-free place, fresh meat should be kept refrigerated). Food and water bowls should preferably be solid, heavy containers that are chew-proof and not prone to spillage. They must be readily accessible and cleaned at least daily. Where dogs leave food uneaten, the food should be removed and disposed of promptly so that it does not spoil or attract vermin or flies. Ideally, cats should be offered their daily food requirements (divided into small portions) several times a day.

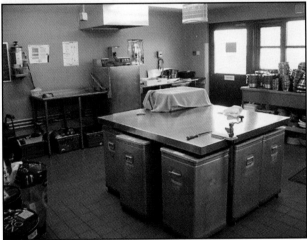

| **12.8** | Separate kitchen area for food preparation for small animals. |

Feeding equipment used within a veterinary practice should be disposable or capable of being sterilized. A wide variety of foodstuffs for the range of species and types of condition being treated should be available. There should be facilities for refrigeration and warming of foodstuffs. See also Chapters 13 and 16.

Exercise

Dogs must have the opportunity for exercise to:

- Allow them to urinate and defecate
- Give them contact with humans and, if appropriate, with other dogs
- Allow muscular activity
- Allow staff to monitor the dog's gait and behaviour.

Exercise can be provided by:

- Allowing dogs access to an exercise area (Figure 12.9) for at least 15 minutes twice daily; and/or

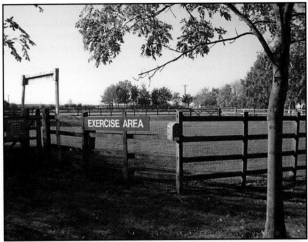

| **12.9** | Exercise area for dogs. Faeces must be removed after each patient. |

- Walking dogs on a lead for at least 15 minutes twice daily.

Very active dogs may require more exercise and old dogs less exercise than specified above.

Cats must have sufficient room to enable them to stretch and to move about freely. Cats should also be monitored for gait and mobility.

Unclaimed animals

Animal boarding establishments should have a policy for dealing with unclaimed animals, giving owners a reasonable opportunity to collect boarded animals.

Staff

All staff should respect the animals and have suitable training and experience in their handling. They should be aware of their responsibilities and competent to carry them out. Cats and dogs require frequent human contact and time should be spent with each animal. Suitable health and safety protocols should be in place and adhered to, ensuring staff safety at all times (see Chapter 2).

Kennel and cattery design
Construction materials

The advantages and disadvantages of the many different materials used for the construction of kennel and cattery units and other animal accommodation are considered in Figure 12.10.

Flooring

Floors of the animal housing areas of kennels and catteries should be made of an impervious material, to facilitate cleaning and drainage. Sealed concrete is ideal. Joints between walls and floors should be curved and impervious.

Drainage

Proper drainage is vital. Solid easy-to-clean channels without covers are recommended. Covered drains gather dirt and are difficult to clean. Kennel and cattery floors should be sloped to enable waste and water to run off.

Material	Advantages	Disadvantages
Concrete	Indestructible. Easily cleaned if sealed and good drainage system. Cool in summer. Easily laid. Relatively inexpensive	Uncomfortable. Planning permission required. Cold in winter. Takes a long time to dry after cleaning. Porous if unsealed
Wood	Inexpensive. Warm. Easy construction. Movable	Not long-lasting or durable. Requires maintenance. Destructible, may be chewed and kicked. Difficult to clean and disinfect (cross-infection risk). Not escape-proof
Fibreglass	Easy to clean. Warm. Indestructible. Durable. Minimal maintenance required	Expensive. Installation difficult. Some disinfectants may cause damage
Stainless steel	Easy to clean. Durable. Indestructible. Minimal maintenance required	Expensive. Cold. Noisy. Installation difficult
Tiles	Hard-wearing. Cool in summer	Cold in winter. Difficult to clean. Tiles may crack. Slippery when wet. Expensive to install
Glass	Easy to clean. Allows natural light in	Expensive (glass should be toughened and double glazed). Breakable
Brick	Insulating. Strong. Easily built. Can paint to seal	Porous (harbours bacteria). Difficult to clean. Not chew-proof
Breeze blocks	Inexpensive. Durable. Good sound-proofing. Insulating	Porous (harbours bacteria). Difficult to clean. Rough. Unattractive
Plastic	Warm. Inexpensive. Easy to clean	Not very strong. May be chewed. Some disinfectants may damage

12.10   Types of construction material used in animal accommodation.

Size of dog and cat housing

Animal housing areas must provide at least enough space for each animal to feed, sleep, sit, lie with limbs extended, stretch and move around. The recommended kennel sizes for short-term housing of dogs are shown in Figure 12.11 and those for cats in Figure 12.12.

Size of dog	Height of unit	Exercise area (floor area)	Sleeping area (floor area)
Up to 60 cm at shoulder	1.85 m	2.46 m²	1.9 m²
Over 60 cm at shoulder	1.85 m	3.35 m²	1.9 m²

12.11   Recommended sizes of dog kennel units for short-term housing.

Number of cats	Height of unit	Exercise area (floor area)	Sleeping area (floor area)
One cat	1.85 m	1.7 m²	0.85 m²
Up to three cats	1.85 m	3.0 m²	1.5 m²

12.12   Recommended sizes of cattery units for short-term housing.

Kennels

Kennels must be separated by solid partitions or chain-wire dividers. The partitions must not allow the dogs to have physical contact with each other, where injury or cross-infection might occur. Any mesh or chain-wire must be of sufficient strength to contain the animals. Mesh size should not exceed 50 mm square and wire should be of at least 2 mm in diameter. Kennels should be designed for ease of cleaning and control of disease and the internal surfaces with which animals have contact must be constructed of impervious, solid, washable materials. Joints and corners should be properly sealed. All kennels should be provided with a raised sleeping area with dry soft bedding material (Figure 12.13).

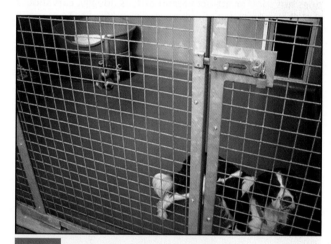

12.13   Kennel with a raised sleeping area.

Catteries

Cats should have access to an exercise area (Figure 12.14) twice daily for a period of no less than 1 hour. Each cat unit should include a night box to allow the cat to withdraw (Figure 12.15). Cats often feel safer if allowed to retreat to higher ground; they may be housed in an area where the bedding is off the ground and accessed via a ladder (Figure 12.16), which is more economical of space and encourages climbing, which forms part of a cat's natural behaviour. Scratching posts, toys, etc. provide exercise and prevent boredom.

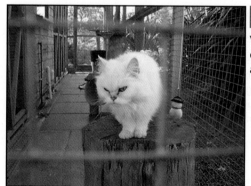

12.14

View of cat exercise area.

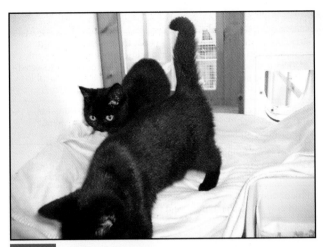

12.15 Night box for cats.

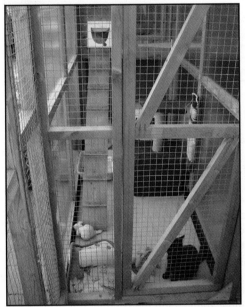

12.16 Cat's ladder access to off-the-ground sleeping area.

Cats must be provided with litter trays. Sufficient suitable litter material, such as commercial cat litter, untreated sawdust or shredded paper, should be provided. Ideally the owner should be asked for information on the type of litter the cat usually uses so that this can be provided. Litter should be changed and litter trays cleaned and disinfected at least daily but ideally every time the litter is soiled.

Heating

Heating and insulation are required in kennel and cattery buildings to:

- Provide warmth and comfort for the dogs and cats
- Allow rapid drying following cleaning and disinfection
- Lower the risk of respiratory diseases by reducing condensation
- Provide comfortable working conditions for staff
- Prevent damage caused by frost or damp.

The use of a maximum/minimum thermometer helps in assessing the variations in temperature throughout the day. There are many methods that can be used to heat whole kennel or cattery blocks or individual units. The types of heating of animal accommodation and their advantages and disadvantages are considered in Figure 12.17.

Lighting

Dogs and cats require light to keep them active during the hours of daylight, providing mental stimulation and avoiding boredom. It is preferable to use natural sources of light wherever possible and to supplement with artificial lighting when needed. Artificial lighting is usually used in addition to natural lighting to facilitate procedures and observation, but it should be noted that artificial lighting produces heat and may cause overheating during hot summer months.

The most common type of artificial lighting consists of fluorescent strip lights with diffusers to avoid shadows. Hanging light bulbs are not recommended. All electricity cables should be encased to keep them waterproof and they should be made inaccessible to the animals. Waterproof switches and sockets should be used.

Type	Advantages	Disadvantages
Central heating	Easily controlled. Safe. Use of thermostats ensure minimum temperature kept constant. Economical	Expensive to install. Requires regular maintenance. Additional heat in individual kennels may be necessary. Requires suitable wall space for fitting. Difficult to clean and disinfect
Electric fan-assisted heating/fan heaters	Convenient. Rapid heating effect	Heater should not be placed too close to animal as overheating may occur. Noisy. Expensive to run. Spread of airborne diseases risk increased. Move dust around
Total air-conditioning/heating	Temperature easily controlled. Humidity can also be controlled. Animals have no potential contact with heating source. Wall space not an issue	Expensive to install. Expensive to run
Underfloor heating	Floors dry quickly. Very comfortable for animals to lie on	If insulation is poor floors can become very hot. Faecal material difficult to remove. Expensive to install and repair
Portable radiators	Mobile. Cheap to purchase	Takes a long time to heat an area. Supervision required. May be knocked over in a busy area. Surface temperature may injure staff or animals if they come into contact. Cables must be protected from animals. Switches and sockets should be waterproof. Sockets in kennels must be covered when not in use
Portable electric fan heaters	Good for boosting the temperature rapidly. Useful as emergency back-up if heating system fails. Can be controlled individually. Heat can be directed towards animals	Heater should not be placed too close to an animal's kennel (overheating). Noisy. Expensive to run. Spread of airborne diseases risk increased. Move dust around. Fire risk

12.17 Types of heating used in animal accommodation.

continues ▶

Type	Advantages	Disadvantages
Infra-red heating lamps	Easy to install. Correct heat can be directed on to an animal's sleeping area. Produces heat without light. Height of lamp can be adjusted to regulate heat reaching the animal. Can be controlled by using thermostats	Requires a socket in each kennel – needs to be waterproof and covered when not in use. Animals may interfere with cables – risk of electric shock. Fire risk. Animal may be either too hot or too cold if incorrectly positioned (use a thermostat)
Heated beds/mats	Enjoyed by animals. Low constant heat. Cheap to buy and run	Damaged by chewing. Risk of electric shock (use circuit breaker). Difficult to clean/disinfect. Only used for supplementary heat. Overheating and burns
Microwaveable pads/ bags	Acrylic durable versions available, which are easy to clean. Quick and easy to use. Remain warm for longer than hot-water bottles	Only used for supplementary heating. Can become too hot if heated for too long. Overheating. Burns if not covered adequately
Hot-water bottles	Cheap. Rapid, direct warmth	Risk of burns/scalds. Water cools rapidly. Used only as supplementary heat source
Incubators	Temperature is easily controlled. Humidity can also be controlled. No risk of burns. Animals easily observable	Only suitable for smaller patients. Not suitable for fractious animals. Expensive
Circulating warm-water beds	Temperature is controllable – do not cause burns. Constant warmth – do not cool. Easily cleaned. Also provides support – good for geriatric or recumbent animals	Damaged by chewing. Risk of electric shock (use circuit breaker). Expensive
Circulating warm-air blankets	Temperature is controllable – do not cause burns. Constant warmth – do not cool as warm air is constantly circulated	Only really suitable for anaesthetized or critical patients as tubing or unit could be interfered with by animal. Relatively difficult to clean. Expensive

12.17   *continued*   Types of heating used in animal accommodation.

During the night, lighting should be dimmed to allow the animals to rest. Most prefer to sleep in a darkened area and cats often prefer to eat when it is dark. The use of screens or blinds may need to be considered for animal housing areas that receive a lot of natural light or direct sunlight, as animals may find it difficult to rest or may become restless very early in the morning. Direct sunlight can cause overheating in summer months.

Ventilation

Good ventilation is vital in kennels and catteries for four reasons:

- To provide clean air for staff and animals by removing odours, fumes (ammonia) and gases (expired carbon dioxide)
- To reduce the risk of cross-contamination of airborne infections
- To control humidity
- To assist in temperature regulation.

Passive ventilation

Fresh air is provided by opening windows, doors and vents. This is an ineffective method of ventilation when used alone within a kennel or cattery environment: there is no control over the number of air changes per hour, draughts are caused, heat will be lost (which is not economical) and there is the risk of animals escaping.

Active ventilation

Active ventilation actively 'pulls in' fresh air and forces out stale air. This dramatically reduces the risk of cross-infection of airborne disease but does not rule it out, so an animal that is suspected of having an infection that can be passed via the airborne or aerosol route should always be isolated.

Active ventilation can be achieved by extractor fans or air-conditioning systems.

Extractor fans can be set to draw air out of or into the unit. Alternatively, passive vents can be used in conjunction with extractor fans: if extractor fans are set to draw air in, passive vents will let air escape because a positive air pressure within the building or area will be caused. If extractor fans are set to suck air out of the building or area, passive vents will allow air in because a negative air pressure will be caused. The movement of air within the facility and individual areas should be carefully considered and ideally be designed to pass fresh air over individual animals and then extract the air from the building before it can be inhaled by other animals.

With air-conditioning systems, induction vents actively push air into each individual kennel unit from an external 'clean' source. The air is then actively extracted by another vent immediately outside the unit (for example, in a corridor). The efficacy of air-conditioning units is reduced by the opening of windows and doors. Air-conditioning units can be incorporated into a heating system so that the exact temperature required can be set. The humidity level can also be controlled. These units are very useful when considering optimum housing conditions for different species, though they are expensive to install and run.

Noise

Design, construction and management of kennels should be such as to minimize noise levels. Dogs should be separated visually to discourage barking at each other and kennels can be designed with this in mind (Figure 12.18).

Cats and small mammals should be housed away from dogs, as they may be disturbed by the noise of barking. Noise barriers such as earth banks and tree belts may be helpful and the site should be large enough to limit any noise disturbance. Double doors and double-glazed windows will limit noise; acoustic tiles may also be used.

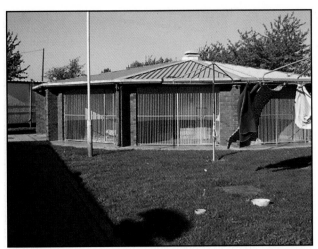

12.18 Parasol kennel. As the dogs cannot see each other, they are less likely to bark.

Security

Kennel and cattery buildings must be kept locked when nobody is in attendance. Each individual kennel, cat cage, module or colony must be fitted with a secure closing device that cannot be opened by the animals held. Where dogs are boarded, a security barrier at least 3 m high should be constructed to prevent the escape of animals or unauthorized entry.

The kennel compound wall may form part of the security barrier. In the case of cats, all buildings in which animals are housed should be fitted with double doors to prevent the loss of any animals that may escape from cages or other facilities.

Other facilities

Each boarding establishment must provide:

- An area for reception
- An area for records storage
- Washing and toilet facilities for staff
- Hygienically maintained facilities for bathing, drying and grooming animals
- An area suitable for cleaning and disinfecting food and water bowls and any other equipment used in the preparation of food
- A hygienic food storage area where there is no risk of contamination of the food by vermin or spoilage by other organisms, and refrigerator space for foods that are likely to spoil at ambient temperatures.

Specialized dog and cat housing

Hospital dog and cat accommodation

Hospital kennels are specifically designed for short-stay patients that are undergoing surgery or treatment. It is for this purpose that the kennels are restrictive, to ensure strict rest and allow good observation. Separate accommodation for hospital patients from any animals being groomed or boarded is recommended and obligatory under the RCVS Practice Standards Scheme.

The RCVS Practice Standards Scheme states that inpatient facilities must be of a suitable size, securable, sturdy, escape-proof, without potentially injurious faults and easily cleanable. Ideally kennels or cages, and their fittings, should be made of non-permeable materials so as to be easily cleaned and disinfected. There must be adequate heating, lighting and ventilation of the hospitalization area. A range of bedding, feedstuffs and clean fresh water must be available. There should be facilities for hospitalization of the full range of species and size of animals routinely admitted. Walk-in kennels should be available for the hospitalization of large-breed dogs (Figure 12.19). Informed consent should be sought for all procedures for which an animal is admitted into a veterinary practice. The veterinary practice should also provide accommodation and have a written policy for the isolation of contagious cases. Figure 12.20 illustrates the minimum recommended sizes for hospital kennels.

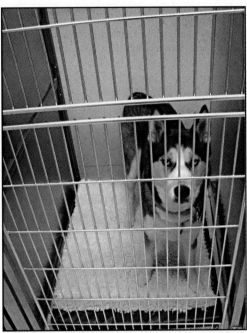

12.19 Walk-in kennels provide accommodation for large-breed dogs in the veterinary practice.

Animal	Height (cm)	Width (cm)	Depth (cm)
Cat	45.72	45.72	72.39
Small dog	45.72	60.96	72.39
Medium dog	76.20	76.20	72.39
Large dog	76.20	121.92	72.39
Giant dog	91.44	152.40	72.39
Walk-in kennel	180	140	110

12.20 Minimum recommended sizes of hospital kennels for dogs and cats.

Whelping accommodation

Anyone running a dog breeding business will require a licence for this purpose. A person is presumed to be carrying on a business if in a 12-month period their bitches give birth (collectively) to 5 litters or more. Bitches owned by different persons who are, for example, part of the same company or family, are all considered to be within the one business even if kept at different locations. Thus, a number of people working together cannot evade the licence requirements by claiming to own different dogs and at different locations. The kennels must be inspected and licensed by the local council and must have a suitable whelping area included in the design.

Special considerations for whelping accommodation

The whelping area must:

- Be small enough for the bitch to feel secure in, yet not too small
- Be quiet and away from ringing telephones and other barking dogs
- Be away from other dogs – the bitch and puppies must be under protective isolation
- Be clean – hygiene should be of utmost importance
- Be escape-proof
- Be warm and comfortable, with bedding in which the bitch can make a nest
- Have additional heating provided for the puppies (e.g. an infrared lamp), which the bitch can move away from should she become too warm
- Give privacy for the bitch but allow observation
- Ideally have a 'cut-out' in one side of the box to prevent the puppies escaping but allow the bitch to leave the box to urinate and feed.

Puppy accommodation

Puppies should be under protective isolation away from other dogs. The accommodation should be escape-proof, with the ability to regulate the temperature of the environment. A stable-type door is ideal, with the bottom half being low enough to allow staff to step over whilst not allowing the puppies to escape.

Dangerous and stray dogs

Accommodation for aggressive animals should be labelled as such to ensure staff safety. Any animal of an unknown disposition should be isolated and observed initially to assess its behaviour. A full history is useful in identifying any specific behaviour traits (see Chapter 11). Any procedure or human behaviour likely to cause aggressive behaviour in an animal should be well communicated to all staff. Staff should ensure their own safety at all times.

It should be remembered that dogs that are extremely friendly and non-aggressive under normal conditions may become aggressive when stressed, in pain or when kennelled. 'Kennel guarding' may occur; dogs become territorially aggressive when placed into the confines of a kennel. In a veterinary hospital it is recommended that all kennelled dogs are fitted with a collar before being put into a kennel. This makes it easier for staff to remove the animal from the kennel should kennel guarding occur. In some practices, dogs will be attached to their kennel door via the use of a long length of indestructible metal chain to ensure that the dog can be removed from the kennel.

Security is very important when housing aggressive animals, and access to the kennels and runs should ideally be from separate service passages with double doors to ensure that the animal does not escape (Figure 12.21). Staff should be provided with a means of personal communication, such as walkie-talkies or mobile-phones, so that they can obtain assistance if necessary.

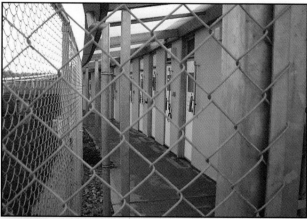

12.21 Double-doored separate service passage for access to kennels and runs.

Equine accommodation

Licensing of equine accommodation

Issues relating to the animal welfare and health and safety of dogs and cats in boarding establishments, described under The Animal Boarding Establishments Act 1963, are similarly covered for horses under the Riding Establishments Act 1964. This is a comprehensive act that relates to the care of horses in riding schools. An annual licence and council inspection is required. There are current discussions within the British Equestrian Federation to extend such licensing to cover livery yards and other equestrian centres such as rescue homes.

Pasture

Under the Animal Welfare Act 2006, many codes of practice cover the keeping of horses and other equids. The simplest form of accommodation for horses, ponies and donkeys is a field; however, there are minimum requirements even for keeping a horse at grass. Section 9 (2) of the act covers environment; this is a guideline and has a lot of helpful advice for the most basic accommodation, which is included in Defra's 'Code of Practice for the Welfare of Horses, Ponies, Donkeys and their Hybrids'.

- All horses must have access to shelter; even the hardiest of breeds need trees, hedges or manmade sheltering from cold winds and flies. Less hardy breeds are probably not well suited to living out all year round; thoroughbred horses should be rugged up and brought in for shelter in harsh weather.
- Permanent stabling should be available to treat any sick/injured animals, and this should have access to electricity.
- There is a minimum amount of pasture that should be allowed for horses permanently out at grass. This should be 1.25–2.50 acres (0.5–1.0 hectares) for horses and ponies, and for donkeys 0.5–1 acre (0.2–0.4 hectares). For animals spending only some time at grass this could be slightly reduced.
- Pasture management should be in place to rotate grazing areas and pick up droppings daily.

- Water should be available to horses at all times. Natural streams may not be suitable as they may be contaminated, and metal baths are not suitable due to their sharp edges. Any water troughs should be cleaned regularly of algae. Horses drink on average 5 litres per 100 kg a day and possibly more in hot weather. Ice must be broken in cold climates.
- A regular worming programme should be in place, to include all horses.
- Fields should be kept clear of poisonous plants, with particular attention to ragwort. Ragwort is subject to the Weeds Act 1959, Ragwort Control Act 2003 and Code of Practice on How to Prevent and Control the Spread of Ragwort 2006. All species of ragwort are poisonous to horses and humans; gloves should therefore be worn to remove ragwort and it should be disposed of by incineration. Cut ragwort is still poisonous to horses and should be removed immediately. Yew and laburnum are also poisonous to horses, and there are many other plants that are potentially dangerous to varying degrees depending on the amount eaten. A list is available in the British Horse Society (BHS) Manual, or on the BHS website.
- Fencing should be 1.25 m high, with the bottom rail 0.5 m above the ground.

Stabling

Stabling can come in many forms and variations, from one or two loose boxes to large barns and even more sophisticated accommodation such as foal high-dependency units. There are some minimum requirements regarding dimensions that are standardized by the BHS (Figure 12.22).

Type/size of horse	Minimum dimensions
Ponies (up to 14.2 hands)	3.05 m x 3.05 m
Horses (up to 16.2 hands)	3.65 m x 3.65 m
Large horses (>16.2 hands)	3.65 m x 4.25 m
Foaling boxes	4.25 m x 4.25 m

12.22 Minimum sizes for equine accommodation.

These figures are just a guide; the horse must also have head room of at least 60–90 cm above its ears.

A yard should have all of the requirements to facilitate the keeping of horses on site, which should include:

- Stabling
- Storage for hay and bedding
- Feed room, this must be rodent-proof
- Access to water
- Parking area
- Secure storage for tack
- Exercise area.

Walls can be made of several materials (see Figure 12.10). Consideration should be given to building materials before construction. Wood may be the cheapest material but it has disadvantages:

- It is prone to being chewed by horses and rodents
- It is susceptible to damp
- It may be harder to disinfect
- It is a fire risk

- It is difficult to eradicate contagious pathogens (e.g. ringworm) or infectious causes of diarrhoea (e.g. *Salmonella* spp.) from wooden structures.

Brickwork is less cost-effective but is easier to keep clean and can be treated with antifungal paint or rubber.

Roofing should be made of heat-resistant materials to prevent overheating in summer and should have insulating properties in winter, preferably with some natural light and guttering. The front should extend approximately 90–100 cm over the front of the stable to protect the horse when it is looking over the door. There should be air vents within the top of the roof, to allow air coming through the windows and door to travel upwards and out of the vents, reducing condensation; this is passive ventilation.

Windows should be placed on the same side as the door to prevent a through draft; they should open outwards and be made of wired safety glass. Small holes at the front and back of the stable can add to the effect, as well as acting as drainage outlets.

Flooring should be have a non-porous, non-slip surface; concrete is ideal and can be covered with rubber, but this should be well sealed to prevent harbouring of bacteria. The floor should slope towards the door so that steam cleaning and disinfection can be carried out easily.

Lighting should be placed centrally to light all parts of the stable and should be good enough to allow procedures to be performed if necessary. Light switches should be outside the stable, tamper-proof from the horse and weather-proof; any electricity supply should be fitted with a circuit breaker in case of damage, to prevent electric shock. Any damage should be reported and isolated immediately.

Heating may need to be increased in the case of sick horses or foals; this can be done with heat lamps, fans, mats or central heating systems.

Doors should have a slide bolt at the top and a kick bolt at the bottom for ease, with an anti-chewing metal strip along the top edge, and should have the facility to hook back to the wall.

Ideally, horses should be fed from the floor. If hay racks or rings are used, they should be of sufficient height to prevent the horse from getting grass seeds in its eyes or putting its feet into a hay net. In a barn situation, there should be some means of preventing the horses in adjacent stables from consuming one another's hay. Water should be given using a method that allows measurement, in a container that is easy to clean and cannot be tipped over. In a foal unit, the water should be raised from the ground to prevent accidental drowning.

Bedding should be non-toxic, low in dust, warm, absorbent, easy to maintain, cost effective and as environmentally friendly as possible. Some examples of equine bedding are included in Figure 12.5. It should be noted that all bedding is only as good as its management, and leaving soiled bedding of any type represents a potential respiratory hazard. Horses that eat their bedding through boredom or hunger may become prone to colic. It is advisable in these situations to choose non-palatable bedding such as cardboard or shavings. High banks and a thick layer of light bedding will go some way to alleviate injury, should a horse become cast in the stable. Rubber matting is particularly useful if it is covered with additional bedding, to provide grip for horses getting up and lying down. It will also reduce the amount of bedding required and thus the size of the muck heap.

Cleaning stables

As a minimum, all stables should be mucked out twice a day (Figure 12.23). Each yard should have designated equipment that is cleaned on a daily basis, to include fork or shavings fork, scoop or shovel, brush and wheel barrow. The best method is to hose down each piece and then soak and/or spray each piece with a suitable disinfectant at the correct concentration at the end of each day.

---

1. Tie the horse up outside the stable if possible, so as to avoid injury from any of the equipment. If the horse has to remain in the stable, the wheelbarrow and any implements should be left outside.
2. Remove water buckets and wash these out before refilling at least daily.
3. Remove hay nets and discard any uneaten hay or haylage.
4. Start at the front of the stable and remove any droppings. Remove any hay/haylage that is uneaten (this will help discourage mice and rats).
5. Fork the bedding up at the sides of the stable, allowing any further droppings to fall and be removed.
6. Remove any urine-soaked bedding. A skip or mucksack can be used to carry the droppings and soiled bedding to the wheelbarrow. Clean bedding should be separated from dirty bedding and put to one side so that it can be re-used.
7. Brush the floor and preferably leave to dry before relaying the bedding and applying fresh bedding on top.
8. The bed can then be put down, using the old material to create the base and adding clean bedding to build up the walls into banks, which help to keep draughts out and protect the horse, to a certain degree, if it rolls from becoming 'cast' (stuck up against a wall). Banks should be removed and replaced on a regular basis to prevent mould spores growing, as these can exacerbate or encourage respiratory disease. The final bed should be thick enough so that when a fork is stabbed into it, the floor cannot be felt.

12.23 How to muck out a stable. The principles of mucking out are the same for straw, shavings, hemp and paper. Peat bedding (which is rarely used because of the environmental impact) is used in a deep litter fashion, where only droppings and urine are removed but the bedding is not thrown up.

After each horse leaves, its stable should be emptied of all bedding and steam-cleaned, then disinfected with a suitable solution. In the case of horses with infections, the stable should then be swabbed for culture, and cleaning repeated if necessary.

All belongings, including rugs, head collar and lead-ropes and grooming brushes, should be washed with a biological washing powder or soaked for the advised length of time with a suitable disinfectant.

Feed and water buckets should be thoroughly cleaned and soaked in disinfectant for the manufacturer's recommended contact time and then rinsed well.

Disposal of equine waste

Normal soiled waste should be disposed of on a muck heap. Any waste contaminated with blood or potentially infectious material should be treated as such and disposed of as hazardous waste (see Chapter 2). Horses that have been admitted as possibly infectious or where infectious disease has been suspected during their stay should have their bedding collected. The animal should be swabbed and samples cultured, and all material kept until they are confirmed clear of disease. Such animals should be isolated (see later) until shown not to be infectious.

Hospital stabling

A routine stable block for the hospital situation needs some basic requirements as a minimum:

- Hand-washing facilities at each yard with soap, hot water and paper towelling (Figure 12.24a,b).
- Alcohol gel dispensers situated at least every three or four stables, for use before and after treatment (Figure 12.24c)
- Separate sinks for making of feeds
- Electricity supply for drip infusion pumps, clippers, X-ray generators and ultrasonography/endoscopy equipment
- Facilities for hanging drips for intravenous fluids (Figure 12.25)
- Heating (Figure 12.26)
- Possibly a sling for compromised patients
- Lighting suitable for examination of wounds and treatments (some areas can be equipped with lighting near the floor to facilitate the examination of the distal limb)
- Separate feeding facilities for each yard (Figure 12.27)
- Individual feed buckets, water buckets, grooming equipment and headcollar/lead rope for each stable (Figure 12.28)
- Separate handling for hazardous, non-hazardous and 'sharps' waste
- Facility to label each patient clearly with its identity and any specific treatments.

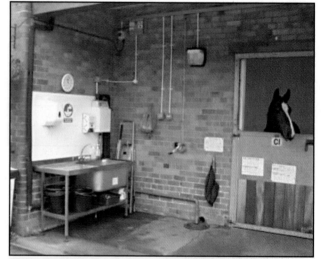
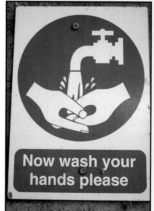
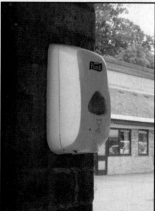

12.24 Hand-washing facilities for equine practice, with reminder sign and gel dispenser.

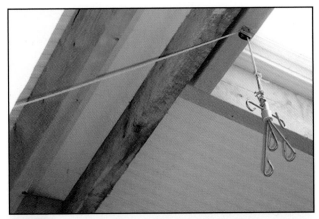

12.25 Facilities for hanging drips for intravenous fluids.

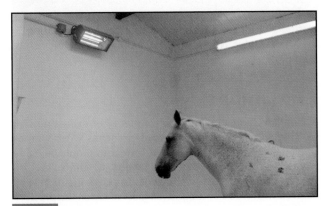

12.26 Heating in an equine unit.

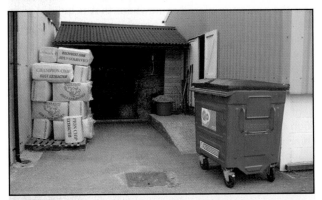

12.27 Equine bedding and feed facilities.

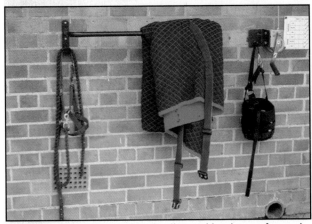

12.28 Separate rug, head collar and lead-rope for each stable.

Specialized stabling

Every animal is an individual with differing requirements and each yard must afford the basic facilities. However, some yards may be equipped for more specialized procedures such as radiation, isolation (see later in chapter) and foal handling units.

Foal stabling

Foal stabling should ideally be in a separate area to the general population and foals should be nursed separately from other cases, or at the very least taken care of before any other case is handled. Facilities will vary greatly from a simple set-up to the most sophisticated hospital that may see many foals each season. The following factors should be considered:

- A separate treatment area (Figure 12.29), with all consumables required kept away from the general population
- A means of separating mare and foal for individual treatment (Figure 12.30)
- Heating, if necessary
- Fluid therapy
- Lighting
- Oxygen cylinder or supply for therapy.

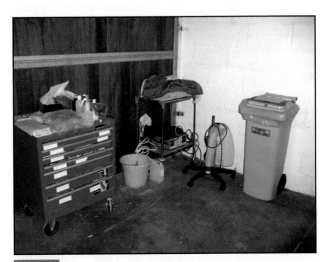

12.29 Foal treatment area.

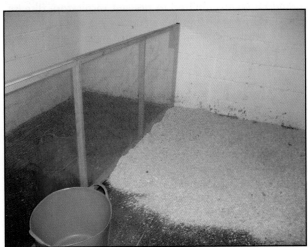

12.30 Simple area for allowing the mare and foal to be nursed individually if required.

Accommodation for exotic pets

Ferrets

Ferrets may be housed indoors or outdoors but should be protected from temperatures above 26°C. They need protection from the rain and draughts, somewhere dry to sleep and plenty of things to prevent boredom, such as tunnels, toys, branches and structures to hide in (e.g. tubes and boxes). They are not good climbers but are very good at burrowing and escaping through small holes. Ferrets quickly learn to use a litter tray. The construction of the cage should ensure an impervious surface, as urine and faeces are strong-smelling. The cage should be tall enough to allow the ferret to stand on its hindlegs. Hay, straw and wood shavings are not recommended for ferrets as they may cause respiratory tract irritation.

Rabbits

The accommodation should be large enough to enable the rabbit to stand on its hindlimbs without its ears touching the top of the cage and to allow the rabbit to stretch, exercise and display normal behaviour. A hutch with access to a grass run is often used. The accommodation should ideally be raised off the ground but incorporate access to grazing for a period every day. Some owners keep their rabbits inside; indoor rabbits should only be allowed to run loose in the house when supervised, as they may chew electrical cables or poisonous house plants. At other times they can be housed in a secure hutch or pen indoors. Outdoor accommodation should provide protection from predation and extremes of heat; temperatures should be kept below 26°C. Mesh tops and bottoms of runs prevent predation, burrowing and escape. The hutch should have a waterproof roof with an overhang and be positioned out of direct sunlight. A darkened area or sleeping box allows the rabbit to retreat and feel secure. Nesting material, such as straw or hay should be provided for females. Boxes or tunnels should also be provided in the run to give cover for an alarmed rabbit. Rabbits easily learn to use litter trays if repeatedly placed in them and this makes the accommodation much more hygienic and easier to clean. Wood- or paper-based litter should be used. The housing area should be well ventilated to prevent respiratory disease. Rabbits can be given toys, tubes and tunnels, and apple wood to gnaw on, to enrich their environment and prevent boredom (Figure 12.31).

Guinea pigs

Guinea pigs should have separate summer and winter accommodation. They are particularly sensitive to damp conditions and it is best to house them indoors in winter. Indoor cages should allow at least 0.2 m² of floor space per animal. In summer a mobile run is ideal, provided there is access to a dry covered area. Pens should be at least 30 cm high to prevent escape and should be covered to prevent predation. A sleeping/nest area with bedding material should always be provided, as well as lots of places for the guinea pigs to hide and retreat to. Temperatures between 12°C and 20°C are ideal, and extremes of temperature should be avoided.

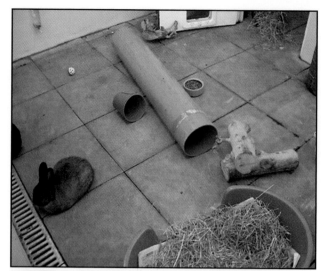

12.31 Enriched environment in accommodation for a rabbit. Note the channel drain for ease of cleaning.

Chinchillas

Accommodation should allow for plenty of exercising. Tall multi-level cages with numerous branches work well as chinchillas like to climb and jump. The cages should be made from small wire mesh rather than wood, as chinchillas love to chew. At least half of the cage's mesh floor should be covered with wood or toughened glass to lessen the pressure on their feet. Newspaper or wood shavings can be placed over the wire mesh. A wooden nest box should be provided and the enclosure placed somewhere that is quiet during the day, as chinchillas are nocturnal, and this is when they will rest. Chinchillas have a unique grooming habit and need access to a dust bath containing chinchilla sand deep enough for the animal to roll around in every day (Figure 12.32). Removing the bath after use keeps it clean of urine and faeces. Branches should be provided for chewing, which aids dental health. A pumice stone is also useful for chewing on. High temperature and high humidity must be avoided as chinchillas prefer cooler temperatures, although damp and draughts must also be avoided.

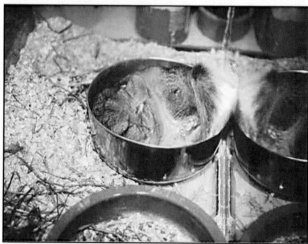

12.32 Shallow bowls of dust give chinchillas an opportunity for a spinning dust bath. (Reproduced from *BSAVA Manual of Exotic Pets, 4th edition*)

Rats, mice, hamsters and gerbils

Rats and mice enjoy climbing and so the accommodation should be tall and provide plenty of opportunity for this. A large aquarium with a wire lid or a cage with a solid plastic bottom and wire top to provide adequate ventilation may be used. Good ventilation and cage hygiene prevent the build-up of ammonia that can cause respiratory disease. Branches may be provided for them to chew as well as climb.

An interesting environment for hamsters can be constructed in a large aquarium (Figure 12.33). Commercial hamster accommodation is available but it should be ensured that this is large enough, chew-proof and adequately ventilated. Deep bedding will allow burrowing – a natural behaviour; and hamsters also require plentiful exercise so a solid-sided exercise wheel is a useful addition.

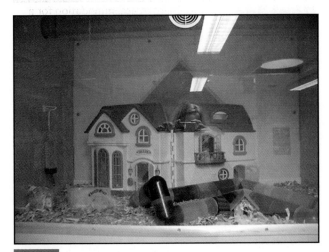

12.33 Aquarium-style hamster accommodation.

Gerbils are ideally housed in an aquarium half-filled with a mixture of peat and straw and furnished with branches, allowing them to dig, chew and explore. Alternatively, the aquarium may be deep littered with shavings, which has the advantage of making soiled bedding easier to see. A wire mesh lid will allow ventilation. Gerbils also enjoy a sand bath. Tanks should be positioned away from direct sunlight and direct heat sources to avoid overheating. Cages should be escape-proof and gnaw-resistant, and should always be well ventilated. Suitable substrates to line the cage include dust-free commercial pet bedding or paper-based cat litter.

All of the small mammals should be provided with a sturdy nest box containing nesting material (shredded paper is preferable to acrylic bedding). Small mammals also appreciate lots of places to hide and retreat to and so their environment should be enriched in this way (Figure 12.34; note also the ventilation considerations of this accommodation). If exercise wheels are used only solid-bottomed wheels should be provided, to prevent fractured limbs.

Chipmunks

Chipmunks do not always adapt well to captivity and commonly develop stereotypical behaviours in anything but the largest enclosures. The best accommodation is a large, secure outdoor enclosure that they cannot dig or chew their way out of. Due to their origin they cope easily with cold temperatures, but they need shelter from hot days and should

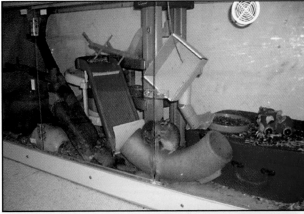

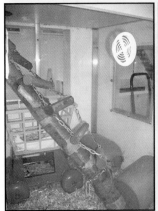

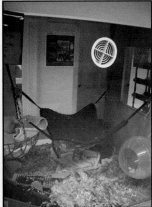

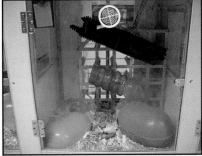

12.34

Accommodation suitable for small mammals. Note the ventilation system in each unit.

be provided with a nest box to retreat to. They should be kept in dry and draught-free conditions, with plenty of branches to climb and opportunity to dig burrows. Their enclosures should be escape-proof. Enclosures for chipmunks should be sited well away from televisions, strip lighting or computer terminals that may emit 50 Hz wavelength radiation, as this frequency can induce manic neurological behavioural problems in this species.

Birds

Birds should ideally be housed in cages that allow free movement and, in the case of smaller birds, flight. The minimum legal requirement is that the bird should be able to stretch its wings in all three dimensions. Caged birds must be allowed out to exercise if their cage is too small for free flying.

Galvanized metal cages are not recommended as they can lead to zinc poisoning. Natural wood perches are best (Figure 12.35) but should be replaced regularly. Sandpaper perch coverings should be avoided, as these can abrade the feet and lead to secondary foot infections. Perches that are too smooth or too small in diameter can lead to overgrown nails and foot lesions. A selection of perches of varying diameters may help prevent foot problems.

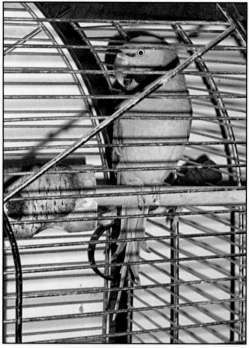

12.35

Birdcage with wooden perches.

Whether the species normally feeds on or off the ground should be taken into consideration.

Aviaries

Aviaries should have deep foundations or a solid concrete base and wire covering the bottom of the aviary to protect against rats and mice. A frost-free shelter should be incorporated, with provision for heating and lighting the shelter during the winter months. Solid roofing material will reduce the possibility of disease spread from wild birds, and a safety (double) door will reduce the possibility of escape. The environmental conditions required by each species should be researched before attempting to set up housing, so that these conditions can be met. These will depend upon where the birds come from, their natural habitat, and the climate.

Reptiles

Reptiles are housed in a controlled environment known as a vivarium (Figure 12.36). The important points to consider when setting up a vivarium are structure, heating, lighting, humidity, ventilation, and furnishing.

Structure

Glass or Perspex aquaria are easy to clean but are often extremely heavy. Custom-built vivaria are made out of melamine-covered chipboard (with the corners sealed with aquarium sealant) or fibreglass and generally have front-opening sliding doors to make access easier. They are generally easier to clean.

Heating

A temperature gradient should be provided across the vivarium. The range should be maintained within the inhabitant's preferred optimum temperature zone (POTZ) to enable the reptile to maintain its preferred body temperature (PBT).

The heating element should be attached to a thermostat and monitored using a separate maximum–minimum thermometer. Overhead heating is a more natural way of supplying heat than heat mats but must be shielded from the reptile: thermal burns are common as reptiles often will not move away from a heat source that is actually burning them.

Bathing facilities should be supplied or the bird should be sprayed regularly to reduce feather dust, maintain plumage and encourage preening.

Caged birds benefit from exposure to either natural or artificial ultraviolet (UV) light on a daily basis; specific UV lights are available for indoor birds. A nest box is often appreciated and cages should be covered at night to allow rest.

Birds should not be kept in the same room as gas fires or in the kitchen, where fumes can cause respiratory problems. These include fumes from Teflon-coated pots and pans, released when the utensils are allowed to become overheated; although these cannot be detected by humans they are rapidly lethal to birds. It is also not recommended that birds are kept by people who smoke.

The cage should ideally be placed high up or at least to the side of the room. The cage should not be so filled with toys that the bird cannot move, but birds often appreciate a few toys and these can be rotated so that the bird does not become bored with them. Parrots are very destructive and their toys should be of the tough acrylic type.

Food and water containers should be placed where the bird can reach them easily and cannot defecate in them.

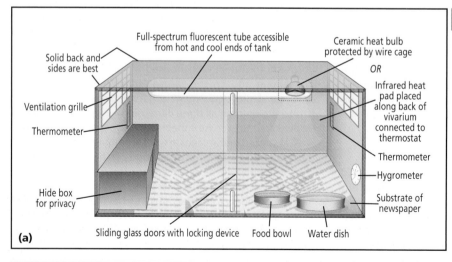

12.36 Reptile environments: **(a)** clinical. *continues* ▶

Full-spectrum fluorescent tube accessible from hot and cool ends of tank

Solid back and sides are best

Ventilation grille

Thermometer

Hide box for privacy

Sliding glass doors with locking device

Food bowl

Water dish

Ceramic heat bulb protected by wire cage

OR

Infrared heat pad placed along back of vivarium connected to thermostat

Thermometer

Hygrometer

Substrate of newspaper

(a)

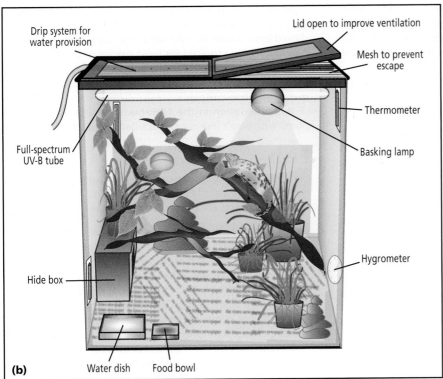

Drip system for water provision

Lid open to improve ventilation

Mesh to prevent escape

Thermometer

Basking lamp

Full-spectrum UV-B tube

Hygrometer

Hide box

(b)

Water dish   Food bowl

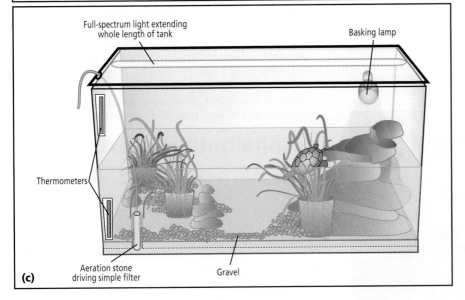

Full-spectrum light extending whole length of tank

Basking lamp

Thermometers

Aeration stone driving simple filter

Gravel

(c)

12.36 *continued* Reptile environments: **(b)** arboreal; **(c)** semi-aquatic.

Lighting

Lighting should be of daylight quality for lizards and chelonians, for activity and foraging. Fluorescent tubes that provide a good daylight spectrum, including ultraviolet (UV-B is specifically required to allow synthesis of vitamin D3 in many reptiles and UV-A is required to stimulate some forms of behaviour, such as breeding and in some cases appetite), should be selected and these should be changed every 6 months, as the UV portion of their spectrum has a limited life.

Reptiles from desert habitats will require a higher light intensity than those from forests.

Humidity and water

Powerful heaters tend to dry the atmosphere, and regular spraying with water is required to maintain a reasonable degree of humidity. This should be carried out regularly, even for desert species, and very often for rainforest species.

A source of water for drinking and bathing should also be provided. It should be noted that many species of reptile (e.g. chameleons and many iguanas) will not drink from bowls, but only from water droplets in the vivarium. This means regular misting of the cage with water, or setting up a drip system to supply continually dripping water, is necessary.

Ventilation

Adequate air vents are essential to ensure good air circulation. If ventilation is poor, an airline powered by a small aquarium pump will encourage the circulation of fresh air.

Furnishing

Arboreal species will require branches for climbing and burrowing species will require sufficient depth of substrate to hide in. Substrates used to line the bottom of the vivarium include bark chippings, peat, aquarium gravel and sand. Sand tends to be used only for desert species of lizard and burrowing species of snake. Sand can cause scale abrasions in snakes.

All species should have hide areas or hide boxes – if possible at least one more hide area than there are reptiles in the tank.

Aquatic or semi-aquatic reptiles and amphibians

The natural history of the species should be researched. It is important when considering housing to know the animal's natural habitat, climate and whether it lives on land, in water or makes use of both.

The requirements for amphibians are similar to those for many aquatic species of reptile. Some amphibians are totally aquatic (e.g. many newts, axolotl); others prefer to have an aquatic and a terrarium area (e.g. many frogs) or just a very moist terrarium (e.g. many members of the toad family).

Aquatic and semi-aquatic species need glass or Perspex aquarium tanks because of the relatively high level of humidity required. Totally aquatic species need a tank equipped as a fish tank, with good water filtration. Terrestrial species need a vivarium similar to that for a reptile but with increased humidity.

Species that need both land and water need an aquaterrarium (Figure 12.37). A glass tank may be used and the land area may be provided by using a piece of glass to separate it from the water, sealed with aquarium sealant. The land area is then filled with soil, moss or gravel. Alternatively, a land area can be provided by building up rocks within the terrarium. In this case it is difficult to provide live plants and there is no area for egg-laying. The rocks should be set securely and ideally glued so that they do not become dislodged.

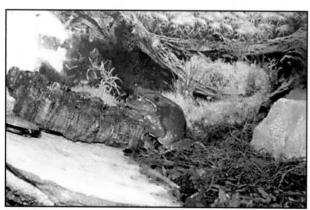

12.37 Frogs require an aqua-terrarium.

Filtration

Where free water is provided it must be changed regularly, or, preferably, an effective aquarium filtration system should be installed, to minimize the build-up of environmental bacteria. If it is necessary to feed reptiles in the water, it is better to move them into a separate tank for feeding as the volume of detritus produced often exceeds the capacity of most filtration devices.

Heating

Some species require heated water, in which case an aquarium heater should be used. The water area must be deep enough to submerge the heater completely and the heater should be protected from the animal to prevent injuries.

Some species need to bask out of water and in this case a basking heat source and a UV-emitting fluorescent lamp should be provided over the land area. Supplemental heating is generally not required for most species of amphibian that originate in temperate climes, but a UV light source is still recommended for anurans (frogs and toads) to prevent metabolic bone disease.

If condensation in the tank becomes a problem, an air pump with an air line can be installed to keep the glass clear.

Fish

Fish need to be kept in a carefully controlled environment (see *BSAVA Manual of Ornamental Fish, 2nd edition*) and the following aspects are particularly important to consider:

- The water for most species of fish should be kept at pH values between 7.0 and 7.5. Water hardness should be >10 mg/ml for most freshwater fish
- Fish require oxygen, either from live plants, diffusion from the surface or by artificial aeration of the water using air pumps. Carbon dioxide is removed from the tank by live plants or the aeration system
- Fish produce ammonia as a waste product of protein metabolism and this must be removed from the tank. Ammonia is used by live plants to build protein but if there are no live plants within the aquarium it must be removed by an under-gravel filter. Bacteria break down nitrogenous waste by converting ammonia to nitrite and then to nitrate; these products need to be kept under control by efficient filtration and should be monitored regularly using a water-testing kit. In general, ammonia is most toxic to fish and its toxicity is exacerbated by higher water temperatures. Nitrites are the next most toxic and nitrates are the least toxic of the three waste products.

Hospitalization of exotic pets

Stress is an important consideration when treating most exotic species kept as pets and should be carefully balanced against the need for hospitalization. Surgical patients should ideally be discharged to their home environment as soon as possible. It may be necessary for owners to be taught how to hand- or syringe-feed their pets and medicate them at home. Owners will usually be more aware of the pet's daily routine and habits and are often more likely to notice abnormal behaviours indicating deterioration of the animal. If hospitalization is considered necessary, the animal's own cage or housing is often the best form of accommodation if it is feasible for it be transported to the veterinary practice. If this is not possible, the natural habitat and behaviour of the species and recommended domestic accommodation as detailed above should be considered and recreated as far as possible in the veterinary environment in order to fulfil the animal's basic needs.

Exotic pets are often natural prey species and should be housed in quiet areas away from dogs and cats to minimize noise and olfactory stressors. Lighting may be subdued and the front of the cage covered to calm them. Most species will appreciate a box or area with plenty of bedding to hide in. Birds should be provided with perches and a water bowl to bathe in. Hay, straw and wood shavings may need to be avoided in animals with wounds or those with respiratory conditions. Rabbits can be hospitalized for a short period of time in a small kennel with newspaper covering the floor and hay or straw provided as bedding, unless contraindicated. Acrylic veterinary bedding may be used. There should be a box where the rabbit can seek cover.

Cleaning and disinfection

Although the size and type of accommodation for animals may differ, the principles of controlling infection within these accommodations are very similar. Cleaning and disinfection are just two of these methods; others are listed below.

Methods of preventing the spread of infection

- Cleaning and disinfection.
- Isolation.
- Barrier nursing.
- Protective clothing.
- Quarantine.
- Treatment.
- Sterilization.
- Vaccination.
- Improved diet.
- Owner compliance.
- Hygiene.
- Ventilation.

Definitions

- **Disinfection** is the removal of microorganisms, but not necessarily all pathogens and their spores (reduction in the number of microbes).
- **Sterilization** is the removal of all microorganisms, including bacterial spores.
- A **disinfectant** is a chemical agent that kills, or prevents the multiplication of, microorganisms on inanimate objects. May also be known as an 'environmental disinfectant'.
- An **antiseptic** is a disinfectant safe to use on living tissue. May also be known as a 'skin disinfectant'.
- **Antisepsis** is the prevention of sepsis, achieved by disinfection. Usually refers to the prevention of infection in living tissues by the use of an antiseptic.
- **Asepsis** is the exclusion of all microorganisms and spores; a sterile state. Achieved by sterilization.
- **-cide** is a suffix meaning kills (e.g. a **bactericide** kills bacteria).
- **-stat** is a suffix meaning preventing growth or multiplication (e.g. a **bacteriostat** prevents further multiplication of bacteria).

Disinfection is a process by which pathogenic microorganisms are destroyed or removed from inanimate objects. It is an important method of controlling the spread of disease within the veterinary practice and is achieved by both physical and chemical actions.

The physical action of scrubbing and cleaning is just as important as the chemical actions of the disinfectants themselves. This is because foreign materials, such as blood and faecal matter, are ideal breeding grounds for pathogens but the efficacy of disinfectants is greatly reduced when used in the presence of organic material. The disinfectants must have direct contact with the microorganisms to destroy them and so the organic materials must first be removed. Only when all the debris has been removed will the actions of the disinfectant be effective. The most efficient method of disinfection is to use chemical disinfection following mechanical cleaning.

Heating is another method of disinfection and way of achieving antisepsis. Microorganisms are destroyed by high temperatures, e.g. during steam-cleaning and machine washing of bedding. The efficacy of chemical disinfectants is also increased by mixing them with warm rather than cold water.

Cleaning a clinical environment

Each area of the practice should be assessed for risk according to the potential for cross-infection. Standard Operating Procedures should then be established for the cleaning and disinfecting of each area according to its risk (Figure 12.38). All staff should be aware of the procedures and potential risks.

---

1. Remove animal from kennel to a safe, secure holding area (not another dog's kennel).
2. Remove all items from the kennel (feeding bowls, bedding, toys, etc.).
3. Remove any gross contamination.
4. Sweep or hose out any hair or debris.
5. Scrub all surfaces of the kennel (including the door) with a detergent or combined detergent/disinfectant.[a]
6. Rinse with water.[a]
7. Apply disinfectant at the correct dilution rate.[a]
8. Allow for contact time of disinfectant.
9. Rinse thoroughly if applicable.
10. Physically dry.
11. Leave to air dry.
12. Return/replace bedding, etc., as necessary.
13. Return animal to kennel.

- All feeding bowls, litter trays, etc., should be washed in detergent (e.g. washing up liquid) rinsed, sprayed with or soaked in disinfectant, rinsed and then dried (alternatively feed bowls may be sterilized using an autoclave or ethylene oxide).
- Bedding should be machine washed at 60°C (most microorganisms will be destroyed).
- Mop heads/cleaning equipment should also be regularly washed and disinfected.

[a] Many of the more recently developed kennel disinfectants are a combination of specialist detergents and disinfectant agents, mixed by manufacturers as part of the active ingredient formulation. This principle potentiates the activity of the disinfectant and accelerates the microbicidal process. When using these products, follow actions 1–5, using the combined detergent/disinfectant instead of a detergent, and cut out steps 6 and 7.

12.38 Example of a Standard Operating Procedure for cleaning a kennel.

- **Low-risk** areas include offices and corridors. They require an easy-to-use product that combines cleaning and disinfection.
- **High-risk** areas include any that may become contaminated by body fluids (e.g. theatres, kennels and consulting rooms).

Certain areas may seem low-risk but the potential for cross-infection is high. An example is the reception area/waiting room – every animal that enters the practice will enter the reception area. Control measures should be put into place: for example, any animal suspected of having a contagious disease should be isolated immediately into a separate area whilst waiting for the veterinary surgeon to attend; and owners of puppies arriving for first vaccinations should be advised not to allow them on the floor of the reception area or to mix with the other animals waiting.

High-risk areas should be thoroughly cleaned and disinfected daily, using a fast-acting, broad-spectrum disinfectant.

- Surfaces and floors should first be cleaned using a detergent to ensure the removal of all organic material, and then cleaned with a suitable disinfectant.
- Walls should be cleaned regularly to a height of 1.5 m with both detergent and disinfectant.
- Mop heads should be machine washed daily and replaced regularly.
- Surfaces in theatres and consulting room tables should also be cleaned *between* patients; any potential contaminants (hair, body fluids, tissue, contaminated instruments and equipment) should be removed and cleaned or disposed of as appropriate.
- Clipper blades should also be cleaned and disinfected between patients.
- Throughout the day surfaces and floors should be spot-cleaned if they become soiled.

The use of daily and weekly cleaning checklists is an effective way of ensuring that all tasks are completed in each area and therefore minimizing the risk of cross-infection within the veterinary practice. Figure 12.39 shows an example of such a cleaning checklist.

Many practices will use one particular agent for main use. The dilution rate may depend upon the intended use, and the manufacturer's datasheet or instructions should always be checked before using any chemical within the veterinary practice. For example, the dilution rate of many disinfectants is halved for high-risk areas (i.e. twice the concentration of disinfectant is used). Too weak a solution will be ineffective,

but too strong a solution would be wasteful and may be harmful to animals and personnel. Practices may consider rotation of disinfectants to avoid resistance of some pathogens to a commonly used disinfectant.

Types of antiseptic and disinfectant

Disinfectants, by their very nature, are toxic. They are designed to kill organisms. There is no such thing as a completely non-toxic disinfectant. Before choosing any disinfectant, it is important to know what organisms are to be killed. Typically, these organisms are viruses, bacteria, fungi or spores. Several factors will influence the selection of a particular type of disinfectant or antiseptic:

- Intended use of the product (environment or living tissue, high- or low-risk area)
- Range of activity against microorganisms
- Contact time
- Safety of staff and animals (i.e. how toxic is it?)
- Corrosive/staining effects
- Ease of use
- Cost and economy of the product
- Ability to be mixed with other products without causing unexpected toxicity
- Stability of the product
- Odour.

There are different classes of disinfectants, based on the types of agent they contain. Figure 12.40 gives examples of the different types of disinfectants and antiseptics. Modern commercial disinfectants often contain more than one of these types to maximize their action.

Consulting room daily cleaning checklist	Date:	
Task		**Initial when completed**
Dispose of hazardous waste and non-hazardous (offensive and domestic) waste accordingly		
Empty hazardous and non-hazardous waste bins, disinfect bins and replace bin bags		
Clean and disinfect/sterilize any used equipment accordingly		
Wipe all surfaces (including walls to a height of 1.5 m) with detergent		
Wipe all surfaces (including walls as before) with disinfectant		
Clean clippers		
Change hand towel		
Change disinfectant and cotton wool in thermometer pot		
Refill disinfectant spray, surgical spirit and antiseptic bottles		
Restock all consumables		
Vacuum floor		
Mop floor with detergent		
Mop floor with disinfectant		

12.39 Example of a cleaning checklist.

Disinfectant class	Examples
Alcohol	70% Isopropyl alcohol
Biguanides Chlorhexidine	Nolvasan, Savlon, Dinex, Hibiscrub
Cationic surfactants Quaternary ammonium compounds	Vetaclean
Halogens and halogen-containing compounds Chlorine-based Iodine-based Halogenated tertiary amines	Sodium hypochlorite (chlorine bleach), Domestos Iodine, Iodophors, Povidone–iodine, Betadine Trigene
Oxidizing agents Peroxides Peroxygen compounds	Hydrogen peroxide Virkon, Vetcide
Phenols and related compounds Phenolics Synthetic phenol	Phenol (carbolic acid), Cresol (cresylic acid), Lysol, Pine tar, Pine oil, Izol, Jeyes Fluid, Chloroxylenols, Dettol
Reducing agents Aldehydes	Glutaraldehyde, Formaldehyde, Cidex, Parvocide, Formula H

12.40 Types of disinfectant.

Types of agents

Alcohol

Alcohol is very effective against bacteria, fungi and some viruses but is not sporicidal. It is non-penetrating and so the skin needs to be cleaned first. It is often used as the final step in the surgical scrub routine of the patient. Alcohol has been proven as an effective surface sanitizer against MRSA. It is more expensive but mixes well with other antiseptics. It is flammable and can be an irritant, as it tends to dry skin.

Chlorhexidine

Chlorhexidine has good activity against Gram-positive bacteria but is less effective against Gram-negative bacteria and mycobacteria. It has a variable antiviral activity and fair antifungal action. It is inactivated by organic matter, soaps and plastics but is unaffected by body fluids. Chlorhexidine is an excellent skin and wound disinfectant and has a residual effect in the tissues.

Quaternary ammonium compounds

QACs have good activity against Gram-positive bacteria but are less effective against Gram-negative bacteria and have no sporicidal action. They have good fungicidal activity but very limited activity against viruses. They are only really suitable for disinfecting low-risk areas and tend to be inactivated by hard water and organic matter.

Chlorine-based halogens

Hypochlorites (bleach) are very effective against viruses, bacteria, fungi and spores. They are cheap but very corrosive and bleaching may occur. They produce strong vapours that can cause airway irritation. Organic matter reduces their efficacy and they deteriorate with storage and exposure to sunlight. They should not be used in the presence of urine as they can produce a noxious gas when mixed together.

Iodine-based halogens

Iodine and iodophors have a broad spectrum of activity against bacteria, viruses and fungi and some action against bacterial spores. They are inactivated by organic matter and may corrode metal and cause staining. Some people may be allergic to iodine. They are used as skin antiseptics and for open wound cleansing.

Halogenated tertiary amines

These contain a quaternary ammonium compound and have a wide range of action against bacteria, fungi, viruses and bacterial spores. They are not inactivated by organic matter and usually contain a detergent. They are irritant at concentrate level but they are generally of low toxicity and have low corrosion effects.

Peroxygen compounds

Peroxygen compounds have a good range of activity against bacteria (except mycobacteria), viruses and fungi and a variable action against bacterial spores. Their efficacy is reduced in the presence of organic material and they are irritant in powder form. They are corrosive to some metals.

Phenols

Phenols (phenolics) may be described as black, white or clear. They have good bacterial and fungal activity but a variable efficacy against viruses. They have a poor action against bacterial spores. They are not easily inactivated by organic material. They are toxic and irritant and should not come into contact with skin.

Phenols are irritant, strong smelling and *highly toxic to cats*. They are absorbed by rubber and plastics and may stain. They are cheap to purchase.

Synthetic phenols have a poor action against Gram-negative bacteria and their efficacy is reduced in the presence of organic matter. They are less irritant and can be inactivated by hard water.

Aldehydes

Glutaraldehyde has a wide range of bacterial, fungal and viral activity and is sporicidal but is slow-acting. It is not in-activated by organic material. It is highly irritant and highly toxic to skin, eyes and respiratory mucosa. This chemical can also cause sensitization, leading to further health problems with continued exposure. Due to its toxic nature, it is not recommended that this product be used as a wash-down disinfectant and should only be used where the necessary precautions to ensure safety of personnel can be taken.

Susceptibility of microbes to disinfection

Some bacteria are naturally more resistant than other bacteria to certain disinfectants. This is known as **intrinsic resistance**. Other, normally sensitive, bacteria can become resistant after exposure to a disinfectant; this is **acquired resistance**. Some viruses also demonstrate intrinsic resistance to disinfectants, but it is unlikely that viruses would develop acquired resistance under natural conditions. Non-enveloped viruses, such as canine parvovirus and feline calicivirus, are more resistant than enveloped viruses such as feline leukaemia virus and feline herpesvirus.

- Bacterial spores are bacterial 'embryos' surrounded by several different layers that make spores extremely resistant to chemical attack.
- Gram-negative bacteria (e.g. *Salmonella*) have a different type of cell wall which acts as a barrier to some disinfectants and so they tend to be more resistant to some disinfectants than Gram-positive bacteria (e.g. *Staphylococcus*).
- Mycobacteria are even more resistant to disinfectants, because of additional waxy layers in the cell wall.
- Plasmids are bacteria that acquire resistance by mutation or acquisition of extra genetic material.

Figure 12.41 shows the susceptibility of microbes to different types of disinfectant and antiseptic.

Precautions and the safe use of disinfectants

- Read the manufacturer's instructions and use as directed.
- Wear protective gloves/clothing and avoid direct contact with skin.
- Only use disinfectants for the purpose recommended by the manufacturer.
- Use the correct dilution for the required purpose according to the manufacturer's instructions.
- Add the disinfectant to the container after filling with the correct amount of water (to reduce inhalation of vapours or possibility of direct contact with concentrated disinfectant).
- Use only freshly made solutions.
- Mix the disinfectant with water at the recommended temperature.
- Leave the disinfectant for the recommended contact time.
- Concentrated disinfectant solutions and powders may be harmful, and so care must be taken when handling these.
- Keep chemicals in their original containers.
- Ensure that all lids are secured.
- Store away from children and animals.
- Do not mix chemicals.
- Minimize skin splashes.
- When spraying disinfectants, use the 'squirt' setting or apply the product with a cloth or sponge to avoid atomizing the disinfectant.
- Only mix enough disinfectant product as is necessary, to avoid introducing excess material into the sewage system.
- Wash hands thoroughly after use.

Disinfectant type	Bactericidal activity	Effectiveness against bacterial spores	Effectiveness against viruses	Effectiveness against fungi
Alcohol	Good. Effective against MRSA	Not active	Variable	Good
Chlorhexidine	Gram-positives: yes. Gram-negatives: less so Poor against mycobacteria	Not active	Variable	Fair
Quaternary ammonium compounds	Gram-positives: yes. Gram-negatives: less so No activity against *Mycobacterium tuberculosis*	Not active	Very limited	Good
Chlorine-based halogens (bleach)	Good	Good	Good	Good
Iodine/iodophors	Good	Some	Good	Good
Halogenated tertiary amines	Good	Good	Good	Good
Peroxygen compounds	Good but poor against mycobacteria	Variable	Good	Good
Phenols	Good	No	Poor	Good
Aldehydes	Good	Good but slow	Good	Good

12.41   Summary of the effectiveness of disinfectants against bacterial, viral and fungal organisms.

Veterinary isolation and barrier nursing

Cleaning and disinfection are obviously of utmost importance when nursing an infectious or potentially infectious patient and strict procedures should be followed for the nursing and care of these patients and the cleaning and disinfection of the isolation facility to ensure the safety of all the animals within the veterinary practice. The first rule should always be: *if there is any doubt as to whether or not an animal has a transmissible disease, it should be isolated immediately, assumed to be infectious and treated as such.* If this rule is not followed, then by the time it is established that the patient is carrying a potentially transmissible disease, that patient has probably entered and contaminated several areas of the practice, contaminated several personnel and been in contact with other animals within the practice. It follows that all reception staff require adequate training to be able to recognize the signs and symptoms of different transmissible diseases. It might be set within practice policy, for example, that any animal presenting for an appointment with vomiting and/or coughing or diarrhoea should be isolated until seen by the veterinary surgeon, as these are common symptoms of many infectious diseases. Practices may carry out a daily isolation risk assessment detailing the level of barrier nursing required for individual cases (Figure 12.42).

RULES and CODES OF PRACTICE

SAFETY PROCEDURES – ISOLATION RISK LEVELS

Level 0: Empty room
- No risk to other patients
- No need for protective clothing

Level 1: Vaccinated pets
- Minimum risk to other patients
- Gloves and apron to be worn when handling

Level 2: Wild animals or animals of unknown vaccination status but apparently healthy (e.g. quarantine)
- Moderate risk to other patients
- All protective clothing to be worn

Level 3: Known infectious or suspected infectious patients
- High risk to other patients
- All protective clothing to be worn and disposed of after use
- Ensure **hand disinfection** is carried out **and footbath** is used

Level 4: Patients with known or suspected zoonoses
- Risk to staff and clients
- All protective clothing must be worn and disposed of after use
- Ensure **hand disinfection** is carried out **and footbath** is used

TODAY'S ISOLATION RISK LEVEL IS: [   ]

12.42   Example of an isolation risk assessment. (Adapted from Isolation Assessment with the permission of Salus Q.P. Ltd)

Definitions

- **Isolation** is the physical separation of the animal suspected of having or proved to have a transmissible infectious disease.
- **Quarantine** is the compulsory isolation (with associated strict protocols) of animals with, or potentially exposed to, infectious diseases. In the case of 'quarantine kennels' this usually applies to notifiable diseases such as rabies. Within ordinary kennels and catteries and in veterinary practices 'quarantine' is used to describe the isolation of all animals with suspected contagious disease or of unknown health status (see Chapter 5).
- **Barrier nursing** creates a 'barrier' between the infectious animal and the nursing staff and other animals (e.g. wearing protective clothing, using separate equipment). This is usually carried out in conjunction with isolating the animal but can be employed alone if no isolation facilities exist.
- **Protective isolation** is the isolation of very susceptible animals (e.g. very young, very old, after surgery, or with compromised immunity) in an attempt to protect them from potential sources of infection.

Small animal isolation procedures

When an animal is admitted to the hospital with a suspected transmissible disease, it should be isolated immediately. The isolation facilities should be labelled as being in use, thus preventing the admittance of other animals into the ward and ensuring that access by staff and the public is restricted.

Visitors should not be allowed into the isolation unit. A method of colour coding might be appropriate so that all staff are immediately aware on glancing at the facility that a contagious case has been admitted. The isolated case should have no contact with other animals.

Equipment for the isolation facility (Figure 12.43) should be collected together so that it is only used within the isolation ward and also to limit the number of times staff have to enter and leave the ward when nursing the patient.

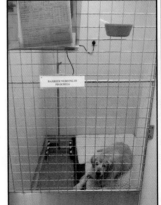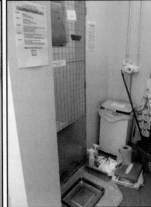

12.43   A self-contained, fully equipped small animal isolation facility. Points to note are: separate designated clinical equipment, PPE, cleaning equipment and waste segregation, together with appropriate isolation notices. (Courtesy of E. Mullineaux)

Equipment for an isolation facility might include:

- Protective clothing, e.g. coveralls, aprons, hoods, clogs, shoe covers, hats, facemasks (for nursing animals with airborne zoonoses, such as psittacosis), gloves, etc.
- Food and water bowls and feeding equipment (e.g. cutlery, jug, scales)
- Litter trays and cat litter
- Thermometer
- Cleaning equipment
- Bucket
- Detergent and disinfectant
- Incontinence pads
- Newspaper
- Bags for hazardous waste
- Stethoscope.

Ideally, one or two members of the nursing staff should be assigned to nursing the isolation case and, if at all possible, should nurse only that patient, to minimize the potential for indirectly passing the infection to other patients. If it is not possible for those members of staff to nurse only that patient, it must be ensured that the infectious case is nursed and treated last, before the other patients are attended to. Under no circumstances should the same personnel nurse both the isolated cases and the very susceptible (i.e. the very young, very old or immunosuppressed).

- A footbath containing a disinfectant effective against the disease being treated should be placed at the entrance to the isolation facility and shoes should be dipped on entering and leaving the isolation ward. The value of this may be minimal, because most disinfectants require a contact time period to allow the disinfectant to work, and so a change of footwear is more appropriate.
- Protective clothing should be donned when entering the ward and should ideally be discarded after use.
- Hands should be thoroughly washed with an appropriate antiseptic on leaving the ward and disposable hand towels should be used to dry hands.

Ventilation within the facility must be considered. The unit should be under mild negative pressure (meaning that air will move into the unit when the door is opened, rather than air rushing out into another ward or area of the practice). This can be achieved by the use of extractor fans, with the fan in the isolation ward set to expel air out of the building and the fan in the room adjoining the facility set to draw air inwards. If active ventilation has been installed, the number of air changes per hour should be increased to 12.

After the contagious case has been discharged, a strict cleaning and disinfection regime must be followed. An example of such a routine is as follows:

- Separate cleaning equipment must be used for the isolation facility (e.g. mop and bucket, cloths) and ideally disposed of after use
- All consumable equipment (newspaper, aprons, gloves, gowns, shoe covers, hats, masks, etc.) should be disposed of as hazardous waste and incinerated
- Ideally all equipment used within the ward should be disposed of, so the use of disposable feeding bowls, gowns/coveralls, bedding (newspaper) etc. is recommended

- Any equipment that is intended to be re-used should ideally be sterilized or, if this is not possible, soaked for 12 hours in a disinfectant known to be effective against the particular contagious disease and then rinsed
- Bedding, gowns, etc. should then be boil-washed after soaking
- All surfaces within the ward should be cleaned with disinfectant (including windows, walls, door handles, all kennels, cupboards, sinks, floors, etc.) and left to soak for 12 hours
- All surfaces should then be rinsed and disinfection repeated and left for a further contact time of 12 hours
- All surfaces should then be rinsed again and allowed to dry.

Equine isolation facilities

The basic considerations for the isolation of horses are similar to those described above for small animals . Figure 12.44 lists the major infectious diseases of horses; suspected or confirmed cases of all of these must be isolated at all times.

Disease/agent	Comments
African horse sickness (orbivirus)	Endemic in sub-saharan Africa; cases seen in zebras in Spain. Carried by midge vectors
Botulism (*Clostridium botulinum*)	Ingested. Affects cows more commonly. May be a problem in big bale silage
Campylobacter jenuni, C. coli, C. fetus	Common bacteria seen in gut of food-producing animals. **Zoonotic**
Contagious equine metritis (CEM) (*Taylorella equigenitalis*)	Sexually transmitted disease. All horses going to stud should be swabbed for this. **Notifiable disease**
Equine herpesviruses (EHV1-5). EHV1: neurological, abortion; EHV1-4: respiratory	Spread by respiratory and sexual routes
Escherichia coli	**Zoonotic**
Dourine (*Trypanosoma equiperdum*)	Sexually transmitted disease. Enzootic in Africa, Asia, south-eastern Europe and South America. Not seen in UK. **Notifiable disease**
Equine infectious anaemia (EIA) (lentivirus)	Spread by horseflies. Can also be spread by saliva, faeces and from ova. **Notifiable disease**
Epizootic lymphangitis (*Histoplasma farciminosum*)	Spread by flies, not commonly seen. **Notifiable disease**
Equine influenza (orthomyxovirus)	Respiratory spread from rugs and brushes
Equine viral arteritis (EVA) (arterivirus)	Transmitted sexually and by respiratory spread
Equine viral encephalomyelitis (EVE) (alphavirus)	Transmitted by mosquitoes; seen in North and South America. **Notifiable disease** and **zoonotic**
Glanders (*Burkholderia mallei*)	Spread by inhalation or through wounds. Eradicated from UK. **Notifiable disease** and **zoonotic**
Salmonellosis (2500 strains of *Salmonella*)	**Zoonotic**

12.44   Examples of infectious diseases of horses where suspected or confirmed cases require isolation.

continues ▶

Disease/agent	Comments
Streptococcus equi zooepidemicus	**Zoonotic**
Strangles (*Streptococcus equi equi*)	Spread by direct contact from tack brushes, feeding bowls, etc.
West Nile disease (flavivirus)	Humans, birds and horses affected. Spread by mosquitoes; seen in Africa and Asia, have been outbreaks in America and Europe. **Notifiable disease** and **zoonotic**
Ringworm (*Trichophyton, Microsporum*)	Survives off the horse on fomites, especially wood. **Zoonotic**

12.44   *continued* Examples of infectious diseases of horses where suspected or confirmed cases require isolation.

In ideal circumstances a separate unit will be available to house potentially infectious patients. If this is not possible then at the very least one or two stables could be set aside. In a purpose-built environment the isolation facility would have a specialist nurse who looked after only these patients; if this is not possible then potentially infectious cases should be nursed last. This area should be isolated from other stables and clearly demarcated as an isolation area (Figure 12.45). Wooden stables are not appropriate for use for horses with infectious diseases, and their floors, walls and ceilings should be constructed of impermeable and easily cleanable materials.

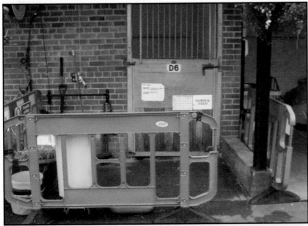

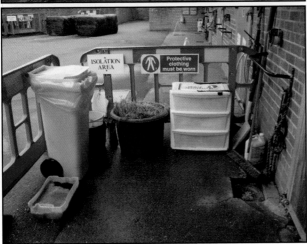

12.45   Basic equine isolation facilities.

The movement of suspect horses, even those apparently without signs of infectious disease, should be avoided. A risk assessment should be made in cases where horses in normal stabling develop signs of contagious disease such as diarrhoea; it may be considered safer to move them to an isolation facility at the onset of clinical signs or, under certain circumstances, to leave them in their original stable.

Additional requirements for isolation stabling include the following:

- A lockable treatment trolley that is easily cleaned after use would be ideal and all necessary consumables should be kept in this trolley and disposed of as hazardous waste. This should include thermometer, stethoscope, watch, treatments and bandages, isolation suits, examination gloves, foot covers and facemasks
- A footbath and alcohol gel
- Hazardous and sharps waste containers
- Large clinical waste bags for bedding. These should be kept separately from other waste until the horse is either deemed free from infection (Figure 12.46), in which case the waste can be disposed of as non-hazardous waste, or is confirmed as infectious, in which case the waste can be disposed of as hazardous waste
- An identifiable strict isolation protocol should be available to all staff.

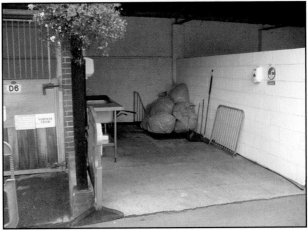

12.46   Hazardous waste is kept separately until swab samples show that the horse is clear of infection.

Acknowledgement

With thanks to the Liverpool University Equine Hospital for their input.

Further reading

Dallas S, Jones M and Mullineaux E (2007) Managing clinical environments, equipment and materials. In: *BSAVA Manual of Practical Veterinary Nursing*, ed. E Mullineaux and M Jones, pp. 76–85. BSAVA Publications, Gloucester

Girling S (2002) *Veterinary Nursing of Exotic Pets*. Blackwell Publishing, Oxford

Meredith A and Johnson-Delaney C (2010) *BSAVA Manual of Exotic Pets*, 5th edn. BSAVA Publications, Gloucester

Useful websites

Animal Boarding Establishments Act 1963. Available from
www.opsi.gov.uk/acts/acts1963/pdf/ukpga_19630043_en.pdf

The Animal Welfare Bill 2006. Available from
www.parliament.uk

British Horse Society (BHS):
www.bhs.org.uk

Defra Code of Practice for the Welfare of Horses, Ponies,
Donkeys and their Hybrids available at: www.defra.gov.uk

Farm Animal Welfare Council (FAWC) (1981):
Riding Establishments Act
Available at: www.opsi.gov.uk/RevisedStatutes/Acts/
ukpga/1964/cukpga_19640070_en_1

RSPCA/BVA Memorandum of Understanding. Available at:
www.bva.co.uk/public/documents/BVAMoU.pdf

Self-assessment questions

1. What is the main legislation governing the housing and boarding of animals?
2. State the minimum recommended sizes of hospital kennel units for dogs and cats, and of stables for horses.
3. List the advantages and disadvantages of different construction materials used for animal accommodation.
4. List the advantages and disadvantages of different animal bedding materials.
5. How much land per horse is recommended by the British Horse Society?
6. Define disinfection.
7. State the principles of cleaning a clinical environment.
8. Describe a suitable procedure for cleaning a kennel and one for a stable.
9. Describe a suitable cleaning procedure of a small animal isolation unit following discharge of a patient that had an infectious disease.
10. In what order would you nurse a routine equine patient, an equine isolation case, and a foal?

Chapter 13

Nutrition and feeding

Isuru Gajanayake, Rachel Lumbis, Gillian Greet and Simon Girling

Learning objectives

After studying this chapter, students should be able to:

- **Describe the process and control of digestion and absorption of nutrients**
- **Recognize the constituents of a balanced diet**
- **Identify and calculate the nutritional needs for a range of species**
- **Describe the differences in energy and macronutrient requirements during the different life stages**
- **Describe the differences in energy and macronutrient requirements for workload**
- **Describe the key nutrients in various disease processes**

Introduction

Nutrition is a fundamental component of health, performance, longevity and disease prevention. It is essential that veterinary nurses have a minimum basic knowledge of this continually evolving field of veterinary medicine in order to play a more active role in the care and welfare of animals.

The provision and delivery of high-quality nutritional care has always been fundamental to the prevention and management of disease. The provision of a **balanced diet** for dogs and cats requires consideration of a number of interlinking factors, namely nutrient content, energy content, digestibility and palatability. A balanced diet maintains a state of metabolic equilibrium, devoid of net gain or loss of nutrients from the body. This is achieved through the supply of key nutrients needed to meet daily requirements, together with the quantity of energy required to sustain the animal's lifestage.

As dietary fat, protein and carbohydrate cannot be absorbed in their natural form through the gastrointestinal tract, they are all useless as nutrients without preliminary digestion. In dogs and cats, chemical digestion of all three nutrients involves the process of hydrolysis and is completed in the small intestine. Enzymes act to transform large food molecules to particles small enough to be absorbed and transferred from the intestinal lumen into the blood or lymphatic system for delivery to tissues throughout the body. All digestive enzymes are designed to act at a specific pH, hence the change throughout the gastrointestinal tract. The anatomy and physiology of the digestive tracts of common species are described in Chapter 3.

Energy

Energy is essential to sustain life, and an animal's energy requirement should be met through metabolism of food. Dietary intake should be sufficient to meet an animal's needs and should produce minimal changes in the energy stored by the body, thus achieving **energy balance**. This is only possible by matching input and output over an extended period. When caloric intake exceeds energy expenditure (positive energy balance), excess energy will be stored primarily as fat, leading to weight gain and obesity. Conversely, another undesirable phenomenon is **catabolism** of body tissue, leading to weight loss and lean body stores, if caloric intake is insufficient to meet energy expenditures (negative energy balance). In order to feed an animal the correct amount of food, knowledge of its energy requirements and energy expenditure is required.

Common measurements of energy

Energy is measured in calories (cal), kilocalories (kcal) and kilojoules (kJ) with 1 kcal equating to 1000 cal or 4.2 kJ. The energy content of a diet is derived from fat (8.7 kcal/g), protein (3.5 kcal/g) and carbohydrate (3.5 kcal/g).

Gross energy (GE) is the total energy released by complete oxidation of food and is usually measured by burning food in an atmosphere of pure oxygen in a calorimeter, an instrument that accurately measures heat released on combustion. No animal is able to utilize the gross energy content of its food, and the extent to which it can be digested and absorbed is known as the **digestible energy (DE)**.

The **digestibility** of any nutrient is a measure of the difference between the amount eaten and the amount lost through faeces. Increasing digestibility leads to a reduction in faecal quantity and subsequent reduced demands on body systems designed to eliminate waste. Only some of the digestible energy is made available to the tissues. The remainder is lost in urine and methane production. The remaining portion that is utilized by the tissues is **metabolizable energy (ME)**. The digestible and metabolizable energy content of foods varies according to species and individual metabolic efficiency.

The energy requirement of the animal, together with the energy density of the food, determines the quantity of food eaten each day and thus the amount of nutrients ingested. Nutrient requirements are usually expressed in terms of ME concentration so that the values are applicable to any type of food or diet regardless of water content, nutrient content or overall energy value. Heat is produced following the intake of a meal as a result of digestion and absorption. This process is known as **meal-induced thermogenesis**.

Net energy (NE) is the metabolizable energy minus the heat increment and is used primarily for maintenance and then production. If there is insufficient energy left after maintenance needs are satisfied, production will not take place.

Energy in relation to other nutrients

Energy density

Animals consume sufficient food to meet their energy requirements (assuming the food is palatable). To ensure that other essential nutrients are eaten in adequate amounts, they should be considered in relation to the energy content or energy density of the diet (Figure 13.1). Ideally, when an animal finishes eating the food provided, sufficient energy should have been consumed and the animal should have met all other nutritional needs.

Bulk-limited diets

If a diet has a low energy density, the animal will continue to eat until its stomach is so full that no further food can be consumed. The animal will stop eating then, even if its energy needs have not been met. It is likely that the diet will also be deficient in other nutrients. The diet is said to be bulk-limited. For example, this type of diet should never be fed to a lactating animal since she will be physically unable to consume enough food to meet her high energy requirements.

Obesity diets are formulated in this way: non-energy nutrient requirements are met with a reduced energy intake. This promotes weight loss through utilization of fat stores, and preserves body protein.

Energy-limited diets

If an animal has an adequate diet and can eat to its energy requirements, the diet is said to be energy-limited. If the diet is then supplemented with additional energy (as in the feeding of titbits) the animal will eat less of the balanced diet and so may become deficient in non-energy nutrients.

Energy expenditure

The **basal metabolic rate (BMR)** is the amount of energy expended by an animal while at rest in a thermoneutral environment with the digestive system inactive and in a post-absorptive state. The release of energy in this state is sufficient only for cellular processes such as respiration, circulation and for organ function.

Factors that determine an animal's BMR include:

- Species
- Bodyweight
- Age
- Hormonal status.

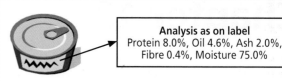

Analysis as on label
Protein 8.0%, Oil 4.6%, Ash 2.0%, Fibre 0.4%, Moisture 75.0%

1. The label is read and the percentage of the energy-producing nutrients noted.
   The percentage of carbohydrate is not usually stated in the typical analysis, unlike protein and fat (oil or lipid) content. It is therefore calculated by adding the percentages of the ingredients given and subtracting this from 100.

   8.0 + 4.6 + 2.0 + 0.4 + 75 = 90

   Therefore, % carbohydrate is 100 – 90 = 10%

2. The percentage content of the nutrients is converted to calorie content.

   Energy produced from fat is 8.7 kcal/g
   Energy produced from protein is 3.5 kcal/g
   Energy produced from carbohydrate is 3.5 kcal/g

   Thus:

   kcal from the fat (oil) per 100 g of the pet food
   = 4.6 × 8.7 = 40 kcal

   kcal from the protein per 100g of the pet food
   = 8.0 × 3.5 = 28 kcal

   kcal from the carbohydrate per 100g of the pet food
   = 10 × 3.5 = 35 kcal

3. The total energy density is calculated by totalling the kcal from the fat, protein and CHO.
   40 + 28 + 35 = 103 kcal per 100 g

4. The energy provided by each nutrient as a percentage of the total energy content is calculated.

   % calories from fat = 40/103 × 100 = 38.8%
   % calories from protein = 28/103 × 100 = 27.2%
   % calories from carbohydrate = 35/103 × 100 = 34%

13.1 Calculation of the energy density of a pet food and the energy of each nutrient as a percentage of the total energy content.

Changes to these factors will, over time, alter the animal's BMR.

Thermogenesis is a process by which the body generates heat, or energy, by increasing the metabolic rate above basal. This rise in metabolic rate is referred to as the thermogenic effect. Dietary-induced thermogenesis (DIT) is the body's way of converting surplus calories directly into heat and can be defined as the increase in energy expenditure above basal metabolic rate. Unlike BMR, DIT can vary significantly and quickly and can cause large daily variations in energy expenditure.

Disparity between the amount of energy consumed and the amount of energy expended by the body will have an adverse effect on bodyweight, growth rate and body composition, namely body fat percentage. Excess energy intake relative to expenditure is common in dogs and cats and will ultimately lead to obesity. In contrast, inadequate energy consumption relative to expenditure will result in cachexia (involuntary weight loss), commonly seen in dogs and cats suffering from cancer and cardiac disease. This accelerated starvation is caused by metabolic alterations and subsequent muscle atrophy, weight loss, weakness and lethargy.

Energy requirements

Calculating the energy requirements for animals has been achieved using a variety of methods including charts, allometric formulae (linking size and energy requirement), linear equations and body surface area (BSA). Ultimately, all of these provide an estimation of energy needs and will require adjustment based on the animal's weight, breed, health status, lifestage, environmental living conditions and activity levels.

Resting Energy Requirement (RER)

The patient's resting energy requirement (RER) is the amount of energy required for maintaining homeostasis while the animal rests quietly in a stress-free, non-fasted, thermoneutral environment.

Calculating RER

RER is calculated using the following formula:

RER = 70 x (bodyweight in kg) $^{0.75}$

For animals weighing between 2 and 30 kg, the following linear formula gives a good approximation of energy needs:

RER = (30 x bodyweight in kg) + 70

In order to calculate the **amount of food** required by an animal, its RER and the metabolizable energy (ME) density of the food need to be determined. The animal's RER is divided by the energy density of the selected diet to determine the amount of food to be fed (Figure 13.2). Every animal is an individual and the calculated energy requirement may therefore need to be altered according to individual requirements and response to feeding.

Traditionally, the RER was multiplied by an illness factor (IF) to account for increases in metabolism associated with different conditions and injuries. Recently, there has been less emphasis on these subjective illness factors and current recommendations are to use more conservative energy estimates to avoid overfeeding. Overfeeding can result in metabolic and gastrointestinal complications, hepatic dysfunction, increased carbon dioxide production, and waning respiratory muscle action. Of the metabolic complications, the development of hyperglycaemia is most common, and possibly the most detrimental.

Maintenance Energy Requirement (MER)

Maintenance energy requirement (MER) is the energy requirement of a moderately active adult animal in a thermoneutral environment. It includes the energy needed for obtaining, digesting and absorbing food in amounts to maintain bodyweight, as well as energy for spontaneous exercise. It does not include the energy required for additional activity (work), gestation, lactation, growth and repair.

Nutrients

The health and viability of an animal is dependent upon an adequate supply of nutrients that the body utilizes as sources of energy or as parts of its metabolic machinery. Knowledge of these nutrients, their requirements and availability, and the consequences of deficiencies and excesses is essential in order to feed animals correctly and provide advice about nutrition and feeding.

Nutrients are food components that help to support life. An **essential nutrient** is one that is required and unable to be synthesized in the body. Consequently, it must be provided as a dietary source.

Energy-producing nutrients:

- Carbohydrate
- Fat
- Protein.

Non-energy-producing nutrients:

- Water
- Minerals
- Vitamins.

Macronutrients are needed in relatively large quantities. **Micronutrients** are needed in smaller quantities.

Macronutrients

Carbohydrate

Carbohydrates are composed of the elements carbon, hydrogen and oxygen and have the basic formula CH_2O. The primary function of carbohydrates is as an energy source, but they may also be converted to body fat and stored. The quality of carbohydrate sources vary. For example, ground whole grains supply high-quality complex carbohydrates, whereas products such as ground wheat or wheat/rice flour grains have been stripped of most of their nutritional benefits. Meat is a poor source of carbohydrate.

A 15 kg adult neutered dog is to be fed a canned food with an energy density of 430 kcal per can. Calculate how many cans should be fed.

1. Calculate the RER for the dog

   (RER x 1.6 = daily energy requirement for a neutered dog – see Energy requirements for different lifestages)

   RER = 70 × (bodyweight in kg) $^{0.75}$ × 1.6 = 70 × 15 $^{0.75}$ × 1.6

   In the absence of a calculator, a simple method to calculate this is:

   a) 15 × 15 × 15 = 3375

      √ 3375 = 58

      √ 58 = 7.6

   b) 7.6 × 70 = 532

   c) 532 × 1.6 = 851.2

2. Calculate the number of cans to be fed.

   The diet contains 430 kcal/can
   RER ÷ energy density = number of cans per day
   851.2 ÷ 430 = 2 cans per day

13.2 Calculation of the quantity of food to be fed. RER = resting energy requirement

Functions of dietary carbohydrate

- Provision of energy (3.5 kcal/g).
- Synthesis of other essential body compounds such as RNA and DNA.
- Source of fibre.

Carbohydrates can be classified as monosaccharides, disaccharides or polysaccharides.

Monosaccharides, commonly referred to as simple sugars, are the simplest form and include glucose, fructose (fruit sugar) and galactose (milk sugar). Glucose circulates in the bloodstream and is the primary form of carbohydrate used for energy.

Disaccharides are composed of two molecules of monosaccharide(s) linked together. Examples include lactose, maltose and sucrose. Digestion of disaccharides is controlled by the activity of specific enzymes (disaccharidases), e.g. sucrase for sucrose, lactase for lactose. The activity of lactase decreases with age in the dog and cat; therefore older animals that consume an excessive amount of milk and other lactose-containing products may develop diarrhoea. Lactose contains glucose and galactose. A deficiency of the enzyme galactosidase, preventing separation of the glucose and galactose molecules and rendering lactose indigestible, causes lactose intolerance in adult animals.

Polysaccharides are more commonly referred to as complex carbohydrates and consist of vast numbers of linked monosaccharide molecules. Polysaccharides are found widely. Examples include starch, glycogen and fibre. Starch is used for energy storage. Dietary fibre or roughage (see below) includes the polysaccharides cellulose, pectin and lignin.

When food is digested, it is mixed with saliva; this contains the enzyme amylase, which hydrolyses starch. This is of particular importance in humans but less important in dogs. Feline saliva lacks amylase and feline pancreatic amylase activity is only 5% of that of dogs. The enterocytes lining the villi of the small intestine contain four enzymes (disaccharidases). The enzymes break down carbohydrates into smaller particles (Figure 13.3). These are then absorbed by enterocytes and rapidly released into the capillaries and transported to the liver. No enzymes capable of hydrolysing complex plant carbohydrate (cellulose) are secreted in the canine or feline digestive tract. Consequently this food is not considered ideal for dogs or cats.

Dietary fibre

Fibre differs from starch in that it resists enzymatic digestion in the small intestine of dogs and cats but is instead subject to bacterial fermentation in the colon. Depending on the type of fibre, it is partly or completely fermented, producing gases (carbon dioxide, methane and hydrogen) and short-chain fatty acids (SCFAs). SCFAs are a significant energy source for the enterocytes and colonocytes of the large intestine.

Functions of dietary fibre

- Increased bulk and water of intestinal contents.
- Low energy content aids the correction and prevention of obesity.
- Regulation of intestinal gut transit time and bowel movements.
- Production of short-chain fatty acids that help to maintain the health of the colon.
- Maintenance of the structural integrity of the gut mucosa.
- Therapeutic uses in the treatment of fibre-responsive diseases.
- Alteration of nutrient absorption and metabolism.

Fibre can be classified as soluble (e.g. pectins) or insoluble (e.g. cellulose and lignin). Whilst fibre is not considered an essential dietary component, both soluble and insoluble

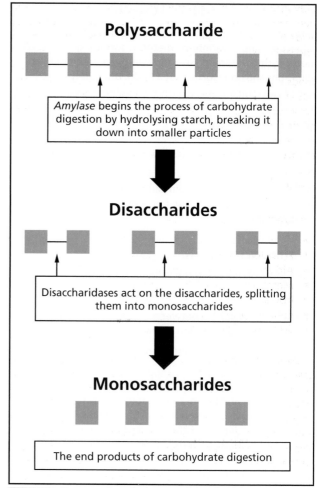

13.3 Enzymes break down polysaccharide carbohydrates into progressively smaller units.

dietary fibre are important and affect the health and function of the gastrointestinal tract. Sources of insoluble fibre can act as bulking (laxative) agents and help prevent constipation. Sources of soluble fibre can also help regulate blood glucose and are of particular importance in diabetic animals.

However, while it is important for animals to consume adequate amounts of fibre, it is also possible to consume too much. Excessive dietary fibre intake can have negative side effects including:

- Flatulence and borborygmi
- Increased bowel movements
- Increased faecal output
- Constipation, due to the bulking effect (particularly if insufficient water is being consumed).

In order to avoid these, any change in diet or increase in fibre intake should be carried out gradually, thus allowing the animal time to adjust.

Fat

Dietary fat is part of a group of compounds known as lipids. Lipids are termed 'fats' if they are solid at room temperature, and 'oils' if they are liquid at room temperature. The most common form of dietary fat is as **triglycerides**, which are composed of one molecule of glycerol and three molecules of fatty acid(s). The physical and nutritional characteristics of the fat are determined by the specific types of fatty acid. These may be saturated, monounsaturated or polyunsaturated, these terms referring to the relative abundance of hydrogen atoms present. Monounsaturated fatty acids have one double bond between the carbon atoms and polyunsaturated fatty acids have two double bonds.

The quality and type of dietary fat used in commercial pet foods is at the discretion of the manufacturer. Lower-grade fats are more difficult for animals to utilize and require more preservatives to stabilize them. Smaller amounts of table-grade (good-quality) fat can deliver the same level of energy as a larger amount of poorer quality tallow fat. Oils are usually from vegetable sources and, unless stated on the label, are normally from varied sources. Vegetable oils are not a source for all of the essential fatty acids.

Functions of dietary fat

- Provision and storage of energy (8.7 kcal/g).
- Provision of essential fatty acids (EFAs).
- Aid absorption of fat-soluble vitamins A, D, E and K.
- Metabolic and structural functions.
- Insulation.
- Enhance palatability.
- Synthesis of hormones (especially steroids).

Dietary fats do not dissolve in the watery content of the gastrointestinal tract. As a result, they are not easily broken down by lipase, a water-soluble digestive enzyme. Thus, fats take longer to digest than carbohydrates or proteins. Digestion begins with the emulsification of fat, which is accomplished under the influence of bile secreted by the liver. The fat globules must be split into smaller particles so that lipase can act on the globule surfaces and break the fats down further into glycerol and fatty acids (Figure 13.4). In the absence of bile secretion, enzymes are less efficient at this process.

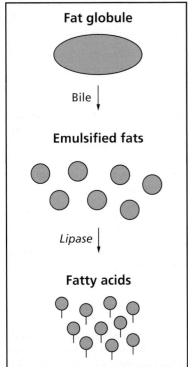

Fat globule

Bile

Emulsified fats

Lipase

Fatty acids

13.4

Digestive breakdown of fats.

Bile salts are also essential to fat digestion and help to separate the fat droplets from surrounding water. Fats are insoluble in water, unlike glycerol and fatty acids, which can be easily absorbed into the body. The fat molecules that are too large to be absorbed into the intestinal cells are split by the pancreatic enzyme lipase. They then enter the lacteals and pass via the lymphatic duct into the venous blood supply. Some fat is utilized directly to release energy and some is stored in adipose tissue for future use. When required, the stored fat is transported to the liver where it is converted and used for energy production.

Essential fatty acids

Dietary fat provides a source of **essential fatty acids** (EFAs), including linoleic acid, linolenic acid and arachidonic acid. The functions of EFAs include acting as constituents of cell membranes, in prostaglandin synthesis and in control of water loss through the skin. In most animals linolenic acid and arachidonic acid can be synthesized from linoleic acid, which is common in vegetable oil and can also be sourced in smaller amounts from poultry and pork fat. An exception to this is the cat which, regardless of the amount of linoleic acid present in the diet, requires a dietary source of arachidonic acid; this can only be found in animal fat. Linolenic acid can be synthesized from linoleic acid by dogs and cats and is therefore not required in dietary fat.

Fatty acid deficiency can impair wound healing and cause a dry coat and scaly skin. It is often the result of consumption of low-fat food or dry food that has undergone prolonged storage, especially under warm or humid conditions. Fatty acids then become rancid and lose their nutritional value.

Protein

Dietary proteins are large, complex molecules composed of long chains of **amino acids** bound together by peptide linkages.

Functions of dietary protein

- Tissue growth and repair.
- Manufacture of hormones and enzymes.
- Source of energy (3.5 kcal/g).
- Protection against infections.
- Transport of oxygen.
- Regulation of metabolism.
- Structural role in cell walls.

Amino acids joined together are called **peptides**; two peptides joined together are a dipeptide, three linked together are a tripeptide, and more than three bonded together are a polypeptide. **Essential amino acids** cannot be synthesized by the body in sufficient quantities and therefore must be supplied in dietary form. **Non-essential amino acids** can be synthesized by the body from other precursors.

Most protein digestion occurs in the upper small intestine, in the duodenum and jejunum. Pepsin, the peptic enzyme of the stomach, begins the digestion of protein molecules by converting them to smaller polypeptides and peptides (Figure 13.5). This splitting of proteins occurs as a result of hydrolysis at the peptide linkages between amino acids. Hydrochloric acid in the stomach combined with stomach contents and secretions from glandular cells, creates an acidic environment that is highly favourable for pepsin activity. Continuous turnover of amino acids results from constant protein digestion. Any surplus amino acids cannot be stored and are therefore excreted via the liver and kidneys in the form of urea.

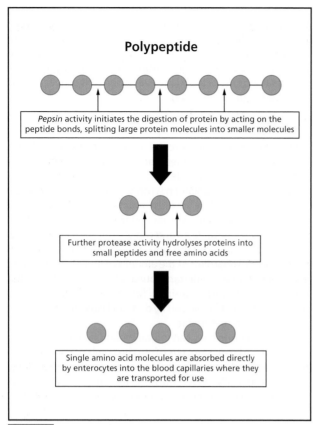

Polypeptide

Pepsin activity initiates the digestion of protein by acting on the peptide bonds, splitting large protein molecules into smaller molecules

Further protease activity hydrolyses proteins into small peptides and free amino acids

Single amino acid molecules are absorbed directly by enterocytes into the blood capillaries where they are transported for use

13.5 Digestive breakdown of proteins.

Biological value (BV)

The quality of a protein is referred to as its biological value (BV) and is defined as the percentage of absorbed protein that is retained by the body. This figure will vary according to the amount and number of essential amino acids that it contains and is dependent on how acceptable, digestible and utilizable the protein is.

Out of the common pet food ingredients, egg is known to be one of the highest quality protein sources (BV approximately 94%). Other high-quality sources include casein (found in cheese), beef, lamb, pork, chicken and liver. Lower-quality sources include soybean, barley, wheat, corn and collagen.

Digestibility and quality of the protein is critical to the body for effective utilization of the food. A poor level of digestibility and a low-quality source changes the significance of the percentage of protein in the food. Highly digestible proteins that contain a sufficient quantity of essential amino acids to satisfy an animal's needs are considered to be of high quality. Those that are either low in digestibility or lacking any essential amino acids are considered to be of low quality.

Water

Water is vital to life and is considered the most important nutrient in terms of the ability to survive. The mammalian body consists of 60–70% water. Deficits of more than a few percent of total body water are incompatible with health, and large water deficits (15–20% of bodyweight) can prove fatal. Water deprivation can lead to death within days, whereas healthy animals can survive without food for a period of weeks. Overconsumption of water is rare in normal healthy animals but may occur in animals offered water *ad libitum* following prolonged dehydration.

Functions of water in the body

- Electrolyte balance.
- Temperature regulation.
- Removal of waste.
- Transport medium for nutrients.
- Major component of blood and lymph.
- Required for chemical reactions involving hydrolysis.
- Regulates oncotic pressure, helping to maintain body shape.

Animals consume water to meet a variety of needs, including physical and social, and individual differences influence the absolute requirement. Factors affecting requirements for water include:

- Polyuria/polydipsia
- Environmental temperature
- Body temperature
- Type and amount of food ingested
- Stress
- Illness or disease and general state of health
- Diarrhoea/vomiting
- Exercise
- Lactation
- Water losses through excretion or evaporation.

Water losses can be replaced either through water derived from metabolism of nutrients or by consumption of water as a liquid or as a portion of the food ingested. Dry foods contain on average 6–10% moisture; semi-moist foods contain on average 24–40% moisture; and canned or moist foods contain on average 80% moisture. Provided that fresh palatable water is freely available to drink and the correct quantity of a complete and balanced diet are fed, most dogs and cats will be able to meet their water requirements and self-regulate their water balance through voluntary oral intake.

Micronutrients
Minerals

Minerals can be further subdivided into **macrominerals** (percentage amounts required in the diet, i.e. parts per hundred) and **microminerals** or **trace elements** (i.e. amounts required in parts per million). The macrominerals include calcium, phosphorus, sodium, chloride, potassium, magnesium and sulphur. The absorption and utilization of minerals from the diet is dependent on many factors, including:

- The amount and form of the mineral in the diet
- The age, sex and species of the animal
- The physiological demand for the mineral
- Environmental factors.

Minerals serve three major functions in the body:

- Structural components, e.g. calcium in bone and teeth
- Body fluid constituents, e.g. sodium in blood
- Catalysts and cofactors for enzymes and hormones, e.g. iodine in thyroid function.

Macrominerals are discussed further below. Provided there is sufficient protein in the diet, there is no dietary requirement for sulphur, as it is obtained from amino acids.

Calcium

Animal products containing bone are good sources of calcium. Dietary calcium is absorbed via an active process in the duodenum and proximal jejunum, and via a passive process in the distal intestine. The absorption, metabolism and excretion of calcium are tightly regulated in the body by parathyroid hormone, vitamin D and calcitonin (see Chapter 3). Vitamin D in particular acts to promote calcium absorption in the proximal duodenum. It is not involved in the passive absorptive process in the distal intestine. Parathyroid hormone is secreted when blood calcium levels are low and leads to the absorption of calcium from the bone, reduced excretion of calcium in the urine and the activation of vitamin D (which then increases calcium uptake in the gut). Calcitonin has an opposing role to reduce the absorption of calcium from bone when the blood concentration of calcium is high. Calcium serves both structural roles (i.e. in bone and teeth) and functional roles (i.e. cellular messaging, blood clotting, muscle and nerve function). Calcium deficiency can lead to growth retardation, reduced bone mineralization and loose teeth, for example. Excessive calcium intake can lead to kidney damage, orthopaedic disease (especially in young large breed dogs) and uroliths containing calcium.

Phosphorus

All meats are high in phosphorus. This nutrient is absorbed from the intestine by a saturable, carrier-mediated process and a non-saturable concentration-dependent process. As with calcium, the absorption and excretion of phosphorus is under the control of parathyroid hormone and vitamin D. In particular, vitamin D enhances the absorption of phosphorus from the gut. However, in contrast to calcium, parathyroid hormone promotes the excretion of phosphorus in the urine rather than reducing its excretion. Phosphorus, like calcium, serves important structural roles in bones and teeth. It is a vital component of nucleic acids (e.g. DNA), cell membranes, ATP (adenosine triphosphate, the basic energy-producing compound) and is also necessary for acid–base balance and oxygen delivery. Phosphorus deficiency can lead to decreased growth, reduced fertility, a dull coat and poor bone mineralization. Excessive phosphorus can cause urolithiasis, soft tissue calcification and secondary hyperparathyroidism.

Magnesium

Foods rich in magnesium include bones, oilseed (e.g. flaxseed) and grains/fibres (e.g. bran). Up to 70% of dietary magnesium is absorbed in the intestine by a carrier-mediated process (when the dietary concentration is low) or by simple diffusion (when the dietary concentration is high). Certain dietary factors (e.g. diets high in fat, protein and calcium) can reduce magnesium absorption. Once absorbed, the kidneys play a central role in magnesium metabolism. For this reason, certain medications (e.g. diuretics) and diseases (e.g. diabetes mellitus) can cause magnesium to be lost through the kidneys as a result of excess urine production. Magnesium has many structural and functional roles in the body. It is the third most common mineral in bone and also serves vital roles in processes such as carbohydrate and lipid metabolism, catalysing enzyme reactions, promoting cellular energy production and in neuromuscular function. Signs of magnesium deficiency include muscle weakness, growth retardation, reduced bone mineralization, neuromuscular hyperactivity (e.g. tetany and seizures) and anorexia. Excess dietary magnesium has been linked to struvite urolithiasis.

Potassium

Foods rich in potassium include grains and fibres (e.g. wheat bran), yeast and soybean. The majority of potassium is absorbed in the upper small intestine by simple diffusion but it is also absorbed to a lesser degree in the lower small intestine and in the large intestine. Potassium is not stored in the body to an appreciable degree and is readily excreted in the urine. The body can therefore become depleted in potassium (hypokalaemia) when excessive potassium is lost by the kidneys (e.g. in polyuric renal failure); conversely, potassium excess (hyperkalaemia) can occur when the kidneys fail to excrete it (e.g. in anuric renal failure).

Potassium is the most important intracellular cation (K^+). It also has many roles in maintaining osmotic and acid–base balance, in nerve function, in muscle (including heart) contraction and in various enzyme systems. Potassium deficiency usually occurs due to excessive (gastrointestinal or renal) loss or reduced intake. The most common signs of potassium deficiency include anorexia, lethargy, weakness, heart rhythm disturbances and neck ventroflexion (in cats). Dietary potassium toxicity is unlikely if kidney function is normal.

Sodium and chloride

Sodium and chloride will be considered together as they are absorbed and metabolized in tandem. Good sources of sodium and chloride include fish, eggs, poultry and whey. The absorption of sodium and chloride occurs primarily in the upper small intestine and is very efficient. Excessive sodium and chloride are excreted in urine. The absorption of calcium and some water-soluble vitamins is linked to sodium absorption. Sodium and chloride are normally tightly regulated in the body via mechanisms that monitor the blood pressure and the tonicity (concentration) of blood. In general, the kidneys are capable of regulating sodium excretion in accordance with the dietary intake. The primary role of sodium and chloride in the body is maintaining the osmotic balance in blood. Additional vital roles include regulation of acid–base and water balance, transmission of nerve impulses and muscle contraction. Deficiency is rare but signs include anorexia and lethargy. Signs of excessive sodium and chloride include thirst, pruritus, constipation and seizures.

Microminerals

Iron

Dietary iron exists in two forms, haem iron (i.e. from haemoglobin and myoglobin in blood and muscle) and non-haem iron (e.g. from grains). Organ meats such as liver and spleen are good sources of haem iron. The absorption of iron is influenced by the iron status of the body, the availability of iron in the diet and the amount of haem *versus* non-haem iron in the diet. Iron is transported in blood by the protein transferrin; when this is saturated, iron is stored firstly as ferritin then as haemosiderin in the liver, bone marrow and spleen. Only a limited amount of iron is excreted from the body. Iron is essential for oxygen transport (in haemoglobin) and also has functions in oxygen activation reactions and in electron transport. Dietary iron deficiency is rare, especially as commercial food is high in iron. Iron deficiency usually occurs due to chronic gastrointestinal blood loss (e.g. endoparasites in the young, bleeding neoplasms in older animals), renal or other external blood loss (e.g. external parasites in the young). Iron deficiency leads to anaemia, a poor coat and ill-thrift. Excessive iron may hinder the absorption of zinc and copper. Clinical signs of iron excess include anorexia and weight loss.

Zinc

Meat and dietary fibre are high in zinc. The absorption of zinc occurs in all parts of the small intestine (and to a lesser degree in the stomach). Zinc absorption is markedly reduced by high levels of dietary phytates (e.g. in cereal-based diets) and calcium. Some zinc is stored in bone but excessive dietary and endogenous zinc are excreted in the faeces. Zinc has many functions in the body, including nucleic acid metabolism, protein synthesis, carbohydrate metabolism, immunity, skin health, growth, reproduction and hormone (e.g. testosterone) production. Dietary deficiency of zinc usually occurs due to the formation of insoluble complexes with phytates and calcium. The signs of zinc deficiency include anorexia, ill-thrift, alopecia, parakeratosis and reduced immunity. Zinc toxicosis usually occurs due to ingestion of metallic foreign bodies containing zinc rather than dietary excess.

Copper

Offal meat (especially ruminant liver) is rich in copper. This metal is absorbed primarily from the small intestine by simple diffusion (when dietary concentrations are high) and by active transport (when concentrations are low). The absorbed copper is transported bound to caeruloplasmin and albumin. In the liver, the copper is metabolized and excess copper is excreted in bile. Copper has several functions in the body, including haemopoiesis, neurotransmitter function and maintenance of connective tissue integrity. Copper also has an antioxidant role. Signs of copper deficiency in cats and dogs include anaemia, reproductive failure, coat depigmentation, skeletal pathology and fetal deformities. Excessive copper can interfere with iron and zinc metabolism and lead to liver damage.

Manganese

Fibre sources and fishmeal are rich in manganese. Absorption of this metal is from the small intestine and can be impaired by excessive dietary phosphorus, iron and cobalt. Excessive manganese is excreted in bile. Manganese acts as an enzyme activator and it also has roles in reproduction, skeletal growth and lipid metabolism. Clinical signs of deficiency include reproductive dysfunction and skeletal deformities. Manganese toxicity is reported in humans with liver failure.

Iodine

Fish, eggs and iodized salts are rich in iodine. The main use for iodine in the body is in thyroid hormone synthesis. Iodine is concentrated inside the thyroid gland. Iodine deficiency leads to inadequate thyroid hormone production and hence hypothyroidism; however, iodine deficiency in cats and dogs is rare. Iodine deficiency can cause congenital hypothyroidism but this is very rare. Iodine toxicity is extremely rare as most species can tolerate a very high intake without adverse side effects.

Selenium

Fish, eggs and liver are good sources of selenium. This element is absorbed in the duodenum but urinary excretion is regulated to counterbalance dietary intake. The main role of selenium in the body is as part of the glutathione peroxidase antioxidant system. This system works in synergy with vitamin E (see below). Selenium also has roles in immune and reproductive function. Selenium deficiency and toxicity have not been reported in dogs and cats. In cattle and humans, deficiency of selenium can lead to muscle disease, reproductive failure and cardiac disease.

Chromium

Chromium is considered to be an ultra-trace element and is ubiquitous in water, soil and living matter. Several studies have shown beneficial effects of chromium in glucose homeostasis.

Boron

Boron is involved in cartilage and bone development and maturation, by influencing parathyroid hormone function. Deficiency of this element can lead to poor growth and anaemia.

Additional trace and ultra-trace elements

Figure 13.6 gives information on additional trace and ultra-trace elements.

Mineral	Functions
Molybdenum	Enzymatic role in oxidation/reduction reactions
Fluoride	Mineralization of bone and teeth
Arsenic	Methionine metabolism
Nickel	Complement system
Silicon	Growth of bone, cartilage and connective tissue
Vanadium	Enzyme systems, cellular glucose uptake, amino acid transport
Cobalt	Part of vitamin B12

13.6 Additional trace and ultra-trace elements.

Vitamins

All vitamins have five basic characteristics:

- They are organic compounds but distinct from the macronutrients
- They are components of the diet
- They are essential for normal physiological function
- An absence causes a deficiency syndrome
- They are not synthesized in the body to a degree that supports normal function.

Vitamins can be subdivided into those that are fat-soluble (vitamins A, D, E and K) and those that are water-soluble (vitamins B and C). Fat-soluble vitamins require bile for their absorption whereas water-soluble vitamins are absorbed via active transport. Fat-soluble vitamins are stored in body fat, making them less prone to deficiencies but more prone to toxicoses. In contrast, water-soluble vitamins are not stored and as a result the body can become depleted in situations such as polyuric renal failure.

Fat-soluble vitamins

Vitamin A

Good sources of vitamin A include fish oils, liver, eggs and dairy products. Plant sources of the vitamin are usually in the form of carotenes (a provitamin that requires activation in the body). Cats are unable to convert beta-carotene to vitamin A and thus require the vitamin in their diet. Carotenoids are more dependent on bile salts for absorption than is vitamin A. The absorbed vitamin is transported to and stored in the liver and then transported in the bloodstream in the form of an ester. Vitamin A is necessary for vision, reproduction, immunity and bone and muscle growth. The classical signs of vitamin A deficiency (hypovitaminosis A) are night blindness and xerophthalmia (dryness of the conjunctiva). In contrast, an excess of vitamin A (hypervitaminosis A) classically manifests in skeletal malformations, including fusion of vertebrae in cats.

Vitamin D

Marine fish and fish oils are particularly good sources of vitamin D. Plants also contain vitamin D but in the ergocalciferol form (rather than the cholecalciferol form found in animals). Cholecalciferol can be produced in the skin of mammals by ultraviolet (sun) light activation of the provitamin. However, this process is inefficient in cats and dogs and a dietary source is necessary. Vitamin D is absorbed from the small intestine by a passive, non-saturable process that is dependent on bile. The absorbed vitamin D is transported in the bloodstream in combination with vitamin D-binding protein that then facilitates distribution of the vitamin to the peripheral tissues. Vitamin D is essential for calcium and phosphorus metabolism and in particular enhances absorption from the intestine and protects against loss of these elements from bone. Clinical signs of vitamin D deficiency include poor bone mineralization (i.e. rickets in young animals, osteomalacia in adults). Decreased serum calcium and phosphorus levels are also noted. Vitamin D excess leads to hypercalcaemia, soft-tissue mineralization and renal failure.

Vitamin E

Vitamin E is only produced in plants and can be found in high concentrations in vegetable oils, seeds and grains. This vitamin is absorbed by a passive and non-saturable process in the intestine. Its absorption is enhanced by simultaneous absorption of fat. The vitamin circulates in the bloodstream bound to lipoproteins and is deposited equally in all tissues of the body. Vitamin E functions primarily as an antioxidant. There are several forms of vitamin E, of which alpha-tocopherol is the most biologically active form. Vitamin E together with selenium is postulated to be the first line of defence against oxidative damage in cells (with the glutathione system forming the second line of defence). Signs of vitamin E deficiency in dogs include degenerative skeletal muscle disease, impaired male reproductive function and failure of gestation. In cats signs include steatitis and myositis. Vitamin E toxicity is rare but high doses can impair the absorption of other fat-soluble vitamins.

Vitamin K

Vitamin K is present in green leafy vegetables in two forms, both of which require activation in the body. Bacteria in the large intestine can also synthesize vitamin K. The vegetable forms of the vitamin (phylloquinone and menaquinone) are absorbed in the small intestine and then transported to the liver, where they are concentrated. The vitamin produced by the bacteria in the colon is absorbed by passive diffusion across the colonic wall. The main function of vitamin K is in the activation of several blood clotting factors and its deficiency leads to signs of coagulopathy. Excessive dietary vitamin K is unlikely to cause signs of toxicity.

Water-soluble vitamins

Vitamin C (ascorbic acid)

Dogs and cats, unlike humans, are able to synthesize vitamin C in their liver; this means that it is not strictly considered to be a vitamin in these species. The absorption of vitamin C in dogs and cats is via a process of passive diffusion. Vitamin C has many functions in the body: it acts as an antioxidant and a free-radical scavenger and also plays roles in collagen synthesis, immunity and in drug and steroid metabolism. An antineoplastic role has also been suggested. Deficiency does not occur in dogs and cats and the risk of toxicity is low.

The B vitamins

These include thiamine (B1), riboflavin (B2), niacin (B3), pyridoxine (B6), pantothenic acid, folate, biotin and cobalamin (B12) (Figure 13.7). Additional information on the B vitamins with recognized clinical deficiency syndromes in dogs and cats is given below.

Vitamin	Dietary sources	Absorption	Functions	Deficiency	Signs of deficiency	Toxicity
Thiamine (B1)	Whole grains, liver, yeast	Jejunum (carrier-mediated)	Enzymatic reactions	Food processing; thiaminases	Anorexia, ill-thrift, muscle weakness, neurological deficits	Very rare
Riboflavin (B2)	Dairy products, meat, eggs, green vegetables, yeast	Upper gastrointestinal tract	Energy metabolism; enzymatic reactions	Uncommon	Cats: dermatitis, erythema, weight loss, cataracts, anorexia, impaired reproduction	Not reported
Niacin (B3)	Yeast, meat, fish, cereals, legumes	Stomach and small intestine	Oxidoreductive reactions; tryptophan metabolism	High corn/grain diet	Pellagra, diarrhoea, dementia, death	Not reported
Pyridoxine (B6)	Meat, whole grain, vegetables, nuts. Widely available	Small intestine	Amino acid, glycogen and lipid metabolism; neurotransmitter biosynthesis; taurine, carnitine and porphyrin biosynthesis	Uncommon	Ill-thrift, muscle weakness, neurological signs (e.g. ataxia), anorexia	Neural damage in experimental studies
Pantothenic acid	Meat, rice, wheat bran, yeast. Widely available	Intestine (energy-dependent)	Energy production and biosynthesis of fatty acids, steroid hormones and cholesterol	Uncommon	Inappetence, poor growth, fatty liver, coma, poor immunity	Non-toxic

13.7 Summary of B vitamins.

continues ▶

Vitamin	Dietary sources	Absorption	Functions	Deficiency	Signs of deficiency	Toxicity
Folate	Liver, egg yolks, green vegetables	Proximal intestine	Nucleotide, phospholipid and methionine biosynthesis; amino acid metabolism; neurotransmitter production; creatinine formation	Gastrointestinal disease	Weight loss, anaemia, anorexia	Not reported
Biotin	Egg yolks, liver, yeast	Intestine	Metabolism of lipids, glucose and amino acids	Very rare: antibiotic therapy; feeding raw egg whites	Dermatitis, poor growth, lethargy, neurological abnormalities	Not reported
Cobalamin (B12)	Meat, milk	Ileum, mediated by pancreatic intrinsic factor	Carbon metabolism; methionine biosynthesis	Gastrointestinal disease	Poor growth, anaemia, neuropathies	Dietary toxicity not reported

13.7 *continued* Summary of B vitamins.

Thiamine is is very labile and is susceptible to destruction by food processing. It can also be inactivated by antagonists such as thiaminases, which can be found in high concentrations in raw fish and shellfish. Thiaminases are destroyed by cooking. Commercial diets are supplemented with the synthetic form of the vitamin. Thiamine is absorbed in the jejunum and transported in red blood cells and dissolved in the plasma. Thiamine is involved in energy production and is necessary for normal nervous system function. Clinical signs of thiamine deficiency include anorexia, ill-thrift, muscle weakness, ataxia and paresis, ventroflexion of the neck (in cats) and cardiac hypertrophy (in dogs). Deficiency states can be confirmed by blood tests (erythrocytic transketolase activity or measurement of blood metabolites). Dietary thiamine toxicity is very rare.

Folate (folic acid) and **cobalamin** are linked in their metabolism. Folic acid refers to the oxidized form of the vitamin (found in supplements) whereas folate refers to the reduced form (found naturally in foods). Cobalamin is the largest and most complex B vitamin and contains a central cobalt ion. Folate is necessary in the daily diet whereas intestinal bacteria can produce cobalamin. Common signs of folate deficiency include weight loss, anaemia and anorexia, whilst cobalamin deficiency is reported to cause poor growth and neuropathies. Deficiencies of these vitamins commonly occur in cats and dogs with enteropathies (e.g. inflammatory bowel disease) or with reduced pancreatic function (e.g. exocrine pancreatic insufficiency). Both of these vitamins can be readily measured in blood to demonstrate deficiency states. In addition to this, serum or urine methylmalonic acid concentration can also be used indirectly to identify cobalamin deficiency. Toxicity has not been reported.

Vitamin-like substances

These include substances that can be considered conditionally essential, i.e. their requirement is dependent on the metabolic state of the animal. Choline and L-carnitine fall into this category, as do carotenoids and bioflavonoids. Carotenoids are found in orange and green vegetables and function mainly as antioxidants. Bioflavanoids are found in red, blue and yellow pigmented compounds and have similar antioxidant properties.

Choline

Choline is synthesized in the liver, and is needed in comparatively larger amounts (compared to vitamins). Although most animals can synthesize choline, young animals require a larger amount than adults. Egg yolks and glandular organs are rich sources. Absorption of choline takes place in the jejunum and ileum by a carrier-mediated process. Choline functions as a structural component in biological membranes, promotes lipid transport and acts as a neurotransmitter (i.e. acetylcholine). Signs of choline deficiency include growth retardation, hepatic lipidosis and renal degeneration. Adverse effects may be possible with over-supplementation.

L-Carnitine

L-Carnitine is necessary in cells to facilitate fatty acid oxidation. This is especially important in cardiac and skeletal muscle. Several compounds including the vitamins pyridoxine and niacin are involved in L-carnitine metabolism. Clinical signs of deficiency include muscle weakness, hypoglycaemia and cardiomyopathy. Toxicity has not been reported in dogs and cats.

Dietary supplements

In recent years various nutritional supplements have come in and out of favour in both the human and veterinary markets.

Supplementation of the **omega-3 fatty acids** docosahexaenoic acid (DHA) and eicosapentaenoic acid (EPA) have gained particular attention. These fatty acids are also termed fish oils, as fish such as sardines, mackerel and salmon are rich in omega-3 fatty acids. The reported beneficial effects are their role in the production of less potent inflammatory mediators. There is some evidence in the veterinary literature that omega-3 fatty acids are beneficial in certain kidney, heart, skin and joint diseases. Human omega-3 fatty acid supplements are used.

Glucosamine and chondroitin have been reported to be useful in orthopaedic diseases such as osteoarthritis. Glucosamine may serve both a structural role (as a component of the cartilage glycosaminoglycan layer) and a functional role (in mediating joint inflammation) in osteoarthritis. Chondroitin is thought to have a synergistic role with glucosamine in reducing osteoarthritic change and ameliorating cartilage damage. Other compounds such as methylsulphonyl methane and green-lipped mussel extracts may also be beneficial in joint disease.

Oxidative damage is important in various diseases but may also occur due to ageing, trauma and with other stresses. Vitamin E, selenium, vitamin C, beta-carotene and other carotenoids and thiols such as *S*-adenosyl methionine are all reported to have **antioxidant** properties. Coenzyme Q$_{10}$ has received particular attention from cardiologists, as its deficiency may lead to cardiomyopathy and also for its antioxidant role in the heart. Although some of these antioxidants have shown beneficial effects in the laboratory, a beneficial effect in patients has yet to be proven.

Probiotics are live organisms (e.g. *Lactobacillus acidophilus*) that provide a beneficial role in health. **Prebiotics** are substances (e.g. lactulose, fructo-oligosaccharides) that act as substrates for beneficial bacteria and thus promote their growth over harmful bacteria. Probiotics and prebiotics are believed to antagonize harmful gut bacteria and also to modulate the immune system of the gut.

Feeding dogs and cats

Carbohydrate requirements of dogs and cats

The metabolic differences between cats and dogs support the classification of cats as obligate carnivores and dogs as omnivores.

The ability to utilize a large amount of dietary carbohydrate is limited in cats and they maintain adequate blood glucose levels when fed low-carbohydrate, high-protein food. They have low levels of the hepatic enzymes glucokinase and hexokinase, both of which act to trap glucose in the liver following delivery from the intestine. In contrast, cats have a strong capability for gluconeogenesis, i.e. production of glucose from amino acids and other compounds. Cats are also deficient in digestive enzymes for carbohydrate absorption. Cats also have lower levels of certain disaccharidases, such as lactase, resulting in impaired digestion of sugars such as lactose (found in milk).

Whilst dogs and cats do not have a minimum dietary requirement for carbohydrates, they do require adequate glucose or glucose precursors (amino acids and glycerol) in order to provide essential fuel. When energy requirements are high, readily digestible carbohydrates and starches should be fed. It is worth noting that sugars may serve to increase palatability for dogs but less so for cats.

Consequences of excessive and inadequate carbohydrate intake are shown in Figure 13.8.

Excessive dietary carbohydrate intake
• Obesity
• Irregular bowel movements (diarrhoea)

Inadequate dietary carbohydrate intake
• Protein will be used to meet energy needs, thus decreasing the amount available for tissue repair and growth
• Lack of energy
• Irregular bowel movements (constipation)

13.8 Consequences of excessive and inadequate carbohydrate intake in dogs and cats.

Fat requirements of dogs and cats

Although not required for health, calories supplied by fat can be more beneficial than those provided by carbohydrate or protein, particularly in cases of high energy demand when increasing dietary fat intake allows for increased energy consumption.

Dogs and cats require dietary fat to enhance absorption of fat-soluble vitamins A, D, E and K. High dietary fat concentration requires increased antioxidant protection, such as added vitamin E. If there are inadequate antioxidants, dietary fats will soon become rancid, resulting in oxidation, reduced palatability and reduced vitamin activity.

Consequences of excessive and inadequate fat intake are shown in Figure 13.9.

Excessive dietary fat intake
• Obesity
• Pansteatitis (yellow fat disease)
• Metabolic and gastrointestinal complications
• Hepatic dysfunction
• Increased carbon dioxide production

Inadequate dietary fat intake
• Fatty acid deficiency
• Lack of energy
• Poor growth
• Poor skin condition
• Impaired fertility
• Anaemia

13.9 Consequences of excessive and inadequate fat intake in dogs and cats.

Protein requirements of dogs and cats

There are 10 **essential amino acids** for dogs and 11 for cats (Figure 13.10).

Cats and dogs are particularly sensitive to a deficiency of the amino acid **arginine**. Following consumption of an arginine-deficient meal, the highly active catabolic enzymes in the liver produce ammonia. Without arginine, ammonia cannot be converted to urea and subsequent ammonia toxicity (hyperammonaemia) occurs within hours, leading to fatality. Signs in cats include vomiting, ataxia, vocalization and hyperactivity. Signs in dogs are similar and include tremors, vomiting, profuse salivation and hyperglycaemia. This condition is rare, however, provided the diet includes a protein source.

Amino acid	Dogs	Cats
Phenylalanine	✓	✓
Valine	✓	✓
Tryptophan	✓	✓
Threonine	✓	✓
Isoleucine	✓	✓
Methionine	✓	✓
Histidine	✓	✓
Arginine	✓	✓
Leucine	✓	✓
Lysine	✓	✓
Taurine	●	✓

13.10 Essential amino acids for dogs and cats. ✓ = essential; ● = not essential.

Cats have a high requirement for **taurine**. Most mammals have the ability to synthesize this from methionine and cystine but the cat's liver has a limited capacity to synthesize taurine and, unlike dogs, it therefore requires a dietary source. The precise amount is influenced by dietary composition and metabolic needs. Commercial pet foods are typically supplemented with taurine in addition to that present in natural ingredients. Taurine can only be sourced in significant quantities from materials of animal origin, thus homemade vegetarian diets and cereal-based dog food can cause taurine deficiency in cats. Taurine is important for normal retinal, cardiac, reproductive, platelet and immune function. Inadequate intake can lead to irreversible blindness, heart problems and impaired reproduction and fetal development. Kittens born to taurine-deficient queens are often small and weak with developmental abnormalities.

Cats fed insufficient **methionine** and **cystine** may show poor growth and crusting skin disease.

Cats require a higher level of **protein** for maintenance than dogs, as their ability to regulate amino acid catabolism is limited, and they have limited capacity to digest carbohydrate (see above). Catabolic enzymes in the liver are designed to manage a high level of dietary protein, regardless of actual intake. They also lack the ability to conserve nitrogen. Additional protein may be required by both species during growth, pregnancy, lactation and tissue repair (see later).

If more protein is consumed than required, the excess cannot be stored. Deamination occurs in the liver: the amino part is converted to urea, which is excreted by the kidneys; the acid part is converted to glycogen or fat and stored as adipose tissue. A high-protein diet may therefore be detrimental to older animals, whose hepatic and renal systems may not function as well as they used to.

The consequences of excessive and inadequate protein intake are shown in Figure 13.11.

Excessive dietary protein intake
• May be detrimental to the health of older animals
• May speed growth
• May be a causal factor in the development of orthopaedic problems in young and large canine breeds

Inadequate dietary protein intake
• Poor growth or weight loss
• Dull hair coat
• Muscle atrophy
• Increased susceptibility to disease
• Anaemia
• Infertility
• Oedema
• Emaciation

13.11   Consequences of excessive and inadequate protein intake in dogs and cats.

Water requirements of dogs and cats

Water requirements are related to maintaining water balance. In a healthy animal, losses are made in:

- Urine (20 ml/kg/day)
- Faeces (10–20 ml/kg/day)
- Respiration and sweating (20 ml/kg/day).

The minimum daily requirement for dogs and cats is considered to be between 40 and 60 ml/kg and can be calculated using the formula: **50 ml x bodyweight (kg).**

Pet food types

It is fundamental that an informed choice of food type is made by pet owners in order to provide a complete and balanced diet appropriate to the lifestage and nutritional requirements of their animals. The majority of novice pet owners will obtain advice on pet care from the supplier or breeder. Consequently, the veterinary profession is often not consulted on important issues such as choosing an appropriate diet. With such a massive consumer market and wide variety of pet diets and types of food available (Figure 13.12), it is imperative that owners receive accurate and comprehensive dietary advice. In order to provide effective information on this topic, veterinary nurses must have knowledge of these requirements together with familiarity of different food types and their ability to satisfy nutritional demands.

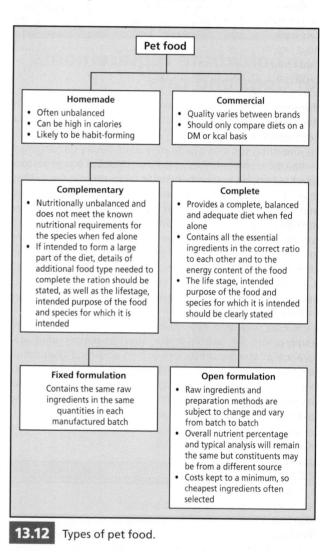

13.12   Types of pet food.

Homemade diets

It is becoming increasingly common for clients to enquire about feeding their pets a homemade diet rather than commercial pet food. Making a suitable homemade diet is time-consuming, demanding and requires a level of nutritional knowledge. Cooking has been shown to alter much of the nutrient content, making some dietary components more readily available (e.g. starches) and others less so (certain vitamins, minerals and proteins). Thus, supplementation is required before homemade diets can be offered as the sole diet. Finding the appropriate balance is not simple and can easily result in the consumption of an unbalanced diet.

Despite the difficulties in producing a balanced homemade diet, there are circumstances when one may be recommended, such as in suspected food allergy or food intolerance. Other reasons may be that no commercial diet is available to meet the needs of a particular patient. If such a diet is recommended for long-term use, a veterinary nutritionist should be consulted.

Unconventional diets

In recent years there has been great interest in using unconventional diets such as raw, vegetarian and BARF (bones and raw food) diets for companion animals. An awareness of the concerns and controversies surrounding their use is important.

Prior to domestication, the diet consumed by dogs and cats was raw food. Dogs were then domesticated for hunting and cats were used to catch vermin. Once cohabiting with humans, dogs ceased to hunt and survived on a diet of leftovers and table scraps, whereas cats continued to eat raw food for a protracted period of time. Much of the present-day justification for feeding a raw food diet stems from the belief that these species are healthier when fed as if still in the wild, and there is the perception that raw food is superior to commercial pet food. In addition, many people are adopting a healthier lifestyle and are demanding the same assurances for their pets.

Raw food proponents support the use of this diet to achieve good health; however, this has not been corroborated by scientific evidence. Claims that raw diets are nutritionally superior to processed foods are unfounded. Feeding trials have not been conducted on the majority of raw food diets; therefore the nutrient content, digestibility and benefit are largely unknown. A raw food diet has yet to be found that meets the criteria for being balanced and complete; however, advocates argue that their regimens are not meant to be balanced on a per meal basis but rather as a long-term dietary regime.

When conversing with advocates of a raw or BARF diet, it is essential to listen to their reasoning for choice and find out why they disapprove of commercially available diets. Any apparent misinformation should be clarified and correct guidance provided. Clients should be educated about the associated risks, including contamination, inadequate nutrient intake, oesophageal or gastrointestinal foreign bodies, and damage to dentition. There may be a public health risk associated with feeding pets a raw food diet and clients should be advised to take care when handling raw meat. To address the bacterial and parasitic risk, the food being offered should be cooked and pets should be treated with an effective anthelmintic.

Feeding a vegetarian diet to cats is not advised. This approach usually stems from owners ascribing their own vegetarian diet preferences to their pet. Whilst dogs can be classified as omnivores, cats are strictly obligate carnivores and are dependent on a supply of animal-derived protein in their diet. Thus, feeding a cat a vegetarian diet long term will cause serious disease. Cats should also not be fed long term on dog food, since it may not meet their specific nutritional requirements. Clients should be educated on the requirements of their cats and the consequences of feeding an inappropriate diet.

Commercial diets

There is a huge variety of pet foods available to pet owners, but it is important to remember that the quality of commercial diets varies significantly between brands. Because commercial pet food is typically mass produced, some individuals have suggested that such foods contain unacceptable levels of harmful chemical preservatives, food colouring agents, pesticides, heavy metals, excess amounts of salt, sugar, over-cooked oils, and meat byproducts not suitable for human consumption. To date, there is no scientific evidence supporting such claims.

The market positioning of pet foods is segmented into generic, private label, grocery and speciality/premium brands (Figure 13.13). Manufacturers may label their products with terms such as premium, ultra premium, natural and holistic. Such terms currently have no official definitions. However, pet foods made using high-quality ingredients and manufactured in accordance with a formula that remains unchanged from one production to the next ('fixed formulation' diets) are considered superior pet foods and are often recommended. In conjunction with strict quality standards for raw materials, this approach ensures quality and consistency by minimizing nutrient variability. They often provide balanced nutrition for each lifestage.

Generic brand
• Plainly packaged • Low cost • May lack palatability resulting in poor acceptability • Often sold through supermarkets
Private label brand
• Manufactured for retail multiples • Manufactured to a given formula • Competitive manufacturing costs • Product quality varies
Grocery brand
• National branded products • Nutritionally adequate for the purpose intended • Formulation critically evaluated • Ingredients and palatability can vary between different branded products from the same manufacturer
Speciality/premium brand
• Fixed formula • Focus on quality • High-quality ingredients • Assessed for nutritional adequacy • Balanced nutrition for each lifestyle • Canned and dry types • May offer a 100% money-back guarantee if owners not 100% satisfied with the product • Often sold through supermarkets, veterinary practices and selected pet retail outlets

13.13   Commercial segmentation of the pet food market.

Veterinary therapeutic diets

Veterinary therapeutic diets are supplied through veterinary surgeons and designed for the dietary treatment or management of dietary problems and pathological conditions, or to achieve a specific dietary requirement (see later). Prescription diets generally undergo many tests to ensure that specifications are met. However, because certain conditions require adjustments that may not be appropriate for healthy animals, it is important to use prescription diets only as directed by a veterinary surgeon. It is important to know that these diets may lack palatability or acceptability, particularly in the advanced stages of illness, and owners may require advice on how to encourage their pet to eat.

Comparison of different food types

Animals consume enough food to meet their energy requirements (assuming the food is palatable). To ensure that essential nutrients are eaten in adequate amounts, they should be considered in relation to the energy content or energy density of the diet (see above).

The nutrient content of different foods is usually expressed in one of the following ways:

- On an as-fed basis
- On a dry matter basis
- On a kilocalorie basis.

These methods provide different values for the same diet as they depend on the moisture content of the diet. In order to guarantee correct nutritional management, it is vital to identify which method has been used to calculate the nutrient content.

Dry matter comparison

If two different foods are to be compared, the nutrient percentages must first be converted to dry matter (DM) figures:

$$\frac{\% \text{ Nutrient}}{\% \text{ Dry matter}} \times 100 = \% \text{ Nutrient on a DM basis}$$

The moisture content of diets varies from 3% in some dry diets up to over 87% in some moist diets (Figure 13.14). For example, if a diet contains 25% moisture, it will contain 75% dry matter (DM).

Classification	Moisture (%)	Dry matter (%)	Packaging and presentation
Moist	60–87+	13–40	Stainless steel cans, aluminium and plastic trays, sachets, plastic and compressed tubes
Semi-moist	25–35	65–75	Cellophane wraps, sachets
Dry	3–11	89–97	Bags and boxes

13.14 Moist *versus* dry pet foods.

Kilocalorie/energy basis comparison

Comparison of nutrient content on an energy basis (Figure 13.15) will provide greater accuracy than comparison on a dry matter basis.

Proximate analysis

Proximate analysis is the most accurate method of determining the nutrient content of a food product using laboratory analysis. By subjecting the diet to a series of tests, the percentage of moisture, fat, protein, soluble carbohydrate, fibre and ash can be determined (Figure 13.16). EC regulations dictate that the concentrations of protein, oil, fibre and ash must be declared as percentages in the product. The Feeding Stuffs Regulations 1991 also require details of the percentage moisture content in the product, if over 14%.

Diet A = 250 kcal ME per 100 g of food, containing 3% protein as fed
Diet B = 500 kcal ME per 100 g of food, containing 3% protein as fed

These diets both appear to contain the same amount of protein; however, closer evaluation reveals a disparity in energy content. Consequently the animal will ingest different amounts of protein.

This can be calculated as follows:

Diet A

Grams of food per 100 kcal $= \frac{100}{250} \times 100 = 40$

Each 40 g of food contains 3% protein as fed

Grams of protein per 100 kcal ME $= \frac{40}{100} \times 3 = 1.2$

Diet A contains 1.2 g protein per 100 kcal ME

Diet B

Grams of food per 100 kcal $= \frac{100}{500} \times 100 = 20$

Each 20 g of food contains 3% protein as fed

Grams of protein per 100 kcal ME $= \frac{20}{100} \times 3 = 0.6$

Diet B contains 0.6 g protein per 100 kcal ME

13.15 Comparison of the nutrient content of two diets on a kilocalorie/energy basis. As Diet B has a higher energy density, the pet eats less food and so consumes less protein.

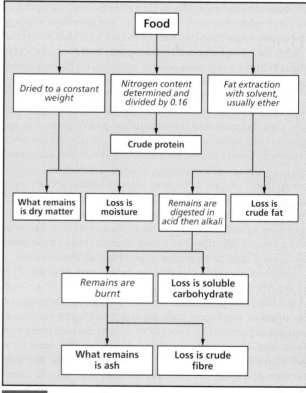

13.16 Proximate analysis process.

Marketing concepts

It is important to recognize that owners will generally choose food according to their own interpretation of what their pet will enjoy, not necessarily considering the nutritional content of the product. Unlike human food products, the final consumer of commercial pet food is not the purchaser. Therefore, when pet food is advertised, all marketing concepts and information regarding content is directed towards the owner or veterinary professional.

- **Anthropomorphism:** Pet foods are increasingly being sold as being similar to human food. Remember that animals' tastes are not the same as ours and their digestive systems are also different.
- **Variety:** This is of great importance to the owner but less so to the pet.
- **All-purpose diets:** All-purpose diets are available mainly in the USA and Asia and are marketed as being suitable for cats and dogs as well as for all lifestages – an erroneous conjecture!
- **Taste and flavour:** This is often used to market the benefits of certain pet foods. It is vital to consider that enhanced palatability is not a criterion of nutritional merit and may lead to excessive intake and obesity. Feeding a variety of flavours can also lead to complications, especially in cases of food sensitivity.
- **Analytical content:** Analytical content is often used on the basis that increasing or decreasing certain nutrients will be of benefit to the animal yet the validity of these claims may be questionable.
- **Health claims:** An increasing number of pet food manufacturers are mirroring the human food industry by incorporating health claims into their marketing strategies and including ingredients such as green tea, glucosamine and chondroitin. One should question whether these are necessary or are being used purely as a marketing tool.

Understanding pet food labels

The pet food label is the primary means by which product information is communicated between a manufacturer or distributor and the buyer. Consumer interest in human food label information has led to an increased awareness of the information available on pet food labels. Owners are now referring to these to assist them in making an informed decision about whether a food will be suitable for their pet.

Similar to food intended for human consumption, animal foods must be correctly labelled. Pet food labels in Europe are divided into two main sections, although the distinction between the two is not as stringent as in the USA. Initial assessment of a particular diet is best determined by looking initially at the principal display panel (section 1). This attracts the buyer's attention and immediately communicates the product's identity:

- Product name
- Manufacturer's name
- Brand name
- Statement of intent
- Nutritional/marketing claim(s)
- Graphics and pictures.

The second section is the information panel (statutory statement) and usually includes the following:

- Directions and description of the product, including the species of animal for which the food is intended and an indication of whether the product is a complete or complementary one

- List of ingredients
- Details of additives – preservatives, antioxidants, colours
- Typical analysis (the average percentage of the nutrient level calculated from several samples) of crude protein, crude fat, crude fibre and ash. Moisture must also be stated if it exceeds 14%
- Address of company responsible for the product
- Best-before date
- Batch number
- Net weight.

Reading and interpreting a pet food label is one way of obtaining information about a pet food; however, labels do not provide information about digestibility and biological value. Contacting the manufacturer or nutrition experts for additional information is the best way to compare the quality of pet foods. Manufacturers often produce manuals and leaflets providing information about their diets. This is usually one of the most accessible sources of information freely available to all members of the veterinary practice team.

Ingredients

Ingredients must be listed on the label in descending order of their predominance by weight according to the product's formulation. Guaranteed analysis assures that *minimum* or *maximum* amounts of the nutrients named can be found in the food but the actual amounts can vary widely. It is often difficult to assess the quality of the ingredients from the label but, as a general rule, cheaper pet foods will often use corn, wheat, soy, byproducts, and meat and bone meal. These ingredients are very inexpensive and often of the poorest nutritional quality. The material of animal origin used by the pet food industry comprises those parts of animals that are either deemed surplus to human consumption or are not normally consumed by people in the UK. Byproducts are basically defined as 'parts other than meat'. These may include internal organs not commonly eaten by humans, such as lungs, spleen and intestines.

Preservatives

The addition of preservatives to pet food serves to protect nutrients from oxidative or microbial damage during use and storage. The primary nutrients that require protection are fats in the form of vegetable oil or animal fat and the fat-soluble vitamins A, D, E and K. Oxidation of fats cannot be reversed and will result in rancidity, loss of calorie content and formation of toxic forms of peroxides that can be harmful to health. In general, the non-vitamin, non-mineral additive content is lowest in moist and frozen foods, since they are preserved by either heat or cold. In comparison, dry food, semi-moist food and treats are known to contain higher amounts.

Manufacturers need to ensure that dry pet foods have a long shelf life to remain edible after shipping and prolonged storage. Consequently, fats are preserved using synthetic or natural preservatives. Some preservatives are added to ingredients or raw materials by the suppliers, and others may be added by the manufacturer. Foods containing chemical additives and artificial preservatives such as butylated hydroxyanisole (BHA) and butylated hydroxytoluene (BHT) may be labelled 'Contains EC permitted preservatives' or 'Contains EU permitted antioxidants'. A more accepted form includes natural antioxidants (primarily vitamins E and C). In addition to being natural preservatives, they also have nutritional benefits. When naturally derived antioxidants are the sole preservative, it is important to observe the best-before date and use the food only within this time frame.

Calculating cost per day

A seemingly cheaper food can be more expensive to feed on a daily basis than one that appears more costly. It is easy for owners to compare the unit price (cost per weight); however, feeding costs are directly related to the energy provided by a given volume of food and the cost of that food volume. True costs of feeding are best reflected by the cost of the food per day or per year or the cost per calorie.

How to calculate cost per day

1. Calculate the animal's MER.
2. Multiply the MER by the relevant factor to calculate daily energy requirement.
3. Select diet and determine the ME density of the food.
4. Divide the energy requirement by the energy density of the chosen diet to determine quantity to be fed per day.
5. Calculate cost per day.

Feeding equine species

The equid is a non-ruminant herbivore with a large and highly developed caecum and colon containing microbes required to ferment and break down the large quantity of fibre in its natural diet (see Chapter 3). The advantage of being a 'hindgut' fermenter is that components in the diet such as protein and simple sugars can be digested and absorbed before fermentation. This is in contrast to the ruminant (see Chapter 3), which ferments virtually all that it ingests in its rumen, including proteins, most of which are broken down to ammonia. However, ruminants have the advantage of being able to absorb the products of fermentation in the small bowel, while in the horse there is very limited intestinal tract left after the colon, which results in less efficient absorption.

Designed to be trickle feeders, horses forage for grass and other herbages in their natural habitat for more than 16 hours per day. Domestication has led to changes, and increasing athletic demands require higher energy levels than their more natural diet can provide. These higher energy demands can be satisfied by utilizing the ability of the stomach and small intestine to digest and absorb more simple sugars, for example those from cereals. However, this can lead to its own digestive and metabolic problems. The teeth of the horse are designed to grind a highly abrasive diet of mainly grass and erupt continuously throughout life. Replacing some of the forage component of the diet with less abrasive food such as cereals can lead to a variety of dental problems. Boredom and stereotypical behaviour can also develop in a horse that is not occupied by feeding for most of its day. For these reasons, feeding the horse has become both an art and a science.

Energy requirement

The energy requirement will depend on many factors including the age and breed of the horse, its temperament, the type and amount of work it is required to do, the climate, the general health of the horse and whether it is pregnant or lactating (see later).

Carbohydrate requirements of horses

Carbohydrates are the major source of fibre and energy in the diet of the horse.

- Non-structural carbohydrates:
  - Glucose, fructose, sucrose and starch are found in legumes and cereal grains. They are broken down to glucose and fructose in the stomach and small intestine and absorbed
  - Fructans (chains of fructose molecules) are found in grasses such as Timothy and fescue. They cannot be broken down or absorbed in the small intestine but pass to the hindgut, where they are fermented to lactic acid
  - Excessive feeding of any of these allows unabsorbed sugars to pass to the hindgut, where rapid fermentation leads to the overproduction of lactic acid, fall in pH, destruction of microbes and the release of toxins implicated in laminitis, colic and endotoxaemia.
- Structural carbohydrates (fibre):
  - Cellulose and hemicellulose are polysaccharides containing up to thousands of linked glucose molecules and are the structural component of the primary cell wall of green plants
  - The polysaccharides pass to the hindgut of the horse, where fermentation by microbes produces volatile fatty acids (VFAs)
  - VFAs are absorbed into the bloodstream and are used as a source of energy immediately or stored as fat.

Fibre

Fibre must make up the major constituent of the horse's diet. This facilitates effective intestinal function and motility, and will also provide the major energy source through the production of VFAs in the hindgut. However, the feeding of cereals may be necessary to meet increasing energy demands by providing more rapidly absorbable sugars.

Grass

Pasture is a good source of forage for horses and, in certain circumstances, can provide most of their nutritional requirements. The nutrient content of the pasture will vary with the species of grasses (influenced by whether it is a permanent pasture or temporary ley), stage of maturity and the season. Grazing is a natural way of feeding, helping to alleviate boredom and allowing a degree of exercise. Feeding from ground level, as with grazing, is the preferred posture, resulting in slower consumption and improved airway drainage. Horses are selective grazers, probably influenced by the palatability and fibrous content of the grasses, resulting in areas of short cropped grass and areas of long tufts of more fibrous grass, which often become latrines. This, along with overgrazing and poor weed management, can severely reduce the quality of a pasture. Regular removal of faeces, harrowing, 'topping' (cutting grass to a uniform length), field rotation and grazing by other species such as sheep will improve the quantity and quality of the grass and also improve parasite control.

Hay

Grass or legume hay can be fed to horses. Grass hay (meadow hay from permanent pastures and seed hay from temporary leys) is usually lower in protein and energy but higher in fibre than legume hay. The nutrient content of grass hay will depend on the species, the stage of maturity and season of the sward when it was cut. Hay has a lower nutritive value than the grass from which it was made, but a horse must eat more grass to obtain the same amount of nutrients because it contains so much water. The nutritional value of hay varies greatly, so it is important to check the quality. High-quality hay is not weathered excessively, is leafy and has very few stems. As a general rule the more mature the grass, the lower the energy and protein levels. For the majority of horses grass hay will satisfy their appetite and provide enough fibre without excess energy or protein. It is important that hay is made from ragwort-free pastures as although horses will avoid this poisonous weed in pasture, they may inadvertently consume it in hay.

Legume hays (such as alfalfa, see Figure 13.17) are higher in protein, energy (due to their non-structural carbohydrate content), calcium and vitamin A than grass hays and contain more protein than any grain. This concentrated source of energy and good-quality protein may be an advantage when fed as part of the ration for young, growing horses, lactating mares and performance horses.

Good-quality hay is usually fed dry but if the dust content is high (as found in poor-quality or old hay) the hay can be soaked before feeding. Soaking hay for long periods of time will remove some of the soluble carbohydrate, which is desirable for obese or laminitis-prone horses. Hay is best fed from the ground, but this will increase wastage. Chaff is chopped hay and can be readily mixed with other feeds, preventing a horse from 'bolting' its grain.

Haylage

This contains grass and other forage plants that are wilted so that the moisture content is between 35 and 45% (55–65% dry matter). Bales of the grass are then compressed to exclude much of the air and sealed into plastic bags. Natural fermentation inside the bag produces lactic acid, reducing the pH, which prevents the development of fungal spores and preserves the grass. The dryness of the material when wrapped limits the extent and length of the fermentation. If the moisture level is >50% the fermentation persists for longer and this may result in very acidic forage with high ammonia levels that is unpalatable to horses. In addition it may allow the proliferation of clostridial bacteria that can cause the usually fatal disease botulism. The pH should be between 4.5 and 5.8 and the ammonia nitrogen level should be <5%. DE should be between 8 and 9 MJ/kg. Up to 90% of the feeding value of fresh pasture can be retained in the preserved grass. Haylage should only be made from ragwort-free pastures.

Sources of additional energy

Working horses require more energy than can be provided by hay or pasture alone and it is necessary to provide concentrates (Figure 13.17). Cereal grains can be fed whole or processed by cracking, rolling, crimping, steam flaking or

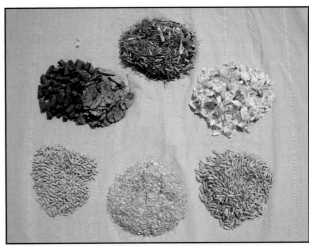

13.17 Sources of additional energy for horses. Clockwise from top: alfalfa hay; flaked maize; oats; bran; barley; and sugar beet pulp (nuts and Speedibeet). (Courtesy of Alison Schwabe)

extruding. Grains are palatable, dense, and usually low in fibre if processed correctly. Concentrates should be fed as a supplement to forage and should be kept at <60% by weight of the total diet.

Oats are a starch-based energy source and the easiest of cereal grains for horses to chew. They have the lowest digestible energy concentration of the commonly fed grains, due to the high crude fibre content (10%) in the outer hull, which helps to reduce the risk of digestive upset if overfeeding occurs. Rolling or crushing does not significantly improve digestibility of the starch in the small intestine, though may be beneficial when feeding foals or aged horses with poor dentition. Like all grains, oats are low in calcium but have a reasonably high level of phosphorus. They are a poor source of vitamins. The quality of the protein they contain is not good because they are deficient in some essential amino acids.

Maize has the highest energy value of all the commonly fed grains as it lacks an outer fibrous hull. It needs to be crushed or cracked for optimum digestibility. Due to its low fibre and high energy content, maize should make up no more than 25% of any grain mix and should be avoided or reduced on rest days. Maize provides a good quantity of vitamin A though is deficient in two amino acids (lysine and tryptophan).

Barley is less palatable than oats or maize. It is intermediate in energy between oats and maize and has a similar protein value to oats. It is relatively low in fibre and can cause digestive upsets if not mixed with sufficient roughage. It is a hard grain and should be rolled and heated before feeding to increase palatability and energy availability.

Bran is made up of the outer covering of the wheat grain and is a byproduct of flour production. It has a poor amino acid balance. Its low calcium and high phosphorus content can lead to an imbalance if not corrected by supplementation. Bran is not an essential horse feed, but is useful for mixing supplements and powders into a feed with molasses; it should be limited to 10% of the feed.

Sugar beet pulp is a byproduct of the sugar refining industry; most of the non-structural carbohydrate has been removed, leaving almost entirely structural carbohydrate or fibre. The energy value is between that of cereals and grass but sugar beet pulp is better used as part of the forage portion of the diet. Dried sugar beet pulp should be soaked prior to feeding or it will swell as it absorbs moisture in the oesophagus or stomach and can cause a major obstruction.

Molassed sugar beet pulp, to which some molasses has been added, contains approximately 20% sugar.

Compound feeds contain mixtures of grains. Feed manufacturers combine various grains and add additional vitamin and mineral supplements to create a mix of predictable nutritional quality, which is simple and convenient to feed. Molasses may be used as a binder to produce a 'coarse mix', which reduces dust and increases palatability (Figure 13.18). Pelleted or extruded feeds (sometimes referred to as 'nuts') may be easier to chew and reduce wastage. None of these compounded diets eliminates the need for forage.

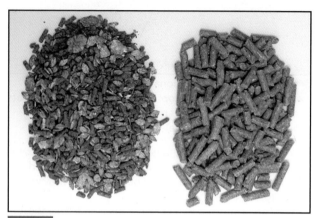

13.18   Coarse mix (left) and pelleted feed (right).

Protein requirements of horses

There are 10 essential amino acids for horses, which must be supplied in the diet: arginine, histadine, leucine, phenylalanine, methionine, isoleucine, lysine, threonine, tryptophan and valine. The mature horse requires only moderate amounts of protein (8–10% of daily ration). Growing horses, pregnant and lactating mares, and aged horses need up to 16% of daily ration (see later). Any excess protein fed will either be converted into carbohydrates and used as a source of energy, or broken down into urea.

Crude protein (CP) contents of common foods are as follows:

- Grass: very variable, ranging from 7 to 23%
- Hay: also variable:
  - Timothy hay 7–11%
  - Alfalfa hay 17–20%
- Maize: 10%
- Oats: 13%
- Barley: 13.5%.

Fat requirements of horses

Fatty acids are an excellent source of energy for muscles if they are adequately supplied with oxygen during exercise. Under these circumstances, the glycogen stored in the liver and muscles is spared and remains available as an energy source for anaerobic activity during periods of greater exertion. A diet high in fat may enable a horse in moderate to heavy work, or a lactating or pregnant mare, to meet their energy requirement without reducing capacity for forage consumption. Additional dietary fat is the most efficient way to increase the energy density of the diet for the high-performance horse. Additional fat can be fed to the underweight horse.

Concentrate mixes with no supplemental fat added will contain 2–2.5% fat. Most commercial feed companies add vegetable oils such as corn or soybean oil to the concentrate mix, to produce a 5–8% fat content. Additional fat can be added in the form of vegetable oil but there is little further benefit if fed at a level >15%.

Water requirements of horses

Clean water should be available to the horse at all times (see also Chapter 12). This can be provided by natural streams (water must be running and not stagnant), water troughs, buckets or automatic water dispensers. Water buckets must be cleaned regularly and the water topped up and changed twice a day. Water buckets allow the water intake of the horse to be monitored but may freeze in the winter and, if knocked over and emptied the horse has no further access to water. Water dispensers allow the horse constant access to water but the amount consumed cannot be monitored.

Water requirements increase as environmental temperature increases; for instance, a rise from 15°C to 20°C will increase water loss by 20% and will therefore increase an adult horse's water requirement by about 5 litres. The effects will be greater in the foal, especially the neonate, due to the greater surface area to body mass ratio and its inability to concentrate urine as efficiently.

Feed composition will also have a major impact on water intake. The resting horse grazing grass with a moisture content of >70% may not need to drink any water, while diets that are dry or high in salt will increase the horse's thirst substantially. Water intake will also vary with workload, age, breed, health, and whether a mare is barren, pregnant or lactating. The signs of inadequate water intake include decreased appetite, especially for dried food, followed by decreased physical activity. Inadequate water intake may increase the risk of intestinal impactions and colic.

Vitamin and mineral requirements of horses

A good-quality well balanced diet should provide a horse with all the minerals and vitamins it requires (Figures 13.19 to 13.21).

Calcium and phosphorus must be present in the diet both in sufficient quantity and in the correct ratio. The ideal Ca:P ratio for the mature horse is 2:1. Grass hay has relatively low levels of both calcium and phosphorus; if combined with cereals, which have a high P:Ca ratio, an imbalance can occur, resulting in calcium being resorbed from the bones. Legume hays have a high Ca:P ratio. A combination of grass, hays (including those containing legumes) and cereals will provide a correct balance.

Dietary supplements

Horses fed proprietary feeds rarely require additional supplements. Health status, individual needs, environmental conditions and workload may necessitate the need for supplementation. An obese horse on a restricted diet to reduce weight or one susceptible to laminitis on restricted or poor quality grazing may benefit from a vitamin and mineral supplement. The most common supplements are oils, vitamins, minerals, salt (in the form of salt blocks), electrolytes and herbs. Supplements are manufactured by feed companies and come in the form of pellets, liquids or powders.

Mineral	Daily maintenance requirement	Functions	Clinical signs of deficiency
Sodium	20 mg/kg BW	Maintaining osmotic balance in blood. Regulation of acid–base and water balance. Transmission of nerve impulses and muscle contraction	Anorexia and lethargy. Deficiency rare.
Chloride	80 mg/kg BW	As for sodium	Deficiency rare.
Potassium	50 mg/kg BW	Most important intracellular cation. Maintaining osmotic and acid–base balance. Nerve and muscle function. Carbohydrate metabolism	Deficiency rare.
Calcium	50 mg/kg BW	Structural: bones and teeth. Functional: cellular messaging, blood clotting, muscle and nerve function	Growth retardation. Reduced bone mineralization
Phosphorus	22–30 mg/kg BW	Structural: bones and teeth. Functional: vital component of nucleic acids, cell membranes and ATP	Poor bone mineralization. Decreased growth. Reduced fertility. Poor coat
Magnesium	15 mg/kg BW	Structural: bone. Functional: carbohydrate and lipid metabolism, catalysing enzyme reactions, cellular energy production, neuromuscular function	Muscle weakness. Growth retardation. Reduced bone mineralization. Neuromuscular hyperactivity

13.19 Essential minerals for horses.

Trace element	Daily maintenance requirement	Functions	Clinical signs of deficiency
Copper	15 mg/kg DM	Many functions. Important in cartilage development in growing horses	Developmental bone disorders in growing horses
Zinc	45 mg/kg DM	Normal cell metabolism. Enzyme activator and antagonist	Widespread physiological effects
Manganese	45 mg/kg DM	Activation of enzymes involved in cartilage formation	Abnormal skeletal development. Reproductive failure
Iron	40 mg/kg DM	Normal haemoglobin and red blood cell production	Anaemia. Deficiency rare; oversupplementation more common
Selenium	0.2 mg/kg DM	Maintenance of normal muscle tissue	Pale, weak muscle in foals. Occasionally white muscle disease in adults. Possible placental irregularities
Cobalt	0.1 mg/kg DM	Synthesis of vitamin B12 in the gut	Impaired vitamin B12 production and hence weight loss, anaemia, reduced growth
Iodine	0.2 mg/kg DM	Synthesis of thyroxine	Cell reaction rate abnormalities

13.20 Essential trace elements for horses.

Vitamin	Daily maintenance requirement or source	Function	Clinical signs of deficiency
Vitamin A	4000 IU/kg DM	Necessary for vision, reproduction, immunity, bone and muscle growth	Night blindness. Deficiency rare
Vitamin D	500 IU/kg DM	Essential for calcium and phosphorus metabolism and absorption from the intestine. Protects against loss of these elements from bone	Poor bone mineralization. Decreased serum calcium and phosphorus levels
Vitamin E	100 IU/kg DM	Primarily as an antioxidant. Works with selenium	Red blood cell fragility. Infertility. Skeletal and heart muscle weakness
Vitamin K	Unknown	Blood clotting	Deficiency rare
Vitamin C	Synthesized in the liver	Antioxidant and free-radical scavenger. Collagen synthesis, immunity, drug and steroid metabolism	Deficiency rare
Choline	Synthesized in the liver although supplement of 0.5–2.0 g/kg DM common	Structural component of membranes. Promotes lipid transport. Neurotransmission (i.e. acetylcholine)	Growth retardation. Hepatic lipidosis. Renal degeneration
Biotin	Unknown. Synthesized by gut microflora	Involved in many enzymatic reactions. Fatty acid, glycogen and protein production	Deficiency very rare. Supplementation may improve poor hoof quality
Thiamine (B1)		Metabolism of carbohydrates. Nervous system function	Bradycardia. Ataxia. Loss of appetite and weight loss. Deficiency rare
Riboflavin (B2)	Synthesized by gut microflora	Energy metabolism. Nervous system function	Deficiency not reported in the horse
Niacin (B3)	Synthesized in the body	Cellular respiration and metabolism	Deficiency very rare
Pantothenic acid	In most cases body can synthesize adequate amounts	Component of coenzymes. Protein, fat and carbohydrate utilization	Deficiency very rare

13.21 Essential vitamins for horses.

continues ▶

Vitamin	Daily maintenance requirement or source	Function	Clinical signs of deficiency
Cobalamin (B12)	Synthesized by gut microflora	Production of red blood cells. Utilization of proteins, fats and carbohydrates	Deficiency very rare. Supplementation may benefit horses in poor health (e.g. anaemia, severe parasitic conditions)
Folate/folic acid	Synthesized by gut microflora but commonly given as supplement of 0.5 mg/kg DM	Formation of red blood cells and cell metabolism. Coenzyme involved in metabolism	Deficiency rare in the horse. Supplementation may benefit some stabled horses

13.21 *continued* Essential vitamins for horses.

Energy density

A horse must consume sufficient food to meet all its nutrient requirements. To ensure that other essential nutrients are eaten in adequate amounts, they should be considered in relation to the energy content or energy density of the diet. When an animal finishes eating the diet, sufficient energy will have been consumed and the animal should have met all other nutritional needs. Figure 13.22 shows how to calculate the daily feed ration for a horse.

---

1. **Weigh the horse**, or estimate the bodyweight by measuring the girth of the horse at expiration using a tape calibrated in kg.
2. **Estimate the total feed capacity of the horse.**
   Total daily ration (kg) = (Bodyweight (kg) / 100) x 2.5
3. **Calculate the energy requirement for maintenance.**
   This is the energy required for a horse doing little or no work and will include most hospitalized horses.

   Energy requirement for maintenance (MJ)

   = 18 + (Bodyweight (kg) / 10)

   So for a 500 kg hospitalized horse, the total feed capacity will be 12.5 kg and the energy requirement 68 MJ of DE.

   Average grass hay contains 9 MJ DE/kg. Thus, for energy requirement the horse requires only 7.6 kg of hay or 60% of its capacity. This should also meet the requirement of 7.5–8.5% crude protein for maintenance.
4. **Calculate the energy requirement for work.**
   Light work (light walking and trotting): Add 1–2 MJ of DE per 50 kg of bodyweight
   Medium work (some cantering, schooling, dressage and jumping): Add 3–4 MJ/50 kg BW
   Hard work (hunting 1–2 days per week):
   Add 5–6 MJ/50 kg BW
   Fast work (eventing, racing): Add 7–8 MJ/50 kg BW
   - A 500 kg horse in light work will need 78–88 MJ of DE or between 8.7 and 9.7 kg of average quality hay, still well within its feed capacity of 12.5 kg of hay. This should also meet the requirement of 7.5–8.5% crude protein for maintenance.
   - A 500 kg horse in fast work will need 138–148 MJ of DE, which would amount to 16.4 kg of average quality hay which is greater than its feed capacity. A proportion of the ration must therefore be replaced by concentrate. For example, 130 MJ of the energy would be supplied by 6.5 kg average-quality hay and 6 kg of oats at 12 MJ/kg. Concentrates should *not* constitute >50% of the ration, leaving at least 50% as forage. Further energy demands could be met by replacing some grass hay by alfalfa hay and/or some oats by maize, or by the addition of a fat component in the ration. The protein requirement of 9.5–10% crude protein for fast work should be met by these combinations.

13.22 Calculating the daily feed ration for a horse.

Feeding exotic pets

Small mammals

Basic energy and macronutrient requirements for rabbits and rodents are given in Figures 13.23 and 13.24.

	Rabbits	Guinea pigs	Hamsters	Gerbils	Rats and mice
Bodyweight (BW)	0.5–7.0 kg	0.75–1.0 kg	85–140 g	50–60 g	20–800 g
Maintenance	110.00	110.00	110.00	110.00	110.00
Growth	190–210	145.00	145.00	145.00	145.00
Gestation	135–200	145.00	145.00	145.00	145.00
Lactation	300.00	165.00	310.00	440.00	440.00

13.23 Basic energy requirements for rabbits and rodents (ME kcal/day) = 110–440 BW $^{0.75}$ where BW is in kg.

	Rabbits	Guinea pigs	Hamsters	Gerbils	Rats and mice
ME (kcal/g)	2–2.4	1.7–2.9	2.5–3.9	2.5–3.7	2.2–3
Protein (%)	12–18	18–20	18–22	17–18	13–20
Fat (%)	2–4	2–4	4–5	6–9	1–5
Fibre (%)	13–24	10–18	4–8	4	4

13.24 Basic macronutrient requirements for rabbits and rodents.

Rabbits

Rabbits are herbivores with a high dietary requirement for fibre. Many commercial rabbit pelleted diets are available (Figure 13.25) but it is still vitally important that rabbits are encouraged to consume significant quantities of freshly grazed grass or dried grass products and hay. This is to ensure that the correct fibre levels (crude fibre levels of >18% with indigestible fibre levels of >12.5% have been quoted) are achieved to encourage normal gastrointestinal motility and dental wear. The silicates present in grasses are particularly abrasive and help to ensure sufficient dental wear. Supervised browsing on other plants may also be encouraged but grass cuttings should not be fed as these may ferment.

Rabbits have an unusual metabolism of calcium, whereby they cannot down-regulate the absorption of calcium from their gut. Instead excess calcium is excreted via the kidneys. Excessive dietary calcium can give rise to urolithiasis (usually calcium carbonate), whereas dietary deficiency (often

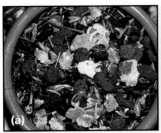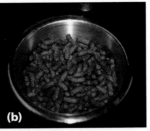

13.25 Commercially available rabbit diets. **(a)** Coarse mix. **(b)** Pelleted diet – this prevents selective feeding. (Reproduced from BSAVA *Manual of Rabbit Medicine and Surgery, 2nd edition*)

exacerbated by a vitamin D deficiency) is a common cause of osteodystrophy, with associated skeletal and tooth defects. Problems can arise in some rabbits fed 'rabbit mixes' because they are selective feeders and may reject the higher-fibre items (often the pellets and hay) in the ration. Most vitamin and mineral supplements are incorporated in the pelleted portion of the diet and rejection of these can produce a diet that is seriously deficient in calcium, vitamin D and other nutrients. Owners should encourage rabbits to eat all ingredients in the ration by offering smaller quantities and refilling the container only when all food has been consumed. Many now believe that pelleted foods, whilst important to provide some of the nutrients that may be absent from forages, should be both homogeneous so the rabbit cannot pick and choose what it wants to eat, and rationed. The rationing of pelleted food is important for several reasons. It ensures that the rabbit turns to forages such as dried grass or hay, which is better for gut and dental health, and it avoids the rabbit being exposed to excess calorie and mineral levels that may lead to obesity, atherosclerosis and urolithiasis. Small volumes of leafy greens and root vegetables such as carrot may be fed but not so much that the rabbit significantly reduces the amount of hay/grass it consumes. Fruit should be avoided as the soluble carbohydrates can lead to osmotic and bacterial diarrhoea.

Rabbits tend to adjust their food intake according to their energy requirements and the energy content of the diet, but adults are likely to eat approximately 30–60 g of dry food per kg of bodyweight (BW) per day. Free access to clean water in bowls should be provided (see Chapter 12) and adults may drink 50–100 ml/kg BW per day. Suspended water bottles may be provided as an alternative but care should be taken to ensure that individuals drink enough if water is *only* provided in this way.

Guinea pigs

Guinea pigs are herbivorous animals and require a dietary source of vitamin C. A deficiency can result in clinical signs of scurvy that include loss of fur, dental disease, swollen painful joints and lethargy. The main types of feed available are pelleted foods or coarse mixes, but these should be formulated specifically for guinea pigs, i.e. have additional vitamin C in them. Rabbit feeds are unsuitable, since they are lower in protein and are not supplemented with vitamin C; also some products contain coccidiostats, which can cause liver or kidney damage in guinea pigs. Some pelleted feeds for guinea pigs contain vitamin C at levels that only just meet the minimum requirements, and prolonged storage (over 3 months) can deplete vitamin C levels in the food. Supplementary vitamin C may be administered in the drinking water (1 g/l), or fresh

fruit and leafy vegetables, which contain high levels of the vitamin, may be added to the diet. Any dietary changes should take place gradually to avoid gastrointestinal upset. The minimum dietary requirement for vitamin C in the guinea pig is 10 mg/kg/day. This will dramatically increase in situations such as pregnancy, growth and disease.

Relatively high levels of fibre are required and a shortage can lead to dental disease and fur chewing, which may result in the formation of hairballs. Gastrointestinal hypomotility may also occur on diets insufficient in crude fibre and lead to bloat. An adequate supply of good quality hay or dried grass products can usually prevent these conditions. Malocclusion can prevent feeding, drinking and swallowing of saliva (slobbers) and can prove fatal, as guinea pigs often develop metabolic ketoacidosis when they cease feeding, as well as developing hypovitaminosis C (scurvy).

Guinea pigs may eat 5–8 g/100 g BW per day. Food may be provided in open bowls on the cage floor but may become contaminated with excreta.

Average daily water intake is 10 ml/100 g BW but this may increase if no succulent foods are fed. Free access to water should be provided. Open water bowls may become contaminated and so inverted water bottles with a small sipper tube are often suspended from the side of the cage slightly above floor level. Fresh water should be provided daily and the water bottle cleaned.

Chinchillas

In the wild, chinchillas eat a wide range of vegetables, but their diet is composed mainly of grasses and seeds. Commercial diets are available but good-quality rabbit or guinea pig diets are also suitable. Good-quality hay should be available *ad libitum* as dental disease due to lack of dental wear is common in chinchillas. The diet may be supplemented with small quantities of dried fruit, nuts, carrot, washed green vegetables and fresh grass. Supplements should be provided in moderation to prevent obesity, bloat, diarrhoea or other gastrointestinal upsets.

Adults may eat approximately 20–40 g/day. Free access to water should be provided from hanging water bottles and it may be advisable to offer an additional water dish until the animal is used to drinking from a bottle.

Gerbils

Gerbils are primarily herbivorous and their natural diet is based on grains and seeds, supplemented with fresh vegetables and roots when these are available. Commercial pelleted foods or seed and grain diets are available for gerbils, or adult gerbils can be fed good-quality rat or mice diets. Some mixes may contain large amounts of sunflower seeds, which are very palatable to gerbils and have a high fat and low calcium content. Gerbils often selectively eat sunflower seeds at the expense of other dietary ingredients but an excessive intake can result in obesity, hypercholesterolaemia (with resultant arterial disease) and calcium deficiency, with associated skeletal problems. The diet should be supplemented with chopped green vegetables, roots and fruit, and if pelleted food is given an appropriate seed mix should also be provided. Average food consumption in the adult is 10–15 g daily.

Like other rodents, gerbils need some hard foods or pieces of wood in their environment to gnaw and so prevent problems with tooth malocclusion. Food dishes should be ceramic, since plastic dishes may be eaten.

Gerbils conserve water efficiently through their ability to concentrate their urine. Most of their water requirement is met from succulent foods and from metabolism of the diet, but free access to clean water should always be provided. Water containers with drinking tubes are best placed outside the cage and should be checked regularly to ensure that they are working. Care should be taken to avoid using water feeders that leak as this leads to increased humidity in the environment, which can encourage skin disease such as red nose in gerbils.

Hamsters

Hamsters are omnivorous. Specific diets are available but most good-quality rat or mouse diets will meet the requirements of the hamster. Commercial pelleted diets or coarse mixes can be supplemented with treat foods such as washed vegetables, seeds, fruits and nuts. Diets rich in simple sugars (glucose, lactose, sucrose, fructose) are best avoided.

Most adults will eat 5–15 g of pelleted feed and drink 15–20 ml of water per day, but free access to water should be offered. Food and water should be provided in heavy dishes that are not easily overturned or contaminated; alternatively, hoppers may be used. Stale food should be removed from the cage to prevent hoarding by the hamster.

Rats and mice

Rats and mice are omnivorous and will eat almost anything. Their nutritional requirements are well documented and commercial pelleted foods or coarse mixes are widely available. The basic ration may be supplemented with small quantities of a variety of foods, particularly vegetable-based materials, and offering these may encourage handling by the owner. Most rats and mice will adjust their energy intake to match their requirements but overfeeding of highly palatable foods can lead to obesity. As a guide, adult rats require 10–20 g/day of dry food, whereas adult mice require 5–10 g/day.

It should be noted that rats in particular are prone to obesity and therefore the feeding of sweet biscuits, cake, etc. should be avoided. In addition, as with other animals, human chocolate should not be fed to rats, as they are prone to chronic progressive nephrosis in later life, which may be exacerbated or induced by the theobromine present in chocolate.

Free access to water should be available from small bowls or suspended water bottles. Adult rats may drink 25–45 ml/day and adult mice may drink 5–7 ml/day.

Ferrets

Ferrets are strict carnivores with high protein and fat requirements. High-fibre diets should be avoided. Ferrets require 35% protein and 20% fat on a dry matter basis, which is higher than for adult cats. Pelleted diets for ferrets are commercially available, or high-quality tinned or dry cat foods may be fed. Dog foods are not appropriate for long-term feeding. Whole carcasses (mice, rabbits, day-old chicks) or chicken heads may occasionally be offered to provide variety or to supplement the diet. If vegetable proteins are fed, urolithiasis and hyper-ammonaemia with resultant fitting may ensue.

Deficiencies are uncommon if a commercial ferret diet is fed, but some home-mixed diets may result in problems. Examples include a diet based purely on meat, which can lead to calcium deficiencies with resultant skeletal and kidney problems. Ferrets, like cats, require preformed arachidonic acid, vitamin A and taurine in their diets, all of which are found in whole meat-based foods and commercial cat and ferret diets.

Food preferences are established early in life and some individuals may resent dietary change. Ferrets should be fed *ad libitum*, as they have high metabolic rates and are prone to conditions such as insulinomas in later life. For this reason, and also because dental disease is common in ferrets, feeding a predominantly dry diet is advisable. Water intake is approximately 75–100 ml/kg per day.

Birds
Cagebirds

Passerine bird species, such as the canary and zebra finch, eat a wide variety of fruit and small seeds to obtain a balanced diet in the wild. Captive birds should be fed a mixture of seeds and fruit that mimic the bird's natural feeding ecology. Similarly, psittacine birds (such as parrots, budgerigars, cockatoos, cockatiels, macaws and parakeets) seek out a natural diet containing a wide range of fruit, shoots and seeds, but in captivity they are commonly fed only seed mixes that are composed predominantly of sunflower seeds, which are high in fat but low in calcium and vitamin A. This type of diet may predispose the bird to obesity or nutritional disorders and the problem is compounded in some individuals that become addicted to sunflower seeds. A particular condition is seen in African Grey parrots (*Psittacus erithacus*) where such a calcium and Vitamin D3-deficient diet can lead to hypocalcaemic episodes with collapse and fitting.

Commercial diets formulated to meet the needs of different types of bird are available (Figure 13.26) but should still be supplemented with fresh fruit and vegetables. All-seed diets are unlikely to be nutritionally complete for birds and careful vitamin/mineral supplementation will be required. Suitable vegetables include romaine lettuce, chickweed, parsley, watercress, sprouted seeds and root vegetables. Suitable fruits include apples, plums, oranges, grapes (in small

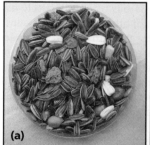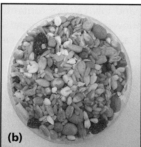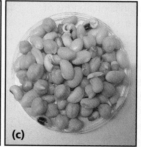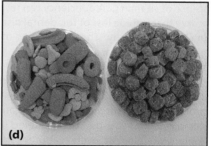

13.26 Commercial cagebird diets. **(a)** Traditional seed diet, with a high proportion of sunflower seed. **(b)** Dehusked seed diet – nutritionally poor. **(c)** Pulse diet, best used as a supplement. **(d)** Two modern pellet feeds for parrots. (Reproduced from *BSAVA Manual of Psittacine Birds, 2nd edition*)

amounts), tomatoes, melon, mango, papaya and pears. Many parrots also relish sprouted seeds such as mung beans or barley/rye grass seeds (owners should ensure that these have not been treated with arsenic, as many commercial lawn seeds are treated with this as an antifungal agent). Millet sprays are often fed to adult budgerigars and should be limited, as they are extremely high in fat and encourage obesity.

Small birds have high metabolic rates and energy requirements, so it is important that a continuous supply of food is available. Empty husks should be blown from the top of the food on a frequent basis to avoid mistakes in judging how much the bird has actually eaten. Food may be provided in seed hoppers but young birds may be fed from the floor of the cage until they are familiar with alternative feeding systems.

Two types of mineral grit, insoluble and soluble, are frequently offered to companion birds as a dietary supplement. Insoluble grit, such as quartz or other forms of silica, remains in the gizzard where it may assist in the mechanical digestion of food and thus improve digestibility of the diet. Some evidence suggests that captive birds such as parrots that dehusk seeds prior to eating them do not actually require insoluble grit in their diets. Indeed, if the diet is deficient in calcium (as so many all-seed diets are) the parrot may over-consume the insoluble grit in an attempt to correct the deficiency and so develop an impaction of the gizzard. Soluble grit, such as oyster shell or cuttlefish, is usually completely digested by birds and provides a valuable supplementary source of minerals, including calcium and phosphorus.

Fresh water should be available at all times.

Birds of prey

Birds of prey are carnivores and in captivity they are usually fed whole chicks, a diet that provides a complete source of nutrition (as it includes the bones and gut contents), though problems may still arise.

Birds of prey are usually 'worked' by their owners in the summer months and should therefore be weighed regularly (at least once weekly) to ensure that the amount fed to them allows them to maintain a steady bodyweight. In general, the larger the bird of prey, the less prey should be fed as a percentage of the bird's bodyweight.

Some falconers feed wild-caught prey to their raptors. Care should be taken, as two main problems can occur. The first is lead poisoning, from any lead shot remaining in the carcass. The second is associated with feeding wild-bird prey such as pigeons, as these may be infected with protozoal parasites such as *Trichomonas* spp. or nematodes such as *Capillaria* spp. The freezing of any wild-caught pigeons and then their thorough thawing before feeding to a bird of prey helps to reduce the risk of transmission of these parasites, but there is still some risk and of course freezing does not remove the dangers of lead poisoning.

Reptiles
Chelonians

Land tortoises are herbivores, whereas terrapins and many of the soft-shelled turtles are carnivores and scavengers.

Newly hatched tortoises start to feed properly once the yolk sac has been absorbed and may be offered a variety of finely chopped fruits, vegetables and pre-soaked specific tortoise pellets. This diet can be supplemented with vitamins and minerals, and food should be offered *ad libitum*. Juvenile and adult tortoises may be fed the same range of foods, but the items do not need to be chopped up and the animals can be housed outdoors in summer, with access to grass and other plants. Food intake is reduced or will stop for up to several weeks prior to hibernation, which occurs when ambient temperature and daylight hours begin to decrease.

Although most water requirements are met from their food, tortoises should be provided with regular access to water. The bowl should be deep enough for them to submerge their nose as well as mouth, as they have no hard palate and so must do this to create suction.

Young terrapins feed in water and it is therefore advisable to have a separate feeding tank from their main housing tank, due to the levels of detritus that build up. Their diet includes small insects, small crustaceans and amphibian eggs and larvae. There are several companies that produce commercial aquatic chelonian pelleted diets. Adult terrapins eat amphibians and fish in the wild and so in captivity whole fish or chopped portions of whole fish should be fed to prevent nutritional imbalance. Herring, sprat, whitebait, sardines, minnows, sand eels, tadpoles or froglets, fresh prawns, shrimps and snails are all suitable foods. It is also possible to feed tinned cat or dog foods, hard-boiled eggs, cheese, earthworms or fresh liver or kidney rubbed in a vitamin/mineral supplement occasionally.

The main deficiencies seen in land-based chelonians are in calcium and vitamin D3. These deficiencies are often exacerbated by diets high in protein and by low environmental humidity, all of which have been implicated in the development of shell deformities such as pyramiding. Tortoises should be provided with a vitamin D3 and calcium supplement, and access to a source of ultraviolet light.

In carnivorous chelonians the main deficiencies are associated with vitamin A and calcium, chiefly in individuals fed an all-meat diet with no supplementation. This can result in shell deformities, kidney damage, and xerophthalmia.

Lizards

Lizards eat a wide variety of foods: different species may be insectivorous, carnivorous, herbivorous, frugivorous or omnivorous, and some species may change their feeding requirements as they mature, e.g. bearded dragons (*Pogona vitticeps*) start out in life as insectivores and become progressively more herbivorous as they mature in the wild. Insectivores (geckos, chameleons, skinks, anoles, lacertids) feed mainly on mealworms, silk-moth larvae, crickets, locusts and wingless fruit flies. However, these insects are relatively deficient in calcium and the insects themselves must first be fed an appropriate nutritional supplement to ensure an adequate intake of supplement by the lizard. Monitors and tegus eat raw eggs, meat, dog food or rodents such as mice or rats. Biotin deficiency can occur due to the avidin content of raw, unfertilized eggs, which can act as an anti-vitamin to biotin; therefore care must be taken when feeding hens' eggs.

Vitamin and mineral supplementation is usually required in diets for captive lizards, particularly calcium and vitamin D3 supplementation in lizards such as iguanas, basilisks, chameleons and water dragons. Access to ultraviolet lighting is also essential, UV-B being necessary to facilitate vitamin D3 synthesis in the lizard's skin (Figure 13.27).

All lizards should have access to fresh water. Some, such as chameleons and a lot of green iguanas, will only drink from water droplets on plants and it is important to mist the tank several times a day. Most lizards should be regularly sprayed with water to prevent skin problems associated with low humidity (see also Chapter 12).

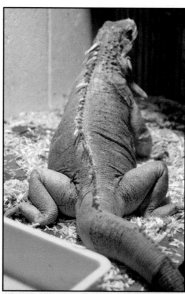

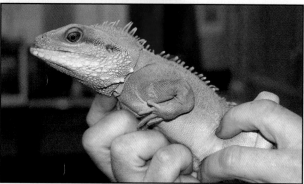

13.27

A deficiency of vitamin D3 can lead to osteodystrophy in lizards. Note the malformed tail (left) and forelimb (below). (Courtesy of Oaklands College, Hertfordshire)

Snakes

Snakes are carnivorous and in captivity will eat rabbits, rats, mice, gerbils, chicks, earthworms, fish, amphibians, lizards or other snakes. The whole carcass is fed, to provide a balanced diet. For humane reasons and to prevent injury to the snake, food is generally offered as dead prey, which may be freshly killed or thawed from frozen.

Certain types of fish, including whitebait, have high thiaminase activity and therefore prolonged feeding without thiamine supplementation can result in thiamine deficiencies. This is particularly common in the fish-eating garter snakes (*Thamnophis* spp.). Supplementation may be given at 35 mg thiamine per kg of food. Cooking the fish to 80°C for 5 minutes will destroy the thiaminases. A garter snake can be converted on to rodent prey by smearing the rodent with the previous fish prey to fool the snake until it regularly accepts the new food.

The quantity of food and frequency of feeding depend on the bodyweight of the snake and surface area of the prey. For example, small garter snakes may require feeding on a daily basis, whereas a large python may require feeding on rabbits once every 2–3 weeks. As a guideline, adult snakes should be fed as often as is required to maintain normal bodyweight. Snakes may not eat for long periods of time and although this is normal at certain times of the year or before a slough, it can result in inanition. Regular weighing is advisable and excessive weight loss may indicate that nutritional support is required. Fluids and easily assimilated foods can be administered by stomach tube.

Water requirements of snakes are low but water should always be provided.

Amphibians

All adult amphibians are carnivores and, since feeding is initiated by the movement of prey, live prey is usually required. Some species may adapt to feeding on dead prey, meat, tinned dog food or even commercial pelleted diets. Raw meat must be supplemented with calcium (10 mg per gram of meat). Captive amphibians should be fed two to three times a week.

Adult frogs and toads feed on insects such as fruit flies, crickets and mealworms; large toads will also eat mice. Aquatic species may eat fish and prepared fish diets. It should also be noted that any amphibian being fed on insects should also receive calcium and vitamin D3 supplementation in the form of a prefeeding/gut-loading powder for the insect or as a dusting powder to prevent metabolic bone disease.

Salamanders eat earthworms, bloodworms, slugs, insects and prepared fish diets. Larval stages are herbivorous and feed on algae initially, or food sprinkled on the water. As they mature, aquatic prey (small crustaceans such as the water flea, *Daphnia* spp.) and then larger insects or animals are eaten.

Ornamental fish

One of the difficulties in feeding ornamental fish is that, with a few exceptions such as the goldfish, they are rarely kept in a single-species environment. Anatomical differences and variations in feeding strategies complicate the formulation of a single diet that will meet all the requirements of a mixed community, which may include representatives of herbivorous, omnivorous and carnivorous fish species.

An adequate delivery of nutrients is essential for the optimum health of the fish, but in a closed aquatic environment overfeeding and poor diet formulation can have a detrimental effect on conditions in the aquarium. Waste, in the form of uneaten food, undigested food and the excreted metabolic breakdown products of protein, will directly pollute the living environment and can pose a serious threat to the health of aquarium fish. To minimize the risk of pollution-induced stress, the diet must be palatable, easily digested, nutritionally balanced and of high biological value. A number of commercial diets are available for ornamental fish. Nutritionally complete diets are marketed as pellets, flakes and granules; other (complementary) foods include certain pond foods and frozen insect larvae, bloodworms and cockles.

Incomplete foods should be fed with care. Although they are useful 'treats' for aquarium fish, an excessive intake may result in dietary imbalance. Live aquatic food, such as *Daphnia* or *Tubifex* spp., is sometimes offered but may represent a disease risk and pre-frozen packs are considered safer. Fish kept in an established pond may feed on the pond's natural flora and fauna, and so complete diets are seldom required. Species that are kept in relatively bare display ponds, such as koi carp, will require a complete diet.

Of the complete diets available, flake formats offer versatility in that they can be floated on the water for surface feeders or submerged to sink slowly for middle and bottom feeders. Since the flakes are easily broken up into smaller pieces, they provide an excellent single food for a range of species and sizes of fish. Granules offer lower leaching of nutrients, because their surface area to volume ratio is larger, and different granule sizes and densities may be used to target different groups of fish in the aquarium.

As a general guideline, fish kept in a community tank should be fed to satiation two or three times per day. This allows close inspection of the fish and the tank on a regular basis. Feeding to satiation involves the continuous addition of small amounts of food to the aquarium until the fish stop feeding eagerly, and is normally achieved in a few minutes or less, depending on the tank size and stocking density.

It should be emphasized that pollution from nitrogenous waste is a considerable threat to the health of fish held in a closed volume of water. Correct diet formulation and feeding regimen can improve protein utilization and help to minimize pollution, but water quality should be maintained through regular water changes or, in the larger aquaria, through the use of filter systems, which must be properly maintained.

Nutrition for different lifestages in dogs and cats

When feeding healthy animals, it is useful to consider the different stages of life separately:

- Neonatal to weaning
- Juvenile (post-weaning to adult)
- Adult
- Senior.

In addition to these lifestages, normal physiological situations where specific nutritional requirements are necessary include **pregnancy** and **lactation**. As many pets are **neutered**, this too may alter nutritional requirements.

The system of lifestage nutrition tailors feeding to optimize longevity, performance and health and to prevent disease. Commercial 'lifestage' diets are widely used.

Energy requirements

The basic calculation of energy requirement is the resting energy requirement (RER) (see above). The daily energy requirement of a healthy animal in different lifestages can then be expressed as a factor of the RER (Figures 13.28 and 13.29).

Lifestage	Energy requirement
Adulthood	
Entire	1.4–1.6 × RER
Neutered	1.2–1.4 × RER
Obese-prone/sedentary	0.8–1.0 × RER
Senior (>7–8 years)	1.1–1.4 × RER
Geriatric (>10–12 years) [a]	1.6 × RER
Breeding	
Early pregnancy	1.6 × RER
At parturition	2.0 × RER
Lactation	2.0–6.0 × RER
Growth	
Growth	2.5 × RER

13.29 Energy requirements of healthy cats during different lifestages as a factor of the resting energy requirement (RER). [a] Tend to have a lower capacity to digest fat.

Lifestage	Energy requirement	Comments
Adulthood		
Entire	1.8 × RER	Dogs housed outside in cold temperatures may require up to 90% additional energy
Neutered	1.6 × RER	Reduced activity levels and possibly increased appetite
Sedentary	1.0 × RER	
Light exercise	2.0 × RER	
Moderate exercise	3.0 × RER	
Heavy exercise	4-8 × RER	Highly athletic dogs such as sled dogs may need up to 15 x RER
Obese-prone	1.4 × RER	
Senior	1.4 × RER	Reduced lean body mass, metabolic rate and body temperature. Increased body fat content
Breeding		
Pregnancy – first two-thirds	1.8 × RER	
Pregnancy – final third	3.0 × RER	
Lactation	(1.9 × RER) + 25% per puppy	Depends on lactation period and number of puppies
Growth		
<4 months of age	3.0 × RER	
50–80% of adult weight	2.5 × RER	
>80% adult weight	1.8–2.0 × RER	

13.28 Energy requirements of healthy dogs during different lifestages as a factor of the resting energy requirement (RER).

Breeding animals

Although there are no specific nutritional requirements during oestrus and ovulation, obese bitches and queens may have a lower ovulation rate, 'silent heats' and prolonged interoestrus intervals. Excess body condition (see Body condition scoring, below) can also impact on gestation and lactation, with smaller litter sizes, insufficient milk production, prolonged labour and increased dystocia reported in obese animals. The energy requirement during the first two-thirds of the pregnancy in the bitch is identical to that of the adult maintenance level; however, in the last third of the pregnancy 3 x RER is recommended (see Figure 13.28). In cats, during gestation up to a 50% increase in energy may be necessary.

The energy requirement during lactation is dependent on the period of lactation and the number in the litter. The process of lactation demands an increased energy intake and energy is also lost to the mother in the milk itself. The energy requirement for a lactating bitch can be estimated from 1.9 x RER plus a further 25% per puppy (i.e. a bitch with four pups will require 3.8 x RER). Peak milk production occurs at about 3–5 weeks of lactation, during which energy provision of up to 8 x RER may be necessary. The energy demands on the bitch and queen can be minimized by introducing food to the young at 3 weeks of age.

Growth

Growth is another physiological state that has a high energy requirement (see Figures 13.28 and 13.29). Growing kittens require about 2.5 x RER as their daily energy requirement: at weaning, kittens need 200 kcal/kg (bodyweight), which gradually declines to about 80 kcal/kg at 10 months of age.

Carbohydrate requirements

Although there are no specific levels of carbohydrate required in dogs, during pregnancy and lactation a carbohydrate allocation of at least 23% is recommended. Athletic dogs and particularly sprinting dogs (e.g. Greyhounds) can benefit from a high-carbohydrate diet.

Pregnant and lactating cats require a minimum of 10% DM carbohydrate as this is known to have a protective effect against weight loss during lactation. Carbohydrate, however, is not required for growing kittens.

Fat requirements

Linoleic acid and linolenic acid are essential in cats and dogs for growth, lipid metabolism and epithelial integrity. An increased fat provision during pregnancy and lactation is helpful to maximize energy provision during these high-demand physiological states.

In healthy adult dogs, a fat content of at least 5% DM is necessary. In geriatric dogs, an increased fat content may help improve energy intake, prevent lean body mass loss and improve diet palatability. In endurance dogs, high-fat diets are desirable as this is the predominant energy source utilized by this group. Fat also improves the energy density of food, which is important in endurance athletes as their performance is limited by the amount of food ingested. In puppies about 10% DM dietary fat is necessary to provide essential fatty acids.

Cats have a special dietary requirement for arachidonic acid. For most cats, 9% DM dietary fat is sufficient but an allocation of 10–35% DM is recommended; 5% of the dietary energy should be provided by linoleic acid and 0.04% by arachidonic acid. Elderly cats can be provided with 10–25% DM dietary fat. In cats prone to obesity, 8–17% DM dietary fat may be more appropriate. Pregnant and lactating queens can be given a higher fat content of 18–35% DM dietary fat to improve performance. A dietary source of the omega-3 fatty acid docosahexaenoic acid is also required for normal retinal development. Growing kittens need 18–35% dietary fat.

Protein requirements

The recommendation for protein allocation in healthy adult dogs is 4–6.5 g of digestible protein per 100 kcal of metabolizable energy or 15–30% DM of crude protein. In older dogs, a mildly reduced protein allocation of 15–23% DM is recommended to minimize the workload on potentially dysfunctional kidneys. In contrast, highly athletic dogs benefit from an increased protein provision.

An increased protein requirement in older cats (to maintain lean body mass, protein synthesis and immune function) is counterbalanced by possible subclinical renal dysfunction, necessitating a reduced protein requirement. A protein provision of 30–45% DM is advised in elderly cats.

In late gestation, the protein requirement of the bitch increases by 40–70%, i.e. to 22–32% DM. In cats, protein deficiency during pregnancy can have a negative impact on kitten health, including lower bodyweight and increased mortality as well as poor immune function, learning behaviour and locomotor development. Taurine is also vital for gestating queens, as its deficiency can lead to abortion and fetal deformities. The taurine content of queens' milk is more than 230 times that of cows' milk; thus milk replacers need to be supplemented with taurine.

The most significant increase in protein requirement is during lactation. This is especially true for bitches, as their milk is high in protein (more than twice that of cows' milk); a protein provision of 19–27% DM or 4.8–6.8 g/100 kcal is recommended during lactation in bitches. Lactation also produces a heavy demand for dietary protein in cats, as a queen in peak lactation produces up to 19 g of milk protein per day; a protein provision of 35–50% DM is recommended for gestation and lactation in queens.

The protein requirement for growth is also high. The protein requirement peaks at weaning, but in general 22–32% DM is recommended for growing dogs. In addition to this, arginine is an essential amino acid in puppies but not adult dogs. Growing kittens need 35–50% DM of protein.

Water requirements

Elderly dogs may have an increased water requirement for medical reasons. The highest water requirement is during lactation, where up to 5–6 litres/day may be necessary. This excessive requirement is especially pertinent to bitches, as they produce comparatively more milk than their human counterparts.

Cats meet the majority of their water requirements from their food but tend to be less sensitive to thirst stimuli. However, they may be less adept at adjusting water intake with changes in the dietary constitution (i.e. changes from moist to dry food).

Calcium and phosphorus requirements

For adult dogs, a dietary calcium provision of 0.5–0.8% DM, phosphorus of 0.4–0.6% DM, and calcium to phosphorus (Ca:P) ratio of about 1:1 is recommended. Adult cats generally require a dietary Ca:P of 0.9:1 to 1.5:1. Older cats require moderate levels of dietary calcium (0.6–1.0% DM) but somewhat reduced phosphorus levels (0.5–0.7% DM) may be indicated.

The demand for calcium and phosphorus increases with gestation, due to fetal skeletal development. However, excessive calcium supplementation during pregnancy can predispose to the development of eclampsia during lactation in the bitch. Therefore, during pregnancy, a calcium allocation of 0.75–1.5% DM and Ca:P ratio of 1.1 to 1.5 is recommended.

The Ca:P balance is most important in growing dogs, as both inadequate and excessive amounts of these nutrients can lead to skeletal disease. In large and giant breeds the risk of over-supplementation is particularly high and a dietary calcium allocation of 0.7–1.2% DM is advised; in small breeds a provision of 0.7–1.7% DM can be safely given. A minimum phosphorus requirement of 0.35% DM is also necessary, leading to a Ca:P ratio of 1:1 to 1.8:1. Growing kittens need 1–1.6% DM of dietary calcium (and Ca:P ratio of 1:1 to 1.5:1) to sustain skeletal growth.

Feeding orphaned puppies and kittens

Newborn animals have high energy demands, with kittens and puppies requiring up to 24 kcal/100 g bodyweight. The ideal method for rearing orphaned animals is to foster them to another lactating bitch or queen (when the age difference between the neonates does not exceed 14 days). Failing this, hand-rearing is possible with the aid of specific milk replacers, as cow or goat milk does not meet the nutritional requirements of puppies and kittens. Orphans should ideally be fed every 2–4 hours when very young but can be fed less often (i.e. every 6 hours) when older.

When caring for orphaned puppies and kittens (see Chapter 26), the provision of heat, humidity, immunity, elimination, sanitation, security and social stimulation also needs to be considered. The physical environment of the puppy and kitten should be warm, draught-free and reasonably humid (50%). Social stimulation should be provided with regular handling. In animals <3 weeks of age, elimination needs to be encouraged by swabbing the perineal region with a warm, moistened cotton ball. As most orphaned kittens and puppies are deprived of colostrum, it is also essential to maintain stringent hygiene practices to prevent infections.

Nutrition for different lifestages in horses

The pregnant mare

The growing fetus makes few demands on the mare during the first 8 months of its development. During this time the mare should be kept fit and healthy, and be fed according to her normal feeding routine. However, the cereal content of the diet should be reduced if workload reduces. Mares in foal can live outside all year round but may need supplements and extra feed when the grass quality and quantity decrease in the winter months.

During the last 3 months of pregnancy the fetus occupies a larger proportion of the mare's abdomen, resulting in reduced capacity for food intake and reduced space for the hindgut. However, the demands of the developing fetus are greater. The energy requirement increases by 10–20% of maintenance during this period, which can be met by supplementation with maize, oats or a proprietary feed for the brood mare. Poor maternal nutrition in the last trimester may result in a weak foal with reduced stores of glycogen in muscle and liver, and in reduced lactation in the mare. Overfeeding should be avoided as this may lead to dystocia due to fetal oversize and/or obesity in the mare. The protein content of the additional feed should be between 16 and 17% to meet the additional demand. A correct Ca:P ratio in the diet is particularly important, and a mixture of grass, hay and grain or the use of a commercial feed will usually supply the correct balance of these minerals.

The lactating mare

The nutritional requirement of the lactating mare is very high and can be compared with the requirement of a racehorse in heavy training. The mare will produce approximately 3.0–3.5% of her bodyweight in milk per day in early lactation and 2.0–2.5% in late lactation. For example, a 500 kg mare will require an additional 45 MJ (a total of 113 MJ) of energy per day during the first 3 months of lactation and 35 MJ (a total of 103 MJ) in the following 3 months. Thus, a diet consisting of 7.5 kg of average quality hay and 4 kg oats will meet her energy demands in early lactation. She also needs about twice as much protein in her diet compared to normal maintenance and this can be met by the use of a concentrate with 16–17% crude protein or by the substitution of legume hay. Inadequate protein will result in reduced milk yield and poor foal growth.

For mares foaling in the spring, good quality pasture can provide all the requirements for energy, protein, calcium and phosphorus.

The foal

Colostrum contains high nutrient levels and is an essential source of immunoglobulins for the foal. The mare does not pass antibodies to the foal across the placenta prior to birth, so the foal must consume a sufficient amount of colostrum to provide adequate disease protection. Colostrum also has a laxative effect on the foal, which assists the expulsion of meconium. The newborn foal should receive at least 4–6 feedings of colostrum from the mare within the first 12 hours after birth and should consume as much as possible during the first 3 days of life. An orphaned foal should receive 2–3 litres of colostrum divided into three or four doses given at hourly intervals. This can be given by bottle or administered via a nasogastric tube.

Foals suckle small volumes of milk frequently, reducing the likelihood of digestive upset. The mare produces around 18–20 litres of milk per day and this will provide all the nutrition in the first few weeks of the foal's life. By 10–21 days the foal should start to nibble at grass, and access to clean good-quality pasture is important. In the case of foals being prepared for early performance (flat racers) or where mares are short of milk, 'creep feed' can be introduced as early as 10 days. A creep feed is one designed specifically to provide additional nutrients for the growing foal but which the mare cannot access. It should be offered well in advance of weaning to help the anatomical and physiological development of the gut, to accustom the foal to concentrates and to facilitate weaning. Foals should receive about 0.5–0.75 kg of creep feed per 100 kg bodyweight. It should have a crude protein content of 16–18%. Adequate amounts of calcium with a Ca:P ratio of at least 1:1 is required, though in rapidly growing foals a ratio of 2:1 is safer.

In other cases no additional feed is needed for many weeks. By 3 months the foal will not receive adequate nutrients from milk alone. Overfeeding, nutrient imbalance and lack of adequate exercise can result in developmental orthopaedic disease such as angular limb deformities, osteochondritis dissecans and subchondral bone cysts, although there is probably a genetic predisposition to these conditions as well.

The weanling

Under natural conditions a mare would wean her foal about a month before her next foal is due, while the weaning age of the domestic foal will vary from 3 to 6 months depending on a variety of circumstances. Weaning can be stressful, especially when it is sudden, as occurs in some management systems. It is important that foals are already adapted to solid food. A foal turned out on good-quality pasture or with access to good-quality hay may require little or no additional concentrate feed. Care should be taken not to overfeed the weanling as this may cause growth-related problems.

The yearling

Yearlings with free access to good-quality grass or hay may not require any additional supplementation or concentrates. If poor-quality grass or hay is provided, concentrates containing 16% protein and appropriate vitamins and minerals may be fed at a rate of 1.25–1.5 kg per 100 kg bodyweight daily. The young growing horse has specialized dietary requirements that will vary according to its future athletic career. A yearling will require high levels of nutrients, especially protein, to build the rapidly growing thoroughbred yearling with its musculoskeletal system being prepared for racing. It will necessitate a diet much higher in protein and minerals than a show cob with a slower rate of maturation.

The geriatric horse

Provided they are able to maintain good bodily condition, most geriatric horses can be fed a maintenance ration without modification. Poor dentition, resulting in reduced mastication of forage, will lead to lowered fibre digestibility and thus reduced energy intake. Where there is loss of body condition, and no other existing disease, the horse should be fed a palatable, easily masticated and digested diet that has a slightly higher protein content (12–16%), maintenance levels of calcium (<1%) and slightly elevated phosphorus (0.4–0.65%), maintaining a Ca:P ratio of close to 1.5:1, and a source of short (chaff) or soaked (sugar beet pulp or grass nuts) fibre.

Athletes

To achieve high performance, horses in training must have adequate levels of energy, protein, vitamins and minerals in their diet. Horses in very heavy work will spend 6–12 hours per week doing strenuous activities, including speed and jumping work. The higher the intensity of the work, the greater the energy requirement will be. In order to satisfy this high energy demand, grain must constitute an ever greater proportion of the total feed capacity. The non-structural carbohydrates from the grain (glucose, sucrose fructose and starch) are digested in the stomach and absorbed by the small intestine, making glucose available for anaerobic respiration.

When the energy demand is very high, the quantity of cereals needed to meet that requirement would overload the stomach and small intestine, allowing unabsorbed sugars to pass to the hindgut where rapid fermentation would lead to the overproduction of lactic acid, a fall in pH, destruction of microbes and the release of toxins, which may result in metabolic disease and laminitis. In order to meet the energy demands of these horses it is necessary to feed fats. Fats are absorbed from the small intestine but are less likely to cause metabolic disturbance. By feeding fat as a source of energy, it is possible to maintain the forage component of the diet at 50% of the total feed capacity. A typical proprietary feed for a 2-year-old racehorse in training will contain around 8% crude fat.

Horses require only a small increase in protein in the diet for optimum production and work performance. It is important to have a balance of amino acids and therefore a source of high-quality protein (soybean rather than oats). A proprietary racehorse ration will contain between 12 and 16% protein.

High-performance horses will lose large amounts of water and electrolytes in sweat. In moderate climates, horses can lose 6–8 litres of sweat per hour, and this loss can increase to 15 l/h in hot climates. Access to water and salt blocks (or the use of added electrolytes) must be allowed to replenish the loss.

Clinical nutrition in dogs and cats

Providing adequate and appropriate nutrition to ill patients is an important aspect of patient management. Comparative studies have shown that nutrition plays a vital role in reducing morbidity, complications and length of hospitalization in human patients. It is logical that this will also hold true for veterinary patients.

Nutritional assessment

The first step in planning a nutritional intervention is to assess the patient's current nutritional status. This is to identify not only the patients who are already malnourished but also those at risk of malnutrition. The assessment should take into consideration historical information (e.g. duration of clinical signs), physical examination findings (e.g. lean body mass) and laboratory parameters (e.g. serum albumin concentration).

Indicators of malnutrition include:

- Unintentional weight loss (>10% of bodyweight)
- Poor coat
- Muscle wasting
- Poor wound healing
- Hypoalbuminaemia.

Patients may not be malnourished at the time of assessment but may still be at high risk of malnourishment (especially if nutrition of that patient is not addressed urgently). In these cases, nutritional intervention can be implemented (e.g. feeding tube placement).

Risk factors for malnutrition include:

- Anorexia for >3 days
- Severe underlying disease (e.g. trauma, sepsis, pancreatitis)
- Large protein losses (e.g. due to gastrointestinal disease, peritonitis).

Body condition scoring

Measurement of bodyweight can be an inaccurate tool in the presence of ascites or when there is excessive body fat together with poor muscle mass. There are also large differences in bodyweight between different dog breeds. Body condition score (BCS) systems utilize both visual and tactile (i.e. palpation) assessment of the body fat content and lean body mass. Generally, 5-point and 9-point scoring systems are in use; with a score of 3/5 and 5/9, respectively,

considered ideal. In the 9-point system (Figures 13.30 and 13.31), each score corresponds to an approximate 10% increase or decrease from the ideal condition (e.g. a BCS of 6/9 would be considered 10% overweight, whereas a score of 3/9 would be considered 20% underweight). Although the 9-point scoring system is preferred as it is validated, it is important to use the same system consistently. Further information on body condition scoring can be found in the *BSAVA Manual of Rehabilitation, Supportive and Palliative Care*.

BODY CONDITION SYSTEM

TOO THIN

1 Ribs, lumbar vertebrae, pelvic bones and all bony prominences evident from a distance. No discernible body fat. Obvious loss of muscle mass.

2 Ribs, lumbar vertebrae and pelvic bones easily visible. No palpable fat. Some evidence of other bony prominence. Minimal loss of muscle mass.

3 Ribs easily palpated and may be visible with no palpable fat. Tops of lumbar vertebrae visible. Pelvic bones becoming prominent. Obvious waist and abdominal tuck.

IDEAL

4 Ribs easily palpable, with minimal fat covering. Waist easily noted, viewed from above. Abdominal tuck evident.

5 Ribs palpable without excess fat covering. Waist observed behind ribs when viewed from above. Abdomen tucked up when viewed from side.

TOO HEAVY

6 Ribs palpable with slight excess fat covering. Waist is discernible viewed from above but is not prominent. Abdominal tuck apparent.

7 Ribs palpable with difficulty; heavy fat cover. Noticeable fat deposits over lumbar area and base of tail. Waist absent or barely visible. Abdominal tuck may be present.

8 Ribs not palpable under very heavy fat cover, or palpable only with significant pressure. Heavy fat deposits over lumbar area and base of tail. Waist absent. No abdominal tuck. Obvious abdominal distention may be present.

9 Massive fat deposits over thorax, spine and base of tail. Waist and abdominal tuck absent. Fat deposits on neck and limbs. Obvious abdominal distention.

The BODY CONDITION SYSTEM was developed at the Nestlé Purina Pet Care Center and has been validated as documented in the following publications:

Mawby D, Bartges JW, Moyers T, et. al. *Comparison of body fat estimates by dual-energy x-ray absorptiometry and deuterium oxide dilution in client owned dogs*. Compendium 2001; 23 (9A): 70

Laflamme DP. *Development and Validation of a Body Condition Score System for Dogs*. Canine Practice July/August 1997; 22:10-15

Kealy, et. al. *Effects of Diet Restriction on Life Span and Age-Related Changes in Dogs*. JAVMA 2002; 220:1315-1320

13.30 Canine body condition scoring chart using 9-point system. (©Nestlé Purina PetCare and reproduced with their permission)

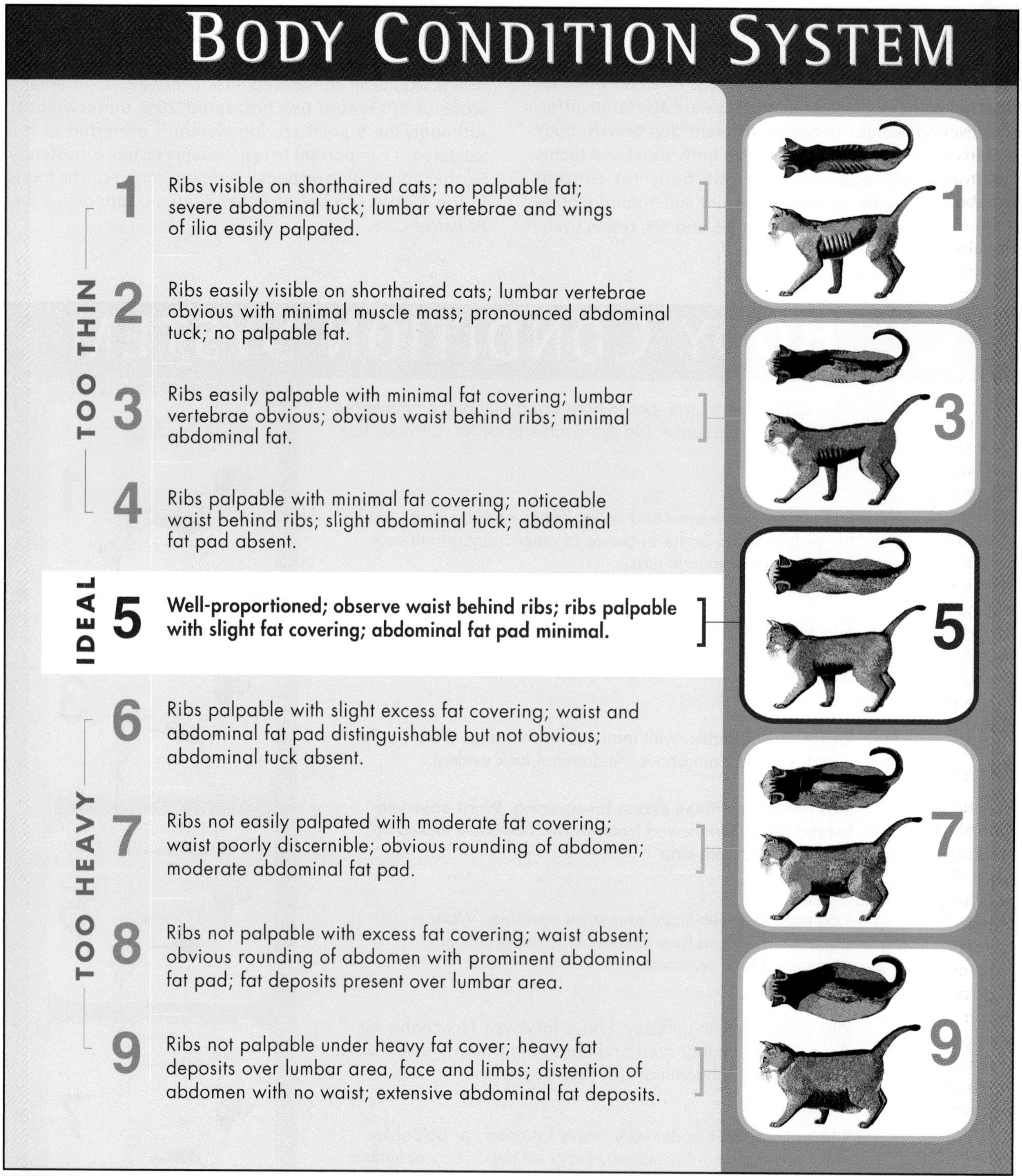

BODY CONDITION SYSTEM

1 Ribs visible on shorthaired cats; no palpable fat; severe abdominal tuck; lumbar vertebrae and wings of ilia easily palpated.

2 Ribs easily visible on shorthaired cats; lumbar vertebrae obvious with minimal muscle mass; pronounced abdominal tuck; no palpable fat.

3 Ribs easily palpable with minimal fat covering; lumbar vertebrae obvious; obvious waist behind ribs; minimal abdominal fat.

4 Ribs palpable with minimal fat covering; noticeable waist behind ribs; slight abdominal tuck; abdominal fat pad absent.

TOO THIN

5 Well-proportioned; observe waist behind ribs; ribs palpable with slight fat covering; abdominal fat pad minimal.

IDEAL

6 Ribs palpable with slight excess fat covering; waist and abdominal fat pad distinguishable but not obvious; abdominal tuck absent.

7 Ribs not easily palpated with moderate fat covering; waist poorly discernible; obvious rounding of abdomen; moderate abdominal fat pad.

8 Ribs not palpable with excess fat covering; waist absent; obvious rounding of abdomen with prominent abdominal fat pad; fat deposits present over lumbar area.

9 Ribs not palpable under heavy fat cover; heavy fat deposits over lumbar area, face and limbs; distention of abdomen with no waist; extensive abdominal fat deposits.

TOO HEAVY

13.31 Feline body condition scoring chart using 9-point system. (©Nestlé Purina PetCare and reproduced with their permission)

Nutrition and specific conditions

In addition to the benefit of providing adequate energy and nutrients to promote immunity, healing and prevent catabolism, nutrition can also have a more direct effect in certain disease conditions. In these situations, adjusting the macronutrients and/or micronutrients of the diet can have a profound effect on the clinical course and prognosis of the disease.

Nutrition and skin disorders

Correct nutrition is important for good skin and coat health. Unbalanced diets such as protein-deficient diets can cause keratinization defects, depigmentation, impaired wound healing and a dry and brittle coat. Similarly, dermal disorders have also been documented in fatty acid deficiency states, as these compounds serve important structural and functional roles in skin. Fatty acid supplements are used in the treatment of some skin conditions.

The micronutrients also play important roles in skin health. For example, copper-deficient diets can cause a loss of normal coloration of the coat, reduced coat density and a dull or rough coat. Perhaps the most recognized nutrient-associated skin diseases are the zinc-responsive dermatoses. These disorders can develop as a result of nutritional deficiencies in zinc provision (e.g. high dietary calcium, phosphate or phytate impair zinc availability in the diet) or due to abnormalities in zinc metabolism. The latter condition is most commonly reported in the Malamute and Siberian Husky breeds where a defect in zinc absorption is suspected. Vitamin A and E are also important in skin health and some dermatological conditions are treated with supplementation of these vitamins.

Adverse reactions to food

These usually manifest as dermal/gastrointestinal disorders. Adverse reactions to food can be categorized as those with an immunological basis (food allergies) and those with a non-immunological basis (food intolerances). Dermatological reactions to food are most commonly due to food allergies. These usually result in pruritic skin disease, sometimes accompanied by concurrent gastrointestinal disease. The most commonly incriminated food allergens in dogs are beef, dairy products and wheat, whilst beef, dairy and fish are implicated in cats. Food sensitivity is investigated by performing a food elimination trial for at least 12 weeks. The diet fed during this period should consist of a single novel protein source or a hydrolysed diet (i.e. a diet that is processed so that the proteins are less likely to incite an immune reaction). Many single-source protein diets and hydrolysed diets are commercially available for this purpose.

Nutrition and orthopaedic disease

Nutrition in early life plays a key role in certain developmental orthopaedic diseases. For example, canine hip dysplasia and osteochondrosis are diseases with a nutritional component. The pathological role of nutrition in these diseases is prior to growth plate closure, especially in large and giant breeds. Two nutritional constituents have been proposed as factors in these disorders, i.e. excessive energy provision during growth and excess calcium in the diet. The provision of a large amount of energy causes rapid skeletal growth which, in turn, can lead to orthopaedic disease via increased biomechanical stresses. Excess calcium intake is known to disrupt endochondral ossification (the process by which bone grows). Based on these observations, feeding *ad libitum* and feeding excessively energy-dense food in large and giant breed dogs is not recommended. A calcium level of 0.7–1.2% DM and Ca:P ratio of 1.2:1 should also be maintained during growth. Deficiencies of other nutrients such as copper, iodine, manganese, zinc and vitamins D and A can also affect skeletal growth and development.

Nutrition is also directly involved in three rare but well characterized skeletal diseases. Nutritional secondary hyperparathyroidism (NSHP) refers to osteopenic skeletal disease and occurs due to diets deficient in calcium, excessive in phosphorus or with an inappropriate Ca:P ratio. For example, feeding puppies and kittens meat-only diets may lead to NSHP, as meat is low in calcium and high in phosphorus. This combination stimulates excessive parathyroid hormone secretion, which in turn causes the resorption of bone. Rickets in young animals (and osteomalacia in adults) are similar skeletal mineralization disorders. These occur due to inadequate dietary calcium, phosphorus or vitamin D. Finally, excessive vitamin A can cause extreme bone deposition and fusion of spinal vertebrae. This has been classically described in cats fed liver-only diets.

Nutrition and dental disease

Periodontal disease is a significant problem in both cats and dogs. Dental disease not only has local consequences in the oral cavity (e.g. gingivitis, pain, tooth loss) but may also have systemic effects on the heart and kidneys. Although dietary factors such as low-protein diets and high levels of calcium and phosphorus can theoretically lead to the development of dental disease, this rarely occurs. Diet can play an important role in the prevention of dental disease. In particular, food texture can play a key role in minimizing plaque development, stimulating beneficial salivary flow and altering the metabolism of plaque-forming bacteria. Foods with enhanced textural characteristics have been shown to prevent the development of periodontal disease.

Nutrition and cardiovascular disease

Taurine and L-carnitine are two nutrients implicated in the development of cardiomyopathy in dogs and cats. Feline taurine deficiency-induced dilated cardiomyopathy (TDDC) was first described in 1987. Since then, commercial diets have been supplemented with taurine and the incidence of this condition has drastically reduced though it is still occasionally noted in cats fed vegetarian diets for example. Taurine-deficient dilated cardiomyopathy has also been reported in dogs fed on diets with very low protein levels. The role of taurine in the heart and the pathogenesis of TDDC are poorly understood. In contrast, it is well recognized that L-carnitine is necessary for the heart to metabolize fatty acids (its primary energy source). Cardiomyopathy due to L-carnitine deficiency is suspected to occur in certain breeds (e.g. Boxers). Unlike taurine, L-carnitine supplements are expensive.

Diet in congestive heart failure

In congestive heart failure (CHF), dietary sodium is an important nutrient of modulation. The current recommendation is for moderate sodium restriction (i.e. 50–80 mg/100 kcal) in mild to moderate CHF and more pronounced sodium restriction (i.e. <50 mg/100 kcal) in severe heart failure. In asymptomatic heart disease, mild sodium restriction (i.e. <100 mg/100 kcal) is advisable, as aggressive sodium restriction when unnecessary can lead to activation of the renin–angiotensin system with deleterious effects. Pet treats (commonly used to administer medication) are usually high in sodium and their salt content must be taken into consideration in heart failure cases. The main drawback of dietary sodium restriction is its negative effect on taste. A diet of high-quality protein can also be beneficial in CHF to prevent lean body mass loss. Potassium and magnesium can both impact negatively on the heart rhythm and contractility when depleted. Omega-3 fatty acids can be helpful to modulate the effects of cardiac cachexia and may also have an anti-arrhythmic effect.

Nutrition and kidney disease

Chronic renal failure (CRF) is a disease where nutritional modulation can have a significant impact on the clinical signs as well as the prognosis. Veterinary studies comparing maintenance diets to those designed for renal failure have shown a positive effect on preventing the onset of uraemia and retarding the progression of this disease.

The hallmarks of renal formulation diets are protein and phosphorus restriction. The main aim of protein restriction is to minimize the load of urea in the body that needs to be excreted by the kidneys. Increased blood urea (due to poor renal excretion) can lead to some of the clinical signs associated with CRF, such as inappetence and vomiting. Generally, 15% DM dietary protein for dogs and 28–30% DM for cats is recommended in renal failure. Phosphorus restriction goes hand in hand with protein restriction as the majority of phosphorus in the diet is in the protein (meat) source. Phosphorus restriction has been shown to reduce progressive renal disease by minimizing the deleterious effects of parathyroid hormone activation (i.e. renal secondary hyperparathyroidism). When diet alone is unable to control the serum phosphate concentration, phosphate-binding agents (e.g. aluminium hydroxide) need to be administered. These medications work by binding to the phosphate in the diet, and so prevent absorption. Phosphate-binding agents will be effective only when used in combination with a phosphorus-restricted diet as the phosphate content of maintenance diets is too high for binders to be effective. Other features of diets designed for renal failure include potassium supplementation, sodium restriction and an alkalizing effect. The main drawback of these diets is their poor palatability. This is compounded by the inappetence typical of CRF patients. Palatability can be improved by increasing the fat content of the diet or by warming the food or adding flavouring agents. Alternatively, a balanced homemade diet can be formulated by consulting a nutritionist.

When renal disease is causing proteinuria but the patient is not azotaemic, moderate dietary protein restriction is recommended. This level of protein restriction can be found in diets designed for senior dogs, as renal formulation diets may have too severe protein restriction. Sodium restriction may also be useful, especially if body cavity effusions are present. There is also good evidence in dogs that omega-3 fatty acids are beneficial in this subset of renal patients.

Nutrition and diabetes mellitus

Canine diabetic diets

Although most endocrine disorders lead to disturbances in metabolism, diabetes mellitus has received the most attention with regard to its dietary manipulation, and dietary fibre has received the most interest with regard to influencing diabetic control in dogs. Fibre can be classified into soluble and insoluble forms. Soluble fibres (e.g. psyllium, oats, barley) form a gel in solution. They delay gastric emptying, delay intestinal transit and are fermented in the colon. Insoluble fibres (e.g. cellulose, wheat, rye) do not form gels and do not affect gastric emptying, but hasten intestinal transit and increase faecal bulk. In diabetic dogs a moderate amount (8–17% DM) of insoluble or mixed dietary fibre is recommended for the possible beneficial effects on glycaemic control. Increased dietary fibre may also be beneficial in overweight diabetic dogs whereas these diets are counterproductive if the dog is underweight.

As diabetes mellitus also involves aberrations in protein and lipid metabolism, adequate but not excessive amounts of these nutrients are indicated for a diabetic dog, e.g. 18–25% DM of high-quality protein and <30% of energy from dietary fat. Several micronutrients are believed to play important roles in diabetic control. In particular, magnesium is thought to be important in glucose homeostasis and this nutrient can be depleted in diabetic animals due to polyuria.

Roles for zinc, manganese, selenium, copper and chromium are also reported. Arguably the most important recommendation is to feed diabetic dogs a consistent amount and type of food, divided into two equal meals to be given at each insulin administration.

Feline diabetic diets

Diets designed for diabetic cats differ from those for dogs in that they have reduced carbohydrate content and increased protein content. These feline diabetic diets have been shown to reduce the insulin requirement and also to increase the possibility of achieving diabetic remission. This is in contrast to the situation in dogs where diabetic remission is rarely achieved, irrespective of the diet, and a reduction in the insulin requirement is not seen with the equivalent (high-fibre) diets. High-protein diets are abundant in the amino acid arginine, which is known to stimulate insulin secretion in cats. The feeding plan is less important in cats and 'grazing' can be instituted instead of meal feeding as this more closely mimics their normal feeding pattern.

Nutrition and gastrointestinal disorders

Gastrointestinal disorders are the most common situation where dietary therapy is considered. In dogs and cats with acute-onset vomiting or diarrhoea, water and electrolytes (such as sodium, chloride and potassium) are the key nutrients of concern. Deficits are addressed by providing intravenous fluid therapy (see Chapter 22). In general, dogs and cats with acute gastrointestinal disturbances are fed a diet of highly digestible protein and carbohydrate (also known as low-residue diets). Although an increased fat content enhances the energy density of diets, a high fat content may not be tolerated in animals with gastrointestinal disorders and thus a moderate fat provision is recommended.

The role of dietary fibre

Fibre source and content are believed to be important in managing gastrointestinal disease. Dietary fibre may have beneficial gastrointestinal effects, especially in the large bowel, where it is thought to normalize colonic motility, prevent toxin absorption, provide a fuel source for cells in the colon, support normal bacterial flora and alter the viscosity of the luminal contents. However, fibre may also reduce nutrient absorption, protein digestibility and the energy density of the food. There is considerable debate about the appropriate fibre type and content for various gastrointestinal disorders. In most cases of acute gastroenteritis a low-fibre diet is recommended; in more chronic situations increased dietary fibre may be beneficial. This is applicable to large intestinal disorders such as chronic colitis, where a response to fibre may be seen. In general, trial and error with various types and amounts of fibre may be necessary to optimize the diet to a particular patient. Dietary fibre may also play a key role in the management of constipation. Likewise, experimentation with various types and contents of fibre may be necessary to find the most suitable option for a particular patient.

Adverse reactions to food

Where an adverse reaction to food is suspected to be the cause of a gastrointestinal disorder, dietary modulation is important. Non-immune reactions to food include food poisoning due to contamination of food with microbes or toxins, reactions to compounds such as histamines (in fish), red blood cell damage due to onion toxicity, and lactose intolerance in adult animals. Food hypersensitivities are generally caused by immune reactions to protein particles. These can lead to chronic gastrointestinal signs (e.g. vomiting, diarrhoea, weight loss, poor appetite) and can also be a significant inciting factor in inflammatory bowel disease. Concurrent allergic dermatological disease may also be present (see above).

A dietary elimination trial with a novel protein source or hydrolysed diet can be performed. Unlike in dermatological food sensitivity disorders, in gastrointestinal disorders patients will normally respond within 4 weeks if a dietary hypersensitivity is responsible.

Gluten-sensitive enteropathy in Irish Setters is not derived from sensitivity to animal protein. Gluten is found in wheat, barley, rye and oats, so diets based on rice and corn are needed to manage these dogs.

Nutrition and pancreatic disorders

Exocrine pancreatic insufficiency

Exocrine pancreatic insufficiency (EPI) and pancreatitis are the main pancreatic disorders necessitating nutritional consideration. As EPI results in an insufficiency of pancreatic enzymes, highly digestible foods are necessary. In general, a moderate fat content (to minimize steatorrhoea) and reduced fibre (to decrease faecal bulk and fat excretion) is recommended. A low-residue gastrointestinal formulation diet may fit these requirements. In some cases, however, continuation of a maintenance-type diet is appropriate. Some experimentation with different diets may be employed to find the most suitable for a particular patient. Most animals with EPI require parenteral vitamin B12 supplementation as absorption of this nutrient is compromised.

Acute pancreatitis

Traditionally, low-fat diets have been recommended to minimize pancreatic stimulation, but there is no evidence to suggest that a moderate fat content is harmful. For this reason, and as low-fat diets are unpalatable (especially in the face of inappetence caused by the disease), a diet of moderate fat content is recommended. Nutrition may need to be provided via a feeding tube or parenterally (see below). Low-fat diets are recommended in dogs that are obese, hypertriglyceridaemic or have recurrent bouts of pancreatitis. It is vital to introduce these poorly palatable low-fat diets only after the dog has recovered from its acute episode. There is no evidence to recommend dietary fat restriction in cats with pancreatitis.

Nutrition and liver disease

Protein is the key nutrient in liver disease. However, not all liver diseases necessitate protein restriction. This is especially pertinent in portosystemic shunting in young animals as unnecessary protein restriction in growing animals can have serious repercussions. In these young patients, diets of moderate protein restriction (but adequate for growth) may be used. A protein allocation of 15–20% DM for dogs and 30–35% DM for cats is generally recommended in patients with portosystemic shunts but more severe protein restriction may be necessary if hepatic encephalopathy is present. In dogs, a protein allocation as low as 8–15% DM may be necessary if hepatic encephalopathy is present, irrespective of the underlying cause (e.g. portosystemic shunt, chronic hepatitis). There is also some evidence to suggest vegetable protein sources (e.g. soya) may be less likely than meat protein sources to cause encephalopathic signs.

A high-carbohydrate and moderate-fat diet is suitable to provide adequate energy. Dietary fibre may be helpful to reduce the absorption of nitrogenous waste in the large intestine. Excessive dietary sodium should be avoided in animals with ascites. Dogs with copper-associated chronic hepatitis have been shown to benefit from copper-restricted diets.

In feline hepatic lipidosis the provision of adequate energy is essential and usually requires a feeding tube, as these patients are invariably anorexic. Diets high in carbohydrate and with moderate protein are recommended unless hepatic encephalopathy is present. In these cases more severe protein restriction is indicated. L-Carnitine supplementation may also be indicated as this nutrient is vital for fatty acid oxidation.

Obesity

The incidence of obesity in cats and dogs is increasing. Obesity should be considered a form of malnutrition, as increased bodyweight can have serious repercussions for health. Human studies have shown that obesity can cause or worsen respiratory, metabolic, cardiac, gastrointestinal, orthopaedic and neoplastic disease. In dogs and cats, obesity can have a significant impact on diseases such as diabetes mellitus, chronic bronchitis, osteoarthritis, tracheal collapse and pancreatitis. Studies have shown that obese dogs live on average 2 years less than their ideal-weight counterparts.

Strategies to manage obesity

A successful weight loss programme should involve careful consideration of the diet, exercise regimen and client education. Feeding a smaller amount of a maintenance diet is unlikely to achieve satisfactory weight loss and may lead to nutrient deficiencies. For this reason, diets designed for weight loss are recommended, as these provide restricted calories but are also supplemented with increased levels of micronutrients to prevent such deficiencies. Diets designed for weight loss tend to be high in fibre and/or protein, both of which are thought to have a satiating effect.

Key elements of a weight management programme

- Prior to starting a weight loss programme, it is important to assess how overweight the patient is by using a body condition scoring system (see above). A complete dietary history to establish the number, quantities and types of meals and treats provided should be obtained.
- Based on this information, an appropriate energy allocation can be made. In general, a safe starting energy allocation is the resting energy requirement (RER) at the starting bodyweight. The daily amount of food can be divided into the usual number of meals the pet is given. A small part of the daily allowance can be allocated for treats during the day.
- It is important to reassess the progress of weight loss with fortnightly weight checks.
- A target weight loss of 1–2 % of the bodyweight per week is ideal. If weight loss is less than this, further calorie restriction is recommended. *continues* ▶

continued

- It is also important to instigate an exercise plan to promote weight loss. This may require 'play-time' with cats and non-traditional approaches such as hydrotherapy in dogs.
- A key aspect in a successful weight loss programme is client education. The health benefits of weight loss must be clearly outlined and owners should be forewarned that the target weight loss may not be achieved for 6–12 months. Diaries and graphs outlining the progress of weight loss may be helpful in maintaining client motivation.

Nutrition and urolithiasis

Certain types of uroliths (struvite, urate and cystine) are amenable to dissolution via dietary and medical management. Recurrence of some uroliths can be prevented by feeding a specific diet. Diets designed for struvite dissolution are acidifying and have reduced magnesium, phosphorus and protein. Diets to prevent oxalate urolithiasis are non-acidifying, have adequate magnesium and phosphorus, and are reduced in protein. Urate dissolution diets are reduced in protein and are alkalizing, whilst cystine urolith dissolution diets are reduced in protein and sodium and are also alkalizing. A factor common to all urolith dissolution and preventive diets is an increase in urine production. Some diets designed for urolith dissolution are severely protein-restricted (e.g. urate dissolution diets) and as such are not appropriate for growing animals or for long-term use in adults.

Nutrition and cancer

Cancer is associated with altered nutrient metabolism. Carbohydrate metabolism is altered and glucose intolerance may be present. Protein metabolism is also affected with loss of lean body mass and plasma proteins. Lipid metabolism is also altered, causing reduced body fat accumulation. With this in mind, animals with cancer should be fed moderate but not excessive amounts of carbohydrate (i.e. <25% DM), increased dietary protein to prevent protein deficiency (i.e. 30–45% DM for dogs and 40–50% for cats) and a large proportion of the energy requirement from fat (i.e. 25-40% DM). The increased fat provision is particularly important, as tumour cells are thought to be less capable of using fat as an energy source.

In addition, omega-3 fatty acid supplementation may be beneficial to inhibit cancer growth and minimize the effects of inflammatory cytokines that cause cancer cachexia. Cancer cachexia is a syndrome characterized by anorexia, nausea and weight loss that is common in human cancer patients. In some situations, cancer therapies such as chemotherapy can compound this situation by causing further nausea and anorexia.

Nutrition and critical illness

Providing adequate nutrition during hospitalization is known to have a significant beneficial effect on outcome in human patients. Likewise in dogs and cats, once the hydration and electrolyte status has been addressed, consideration should be given to addressing the nutritional needs of the animal. Providing adequate calories is essential in preventing catabolism of lean body mass, in maximizing healing and immunity, and preventing muscle weakness. It is a misconception that overweight or obese animals are better able to tolerate malnutrition due to their abundant body fat stores as, during illness, the body preferentially catabolizes lean body mass (rather than body fat stores) for energy production.

In general, unless the disease dictates otherwise, hospitalized dogs should be provided with 4–6 g protein/100 kcal (15–25% of total energy requirement) and hospitalized cats should be provided with at least 6 g protein/100 kcal (25–35% of total energy requirements). Other nutritional requirements will depend upon the patient's underlying disease, clinical signs and laboratory parameters.

The energy goal for hospitalized patients is to provide the resting energy requirement (RER). This amount should be delivered gradually over 2–3 days, depending on the duration of anorexia and tolerance to this provision. A continual decline in bodyweight or body condition should prompt the clinician to reassess and perhaps modify the nutritional plan (e.g. increasing the calories provided by 25%). Previous recommendations to provide increased energy in certain disease states (termed illness factors) are no longer recommended due to the risk of associated metabolic complications such a hyperglycaemia, hepatic dysfunction and hypertriglyceridaemia.

Re-feeding syndrome is an uncommon yet potentially devastating complication caused by providing rapid and excessive nourishment in patients following prolonged periods of anorexia. In this condition, the sudden provision of food leads to metabolic imbalances such as hypokalaemia and hypophosphataemia, both of which can then lead to severe cardiovascular (arrhythmias), neurological (seizures) and haematological (anaemia) consequences. Re-feeding syndrome can be prevented by slow introduction of nutrition where prolonged anorexia has been present (e.g. 33% of the daily energy requirement on day 1, 66% on day 2 and 100% thereafter) and by closely monitoring for these metabolic derangements.

Nutritional interventions

Once nutritional intervention is deemed appropriate for a patient, a decision has to be made as to the most appropriate type and route of delivery. Even when parenteral (i.e. intravenous) nutrition is available, enteral (i.e. gastrointestinal) nutrition is preferred due to its beneficial effects on the gastrointestinal tract, fewer complications and reduced cost. Feeding tubes are used widely in general veterinary practice; however, parenteral nutrition is still generally confined to referral institutions.

Appetite stimulants

Force-feeding dogs and cats is usually poorly tolerated and can lead to food aversion or more serious complications such as aspiration pneumonia. Feeding tubes are preferred (see below).

Appetite stimulants have traditionally been used to combat anorexia, especially in cats, but there is no published evidence of their effectiveness in ensuring long-term adequate food intake. Medications such as cyproheptadine and diazepam can result in a rapid improvement in appetite, but the appetite-stimulating effect tends to be short-lived and ultimately the nutritional goals of the patient are not met. In addition, these medications can cause complications such as sedation (cyproheptadine) and liver necrosis (diazepam). For these reasons, appetite stimulants should not be used instead of feeding tubes or parenteral nutrition.

Feeding tubes

The provision of enteral nutrition via feeding tubes is widely utilized in general veterinary practice.

The four main types of feeding tube are:

- Naso-oesophageal
- Oesophagostomy
- Gastrostomy
- Jejunostomy.

Each has distinct features with regard to placement, use and complications.

Choice of feeding tube

- **Patient factors:**
  - Duration of intended intervention
  - Underlying disease
  - Necessity/safety of anaesthesia
  - Tolerance of tube.
- **Technical factors:**
  - Clinician experience
  - Risk of complications
  - Invasiveness
  - Type of diet to be used.
- **Owner factors:**
  - Cost
  - Willingness to use at home.

Naso-oesophageal feeding tubes

Naso-oesophageal (N-O) feeding tubes are placed via the nasal cavity into the oesophagus or stomach. These are the least technically challenging to place and can be placed with the aid of topical (nasal) anaesthesia and/or light sedation. N-O tubes are usually well tolerated in the short term (i.e. 3–5 days) but their use is limited by the small bore of the tube (and thus the type of diet that can be used). They are useful in patients that can tolerate gastrointestinal feeding but are not sufficiently stable to undergo general anaesthesia (Figure 13.32). In such patients N-O feeding can provide nutrition for 3–5 days, after which another feeding tube can placed if

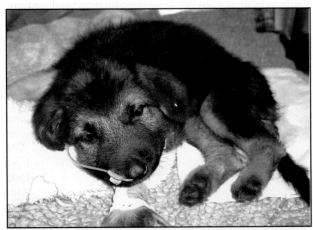

13.32 A naso-oesophageal feeding tube in place in a puppy. (Courtesy of Johan Schoeman and Parvo Isolation Unit, Onderstepoort Veterinary Academic Hospital, Pretoria. Reproduced from *BSAVA Manual of Rehabilitation, Supportive and Palliative Care: Case Studies in Patient Management*)

necessary. N-O tubes are generally contraindicated in animals that are vomiting or have reduced mentation. The tubes are usually made of PVC and sizes typically used are 5–6 Fr in cats and 8-10 Fr in dogs.

Due to the small bore of these tubes, liquid diets must be used. Such diets are high in protein and sodium and are therefore contraindicated in heart, kidney and liver failure. To calculate the amount to feed, the patient's daily energy requirement (usually its RER) is divided by the energy density of the diet (e.g. Fortol C+ (Arnolds) has 1 kcal/ml and Enteral-Care (Formula V) has 1.2 kcal/ml). This total daily volume is then divided into the number of meals fed during the day, with each meal volume ideally not exceeding 10 ml/kg. In some circumstances, the feeding can be provided as a constant rate infusion (CRI) (with the aid of a syringe driver or intravenous pump) so that gastric overdistension does not occur. Patients receiving CRI feeding require continual monitoring.

Oesophagostomy feeding tubes

Oesophagostomy (O) tubes have revolutionized enteral feeding due to their versatility, patient tolerance and relative ease of placement (Figures 13.33). O tubes have superseded the use of pharyngostomy feeding tubes as the latter are associated with patient discomfort and an unacceptable rate of complications. General anaesthesia is required to place an O tube; however, the placement technique is not challenging and specialized equipment is not necessary. O tubes are usually well tolerated (especially by cats) and animals can eat in spite of them. They are generally used for short- to mid-term nutritional intervention (i.e. 3–4 weeks) but can be used for prolonged periods (including for home feeding).

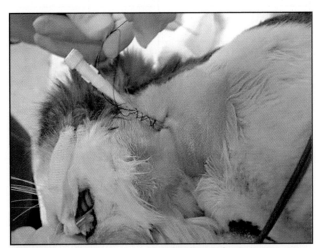

13.33 An oesophagostomy feeding tube in a cat, secured with a Chinese finger-trap suture.

Although O tubes made from different materials are commercially available, silicon feeding tubes are recommended for their flexibility and biocompatibility. One of the main advantages of O tubes is the relatively large diameter (typically 14 Fr for cats and 19 Fr for dogs), which enables the use of many different types of diets. Liquid diets (see above), instant powdered diets or even liquidized canned diets can be used with these tubes. To prevent blockages, it is recommended that an extra exit hole is made in the side of the tube prior to placement. O tubes can be used immediately after placement (although the patient should fully recover from anaesthesia before feeding) and can be removed at any time. Most owners can be taught how to feed their pet at home using these tubes.

When using instant powdered diets (e.g. Instant Convalescence Support, Royal Canin) the daily energy requirement of the patient (usually its RER) is divided by the energy density of the diet (i.e. 4.73 kcal/g for Instant Convalescence Support). This amount of powder is then dissolved in three times that volume of water. For example: a 5 kg cat with RER 234 kcal/day will need 50 g (i.e. 234 kcal ÷ 4.73 kcal/g) of the diet per day. This is dissolved in three times that volume of water, i.e. 150 ml. This daily amount is then divided into an appropriate number of meals during the day, so that each individual meal size does not exceed 10 ml/kg.

Due to the relatively large diameter of these tubes liquidized canned diets can be used. This is particularly helpful in situations where the specific dietary requirements of a patient (e.g. renal or liver failure) cannot be met by the liquid or instant diets. The canned diet must be liquidized in a blender (for at least 5 mins) with a defined amount of water to produce slurry that will easily pass through the tube (Figures 13.34 and 13.35). It is important to strain the slurry prior to feeding to prevent tube blockages.

Diet (manufacturer)	Can size (g)	Water volume to add (ml)	Energy density (kcal/ml)
FP (Eukanuba)	400	120	0.9
a/d (Hill's)	156	25	1.0
i/d (Hill's)	370	330	0.7
k/d (Hill's)	370	360	0.7
EN (Purina)	415	290	0.6
NF (Purina)	400	320	0.6
Renal (Royal Canin)	430	360	0.8

13.34   Dilution factors for a selection of canned canine diets for use with a 19 Fr oesophagostomy feeding tube.

Diet (manufacturer)	Can size (g)	Water volume to add (ml)	Energy density (kcal/ml)
a/d (Hill's)	156	25	1.0
d/d (Hill's)	156	80	1.0
i/d (Hill's)	156	40	1.0
k/d (Hill's)	156	30	1.0
l/d (Hill's)	156	40	0.9
Renal (Royal Canin)	100	25	1.1

13.35   Dilution factors for a selection of canned feline diets for use with a 14 Fr oesophagostomy feeding tube.

Gastrostomy feeding tubes

Gastrostomy feeding tubes can be placed surgically or via endoscopy (percutaneous endoscopically placed gastrostomy (PEG) tubes (Figure 13.36)). Tubes may be placed at the time of another surgical procedure such as an exploratory laparotomy. PEG tubes require flexible video-endoscopy and are technically challenging to place. Typically gastrostomy tube sizes are 15 Fr for cats and small dogs and 19 Fr for medium to large dogs. PEG tubes can be bought as a complete kit or can be modified from a gastrostomy tube. Although oesophagostomy feeding tubes are safer and easier to place, there are clinical situations (e.g. megaoesophagus or oesophagitis) where gastrostomy feeding tubes are preferred.

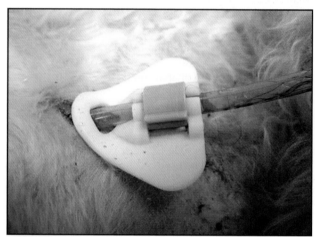

13.36   Percutaneous endoscopically placed gastrostomy (PEG) feeding tube.

Once placed, PEG tubes must not be removed for at least 10–14 days (or longer in hypoproteinaemic or immune-compromised patients) in order that a seal can form between the gastric and abdominal walls. Removal of the tube prior to this (intentionally or due to self trauma) can result in septic peritonitis. Due to the large bore of the tubes, both instant convalescence diets and liquidized canned diets can be used. As with oesophagostomy tubes, PEG tubes can also be used by the owner at home. In cases of prolonged use, the gastrostomy tube can be modified to a low-profile feeding tube. In medium to small dogs PEG tube removal requires endoscopy to retrieve the 'stopper' from the stomach (Fig 13.37), whereas in larger dogs this can be left to pass with the faeces.

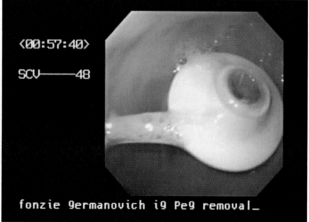

13.37   Endoscopic view of a PEG tube prior to removal of the stopper.

Jejunostomy feeding tubes

Jejunostomy tubes (J tubes) bypass the oesophagus and stomach and are placed directly into the small intestine. J tubes are usually placed surgically, although endoscopic placement techniques have been described. These tubes are technically challenging to place and can be associated with serious complications. The indications for these tubes are limited to situations such as following major pancreatic, proximal gastrointestinal or biliary tract surgery. J tube feeding should be performed as a constant rate infusion (rather than bolus feeding) with a liquid diet to mimic the normal physiology of the intestine.

Administering food

In general, 50% of the daily energy requirement is administered on the first day and if this is tolerated the full amount is given from the second day on. If bolus feeding is used (rather than CRI), the total daily food volume is divided into 4–6 meals per day. The number of meals given is calculated so that each individual meal volume does not exceed 10 ml/kg, as this can lead to gastric overdistension.

The tube should be flushed with a small volume of water (5 ml) prior to use to ensure patency and positioning. After each meal the tube is flushed again (with 10 ml for liquid diets and 20 ml for liquidized diets) to prevent food material blocking the tube. These flush volumes must be taken into consideration when determining appropriate meal sizes.

Administering medications

Drugs can also be administered via feeding tubes, but some steps should be taken to avoid drug interactions or tube complications:

- Ideally give medications separately to food
- Give one medication at a time and flush the tube in between
- Use a liquid form of the medication whenever available
- Tablets must be crushed to a fine powder and mixed with water
- Open capsules to mix powder/granules with water
- Some medications (e.g. sucralfate, aluminium hydroxide) should never be delivered via feeding tubes
- Always deliver antacids, tetracyclines and quinolones separately to food.

Tube blockages and obstructions

Prevention is the key to managing tube blockages. Diets should be properly prepared (e.g. canned diets adequately liquidized) and the tube flushed with the recommended amount of water after feeding. Minor blockages can be managed by repeated flushing and suction with warm water or by instilling a carbonated soft drink in the tube for about 1 hour followed by flushing. Alternative techniques using pancreatic enzymes and sodium bicarbonate have also been described but with mixed success.

Tube care

A non-adhesive dressing with antibiotic ointment can be used to cover the stoma site of oesophagostomy, gastrostomy and jejunostomy tubes. The tube exit site is then covered with a light bandage (Figure 13.38). For gastrostomy tubes, stockinette can be used instead of a bandage, provided the animal cannot reach the tube. Elizabethan collars may be necessary to prevent damage to the tube. For the first few

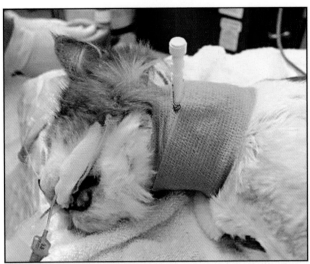

13.38 The oesophagostomy feeding tube is covered with a light dressing.

days after tube placement daily bandage changes are recommended; after this, bandage changes every 2–3 days are sufficient in most cases.

Feeding at home

Most owners can be taught how to feed their pets at home using feeding tubes. In these situations, it is necessary to provide detailed written instructions on food preparation and administration, as well as a clear demonstration of the feeding protocol prior to discharge. Owners should be advised to monitor their pet for signs of vomiting (after feeding), coughing, discomfort, dyspnoea, abdominal distension or discharge from the stoma and to contact the veterinary practice if any of these occur.

Complications

While feeding tubes are generally highly beneficial to anorexic patients, no technique is entirely without risk of complications. These aspects need to be considered when deciding how to proceed and patients should be monitored closely so that significant complications are not overlooked.

Parenteral nutrition

Parenteral nutrition (PN) is the provision of an animal's nutritional requirements intravenously. It is being used more frequently, especially in referral hospitals.

PN solutions usually contain carbohydrate (glucose), protein (amino acid) and lipid components. In total parenteral nutrition (TPN) the animal's entire energy requirement is provided intravenously, whereas partial parenteral nutrition (PPN) solutions supply only a proportion (typically 40–70%) of the energy requirement. PN solutions are usually administered centrally (i.e. via a jugular catheter) but can also be administered peripherally if the osmolality is not excessive. TPN solutions are usually tailor-made to a patient's nutritional requirements and require proficiency in formulation and administration (Figure 13.39). Readymade PN solutions (usually containing protein and carbohydrate sources only) are also available.

The administration of PN requires proficiency in catheter placement (i.e. jugular catheter or long-stay peripheral catheter) and the provision for monitoring these patients. Catheters for PN should be placed and managed aseptically.

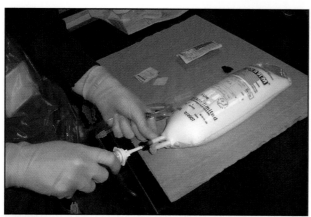

13.39 Preparation of parenteral nutrition in an aseptic manner prior to administration.

Although metabolic (e.g. hyperglycaemia, hypertriglycerid-aemia), mechanical (e.g. thrombophlebitis) and septic complications are possible with PN, this form of nutrition has been unfairly criticized for being associated with a high complication rate. However, it is imperative that if PN is to be administered, patients should be monitored closely and any complications dealt with promptly and appropriately.

Clinical nutrition in horses

Nutritional assessment

Assessing bodily condition and giving the horse a body condition score (Figure 13.40) is the best way to monitor nutrient intake, which can then be adjusted as required.

Nutrition for specific disease conditions

Laminitis

Laminitis is a painful inflammatory condition of the foot, caused by damage and disruption to the laminae, and is a major cause of lameness in horses. The cascade of events leading to laminitis is complex, but one of the initiating factors is excess sugar and starch in the diet. These overload the stomach and small intestine, allowing unabsorbed sugars to pass to the hindgut where rapid fermentation leads to the overproduction of lactic acid, a fall in pH, destruction of microbes and the release of toxins. Fructans cannot be digested or absorbed in the small intestine and will always pass into the hindgut where they will be fermented. Horses and ponies that are chronically overweight may be at increased risk from the disease due to the development of insulin resistance and the effect on blood sugar levels.

Horses and ponies susceptible to laminitis should have their weight carefully controlled. Access to grass during the growing season should be restricted, or even denied, to these animals due to the variable and unpredictable nature of fructan accumulation in pasture. Under certain conditions, which include low temperatures combined with bright sunlight, the grass will create more sugars by photosynthesis than it uses in respiration and the excess is stored as fructans. If some grazing is unavoidable, horses should be turned out late at night or very early in the morning and removed by mid morning as fructan levels are likely to be at their lowest at these times. Alternatively, a grazing muzzle can be used during the high-risk periods. These can be designed with a small opening, allowing the horse some access to grass without limiting water intake. Poorly managed pastures and recently cut hay stubble will contain more 'stemmy' grass, and fructans are stored in the stem.

Susceptible animals should be fed highly digestible fibre feeds that are low in sugar or starch. Feeding little and often will mimic natural grazing behaviour and ensure that any sugars and starch are fully digested in the small intestine. Regular exercise is also important to reduce risk. If more energy is required for additional work or weight gain, feeds are used that are high in fibre with a low starch content, and oil is added, e.g. soya oil which contains no sugars or starch.

Proprietary feeds are available for horses prone to laminitis. These are usually a high-fibre, low-energy formulation balanced for protein, minerals and vitamins.

Metabolic disorders

Equine Cushing's disease, equine metabolic syndrome, osteo-chondritis dissecans, recurrent equine rhabdomyolysis and polysaccharide storage myopathy are disorders that can be

Condition score	Pelvis	Ribs and back	Neck
0 Very thin	Pelvic bones clearly projecting. No evidence of fatty tissue between skin and bone	Dorsal and transverse spinous processes clearly visible. Skin taut over ribs	Bone structure easily felt
1 Thin	Pelvis well defined, no fat covering but the skin is supple	Dorsal spinous processes easily felt. Some fat covering over transverse processes	Bone structure can be felt
2 Fair	Pelvis easily felt but with some fat covering	Spinous processes not visible but can be felt. Some fat covering. Ribs just visible	Some fat covering bone structure
3 Good	Round appearance to pelvic area. Can palpate pelvic bones with firm pressure. Supple skin with good layer of subcutaneous fat	Spinous processes only felt on firm pressure. Ribs just visible	Contour of neck flows smoothly into shoulder
4 Fat	Cannot palpate pelvic bones	Spinous processes and ribs only felt on firm pressure	Wide and firm to touch. Fat deposits starting to form crest
5 Very fat	Cannot palpate pelvic bones and skin is taut	Spinous processes and ribs cannot be felt. Evidence of fat pads over the shoulder	Wide and firm to touch. Crest evident

13.40 Body condition scoring for horses.

caused or exacerbated by excessive energy intake. They can be managed by careful regulation of both the amount and the source of energy provided. Excessive consumption of carbohydrates is one of the major causes of these problems in the horse.

Respiratory diseases

Hay and straw bedding are primary sources of airborne allergens (dusts, moulds, fungi) implicated in the aetiology of allergic respiratory disease and therefore attention to feeding and housing management (see Chapters 12 and 16) is essential for long-term control of these conditions. Ideally, affected horses should be housed outside or in well ventilated barns on dust-free bedding. Hay should either be replaced by haylage or be soaked (completely immersed in water for a minimum of 5 minutes – prolonged soaking, however, leaches nutrients from the hay).

Nutritional interventions

If **reduced appetite** is a problem, it may be stimulated by offering fresh grass, molassed feed, succulents (carrots, apples, etc.) and haylage. Energy-dense feeds (>8–10 MJ DE/kg) should be given where feed intake is reduced. Treatment of a primary problem, for example the use of non-steroidal anti-inflammatory drugs to reduce temperature or control pain, is also essential to restore normal appetite.

Horses suffering from **trauma, sepsis or severe burns** need a high level of protein (12–16%) in their diet.

Horses with **hepatic failure** should be fed soybean or linseed meal in addition to grass hay to meet maintenance protein requirements, as they contain the correct type and ratio of amino acids. Vitamins A, C, and E should also be supplemented. With severe liver dysfunction, reduced gluconeogenesis will result in hypoglycemia. A diet containing highly digestible starches will help maintain blood glucose levels.

Horses with **reduced renal function** should have their intake of protein, calcium, and phosphorus reduced. Pasture or grass hay are ideal as soluble carbohydrates, protein and mineral levels are all comparatively low. A vitamin-only (*not vitamin and mineral*) supplement can be fed.

Following **large intestinal surgery**, horses can usually be offered high-quality feed within 24 hours. It may be necessary to reduce the fibre content if a resection has been performed. After surgical **resection of the small intestine**, horses should be fasted for 1–3 days and then offered low-residue diets while the bowel recovers motility. With **small intestinal diseases** generally, the digestive function of the large bowel must ultimately be optimized. This can be achieved by feeding a highly digestible fibre source such as alfalfa, beet pulp or soybean, restricted grain, and the use of vegetable oil to meet energy requirements.

Horses with **diarrhoea** should not be deprived of oral feed (either eaten voluntarily or administered by nasogastric tube) for prolonged periods of time, unless there is gastric distension or reflux, as fasting will adversely affect bowel function and delay recovery. Diarrhoea in the adult is usually due to large intestinal dysfunction such as colitis secondary to *Salmonella* spp. or clostridial infection. In the acute phase, many horses will be inappetent and may need enteral nutritional support if this is prolonged. The ability of the small intestine to digest and absorb nutrients is usually unaffected and therefore low-residue diets with highly digestible sources of carbohydrate, protein and fat should be fed. As appetite improves, hay and other sources of fermentable fibre should be fed. Yoghurt cultures or commercially available probiotic preparations are often administered to encourage the re-establishment of normal microbial flora. There should be a gradual return to a regular diet over a 1–2 week period.

Nutritional support for the sick horse

Some horses may be unable to feed themselves adequately due to a variety of medical problems or with certain head or neck injuries. Adult horses can tolerate 2–3 days of feed deprivation provided they remain hydrated either by drinking water or by administration of fluids via nasogastric tube or intravenously. If the illness is more prolonged, nutritional support may be required and can be delivered by the enteral or parenteral (intravenous) route. Enteral feeding is either voluntary or assisted. The method of nutritional support given to a sick animal will depend on the ability of the horse to voluntarily consume food and water, the nature and duration of the illness, and the economics of the situation. Although total parenteral nutrition (TPN) is frequently used in sick neonatal foals, the cost is usually prohibitive in mature horses, and assisted enteral feeding becomes the most cost-effective means for delivery of nutritional support. More importantly, a prolonged period of TPN is associated with atrophy of the intestinal mucosa in the adult; therefore, a further advantage of enteral feeding is the maintenance of intestinal health and function and the promotion of gut maturation in the foal.

Assisted enteral feeding

Food is delivered via the oesophagus directly into the stomach by a nasogastric tube. Indications include:

- The inappetent horse with a functional gastrointestinal tract
- The horse that is willing to eat but cannot due to oral, pharyngeal or oesophageal problems (e.g. severe fractures of the jaw, pharyngeal paralysis)
- Foals that have not received colostrum
- Foals unable or unwilling to suck.

Feed is delivered via a nasogastric tube or a surgically positioned oesophagostomy tube. An oesophagostomy tube is used only when the nasal passages, pharynx, or proximal oesophagus must be bypassed. There is a high complication rate and the technique should only be employed when tube feeding is anticipated for 10 days or more and should be a last resort. The use of a nasogastric tube for assisted feeding can also have complications. In some horses the repeated passing of a tube may be traumatic while others are not tolerant of an indwelling tube, which may cause rhinitis, pharyngitis and ulceration of the oesophageal mucosa if use is prolonged.

Nasogastric tube

The technique for passing a nasogastric tube is shown over the page; the degree of restraint required will depend on the temperament and state of the horse. Recumbent horses should only be fed while held in the sternal position. The position of the tube should be checked before each feeding and it must be flushed with warm water both before and after each feeding.

Passing a nasogastric feeding tube into a horse

1. Select a nasogastric tube of suitable size and mark it at locations that approximate to the pharynx and stomach of the horse, such that the tip can be located as the tube passes through the nose, pharynx and oesophagus.

2. Stand level with the horse's nose and insert the lubricated nasogastric tube into the horse's nostril in a ventral and medial position, pushing it gently into the ventral meatus. It is almost always passage of a tube through the first 10 cm of the nasal passages that causes most resentment. The middle nasal meatus, which is immediately dorsal to this, must be avoided.

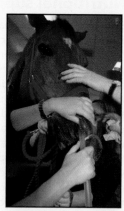

3. Advance the tube slowly; resistance will be felt at the pharynx.

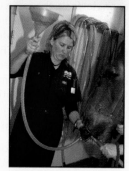

4. Encourage swallowing by flexing the horse's neck and touching the pharynx with the tube. Advance the tube quickly but gently into the oesophagus when swallowing occurs. If the horse does not swallow immediately, gentle movement and rotation of the tube back and forth will encourage swallowing.

5. Confirm that the tube is in the oesophagus using the following techniques before advancing any further:
   - The tube should be seen sliding in the oesophagus when it is moved back and forth (usually on the left side of the neck)
   - Blowing through the tube should create a bubble of air that can be seen in the oesophagus
   - Sucking on the tube should result in negative pressure
   - When advancing the tube down the oesophagus a degree of resistance should be felt (no resistance will be felt if the tube is in the trachea)
   - If the tube is in the trachea it can be rattled by rapid side-to-side movement of the trachea. If this is the case, the tube must be withdrawn immediately and the horse encouraged to swallow the tube as described above
   - If the horse coughs paroxysmally the tube should be removed unless there is 100% certainty of the tube's position in the stomach.

6. Once the tube is confirmed to be in the oesophagus, gently blow through the tube as it is advanced to ease passage into the stomach. Confirm the tube is positioned in the stomach by listening for gastrointestinal sounds at the end of the tube and smelling for gastric contents.

Pelleted complete horse feed can be pulverized in a kitchen blender and mixed with water just prior to feeding. However, prolonged soaking of complete pellets until a gruel-like consistency is reached has been found to be the most successful. Large volumes of water are required to reduce the viscosity of the mixture so that it can be administered via the tube; blockages are frequent. Vegetable oil can be added to increase the energy content or soybean meal added to increase protein. The addition of alfalfa meal into the blend will increase the fibre content. Tolerance to liquid diets is best when small volumes are delivered frequently.

Parenteral nutrition

Parenteral nutrition can be a valuable aid in supplying energy and nutrients to critically ill horses or to those temporarily unable to ingest adequate feed to meet their energy requirements. However, the expense of TPN often precludes its use in adult horses and is more commonly used in foals. Major contributors to the cost of providing parenteral nutrition are the laboratory tests performed in order to minimize the occurrence of complications, and the nursing care required. Partial parenteral nutrition (PPN) may revive an anorectic, malnourished animal sufficiently to initiate recovery. It is advantageous to supply even a small amount of enteral nutrition if this can be tolerated.

Indications for parenteral nutrition in horses

- Foals without a sucking reflex.
- Foals with immature/compromised gastrointestinal tract.
- Animals with gastrointestinal disorders that preclude enteral feeding (very rare).
- Horses that require more energy than can be provided by enteral feeds alone.

Administration

Prior to the administration of any parenteral nutrition it is very important to have clear protocols in place for the strict aseptic handling of intravenous lines and nutrition products, as well as patient monitoring and record keeping in order to avoid as many complications as possible. Most equine patients given either PPN or TPN are compromised neonates at high risk of sepsis. Stringent aseptic technique is required to prevent microbial contamination of the nutrition solution. A non-thrombogenic polyurethane catheter is placed aseptically into a dedicated vein (usually the jugular) to prevent any precipitation or other chemical reactions with medications or additives to poly-ionic fluids. Once in position, a spiral giving set can be attached to the TPN bag and to the catheter via an extension set. Non-TPN fluids should be run through a separate intravenous line to assist in maintaining sterility. During treatment, the catheter site should be checked for signs of infection and the catheter for patency. The TPN bag must be protected from light, which will cause it to degrade.

Potential complications of parenteral nutrition are:

- Risk of thrombophlebitis and sepsis of the catheter site
- Intolerance to glucose or lipids
- Gastrointestinal atrophy
- Decrease in gastric pH, increasing the risk of gastric ulcer development. Anti-ulcer medication is essential in foals.

Acknowledgement

The authors and editors would like to thank Emma Rees and Deirdre Carson for their help with the equine content of this chapter.

Further reading

Agar S (2001) *Small Animal Nutrition*. Butterworth-Heinemann, Oxford

Bercier DL (2003) How to use parenteral nutrition in practice. *49th Annual Convention of the American Association of Equine Practitioners 2003*

Chan DL (2007) Nutritional support for the critically ill patient. In: *Small Animal Emergency and Critical Care for Veterinary Technicians, 2nd edn*, ed. AM Battaglia, pp. 85–108. Saunders Elsevier, St. Louis

Coumbe K (2001) *Equine Veterinary Nursing Manual*. Blackwell Science, Oxford

Davies Z (2009) *Introduction to Horse Nutrition*. Blackwell Publishing, Oxford

European Pet Food Industry Federation (FEDIAF) (2008): *Nutritional guidelines for complete and complementary pet food for cats and dogs* (updated September 2008). Available at: www.fediaf.org

Frape D (2004) *Equine Nutrition and Feeding, 2nd edn*. Blackwell Science, Oxford

Hand MS, Thatcher CD, Remillard RL *et al.* (2010) *Small Animal Clinical Nutrition, 5th edn*. Mark Morris Institute, Topeka, KS

Hardy J (2003) Nutritional support and nursing care of the adult horse in intensive care. *Clinical Techniques in Equine Practice* **2**, 193–198

Kirk CA (2006) Dietary management and nutrition. *Veterinary Clinics of North America: Small Animal Practice* **36**(6), 1183–1401

Lumbis R and Chan DL (2008) Clinical nutrition. In: *BSAVA Manual of Canine and Feline Advanced Veterinary Nursing, 2nd edn*, ed. A. Hotston Moore and S. Rudd, pp.54–71. BSAVA Publications, Gloucester

Pagan JD (2000) *Advances in Equine Nutrition, 2nd edn*. Nottingham University Press

Pilliner S (1999) *Horse Nutrition and Feeding, 2nd edn*. Blackwell Science, Oxford

Watson P and Chan DL (2010) Principles of clinical nutrition. In: *BSAVA Manual of Rehabilitation, Supportive and Palliative Care: Case Studies in Patient Management*, ed. P Watson and S Lindley, pp. 42–59. BSAVA Publications, Gloucester

Weyenberg S, Hesta M, Kalmar ID, Vandermeiren J and Janssens GPJ (2009) Nutritional management of laminitis in a horse. *Veterinary Record* **164**, 694–695

Wortinger A (2007) *Nutrition for Veterinary Technicians and Nurses*. Wiley-Blackwell, Iowa

Useful websites

Association of American Feed Control Officials (AAFCO): www.aafco.org

AAFCO provides a mechanism for developing and implementing uniform and equitable laws, regulations, standards and enforcement policies for regulating the manufacture, distribution and sale of animal feeds; this results in safe, effective, and useful feeds in the USA.

Department for Environment, Food and Rural Affairs (DEFRA): www.defra.gov.uk

The UK government department responsible for the environment, for food and farming, and for rural matters.

Food Standards Agency: www.food.gov.uk

An independent Government department set up by an Act of Parliament in 2000 to protect the public's health and consumer interests in relation to food.

Pet Food Manufacturers Association (PFMA): www.pfma.org.uk

PFMA is the principal trade association for the prepared pet food industry and can provide both the pet owner and pet profession with information on small animal nutrition in addition to the latest news from the pet food industry. Individual manufacturers of speciality, premium or super premium diets and veterinary therapeutic diets often have their own websites and diet manuals that provide information on their products.

Self-assessment questions

1. Explain the meaning of the resting energy requirement of an animal.
2. How does the protein and energy requirement during growth compare to that of adulthood?
3. Name three factors that will influence a horse's nutritional requirement.
4. When would a novel protein source diet in domestic pets be indicated?
5. Name two diseases in domestic pets where dietary protein restriction will be beneficial.
6. Briefly describe the process of fat digestion and absorption.
7. Why is it inappropriate to feed cats a vegetarian diet?
8. What are the dangers of increasing the proportion of grain to meet the energy requirement of a horse in heavy work? How can these be avoided?
9. Name two factors that contribute to obesity in exotic pets.
10. What are the indications for parental nutrition and what are the possible complications?
11. How do you confirm that a nasogastric tube in the horse is correctly positioned?

Chapter 14

The nursing process, nursing models and care plans

Andrea Jeffery
with clinical application of models by **Stuart Ford-Fennah**

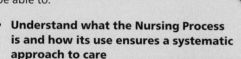

Learning objectives

After studying this chapter, students should be able to:

- **Understand what the Nursing Process is and how its use ensures a systematic approach to care**
- **Understand the difference between the Medical (Biomedical) Model and the Nursing-focused Model**
- **Explain the key principles of a range of nursing models, including the Roper, Logan and Tierney and Orem models and models for veterinary nursing, and how they might be applied to improve patient care**

Introduction

In defining a professional role for veterinary nurses, one of the first steps has been to introduce the **nursing process** and **models of nursing** into the veterinary nursing syllabus, emphasizing the importance of developing up-to-date evidence-based nursing practice through the implementation of care plans, in which the nursing care of veterinary patients is systematically planned and delivered by nurses. The effectiveness of the care given is then evaluated by the whole team, including the veterinary surgeon.

The history of nursing

Florence Nightingale, as long ago as 1859, was of the opinion that medicine and nursing should be clearly differentiated from each other, and yet in the 1970s doctors were still being asked to lecture to nurses about nursing. Even today, in the 21st century, veterinary surgeons lecture nurses about nursing. Peplau in 1987 argued that those who teach control the content of the occupation. It is therefore important that other veterinary nurses and not just veterinary surgeons deliver the education of veterinary nurses regarding patient care.

The Medical (Biomedical) Model

According to Aggleton and Chalmers (2000), within the Medical Model (also referred to as the Biomedical Model) (Figure 14.1) the patient is seen as a complex set of anatomical parts and physiological systems. This model emphasizes anatomical, physiological and biochemical malfunctions as the causes of ill health and, by doing so, it encourages a disease-oriented approach to the patient. The primary role of the veterinary surgeon is to diagnose and treat disease, and they may therefore have a disease-oriented approach to a patient. The veterinary team, and veterinary nurses in particular, however, should see their patients as unique individuals and take a holistic (nursing each animal as a 'whole' individual rather than the disease it has been admitted with) patient-oriented approach to the nursing care they deliver. Veterinary nurses should still be fully aware of, and have a good understanding of, the clinical problem that the patient has, as this will inform the care delivered.

It was disenchantment with the Medical Model that brought about the development of nursing theories and models of care. Nurses believed that the medical, disease-oriented model was not a focus for nursing and, as the quest began for professional recognition of nursing practitioners in their own right, the emphasis on nursing care expanded.

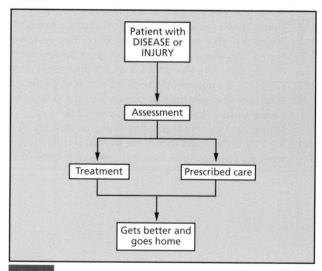

14.1 The Medical Model.

The nursing process

The nursing process is the key to professional nursing, as it enables nurses to provide organized, structured and holistic care to patients. By nursing in this way it is hoped that the care provided addresses the individual patient's needs, rather than focusing on the disease or clinical problem the patient has been admitted with.

The nursing process is a cyclical process, which provides a structure to the way in which nursing care for the patient is planned. The 'process of nursing', as currently used to plan and deliver patient care, is encapsulated in Figure 14.2.

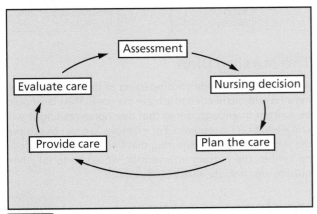

14.2   The process of nursing.

In contrast, Figure 14.3 illustrates the 'nursing process'. There is very little difference between the diagrams, but one difference is the insertion of the additional stage that occurs between Assessment and Planning: the 'nursing diagnosis'. This was introduced later in the development of the nursing process and is not always included in nursing textbooks on the subject. It refers to the **nursing decision** that is made, with regard to what care is given to patients. The nursing diagnosis is an important element of the nursing process; after all, the care of a patient cannot be planned if no decision has been made on what that care should be. In this way the nurse is making a diagnosis of the patient's individual needs based on its care requirements, which are ascertained by using a systematic approach involving a detailed patient assessment.

Following the nursing process will ensure that nurses have a systematic approach to the delivery of care.

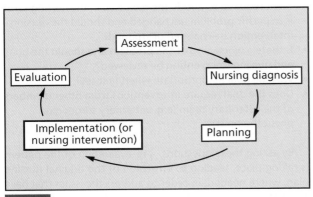

14.3   The nursing process.

Assessment

Assessment will clearly establish the individual needs of the patient. It is only once a patient assessment has been carried out that effective care can be given.

1. Collect the necessary information systematically from your own observations and from the client and other team members.
2. Review the collected information.
3. Identify actual and potential nursing problems.
4. Identify priorities among the problems.

It is important to remember at this point that the nursing process and models of care can be used to provide holistic nursing care to all species seen within general practice, from rabbits to horses. However, for the purpose of this chapter the majority of examples given are either canine or feline patients.

> ### Case example: Ben, a dog with polyuria/polydipsia
>
> Ben Jones is an 11-year-old male neutered Golden Retriever. He has been admitted to the hospital by the veterinary surgeon for investigation of lethargy, polydipsia and polyuria, which he has had for several days. The veterinary surgeon has requested that he is kennelled for observation and that preliminary urine and blood tests are carried out to investigate the cause of the problem.

The admitting veterinary surgeon will have provided some information but is likely to have asked questions with a disease-focused approach. This means that additional information is likely to be required from the client and from patient observation in order to carry out a more detailed assessment of the dog and the problems he has. Gathering information about a patient is very important as it sets the scene for any action to be taken:

- Wrong information → wrong action
- Lack of information → inadequate action.

There may not always be the opportunity to do this during the admission of the patient (or it may not feel like the right time). If a face-to-face conversation with the owner does not take place, it may be possible to telephone the owner at a later time on the day of admission, as a follow-up.

At whatever point the nurse decides to carry out the interview, it is important that the owner knows that the nurse is asking these additional questions to help them to plan the pet's care.

The conversation with the owner, along with the information from the admitting veterinary surgeon, is essential as it is important to know what is 'normal' for each patient. Knowing what the patient's 'normal' routines, behaviour and preferences are will ensure that the nurse's approach to the care of patients is as individualized as possible. Gathering this information could make a significant difference to the care delivered.

Ben: Assessment

It is already known from the admitting veterinary surgeon that Ben has exercise intolerance, polydipsia and polyuria. However, if a veterinary nurse had spoken to the dog's owners they might have found out that Ben is deaf in his left ear, eats one meal per day, in the evening, and will only urinate and defecate on concrete and not on grass. All of this information will be important for Ben's stay in hospital.

Nursing diagnosis

As discussed earlier, nursing diagnosis differs from medical diagnosis in that it is not concerned with making a judgement about disease but rather with the nursing intervention needed by the patient to provide it with the most appropriate nursing care.

There may occasionally be some overlap but it is extremely important to understand the difference between a clinical veterinary diagnosis, which is not within the remit of nursing, and a nursing diagnosis, which obviously is.

Planning

After the assessment phase of the nursing process, where all the information is gathered, comes the **planning** stage. This involves making plans to overcome the nursing problems that have been identified.

Planning may begin by considering the aims of nursing:

- To solve identified actual problems
- To prevent identified potential problems becoming actual
- To alleviate any problems that cannot be solved
- To help the patient and client cope positively with problems that cannot be solved or alleviated
- To prevent recurrence of a treated problem
- To help make the patient as comfortable as possible, even when death is inevitable.

The veterinary surgeon has made a diagnosis of diabetes mellitus. Planning Ben's nursing can now be carried out, using all the information that has been collected.

The **actual problems** identified for Ben are:

- Exercise intolerance
- Polydipsia/polyuria due to unstable diabetes mellitus
- Unilateral deafness due to age-related degeneration.

The **potential problems** identified if the actual problems are not solved include:

- Weight loss
- Dehydration
- Hypoglycaemia.

Setting goals

A goal must be set for each actual and potential problem identified during the initial assessment, and a distinction should be made between short-term and long-term goals. It is important that any goals set should be stated in terms of outcomes that can be observed, measured or tested, so that effective evaluation can then be carried out.

Short-term goals for Ben while his diabetes is stabilized			
Problem	**Short-term goal/outcome**	**Timing**	**Nursing intervention**
Polydipsia	Prevent dehydration	At all times	Provide fresh drinking water at all times. Measure fluid intake
Polyuria	Ensure Ben has the opportunity to urinate regularly	Every hour	Take Ben into an outside concrete run to allow him opportunity to urinate

The nursing plan

A plan should be made encompassing all the proposed nursing interventions needed to achieve the goals. This plan should be written in enough detail that any nurse reading it will know what care is required. For example, in order to achieve the short-term goal of ensuring that Ben does not urinate in his kennel, the nursing intervention would be to take him outside, on concrete, every 60 minutes.

Implementation

Implementing the nursing plan is the **doing** stage of the nursing process, otherwise known as the **nursing intervention**. It is important that nurses make it clear what decision-making has taken place, in order to justify the nursing intervention. All of this information should be recorded clearly and indelibly on the patient care plan.

Evaluation

This is a vital part of the nursing process. It is difficult to justify planning and implementing nursing interventions if the outcomes cannot be shown to have benefited either the patient or the client in some way. Evaluation involves reflecting upon the nursing process and the outcomes achieved by it. Evaluation is a difficult process. As a nurse, one hopes that the evaluation will show that all the nursing goals have been achieved. If this is not the case, the following questions need to be asked (adapted from Luker (1989) in Kratz, 1989):

- Has the goal set for the patient been partially achieved?
- Is more information from the veterinary surgeon or the client required to decide the next step in the nursing care?
- Is a specific problem unchanged and should the nursing intervention be changed or stopped?
- Is there a worsening of the problem and should the goal and nursing intervention be reviewed?
- Was the goal inappropriate when first set?
- Does the goal require interventions from other members of the veterinary team (e.g. veterinary surgeon or physiotherapist)?

By asking these questions, a re-evaluation of the patient is taking place, leading to a revision of the original nursing plan, where needed, in order to address the issues that have become apparent. Any changes required are recorded on the care plan and the whole process begins again.

Models of nursing

The nursing process offers a **systematic approach** to care but is limited in its *function* unless it is integrated into a nursing model/framework.

According to Aggleton and Chalmers (2000) the nursing process:

- Encourages nurses to assess but does not tell them what to look for
- Advocates planning but does not say what form the care plan should take
- Talks of intervention but does not specify what might be appropriate interventions
- Calls for evaluation without specifying the standards against which comparisons should be made.

This is where nursing models come in. **Nursing models provide the nurse with key pointers regarding patient assessment, care planning, the type of interventions that are appropriate and, finally, evaluation.** Together with the nursing process, they provide detailed guidance for the steps that need to be taken when delivering nursing care.

Models are systematically constructed. This means that they have been developed logically and can be adapted to meet specific patient requirements. They also act as guides for nursing practice by providing a framework in which to deliver nursing care.

There are a number of published nursing models developed by human-centred nursing theorists, two of which will be discussed later in the chapter; these are the Roper, Logan and Tierney Model, which focuses on the twelve activities of living, and the Orem Self-care Model, which focuses on the patient's self-care requisites (how much the patient can still do for itself).

The **Ability Model** is an adaptation of both of these models, with the assessment phase focusing on the 'abilities' of the individual animal, no matter which species it belongs to.

The Ability Model

Figure 14.4 provides a visual representation of the Ability Model, showing the three key components:

- The **ten abilities**: Orpet and Jeffery (2007) believe that if the animal is able to achieve these it can be deemed 'healthy'
- **Lifespan**: This will be an influencing factor; it is important to know where, within the lifespan, the patient sits when carrying out an assessment
- **Key influencing factors**: These include cultural, financial and owner compliance factors, which may impact on the patient and its abilities.

Assessment

Ideally, the initial assessment of the patient should take the form of a questionnaire that the owner completes before or during the admission of their animal. Giving the questionnaire to the clients prior to admission provides them with the opportunity to think clearly about their answers and often makes them feel that the practice values their pets and the care given to them.

The information needed for the assessment is based on the ten abilities of the animal (Figure 14.5).

It is important to remember that the way in which questions are asked and the environment in which questioning takes place is very important. Open questions are likely to gain more information about the patient than closed questions. For example, with Ben the Golden Retriever, 'Does Ben eat adequately?' would probably result in a yes/no answer. However, 'What does Ben normally eat? How much does he eat and at what times?' will hopefully give a better idea of the dog's routine. It is important to consider where the assessment is done, e.g. on the phone before admission or in a room away from the busy reception area, so that attention can be focused on the owner and what they are saying, without any distractions.

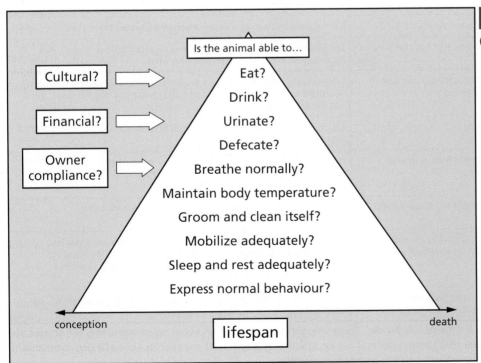

14.4 The Orpet and Jeffery Ability Model.

(© Orpet and Jeffrey, 2007)

Is the animal able to....	Questions to ask the owner	Rationale for question
Eat adequate amounts?	What does the patient normally eat?	To get the patient back to eating normal food
	How much, how often and when?	Calculation of basal or maintenance energy requirement may be necessary to maintain bodyweight (see Chapter 13)
	Does the patient prefer any particular type of bowl?	Brachycephalic cats (e.g. Persians) often prefer flat bowls. Cats generally prefer china or ceramic rather than plastic bowls
Drink adequate amounts?	How much does the patient normally drink?	This will vary from animal to animal. It may depend on whether the animal's normal diet is wet or dry
	Does the patient often drink water from containers outside, e.g. collected rain water?	The type of water can be important. Cats may drink from a dripping tap. Rabbits and other small mammals may drink from a bottle or bowl
Urinate normally?	Where does the patient normally urinate?	Patients may show different preferences. Inside or outside? Does a cat use a litter tray? What type of litter? Does a dog urinate on walks? Always on grass or on concrete?
	Does the owner use any commands for urination?	Used in well trained animals
	Does the patient have any problems urinating?	Does the patient have arthritis? Joint stiffness can affect how the animal urinates
Defecate normally?	How often does the patient defecate per day and when?	How often the animal defecates can depend on its diet
	Where is this usually done and on what?	Some dogs have preferences on where they urinate/defecate. Likewise, cats may have a preference for the type of substrate used in their litter tray
Breathe normally?	Does the patient have any problems breathing?	This may be linked to exercise. There may be underlying disease, including allergy
	Does the patient often snore while sleeping?	Facial conformity of the animal may result in breathing difficulties, e.g. Persians or Pugs
Maintain body temperature?	Do you think the patient feels the cold? Do they have a coat in colder weather?	Very young and old animals may not be able to regulate their temperature effectively
	Where does the animal normally sleep?	Animals may show preferences, for example for warmer or cooler places (e.g. kitchen floor)
Mobilize adequately?	Does the patient have any problems walking?	Difficulties in mobility may affect care routines. These may be identified by simply watching the animal walk. With cats sitting in baskets, however, it may not be possible to assess
	Can they get into the car easily or get upstairs?	Older animals may suffer from stiff joints and arthritis, which limits their normal routine
Groom and clean itself?	Does the patient normally groom itself?	Cats often spend a long time grooming and washing themselves
	Do you normally groom or bath the patient? If so, how often?	Long-haired animals are often groomed regularly by their owners. It is important to know how often and with what
Sleep and rest adequately?	How much sleep does the patient have during a 24-hour period?	Dogs actually spend a lot of time sleeping despite what owners think. Cats are often nocturnal, hunting at night and sleeping all day. However, this is not something the owner will usually monitor
Express normal behaviour?	Is the patient neutered? If female, when was her last season?	Un-neutered animals can display certain behaviours associated with sex hormones
	How does the patient behave toward strangers or other animals?	It is important to try and ascertain whether the animal displays any aggressive behaviour. Be aware you may not always get accurate information on this from owners
	Does the patient have any favourite toys, chews, etc.?	Toys can help settle the animal into the hospital environment
	Does the patient respond to any particular commands for certain activities?	Police dogs and guide dogs may have certain commands – it may be necessary to know these in advance. Many dogs have a command for urinating or defecating – this may also be useful for dogs in strange environments away from the owners
	Does the animal suffer from any sight or hearing impairment?	Often associated with old age – important to know as the animal will be unsettled even more in a strange environment

14.5 Assessment framework for the Ability Model. These are questions to ask the owner when admitting the animal. It is important to remember that these questions can be asked of the owner of any species kept as a pet, including horses and exotic pets, although they might need to be adapted slightly.

Patient assessment form for Ben

Date of Admission: 15 February 2011	**Date of nursing assessment:** 15 February 2011
Case No. 1900210	**Patient Name:** Ben **Breed:** Golden Retriever **Sex:** Male, neutered

Owner:
Address:
Contact No.:

Clinical summary (reason for admission): Investigation into polyuria and polydipsia, lethargy, inappetent	**Owner's perception of problem:** Excessive drinking and urination, no energy and not eating

Previous history (surgery, disease, vaccination status, allergies):   Castrated 2000, vaccinations up-to-date

T 38°C	**Current medication**
P 80 beats/min	
R 20 breaths/min	None yet – to be prescribed by VS once blood tests and urinalysis carried out
MM pale pink	
CRT <2 s	
Weight 37 kg	

Life stage:

Age: 11 years   neonate   adult   geriatric

Assessment of activities of living

Ability	Usual routine	Actual problems	Potential problems
Eat adequate amount	Eats 1 tin of Chappie with mixer in evenings	Not eating	Weight loss
Drink adequate amounts	Approx. 500 ml/day	Drinking 1–2 litres/day	Dehydration if water not replenished
Urinate normally	Outside 3 times a day on concrete	Increased to 7–8 times a day	Urination in kennel if not taken out hourly
Defecate normally	Outside once daily, early morning		
Breathe normally	Normal		
Maintain body temperature	No problems – sleeps in bed on tiled kitchen floor		Patient may be too warm in hospital kennels
Groom itself	Owner grooms weekly	None	Matted coat if not groomed
Mobilize adequately	Goes for walks at 7am and 4pm, about 40 mins each	Has not wanted to walk, very slow and not interested in anything	Stiffness and muscle weakness
Sleep/rest	No problems – indoors mostly	Very lethargic, has not wanted to get up for walks	
Express normal behaviour	Normally active. **Use a whistle to call him as he is deaf in left ear**	Deafness. Not willing to exercise	Not able to hear staff approaching. Boredom

A further example of a completed patient assessment form (Jess) can be found at the end of this chapter (page 358).

The next stage of the nursing assessment concerns what the animal is able or not able to do once it has been admitted. This uses the same 'checklist' of ten abilities from the model.

The care plan

The information gained from the assessment can be used to identify *actual* problems. It is also important to consider *potential* problems that may occur, so that they can be prevented. Once the problems have been identified and prioritized, the goals and nursing interventions can be decided.

Implementing the care plan

Detail in the care plan is important; everyone needs to know exactly what the nursing intervention is, how often care should be implemented and how much care is required.

Evaluation

In order to evaluate effectively, the assessment phase should be carried out again. For each of the ten abilities, the animal should be assessed on what it can now do or still not do by itself. Hopefully the nursing interventions have worked and the animal is now more 'able' than when admitted. If not, the care given should be looked into and the plan adjusted as necessary.

Care plan for Ben

Patient Name: Ben | **Date:** 15 February 2011

Date	Problem	Short-term goal	Nursing intervention	Reassess/ evaluation	Review time/date
15 February	Not eating	To eat 1 tin of Chappie per day	Tempt to eat by hand-feeding, warming food	Has eaten half a tin of Chappie	16 February 2011
15 February	Drinking excessively	Ensure hydration status is maintained	Assess hydration status and check hourly that water bowl is full	Hydration status maintained	16 February 2011
15 February	Excessive urination	Ensure patient has opportunity to urinate regularly	Take dog out hourly into concrete run	Urinated 8 times, no soiling of kennel	16 February 2011
15 February	Normal behaviour affected by condition	Encourage as far as possible normal behaviour	Regular contact with nursing staff, not just when feeding or medicating. Assess pain relief requirements		Ongoing during stay

Ben was diagnosed with diabetes mellitus and his condition was stabilized using insulin. The problems he had on admission associated with the disease were solved once the treatment began.

Influencing factors

The life stage

The assessment and consequent nursing care that is carried out may be affected by other factors. The life stage of the animal is an important factor to consider. Even healthy neonates are unable to feed, drink, keep warm or mobilize by themselves. Geriatrics may have weaker senses purely because they are old, and mobility may be decreased due to arthritis.

Cultural differences

These may affect the care given to the animal. It is important to consider the role that the pet plays in the owner's life, e.g. whether it is a working animal, a family pet, or used for breeding. It may be that the owner does not believe in euthanasia, or their religious beliefs may stop them consenting to a blood transfusion. It is important to understand and respect these beliefs, remembering that the welfare of the animal should remain the number one concern.

Financial implications

Financial implications may prevent the required care from taking place. In this situation, alternatives should be explored. For example, where full physiotherapy and hydrotherapy is recommended but is too expensive for the client, the veterinary nurse may be able to teach the owner some basic care techniques or rehabilitation methods. Nursing involves not only caring for the patient, but liaising with the owner regarding the nursing care given. The veterinary nurse's role is vital in maintaining the communication between the client and the practice (see Chapter 9). Veterinary nurses often speak to clients to reassure them of how their pet is progressing in the hospital. Once the animal goes home, the veterinary nurse must ensure the owner is competent at administering any further care required.

Alternative solutions to a problem may need to be explored. For example, it is unrealistic for a Dobermann with a hindlimb amputation to negotiate four flights of stairs in a block of flats with a 70-year-old owner. The influencing factors should always be considered when creating the care plan for the animal, and adjustments made appropriately for when the animal is to return home.

The Roper, Logan and Tierney Model

The Roper, Logan and Tierney Model of nursing is made up of five parts:

1. Activities of living
2. The patient's lifespan
3. Dependence–independence continuum
4. Factors influencing the activities of living
5. Individuality in living.

Part one: Activities of living

According to Roper, Logan and Tierney these are the central components of the model. There are twelve activities of living:

The twelve activities of living

- Maintaining a safe environment.
- Communicating.
- Breathing.
- Eating and drinking.
- Eliminating.
- Personal cleansing and dressing (grooming).
- Controlling body temperature.
- Mobilizing.
- Working and playing.
- Expressing sexuality.
- Sleeping.
- Dying.

If a client were asked to describe what each day involved for their pet, most people would include some or all of the functions listed above. This is why they are called 'activities of living' (ALs).

Roper reports that when this model was first introduced in 1980, the inclusion of 'expression of sexuality' as an AL was greeted by surprise, but is less likely to cause a problem within the veterinary field. Also the fact that 'dying' was considered an AL was unusual at this time, but in veterinary science euthanasia is something that a client can opt for when and if it is needed, which makes this an important activity when this model is applied to veterinary patients.

Part two: Lifespan

Each animal has a lifespan from birth to death and is likely to have stages along the way of neonate, kitten/puppy/foal, adolescent, adult, senior (geriatric). Some may die before they reach old age.

Within the care plan, the 'lifespan' is represented as a diagram showing a unidirectional arrow from birth to death:

Neonate ————→ Geriatric

It is added at the beginning of the care plan in order that a particular patient's position can be plotted on it, and their age can be seen at a glance. It is important that nurses have a visual reminder of the patient's age when they consider each of the ALs for any particular patient.

Part three: Dependence–independence continuum

This part of the model is closely related to lifespan and to the ALs:

Total dependence (D) ————→ Total independence (I)

It acknowledges that there are times in life when a patient cannot perform certain ALs independently. Each patient will have a dependence–independence continuum for each AL and the patient's position can be plotted on each of these to provide an impression of that patient's degree of dependence or independence. Throughout the patient's stay, its position on each continuum will be plotted more than once; the patient should become less dependent during its stay at hospital, as the problem for which it has been admitted resolves.

Some examples of how the Roper, Logan and Tierney model can be applied to feline, equine and rabbit patients are given at the end of this chapter (pages 359–363).

Part four: Factors influencing the activities of living

Five main factors influence the ALs and should be considered when preparing a care plan for each individual patient:

- Biological
- Psychological
- Sociocultural
- Environmental
- Politicoeconomic.

Biological

It is important to be aware of the biological state of the patient's body and how this might influence any of the ALs. The veterinary nurse must be familiar with the anatomy and physiology of both the healthy and sick animal in order to understand the impact of a disease on an animal within their care.

Psychological

The impact of psychological stresses on the ALs can be significant. For example, a veterinary patient that is separated from its owner may become withdrawn, refuse to eat and drink, and be unable to sleep, all of which will have a detrimental effect on its health and an impact on the ALs.

Sociocultural

It is important that nurses have knowledge of sociocultural factors and how they may influence ALs. It may appear on first reading that this is not appropriate when nursing veterinary patients, but the relevance becomes apparent when considered in the context of the owner:

- The client: Cultural idiosyncrasies of the client need to be considered in relation to the Activities of Living
- The patient: Some animals are herd animals. A donkey may become 'lonely' and withdrawn without a companion.

Environmental

The environment in which the patient is housed (see Chapter 12) may influence its ALs.

- The atmosphere – light and sound waves. For example, bright light can be very tiring for an ill patient, as can the noise of a busy ward with the radio on. Both of these may even prevent the patient from resting or sleeping.
- The atmosphere – organic and inorganic. For example, dust may irritate an atopic patient and pathogenic microorganisms are a risk to all patients, in particular those who are elderly, immunosuppressed or recovering from major surgery.
- The built environment. For example, the veterinary practice kennels and all other areas must be safe in order that the first AL ('maintain a safe environment') can be achieved.

Politicoeconomic

There are two parts to this:

- Health and economic status. This relates to the client more than the patient in a veterinary context; it is likely that the economic status of the client may influence the ALs.
- Health and world economy. Recession will have an impact on the amount that clients will spend and that veterinary surgeons will invest in staff and equipment; this may impact on the care of the veterinary patient.

Part five: Individuality in living

The ALs are the main concept of this model. Although every patient is likely to carry out these activities, each patient may do them differently, thus expressing themselves as an individual. For example, a cat may eat in a very different way to a dog.

Relationship between the component parts of the model

Figure 14.6 shows how the component parts relate to one another and the significance of each in the construction of the Roper, Logan and Tierney Model of Nursing.

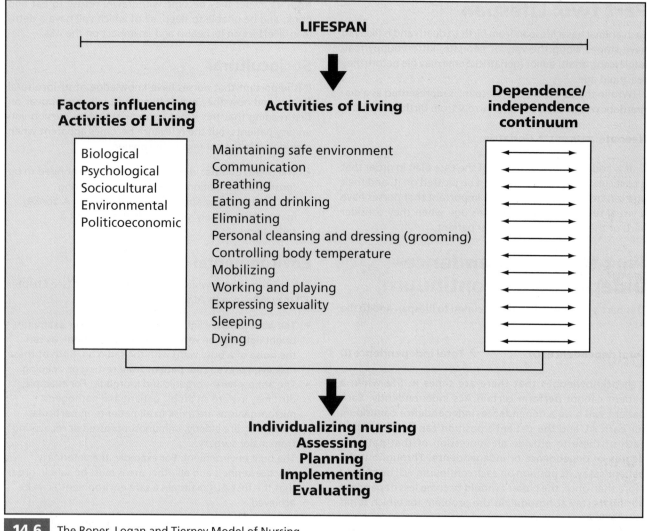

14.6 The Roper, Logan and Tierney Model of Nursing.

Orem's Model

Dorothea Orem's views on nursing science are the basis for understanding how empirical nursing evidence is gathered and interpreted. Her quest for greater understanding of the nature of nursing focused on three questions:

- What do nurses do, and what should nurses do, as practitioners of nursing?
- Why do nurses do what they do?
- What are the results of nursing interventions?

Orem's model of nursing focuses on the key idea that an individual is self-caring if they can manage the following effectively:

- Support of life processes and normal functioning
- Maintenance of normal growth and development
- Prevention and control of disease and injury
- Prevention of, or compensation for, disability
- Promotion of wellbeing.

According to Cavanagh (1991), central to Orem's concept of self-care is the concept that care is being initiated voluntarily and deliberately by an individual. Self-care is the practice of activities that will maintain life and health and will promote wellbeing.

Universal self-care requisites

Essential to Orem's model are the eight 'universal self-care requisites', which are activities that must be performed in order to achieve self-care:

Orem's universal self-care requisites

- The maintenance of a sufficient intake of air.
- The maintenance of a sufficient intake of water.
- The maintenance of a sufficient intake of food.
- Satisfactory elimination functions.
- The maintenance of a balance between activity and rest.
- The maintenance of a balance between solitude and social integration.
- The prevention of hazards to life, wellbeing and functioning.
- The promotion of functioning and development within social groups and the desire to be normal (normality).

These self-care requisites are essential tasks that an individual must be able to manage in order to care for themselves. As with Roper, Logan and Tierney's ALs, these are all requisites that an animal can achieve, but some of the self-care requisites may be easier for wild animals than for domesticated ones. For example, intake of food may be difficult if the domesticated animal is reliant on an owner to feed it and it has no freedom to scavenge or hunt.

The idea of balancing demands and abilities (Figure 14.7) is central to Orem's model.

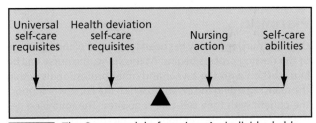

14.7 The Orem model of nursing. A healthy individual: self-care abilities meet self-care requisites.

Developmental self-care requisites

Orem identified a second kind of requisite found in special circumstances associated with development.

Orem's specific developmental self-care requisites

- Interuterine life and birth.
- Neonatal life.
- Infancy.
- The developmental stages of childhood (for which substitute puppy, kitten, foal, etc.), adolescence and early adulthood.
- The developmental stages of adulthood.
- Pregnancy.

It is at this point that Orem differs from Roper, Logan and Tierney, as the lifespan within the Roper, Logan and Tierney Model begins with the neonate and does not consider interuterine life as Orem does. Orem argues that at each of these stages universal self-care requisites must also be considered (Figure 14.8). An example of a specific developmental self-care requisite would be temperature regulation in a neonate. An adult may be able to control its own body temperature but a neonate may not.

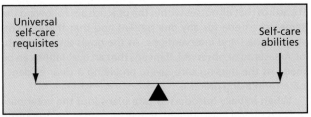

14.8 The Orem model of nursing. An individual with additional developmental self-care requisites is in need of intervention.

Health-deviation self-care requisites

There are times when an individual is ill, becomes injured, has disabilities or is under medical care. In these circumstances, the following additional healthcare demands are placed upon them:

- Seeking and securing appropriate medical assistance
- Being aware of and attending to the effects and results of pathological conditions and states
- Effectively carrying out medically prescribed treatment
- Being aware of, and attending to, the discomforting and deleterious effects of medically prescribed treatment
- Modifying self-image in accepting oneself as being in a particular state of health
- Learning to live with the effects of pathological conditions and states.

The owner may act for the animal in order that some of the additional health-care demands are achieved, and an individual animal may experience a change in the status of their health but still be able to meet the universal and health-deviation self-care requisites (Figure 14.9).

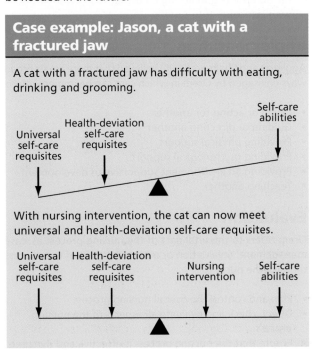

14.9 The Orem model of nursing. An individual able to meet all requisites with nursing assistance.

However, a situation could exist where the total demand placed on an animal exceeds its ability to meet it. In this situation an individual will need nursing intervention in order to enable it to meet its self-care needs. The nurse needs to assess which interventions are needed immediately and which might be needed in the future.

Case example: Jason, a cat with a fractured jaw

A cat with a fractured jaw has difficulty with eating, drinking and grooming.

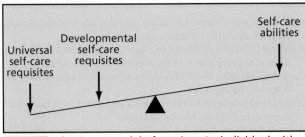

With nursing intervention, the cat can now meet universal and health-deviation self-care requisites.

Putting the theory into practice

Cavanagh (1991) suggested that there is no single 'correct' way of setting out a care plan based upon Orem's model. Instead, the nurse must take the ideas that Orem presents and develop a plan to meet the needs of each patient. This takes confidence as a nurse, but this is a model that can be adapted to meet the needs of veterinary practice while still individualizing care of the patient. If this is the model that is used in practice, it is vital that each stage is recorded to ensure all who read the plan are able to understand and follow it. The nursing process is a vital part of the model and is the basis of the care plan for any individual patient. An example of a completed care plan, demonstrating the application of the model to the case example, Jason, is given at the end of this chapter (page 364).

Interpretation of language used within Orem's Model

Assessment

Orem does not often refer to 'assessment' but chooses to use 'nursing history' instead.

Planning

Once the nursing history has been taken, the 'planning' stage of the nursing process begins. At this stage, the nurse will be in discussion with the owner and other professionals within the team regarding the extent to which the nurse will support the patient with their self-care requisites. The following degrees of nursing intervention might be considered.

- **Wholly compensatory** – the patient and client are completely dependent on the veterinary nurse (e.g. a paraplegic dog)
- **Partially compensatory** – the nurse and patient and client working together to meet the self-care requisites (e.g. a dog with a long bone fracture)
- **Supportive/educative** – the nurse is there for support/reassurance (e.g. teaching an owner to inject their pet with insulin).

Implementation

Aggleton and Chalmers (2000) believed that there are six broad ways envisaged by Orem in which care can be implemented:

- Doing or acting for another
- Guiding or directing another
- Providing physical support
- Providing psychological support
- Providing an environment supportive of development
- Teaching another.

Evaluation

Orem refers to this vital part of the nursing process as 'case management' (evaluation or audit). This part of the process requires the nurse to:

- Plan and control the overall nursing process
- Direct, check and evaluate all aspects of the nursing process
- Ensure that the nursing process is effective and dynamic.

Using models of nursing in a clinical veterinary environment

The use of a nursing model in which the nursing process is embedded is vital when delivering nursing care to patients. It ensures that all nurses within the practice are following the same set criteria for any one patient and that there are recorded goals and interventions. As the goals set are able to be measured or observed, it means that an evaluation can be made of the nursing care given, providing a clear evidence base for nursing practice.

When initially introducing care plans into the veterinary nursing clinical environment, it may be seen to be producing yet more paperwork for nurses to complete on a day-to-day basis. It is therefore important to emphasize the rationale for nurse care planning and the nursing process.

Some nurses will argue that they perform care planning and evaluation automatically; for example if a patient does not eat one type of diet attempts are made at tempting them with another. However, in a clinical setting in which numerous nurses may be caring for a single patient, there may be a lack of continuity of this care.

Following on from the diet example, a nurse may have found that a patient refuses to eat diet 1, but does eat diet 2. However, if this information is not recorded anywhere and the nurses then change shifts, a second nurse may give diet 1, and unsurprisingly find that the patient does not eat this. This lack of communication is likely to compromise patient care.

If a care plan had been implemented in this situation, with documentation of the nursing process, the second nurse would be aware that the patient does not eat diet 1 and instead prefers diet 2. The use of a care plan will ensure there is continuity of care throughout conventional 'handovers', with individual nurses and the nursing team as a whole providing a high level of care tailored to a patient's individual needs. Where care plans are implemented, clinical outcomes may be improved and recovery from illness shortened.

Patient admission is usually the time when the nurse asks the client questions about their pet and is the most effective time for assessment to be carried out.

References and further reading

Aggleton P and Chalmers H (2000). *Nursing Models and Nursing Practice, 2nd edn.* Palgrave, Basingstoke

Benner P (1984) *From Novice to Expert: Excellence and Power in Clinical Nursing Practice.* Addison-Wesley, Menlo Park, CA

Cavanagh SJ (1991) *Orem's Model in Action, 3rd edn.* Macmillan, Palgrave, Basingstoke

Chin PL and Kramer MK (1995) *Theory and Nursing: A Systematic Approach, 4th edn.* Mosby, St Louis

Holland K (2003) *Applying the Roper-Logan-Tierney Model in Practice: Elements of Nursing.* Churchill Livingstone

Jeffery A (2006) Moving away from the medical model. *Veterinary Nursing Journal* **21**, 9

Jeffery AK and Orpet HA (2007) Holistic Nursing. *BSAVA Congress Scientific Proceedings: Nursing Programme*, 4–5

Joiner T (2000) An holistic approach to nursing. *Veterinary Nursing* **15**, 4

Kratz C (1979) *The Nursing Process*. Baillière Tindall, London

Luker KM (1989) Evaluating nursing care. In: *The Nursing Process*, ed. CR Kratz, 124–146. Baillière Tindall, London

McGee P (1998) *Models of Nursing in Practice, a Pattern for Practical Care*. Stanley Thornes Ltd, Cheltenham

Murry ME and Atkinson LD (1994) *Understanding the Nursing Process, 5th edn*. McGraw–Hill, New York

Orpet H and Jeffery A (2006) Moving towards a more holistic approach. *Veterinary Nursing Journal* **26**, 5

Orpet H and Jeffery A (2007) *BSAVA Congress Proceedings*

Peate I (2006) *The Compendium of Clinical Skills for Student Nurses*. Wiley

Pearson A, Vaughan B and Fitzgerald M (2004) *Nursing Models for Practice*. Butterworth-Heinemann, Oxford

Roper N, Logan W and Tierney A (1993) *The Elements of Nursing: A Model for Nursing Based on a Model for Living*. Churchill Livingstone, Edinburgh

Roper N, Logan W and Tierney A (2002) *The Elements of Nursing, 4th edn*. Churchill Livingstone, Edinburgh

Walsh M (1997) *Models and Critical Pathways in Clinical Nursing: Conceptual Frameworks for Care Planning*. Baillière Tindall, London

Wilkinson J (1996) *Nursing Process: A Critical Thinking Approach*. Addison-Wesley, Menlo Park, CA

Self-assessment questions

1. What are the key components of the Medical (Biomedical) model?
2. Name the five stages of the Nursing Process.
3. At which stage of the Nursing Process does the nurse plan the patient care?
4. Why is it important to set goals for patients that can be measured in some way?
5. What are the key questions that the nurse needs to ask themselves during the evaluation stage of the Nursing Process?
6. List the 5 components of the Roper, Logan and Tierney Model.
7. With regard to the Roper, Logan and Tierney Model, what is the purpose of the dependence–independence continuum?
8. Orem refers to the patients 'self-care requisites'; how many of these are there?
9. List the three key components of the Orpet and Jeffery Ability Model.
10. With regard to the Orpet and Jeffery Ability Model, why is the initial patient assessment important in patient care delivery?

More patient examples ▶

Date of Admission: 4/2/11		Date of nursing assessment: 5/2/11	
Case No. 12345		Patient Name: Jess Breed: Basset Hound **Sex:** Female, entire	
Owner: Address: Contact No.			
Clinical summary (reason for admission): Road Traffic Accident. Subsequent fractured pelvis and growth plate fracture		Owners' perception of problem: Owners are aware how serious the injuries are and are expecting Jess to have a long recovery.	
Previous history (surgery, disease, vaccination status, allergies): Up-to-date vaccines and preventive parasite treatment. No other known problems			
T 38.7 °C		**Current medication** Morphine Meloxicam Amoxicillin/Clavulanate IVFT – Hartmann's 2 ml/kg/h (maintenance)	
P 88 beats/min			
R 28 breaths/min			
MM pink			
CRT >2 s			
Weight 15.3 kg			

Life stage:
Age: 7 months

neonate — adult ——————→ geriatric

Assessment of activities of living

Ability	Usual routine	Actual problems	Potential problems	Long-term goals
Eat adequate amount	Fed twice daily	Anorexic	Unable to maintain body condition	Provide nutrition to prevent loss of body condition
Drink adequate amounts	Water available at all times	Unable to move to water bowl	Inadequate fluid intake	Provide access to oral fluids at all times
Urinate normally	Goes out 4 times a day. Has command 'Go toilets'	Fractures prevent Jess walking, therefore difficult to take out	Urine retention, discomfort	Enable Jess to carry out normal routine
Defecate normally	As above. Usually passes am and pm	Fractures prevent Jess walking, therefore difficult to take outside	Morphine may cause reduced gut motility and constipation	Freedom from constipation and provide normal routine
Breathe normally	Normal for breed	None at present	Morphine may alter respiratory rate and depth	Maintain normal
Maintain body temperature	Usually sleeps in kitchen at home	Temperature high end of normal	Warmer in hospital than at home, may increase body temperature	Monitor and maintain normal range
Groom itself	Owner grooms weekly, occasional baths	Damage to coat from incident	Wounds and sores where no fur covering	Keep coat clean and enable wounds to heal
Mobilize adequately	Normally walked twice daily	Fractures impede movement of hindquarters	Decubitus ulcers (pressure sores), constipation, hypostatic pneumonia	Prevent, reduce potential problems occurring
Sleep/rest	Normally sleeps afternoons and night-time	Hospital active throughout day, so Jess unable to have quiet time	Jess cannot sleep in active noisy environment	Allow rest time between medications and checks
Express normal behaviour	Usually playful puppy	Unable to play due to injuries	May become depressed	Ensure adequate pain relief is provided at all times. Provide stimulation between rest periods

Patient assessment form for the Ability Model. Completed as for patient example, Jess.

Client questioned by: Nurse X	Date: 8/3/11
Patient details: A 7-month-old female neutered DSH cat	
Diagnosed condition/clinical signs: Upper respiratory tract infection (suspect cat 'flu) **Unvaccinated**	
Life stage: Neonate ──X──────────────────────────────────▶ Geriatric	

Area	Client responses
Breathing	No problems normally but has been snuffly over the last week
Drinking	Has access all day, owner doesn't think she drinks much normally
Eating	Normal food = complete dry food – owner will bring the bag in to be used during hospitalization, usually fed twice daily
Defecating	Normally passes twice daily (morning and evening) in her litter tray
Urinating	Usually goes out daily but uses litter tray with pine-based litter
Controlled body temperature	Bella lives and sleeps inside, she has her bed in the kitchen next to the ratidator
Mobilization	Normally very lively and goes out and plays daily, enjoys playing with a 'mouse on a stick'
Sleeping	Bella will come inside each evening normally and sleep in the kitchen
Grooming	Short-coated, groomed once a week, usually grooms herself well
Playing	Bella has lots of toys and is very good with children, likes cuddles and other close contact affection
Pain	Bella has no history of showing pain but the owner reports her to be quite stalwart

Initial patient evaluation for respiratory case Bella, using an adaptation of the Roper, Logan and Tierney Model.

Patient details: A 7-month-old female neutered DSH cat, with upper respiratory tract infection		Date: 8/3/11	Reassessment date: 9.3.11
Area	**Presenting problems**	**Goals**	**Considerations/potential problems**
Breathing	Respiratory mucus obstructing nares	Keep airways clear	May obstruct and cause dyspnoea
Drinking	Difficult if nares obstructed	Maintain normal intake	Obstructed nares → may not drink due to dyspnoea Reduced intake → dehydration
Eating	Anorexic	Tempt to eat	Blocked nares → reduced olfactory function
Defecating	Anorexia	Keep regular	Reduced food input → reduced defecation Reduced mobility
Urinating	None	Keep regular	Reduced drinking → dehydration
Controlling body temperature	Pyrexia	Keep normothermic	Pyrexia exacerbates anorexia
Mobilization	Hospitalized in isolation ward	Allow normal activity	Reduced mobility Become depressed
Sleeping	Busy hospital ward prevents rest	Allow rest periods	Reduced sleep
Grooming	Unwilling to groom – obstructed nares	Allow to groom	Knotted fur, reduced coat condition
Playing	In isolation ward	Provide stimuli	Become depressed
Pain	Uncomfortable eyes	Keep eyes clean from discharge	Depressed, anorexic

Actual and potential problems for URTI case Bella.

Patient details: A 7-month-old female neutered DSH cat, with upper respiratory tract infection	
Area	**Intervention**
Breathing	Clean nares with damp cotton wool twice daily, use cotton wool buds if required Steam bath twice daily
Drinking	Monitor water intake
Eating	Provide own food and other tasty more strong-smelling foods
Defecating	Monitor and encourage food intake
Urinating	Monitor frequency
Controlling body temperature	Monitor temperature daily
Mobilization	Provide largest kennel possible in the isolation area, provide toys and attention to encourage movement
Sleeping	Provide rest periods by grouping check and medications together, keep environment quiet and turn off lights at night
Grooming	Encourage grooming; groom with brushes and damp paper towel q8h – try and perform at same time as checks and medications
Playing	Provide mental stimulus with toys and provide attention and mental stimulus
Pain	Clean eyes q12h with damp cotton wool and monitor for discomfort

Nursing interventions for URTI case Bella.

Patient details: A 7-month-old female neutered DSH cat, with upper respiratory tract infection	Date: 9.3.11
Area	**Evaluation of nursing interventions**
Breathing	Twice-daily cleaning working well at the moment, some reddening to the nose so care when cleaning Goal reached (Y)/ N
Drinking	Currently drinking 45 ml/kg/day Goal reached (Y)/ N
Eating	Currently eating pilchards in tomato sauce Goal reached (Y)/ N
Defecating	Hasn't passed any faeces over last 24 hrs; this could be because Bella hasn't eaten well for a number of days prior to hospitalization. Continue tempting to eat Goal reached Y /(N)
Urinating	Urinating twice a day at the moment Goal reached (Y)/ N
Controlling body temperature	Pyrexia has subsided with medications and treatment – continue to monitor Goal reached (Y)/ N
Mobilization	Normal activity not able to be met due to isolation. Continue to provide attention and affection at checks and medication times. Goal not met as isolation kennels too small, but is actively playing in the kennel Goal reached Y /(N)
Sleeping	Medications and checks at the same time so able to have rest periods. Also isolation is being kept quiet. Lights turned off overnight to allow sleeping Goal reached (Y)/ N
Grooming	Grooming going well, likes the rubber brush and the hand pad. Observed grooming herself Goal reached (Y)/ N
Playing	Enjoying the toys, wind-up mouse seems to provide amusement, owner has also brought in own toys Goal reached (Y)/ N
Pain	Eyes seem more comfortable, twice-daily cleaning seems to be adequate Goal reached (Y)/ N

Re-evaluation for URTI case Bella.

Patient Details: 8-year-old Belgian Warmblood mare admitted with colic

Patient's position on lifespan: Neonate ← | → Geriatric

Activity of living	Nursing assessment of patient ability to carry out activity of living	D=dependent I = independent	Patient problem potential/ actual	Nursing goals	Nursing interventions	Evaluation
Maintaining a safe environment	The horse is unable to maintain its own safe environment and therefore should have a quiet stable containing a deep shavings bed or similar bedding and access to water. Ensure the patient has space to roll	D ← | → I	Colic may result in patient rolling and injuring herself (Potential)	To ensure that the horse has a safe and comfortable stable in a quiet area away from the other busier areas of the practice to minimize stress and to promote recovery from colic	Observe horse every 15 minutes to ensure she is safe within her stable environment. Stable should be away from other horses and excess noise to minimize stress.	A safe and comfortable environment was maintained and the horse was regularly monitored
Communicating	The horse was able to communicate pain and discomfort	D ← | → I		To be able to interpret and effectively act upon the behavioural signs shown by the horse	To observe the patient behaviour every 15 minutes, record it and report any changes in behaviour to the vet in charge.	The horse was pawing the ground, rolling, looking at flanks and sweating until the signs of colic subsided
Breathing	The horse has an increased respiratory rate	D ← | → I	The patient's respiratory rate is high (Actual)	To reduce the respiratory rate to within normal parameters	To monitor respiration every 15 minutes and record it	The respiratory rate was increased on arrival at the practice but lowered following administration of anti-inflammatory drugs and analgesics
Eating and drinking	The horse was able to drink but food was withheld due to colic	D ← |→ I	The patient is unable to eat due to colic (Actual)	After signs of colic, feed little and often until feeding back to normal. Fluid intake to remain at normal maintenance intake	Record fluid intake and urinary output. Record faecal output every 15 minutes	The mare was subdued and no hay was given until droppings were passed
Eliminating	On arrival at the practice, the horse was not passing droppings due to colic	D ←| → I	Actual	To ensure that normal droppings are passed, to show that the gut function is correct	To observe defecation pattern and record, inform vet if droppings not produced and administer further gut stimulants as directed	The horse did not pass faeces so a gut stimulant was administered and an analgesic to aid with pain relief. Liquid paraffin was given to the horse via a nasogastric tube
Personal cleansing (grooming)	The horse was unable to groom itself, therefore will need grooming once colic is stabilized	D ◄| ► I	Actual	To ensure that the horse stays clean and dry throughout hospitalization and the coat remains in good condition	Clean any stable stains. Apply a sweat rug to avoid chilling, groom daily once colic has subsided	A rug was applied once the horse had stopped rolling
Controlling body temperature	Horse's temperature is raised and the patient can not maintain normal body temperature	D ◄|► I	Actual	To reduce temperature to within normal range by providing prescribed analgesia	Monitor and record temperature, pulse and respiration rate every 15 minutes until the horse remains stable.	Temperature was reduced to normal ranges and stabilized once pain and gut movement were controlled, as were the pulse and respiratory rates
Mobilizing	The horse kept rolling due to colic and therefore could not mobilize normally	D ← |► I	Actual	To ensure that on recovery from colic the mare is able to mobilize normally	Provide a comfortable well padded stable environment for the mare, to minimize the risk of injury during episodes of colic	The mare recovered well without any injuries
Working and playing	The horse was unable to exhibit normal behaviour due to spasmodic colic	D ◄| ► I	Actual	To ensure that the mare recovers well and has no further episodes of colic	Provide a comfortable well padded stable environment for the mare to minimize the risk of injury during episodes of colic	The horse was quiet following the colic episode and did not show any interest in wanting to play. She was less active than normal
Expressing sexuality	The mare had no problems in showing sexuality prior to colic	D ← |► I	Actual	N/A	N/A	N/A

Nursing care plan for an equine patient, using the Roper, Logan and Tierney model.

continues ▶

Patient Details: 8-year-old Belgian Warmblood mare admitted with colic

Patient's position on lifespan: Neonate ◄————┼————► Geriatric

Activity of living	Nursing assessment of patient ability to carry out activity of living	D=dependent I = independent	Patient problem potential/ actual	Nursing goals	Nursing interventions	Evaluation
Sleeping	The horse was unable to rest on admission due to colic	D ◄—┼—► I	Actual	Ensure that a comfortable stable is provided in a quiet area away from noise and distraction	Provide a deep bed and observe patient every 15 minutes to ensure that the medications provided to the patient for treatment of colic are effective and enable the patient to remain pain free	The horse was able to rest and sleep once she responded to treatment
Dying	Colic is a high-risk medical condition and there was a risk on admission that the mare could die from the colic	D ◄—┼—► I	Potential	To ensure that the horse is monitored closely and treatment given to ensure recovery from colic	Observe patient every 15 minutes and carry out monitoring of vital signs and patient's response to medication	The mare responded to treatment and had a good recovery from the colic

continued **Nursing care plan for an equine patient, using the Roper, Logan and Tierney model.**

Patient Details: A 1-year-old male Dutch rabbit due to have an elective castration

Patient's position on lifespan: Neonate ◄————┼————► Geriatric

Activity of living	Nursing assessment of patient ability to carry out activity of living	D=dependent I = independent	Patient problem Potential/actual	Nursing goals	Nursing interventions	Evaluation
Maintaining a safe environment	The rabbit is unable to do this himself and must be provided with a quiet kennel containing a bed, hay, food and a water bottle or bowl	D ◄—┼—► I	Potential	To ensure that the rabbit has a safe and comfortable cage in a quieter area away from other noisy animals, to minimize stress and allow recovery from anaesthesia	Place the rabbit away from dogs, cats and excess noise, to minimize stress	A safe and comfortable environment was maintained and no problems occurred
Communicating	The rabbit is able to use physical ways of communicating which are interpreted by the nurse based on the owner information	D ◄———┼—► I		To be able to understand the signs given by the rabbit	Observe and record patient behaviour to ensure there are no changes	On recovery, the rabbit showed signs of being distressed and an increased respiration rate. A towel was placed over the front of the cage to darken it and to make the rabbit feel safer. The patient was observed every 15 minutes until distress subsided
Breathing	The rabbit is a young healthy rabbit with a normal respiratory pattern	D ◄———┼—► I	Potential	Respiratory function to be maintained within normal parameters	To monitor respiration rate in the peri-operative period and to ensure that it remains within normal parameters	The respiratory rate stayed within normal parameters with no complications whilst in surgery. During initial stages of recovery it did increase but returned to normal within 30 minutes
Eating and drinking	The rabbit was able to eat and drink normally on admission	D ◄—┼—► I	Potential	To ensure on recovery that the rabbit eats and also passes faeces normally	In line with current guidelines, the rabbit was not starved prior to surgery. Encourage eating. Offer dandelions to stimulate feeding, or syringe feed if required	After surgery, the rabbit recovered and ate with encouragement No faeces passed

Nursing care plan for a rabbit, using the Roper, Logan and Tierney model.

continues ►

Patient Details: A 1-year-old male Dutch rabbit due to have an elective castration

Patient's position on lifespan: Neonate ←————————→ Geriatric

Activity of living	Nursing assessment of patient ability to carry out activity of living	D=dependent I = independent	Patient problem Potential/actual	Nursing goals	Nursing interventions	Evaluation
Eliminating	The rabbit was fit, healthy and had no difficulties in toileting or any previous history of problems	D ←——┼—► I	Potential	To ensure that toileting remains normal during stay	Observe for and record faecal output to show that the gut function is correct. Inform VS if not and administer faecal stimulant as directed	The rabbit had not passed faeces, so a gut stimulant was administered
Personal cleansing (grooming)	The rabbit was in good condition and was able to groom itself	D ←———┼—► I	Potential	To ensure that the rabbit stays clean and dry throughout his stay and coat remains in good condition	Clean any eliminations accordingly to reduce any contamination to the surgical wound	The rabbit did not eliminate throughout his stay and therefore no assistance was required in keeping coat clean
Controlling body temperature	Prior to surgery the rabbit's temperature was within normal limits.	D ←———┼—► I	Potential	To ensure that normal parameters are maintained throughout the surgery and post surgery	Monitor temperature pulse and respiration rate every 15–30 minutes during the perioperative period (as directed by vet) to ensure that the rabbit maintains his body temperature, pulse and respiration rate within normal ranges and he doesn't become hypothermic. Supply external heat sources if required	The rabbit maintained normal body temperature throughout and post surgery. However, external heat sources were supplied until he had fully recovered from anaesthesia
Mobilizing	The rabbit has no problems in his mobility	D ←————┼► I	Potential	To ensure that the rabbit recovers well and gains full mobility following surgery	Provide a padded environment for the rabbit to recover in and to avoid any bumps or knocks. Ensure patient is able to mobilize fully	The rabbit recovered well without any injuries
Working and playing	A young active rabbit with no problems in playing etc.	D ←————┼► I	Potential	To ensure that the rabbit recovers well but limit activity following surgery	Provide a less active environment to discourage play	The rabbit was lethargic following the surgery and did not show any interest in wanting to play. He was less active
Expressing sexuality	The rabbit was showing evidence of sexual activity prior to surgery	D ←———┼—► I		N/A	N/A	The rabbit had an elective procedure to eliminate this
Sleeping	Needs to be provided with a quiet environment for him to be able to sleep	D ←┼———► I	Potential	Ensure that a comfortable environment is provided in a quiet area away from noise and distraction, to enable rabbit to rest and sleep	A quiet dark bed was provided and also a heat pad so that the rabbit could rest and recover from surgery in a warm comfortable environment	The rabbit was stressed following surgery but a quiet cage was provided, allowing him to sleep
Dying	On admission the rabbit was young fit and healthy	D ←┼———► I	Although the rabbit is young, there is a risk with general anaesthetic, and handling can cause stress levels to rise. (Potential)	To ensure that the rabbit is monitored closely under anaesthetic to avoid any potential problems arising and makes a full recovery	The patient was monitored every 5 minutes using the following anaesthetic monitoring equipment: oesophageal stethoscope, pulse ox, ECG, to ensure that its vital signs remained within normal range during the surgical procedure	The patient was stable during anaesthesia and recovered well

continued Nursing care plan for a rabbit, using the Roper, Logan and Tierney model.

Patient details:	12-month-old neutered male, DSH cat			
Reason for admission:	Fractured jaw			

Universal self-care requisites	Self-care abilities	Self-care limitations	Patient actions	Nursing actions
Maintain intake of air	Breathes without difficulty	Unable to groom/clean therefore food sticks to nose	Breathes well when nostrils clear	Ensure nostrils remain clear during and after feeding Assess respiratory adequacy
Maintain intake of water	Can put mouth down to water bowl and lap water	Difficulty in drinking from a high-sided bowl	Drinking Swallowing	Provide water in a shallow bowl Keep a fluid balance chart Observe for signs of dehydration
Maintain intake of food	Can put mouth down to food bowl	Unable to prehend food	Can swallow when food in mouth	Ensure food is in manageable form Assist with feeding Maintain a record of food eaten
Manage elimination	All	Normally urinates outside in soil	Use litter tray to urinate and defecate	Provide litter tray containing soil Keep a record of urinary/faecal output
Balance activity and rest	Is able to rest and sleep	Unable to have free access	Walk around kennel Rest and sleep on Vetbed	Provide a large kennel Provide an environment for rest/ sleep when required
Balance solitude and social intergration	Is able to communicate through body language	Unable to purr or meow due to fracture Unable to communicate with brother		Provide regular nursing attention Organize for family, including children to visit
Prevention of hazards to life, wellbeing and functioning	Possesses pain sensation Can hear and see	Cannot maintain safety of environment		Monitor vital signs and assess patient for changes in physical and psychological condition
Normalcy	Is able to communicate through body language	Unable to vocalize	Interact with staff, family and other animals	Provide an environment in which he feels at ease

Nursing care plan for a cat Jason, using Orem's model.

Chapter 15

Observation and assessment of the patient

Lucy Goddard and Catherine Phillips

Learning objectives

After studying this chapter, students should be able to:

- **Describe the procedure for performing a complete health check on dogs, cats, exotic pets and horses admitted for hospitalization**
- **Know how to measure and monitor vital signs and understand the range of normal clinical parameters in animals**
- **Recognize the possible causes of abnormalities in hospitalized patients**
- **Apply the knowledge of normal and abnormal appearance of animals to evaluate the condition of patients receiving nursing care**
- **Recognize signs of stress and pain in hospitalized patients and demonstrate methods to minimize the detrimental effects these can have upon the patient**

Patient observation

Veterinary nurses are important members of the veterinary team that will care for the patient while it is within the veterinary practice. Nursing observations on the patient's health status at admission, during its adaptation to a hospital environment and throughout treatment will all provide valuable information to the veterinary surgeon on the animal's clinical condition, wellbeing and progress. It is necessary for the veterinary nurse to be able to recognize normality and abnormality in the appearance, demeanour and behaviour of any species of patient that is in his/her care. Observation can commence from the time the patient enters the practice.

Initial observations

- Dogs that enter the reception area can be observed for interaction with new surroundings, unfamiliar people and other animals.
- Horses can be assessed as they are unloaded from vehicles. ▶

- Such observation can provide information on the animal's character and behaviour, such as excitement, aggression or anxiety within a strange environment.
- Observations from afar may also reveal information on an animal's presenting condition, such as lameness, or the patient's basic physical state and urgency of condition, such as difficulty in breathing or a bleeding wound that may require prompt veterinary attention.
- Cats and small animals that are transported within secure carriers may not be easily visible due to the design of the carrier but, where possible, smaller patients should be observed to ensure that they are not exhibiting signs of excessive stress due to travelling or presenting illness.
- Cats and small animals that are observed 'mouth breathing' could indicate stress or severe respiratory distress and should be given immediate attention.

Adaptation to the hospital environment

Different species and breeds of animal will respond and adapt to being in a hospital environment in different ways. It is important to address the needs of each patient as an individual and provide care and accommodation that will meet their nursing care needs. Rabbits, small animals and birds require special consideration as they may feel extremely vulnerable outside their normal environment. This unfamiliar environment can cause animals to behave in a way that may be quite out of character; normally well behaved animals may become difficult to handle, unexpectedly aggressive or submissive. Some patients may display behavioural traits such as kennel guarding when confined within an enclosed space. 'Vices' in horses are well recognized and include box walking, weaving, wind-sucking and crib biting. Such stereotypical behaviours are more frequently observed in stressed equine hospital patients.

Stress reduction

Stress in veterinary patients should not be overlooked; a change in routine and environment can be a stressful time for the patient, and measures should be taken to reduce or control this. Stress and anxiety may have detrimental effects on the patient's health whilst it is hospitalized and can result in inappetence, altered biochemical parameters and prolonged recovery times, as well as making patients restless and unsettled.

An unsettled patient should be assessed for any obvious reason that could explain such behaviour; for example, some dogs may become agitated or vocal if they need to urinate or defecate. Even just one unsettled and stressed patient within a ward will have an effect upon the other patients within the nearby area. A noisy ward of barking dogs can become very stressful for staff and patients alike. There are many ways in which the veterinary nurse can try to minimize stress within the hospital environment, e.g. by helping to promote normal patient behaviour and segregating species appropriately. Horses, however, may benefit from seeing other horses and will settle more easily into a new environment.

Rabbits, rodents and birds will benefit from being housed away from dogs and cats, as the majority of these species are 'prey' animals that would normally rely on their 'flight or fight' response when in a potentially dangerous situation. They may become anxious if in close proximity to the noise and smells of other patients, especially when they have no means of escape due to the confinement of a kennel or cage.

Housing small mammals or birds in their own cages may be beneficial if they allow observation of the patient. Considerations should be made for patients who are very young or elderly, as they may not be able to adapt to a change in routine and environment as easily as other patients.

Promotion of normal patient behaviour

Admission questionnaires

A short questionnaire completed by the animal's owner at the time of admittance to the hospital can provide important information on their pet's normal behaviour and routines at home. This is in addition to general admission information (see Chapter 12) and may help to differentiate normal from abnormal behaviour for each individual patient and to identify measures that can be implemented to aid in providing familiar surroundings.

Questionnaires can be designed for each species of patient that may be admitted to the hospital; examples for dogs, cats and horses are given at the end of this chapter.

For small mammal and other exotic pets, questions asked should address:

- Type of water bottles or bowls normally used
- Usual bedding material
- Normal and favourite foods
- How easily the pet may be handled.

As is described in Chapter 14 the information gained about the animal can be useful to the nursing team once the patient is within the hospital environment. To give an example: on admission to the hospital it is observed that a cat does not eat the wet food placed towards the front of its cage; however, with additional information provided by the owner on the cat's normal behaviour at home it emerges that the cat is shy of new people and prefers to graze on dry biscuits throughout the day. With this information, biscuits can be left at the back of the cage and the cat can be provided with an area to hide away in, making it feel more secure and more likely to eat.

Inpatient behaviour

Animals will sense the mood and attitude of staff working closely around them, and a calm and quiet approach will be beneficial for patients and staff alike.

Cats

Cats especially can become very unsettled by a stressful environment, but a few simple 'rules' for the cat ward can easily help to make a cat-friendly environment.

Calm and happy cat wards

- No dogs.
- Avoid cats facing each other.
- Reduce noise, banging doors, lots of people.
- Avoid kennels at floor level.
- Place cats in baskets on a table and cover the basket with a towel.
- Use boxes or covered beds for cats to shelter in (Figure 15.1).
- Gentle handling.
- Calm atmosphere, quiet radio and calm nurses.
- Use of feline pheromones.

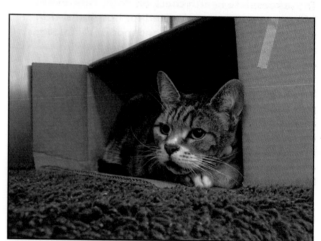

15.1   Relaxed hospitalized cat settled within a cardboard box.

The use of pheromones to modify the behaviour of animals within the hospital setting (pheromonatherapy) can be useful to help reduce stress in the cat. Synthetic versions of two naturally occurring facial pheromones (F3 and F4) are commercially available, commonly used in a spray or plug-in diffuser form. Environmental application within the entire ward can be achieved with the use of a diffuser (Figure 15.2). The environmental use of pheromones may improve the demeanour, appetite and ability to adapt to the stresses that a strange environment can cause to feline patients. Sprays may also be applied directly on to objects prior to admission, such as bedding and carrying baskets, or to the person who is about to handle the cat.

Dogs

Dog-appeasing pheromone (DAP) diffusers are available for canine wards. The synthetic pheromone can help to reduce stress and anxiety within the kennel environment. Appeasing pheromones may help to make dogs feel more calm and safe. DAP sprays and collars are also available.

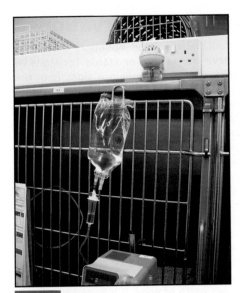

15.2   Pheromone diffuser used in a cat ward.

Equine patients

The veterinary nurse within an equine hospital environment is likely to need to manage some challenging equine behaviours. It must be remembered that horses are herd animals and are therefore better housed in a position where they have company and, ideally, the ability to see other equine patients. Stallions should be housed away from cycling mares, particularly breeding mares with foals at foot. Some stallions may be provided with their own 'stallion handler' to remain with the animal at all times during its hospitalization. There are chemical sprays that can be applied to the handler to calm horses, though these have variable success. It is advised that donkeys are housed with a companion and, consequently, stables must be of a suitable size to allow for this (see Chapter 12).

Patients requiring special consideration

Some patients admitted to the hospital may be critically ill or have conditions that may require them to be hospitalized in a separate area from other patients. Patients that are suspected of having, or proven to have, a contagious disease may need to be admitted for hospitalization. Physical segregation of the patient into a self-contained ward will eliminate the potential for transmission of a contagious disease to other patients via contact between animals. Barrier nursing of the patient will need to be implemented to prevent spread of infection. (See also Chapters 5 and 12.)

Patients that are admitted due to seizure activity, whether continuous as in status epilepticus or intermittent, should be hospitalized in an area that is quiet and, preferably, dimly lit. Frequent or continuous monitoring of the patient will be required, and the area should not be too remote from other personnel and assistance.

Seriously ill patients and those with potentially life-threatening conditions (e.g. pneumothorax, severe haemorrhage, gastric torsion volvulus (GVD)) should be admitted directly into an area where immediate attention can be given. These patients may require one-to-one constant nursing, as changes in their condition may occur quickly, and they often require high levels of nursing care (see Chapter 21).

Assessment of the patient

On admittance, patients will normally have had a full history taken to gain as much information about the patient as is available. A thorough physical examination, as described below, will allow useful information to be gained on the animal's physical status and will provide baseline parameters, such as temperature, respiratory rate, heart rate and pulse quality. During the patient's stay these parameters will be re-evaluated at regular intervals. All observations made should be recorded and these will form part of the patient's general hospital care record (see Chapter 16). Patients with an apparently obvious disease should still undergo a full examination and assessment of every body system, as concurrent issues may be identified. Treatment and nursing plans will address all areas of the patient, not just the specific illness or injury identified (see Chapter 14).

Initial observation

The patient should initially be observed from afar; mental alertness, response to surroundings, body posture, gait, body condition, and coat quality can all be assessed in this way. The observation of the equine patient should begin from standing outside the stable (Figure 15.3) or before entering a horsebox. The animal's environment, kennel or stable, will also provide useful information as to its condition and any changes since it was last observed.

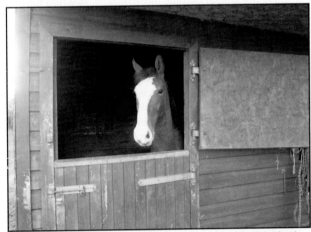

15.3   Horses should first be observed from outside the stable. In this case the horse is standing, bright and alert, aware and interested in the observer.

Respiration rate and effort should be noted prior to any restraint of the patient, as excitement and nervousness may produce inaccurate rates. Heart rate may also be elevated by an autonomic response to a stressful situation. Measuring the respiration rate of cats, rabbits and small mammals may be possible while they are still contained in carrying baskets, if they are settled prior to examination.

Patient mentation

The patient's mental state should be considered as much as parameters such as temperature, pulse and respiration. Although this assessment is subjective to the person assessing the animal, improvement or deterioration in the patient's condition may be detected. Bright, alert and responsive (BAR) or quiet, alert and responsive (QAR) are basic terms that can be noted on the patient's records. Some animals may appear to be withdrawn and quiet in a kennelled environment; this may be due to fear, stress or pain. Variations in species, breed and age must be considered.

- Observation of mentation in exotic species such as reptiles is hard to assess, as interaction with humans is usually limited.
- Small mammals, such as hamsters, rabbits and guinea pigs, and also birds are more sociable and may be used to interaction with humans, and changes in demeanour and behaviour can be recognized more easily.
- A normal horse should be bright, alert and responsive to its surroundings and to its handlers. Horses will rarely lie down whilst there is activity in their environment and most horses will spend a large proportion of their time, given the option, in grazing or eating activities. A normal horse will move around its stable regularly and with ease.

The patient's response to stimulation should be assessed.

Response to stimulation
- Does the animal respond to the observer's presence?
- Does the animal respond to verbal communication (if appropriate for the species)?
- Is the animal more responsive outside exercising than sitting in its kennel/cage?
- Does the animal become more responsive when food is offered?
- Does the animal respond to contact, such as grooming?

By assessing the response to these situations, more information can be obtained about the animal and an assessment made. This information should be reassessed, at least once a day, and any changes noted. **Patients with neurological conditions such as head trauma or brain tumours must be assessed for changes in mentation much more frequently,** as subtle changes could indicate that fatal deterioration is occurring (see Chapter 21).

Young animals

Depending upon their species and age, small animal neonates will tend to have cycles of activity (eating, playing, urinating, defecating) interspersed with periods of (often deep) sleep. Careful observation is necessary to ensure that a normal pattern is followed.

The behaviour of a foal is usually quite different to that of an adult horse. A young foal should follow a frequently repeated cycle of suckling from the mare, urination and recumbent sleep. **Deviation from this normal pattern of activity is often an indicator of abnormality; under these circumstances a veterinary surgeon should be involved without delay.** The monitoring of all hospitalized foals, whether they are patients or are merely accompanying a mare that is a patient, is important. Consideration must be given not only to normal behaviours, as described above, but also to denying the foal access to a mare's oral medication, ensuring limb health in young foals if the mare cannot be turned out and to gastric ulcer prophylaxis.

Environmental observations

Prior to cleaning out patient accommodation, the nurses should first observe the kennel or stable for signs of abnormality. These may include obvious signs (e.g. the presence of vomit or diarrhoeal faeces in a patient with gastrointestinal problems) or less obvious ones (e.g. disturbed bedding and litter trays in animals known to be at risk of neurological signs). The presence of faeces, urine, uneaten food and remaining water should all be recorded.

For horses, environmental observations should include the condition of the bed (noting any excessive disruption) and any indicators of disturbance to the stable (including any fresh damage to the stable construction or signs of faecal contamination to the stable walls). The patient's bed will usually need to be disturbed by the observer to assess urinary output. Faecal output can be easily monitored by noting the nature and volume. It would be normal to expect to find several piles of faeces in the stable in the morning and an easily observable wet patch of urine. It is important also to note how much feed has been consumed (based on a knowledge of what has been given) and how much water has been drunk (by observing the water bucket).

Physical examination

A methodical approach should be taken to ensure that a thorough examination is performed and a thorough record made. Following the general overview of the patient, as above, the 'hands on' examination may then start with the animal's head and progress towards the tail region. A physical examination chart can be used as a visual reminder to ensure that all areas of the patient are assessed and information recorded; an example for an equine patient is given at the end of this chapter.

Handling and restraint

Handling techniques for dogs, cats, horses and exotic pets are described in Chapter 10 and should be adopted fully for the safety of both the animal and handler. The physical examination of small mammals, birds and reptiles requires special consideration, as many of these patients may not be used to regular handling. These patients will be susceptible to stress from travelling to the hospital, change in environment and being handled in an unfamiliar way. In horses, gentle restraint with a head collar should be used; however, a bridle or a bit may be necessary, particularly if a horse is examined outside its stable. A gentle yet confident approach should be adopted to complete the examination thoroughly and quickly.

Head and oral cavity
Head

The patient's head posture should be upright, with no deviation to either side (no head tilt). The musculature of the head should be symmetrical and normal for the species and breed. The surface of the skull, periorbital area, zygomatic arches, maxilla and mandibles should be palpated for any abnormalities such as masses or swelling. Patients with suspected head trauma should be examined carefully, as any inadvertent depression of skull fractures may result in brain compression. Cheek pouches of hamsters should be examined to ensure that they are not impacted.

Nares and upper respiratory tract

The nares should be slightly moist with no discharge. Airflow should be patent through each nostril (a few cotton wool fibres can be held in front of each nostril and observed for movement). Cats and rabbits are obligate nasal breathers and mouth breathing for these species often indicates severe respiratory compromise.

Upper respiratory noise, **stertor** (noise on inspiration; snoring) and **stridor** (noise on expiration), can often indicate partial obstruction of the airway. Some breeds of dog, e.g. Cavalier King Charles Spaniels, are particularly predisposed to airway problems such as elongated soft palates. Horses that may have undergone upper airway surgery to improve performance may present with an unusual sounding whinny. Horses suffering upper respiratory tract abnormalities may present with whistling or roaring noises on inspiration, normally during fast exercise. Expiratory noises, such as gurgling, may suggest epiglottic or soft palate abnormalities, or an upper respiratory tract infection.

Oral cavity

The jaws should be able to be opened without difficulty and examined for any misalignment; the tongue, teeth and oral cavity can then be inspected.

The tongue should be examined for any ulcerated areas; rabbits especially can develop ulcers due to cheek teeth malocclusion. Gentle examination can be performed using an auriscope to view such lesions and the teeth edges (Figure 15.4). Lacerations and masses may also be seen when examining the tongue. Teeth should be examined for evidence of

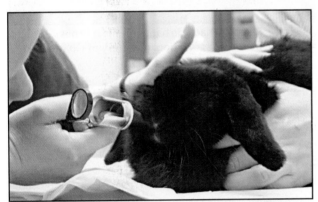

15.4   Using an auriscope to examine the mouth in a conscious rabbit. (Photography by J. Bosley; © Quantock Veterinary Hospital).

dental disease, such as tartar, bleeding or receding gums, odour and fractured or missing teeth. The hard and soft palate should be inspected for congenital deformities, such as cleft palate in neonates, wounds and foreign bodies.

The skin and hair around the mandible should be examined for signs of excess salivation (indicative of dental problems in small mammals) or skin fold pyoderma, which is often seen in breeds with large or excessive skin folds, such as St Bernards and Springer Spaniels.

The examination of the equine mouth is described in Chapter 10; excess salivation, pain or dropping of food (quidding), should all be noted. Dental disease and treatment in small animals is covered in Chapter 27.

Mucous membranes

The mucous membranes of the oral cavity can provide important information on several body systems of the patient. The gums and insides of the lips should feel moist; dry or tacky membranes can indicate dehydration (Figure 15.5).

Generally, mucous membranes should be pink (Figure 15.6), indicating good blood perfusion to the patient's peripheral tissues. Some healthy animals have pigmented mucous membranes; e.g. Chow Chows have almost completely dark pigmented mucous membranes and tongue, which is usual for the breed. **Mucous membranes in healthy cats are noticeably paler than in healthy dogs.** In horses, abnormal mucous membrane colour may be associated with endotoxaemia, purpura haemorrhagica and other medical disorders.

Mucous membrane colour

- **Pale** membranes are indicative of poor perfusion; this may be seen in patients with circulatory collapse, haemorrhage, anaemia or severe vasoconstriction.
- **Red** ('congested') membranes (Figure 15.7) may indicate sepsis, fever, congestion, causes of extensive tissue damage or excitement.
- **Blue or purple** membranes (cyanosis) indicate severe hypoxaemia (lack of oxygen in the blood); this could be caused by respiratory difficulty, and immediate action must be taken to increase the patient's oxygen saturation.
- **Yellow** membranes (icterus/jaundice) may be due to liver disease, bile flow obstruction or an increase in red blood cell destruction and circulating bilirubin, or by neonatal isoerythrolysis in equine neonates. Clinically normal horses at grass may occasionally appear to have icteric mucous membranes.

continues ▶

Estimation of dehydration (% bodyweight)	Moisture status of mucous membranes	Skin turgor	Capillary refill time (CRT)	Eye position	Heart rate
<5%	Moist	Normal	1–2 seconds	Normal	Normal rate
5–8%	Tacky	Slight tenting	Slightly prolonged	Slightly sunken	Normal to slight tachycardia
8–10%	Dry	Moderate tenting	Prolonged	Sunken within orbit	Tachycardia
10–12%	Dry	Tenting remains in place	Prolonged >2 seconds	Sunken within orbit	Tachycardia and signs of shock
12–15%	Dry	Tenting remains in place	Prolonged >2 seconds	Sunken within orbit	Shock, collapse, unconsciousness, death

15.5   Physical examination indicators used to estimate hydration status.

continued

- **Orange** membranes may be seen after administration of synthetic haemoglobin products.
- **Chocolate brown** mucous membranes in dogs and cats are indicative of paracetamol poisoning. Cats are unable to metabolize paracetamol and toxicity therefore occurs after consumption of even low doses.
- **Cherry red** membranes are seen in patients suffering from carbon monoxide poisoning, for example as a result of exposure to car exhaust or fire fumes.

Petechiae may be observed on the mucous membranes of patients with clotting disorders such as von Willebrand's disease or with rodenticide poisoning; these pinpoint, round purplish spots are caused by submucosal haemorrhage (Figure 15.8).

Capillary refill time

Capillary refill time (CRT) is a very useful guide to a patient's circulation status. Pressure is applied to the patient's gum, preferably above the canine tooth (usually the incisor or canine teeth in horses), with a clean finger; this will push the blood out of the capillaries, causing a blanching of the tissue (Figure 15.9). The time is then noted for the pink colour to return to the tissue. A normal CRT is 1–2 seconds. Prolonged times can indicate poor perfusion due to hypovolaemia, dehydration (see Figure 15.5), heart failure or shock. Patients with severe sepsis and fever may demonstrate a fast CRT.

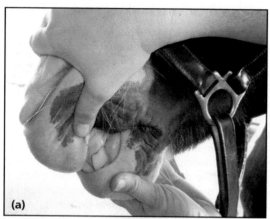

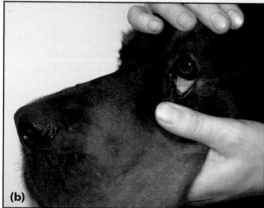

15.6 **(a)** Normal pink gingival mucous membranes in a horse. **(b)** Normal pink conjunctival mucous membranes in a dog.

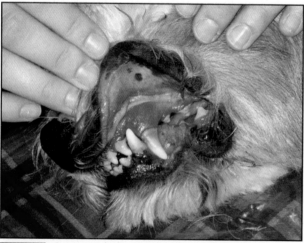

15.7 Congested mucous membranes due to polycythaemia. (Courtesy of N. Whitley)

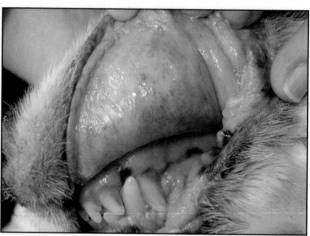

15.8 Petechial haemorrhages on the mucous membranes of a dog. (Courtesy of I. Battersby)

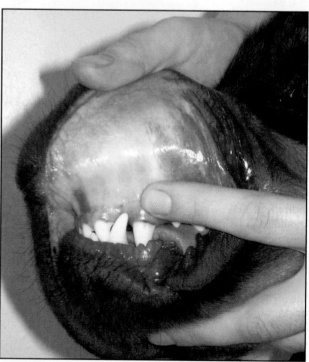

15.9 Capillary refill time is assessed by first applying finger pressure to the gum above the canine tooth, then releasing it.

Eyes

The ocular surface is very delicate and the smallest scratch can develop into a painful ulcer. Examination of the eyes must be performed gently, and the surface of the cornea must not be touched.

The patient's eyes should be open, with no squinting of the eyelids (**blepharospasm**). Both eyes should be of the same size and neither eye should protrude more than the other; an enlarged globe may be indicative of glaucoma, a condition where intraocular pressure is raised. Eyes that are sunken within the orbits may be seen in patients suffering from dehydration (see Figure 15.5) or in patients with excessive muscle wastage, as seen in cachexic patients.

Exophthalmos is the term used to describe an abnormal protrusion of the globe. It may be seen with orbital masses or abscesses in small mammals with dental disease. **Proptosis** (prolapse of the globe) is a condition that requires urgent veterinary attention to preserve the eye (see Chapter 21).

Observation should be made of any discharge from the eyes. In all species **conjunctivitis** may be caused by bacterial, viral, fungal or parasitic infection. The presence of foreign bodies, such as grass awns, or even irritation by flies may lead to ocular inflammation and discharge. Consistency of the discharge and which eye is affected should be noted; cleaning of the discharge may need to be postponed until the clinician has examined the patient. This can be particularly important if the patient has undergone recent intraocular surgery, as a clear discharge may indicate leakage of fluid from the anterior chamber of the globe if sutures have failed. Ocular discharge in small mammals can indicate dental problems. Tear duct orientation can be affected by the abnormal growth of cheek teeth and incisor roots, producing abnormal tear flow (increased or reduced) and purulent discharge from the tear ducts.

Irritation can also be caused to the ocular surface by abnormal anatomy of the eyelids. **Entropion** (internal rotation of the eyelid margins) and **ectropion** (outwards rotation) can lead to inflammation of the cornea (**keratitis**). Corneal ulceration can also be caused by the presence of **distichia**, an additional row of eyelashes that rub against the globe.

The third eyelid or **nictitating membrane** should be assessed; this fold of conjunctiva is attached to the medial canthus and moves across the eye when the eyelids are closed. In normal healthy patients it is normally not visible, but may become obvious if the globe is depressed within the orbit, as can be seen with dehydration. Unwell cats often have a visible nictitating membrane and this as a non-specific sign of ill health.

Size and location of the pupil should be assessed. Pupils should be of the same size; unequal pupils (**anisocoria**) can indicate abnormal neurological signs (Figure 15.10). Pupils should respond to a pupillary light reflex; normal pupils will constrict in the presence of a bright light being shone into them and then return to normal when the light is withdrawn. In horses, it may be possible to identify an additional fold (usually seen as small almost circular bodies) to the iris called the corpora nigra. It is thought that this additional tissue may contribute to the amount of light that enters the equine eye.

Ocular conjunctiva can be used to assess mucous membrane colour (see Figure 15.6b); this may be useful in patients with pigmented oral membranes.

Ocular sclera can be examined for abnormal coloration, such as jaundice/icterus (Figure 15.11) or haemorrhage (Figure 15.12).

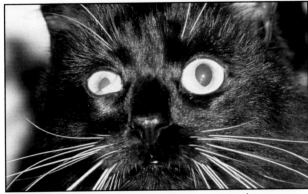

15.10 Anisocoria in a cat with Horner's syndrome. (Courtesy of Dr D. Gould)

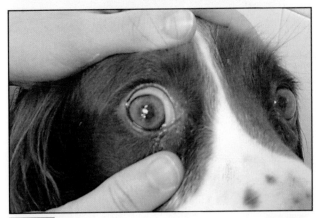

15.11 Icteric sclera in a dog. (Courtesy of I. Battersby)

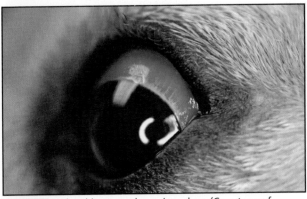

15.12 Scleral haemorrhage in a dog. (Courtesy of Dr N. Whitley)

Lymph nodes

Peripheral lymph nodes (see Chapter 3) should be palpated for evidence of enlargement. Submandibular, prescapular and popliteal nodes can normally be located in the dog and cat; axillary and inguinal nodes may only be palpable when enlarged. In the horse, the retropharyngeal lymph nodes are also commonly increased in size when respiratory infection is present.

Rabbits have smaller lymph nodes than dogs and cats and they may be palpable in the prescapular, submandibular and popliteal areas. Reptiles and most bird species do not have recognizable lymph nodes, although lymphatic tissue is found within internal organs. Lymphadenopathies (diseases of the lymph nodes) produce enlargement and may indicate infection or neoplasia, which may be localized or systemic.

Ears, skin, hair and feathers

Ears

Ear pinnae should be examined for scratches, wounds and swelling, such as haematoma. The vertical ear canal can be checked for signs of inflammation (Figure 15.13), wax, purulent discharge, foreign bodies, and ectoparasites (see Chapter 7) such as ear mites. Rabbits are prone to ear mites (*Psoroptes cuniculi*), which may result in large accumulations of exudative crusts within the ear canal. Horses may also occasionally be infected with psoroptic mites. Odour may be indicative of infections such as *Malassezia* and *Pseudomonas*.

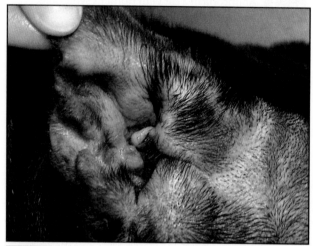

15.13   Otitis externa in a dog. (Courtesy of J. Bray)

Skin

In mammals, overall haircoat quality can be assessed in the initial evaluation of the patient from afar. Areas of thinner coat or hair loss (**alopecia**) may be identified and may be signs of endocrine disease. Syrian hamsters can have darkly pigmented areas on their flanks due to glandular secretions; older animals may also have an area of alopecia over this area, which is normal. In comparison, an unusually long and curly coat on older ponies may be indicative of equine Cushing's disease, an endocrine condition caused by a degenerative disease of the brainstem that brings about the overproduction of cortisone from the adrenal gland. Equine patients showing areas of thinner or patchy hair loss must be considered with caution, as this could be a sign of a fungal infection.

The skin should be examined for dryness, scaliness, greasiness and evidence of macroscopic ectoparasite infestation, such as fleas, flea dirt, lice and ticks (see Chapter 7).

In birds, feathers should be examined for evidence of damage, areas of missing feathers or irregular moulting. The skin should be examined for wounds, inflammation and signs of infection, such as pustules and redness. Microscopic ectoparasites, such as demodectic, chorioptic and sarcoptic mites, may cause skin lesions that will require further diagnostic procedures (see Chapter 19).

Evaluation of skin elasticity can give an indication on the animal's hydration status. A normally hydrated animal's skin will fall back into place when released. Skin tenting indicates a degree of dehydration; elasticity of the skin and return to the normal position will reduce as the dehydration worsens (see Figure 15.5).

Forelimbs

The patient's degree of movement and gait may indicate areas that require further investigation. In small animals, the range of movement, flexion, extension and rotation of the forelimbs should be noted, as well as any muscle wastage (**atrophy**). The limbs and joints should be gently palpated for signs of discomfort, swelling and abnormal sounds (**crepitus**) that might indicate dislocation or fracture. The feet, pads and claws should be examined for wounds, abrasions and foreign bodies. Frayed and torn nails may indicate involvement in road traffic accidents. **Proprioception** tests may be performed to evaluate the animal's neurological function.

In horses, the dorsal wall of the hoof should be palpated for assessment of increased heat, which may be found in patients suffering from conditions such as laminitis, fracture of the pedal bone or penetration of the navicular bursa by a foreign body. Digital pulses should be assessed by palpation of the palmar digital arteries (see 'Pulse' below). A general assessment of any abnormal swellings in the limbs should be made. Once this has been done with the horse standing, the case-specific observations (such as assessment of lameness) should be carried out. This is normally observed by walking the horse over a short distance from the stable, if it is safe and appropriate to do so. Specific signs of limb pain are listed under 'Pain assessment', see later.

Thorax

Respiration rate and effort can be recorded if not previously assessed prior to the physical examination. Examination of the thorax should include palpation of the thoracic vertebrae, sternum and ribs. In horses it is vital that the animal's rug is removed daily to make accurate observations.

The ease of **palpation** of the ribs is often used as an indication of an animal's body condition; only gentle palpation should be necessary. Palpation of the ribs in an overweight patient will prove difficult, or unachievable, without an increased amount of digital pressure being applied.

The **heartbeat** can be located between ribs three and six, on the left side of the ventral chest; in horses this is just behind the elbow in the region of the girth. Auscultation of the heart and lungs can be performed using a stethoscope (see below). Palpation of the heartbeat may be carried out in small mammals, cats and smaller dogs with narrow chests. Auscultation of the lung fields should be performed to detect abnormal lung sounds, such as **crackles** and **rales**, which may indicate thoracic pathology such as pneumonia, pulmonary oedema or bronchitis (see later).

Abdomen

The abdomen should be assessed visually for distension. Ascitic fluid or haemorrhage within the abdominal cavity, gas within the stomach, a gravid (pregnant) uterus or very full bladder may all cause the abdomen to appear distended.

In small animals, gentle **palpation** can be performed to evaluate the cause of the distension. Light pressure is applied using flattened fingers, with one hand on either side of the abdomen; internal structures may be located. Abnormal structures, masses and painful or tender areas may be detected in this way. Deeper internal organs, such as kidneys, liver and intestines, can also be palpated, although care should be taken with the amount of pressure applied. Patients that are tense or obese may be difficult to assess. Mammary tissue may also be palpated for abnormalities. In horses, the abdomen should additionally be assessed by auscultation (see below) of intestinal sounds.

Care is required when handling the abdomen of birds; a lack of diaphragm means that the abdominal muscles are required for respiration and so constriction of a bird's abdomen during restraint for examination could restrict its ability to breathe.

Pelvis and hindlimbs

In small animals, the patient's gait and the range of movement of its hindlimbs should be observed. Musculature, flexion, extension and rotation of the limb should be noted. The limbs and joints are palpated for signs of discomfort or swelling (see 'Forelimbs'). Popliteal lymph nodes can be palpated on the caudal aspect of the limb within the gastrocnemius muscle caudal to the stifle. The femoral pulse can be palpated on the medial aspect of the hindlimb as the femoral artery passes over the proximal femur. The skin of the medial hindlimbs and ventral abdomen should be examined for signs of irritation that could be associated with ectoparasites or soiling.

The hindlimbs of horses should be examined as described above for the forelimbs. It is important to observe or palpate equine limbs for any obvious soft tissue swellings or heat in the region of the tendons and ligaments, as well as checking for any joint or tendon sheath distension; these should be noted and reported immediately.

The limbs of birds should be examined for evidence of raised keratinous scales or swollen toes, which may indicate diseases such as 'scaly leg' or 'bumble foot', which require treatment.

Tail

The tail should be examined to ensure that voluntary movement is present, and that there are no wounds or damage to the tail tip. Lizards must never be restrained by their tails, as shedding of the tail (**autotomy**) is a protective mechanism in some species. The tail tips of rats and mice can also be easily damaged through inappropriate handling (see Chapter 10). Some small mammals and birds have a glandular area just above the tail that can appear greasy; this is normal for these species. The 'dock' of a horse (the area at the top of the tail) should be checked for any signs of irritation or tissue inflammation.

Anus and perineum

The anus should be examined for signs of soiling, discharge or disease, such as masses or furunculosis. Anal glands situated on either side of the anus in carnivores should be examined for signs of swelling or infection. The area of the perineum should be examined for signs of inflammation or swelling, as may be seen with perineal ruptures. Hamsters that have 'wet tail' will have evidence of wetness and diarrhoea around the perianal area. The patient's rectal temperature could be taken at this stage (see below).

Reproductive organs

External genitalia should be examined; small mammals should be supported correctly during examination to prevent spinal injuries. Entire male animals should have two descended testes within the scrotum; the penis should be examined for injuries or abnormal discharge. The sheath of a gelding or stallion should be regularly checked for any abnormalities, such as swelling or discharge.

Female animals should be examined for discharge or swelling of the vulva. In the bitch, vaginal discharge is associated with the normal reproductive cycle, and swelling of the vulva will also be obvious in stages of the oestrous cycle. Abnormal discharges should be noted; purulent discharge in entire middle-aged bitches may be associated with an infection of the uterus (**pyometra**). Imminent parturition can be indicated by clear or blood-stained discharge in the bitch and by brown discharge in the queen, whereas a discharge that is green/black and odorous may indicate the death of unborn fetuses or postpartum infection (see Chapter 26). The genital openings of mares should be observed for any obvious discharge or swelling, as this may be indicative of infection. It is important to note that some breeding mares may have undergone Caslick's surgery (suturing of the vulva due to poor conformational structure) and these sutures may be encountered during routine clinical examination. Again careful observation for swelling and discharge is required and it is important that the sutures are removed before foaling.

Rabbits with myxomatosis have oedema (swelling) of the anal and genital openings. In birds that are egg-bound, palpation of the egg may be possible if it is within the lower reproductive tract. Prolapse of the cloaca may indicate egg-binding in snakes.

Physiological assessment

Normal bodily functions should be observed and assessed for variations and abnormal changes.

Changes in urination and thirst

Colour, smell, turbidity (cloudiness) and volume of urine should be noted on the patient's records. Urine samples should be obtained for complete analysis (see Chapter 19) when any form of urinary dysfunction is evident. Urinalysis can be performed on samples of avian urine but care must be taken to avoid contamination with the faecal portion of the dropping.

Urine production

- A dog, cat or horse with normal renal function should produce 1–2 ml/kg/h of urine; this rate will fall slightly overnight.
- Reduced urine production (**oliguria**) may be due to conditions such as dehydration, hypovolaemia and acute renal failure; a volume of <0.5 ml/kg/h should be investigated and intravenous fluid therapy may need to be instigated.

Accurate measurement of urine production can only be achieved by placement of an indwelling urinary catheter and collecting system. Lack of urine production (**anuria**) can be very serious; causes such as damage to the urinary tract, a ruptured bladder or urinary obstruction (seen with urolithiasis, i.e. urinary stones and calculi) and acute renal failure, can lead to other metabolic abnormalities that may be life-threatening. Patients may be observed to have difficulty urinating (**dysuria**). Urine should be passed freely with no straining or discomfort.

Urine appearance

The colour and consistency of urine produced should be noted.

- Blood in the urine (**haematuria**) may be visible; cystitis, trauma to the urinary tract, neoplasia and infection may all be possible causes.
- Rabbit urine contains plant pigments (porphyrins) that cause the colour of normal urine to vary from dark yellow to red; this can be mistaken for haematuria.
- Guinea pig urine is pigmented yellow and cloudy, as is urine from the female chinchilla.
- Normal equine urine appears yellow in colour, the shade varying with hydration status. The presence of calcium carbonate crystals is normal in horses and explains the cloudy appearance of the urine.

Thirst

Increased urine production (**polyuria**, PU) is usually accompanied by an increased thirst (**polydipsia**, PD). Many conditions present with both PU and PD as clinical signs, e.g. diabetes mellitus, diabetes insipidus, Cushing's disease and pyometra. Some medications, such as corticosteroids, will also make a patient become 'PU/PD'.

Voluntary water intake will vary with species and the diet fed to each animal. The maintenance water requirement for dogs, cats and horses is noted as 50 ml/kg/24 h. This can be used to estimate the amount of water each patient should consume a day.

Patients suspected of being polydipsic should have their water consumption measured. A measured amount of water is offered to the animal and replaced when drunk; a chart can be kept to record the total amount of water drunk over a specific period of time (normally 12 or 24 hours). Periods of exercise, and quantity and type of food eaten should also be recorded and taken into consideration when totalling the quantity of water drunk.

Changes in defecation

The amount and consistency of faeces passed by the patient should be observed and recorded.

Faecal appearance

Normal faeces vary considerably between species, especially in exotic pets (Figure 15.14).

Examination of colour, smell, shape and consistency can be done macroscopically.

- Black faeces (**melaena**) can indicate bleeding into the upper gastrointestinal tract.
- Fresh blood in faeces (**haematochezia**) is indicative of bleeding occurring in the lower bowel.

Further, microscopic, investigation may be required to assess the presence of microorganisms and parasites (see Chapters 8 and 19).

Diarrhoea

Diarrhoea is an increase in liquidity of faeces, which are normally passed more frequently. Some patients may appear systemically well apart from passing loose faeces. The causes of diarrhoea are multiple and include irritation of the intestinal mucosa, dietary causes, inflammatory conditions, bacterial infections (e.g. *Escherichia coli*, *Campylobacter*), endoparasites and viral diseases (e.g. parvovirus infection). Patients suspected of having an infectious or zoonotic cause for the diarrhoea must be barrier nursed to prevent cross-contamination to other patients and to staff handling the patient; all contaminated bedding materials must be thoroughly washed and contaminated and faeces disposed of in the correct manner. Stress can also be a contributing factor in hospitalized animals developing diarrhoea. Diarrhoea may originate from either the large or the small intestine.

Patients with diarrhoea should be given plenty of opportunities to go outside, as many will not want to soil their beds. Patients should be kept clean, and regular examination of the anus and perineal region is required to ensure that the animal does not become soiled as this can lead to skin sores. Good hygiene protocols should be implemented to avoid cross-contamination.

Dehydration can occur due to the increased fluid loss with each motion; intravenous fluid therapy may be required (this is especially important in small mammals such as rabbits and in equine neonates), as well as analgesia and spasmolytic agents for patients with abdominal pain.

Constipation

Constipation is difficulty in passing faeces, which can lead to straining (**tenesmus**). Hard and dry faecal material may build up within the colon or rectum, causing **impaction**. Constipation may be caused by many factors including ingestion of foreign material (e.g. bones and hair), drug treatment, and neoplasia. Environmental factors, such as changes in routine for dogs and

Patient type	Appearance of normal faeces	Appearance of abnormal faeces	Possible causes of abnormality
Rabbits	Round dry pellets or soft, mucus-covered caecotrophs	Presence of dark and sticky caecotrophs around anus; diarrhoea or loose faeces	Enteritis; change in diet; lack of consumption of caecotrophs may indicate illness/intestinal stasis
Guinea pigs	Oval pellets (medium to dark brown); caecotrophs (aromatic greenish pellets)	Clumped pellets; smaller pellets; pitted pellets; diarrhoea	Reduced food intake; intestinal bacterial overgrowth; parasitic or bacterial infection
Hamsters	Small, oval, brown pellets, moist to dry	Soft consistency; diarrhoea around anus and/or abdomen	Insufficient foods high in moisture, such as greens and fruit; proliferative ileitis ('wet tail')
Birds	Three components: urine (clear, watery portion); solid urate (white); faeces (colour dependent on diet, light brown to black in liquid or tubular form)	Colour change of urate to yellow or green; diarrhoea	May indicate malnutrition or liver disease; change in diet; endoparasites
Reptiles	Formed faeces with chalky, solid urates (urinary waste)	Diarrhoea	*Salmonella*; endoparasites

15.14   Characteristics of normal and abnormal faeces from some exotic pets.

outside cats having to use litter trays, may also stop the animal from passing faeces.

Variation in faecal output in horses can occur associated with: hospitalization, where there is reduced access to exercise; eating stabled bedding; or a change in the fibre content of the diet. These can ultimately lead to impaction. Reduced faecal output may also be associated with medical and surgical conditions, including the various causes of colic and grass sickness.

Changes in appetite

A change in the patient's appetite is commonly encountered in hospitalized animals. Changes in environment and routine, disease processes, medication and diet offered, may all cause alterations in the animal's feeding patterns. Loss of appetite (**inappetence**) may often be the first sign an owner notices to indicate that their pet is unwell. There are many reasons that an animal may not eat.

- Dental disease is a common cause of inappetence in cats, dogs, rabbits and horses.
- Difficulty in eating (**dysphagia**) may be due to pain, ulceration or trauma to the mouth.
- Nausea and loss of smell due to nasal disease may be a significant factor, especially in the cat, as this is an important factor when encouraging a patient to eat.

Disease processes such as unstable diabetes mellitus and hyperthyroidism in cats will give them a voracious appetite. Medication such as corticosteroids will also increase appetite, as well as thirst.

Pica is the name given to the craving of unnatural foodstuffs, such as cotton wool, sawdust shavings or faeces (**coprophagia**). The eating of these unusual items may be due to a dietary imbalance, but may just be an unwanted behaviour trait.

Occurrence of vomiting

It is important to determine whether a patient is vomiting or regurgitating. Patients that are suspected of either should be observed frequently, as both vomiting and regurgitation have the risk of the patient aspirating food particles or fluid that could lead to aspiration pneumonia.

- **Vomiting** is the forceful evacuation of stomach contents through the mouth, with active retching and abdominal contractions. Patients often demonstrate signs of nausea, such as hypersalivation and licking their lips, prior to vomiting. Common causes of vomiting include gastric foreign bodies, gastritis, gastric dilatation, poisons and systemic disease such as renal and hepatic failure or pancreatitis.
- **Regurgitation** is the passive movement of food and or liquid back into the mouth with no warning. Regurgitation may occur due to megaoesophagus, oesophagitis, oesophageal strictures or vascular ring anomaly.

Many small animals and exotic pets, as well as the equine species, are physically unable to vomit. Some conditions of the equine patient may lead to the passage of stomach contents out of the stomach with exit via the nose; this process is termed **spontaneous nasogastric reflux** and these cases should be investigated thoroughly as a matter of urgency.

- Rabbits, guinea pigs and rats are unable to vomit.
- The movement of food from within a hamster's pouch may be mistaken for regurgitation.
- Birds can both vomit partially digested or digested food

from the proventriculus and regurgitate food from the crop. Vomiting is abnormal for birds, whereas regurgitation may be normal behaviour.

- Lizards are able to regurgitate/vomit food; this may occur due to illness or be because the food is too large or spoiled. Stresses, such as disturbing or moving the animal soon after eating, may induce a lizard to regurgitate/vomit (the exact process may be hard to differentiate and may be judged by the time after feeding).

The amount and frequency of the vomiting episodes should be noted, and vomitus should be examined for blood and evidence of foreign materials. Vomit may contain more than just food stuff and bile. Vomiting of material that contains blood is known as **haematemesis**. Forceful projectile vomiting without retching is indicative of pyloric obstruction. The vomiting of faecal matter is termed **stercoraceous** vomiting. Excessive vomiting can be very tiring and distressing for the patient; nurses should ensure that the animal is kept clean and their mouth is gently cleaned. Vomiting can cause severe electrolyte disturbances and patients will often require intravenous fluid therapy and electrolyte supplementation.

Patients that are regurgitating should be observed to detect whether there is any pattern to the time they regurgitate. Food material may remain within the oesophagus for an extended period of time after eating.

The nursing management of the vomiting patient is described further in Chapters 17 and 20.

Occurrence of coughing

Patients that are presented with coughing should first be assessed to ensure that it is not of a contagious origin (e.g. kennel cough in dogs, herpesvirus infection or influenza in the horse); such patients, if admitted, will require isolation. The cough reflex is initiated by sensitivity of the respiratory mucosa and is used for clearing the respiratory passages of foreign matter. Inflammation and irritation can also induce a cough reflex. In horses, non-infectious lower respiratory tract diseases such as chronic obstructive pulmonary disease (COPD) may result in coughing. These are usually caused by a hypersensitivity to the environment, particularly to fungal spores and other small particles in stable bedding and hay, or may be associated with summer allergies in horses at grass.

Certain conditions are associated with coughing, such as right-sided heart failure, canine distemper, bronchitis, lungworm and collapsing trachea. Types of cough can vary and patients should be observed to distinguish whether the cough is moist and productive, or harsh and dry. Patients that develop a cough while hospitalized should be reported to the clinician immediately, especially if they are receiving intravenous fluid therapy or have a condition such as megaoesophagus and are prone to regurgitation. If an infectious cause is suspected, the patient must be isolated immediately. Pulmonary oedema and inspiration pneumonia may be possible causes of unexpected coughing. Coughing may be associated with other changes in respiration (see below).

Pain assessment

The stress that may be caused to animals upon hospitalization has been discussed earlier. Uncontrolled pain should be considered as one reason why an animal may appear to be unsettled. Different species and ages of patients show signs of pain in different ways, and pain recognition can be especially difficult in 'prey' species. Pain assessment and evaluation of signs are subjective and can be challenging. Recognition of signs of pain in all species of patient is an essential role of the veterinary nurse. Pain has no positive effects for patients, and assessment and treatment of pain in the hospitalized patient is an essential part of patient care. The detrimental effects of pain will prolong a patient's recovery and the return to normal behaviour and function:

- An animal with chest pain may alter its respiratory effort
- Abdominal pain will make a patient's abdomen tense and it may be reluctant to move
- Oral pain will prevent patients from obtaining the vital nutrition they need for recovery.

Providing pain relief (analgesia) is an ethical and responsible action (see Chapter 23). Identifying pain in animals and monitoring responses to analgesic drugs can be challenging but some general indicators can be used.

Effects and signs of pain in animals:

- Increased anxiety, fear and restlessness
- Vocalization
- Subdued, depressed, lack of response to stimulation
- Reluctance to move
- Abnormal posture and movement
- Aggression
- Abnormal urination/defecation or reluctance to urinate/defecate
- Inappetence
- Wound interference and self-trauma.

In all species, good nursing measures can help to alleviate pain and suffering in patients.

- Care should be taken to provide dry, comfortable bedding that can support the patient's limbs if required.
- Padding should be used to reduce pressure on painful areas and prevent decubitus ulcer formation.
- Regular mental stimulation and changes in positioning and view can alleviate boredom for the patient.
- Discharges from eyes and nose should be cleaned, and animals that cannot groom themselves should be washed and groomed.

- Physiotherapy can be performed to improve circulation, reduce muscle cramp and promote movement (see Chapter 20); this also provides the patient with human contact and TLC.

Indicators of pain in horses include:
Abdominal pain:
- Flank watching
- Rolling
- Lip curling
- Stretching as if to urinate
- Inappetence
- Teeth grinding
- Sweating
- Lying down and getting up frequently
- Penile erection.

Limb pain:
- Observable lameness on movement
- Failure to bear weight fully
- Weight shifting
- Persistently resting a limb
- Standing with a limb persistently in an abnormal position (usually forward of its natural weight-bearing position).

Monitoring: temperature, pulse and respiration

The vital clinical signs of temperature, pulse and respiration (Figures 15.15, 15.16 and 15.17) should be regularly monitored whilst a patient is hospitalized. If the patient is nervous or unused to handling, then measurement of these parameters may be performed independent of a more general physical examination, as pulse and respiratory rates may become elevated associated with handling.

Species	Body temperature (°C)	Heart rate (beats/min)	Respiratory rate (breaths/min)
Dog	38.3–39.2	70–140	10–30
Cat	38.2–38.6	100–200	20–30
Horse	37.2–38.9	30–40	12–20
Ferret	37.8–40	200–250	33–36
Domestic rabbit	38.5–40	130–325	30–60
Chinchilla	37–38	200–350	40–80
Guinea pig	37.2–39.5	230–380	90–150
Chipmunk	38 (during torpor, a few degrees above ambient)	264–296 (during torpor, may drop to 3–6)	75 (during torpor, may drop to <1 and is barely detectable)
Gerbil	37.4–39	260–600	85–160
Hamster (Russian)	36–38	300–460	60–80
Hamster (Syrian)	36.2–37.5	300–470	40–110
Rat	38	310–500	70–150
Mouse	37.5	420–700	100–250

15.15   Normal range of vital signs in the dog, cat, horse and some common small mammal pets.

Species	Body temperature (°C)	Heart rate (beats/min)	Respiratory rate (breaths/min)
African grey parrot	40–42	100–300	15–45
Cockatiel	40–42	150–350	40–50
Lovebird	40–42	250–400	60–100
Budgerigar	40–42	260–400	60–100

15.16 Normal range of vital signs seen in some common bird species. (Values taken from Girling (2003), the *BSAVA Manual of Exotic Pets, 5th edn* and the *BSAVA Manual of Advanced Veterinary Nursing*).

Species	Preferred optimal temperature range (°C)	Heart rate (beats/min)	Respiratory rate (breaths/min)
Cornsnake	25–30	40–50	6–10
Royal python	25–30	30–50	6–10
Green iguana	26–36	30–60	10–30
Leopard gecko	23–30	40–80	20–50

15.17 Normal range of vital signs seen in some common reptile species. (Values taken from Girling (2003), the *BSAVA Manual of Exotic Pets, 5th edn* and the *BSAVA Manual of Advanced Veterinary Nursing*)

Temperature

Temperature measurement in conscious patients is usually taken rectally; some alternative sites may be used if this route is not possible due to surgical or trauma sites or due to lack of patient cooperation. The axilla and external ear canal (Figure 15.18) are alternative sites, although readings made in these areas may not be as accurate as a rectal value. Specific aural thermometers are available and can provide fast readings.

Digital thermometers (Figure 15.19) are safe and robust; disposable covers should ideally be used to avoid patient cross-contamination. Glass mercury thermometers have largely been superseded by the use of faster and safer digital thermometers. The health and safety implications of mercury thermometers should be considered if the thermometer breaks, as broken glass and leakage of mercury are hazardous. A kink in the mercury channel prevents the mercury from returning to the bulb once the temperature has been recorded and the thermometer requires 'shaking down' to return the mercury to the bulb prior to use; this is the most common time for the thermometer to be broken.

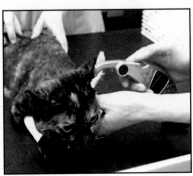

15.18 Use of an aural thermometer in a cat (Photography by J. Bosley; © Quantock Veterinary Hospital).

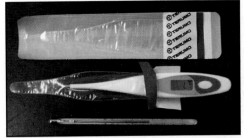

15.19 Thermometers. From the top: thermometer cover; digital thermometer with cover; mercury thermometer.

- Care should be taken when taking rectal temperatures of small mammals; adequate restraint must be used to avoid struggling by the patient causing thermometer injury.
- Birds have delicate cloacal openings and trauma to the gastrointestinal tract must be avoided.
- Reptiles are **exothermic** (see Chapter 3) and therefore rely on environmental temperature to determine their body temperature.

Procedure to record rectal temperature using a digital thermometer

1. Ensure the thermometer is clean prior to use; antibacterial wipes or dilute chlorhexidine-soaked cotton wool swabs can be used to clean the thermometer, but do **not** leave in constant soak.
2. Apply a disposable thermometer cover (if available).
3. A small amount of lubricant, such as a veterinary obstetrical gel, may be applied to the bulb of the thermometer.
4. Restrain the patient, to prevent inaccurate readings from patient movement and possible thermometer trauma.
5. For horses, the operator should stand to one side of the patient's hindlegs, while lifting the tail gently.
6. Insert the thermometer into the rectum, using a gentle twisting motion, and position the tip against the dorsal rectal wall to avoid insertion into faecal matter
7. Hold the thermometer in place for 30–60 seconds (or as recommended by the manufacturer) or until bleeping denotes a constant temperature has been recorded. **Never let go of the thermometer during the procedure.**
8. Gently remove the thermometer and clean it, or remove and discard the cover.
9. Read and record the temperature.

Interpretation of temperature measurements

Temperature can be measured in degrees Celsius (°C) or degrees Fahrenheit (°F); both values may still be used, although Celsius is now the standard unit of measurement.

Temperature conversion

- °C to °F: Multiply by 9, divide by 5, add 32
- °F to °C: Subtract 32, multiply by 5, divide by 9

An elevated temperature may be due to fever (**pyrexia**), pain or hyperthermia.

- **Fever** is caused by infectious diseases, drug reactions and neoplasia, which release pyrogens that raise the thermoregulatory set point in the hypothalamus.
- **Hyperthermia** occurs when the hypothalamic thermoregulatory set point is not changed, but mechanisms of heat loss are unable to respond to temperature rise. This occurs from high environmental temperatures (heat stroke), increased muscle activity from seizures and exercise, and increased metabolic rate from pain and stress.

A low temperature (**hypothermia**) may be seen in connection with:

- Chronic disease and illness
- Heat loss during anaesthesia and recovery
- Exposure or drowning.

Hypothermia is also seen in neonatal and paediatric patients that cannot regulate their own body temperature when environmental temperature is too low, as well as in depressed, moribund and comatose patients. It may also be due to inaccurate recording of temperature (user error).

Pulse

Assessment of pulse rate and quality will help to evaluate the efficacy and condition of an animal's cardiovascular system. Pulse waves can be palpated at areas where an artery runs close to the peripheral tissue. The rhythmical wave corresponds to blood being ejected from the left ventricle of the heart and travelling through the arterial circulation. In the dog and cat, peripheral pulses can be assessed at various sites (Figure 15.20). Palpation and recording of a pulse rate can be difficult in some patients, e.g. those that are trembling. Obtaining pulse rates from cats and small mammals can also take some practice, due to their faster pulse rates. Auscultation of the heart rate using a stethoscope can be useful in these animals.

Common pulse points in small animals

- Lingual artery – ventral surface of the tongue (not advised in the rabbit as excessive palpation of the tongue may cause swelling).
- Carpal artery – palmar aspect of carpus.
- Femoral artery – medial aspect of proximal femur.
- Coccygeal artery – ventral aspect of tail base.
- Dorsal metatarsal artery (as shown) – medial aspect of tarsus.

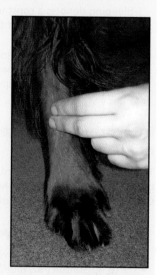

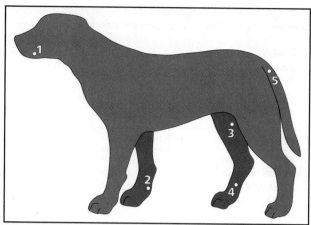

15.20 Common pulse point locations in the dog: 1. lingual; 2. carpal; 3. femoral; 4. dorsal metatarsal; 5. coccygeal.

Common pulse points in horses

- Ventral ramus of the mandible in the horse – where the facial artery passes over the angle of the jaw.

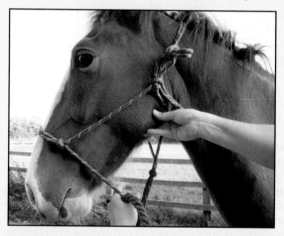

- Transverse facial artery in the horse.
- Palmar digital arteries in the horse – located medially and laterally towards the palmar aspect of the fetlock or pastern.

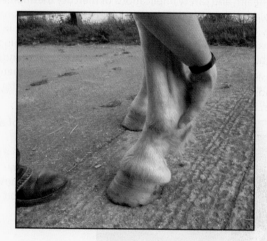

- Radial artery in the horse.

It is useful to assess the **pulse quality** (strength and speed of pulse duration), as well as rate, to detect abnormalities.

- **Sinus arrhythmia**: normal variation in pulse rate; the pulse speeds up on inspiration and decreases on expiration.
- **Tachycardia**: increased heart and pulse rate. May be seen with exercise, stress, disease processes, hypovolaemia and drug administration (e.g. atropine).
- **Bradycardia**: reduced heart and pulse rate. This is either drug-induced or is seen in animals that are asleep, extremely fit, or suffering from cardiac arrhythmias. Exotic animals in hibernation during winter will have low pulse rates.
- **Weak** pulses may indicate reduced circulating blood volume or cardiac disease.
- Pulses that are strong and jerky (**hyperdynamic**) can indicate temporary compensatory mechanisms for reduced circulating volume or certain congenital cardiac anomalies, such as patent ductus arteriosus.
- A pulse rate that does not correspond to the heart rate indicates that a **pulse deficit** is present. Electrocardiography should be performed to gain more information regarding the abnormal rhythm.

Auscultation using a stethoscope

Auscultation (listening for sounds produced within the body) is a useful skill that veterinary nurses can perform in conjunction with a physical examination. Auscultation may be performed on the heart, lung fields and abdomen. A stethoscope is routinely used to amplify the sounds and allow more detailed information to be gained when listening to subtle sounds. Abdominal auscultation can be used to determine whether intestinal peristalsis is present; absence of gut noises, especially in rabbits and horses, can be indicative of intestinal stasis.

Stethoscopes

Stethoscopes have earpieces that should sit within the operator's ears in a forward facing direction. Binaurals or ear tubes connect the earpieces to the tubing that transmits sounds from the head of the stethoscope to the earpieces. The head of the stethoscope may be double- or single-sided (Figure 15.21) and may vary in size according to the size of patient and area to be ausculta ted. Double-sided stethoscopes contain a flat diaphragm and a cup-shaped bell side. The head rotates, allowing one or the other side to be used. The flat diaphragm is used for detecting high-frequency sounds, such as the heartbeat. The cup-shaped bell side is used to detect lower pitched sounds, as may be produced by lung fields. Single-sided stethoscopes rely on a variation of pressure that is applied to the head by the user to detect differently pitched sounds: light pressure applied to the head of the stethoscope when against the animal will detect low-pitch sounds; and

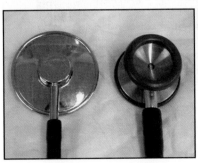

15.21 Single-sided (left) and double-sided (right) stethoscope heads.

application of firmer pressure will allow detection of higher pitched sounds. Stethoscopes can be expensive items and care should be taken that they do not become damaged. The diaphragm is fragile and can become perforated. The head of the stethoscope should be cleaned after use to avoid cross-contamination between patients; antimicrobial wipes are ideal as stethoscopes should not be submerged or soaked.

Technique

Procedure for auscultation

1. Locate the heartbeat between the third and sixth ribs on the left side of the ventral chest. In the horse, this is typically directly behind the left elbow.
2. Hold the diaphragm of the stethoscope gently against the patient's chest and move it cranially, caudally and ventrally to cover the base and apex of the heart. The heart rate should be monitored over at least 1 minute to establish a beats per minute reading. Note the rate, rhythm, intensity and clarity of the heartbeat.

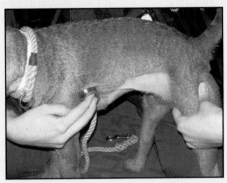

3. If physically possible, palpate the patient's pulse simultaneously to ensure that there is no pulse deficit (heart sounds with no accompanying pulse produced), as this could indicate that the patient has a cardiac arrhythmia (Figure 15.22).
4. Auscultation should also be performed from the right side of the chest – although not as clear, different heart sounds or murmurs may be heard.
5. Then auscultate the cranial and caudal lung fields, dorsally, medially and ventrally at inspiration and expiration, to detect abnormal lung sounds.

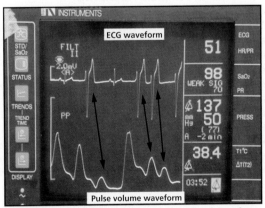

15.22 ECG trace showing reduced pulse volume associated with ventricular premature complex (VPC).

Abdominal auscultation in horses

An assessment of intestinal sounds may be conducted in a horse with a gastrointestinal problem. Familiarity with normal respiratory and intestinal sounds is important before assessing clinical patients. Note that borborygmi are an unreliable indicator of abdominal problems. Absence of sounds is potentially very serious.

Horses are routinely auscultated over four quadrants: the upper and lower right and left flank areas. These relate to specific parts of the equine gastrointestinal tract; for example, auscultation of the right side will identify sounds from the caecum. It is usual to grade the presence of intestinal sounds.

Upper left quadrant (small intestine) +++	Upper right quadrant (large intestine and caecum) +
Lower left quadrant (large intestine) ++	Lower right quadrant (large intestine) +++

+ indicates the presence of gut sounds; the more +s, the greater is the frequency of sounds recorded in the *normal* equine patient.

Respiration

The natural movement of the chest is to expand on inspiration and to contract on expiration. The number of breaths the animal takes per minute (respiratory rate), counted on either inspiration or expiration, should be recorded whilst it is in a calm state so as not to give incorrect values. The amount of effort that the patient takes to draw in one breath (tidal volume) should also be observed. A patient with respiratory difficulty may have to exert more effort to inspire, and the amount of movement made by the patient's chest will be exaggerated; abdominal movement may also be noted in animals in severe respiratory difficulty. If observed, these signs should be reported to the clinician immediately.

Abnormal respiration

- An increased respiratory rate **(tachypnoea)** may be observed in animals that are excited or following exercise. Thoracic pathology (such as pneumothorax), stress, pain and fear may be other causes.
- A reduced respiratory rate **(bradypnoea)** is seen in relaxed and sleeping patients. Brain and neck trauma can also affect an animal's ability to ventilate normally.
- Difficult or laboured breathing **(dyspnoea)** may be caused by obstruction or disease of the respiratory tract, lung pathology, increased pressure upon the diaphragm from abdominal organs, or trauma to the thorax.
- **Paradoxical** (different from what is expected) movements may result from a severe traumatic injury to the chest, where ribs become broken and free-moving from the rest of the rib cage (flail chest).

Further reading

Bowden C and Masters J (2003) *Textbook of Veterinary Medical Nursing.* Butterworth Heinemann/Elsevier, Oxford

Combe K (2001) *Equine Veterinary Nursing Manual.* Blackwell Publishing, Oxford

Girling S (2003) *Veterinary Nursing of Exotic Pets.* Blackwell Publishing, Oxford

Higgins A and Snyder J (2006) *The Equine Manual.* Elsevier Saunders, Philadelphia

Meredith A, Redrobe S and Mullineaux E (2008) General care and management of other pets and wildlife. In: *BSAVA Manual of Practical Animal Care,* ed. P Hotston Moore and A Hughes, pp.123–137. BSAVA Publications, Gloucester

Mills D. Feline pheromones and pheromonatherapy. *FAB Feline Advisory Bureau* http://www.fabcats.org/behaviour/spraying/pheromonatherapy.html

---

Self-assessment questions

1. What things should be considered in an attempt to minimize any stress when hospitalizing small animals, horses, birds and exotic animals?
2. Why is it important to perform a complete examination of the patient on admission, even if the presenting complaint is known?
3. Make a systematic list of the parts of the body to be examined in a full clinical examination.
4. What is considered to be normal mucous membrane colour? List some abnormal colours of mucous membranes and state what they might be indicative of.
5. Where is the best site for assessing capillary refill time and what information can CRT provide regarding the animal's health status?
6. What clinical parameters can be used to help assess the degree of dehydration of a patient?
7. List some causes of coughing in horses.
8. Comfort can be provided to animals using prescribed pain-relieving drugs. What other nursing methods can be employed?
9. Where might you take the pulse of a dog and a horse? What might a weak pulse indicate?
10. What methods of assessing cardiac function are included in a routine clinical examination?

Examples of client questionnaires and clinical assessment form ▶

Client Questionnaire – Canine Patients

It would be helpful if you could take a few minutes to tell us a little bit about your dog. Coming into hospital can be a stressful time, and some dogs will develop behaviours or signs that can affect our interpretation of their recovery from disease or surgery. By knowing more about your dog's general routines and personality, we will be able to care more for his/her individual needs during his/her stay with us.

Dog's name.. Your surname:...

Personality

How does your dog get on with people?..

How does your dog get on with other dogs?..

....

Is your dog shy at home?...

Does your dog get stressed easily?...

Other comments:..

....

Toilet habits

Where does your dog prefer to urinate at home?　　Anywhere ☐　　Grass ☐　　Gravel ☐　Bushes ☐

Will your dog go to the toilet when walked on lead?　　　　　　　　Yes ☐　　No ☐

Toilet command (if any)...

Other comments:..

....

Diet

What is your dog's normal diet?..

What is your dog's favourite snack?..

Would you be surprised if your dog chose not to eat while in hospital?　Yes ☐　　No ☐

How often do you feed your dog?..

Other comments:..

....

Vaccinations

Are your dog's vaccinations current?　　　　　　　　　　　Yes ☐　　No ☐

When did your dog last receive a kennel cough vaccine (given into the nose)?....................................

*Note: If your dog has **not** received kennel cough vaccination within the last six months, it is our policy to administer this to all dogs that are in sufficiently good health and are likely to stay 3 nights or more. There is no charge for this vaccination. Although this will not eliminate the chance of your dog developing kennel cough, we have found it does reduce the incidence of outbreaks within our hospital. **If you would rather your dog did NOT receive this vaccination, please speak with your clinician during the consultation.***

Example of a client questionnaire for admission of canine patients. (Courtesy of Davies Veterinary Specialists)

Client Questionnaire – Feline Patients

Coming into hospital can be a stressful time, and some cats will develop behaviours or signs that can affect our interpretation of their recovery from disease or surgery. By knowing more about your cat's general routines and personality, we will be able to care more for his/her individual needs during his/her stay with us.

We try and provide our cat patients with an environment which attempts to reduce the stress they may experience while in hospital. They are kept in a ward away from dogs, and noise in the ward is kept to a minimum. Soft classical music is also played, as this has been shown to have a calming effect. Timid cats may have a box in their cage where they can hide away if they wish. Feline pheromone sprays and 'plug-ins' are used throughout the ward as these have also been shown to reduce anxiety.

It would be helpful if you could take a few minutes to tell us a little bit about your cat.

Cat's name ....   **Your surname:**..

Personality

How does your cat get on with people?..

What type of bedding does your cat prefer?..

Does your cat like being groomed?..

Other comments:..

....

Toilet habits

Will your cat use a litter tray? ....   Yes ☐   No ☐

What type of cat litter does your cat prefer? ....   Soil ☐   Woodchip ☐   Gravel ☐

Other comments:..

....

Diet

What does your cat normally eat?..

Does your cat prefer to be offered single meals, or does he/she prefer to 'graze' through the day?................

....

What is your cat's favourite treat? ....

Does your cat drink out of a water bowl?.......................   Yes ☐   No ☐

Other comments:..

....

Vaccinations

Are your cat's vaccinations current? ....   Yes ☐   No ☐

Example of a client questionnaire for admission of feline patients. (Courtesy of Davies Veterinary Specialists)

Client Questionnaire – Equine Patients

Horse's name: ....
(If your horse is insured we <u>must</u> have the <u>correct</u> spelling of the name known to the insurance company)

Owner's Name: ....

Contact tel. no: ....

Feeding requirements:

Hay   ☐   Haylage ☐   Soaked hay ☐

Due to the fact that most lame horses are not in full work, we feed them a mixture of non-heating pasture mix and chaff. If you have any special feeding requirements please detail below:

....
....
....

Items left with horse:

Headcollar	☐	Lead rope	☐
Rugs – No.	☐	Rug description	
Saddle	☐	Bridle	☐
Stable bandages	☐	Travel bandages/boots	☐

Any other items (please detail)

....
....

N.B. If applicable, please give any information we may need to help us treat your horse, e.g. difficult to inject, kicks, bites

....
....

Example of a client questionnaire for admission of equine patients. (Courtesy of Lynn Irving, Rossdale's Diagnostic Centre)

Patient details: _____

Initial assessment:

General demeanour: Bright and alert   Quiet   Depressed
Body condition: (Emaciated)   1   2   3   4   5   (Obese)
Other comments (including scars and wounds):

Head and neck:

	Normal	Abnormal (describe)
Ears	❏	_____
Eyes	❏	_____
Facial symmetry	❏	_____
Nasal airflow	❏	_____
Nasal discharge	❏	_____
Submandibular lymph nodes	❏	_____
Jugular vein patency	❏	_____
Skin lesions/Scars	Yes/No	If yes, describe _____

Thorax:

Respiratory rate: _____ bpm

Heart rate: _____ bpm

Regular heart rhythm   Yes/No   If no, describe _____

Heart murmurs:

Left   Yes/No   If yes, describe _____

Right   Yes/No   If yes, describe _____

Auscultation of lung fields:

Left   Normal/Abnormal   If abnormal, describe _____

Right   Normal/Abnormal   If abnormal, describe _____

Evidence of a heave line?   Yes/No

Skin lesions/Scars: Yes/No   If yes, describe _____

Abdomen:

Auscultation:

Skin lesions/Scars (including previous surgical scars):   Yes/No   If yes, describe _____

Ventral oedema?   Yes/No   If yes, describe the extent _____

Perineum/Urogenital:

Rectal temperature: _____ °C

Anal tone: Normal/Abnormal

Penis/Prepuce: Normal/Abnormal   Discharge/swelling?   Describe _____

Vulva: Normal/Abnormal   Discharge/skin lesions? Describe _____

Urination: Normal/Abnormal   If abnormal, describe _____
(if observed)

Limbs:

Any effusion of synovial structures/other swellings or scars should be noted.

Forelimbs:	LEFT	RIGHT	Describe abnormalities
Shoulder/Elbow:	❏	❏	_____
Carpus	❏	❏	_____
Metacarpus – (Flexor tendons)	❏	❏	_____
Metacarpus – (Digital flexor tendon sheath)	❏	❏	_____
Fetlock	❏	❏	_____
Pastern	❏	❏	_____
Distal interphalangeal joint (coffin joint)	❏	❏	_____
Digital pulses	❏	❏	_____
Hooves	❏	❏	_____

Hindlimbs:			
Pelvic symmetry	❏	❏	_____
Stifles	❏	❏	_____
Hocks	❏	❏	_____
Metatarsus (Flexor tendons)	❏	❏	_____
Metatarsus (DFTS)	❏	❏	_____
Fetlock	❏	❏	_____
Pastern	❏	❏	_____
Distal interphalangeal joint (coffin joint)	❏	❏	_____
Digital pulses	❏	❏	_____
Hooves	❏	❏	_____

AT WALK: Any lameness present?   Yes/No   Limb(s) affected: _____   Grade: _____ /10

Signed:_____

Date:_____

Example of a clinical examination chart for an equine patient. (Courtesy of the University of Liverpool)

Chapter 16

Essential patient care

Lucy Goddard and Lynn Irving

Learning objectives

After studying this chapter, students should be able to:

- **Recognize the basic requirements for hospitalized animals**
- **Describe how these requirements can be provided**
- **Recognize normal and abnormal behaviour in hospitalized patients**
- **Describe the important points of a daily care routine for hospitalized patients**
- **Describe different methods of identification for patients within the hospital or veterinary practice and explain why their use is important**
- **Understand the types of records that are kept for hospitalized patients and why accurate and up-to-date record keeping is essential for patient care**
- **Explain why patient hygiene and grooming is an important part of the daily care routine**
- **Understand the requirements for bathing, grooming and foot care in different species**

Care of hospitalized patients

Patients that have been admitted to the veterinary hospital or practice for treatment or investigations may be hospitalized for times varying from just a few hours to some weeks. Regardless of the length of stay, the patient's essential requirements must be addressed. As well as treating patients for their presenting condition, the whole animal must be considered during the hospitalization period. A nursing care plan should be formulated and followed for each patient (see Chapter 14). This ensures that each patient's individual needs will be fulfilled, and that the patient receives the nursing care it requires.

Every patient has basic requirements that need to be addressed during the period of hospitalization:

- Comfort and warmth
- Protection from disease (hygiene)
- Nutrition (food and water)
- Safe environment, free from distress fear and pain
- Ability to express normal behaviour and mental stimulation
- Exercise (if appropriate) and opportunity to urinate and defaecate way from the sleeping area.

Comfort

On admittance to the hospital, each patient should be assigned a kennel or stable. Thought should be given to the species and breed of patient, as well as the reason for admittance.

As described in Chapter 15, hospitalization can be a stressful time for patients. Placing cats and small animals in close proximity to dogs or in a noisy area may increase anxiety in these patients, which can inhibit normal behaviour such as eating and sleeping. 'Igloo' style beds (see Chapter 12) provide a comfortable area of security within a kennel for cats. As herd animals, horses or donkeys may become stressed if they are stabled on their own, without other equine patients in the hospital, especially if they are used to living with others.

General accommodation requirements for the various species are described in Chapter 12. All patients should have room to move around in their enclosure and enough space to allow food and water bowls and litter trays (if applicable) to be placed in an area away from the bed.

Suitable bedding should be provided for each species of patient (see Chapter 12). A range of materials should be available to meet potentially changing needs, for example in **small animals**:

- Metal kennels should be lined with insulating materials to avoid the patient coming into contact with the cold surface
- Arthritic patients should be provided with thick comfortable bedding
- Recumbent patients may benefit from additional padding such as waterproof foam mattresses, as well as normal bedding materials (Figure 16.1), to prevent pressure sores and decubitus ulcer (deep, slow-healing ulcers) formation
- Veterinary fleece bedding (e.g. Vetbed) is soft and comfortable and allows fluid to pass through and be

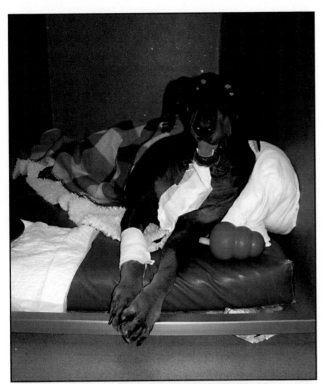

16.1 This Dobermann has been provided with a supportive mattress, warm bedding and a chew toy.

absorbed by the base layer; this helps to keep the patient dry
- Wood shavings and chopped paper are suitable for small mammals; however, care should be taken if using shredded paper as long strips can become wound around the patient's limbs.

Additional bedding such as pillows and duvets can be useful positioning aids for raising a patient's head or providing support for patients that would benefit from being positioned in an alternative recumbency. Patients admitted with fractured limbs, wounds or after trauma should be given sufficient bedding and positioned with the affected limb/area uppermost, supported with additional padding to avoid rotation and movement of the area. Paraplegic patients may often feel anxious and distressed if their lack of mobility has been of acute onset. If appropriate, the patient's head can be raised slightly to allow it to look around its surroundings when placed in lateral recumbency in a kennel.

Most horses admitted to a veterinary clinic or hospital will be stabled for the duration of their stay. Their comfort can be maintained by provision of a stable of appropriate size and suitable bedding material (see Chapter 12). A mare with a foal at foot should be accommodated in a stable of suitable size for their care. It is preferable to keep breeding stallions away from other types of horse, especially mares during the breeding season. Decisions regarding additional stable features, such as a top door with bars or windows that can be blackened, should be made on admission, following discussion with the owner regarding the horse's temperament (see Chapter 15). This avoids moving the horse during or after treatment. Ideally, a horse will stay in the same stable until its discharge, when the stable can then be cleared out completely, keeping the risk of cross-infection to a minimum. Horses thrive on

routine: a hospitalization plan should be designed to ensure the horse remains as comfortable and settled as possible during its stay.

The choice of bedding material for horses is dependent upon several individual factors (see Chapter 12). In a hospital situation, medical problems are significant determining factors in the choice of bedding:

- Horses with open wounds are better stabled on paper
- Deep beds are essential for horses with sore feet, in order to cushion the weight of the horse. Ideally, rubber matting should be laid as a primary layer under bedding to further prevent foot concussion
- A thick, dry, clean bed also allows the horse to rest properly
- Some horses, especially those with laminitis, spend a lot of their time during the treatment stage lying down, as they find this more comfortable than constantly standing. Providing an environment that allows the horse to feel at ease enough to lie down is very important
- Pre-existing respiratory conditions, such as recurrent airway obstruction (RAO), may also influence the choice of bedding, as they require the horse to be kept in a dust-free environment.

Warmth

Wards should be kept at a constant temperature between 18 and 22°C, and care should be taken that patients are not positioned in a draught. Patients that are admitted for hospitalization may require supplementary warmth due to their presenting condition/illness or age, or because of procedures that are performed during their stay (e.g. sedation, anaesthesia). Some patients may have abnormally low temperatures on admittance, e.g. those that are collapsed, shocked or have severe illness. Very young patients (neonates) are unable to control their own body temperature and rely on environmental temperature control for the initial few days of life. A temperature of 25–30°C is recommended; this can then be reduced to 22°C as long as it can be kept constant and measures are taken to prevent draughts. Even healthy patients that are hospitalized for routine procedures may require supplementary warmth. Patients that have received premedication prior to surgery should be monitored to ensure that they do not become cold prior to their procedure, and supplementary warmth will be required in the recovery period once the patient is returned to the ward. General methods of managing environmental temperature are described in Chapter 12. Methods of providing additional warmth to hospitalized small animal patients are given below.

Sources of supplementary warmth for small animals

- **Blankets, towels and bedding** can be used to provide an insulated area for the patient to lie on. Patients can be covered with additional bedding to prevent heat loss, but this is not an effective way to replace heat in a patient that is already cold. Care should be taken to ensure that the patient is not lying on bedding that has become wet due to urination.
- **Incubators** (Figure 16.2) are thermostatically

continues ▶

continued

controlled to provide the desired level of warmth; they are ideal for smaller patients and provide a warm, confined area that allows easy observation of the patient. This can be very useful for patients recovering from anaesthesia and those that are critically ill and need constant supervision.

- **Heat pads** (Figure 16.3) are water-resistant electrically heated flat pads that warm up to a pre-set temperature (often quite hot); care should be taken that they are always well covered with bedding so that the patient cannot come into direct contact with the pad. They should be used with caution with recumbent patients as they can cause thermal burns; any patient should be turned frequently whilst heat pads are being used. The electrical wire is a potential electrocution hazard and should not be used with animals that have a tendency to chew items.

- **Hot water bottles** can be used for small mammals and for puppies and kittens. They are cheap and easy to use, although care should be taken not to use boiling water and to ensure that the seal is fully watertight before use. Cooling of the contents will occur and so regular refilling will be required. The bottle should always be covered with a towel or bedding to prevent thermal burns and there is a risk of leakage and scalding if the bottle should burst or if it is chewed.

- **Microwaveable pads and bags** can be of use as they will stay warmer for a longer period of time than hot water bottles. Care should be taken not to overheat them as they can become very hot and risk burning a patient, especially if recumbent.

- **Warmed fluid bags and 'hot hands'** (gloves filled with warmed water) (Figure 16.4) are of limited use for patients that are mobile, as there is a high risk of puncture resulting in leakage of warmed water on to the patient. They can be useful for recumbent or anaesthetized patients when heated for a short period of time to make them warm; they can then be placed around a patient due to their flexible nature. Care should be taken not to make these items too hot, as they can cause thermal burns if placed close to the patient. Towels or bubble wrap can be used as thermal protection. A food dye added to the fluid bag will be a visual aid to alert staff that it is not to be infused. Fluid bags can be reheated multiple times, but 'hot hands' should be discarded when cooled.

- **Heat lamps** should be used with caution. They must be used with extreme care if the animal is recumbent and unable to move away from the heat. Lamps can become very hot and there is a risk of overheating the patient, contact burns if the bulb is touched, and shattering of the bulb if it comes into contact with water. Heat lamps should only be used in areas where constant supervision can be provided.

- **Circulating warmed air systems** (Figure 16.5) are now commonly available for purchase or hire. These systems provide a safe, thermoregulated source of warmed air that is circulated through a special blanket, allowing the air to escape through small holes and circulate around the patient. Various sized blankets are available for different sizes of patient and can be positioned either under or over the patient. These systems are extremely effective.

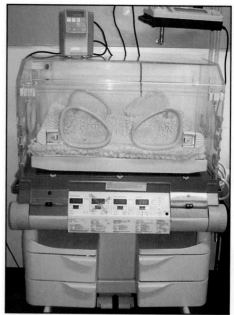

16.2 An incubator suitable for warming veterinary patients.

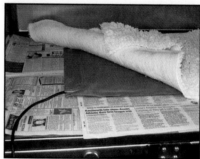

16.3 A heat pad placed under fleece bedding.

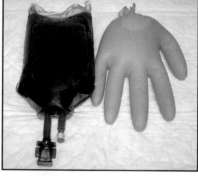

16.4 Fluid bags and gloves filled with warm water may be useful for short-term use in warming recumbent or anaesthetized patients.

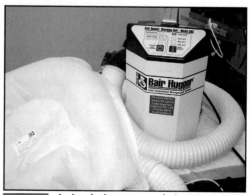

16.5 A circulating warmed air system is an efficient way to provide supplementary warmth.

Rugging of horses

On admission, the owner should be asked about the horse's usual requirement for rugging. This ensures that the horse remains warm, even in inclement weather. Choice of rug is also determined by hospital environmental temperature. The thickness of a rug is usually indicated by a description of its weight. There are many different types of rugs available, but essentially they fall into two categories: outdoor and indoor.

Outdoor rugs (Figure 16.6) are waterproof, vary in thickness and are used when the horses are out in paddocks rather than stabled. There are several different types of outdoor rugs and normally the rug is chosen depending on the weather.

- The **New Zealand rug** is made of heavy-duty waterproof material lined with quilt or cotton. This type of rug has largely been superseded by turnout rugs in a variety of synthetic modern fabrics.
- **Turnout rugs** vary in thickness and may or may not have a half or full neck piece. They are waterproof and various types exist in modern synthetic fabrics.

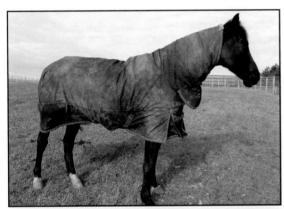
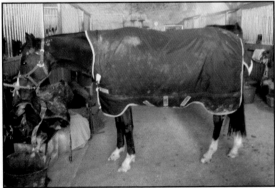

16.6   Outdoor rugs.

Indoor rugs are for horses to wear when inside a stable. There are several different types, but the most commonly used in hospital environments include:

- The **fleece rug** (e.g. Thermatex) (Figure 16.7a), which wicks any moisture out of the horse's coat and creates a film on the outer layer of the rug. This type of rug is used after surgery to dry the horse. Once dry, the horse is then rugged depending on the temperature
- The **summer sheet** (Figure 16.7b), which is made of cotton or fleece and is a thin rug that is used to keep the chill off the horse's back

- The **stable rug** (Figure 16.7c), which is available in a range of thicknesses and can have a neckpiece attached. This sort of rug is used for horses that are either clipped or sick and therefore need extra help keeping their temperature within the normal limits.

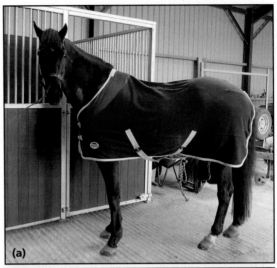

(a)

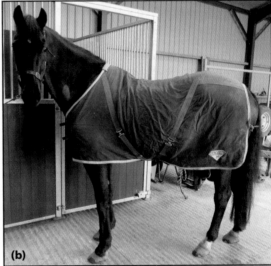

(b)

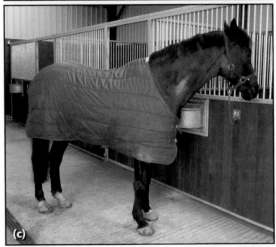

(c)

16.7   Indoor rugs. **(a)** Fleece rug, ideal for use after exercise or competition, and also used after surgery. **(b)** Summer sheet, ideal for summer evenings or after exercise. **(c)** Stable rug, essential in cold weather for horses that are clipped, and it can also be used after surgery. (Courtesy of E. Mullineaux)

Hygiene

Strict hygiene and cleaning protocols should be followed when nursing animals within a hospital environment. Patients within the hospital may be awaiting elective surgery, recovering from elective and non-elective surgeries, systemically unwell or possibly immunosuppressed due to illness or drug therapy. Patients with possible contagious diseases or contaminated wounds should be hospitalized away from other patients and barrier nursing employed to protect other patients and the affected animal from cross-contamination (see Chapter 12). All staff must adhere to measures put into place to prevent patient cross-contamination and hospital acquired infection (HAI) occurring. Good hand washing technique and use of personal protective equipment (PPE) should be implemented when treating patients. Information on the fundamental principles of infection are given in Chapter 5 and the principles of cleaning and disinfection in Chapter 12.

Ward hygiene

The routine cleaning of small animal patient kennels on a daily basis with suitable disinfectant, even when they are not physically soiled, promotes a clean sanitary environment. All communal ward areas should be kept tidy and clean, bins should be emptied regularly, and odorous waste disposed of outside of the ward. Ventilation, provided by either active air circulation or passive movement by opening of windows, will reduce airborne particles within a confined environment, remove smells and assist with climate control within the ward. Care should be taken that patients are not positioned in a draught. Soiled bedding material should be disposed of as hazardous waste or washed appropriately to eliminate the source of contamination. Items that could be potential fomites, such as food bowls, toys, leads and harnesses, should be washed or sterilized in a way appropriate for the item. For information on basic stable hygiene see Chapter 12.

Patient hygiene

Patients should be physically examined for abnormal discharges; aural, ocular, nasal, oral or genital. Any abnormalities should be noted on the patient's daily hospital record and the clinician informed. Some discharges, especially ocular, should not be cleaned until directed by the clinician (see Chapter 15); once directed to do so, discharges should be removed with damp swabs or cotton wool.

Patients that are polyuric (increased urination) or that have diarrhoea should be examined around the perineal area, tail and hindlimbs to ensure there is no soiling of the coat or skin. Urine should be washed from the animal as soon as soiling has occurred, to prevent urine scalding of the skin. The patient should then be bathed as soon as possible, to avoid skin irritation and for its wellbeing. Some patients can become distressed as a result of soiling in their kennels and upon themselves.

Vomit, regurgitated material and excessive salivation should be cleaned from around the patient's mouth with damp swabs. Patients with oral fractures should have their faces gently washed with damp swabs and be groomed daily, as they are often unable to clean themselves due to their injury. These patients are often very receptive to this attention and 'TLC' is a very important part of their recuperation. Information on patient bathing and grooming is given later in this chapter.

Patients that are left in contact with wet or dirty bedding are more likely to develop skin irritation that could progress to scalding and ulceration of the skin. Even non-offensive soiling, such as spilt water bowls and leakage of intravenous fluids on to bedding, should be attended to promptly. Decubitus ulcers can develop on bony prominences and areas that are in constant contact with bedding, due to continuous recumbency. Soiled bedding is more abrasive and will increase skin irritation, exacerbating a potential problem. Patients that are in an unclean environment are at greater risk of contracting a hospital-acquired infection (HAI), such as wound or skin infection. Bandages and dressings that become wet must be replaced to prevent strike-through to wounds and prevent sores occurring. Many hospitalized patients may have indwelling intravenous catheters, surgical drains, feeding tubes and wounds; all of these sites must be maintained in a dry aseptic way to prevent contamination (see Chapter 17).

Surgical wounds, abrasions, wound and chest drains, feeding tubes and intravenous catheter insertions should all be examined at least twice a day for abnormal discharges, seroma formation and evidence of patient interference (see Chapter 17). Discharges should be cleaned without disturbing the sutures or wound and covered with sterile dressings or clean bandages. Gloves should always be worn when attending to wounds and drains. A water-resistant barrier, such as Vaseline, can be useful to protect the skin against constant wound discharge from passive wound drains or moisture, such as that caused by urinary or faecal incontinence.

Feeding

Every patient requires the appropriate nutrition for its species, breed, life stage and health status. Good nutrition is required for basic metabolic function (see Chapter 13). Patients that are unwell, recovering from surgery or trauma or have neoplasia will all have additional nutritional requirements to facilitate tissue repair and convalescence.

Monitoring food intake

Patients that are admitted to the hospital should have an individual daily energy requirement calculated on the basis of their bodyweight, age and illness. This allows an appropriate diet to be selected and the daily volume of food required to be calculated. Knowing the volume of food a patient needs to consume daily to meet its nutritional requirement makes it easier to monitor whether it is consuming the vital nutrition required. Food charts (Figure 16.8) can be a useful way to keep a visual check on the amount of food a patient is voluntarily consuming. Information on the type of food, the time it is given and the amount consumed can all be recorded on the chart; this allows a patient's food intake over a period of days to be monitored easily.

The amount of food consumed by exotic pets may be harder to assess than that consumed by dogs and cats, although using small amounts of food that are pre-measured or weighed assists with this process. Fresh food, such as vegetable and fruit, can be visually examined to determine whether the patient has eaten any of it. The dry diet that is often offered may be harder to monitor as these patients may scatter or store food, making it difficult to determine whether any has been consumed unless the patient is observed actually eating it. Rabbits can sometimes appear to be masticating (chewing) food but close observation is required to ensure that they are really ingesting it. Observation of the

Davies
Veterinary Specialists

Label   Kennel No:_____

IN PATIENT FEEDING CHART

Admission weight:	Date admitted:	Normal Diet:

Feeding Calculation Area

Diet Selected:_____Illness factor:_____Daily Energy Requirement (RDI):_____

Daily amount to be fed:_____Number of feeds:_____Quantity of food req'd (each meal):_____

Daily food intake chart (indicate amount eaten e.g. ◗ = ¾ eaten)

Mealtime		Admit Day						
Comments (e.g. NBM, Sx, Procedures)								
1 Time ____	% eaten	◯	◯	◯	◯	◯	◯	◯
	Food type							
2 Time ____	% eaten	◯	◯	◯	◯	◯	◯	◯
	Food type							
3 Time ____	% eaten	◯	◯	◯	◯	◯	◯	◯
	Food type							
4 Time ____	% eaten	◯	◯	◯	◯	◯	◯	◯
	Food type							
% RDI eaten								

Comments:_____
_____
_____
_____
_____
_____
_____
_____
_____

16.8 An example of an inpatient feeding chart. (Courtesy of Davies Veterinary Specialists)

amount and type of faeces an exotic pet passes may be one of the only indications that it is efficiently consuming food whist hospitalized.

Rabbits especially should have a record kept of the amount of faecal pellets passed; these should be cleaned away as soon as they are noticed in the kennel so that further production can be noted. It is important that rabbits consume the caecotroph pellets that are passed at night; these soft, mucus-covered pellets are swallowed straight from the anus and contain important nutrients that require a second passing through the gut in order to be absorbed (see Chapter 3). Patients that do not consume caecotrophs are at higher risk of developing gut stasis. A rabbit's anal area should be examined daily to ensure that the soft caecotroph pellets have not become stuck around the anus. Patients that are not consuming the important caecotrophs will need nutritional supplementation to ensure that intestinal stasis does not occur.

Changes in appetite

A change in appetite can sometimes be one of the first signs an owner may notice to alert them that their pet is feeling unwell, and a willingness to eat is often used to assess the progress of hospitalized animals. Patients may be hospitalized due to anorexia (loss of appetite for food); investigations are then undertaken to find the cause, or underlying illness of the patient. Some illnesses and conditions may physically stop the patient from being able to eat normally, such as oral and nasal masses (nasal obstruction makes it difficult for patients to breathe and eat simultaneously), fractured mandibles or megaoesophagus. In these cases, feeding tubes, such as naso-oesophageal, oesophagostomy and percutaneous endo-scopically placed gastrostomy (PEG) tubes (see Chapter 13), may need to be placed to facilitate feeding. Patients that are anxious or are stressed by the hospitalized environment may be reluctant to eat. Pain may also cause patients to be anorexic and this should be a particular consideration following surgical procedures.

Choice of diet

The diet a patient is offered may be chosen because it is appropriate for that patient's specific condition, such as renal or hepatic dysfunction. If a patient has no specific dietary requirements the diet chosen should be similar, whenever possible, to what the patient normally eats at home. Information on the patient's normal diet and feeding routine should be collected when the patient is admitted (see Chapters 14 and 15). This information can also highlight any foods that should be avoided, due to sensitivity or patient preference.

Communication with the owner regarding diet is essential when admitting horses to a hospital environment, as marked dietary changes can lead to the development of colic; it must be remembered that stabled horses are prone to colic and those involved in their care must be aware of the signs.

Feeding considerations

Some patients may need no encouragement to eat their daily nutritional requirement; this may be due to species, breed, age, demeanour, or appetite changes due to drug therapy. However, there are often many patients in the hospital that may not be so keen to eat, and various nursing considerations can be implemented to encourage voluntary food intake.

Encouraging feeding

- Reduce stressors, such as noise and different species in the same ward.
- Ensure the animal is not in pain; administer analgesia if required.
- Offer the patient its normal diet or favourite foods.
- Increase palatability by warming foods.
- Do not place cats' food and water bowls near their litter trays.
- Use wide shallow bowls for small mammals; being able to see over the bowl whilst eating can decrease their feeling of vulnerability.
- Be aware that some dogs will prefer to eat outside their kennels.
- For cats, who may prefer privacy, cover the kennel or provide a box to hide in and place a food bowl in the box.
- Spend time with the patient, encourage it to eat by talking, stroking and offering food by hand.
- Remove food if the patient seems physically repelled by food (turns its head or body to the food) and try again later.
- Offer a small selection of food, but do not overwhelm the patient with multiple dishes of food in the kennel.
- Remove any uneaten food from dogs after a short period of time; cats and horses may graze, so food can be left for a longer time.

Assisted feeding

The term 'assisted feeding' is now generally used in connection with patients that have had feeding tubes placed and where their nutritional requirements are divided into frequent small meals. As a patient starts to eat voluntarily again (if possible), tube feeds are reduced or used to supplement the patient's voluntary intake (see Chapter 13).

If a patient continues to refrain from voluntary feeding after all the nursing considerations above have been tried, syringe- or spoon-feeding may be used to initiate voluntary feeding but is often not well tolerated and should cease if the patient becomes distressed, as there is a risk of aspiration pneumonia if food is inadvertently inhaled. Syringe/spoon-feeding is unlikely to meet the patient's nutritional requirements if used as the sole method of feeding.

In some cases, placing food on a patient's paws may be used to instigate licking of the food and then hopefully stimulate eating. However, this method may just distress the patient; cats especially do not like to be unclean and so this method may only serve to reinforce an aversion to food.

Appetite stimulants

Anorexia is not normally a primary condition, and investigation into the underlying cause of the patient's inappetence is required if the patient persistently refuses to eat. If the patient is still reluctant to eat after diagnosis and treatment have been implemented, the use of appetite-stimulating drugs such as diazepam or mirtazapine may be appropriate, although some drugs may have side effects if used long term. The use of feeding tubes may be a more beneficial way to manage an anorexic patient until it begins to eat voluntarily.

Water consumption

All patients should be offered free access to water while they are hospitalized (unless directed otherwise by the clinician). Even patients that are scheduled for anaesthesia may not need to have water withdrawn until premedication is administered prior to the procedure. There are many factors that may alter the amount of water a patient consumes, for example: water intake will alter with the type of diet fed – tinned diets have a high moisture content and patients may not drink as much as those on a completely dry diet; dogs that are excited or nervous may pant excessively and have increased respiratory losses and therefore drink more. Patients may be admitted for investigation into excessive thirst (polydipsia), and the amount of water they consume may need to be monitored (see Chapter 15).

Small mammals should be offered water in a way that is familiar to them, either by bottle or bowl. Some cats may prefer to drink from running water, or dripping taps rather than a still bowl; water fountains (Figure 16.9) can be useful for these patients. This information should be obtained from owners as part of the nursing admission process (see Chapter 15).

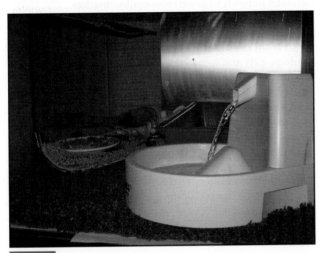

16.9 A drinking water fountain for cats.

Fresh water should always be available for horses that are allowed it; those under a nil by mouth regime should receive at least maintenance fluid and electrolyte requirements by the intravenous route. Automatic water drinkers are not ideal for hospitalized horses in which it is important to monitor water intake, especially before and after surgery. Horses used to being kept outdoors or recently in full work can suffer from colonic impaction when stabled, so daily water intake and faecal output should be monitored closely and recorded. Small horses and ponies must have access to water mangers; these must therefore be placed at an appropriate height.

Special considerations for older animals

Older animals may not adapt as quickly to a change in routine and environment as younger ones. Many older patients would normally sleep for an extended time at home and acclimatization to a possibly busy and noisy ward may take a little longer than for younger, more outgoing patients. Older patients should be handled gently, as many may have a degree of osteoarthritic change, and assistance may be required for climbing stairs and moving in and out of kennels if there is a raised step.

Older patients may suffer from deterioration in sight and hearing, which may increase anxiety when they are in unfamiliar surroundings. Special consideration should be given to patients who have reduced vision: a harness or short lead should be used, to allow the patient to be guided through doors and when exercising. Animals that have lost their sight gradually will often have adapted to their reduced vision, but patients that have become acutely blind can be distressed and disorientated when walking.

The patient should be spoken to as it is approached and handled; continuous vocal encouragement will give the patient a guide as to where the handler is and in which direction it is expected to go. All unexpected procedures, such as injections or the application of eye drops, should be performed slowly, once the patient is aware that it is being handled and examined, so as not to startle or alarm. Patients that have a degree of deafness may require visual guidance; hand signals may help the patient to get a sense of what it is being asked to do and a gentle, calm approach can prevent it becoming anxious during handling and procedures.

Behaviour of hospitalized patients

As described in Chapter 15, admission to a hospital environment can be a very stressful and unsettling time for animals. Not all patients will adapt easily to a change in routine, unfamiliar surroundings and confinement. Patients that are feeling unwell may become anxious and withdrawn; some patients may be scared or feel threatened by the change in surroundings and by having other animals in close proximity; some may show warning signs of aggression or become submissive when handled; while others may become excited. Every effort should be made by nursing staff to interact with every patient.

Spending time with patients, talking to them, stroking, grooming, gaining their confidence and 'making friends' will all help to stimulate, comfort and reassure them. Patients that are comfortable and happy in their surroundings will usually be relaxed and exhibit normal behaviour such as feeding, grooming, sleeping and interaction with people.

Recognizing pain

Pain can have a major effect on physiological parameters and should be considered as a possible cause of behavioural changes. Signs of pain are described in Chapters 15 and 21. Pain can be hard to assess and different species may mask signs of pain as a protective behaviour; for example, 'prey animals' such as rabbits may not express signs of pain because this would make them appear vulnerable and attract predators. Cats also may modify their behaviour if they are housed close to dogs and feel threatened. Variations within breeds will also be seen: a Greyhound and a Labrador may react quite differently when administered a subcutaneous injection. Differences in behaviour cannot be used to judge accurately the degree of pain an animal is experiencing. Some patients may appear to have a very dramatic response to pain; however, the patient that is stoical or sits motionless may be experiencing just as much pain as the animal that is vocalizing and pacing around its kennel. Nurses should assess all patients for signs of pain and pass on any observations to the clinician, as well as recording findings on the patient's hospital form.

Promoting normal behaviour

Using known commands

Most dogs have been taught to respond to basic training commands by their owners; if possible, these basic commands should be used while the patient is within the hospitalized environment. Most dogs are used to being told a command and will follow with the appropriate learnt response; this allows the animal to behave in a way that is familiar to it. Use of commands will help provide an element of normality for the patient within a strange environment and can also be useful for nurses when handling and restraining patients.

Exercise

Although interaction with other hospitalized patients should be avoided due to the possibility of cross-contamination, time spent out of the kennel can further stimulate patients. Outdoor or out of kennel exercise, fresh air, and 'a change of scene', even for non-ambulatory patients (Figure 16.10), should be encouraged. Dogs should be given the chance to

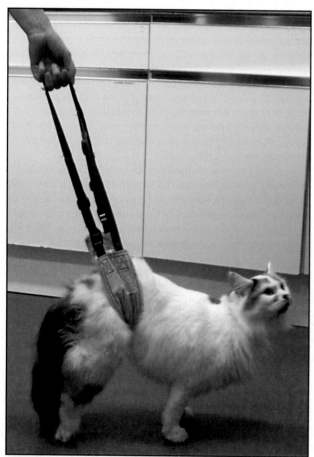

16.10 Providing support whilst standing can enable a paraplegic animal to spend time outside its cage.

urinate and defecate at regular intervals throughout the day; many patients will not like to soil their bedding area and may become vocal or restless when they need to go to the toilet. Patients that are polyuric (due to intravenous fluid therapy, steroidal medication or diseases such as diabetes mellitus or diabetes insipidus) will need to go outside more regularly.

Human interaction

Patient stimulation and interaction with people is important whilst patients are hospitalized. Confinement within a kennel or cage must lead to a degree of boredom, especially when the period of hospitalization is extended.

All patients, but especially those that are young, recumbent or 'intelligent' (e.g. parrots), may benefit from human contact and the use of toys (see Figure 16.1) that promote normal behaviour. Educational toys, such as those that release food as a reward if they are moved around, and indestructible toys can all aid in patient stimulation. Thought must be given to the practicalities of admitting patients with their own toys from home, as there is a chance these could get lost or damaged. Toys within the practice must be cleaned effectively between patients to avoid cross-contamination.

Patients that are not responding well to the hospital environment and are subdued or anorexic may benefit from a visit from their owners; this is more likely to be the case for dogs, cats and some well bonded horses. Some patients may be hospitalized for extended periods and owners may request to visit their pet. For many patients, visiting is a positive experience for both patient and owner; a familiar face and voice can provide vital mental stimulation for the patient.

Anorexic patients may be tempted to eat whilst spending time with their owners. Some patients can become distressed and subdued once their owners have left, and each patient should be considered individually as to whether visiting is advisable.

Rest

It is also important that patients are given the chance to rest and have undisturbed sleep. Wards are often busy, noisy places and many hospitals have staff covering night shifts, which can interfere with the normal day and night pattern an animal may be used to. Critical patients that require high levels of monitoring, or patients that are undergoing diagnostic tests such as hourly blood glucose curves, will need a time when they can sleep. Owners often report that their pets are exhausted for a few days following a period of hospitalization.

Daily routine

It can be helpful to have a daily hospital routine of times when patients are fed, medicated, walked and left to rest; this will need to be adapted to each patient. Suitable records should be kept to record this basic inpatient care information as well as clinical information (Figure 16.11). In some instances, care forms may be tailored to specific problems such as equine colic (Figure 16.12). More information on recording clinical parameters is given in Chapter 15.

Davies
Veterinary Specialists

Standard Hospital Chart

Today's date:	
Hospital Day No:	
Kennel No:	
Admit Weight:	
Today's weight:	

Intrac status: A B C	Vet X-rays: ☐ Vet CD: ☐	Day Case: Yes ☐ No ☐

Reason for admission:

Admitted with:

Known allergies/Drug reactions:

Normal diet:

Diagnosis/Procedures performed:

Cautions:

Time of Event							Overnight Observations				Pre-rounds
							2300	0100	0300	0500	0700
Clinical assessment											
Temperature (°C)											
Pulse rate/character											
Respiratory rate											
Pain score (see chart)											
Time taken out											
Faeces											
Urine											

IV catheter care	Size	Location		Day No

Today's Evaluation:

Today's Plan:

Medication (BID/TID treatments shaded)																						Overnight Medications			
Name of Drug	Freq.	Dose	Route	07 00	08 00	09 00	10 00	11 00	12 00	13 00	14 00	15 00	16 00	17 00	18 00	19 00	20 00	21 00	23 00	01 00	03 00	05 00

Fluid Therapy Rate	Fluid Type			
Flush IV: am ☐ pm ☐	Fluid Additives			

Anaesthesia	Premed drug1	Dose	Given? ☐ (Time/Sign)	Pre-op drugs
Starve? Yes / No	Premed drug 2	Dose:		

Anaesthesia Warnings:		See anaesthesia chart ☐

Daily Task List		Orders for (pre-rounds)
Check wound: ☐ (comment over):		Starve? YES / NO
Speak to owner (circle): Vet / Nurse		

16.11 Example of a hospitalization form. (Courtesy of Davies Veterinary Specialists)

		TPR			MM./CRT	GUT		PARAMETERS				FAECES O,N,S,D,	REFLEX	PAIN	FLUIDS	FLUID RATE	FLUID ADDITITIVES	COMMENTS
DATE	TIME	T	P	R		L	R	PCV	TP	GLUCOSE	LACTATE							

HORSE NAME: PAGE No.

16.12 Example of an equine colic intensive care form. (Courtesy of Rossdale and partners)

Daily tasks

- **Record temperature, pulse and respiration (TPR).** These essential parameters should be recorded while the patient is in a calm state (prior to exercise) in order to obtain accurate measurements.
- **Record bodyweight.** This will highlight any changes during the period of hospitalization, possibly due to anorexia or fluid accumulation.
- **Evaluate mental state** of the patient. Is the animal bright, responsive, disorientated, depressed, etc.? These subjective findings can help to determine whether a patient is progressing or deteriorating.
- **Opportunity to exercise and eliminate outside the kennel.** Dogs should be taken outside 3–4 times daily if appropriate; other patients should be provided with litter trays or areas of the kennel that are away from the bedding area.
- **Observation of wounds** should be performed at least once daily for signs of swelling, discharge, dehiscence, or interference. Dressings or bandages should be changed as necessary.
- **Monitoring for signs of pain or discomfort** should be performed continuously throughout the day and the clinician informed of any change in the patient's condition.
- **Medication** should be administered at the appropriate times and in the correct way (see Chapter 8).
- **Provide nutritional requirements** (unless nil per mouth). The correct food should be provided and a record kept specifying what food has been offered and the quantity consumed.
- **Correct care of intravenous catheters.** Peripheral ▶

intravenous catheters should be flushed twice daily to ensure patency, and insertion sites inspected for signs of contamination. Catheters should be removed and replaced in another location if necessary (see Chapter 17).
- **Appropriate care of wound or cavity drains and feeding tubes.** Insertion sites should be checked at least twice daily and bandaged as necessary. Draining fluids (Figure 16.13) should be recorded.
- **Maintain patient hygiene.** All patients should be examined for areas of soiling of their coats, and bathed and groomed as necessary.
- **Routine equine foot care** – including picking out feet (see later).
- **Physiotherapy** – should be performed on recumbent or inactive patients, usually 2–4 times daily.

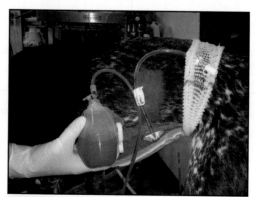

16.13 A surgical drain should be emptied as necessary and the total volume of fluid collected should be recorded for every 24-hour period.

Identification of patients

It is vital that every patient admitted to the hospital can be identified and distinguished from other patients, in order to avoid confusion.

Name bands and tags

Paper or plastic name bands can be used effectively in both dogs (Figure 16.14) and cats. A name band should be placed on the patient, normally around its neck, as soon as it is admitted to the hospital (see Chapter 12). This should contain information such as the patient's full name and the veterinary practice's name and telephone number, written in indelible ink. Patients' own collars can be an unreliable way to identify the animal; tags (if present) may be hard to read, belong to other pets or contain details that are not current, which could lead to confusion. If a name band has to be removed for surgery it should be replaced in another location, such as above the hock, immediately. This identification not only allows staff to check the correct patient is being treated, it also provides identification and contact details should the patient escape from the veterinary practice.

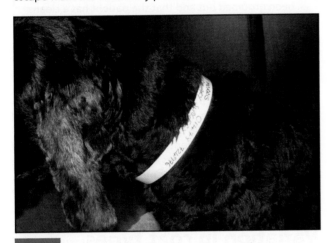

16.14   A patient identification collar on a dog.

Horses should be identified on admission and any items the owner is leaving behind should also be labelled and noted on the case record. Identification bracelets or tags can be attached to the horse's headcollar, rugs and any other items. Headcollars are normally removed once the horses are in the stables, so a plait is placed in the mane near the withers and an identification tag can be attached there (Figure 16.15), allowing identification even without the headcollar. If the horse has a hogged mane, the identification tag is placed in the tail instead. There are some horses that do not have their headcollars removed, for example; stallions, colts, yearlings, weanlings and foals. This is due to the behaviour of these animals making it safer to leave the headcollar on at all times. Care must be taken when horses arrive with headcollars that have already been labelled, as the name on the headcollar often does not match that of the horse that is wearing it; taping over the name-tag on the headcollar will remove any possibility of confusion. Name cards should be placed on the stable door, stating the horse's name, age, sex and reason for hospitalization.

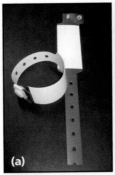 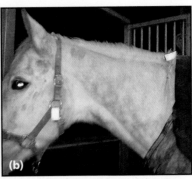

16.15   **(a)** Equine identification tags. **(b)** Identification tags on a horse's mane and head collar.

Other methods

Different breeds of dogs, cats, horses and small pets should be recognized by the veterinary nurse (see Appendix 1). There should be no confusion, for example, between a Birman cat and a Burmese cat, or a Border Collie dog and a Bearded Collie dog. Additional identifying marks should be recorded on consent forms and in the patient's notes. This may be important if two sibling cats that are almost identical are admitted for procedures; nurses must be able to distinguish between each cat so that accurate records can be kept for each patient.

Permanent methods of identification

- **Microchips** have a unique identification number that cannot be lost or altered once implanted under the skin of the animal.
  - In dogs and cats, the microchip is placed subcutaneously between the scapulae in the dorsal midline. Microchips are a requirement of the PETS passport scheme prior to rabies vaccination (see Chapter 5). They are also required for some canine health schemes.
  - In horses, the microchip is placed in the mid neck, between the poll and the withers, on the left hand side, into the nuchal ligament. Since July 2009 microchipping of horses has been a requirement when any new equine passport is applied for. Also since 1999 all racehorses have been microchipped to ensure the correct identity of the horse that is raced.
  - Microchips are also commonly used in exotic species and may form part of legal restrictions for the importation of such animals. The accepted sites for microchipping vary between species and should be checked with the regulatory authorities or microchip suppliers prior to placement.
  - There are several brands of microchip; only those that are of a recognized international standard (ISO) are suitable for pet importation and exportation schemes, such as the Pet Travel Scheme (PETS).
  - For most owners, the main purpose of a microchip is to aid the recovery of their pet if it gets lost or is stolen. The individual microchip number, together with patient and owner information, is held on a

continues ▶

continued

central databank, which allows animals to be traced back to their registered owners.

- **Tattoos** are not used routinely in domestic species in the UK. They are, however, used on laboratory animals and racing Greyhounds. Animals imported from outside the UK may have tattoo marks within their right ears, containing information on where they were bred and as identification.
- **Freeze branding** is a form of identification used in horses and other large animals. It has the advantages over microchipping that it is easily visible, allowing easy identification, and may act as a theft deterrent. The cold brand destroys hair pigment follicles so that hair regrows white at the brand site. Freeze brands are still used in some horses, although the need for microchipping as part of the equine passport requirements may have reduced their use.
- **Hot branding** of horses and ponies is considered by most veterinary and welfare organizations in the UK to be inhumane and unethical; the procedure has been banned in Scotland.

Microchip or tattoo identification may need to be verified prior to a procedure being performed to ensure the identification of the animal. Since January 2010 the BVA canine health schemes for hips, elbows and eyes require that the animal is permanently identified. Other forms of documentation may also be examined at the time a patient is admitted to the hospital. Proof of the patient's vaccination status may be required in some instances. Vaccination status is essential information that will need to be known when unwell patients are admitted to the hospital, as this may aid in differential diagnosis and determine the location in which the patient is kennelled in case an infectious disease is suspected.

Grooming and bathing

Maintaining the cleanliness of a patient is essential to its clinical care and wellbeing. Such care may include bathing, grooming and clipping of the haircoat. Grooming should be performed on a regular basis and not only when soiling makes it essential. Self-grooming is often part of an animal's natural behaviour; observing a patient grooming itself suggests that it is relaxed and comfortable within the hospitalized environment. Stressed, anxious and unwell patients are less likely to groom themselves. Some species have special requirements within their cage to allow them to groom. For example, a chinchilla's fine dense fur can become matted if it is in a damp environment; fine pumice sand baths should be provided for the animals to use (see Chapter 12).

Reasons for grooming/bathing patients include:

- It maintains patient cleanliness, reducing the risk of sores and infection
- It provides mental stimulation, contact and bonding with the patient. It can help to reduce anxiety and

  ▶

fear, and may encourage normal behaviour such as voluntary feeding, especially in cats
- Grooming can be performed in a systematic way, allowing the whole animal to be examined for:
  - Skin and coat changes, such as hair loss, pyoderma, ectoparasites and skin masses
  - Discharges from ears, mouth and genitalia
  - Signs of skin irritation or abnormal wound healing
- Bathing can be used as treatment for specific skin conditions; medicated shampoos and washes may be used
- Grooming may be necessary prior to elective surgery (especially orthopaedic), e.g. bathing or clipping of a patient's coat, especially in breeds with thick double coats (e.g. Newfoundland). The removal of dirt, dead hair and skin scurf may help to reduce the risk of postoperative complications. Bathing and clipping will also disturb the natural skin flora and need to be performed a few days prior to surgery to allow the skin to settle before surgery is performed
- Regular grooming and bathing ensures the patient is in a presentable condition for discharge from the hospital. Ongoing care should have been performed regularly during the period of hospitalization, but this final preparation ensures that matts and tangles have been groomed out and that the patient has a clean face and perineal area. Owners are very aware of the condition of their pet, and a patient discharged in a clean and tidy way shows that a professional, caring service has been provided.

The grooming and bathing of animals is a skilled job. Veterinary nurses must be able to perform basic grooming and bathing tasks to maintain the cleanliness and hygienic condition of hospitalized patients. The clipping, stripping and de-matting of animals requires advanced knowledge and the correct use of grooming tools. Professional grooming courses, books and information are available for people who wish to extend their skills in animal grooming.

Variation in coat types

There is a wide variation in coat type amongst the breeds of many species, and many breeds are recognized as much by their coat as by their size, build and head shape. The coat type of a patient will influence the amount of grooming and care required to keep it in good condition. In practical terms, patients with longer, thicker coats may be more prone to soiling and require more intensive grooming to maintain cleanliness and condition.

Canine coat types can be divided into five sorts:

- **Double coat** – long topcoat with a thick, soft undercoat. Some of the breeds with this type of coat may be trimmed into a short style to aid coat care and cleanliness. Breed examples include: German Shepherd Dogs, Rough Collies, Old English Sheepdogs and Lhasa Apsos
- **Silky coat** – varies in length from medium to long with a fine texture. Breed examples include: Afghan Hounds, setters, Bearded Collies and most spaniels
- **Smooth coat** – short length and close to the body; minimal maintenance required to keep clean. Breed examples include: Dobermanns, Boxers, some Dachshunds and Staffordshire Bull Terriers

- **Wire coat** – topcoat is harsh and thick with a softer undercoat; some breeds require 'hand-stripping' to maintain the correct coat condition. Many breeds may just be clipped to keep them clean and easier to manage. Breed examples include: Border Terriers, Norfolk Terriers, West Highland White Terriers and Wire-haired Dachshunds
- **Wool coat** – many breeds could be described as having woolly type coats; many may require special trimming, washing and drying techniques. Breed examples include: Poodles, Curly Coated Retrievers, Bichon Frises and Irish Water Spaniels.

Cats' coat types are broadly divided into two sorts: **long hair** and **short hair**. The coats are made up of different types of hair:

- **Guard hairs** – long, coarse hairs that make up the outer coat layer; they taper to a point to protect the undercoat. They are connected to the autonomic nervous system and respond to sensory information (fight and flight response)
- **Awn hairs** – intermediate length hair, shorter than guard hairs and longer than down hair. Most visible part of the coat, helps with insulation and protects the down hairs
- **Down hair** – fine, soft fluffy hair that is closest to the skin, helps to trap air and insulate the animal.

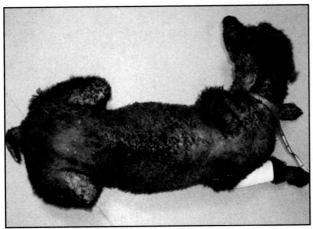

16.16 Poor coat quality in a dog with hyperadrenocorticism. (Courtesy of P. Ibarrola)

The amount and distribution of the types of hair that make up the animal's coat will differ with breed variation; for example, the Sphynx cat, which is known as hairless, actually has a very fine covering of down hair, and cats with curly coats will have curly awn hairs but no guard hairs.

Changes in the coat of animals occur with the natural seasonal changes in daylight. Spring days will initiate the production of a less dense summer coat and the shedding of the animal's winter coat. In the autumn the reverse occurs, preparing the animal for the colder weather by growth of a thicker winter coat and the shedding of the summer coat. Seasonal coat changes are more noticeable in animals that are housed outdoors. Most domestic dogs that live within a heated environment will shed their coat throughout the year, with an increase in spring and autumn. Seasonal changes affect the need for clipping (see below) and rugging (see above) of horses.

Coat changes can also occur due to endocrine disturbance such as hyperadrenocorticism (Cushing's syndrome) (Figure 16.16) and hypothyroidism, seen most commonly in dogs. Animals that are unwell or fed a nutritionally inadequate diet may have a dull and dry coat appearance and condition.

Grooming small animals

There is a wide range of grooming equipment available, but a basic selection of brushes and combs will be sufficient for the grooming needs of most small animal patients (Figure 16.17).

Dedicated grooming areas and specialized equipment such as grooming tables and walk-in baths are not normally found within veterinary practices. Larger patients may be groomed in a quiet area of the ward; small and recumbent patients may be groomed within their own kennels. It should be remembered that some patients may be feeling unwell, uncomfortable or require careful handling due to surgery or medical conditions. The patient's temperament and patience should be assessed to avoid causing distress to the patient and injury to the groomer. The patient's coat type should be assessed, noting areas that need extra attention and areas that should be avoided or groomed with care (e.g. areas of skin irritation, wounds or areas around skin masses, such as warts). The appropriate types of brushes and combs should be selected for the patient's coat type. De-matting tools should only be used by individuals experienced in their use, as the correct technique is required to remove matts safely without causing cuts or damage to the skin.

Equipment	Features and use
Slicker brush	Can be used with all coat types except smooth coats. Fine directional bent pins remove loose hair. Correct use of the brush is required to avoid skin abrasion by the pins. Only light pressure should be applied to a brush that is positioned flatly against the coat in small sections to allow access to the undercoat. The pins on new brushes can be harsh and care should be taken not to damage the skin until the pins have 'relaxed'
Deep pin brush	Long metal pins with rounded ends that protect the skin. Useful for thick double coats and long silky coats

16.17 Small animal grooming equipment.

continues ▶

Equipment	Features and use
Soft-bore bristle brush	Often found on the reverse side of a deep pin brush. Firm bristles good for wire coats and removing dried dirt from short coats, less useful for thicker longer coats as bristles may be too dense to separate coat
Combs	Variety of wire-toothed combs, with variation in tooth position and length. Suitable for all coats except smooth coats. Usually used after brushing to smooth coat and remove remaining knots, especially in longer coats
Rubber comb	Used in smooth-coated breeds to remove undercoat and smooth the topcoat
Shedding blade	Used to remove dead hair and hairs on the verge of shedding. Useful on short- and longer-coated breeds. Smaller blades can be used for cats. Double-sided with different sized teeth. Excessive pressure should be avoided so as not to damage the skin
Undercoat rake	Used with thicker and double coats to remove dead undercoat and untangle small knots and matts. Light pressure should be used as the metal pins can be abrasive if pulled along the skin
Coat king	Used for thinning out coats. A selection of different sized blades is available with variable sized teeth. Mostly used by professional groomers as care is needed not to remove too much coat
Matt breaker	These tools break through knots and matts, they should not pull them out. Care is required as teeth and blades may cut the skin if used incorrectly
Stripping stone	Light 'airy' pumice type stone that is used for hand stripping wire-coated breeds
Scissors	Wide variety of sizes and styles are available. From top to bottom: safety scissors, with rounded ends for trimming around delicate areas; thinning scissors, used with thicker coats; trimming scissors, used for finishing coats
Electric and battery clippers	Can be used to trim fur and remove matts safely that are tight to the skin. Avoid using against the skin for extended periods of time as the clipper blade can become hot. Keep clean and well lubricated
Nail clippers	A wide variety of nail clippers is available. Heavy duty clippers may be required for larger breeds' nails. Sharp cutting types may be preferable to guillotine style cutters, which tend to squash the nail when it is cut

16.17   *continued* Small animal grooming equipment.

Grooming and clipping horses

Grooming

Horses should be groomed daily to remove any dead hair, dirt and skin. Grooming is also a good way to improve a horse's demeanour, as most horses appear to enjoy being groomed. Grooming may be limited by, for example, open wounds or drains.

Grooming a horse provides a valuable opportunity for assessing a patient's overall wellbeing and its ability to cope with hospitalization. It is also a good opportunity to assess pain management and determine whether the level of any analgesia is appropriate. The animal's case records should be completed appropriately at this time.

There are several components of a grooming kit, including many different types of brushes and combs. The **dandy brush** (Figure 16.18a) has firm bristles and is used to remove dry mud and dead hair; it should not be used on sensitive parts of the horse as the horse may find it uncomfortable. The **body brush** (Figure 16.18a) has soft bristles and can be used anywhere on the horse; it is particularly useful for sensitive horses and around the face. The **curry comb** (Figure 16.18b) comes in different materials, from rubber to metal, and is used for removing dead hair, especially when the horse's coat is changing. It is also used to clean the body brush of hair. The **mane comb** is used for brushing the mane and removing any tangles or knots in the hair. **Stable rubbers, sponges** (Figure 16.19) or whisps are used at the end of a grooming session to massage the horse's muscles and leave the horse's coat smooth and shiny. Other items of a grooming kit may include mane and tail conditioner, mane pulling comb, hoof ointment, sponges for the eyes and nostrils.

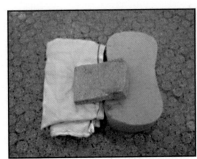

16.19 Equine grooming sponges.

How to groom a horse

1. Begin at the top of the neck, working down and over the main trunk of the body with the body brush. The legs can then be brushed using the dandy brush if required, to remove any dry mud. This routine should be carried out on both sides of the horse.
2. Move on to the face, using the body brush.
3. The mane and tail should then be brushed, using the mane comb for the mane and the body brush for the tail. A dandy brush should *not* be used on the tail as it will damage the hair.
4. Two different sponges should then be used: one for the nostrils and eyes, to remove any discharge or mucus, and the other for the anus and under the tail, the sponges should be labelled to avoid mixing them up.
5. Finish the body by using a whisp or stable rubber to massage the main trunk of the body, leaving it shiny and clean.
6. Pick the feet out (see below).

Clipping

As the weather changes, the horse's coat adapts to the temperature by losing hair or growing a thicker layer. Horse owners support their animals during such changes by using rugs (see above) and providing shelter when it is very cold. Sweat produced on exertion can leave the horse cold and wet following exercise during the colder months. A more comfortable environment for the horse can be achieved by clipping the hair in winter. Different types of clip are used, depending on the horse's lifestyle and exercise regime (Figure 16.20).

- **Trace clip:** This involves removing hair from the underside of the neck and abdomen. This clip originates from the carriage horse; the clip followed the lines of the harness. The hair is left on the topside of the body and legs for warmth. This type of clip is now used for horses in light work. There are two types of the trace clip: the high and low trace clip. The type used depends on the horse's workload. More hair is removed for a 'high' clip; this clip is nearer to a full clip and so is used for horses with a higher workload. This clip will still allow the horse to live outside.
- **Blanket clip** (Figure 16.20b): This is similar to the trace clip but also involves the removal of hair from the neck and the flanks, leaving a blanket-shaped area of coat over the back and hindquarters. This clip is used for horses in medium type work (e.g. those that take part in the occasional show) and again still allows the horse to be turned out.

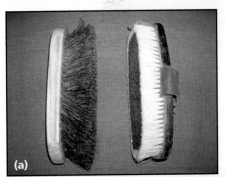

(a)

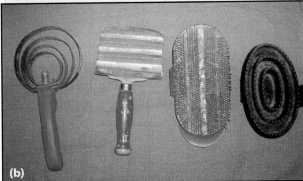

(b)

16.18 Depending on the type of coat, these pieces of the equine grooming kit are used for removing dead hair and mud. **(a)** Brushes: (left) dandy brush used for removing dirt and hair from the horse's legs; (right) body brush. **(b)** Curry combs: (from left to right) mud stripper, metal curry comb, plastic curry comb, rubber curry comb.

- **Hunter clip**: This clip involves removing all the hair from the body, leaving only the legs and a small area where the saddle sits. This type of clip is for horses in heavy work often involving mud, e.g. cross-country riding. This clip facilitates easy cleaning and drying of the horse after exercise.
- **Full clip** (Figure 16.20c): This involves removing all the hair from the body and legs. This clip is for horses in full competition work. Careful stable management is required when a horse is fully clipped; they must be rugged at all times and monitored for any rubs or sores, which may be more likely due to the reduced hair coat.

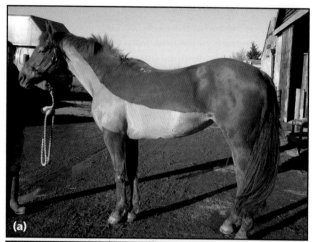

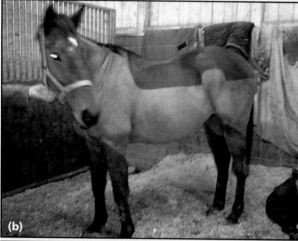

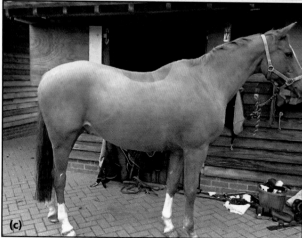

16.20 Equine clips: **(a)** chaser clip (similar to trace but flank coat left intact); **(b)** blanket clip; **(c)** full clip.

Before starting to clip:

- The horse should be groomed and, if necessary, given a bath (see below), as dirt and grime will blunt the clipper blades. The horse should be dry before clipping commences
- All equipment required must be made ready; this includes a well maintained pair of clippers that have newly sharpened blades in place, a brush and clipper oil (Figure 16.21).
- The horse may need to be restrained using a bridle or twitch (see Chapter 10). It is safest to have an assistant hold the horse while it is being clipped; however, if the horse is familiar and confident with being clipped it may be tied up in a secure area
- If necessary, the clip can be marked with chalk or a black marker to ensure that lines remain straight.

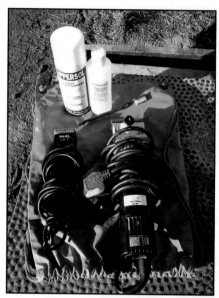

16.21 Equine clipping equipment.

When clipping a horse for the first time, the clippers should be introduced with care. The clippers should first be run over the horse's body when they are turned off. Once this has been done successfully, the clippers should be turned on and again run over the horse's body, so that it can feel the vibrations coming from the clipper. Some horses, no matter how much time and effort is put in, will not tolerate being clipped and may require sedation by a veterinary surgeon; it is safer to sedate the horse than risk someone getting hurt.

How to clip a horse

- Clipping should begin at the head and work back towards the tail, with the clipper blades placed flat to the horse's coat.
- The blades should glide over the hair; if too much pressure is applied 'tram lines' will be obvious on the skin.
- When clipping around the head and ears, a small pair of finishing clippers should be used to make the experience as pleasant as possible for the horse.
- Once finished, the horse should be given a thorough groom to remove any loose hair and then rugged immediately.

Bathing patients

Bathing may be required to remove coat soiling, maintaining the patient's cleanliness whilst it is hospitalized. Bathing may also be required to apply treatments to a patient's skin and coat, such as washes for demodectic or sarcoptic mange, and medicated shampoos for skin conditions such as *Malassezia* infection and skin hypersensitivities. Some animals may have coat contamination from substances, such as engine oil, which may be difficult to remove and so require special treatments. Care should be taken with the removal of possible toxic substances as the use of detergents to aid removal may increase absorption of the toxic substance through the skin.

Some patients may require bathing of only specific areas, such as feet, perineal area (commonly a problem in pet rabbits) or skin folds around the mouth to treat skin fold dermatitis (this often affects dog breeds with excessive jowl skin, such as spaniels and St Bernards). Each patient should be assessed individually prior to bathing, as complete bathing of some patients may be contraindicated in certain circumstances, for example:

- In the initial days after surgery, to reduce the possibility of introducing infection to the wound
- In patients with dressings or wounds such as skin grafts that require minimal disturbance and the area to be kept dry
- In patients with unstabilized fractures
- In the initial days after extensive orthopaedic procedures such as total hip replacements; if the patient struggled or slipped in a bath, dislocation of the joint could occur
- In weak, very unwell or dyspnoeic patients, where stress could exacerbate their condition.

In such cases, cleanliness can be maintained by 'bedbathing' the patient using a bowl of warm water and cotton wool. Damp cotton wool swabs can also be used to clean ocular and nasal discharges. Animals with facial injuries and small animal patients (especially cats) wearing Elizabethan collars should be cleaned frequently.

Bathing small animal patients

Depending on the size of the patient and the facilities available, bathing can be performed in a sink or bath or using a 'tub table' bath, where the patient is placed upon a metal grid supported above the bath (Figure 16.22).

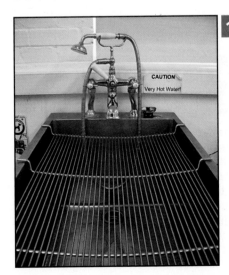

16.22 A 'tub table'.

All items required, including towels, shampoo, and bathing implements such as sponges or jugs, should be prepared prior to placing the patient within or on the bath. All baths should have a non-slip bottom to avoid accidental injury to the patient. Smaller patients such as cats and rabbits should be properly restrained to avoid injury occurring if the patient struggles. Care should be taken when lifting large patients into a bath to avoid injury to handlers. Personal protective equipment (PPE) should be worn that is appropriate for the shampoo or medicated washes that are being used. Water temperature should be monitored during use to avoid extremes of temperature.

Bathing a dog

1. Restrain the dog using a slip lead that is held by the groomer or an assistant. Patients should never be tied to the bath in case they try to jump out, causing injury or possible strangulation.
2. Wet the patient's coat thoroughly using a shower head or jugs of water.
3. Apply the shampoo and massage it into the coat, avoiding the face (medicated washes should be applied with a damp sponge of solution around the face, preventing the substance from running into the patient's eyes, ears or mouth). Leave the shampoo or wash on for the appropriate contact time, as directed by the manufacturer's recommendations. Gently holding the dog's muzzle will stop it shaking itself, preventing possible introduction of shampoo into its own or the handler's face.
4. Rinse the patient thoroughly, working from the upper body down to the underneath and legs; excess water can be squeezed from the coat.
5. Lift the patient out of the bath or move it on to a non-slip absorbent surface to be towel-dried. A hairdryer can be used to dry the patient if tolerated; care should be taken not to burn the patient by holding the dryer too close.
6. Once fully dry, the coat can be brushed through and the patient returned to a warm, draught-free environment.

Bathing the equine patient

Horses may need to be bathed for similar reasons to small mammals; however, their size necessitates that the process is a little different. Having all the equipment to hand (Figure 16.23) before starting the bathing procedure makes everything run much more smoothly.

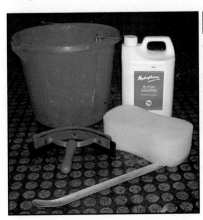

16.23 Equine bathing equipment: a bucket, sweat scrapers, shampoo and a sponge.

Bathing a horse

1. All equipment needed to bath the horse should be prepared and placed in the washing area; this includes shampoo, sponges, sweat scraper, towels, and access to hot and cold water.
2. Paint the horse's hooves with a hoof ointment; this will seal them and prevent them from drying out, which can happen if they are soaked with water during the bathing session.
3. Wet the legs thoroughly and apply the shampoo either by adding it to the water or applying it to the sponge.
4. Massage the legs, working up and down, and working the shampoo through the hair to break down any grease. Move up the forelegs, over the shoulder and neck (including the mane) and over the back (including the tail), keeping the hair moist and massaging in the shampoo. Continue in this manner until the back legs have been shampooed. A separate sponge should be used for around the anus and the area between the back legs.
5. Clean the mane and tail again, applying the shampoo to the wet hair and gently rubbing it through the hair, right down to the roots.
6. The face should be the last area to be washed, using a sponge in order to prevent any shampoo getting into the horse's eyes or any water entering the ears.
7. Remove the shampoo – a hose is the easiest way. Alternatively, buckets of water may be poured over the horse.
8. Repeat steps 3 to 7.
9. At the end of the bathing session, rinse the horse until there is no evidence of any soapy residue in the hair. Care should be taken to double-check the abdomen and heels for any shampoo residue, as the water runs and collects in these areas. Any residual shampoo can cause irritation of the skin.
10. Remove excess water with the sweat scraper on the main body and neck. Towels should be used to dry off the horse's legs and face.
11. Once the bathing session is finished, walk the horse for 10 minutes and hand graze (i.e. graze on a headcollar and lead rope) if the weather is warm, to dry the coat out completely. If the weather is not sufficiently warm, the horse should be rugged up with a fleece rug to help wick the last of the moisture away from the horse's skin. Once dry, this rug should be removed and the horse re-rugged with a dry rug if necessary and put in a stable to relax. If a solarium is available, the horse can dry out and relax under the heat lamps.

Small animal nail clipping

The trimming of a patient's nails is often a task that is performed by the veterinary nurse. Claws may be trimmed for patient comfort when walking, as an aid to managing unwanted behaviour such as scratching furniture, or to aid safe handling of the animal.

- Correct restraint should be used when handling pets for nail clipping and an additional person may be required. Birds and rodents may benefit from being restrained within a towel to prevent damage to both the animal and handler.
- The patient's digit should be firmly held and the nail examined to determine whether trimming is required. The hard part of the nail is an extension of the epidermis and varies in colour from transparent to pigmented. Beneath this is the dermis, which provides the blood and nerve supply to the nail. Care must be taken when trimming nails not to cut into the dermis as this will cause bleeding from the nail and will be painful to the patient. Transparent nails often allow a visual border of the dermis, which aids in deciding how far to cut the nail (Figure 16.24). The clipping of pigmented nails should be performed with care; a small amount can be cut and the nail then examined to decide whether it should be trimmed further.
- Specialized nail clippers of various sizes are available and an appropriate size and strength clipper should be used for each patient. For example, the nails of a hamster will require a small, delicate clipper to allow accuracy when clipping, whereas the nails of a Great Dane will require sharp heavy-duty clippers that are strong enough to cut the nail cleanly without crushing it.

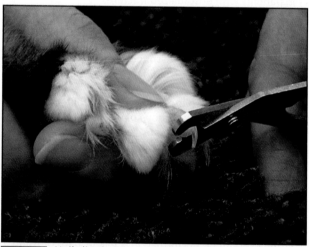

16.24 Nail clipping in a cat. Transparent nails allow visual assessment of how far to clip.

Foot care of equine patients

Hoof care should be a regular part of an inpatient's regime, involving daily cleaning and picking out of the feet, and treatment of any disease or injury when required. An appropriately trained person can carry out day-to-day care, but it is also essential to seek expert input from a farrier and veterinary surgeon. Hoof care is extremely important; badly neglected feet (Figure 16.25a) can lead to severe problems, necessitating euthanasia in some cases.

The equine hoof has evolved to cope with varying conditions, climates and surfaces. The rate of hoof growth and

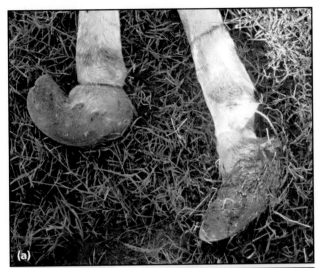

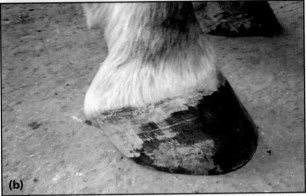

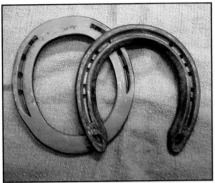

16.26 The oval shoe is an egg bar shoe, most commonly used for horses with foot problems such as laminitis. The standard U-shaped horse shoe is more common and can be put on any general purpose horse without foot problems.

16.25 **(a)** Badly neglected feet: the hoof wall and sole are badly overgrown so that the toe is long and curved upwards. Feet with this severity of overgrowth would be a welfare concern in breach of the Codes of Welfare for Horses and the Animal Welfare Act. **(b)** A well maintained and shod foot: the edges of the hoof are smooth and round, the toe is not overlong, and the shod sole makes flat contact with the ground.

wear may also be affected by breed, age and workload. The need to shoe horses is also determined by these factors. In addition, there are clinical situations in which shoes may benefit equine patients, such as in the management of laminitis. Attaching a shoe to a horse's hoof lifts the sole off the ground, protecting it from wear, damage and injury. Most horseshoes are U-shaped and made of steel (Figure 16.26), but materials can differ depending on the requirement. For example, aluminium shoes are used for racing because they are light but strong. Each shoe should be made to fit each individual horse's foot (Figure 16.25b), as every hoof is slightly different in conformation or size. Shoes are secured in place by nails or glue, depending on the material from which the shoe is made. There are many types of remedial shoe, each designed to suit a particular purpose. An example is the 'egg bar' shoe (Figure 16.26), which is oval in shape and designed to extend the heel area, providing better support for weight bearing at the heel. This is a very valuable type of shoe for horses with a broken back hoof–pastern axis (i.e. with a long toe and low heel conformation), or those with heel pain caused by navicular syndrome.

To ensure a horse's feet are being correctly looked after, knowledge of equine foot anatomy and physiology is essential

(see Chapter 3). Trimming by a registered farrier should be carried out every 4–6 weeks, but varies according to the horse's lifestyle and workload. Even unshod horses living out in a field, or those that are retired, need regular hoof maintenance.

Daily care of the horse's feet should include picking out the hoof, brushing out the hoof, ensuring no foreign bodies are in the hoof, checking for damage to the hoof, assessing soundness of the horse and applying any hoof treatment as required. Appropriate handling should be used at all times (see Chapter 10).

'Picking out' horses' feet

Picking out a horse's feet is an easy task if performed regularly. From a young age, horses should be encouraged to allow people to pick up and examine their feet. The correct technique should be used to pick up the feet (see Chapter 10).

How to 'pick out' a horse's feet

1. Begin on the left (near) side on a forelimb. Start by running your hand down the back of the leg. As you come to the cannon bone start to apply digital pressure. As you reach the fetlock the horse should then pick up its foot. If the horse has feathers, you can take hold of these to help you pick the foot up. Cupping the hoof in your hand, ensure you have a firm hold before you start picking out the feet.

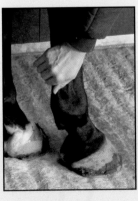

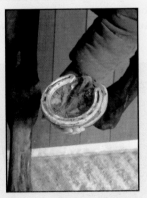

2. Scrape out the mud and debris using a hoof pick.
3. Ensure that you always scrape the hoof pick downwards and away from yourself.

continues ▶

continued

WARNING: Never turn a hoof pick round and scrape towards yourself. You could end up sticking the pick into your hand or getting a piece of foreign material in your eye.

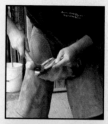

4. Use the brush on the hoof pick to clean out the sole, leaving a clean dry area. This is important as the sole and frog may become soft in wet weather or if the horse has been standing on wet bedding for too long.

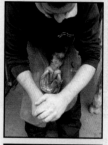

5. Hydrogen peroxide, formalin or iodine solution can be used to harden the sole and help maintain a healthier hoof.

6. Once the foot of the left (near) side forelimb has been picked out, move on to the hindlimb of the same side.

7. Repeat this method on the right (far) side (as illustrated). In some instances, a horse may be trained to have all four feet picked out from the near side to save time; however, this is not the safest way.

Removing a shoe

In the absence of a farrier, a veterinary nurse may remove a horse's shoe under the guidance of a veterinary surgeon. For example, removal of the shoe is essential prior to imaging of the foot, as metal will result in artefacts in radiographs and potential damage to MRI equipment.

Specialized equipment is needed to remove a shoe, including a buffer, a shoeing hammer, a nail puller and farrier pulloffs/pincers (Figure 16.27). A farrier's leather apron is valuable to protect clothing and legs from raised clenches (the bent over ends of the nails), especially if the horse pulls its leg away during removal. Nail pullers are very helpful but must only be used once the clinches have been well 'knocked up'. The affected hoof must be picked up correctly (see Chapter 10). Safety should be foremost; heavy metal tools are used for removing shoes and these should always be grasped firmly throughout the procedure. With the hoof firmly secured between the nurse's legs, the process should be well controlled and undaunting in a well behaved patient.

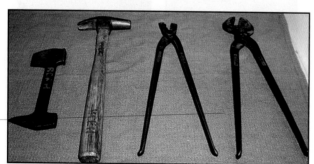

16.27 Tools for removing a shoe: (from left to right) buffer, shoeing hammer, nail puller and farrier pulloffs/pincers.

How to remove a horse's shoe

1. Raise the clinches by using the blade of the buffer. Place the blade under each clinch and using the hammer hit the buffer to ease the blade under the clinch and raise it away from the hoof. Do this with each clinch around the whole foot.

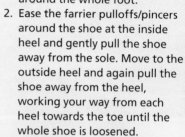

2. Ease the farrier pulloffs/pincers around the shoe at the inside heel and gently pull the shoe away from the sole. Move to the outside heel and again pull the shoe away from the heel, working your way from each heel towards the toe until the whole shoe is loosened.

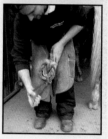

3. Use the farrier pulloffs/pincers to take hold of the shoe at the toe and pull backwards towards the hoof. The shoe should come away completely from the hoof, removing intact nails and leaving no bits behind in the hoof. Any nail that is left behind can be removed using a hoof knife.

Other farriery equipment that may be used within a hospital by the veterinary surgeon on horses' feet include:

- **Hoof knives** (Figure 16.28) – these come in different styles and sizes and may be curved or looped. Hoof knives also come with left- or right-handed handles for ease of use. They are used to remove dirty or abnormal sole and frog when cleaning the foot out prior to surgery or radiography and to look for abscesses within the hoof capsule. Hoof knives must be cleaned and dried after each use and, most importantly, they must be sharpened regularly.

- **Hoof rasps** – these usually have a wooden handle and teeth on both sides; the teeth are bigger on one side, which is used for levelling the sole and removing larger amounts of hoof, and smaller teeth on the other side, which are used to create a smooth finish. The rasp is also the tool used most commonly in foals treated for flexural limb deformities such as 'club foot'.

- **Farrier nippers** – these are used to remove large wedges of outer hoof wall when trimming the hoof. They must never be used for pulling off shoes, as this blunts their sharpened edge blades, which differentiate the tool from pulloffs/pincers. Farrier pull-offs/pincers have knobs at the end of their blades, which allows them to be differentiated from pincers

- **Hoof testers** (Figure 16.29) – this is one of the tools most commonly used by veterinary surgeons. Horses respond to pressure over painful areas of hoof, allowing location of focal pain and directing the veterinary surgeon to a soft area from which pus may be released. Sometimes an abscess might reveal pus when hoof tester pressure is applied to the affected area (see Common foot conditions below).

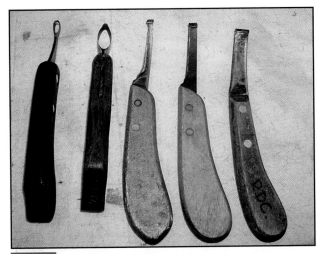

16.28 Selection of hoof knives.

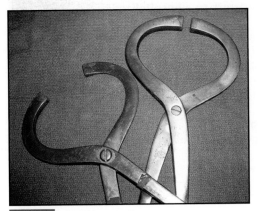

16.29 Hoof testers.

Common foot conditions in horses

It is useful for the veterinary nurse to understand some of the common foot conditions of the horse in order to best manage those animals under their care.

Abscesses can result from penetrating injuries, a bruised sole or badly fitting shoes. Abscesses can be easily diagnosed using hoof testers. The hoof should be held as for removing a shoe, and hoof testers used to examine the whole of the hoof. When pressure is applied to the area affected by the abscess the horse will react, usually by pulling the foot away, as it is painful. Sometimes the abscess will burst during the examination; at this point, the veterinary surgeon can use hoof knives to pare out the affected area. A poultice should be applied to draw out the infection, and changed daily until there is no discharge on the dressing. Poultices can be applied wet or dry. The foot should remain covered until the farrier or the veterinary surgeon is happy with the horse's clinical progress.

Penetration injuries can be fatal due to the fact that three synovial structures can be reached through the sole of the foot: the navicular bursa, the coffin joint and the deep digital flexor tendon sheath. When a horse has a penetration injury, radiographs are usually taken to identify the point at which the foreign body has entered the foot; this allows the veterinary surgeon to assess the severity of the injury.

Preparing the foot for surgery

Thoroughly preparing a foot for surgery is very important, particularly if an aseptic procedure is to be performed, because the foot is usually a dirty area. Preparation is often carried out the day prior to surgery and the clean foot is then often kept overnight in an iodine-soaked bandage. It should be noted that iodine is a radiodense element and can obscure any radiographic images that may be taken during or immediately after surgery. To prepare a foot for surgery it should first be picked out to remove any bedding and debris. An iodine-based scrub should then be used, followed by a hoof knife to scrape away dirty or abnormal sole and frog, removing any remaining dirt. This will leave a clean foot ready for surgery. To make the veterinary surgeon's job easier, a soak boot can be placed over the foot in order to soften the hoof slightly, making it easier for the veterinary surgeon to handle it during surgery.

How to make a soak boot

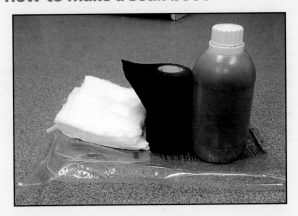

1. Pack swabs, wetted with an iodine-based scrub, into the foot.
2. Place the foot into a 5 litre fluid bag with the top cut off
3. Pour iodine solution into the bag until the hoof is covered
4. Seal the fluid bag using a cohesive dressing, such as Vetrap, and secure it to the leg.
5. The soak boot is normally put on the night before or the morning of the surgery, allowing time for the hoof to soften.

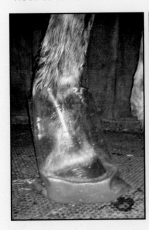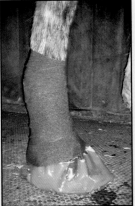

Acknowledgement

The editor (EM) would like to thank Liz Anne Dobson and 'Rio' for some of the photos in this chapter.

Further reading

Brega J (2007) *Essential Equine Studies: Injury, Disease and Equine Nursing: Book 3*. JA Allen & Co Ltd, London

British Horse Society (2005) *BHS Complete Horse and Pony Care*. Collins, UK

Curtis S (2002) *Corrective Farriery – A Textbook of Remedial Horseshoeing*. R &W Publications, Newmarket

Dallas S, North D and Angus J (2006) *Grooming Manual for the Dog and Cat*. Blackwell Publishing, Oxford

Flecknell P and Waterman-Pearson A (2000) *Pain Management in Animals*. WB Saunders, London

Girling S (2003) *Veterinary Nursing of Exotic Pets*. Blackwell Publishing, Oxford

Hughes A and Soloman-Kretay J (2007) General care and management of the dog. *BSAVA Manual of Practical Animal Care*, ed. P Hotson Moore and A Hughes, pp. 14–31. BSAVA Publications, Gloucester

Masters J and Willoughby K (2007) General care and management of the cat. *BSAVA Manual of Practical Animal Care*, ed. P Hotson Moore and A Hughes, pp. 32–52. BSAVA Publications, Gloucester

Self-assessment questions

1. List four methods that could be used to provide supplementary warmth to a hospitalized patient.
2. What potential problems could occur if a recumbent patient urinates on its bedding?
3. List some considerations that could influence the voluntary food intake of a hospitalized patient.
4. Why is it advantageous for the veterinary nurse to have information regarding a patient's normal behaviour prior to its admission to the hospital?
5. What benefits does exercising a patient out of its kennel or stable provide?
6. What methods of identification can be used for horses?
7. Why is patient identification essential within the veterinary hospital?
8. Grooming and bathing of a patient is required if coat soiling has occurred, but what other reasons are there for grooming of patients?
9. Name the farrier tools required for removing a shoe from a horse.
10. How would you prepare a horse's foot for surgery?

Chapter 17

Principles of general nursing

Sharon Chandler and Lucy Middlecote

Learning objectives

After studying this chapter, students should be able to:

- **Understand the reasons for bandaging and the principles of basic bandage selection, application and care**
- **Select appropriate dressing materials and bandages for a range of conditions and species**
- **Apply standard bandaging techniques to the limbs, head, body and tail of animals**
- **Describe methods for local applications of heat and cold**
- **Describe the general nursing requirements for a range of patients, including those that are geriatric, vomiting, soiled, recumbent, comatose, critically ill or neonatal**
- **Select equipment for, and carry out, enemas**
- **Select appropriate equipment for urinary catheterization**
- **Describe procedures for placement of urinary catheters and their management**
- Monitor for and recognize bandage-related problems
- Instruct owners on care and observation of the bandage
- Assist with application of specialized bandages.

Bandaging and dressings

The ability to place an effective bandage can make the difference between success and failure for any given surgical or non-surgical wound. Indeed, bandages can *create* wounds, or make existing wounds worse, if applied incorrectly or without due care. To be able to apply appropriate dressings and bandages it is essential to have knowledge of the way in which wounds heal, as this will affect how they are managed (see Chapter 25).

Veterinary nurses should be able to:

- Recognize types of wound
- Select correct materials appropriate to dress the wound
- For standard, uncomplicated applications, apply materials in the correct order and manner, resulting in an effective bandage

Reasons to bandage

Bandaging is used to hold dressings in place on any area of the patient. Other reasons for bandaging include:

- Support for:
  - Fractures or dislocations
  - Sprains or strains
  - Healing wounds
- Protection against:
  - Self-mutilation
  - Infection
  - Environment
  - Further injury
- Pressure to:
  - Arrest haemorrhage
  - Prevent or control swelling
- Immobilization to:
  - Restrict joint movement
  - Restrict movement at fracture site
  - Provide comfort and pain relief.

Bandaging materials

Dressings

Dressings are applied before any other materials, directly to the wound. They prevent subsequent layers from sticking to, or contaminating, the area. Dressings are invariably sterile and need careful handling. There are many different dressings available (Figure 17.1). More information on the uses of different dressing types in small animals is given in Chapter 25.

Padding, conforming and protective materials

Types of padding material are described in Figure 17.2. Conforming materials (Figure 17.3) are supplied in two basic varieties: those with an elastic/latex component and those without. Each manufacturer uses a different design, construction and proportion of elastic/latex. Protective materials may be adhesive or cohesive (Figure 17.4).

Dressing type	Description	Uses
Dry	Plain gauze swabs	Debridement of wounds
Impregnated	Petroleum gel Antibiotic	Superficial open wounds
Semi-occlusive	Usually with a layer of permeable non-stick material on one or both sides and a central absorbent core May have adhesive section round edge to enable accurate, stable placement	Surgical wounds Wounds with mild to moderate discharges
Absorbent	Made of various materials Usually thicker and often with a coloured side that faces the wound May have adhesive section round edge to enable accurate placement	Large wounds where there is a large amount of exudate; helps to remove fluid from wound area whilst preventing drying at the wound surface
Gels	Gel-based; or gels with no base that need to be used in conjunction with other dressings	Where maintenance of moisture is essential (granulating wounds) Where there is a large deficit beneath skin level that is difficult to dress in any other manner
Others	Silver-impregnated Iodine-impregnated	Properties proven to help to prevent infections and encourage speed of healing

17.1 Types of dressing.

Type	Description	Uses/comments
Cotton wool	Natural or man-made absorbent material in rolls	Can be used as sole padding material in most bandages Can be difficult to apply compared with others
Padding bandage	Natural absorbent material supplied in rolls of various sizes	Preferable to cotton wool in most cases due to ease of application Particularly good for limbs
Synthetic padding	Supplied in rolls of various sizes Thinner and lighter	Good where less bulk is needed (e.g. under casts, smaller patients) Can cause sweating and is not so absorbent
Foam	Variety of thicknesses	Useful when external fixators are bandaged or under drains etc.
Cotton wool/gauze	Cotton wool sandwiched between gauze layers Supplied in rolls	Very useful for abdomens and thorax bandages Holes may be cut to accommodate legs and prepuce

17.2 Types of padding.

Type	Description	Uses/comments
Loose open weave	Has no elastic component but loose weave aids conforming property (e.g. Crinx)	Can be used to hold padding to any area of the body
Conforming	Has an elastic component	Can be placed too tightly – care needs to be taken during application, especially if not a lot of padding underneath: blood/fluid flow can be compromised, resulting in swelling or death of tissue
Tubular	Bandage supplied in a tube construction	Under casts and on abdomens and thorax Holes can be cut for legs/prepuce etc.
Crepe	Washable cotton fibre material on a role	Not commonly used but may be useful to hold small dressings in place on thorax etc.

17.3 Conforming materials.

Type	Description	Uses/comments
Adhesive	Thick cotton-based material with an adhesive side. Supplied in rolls of various widths	Good for foot bandages (due to thickness). Avoid applying direct to skin and hair
Cohesive	Latex-containing material that 'sticks' to itself but not to skin or hair. Supplied in rolls of various widths, colours and designs	Most commonly used protective material. Performs well and can be used in any bandaging. *Care must be taken as the latex component has a 'memory' and will tighten once in place, especially if stretched too much during application*

17.4 Description and uses of adhesive and cohesive protective materials.

Basic principles of bandaging

Basic bandaging formula

- Initial layer – dressing.
- Primary layer – padding (comfort/support/absorption).
- Secondary layer – conforming (strength/contouring/security).
- Tertiary layer – protection (conforming/strength).

Rules for bandaging

- Avoid departing from the basic bandaging formula wherever possible.
- Never leave more than the tips of the toes out on limb bandages.
- Check and change bandages regularly.
- Always attempt to include a padding layer to provide comfort.
- Avoid sticking adhesive material to the skin to prevent bandage slippage – poorly applied previous layers will tend to 'slip' below the adhesive bandage, causing 'drag' on the skin, which may result in skin sores or more serious complications.
- Never exchange firmness for tightness in order to achieve the aim of the bandage.

Bandaging assessment

To ensure correct selection and application, three questions should be asked during the bandaging procedure:

- Is the bandage achieving the aim (e.g. no slipping; immobilizing correct joint)?
- Is the bandage comfortable (e.g. no chewing/interference by the patient)?
- Is the bandage sensible (e.g. the patient can move/breathe easily)?

These assessment questions apply equally to all species.

Care of bandages and dressings

Once the bandage has been applied, constant checks should be maintained until it is removed.

- The bandage should be checked to ensure that it is not uncomfortable or too tight.
- Any evidence of odour, oedema, discharge, skin irritation, or wetness due to the wound itself (discharges or blood) should be investigated – usually by changing the bandage.
- It is important that the dressing does not become soiled or wet from environmental factors (e.g. urine, water, mud). The dressing should be covered with a protective covering when the patient is taken outside; there are commercial 'booties' available but empty, dried and adapted drip bags are durable and work well as a protective 'do-it-yourself' boot.

Constant chewing or licking at the bandage by the patient should be discouraged, but patient interference can indicate that the bandage is uncomfortable, causing irritation or causing pain and should be investigated. If there appears to be nothing wrong and the behaviour persists, one of the following measures may be tried depending on the species involved:

- Elizabethan collar (Figure 17.5). Tiny commercial collars are available for small mammals and birds, although these can be made easily and more cheaply from unwanted/old X-ray film
- Training and reward, as appropriate
- Provision of toys
- Muzzle
- Application of commercial foul-tasting substance to dressing
- Sedation
- Cross-tying of equine patients (see later).

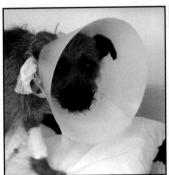

17.5 The Elizabethan collar prevents this dog from interfering with its bandages.

Common bandaging techniques for dogs and cats

Limb

Limb bandages are commonly required in general veterinary practice. They can be used for the distal portion of the limb only (e.g. for cut pads, dew claw removal) or for the entire limb (e.g. many surgical procedures or trauma).

Procedure for limb and foot bandage

1. Ensure the patient is suitably restrained.
2. Place cotton wool padding between the patient's toes, pads and dew claws to absorb sweat and prevent irritation (Figure 17.6a)
3. Apply a layer of cotton wool or soft dressing material around the foot. If using pre-rolled padding bandage apply it longitudinally to the cranial and caudal surfaces of the limb (Figure 17.6b).
4. Wind it around the foot in a figure-of-eight pattern.
5. Continue up the limb.
6. Apply the conforming bandage, similarly, longitudinally to the cranial and caudal surface of the limb.
7. Wind the conforming bandage around the foot in a figure-of-eight pattern, ensuring even tension throughout (Figures 17.6c,d).
8. Continue up the limb.
9. Anchor the bandage over the hock, carpus or olecranon as appropriate. The anchor point on full hindlimb bandages is more difficult as stifle movement encourages slippage rather than helping to prevent it; the key here is to ensure sufficient padding material is used to allow safe compression with conforming bandage to create a firm but not constricting result.
10. Apply the protective layer (Figure 17.6e) in the same manner.

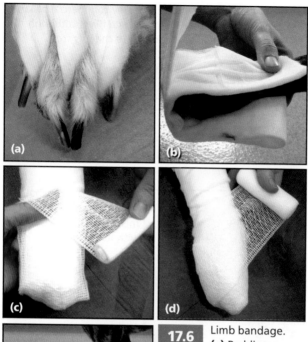

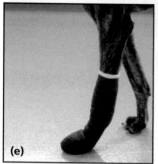

17.6 Limb bandage. **(a)** Padding between the toes. **(b)** Pre-rolled padding bandage is applied longitudinally. **(c,d)** Figure-of-eight pattern shown for conforming bandage. **(e)** Bandage with final protective cohesive layer.

This method of limb dressing encloses the digits. Alternatively, the very tips of the toes can be left out of the bandage to enable peripheral circulation to be monitored. In these cases the bandage at each stage is simply started by passing the bandage around the foot excluding the toes. Either technique is acceptable and effective.

WARNING

Only the very tips of the toes should be seen. Avoid leaving the whole foot out of a limb bandage; the foot invariably swells and such bandages are prone to significant slippage.

Ear

Ear bandages are used either to help arrest haemorrhage or to keep dressings in place. They may be used after some surgical procedures (e.g. aural resections), but recent thinking is that surgical ear wounds are best left open to the air. The commonest reason for bandaging is trauma. Either one ear or both ears may be bandaged.

Procedure for bandaging a single ear

1. Place a pad of cotton wool on the top of the patient's head.
2. Apply appropriate dressings to any wounds on the pinna and then fold the ear back on to the pad (Figure 17.7a).

3. Place a further pad of cotton wool over the ear.
4. Apply padding (cotton wool) around the head or, if using a pre-rolled padding bandage apply this in a figure-of-eight pattern around the opposite ear (Figure 17.7b,c).
5. Apply conforming bandage as in step 4, ensuring the padding stays proud of the conforming layer to prevent constriction or rubbing.
6. Cover the bandage with adhesive tape or cohesive bandage (Figure 17.7d).
7. Anchor the bandage using the opposite ear. If applying to a patient with small ears or ears that lie flat to the head (e.g. Greyhounds) it may be advantageous to include both ears.

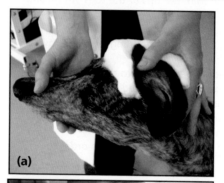

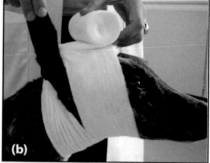

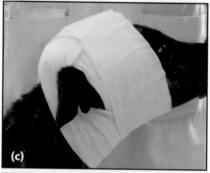

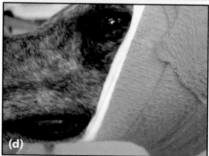

17.7 Ear bandage. **(a)** Ear pinna folded back on to padded head. **(b,c)** Pre-rolled padding bandage is applied in a figure-of-eight pattern around the opposite ear. **(d)** Cohesive bandage in place.

After application, the patient should be observed for a few minutes to ensure that the bandage is not too tight and causing breathing difficulties. The aim is to have the bandage as far forward as possible (without interfering with sight), otherwise it will slip backwards and its role be compromised. Checking that two fingers can be passed under the edges of the bandage ensures it has not been applied too tightly.

Chest and abdomen

The chest bandage is prevented from slipping by passing the bandaging materials between the front legs in a figure-of-eight fashion, resulting in a cross-over of bandages between the forelimbs on the ventral surface (Figure 17.8).

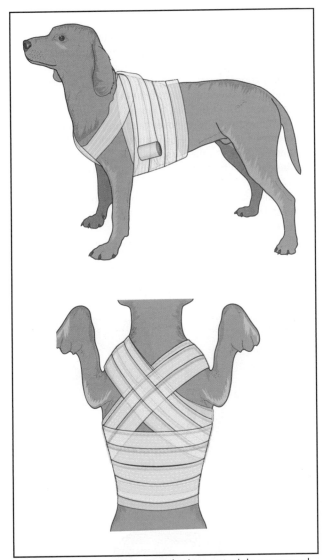

17.8 Chest bandage. Bandaging materials are passed between the front legs, in a figure-of-eight pattern, to prevent the chest bandage from slipping. (Reproduced from the *BSAVA Manual of Practical Veterinary Nursing*)

If cohesive bandage is used it must *not* be placed too tightly, as tightness may result in the patient having difficulty in breathing. Adhesive material should be avoided as it tends to make the patient very hot and has minimal ability to expand and retract with respiration.

The abdomen is difficult to bandage in dogs due to the relative narrowness of the area compared to the thorax.

'Bunching' of material tends to occur and the only way to help prevent this is to extend a chest bandage down over the abdomen. This works well in round-chested breeds (e.g. Dachshunds) but less well in deep-chested breeds (e.g. Dobermanns). Padding layers can simply be laid around the abdomen and secured with conforming and protective layers, or Gamgee can be used and secured with tape.

Dressings on the chest and abdomen can be given extra assistance to stay in place by tubular 'stretchy' vests; there are a variety of these available (Figure 17.9).

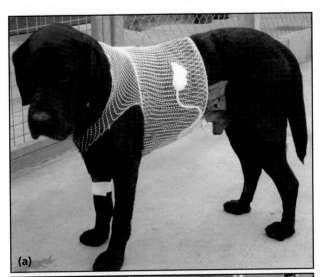
(a)

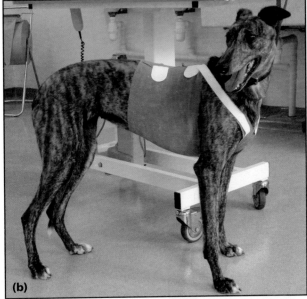
(b)

17.9 A variety of vests are available to assist in holding chest and abdomen dressings in place. **(a)** Stockinette vest. **(b)** Commercial tapeless vest.

Tail

The tail occasionally needs a *light* bandage to arrest haemorrhage, to keep a dressing in place or to protect the tail tip from injury. Tail bandages are difficult to keep in place but are applied in much the same manner as a limb bandage. Opinions differ as to technique, but avoiding excessively heavy padding is always wise. Flicking hair into some turns of the initial layer of bandage can help to hold it in place. Some people prefer to avoid bandaging the tail if possible, opting for the use of plastic tubes to protect tail tip injuries (tape can be minimally used to attach the tube to the tail) or of dressings that have an adhesive surround, e.g. Primapore (Smith and Nephew).

Procedure for bandaging a tail

1. Place a dressing on the wound if required.
2. Apply a light synthetic padding bandage, longitudinally to the cranial and then the caudal surface of the tail tip (Figure 17.10a).
3. Change the orientation of the bandage and pass it horizontally around the tail (Figure 17.10b).
4. Continue to bandage around the tail tip in a figure-of-eight pattern (Figure 17.10c,d), resulting in a neat compact tail tip.
5. Proceed to wind the bandage around the tail, moving cranially (Figure 17.10e). At each turn of the bandage, flick a little hair out from under the previous turn and include this in the next turn of bandage. This will aid the 'grip' of the bandage on to the tail and will help to prevent the bandage from simply sliding off.
6. Repeat with a conforming bandage and a final protective layer. Flicking of hair is obviously only possible in the primary bandage layer.

Specialized bandaging techniques

The four most common special techniques are:

- **Ehmer sling**: to support the hindlimb following reduction of hip luxation (surgical or non-surgical)
- **Velpeau sling**: to support the shoulder joint following luxation or surgery
- **Robert Jones bandage**: to provide support and immobilization to fractured limbs in a first aid situation or following surgery
- **Spica bandage**: to immobilize the forelimb, in particular the elbow joint and associated bones.

Procedure for Ehmer sling

1. Apply padding material to the metatarsus and stifle.
2. Flex the leg and rotate the foot inwards; this will engage the hip joint into the acetabulum.
3. Apply cohesive bandage (some veterinary surgeons prefer adhesive tape) to the metatarsus, bringing it medial to the stifle joint (Figure 17.11a).
4. Continue the bandage over the thigh and back to the metatarsus in a figure-of-eight motion; the bandage passes medial to the tarsal joint (Figure 17.11b).
5. Repeat until full support of the hip is achieved (Figure 17.11c).
6. Padding can be applied at 'high friction' points to try and avoid excessive discomfort and help avoid injury to skin.
7. This dressing is usually kept in place for 4–5 days.

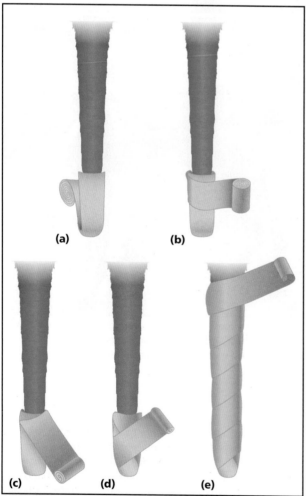

17.10   Tail bandages are applied using longitudinal, horizontal and figure-of-eight stages for each layer.

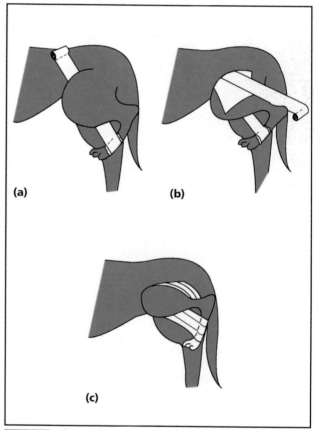

17.11   Ehmer sling. Applying the cohesive bandage. Padding may be used between the flexed leg and the body to aid comfort and avoid friction problems.

Procedure for Velpeau sling

1. Apply a layer of padding material to the foot and carpus and around the torso (this is easier if pre-rolled padding is used rather than cotton wool).
2. Secure the padding layer with conforming or cohesive bandage, ensuring that the bandage emerges in a cranial direction on the lateral side of the foot, in order to provide 'lift' to the limb (Figure 17.12a).
3. Hold the leg in flexion and take the bandage over the shoulder and around the chest, returning to complete a full circle around the torso.
4. Repeat until full support of the shoulder is achieved.
5. Apply cohesive bandage to cover other layers (Figure 17.12b).

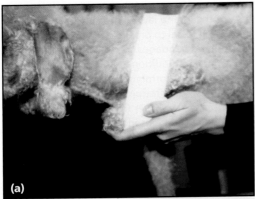

(a)

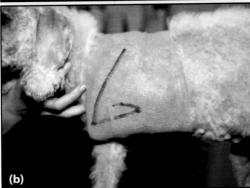

(b)

17.12 Velpeau sling. **(a)** Bandaging provides lift to the limb. **(b)** Final cohesive layer in place. The arrow is drawn on to indicate the position of the limb under the bandage.

Procedure for Robert Jones bandage

1. Apply zinc oxide traction tapes to the dorsal and ventral surfaces of the foot (commonly referred to as 'stirrups') (Figure 17.13a).
2. Using cotton wool from a roll, take a large length and wrap it lightly around the leg and foot. A large quantity should be used to support the limb (Figure 17.13b).
3. Apply conforming bandage firmly over the cotton wool padding. The aim is to compress the cotton wool so that it conforms to the leg contours. The deep layer of cotton wool incorporates a lot of air and it takes some effort when applying this layer to achieve adequate conformity. ▶

4. Incorporate the traction tapes into the bandage to prevent slipping (Figure 17.13c).
5. The toes should be visible so that checks may be made for evidence of oedema or abnormal changes in temperature (Figure 17.13d). Occasionally the toes are included in the bandage.
6. Cover the bandage with cohesive bandage for protection and extra support (Figure 17.13e).
7. The bandage may be kept in place for up to 2 weeks.

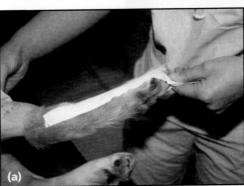

(a)

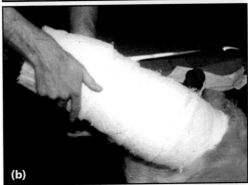

(b)

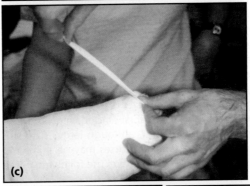

(c)

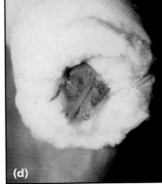

(d)

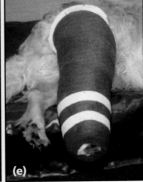

(e)

17.13 Robert Jones bandage. **(a)** Applying traction tapes. **(b)** Cotton wool around the limb. **(c)** The traction tapes are incorporated into the bandage. **(d)** Exposed toes. **(e)** Cohesive bandage in place.

Spica bandage

This specialized bandage is used to immobilize the elbow joint or associated bones (e.g. scapula, humerus, proximal radius and ulna). It involves taking the bandaging material up and over the cranial thorax, before placing a figure-of-eight bandage around the opposite leg (Figure 17.14).

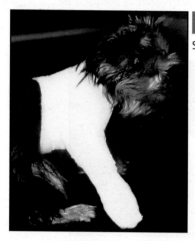

17.14

Spica bandage in place.

Bandaging and wound care in horses

The general principles of wound care and bandage management in horses are similar to those for other species, and will depend upon the location and severity of the wound. Closed wounds such as bruising and haematomas usually require little intervention, whereas open wounds including abrasions, punctures, incisions, proud flesh and lacerations often require more treatment and care. The purpose of wound care is to enable primary wound closure or to encourage healthy granulation tissue and healing, and to prevent infection (see Chapter 25). Excessive granulation tissue can, however, cause problems in horses (and, to a lesser extent, in ponies) as it may form rapidly, particularly in wounds to the limbs. Regular monitoring and observation of all wounds must be carried out in order to prevent excessive granulation tissue from developing; it is not uncommon for surgical excision of granulation tissue to be required.

Bandaging materials used in horses include most of those discussed earlier in the chapter, although larger sizes are generally required. Bandages in horses may be light and simple (Figure 17.15), e.g. for short-term use following nerve

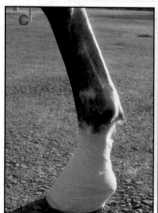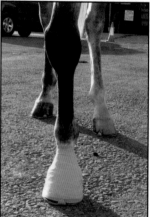

17.15   A light bandage on the hoof of an equine patient.

blocks or for more superficial wounds. Larger bandages (Figures 17.16 and 17.17) are usually for more serious wounds, e.g. those that are exudative or those requiring added support. It is often helpful to use an adherent/adhesive material to secure the bandage at the top and bottom, to prevent movement or slippage and to prevent any debris from entering inside the bandage. Such materials must, however, be applied in such a way that they are not too tight, and must be removed very carefully so as not to damage the patient's skin.

Procedure for applying a larger/ multi-layered bandage to a horse

1. Secure the sterile dressing in place with the initial padding layer (soft cotton bandage) (Figure 17.16a).
2. Apply the initial padding layer to the limb, from distal to proximal (Figure 17.16b,c).
3. Apply a second padding layer (cotton wool) to the limb, again from distal to proximal (Figure 17.16d,e).
4. Apply conforming bandage in a similar fashion (Figure 17.16f,g). (NB Additional multiple layers (cotton wool then conforming bandage) can be repeated at this stage if required.)
5. Apply the outer/tertiary layer (Figure 17.16h,i). (NB An adhesive bandage can be used to secure the top and bottom of the bandage if required.)

Common bandaging techniques for horses

Head

Wounds on the equine head are not easy to bandage and it is common practice to leave them undressed unless absolutely necessary. If head dressings are used it is important that the patient's eyes, nostrils and mouth are not obstructed by the bandage, and that the horse is still able to eat easily. A 'donut' bandage can be used to reduce the risk of further trauma to ocular wounds and wounds around the eye. Alternatively, wounds to the head or eye area can be dressed with bandage stents sutured over the site of the wound.

Body

Belly bands and stents can be useful for wounds on the body, although these areas are difficult to bandage. Adhesive dressings can also be used where required, although how long they stay in place is usually dependent on the area on which they are used.

Upper limb

It is fairly uncommon practice to cover the upper limb areas of horses as they are difficult to bandage; however, retaining straps or suturing of dressings or stents to the skin can sometimes be useful. Adhesive dressings can also be used, although they rarely stay in place for long periods of time.

Hock

Wounds on the point or the dorsal aspect of the hock are particularly hard to dress because of the amount of movement in these areas. Various commercial human dressings and adhesive dressings can be adapted and normally stay in place if the rest of the bandage is applied appropriately. The particularly vulnerable areas of the hock (common calcanean tendon

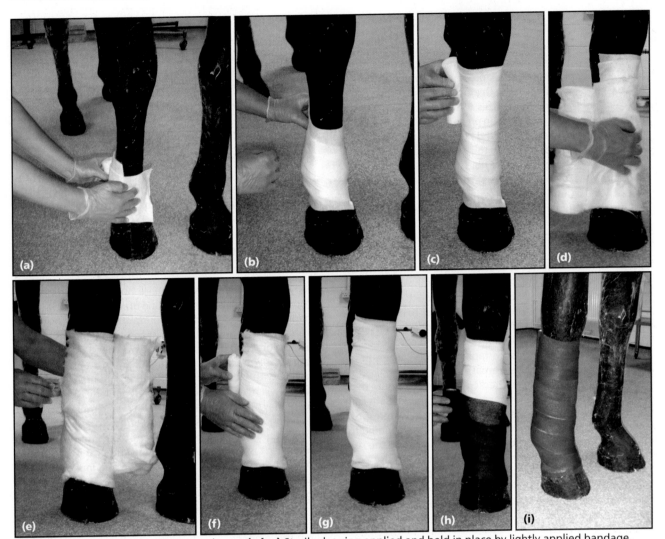

17.16 Multi-layered bandage on a horse. **(a,b,c)** Sterile dressing applied and held in place by lightly applied bandage. Layers of cotton wool **(d,e)**, conforming bandage **(f,g)** and the outer covering **(h,i)** are applied to the limb in a distal to proximal direction.

area, dorsal aspect of the hock below the tarsometatarsal joint, and the point of the hock) are all potentially at risk from bandaging trauma if an inappropriate or tight bandage is placed. In order to reduce trauma to these areas, a figure-of-eight bandaging technique can be utilized so that there is no tension on the calcanean tendon area, and the point of the hock is left as free as possible. To reduce risk, it may sometimes be more appropriate to utilize a pressage bandage for this area (see below).

Carpus

Although horses tend to tolerate immobilization of the carpus ('knee') better than the hock, it is also a vulnerable area. The skin covering the bone in this area is very thin, so there is a risk of damage as a result of bandaging. The skin over the accessory carpal bone is particularly prone to damage if it is covered because of the pressure that is put upon it during movement of the carpus. Trauma caused by bandaging can be prevented by ensuring that the accessory carpal is left uncovered or by relieving pressure over the area (Figure 17.17). A figure-of-eight bandaging technique is recommended as this allows the accessory carpal to remain uncovered. To reduce the risk it may sometimes be more appropriate to utilize a pressage bandage for this area (see below).

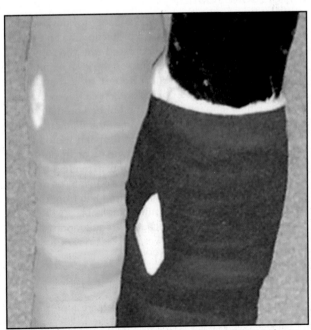

17.17 To prevent trauma from a knee bandage, the pressure can be released by carefully incising the conforming bandage layer over the accessory carpal bone.

Pressage bandage

The pressage bandage is a method of applying even pressure to wounds in horses in order to reduce oedema, exudation and proud flesh. A pressage bandage is a re-usable elasticated stocking with a zip fastening. Pressages are available in a range of sizes for the hock, knee and fetlock region, and provide even pressure over the dressing and padding layer(s). In hock and knee areas it is useful to apply a stable bandage below the pressage bandage and an adhesive bandage above, to hold it in place and prevent slipping. Pressage bandages are particularly useful for more superficial wounds and following surgical procedures where the wound is minimal and exudate is not heavy.

Foot

In order to reduce the risk of foot bandages moving upwards over the pastern area, dressings should incorporate both the heel and sole of the foot. Strong tape (e.g. 'duct' tape/nylon tape) can be used to reinforce the bandage, or to make a 'toe and sole pad', which should stop the horse wearing through the bandage. It is important that the skin and coronet band are not incorporated into such taping, as this can result in trauma and irritation to these areas.

Foot bandages need to be checked regularly to ensure that they are intact and have not become wet or soiled. Bags can be used to cover foot bandages and make them waterproof, although this is not recommended long term as they tend to cause the foot to become hot and sweaty, increasing the risk of further problems. In certain circumstances the use of a hospital plate fitted to an egg bar shoe may make the application of dressings to the sole much easier and may also reduce the cost due to the need for less frequent repeated bandage application.

Specialized equine bandaging techniques

Robert Jones Bandage

As in small animals, a Robert Jones Bandage provides increased limb immobilization, stability and protection. It can be used with or without a splint support placed over the top of the outside of the bandage, depending on the level of immobilization and support required. A Robert Jones bandage is multi-layered to increase rigidity and spread even pressure over the whole limb region, and the finished product should result in a bandage that is three times the diameter of the normal leg. The bandage should be firm and should sound like a ripe melon when tapped. Depending on its purpose, a Robert Jones bandage will be **half limb**, extending from the floor up to the proximal metacarpus (forelimb) or proximal metatarsus (hindlimb), or **full limb**, extending from the floor up to the elbow (forelimb) or stifle (hindlimb).

A half limb Robert Jones bandage will require approximately:

- 4–5 rolls of 500 g cotton wool
- 8–10 conforming bandages
- 2–3 self-adherent bandages.

A full limb Robert Jones bandage will require approximately:

- 10 rolls of 500 g cotton wool
- 20 conforming bandages
- 4–6 self-adherent bandages.

Splinting

A Robert Jones bandage can be used in combination with splinting to aid immobilization of wounds, to support both open and closed fractures, and to stabilize limbs prior to travelling and/or surgery. The splint is applied over the top of the bandage and secured in place with an adhesive bandage. Ideally a splint should immobilize the joints above and below the area that is damaged. A splint should be lightweight, strong and rigid. Many practices utilize various materials such as wood or plastic guttering to act as splints, and these usually work well as long as they are cut to an appropriate length and the ends are padded to provide protection. Commercial splints are also available to aid stabilization of fractures below the distal metacarpus/metatarsus.

Management of bandages in equine patients

Many equine patients will require hospitalization and appropriate care whilst bandages and dressings are in place (see Chapters 12 and 16). Additional precautions may be necessary to prevent self-trauma during this time. Most patients tolerate having a dressing in place but some may need to wear a neck cradle or be muzzled or cross-tied in order to prevent interference with bandages and dressings. A patient wearing a muzzle will need to have it removed regularly to allow feeding, or may need to be muzzled only when it runs out of food; providing such patients with *ad libitum* forage may deter them from interference. If a patient does interfere with its bandage, it is first worth assessing whether it is uncomfortable and, if so, ascertaining the reason and implementing a treatment for this before a decision to use an anti-interference device is made.

It is sometimes necessary to cross-tie an equine patient in order to prevent interference with the bandage, or to limit movement.

Cross-tying a horse

- By limiting side-to-side motion, cross-ties diminish the likelihood of movement, as well as making it very difficult for the horse to lie down, which can be useful for recovery from injuries such as fractures.
- The horse is tied up by both sides of its head. The rope/tie on either side should extend from the horse's headcollar and be attached to bailer twine or similar material that will break. This is attached to a tie ring that is, in turn, attached to a sturdy wall, rail or post. The clips used to attach the ropes/ties should allow for quick release in case the horse should panic.
- Light chains are sometimes used in place of ropes but this must be done with caution: if a panicking horse breaks free with chains attached, the chains can swing and cause injury to both horse and handler.

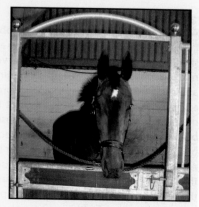

For a cross-tied horse, it is imperative that water buckets and feed are still easily accessible. It is recommended that the patient is untied and fed from the floor (under supervision) at frequent intervals, as this can aid drainage of fluid that may build up as a result of having the head tied in an upright position and can help to prevent lower respiratory problems such as pleurisy from occurring. Frequent monitoring of body temperature is especially important for a cross-tied patient because they are unable to move around and keep themselves warm; extra rugs and stable bandages may be required. It is also imperative that urinary and particularly faecal output are carefully monitored, as gut motility may be slowed with limited/restricted access to movement and box-rested and cross-tied patients may therefore be at increased risk from impaction colic. Nasogastric intubation with an electrolyte solution may be helpful in reducing gastrointestinal impactions in horses receiving box rest.

Bandaging exotic pets

The basic bandaging principles described above may be applied to small mammals, birds and other exotic pets, although a certain amount of creativity is often required to ensure the aim of the bandage is achieved. All the dressing types mentioned above are appropriate for use in small patients, although they are often too large and must therefore be cut to size. Rolls of bandage can be cut in half with a sharp knife to provide a more suitable size for easier application. Adhesive tape to secure dressings and bandages may be appropriate in small animals. Imaginative use of non-veterinary products, e.g. the use of lollypop sticks as splints, is common and can be very successful. Specific bandaging techniques are used to support the wings of injured birds (see *BSAVA Manual of Wildlife Casualties*).

Local applications of heat and cold

The application of heat causes vasodilation and therefore increased blood supply to the affected area. This will provide white blood cells for wound healing and assist in fluid removal from the area. Heat may be provided by applying cotton wool soaked in hot water or by means of a poultice prepared with medicants such as kaolin; re-useable hot and cold packs (Figure 17.18) are also widely available.

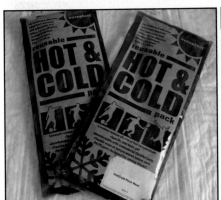

17.18

Re-useable hot and cold packs.

The application of heat is indicated in cases of:

- Oedema
- Infected wounds
- Abscesses.

Cold may be provided by applying gauze soaked in cold water or an ice pack. Burns and scalds should be flushed with cold water from the tap. The cold application will cause vasoconstriction, therefore reducing heat and blood loss. The application of cold is indicated in cases of:

- Swelling
- Pain
- Haemorrhage
- Minor burns and scalds
- Heatstroke.

Enemas

An enema is a liquid substance placed into the rectum and colon of a patient. The enema is not intended to flush colonic contents but to distend the rectum and distal colon gently, initiating normal expulsive reflexes.

Reasons for administering an enema

- **For emptying the rectum:**
  - To relieve constipation or impaction
  - As preparation for radiographic studies. The colon and rectum overlie abdominal structures and will obscure them if they are not emptied
  - As part of a radiographic contrast study
  - To enable the administration of drugs
  - In preparation for endoscopic examination.
- **As a diagnostic aid:** Barium sulphate enemas can be given to outline the rectal and colonic walls in radiographs. After the radiography the patient will need to evacuate the barium, so a quick retreat to the outside is strongly advised.
- **For administration of medication:** The colon has a large capacity for absorption. It is therefore a good route for the administration of soluble drugs, but it is rarely used in veterinary medicine due to lack of patient cooperation. One good example, however, is the administration of rectal diazepam (Figure 17.19) in seizuring patients, where oral medication is dangerous and gaining intravenous access may well be extremely difficult and not possible for owners to administer.

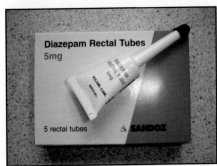

17.19

Diazepam rectal tubes.

Solutions used

- **Water:** Warm tap water is the preferred solution. It is readily available, non-toxic and non-irritant. In addition, any cleaning of the perianal area is reasonably straightforward.
- **Liquid paraffin:** This is readily available and reasonably cheap. Cleaning the patient after the enema can be difficult, since liquid paraffin is oil-based and not water-soluble. The patient must be bathed with shampoo to remove the paraffin.
- **Mineral oil:** This has the same disadvantages as liquid paraffin and is more expensive. However, oil-based substances are an advantage when treating a constipated patient. The oil helps to soften and lubricate the faecal masses and allows easier evacuation of the bowel.
- **Saline (phosphate enema):** This is usually available as manufactured sachets with phosphate included. They promote defecation as they are osmotically active, promoting water retention in the colon. These enemas should be used with care in small (<15 kg) and young patients because their excessive use can result in unwanted absorption of certain ions, resulting in system toxicity.
- **Ready-to-use mini-enema:** A proprietary brand of miniature enema is introduced into the rectum by an attached nozzle. It is extremely useful in cats, the procedure being no more stressful than using a rectal thermometer.
- **Gastrointestinal cleaning agents:** These are laxatives rather than enemas but can be used for bowel clearance for all the same indications. These agents are given orally, and defecation occurs rapidly after administration. Stomach tubing may be required to administer the fluid, as they are flavoured for the human market, so dogs, for example, are usually unwilling to drink them.
- **Miscellaneous substances:** The following variations are either more expensive or largely outdated and have no advantages over solutions already mentioned:
  - Glycerine and water
  - Olive oil and water
  - Obstetric lubricant
  - Soft soap (may cause mucosal irritation).

Equipment

The basic equipment includes enema solution, gloves, lubricant (e.g. K-Y jelly) and any of the following: can and tubing, Higginson syringe, barium solution, syringe and catheter (Figure 17.20).

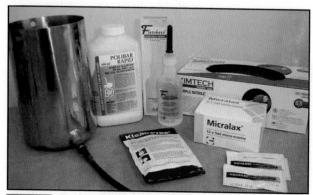

17.20 Equipment for enemas: can and tubing; proprietary enemas; gloves.

Administration of an enema

Figure 17.21 gives guidance on the volumes of solution used when administering an enema.

Solution	Volume used (ml/kg)	Frequency
Water	5–10	Every 20–30 minutes if necessary
Liquid paraffin	2–3	Every 1–2 hours
Saline solution	1–2	Do not repeat for 12 hours
Barium sulphate	5–10	Single administration
Klean Prep	20	Single administration
Laxative fluids	5–10	Single administration

17.21 Enema solutions and volumes.

Giving an enema to a dog or cat

This method requires two people.

1. Prepare all equipment.
2. The assistant restrains the patient in a suitable area; this is preferably outdoors, where cleaning will be easier.
3. Lubricate the end of the tube or nozzle.
4. Elevate the patient's tail and place the tube into the anus. Rotate gently until access to the rectum is achieved (this is easy in the dog but occasionally more difficult in the cat).
5. Advance the tube into the rectum.
6. Stand to the side of the patient and allow fluid to run into the rectum by gravity, or gently pump/syringe in fluid.
7. Allow dogs free exercise to evacuate bowels and supply cats with litter trays and an adequately sized cage.

Administration of an enema to a foal

One of the most common indications for administering an enema to an equine patient is meconium impaction in the foal (see Chapter 26).

It is imperative that these patients are handled and restrained appropriately. At this stage, neonates are likely to be vulnerable and react severely to stressful situations; it is therefore important that they are handled sympathetically. In order to reduce stress levels, foals should be kept in full view of, and if possible have contact with, their dam. Safety, however, must be taken into account and so it is usually sensible to restrain the dam as well as the foal, or to incorporate a partition (whereby the mare and the foal can still see each other) between the mare and foal so that the risk of injury to handlers is reduced. Appropriate PPE should be worn, based on a risk assessment (see Chapters 2 and 10).

Commercial **phosphate enemas** can be administered as a prophylactic treatment if deemed necessary. The foal should be restrained either standing or in lateral recumbency. The protective seal is removed from the enema bottle and the pre-lubricated tip carefully inserted into the foal's rectum. The bottle is then gently squeezed to release the contents.

Mild impaction should also respond to administration of a **gravity enema** using 0.5–1.0 litre of warm soapy water, which may be mixed with a rectal lubricant. The foal should be restrained as above, and the gravity enema then infused slowly into the rectum through a soft flexible Foley catheter.

If the above are not successful then administration of an acetylcysteine **retention enema** may be indicated. This enema assists in making the outer surface of the meconium slippery and easier to pass. For administration, the foal needs to be restrained in a recumbent position or sedated. A soft, flexible Foley catheter is inserted 2.5–5 cm (1–2 inches) into the rectum and the balloon cuff inflated with no more than 30 ml of air. A 4% solution of acetylcysteine (6 g acetylcysteine powder in 150 ml water) is slowly infused into the rectum via the catheter, and the catheter clamped so that the solution can remain in the rectum for 20–40 minutes. After this time the clamp is removed, the cuff deflated, the catheter removed, and the foal set free to move around.

Following administration of any type of enema, the foal must be monitored closely to ensure complete passage of the retained meconium. A good indication of this is that the normal 'milk faeces' are then passed.

Urinary catheterization

A catheter is a tubular instrument (usually flexible) that is passed through body channels for the withdrawal of fluids from (or the introduction of fluids into) a body cavity. A urinary catheter is one placed into the urinary bladder.

Reasons for urinary catheterization include:

- To obtain a (sterile) urine sample when a patient will not urinate when required. This may be because the patient is only at the practice for short periods, e.g. at consultation, or timed urine samples are required, e.g. water deprivation test. Obtaining a midstream urine sample (MUS) can be difficult as some male dogs void little and often during exercise. Culture and sensitivity testing requires sterile urine collection
- To empty the urinary bladder:
  - Before abdominal, vaginal and urethral surgery
  - Before some types of bladder/penile surgery
  - For equine patients, during/following a general anaesthetic, to reduce the risk of urine contamination or to help reduce the risk of the horse attempting to stand too quickly
  - Before a pneumocystogram
  - When there is a partial obstruction or inability to urinate but a catheter can be passed into the bladder (e.g. due to prostatic enlargement)
- To introduce contrast agents for radiography
- To maintain constant, controlled bladder drainage (indwelling catheters):
  - In the recumbent or incontinent patient to prevent soiling
  - After bladder surgery, to avoid over-distension of the bladder, thereby reducing tension on the ▶

suture line and helping to provide optimum healing conditions for the operative site
- For retrograde flushing (the use of fluid pressure to dislodge particles causing an obstruction: a urinary catheter is placed caudal to the particle and water or sterile saline used to dislodge the calculi from the urethra back into the bladder). Hydropulsion can be used to relieve a partial blockage in an emergency situation
- To maintain a patent urethra:
  - In male cats suffering from feline lower urinary tract disease (FLUTD) – a catheter may be placed to maintain bladder drainage whilst treatment or dietary management is initiated; catheter placement also allows flushing of the bladder with solutions that may dissolve struvite crystals
  - Where dysuria or anuria is present but surgery is delayed due to the patient being in a poor condition for surgery (e.g. raised blood urea levels, electrolyte imbalance)
- To monitor urine output:
  - Essential in patients with renal failure receiving intravenous fluids
  - If the patient is in intensive care
  - After renal surgery, to ensure adequate production of urine (minimum urine output should be 2 ml/kg bodyweight/hour)
- To introduce drugs.

Patient resistance to catheterization is common in bitches, queens and tomcats. Sedation or general anaesthesia may be required.

Types of urinary catheter

Most catheters manufactured for the veterinary market (Figures 17.22 and 17.23) are supplied individually, double wrapped, with an inner nylon and outer paper or plastic sleeve. The catheters are ready for use, having been sterilized by either ethylene oxide gas or gamma radiation.

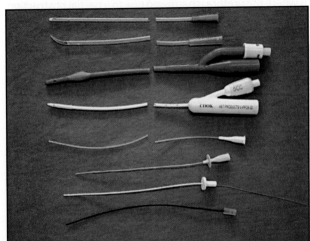

17.22 Urinary catheters. From top to bottom: dog catheter (flexible grade nylon/polyamide); Tieman's; latex Foley; silicone Foley; cat catheter (flexible grade/polyamide); Jackson cat; silicone cat; Teflon cat. Central sections have been removed from some to show the ends of the tubes.

Type	Species	Sex	Material	Indwelling	Sizes (FG)	Length (cm)	Luer fitting
Dog catheter	Dog	Male and female	Flexible grade of nylon (polyamide)	No but can be adapted to be indwelling	6–10	50–60	Yes
Silicone Foley	Dog	Male and female	Flexible medical grade silicone	Yes	5–10	30 and 55	No
Tieman's	Dog	Female	PVC (polyvinyl chloride)	No	8–12	43	Yes
Foley	Dog	Female	Teflon-coated latex	Yes	8–16	30–40	No
Cat catheter	Cat	Male and female	Flexible grade of nylon	No	3 and 4	30.5	Yes
Jackson cat catheter	Cat	Male and female	Flexible grade of nylon	Yes	3 and 4	11	Yes
Silicone cat catheter	Cat	Male	Medical grade silicone	Yes	3.5	12	Yes
Slippery Sam catheter	Cat	Male	PTFE (Teflon)	Yes	3–3.5	14 and 11	Yes

17.23   Types of urinary catheter.

Silicone Foley catheters may come non-sterile and require sterilization by autoclave or ethylene oxide. Metal bitch catheters are now very outdated and their use is not recommended.

With the exception of silicone catheters (which may be re-sterilized in the autoclave), urinary catheters are designed for single use only. The cleaning and re-use of catheters is generally not recommended.

Dog catheters

Plastic dog catheters

These have a rounded tip, behind which are two oval drainage holes (one at each side). They are designed for single use in the male dog and can be used as indwelling catheters.

The largest gauge appropriate for the patient's size should be chosen. If the gauge is too small, the tip of the catheter has a tendency to 'catch' in the urethral epithelium and bend. This may cause significant urethral trauma. The only exception is where the urethra is narrowed due to a partial obstruction, such as an enlarged prostate, or a stricture. In these cases, there is no option other than to use a catheter that would otherwise be too small for the patient.

A second disadvantage of using small catheters in large patients is that the patient is stimulated to urinate when the catheter is introduced into the urethra, and urine will flow around the catheter as well as through the lumen.

Many people prefer to use dog catheters to catheterize bitches. They have no curved tip but are much firmer, providing more control for insertion into the urethral orifice, particularly when digital catheterization is used. This extra rigidity far outweighs the advantage of the curved tip of the Tieman's catheter (see also below).

Foley silicone catheter

These catheters are exactly the same in design as a standard latex bitch Foley (see below). For dogs, a longer length is obviously selected. The catheter is very flexible but, despite this, will advance up the curved male urethra into the bladder where the retaining balloon can be inflated, thus creating an indwelling male dog catheter. Wire-guide stylets are available,

which pass up the centre of the catheter to assist in catheter introduction if required. It is the microscopic 'smoothness' of the medical-grade silicone that enables these catheters to be passed up the male urethra. Silicone is inert and causes no mucosal irritation.

All lubricants are compatible with these catheters.

Bitch catheters

Tieman's catheter

Designed for catheterization of the human male, these catheters became popular for use in the bitch due to their curved tip. The moulded tip was found to be advantageous when placing it into the urethral orifice. However, the rest of the catheter is so soft and flexible that the amount of control over the tip is negligible. This makes placing the catheter into the urethral orifice a very difficult task. The excessive length of the catheter is a further disadvantage. These catheters are now rarely used in the veterinary patient.

Latex Foley indwelling bitch catheter

Foley catheters incorporate an inflatable balloon behind the drainage holes at the tip of the catheter. The balloon is inflated after placement of the catheter into the bladder, making it an indwelling catheter.

Foley catheters are produced for the human market, but suitable sizes are available for use in most bitches except very tiny puppies. They cannot be used in cats or the male dog (unless in conjunction with a urethrostomy). The balloon is inflated (usually with sterile water or saline) via a channel built into the wall of the catheter, which ends in a side arm and a one-way valve. The catheter is removed by deflating the balloon through the same side arm. These latex catheters must not be re-used: the balloon is weakened after use and cannot be relied upon to function correctly if re-used.

Latex Foley catheters are very flexible, which provides maximum patient comfort but causes a problem when introducing them. Placement is achieved by the use of a rigid metal stylet or probe laid beside the catheter with the point secured in one of the drainage holes at the catheter's tip (Figure 17.24). The stylet is removed once the balloon is inflated.

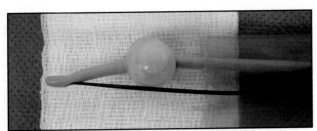

17.24 Tip of Foley catheter showing the balloon inflated and the metal stylet.

Latex Foley catheters must not be lubricated with petroleum-based ointments or lubricants, as this will damage the latex rubber, increasing the chance of the balloon bursting on inflation.

The absence of a Luer mount in this catheter may cause problems for continuous collection of urine, but urine collection bags with appropriate connectors are available from medical suppliers. If these bags cannot be supplied, the catheter must have an adapter placed so that drip bags can be used for urine collection. Unless 3 litre drip bags are employed, frequent emptying will be required in most dogs. It would be unwise to leave a large dog with only a 1 litre collection bag attached overnight.

An alternative is to place a bung in the catheter and drain the bladder at regular intervals with a spigot or a catheter-tipped 50 ml syringe (Figure 17.25). This method may be acceptable for a recumbent patient but not, for example, after bladder surgery, where continuous drainage is required to prevent extension of the bladder wall.

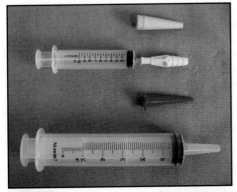

17.25 Spigots and catheter-tipped syringes.

Silicone indwelling Foley catheter

This can be used in the bitch (at shorter lengths) as for the male. These catheters still require a stylet for correct placement in the bitch. The silicone Foley is inert, causing little mucosal irritation, and may be preferable for use in patients with wounds near the urethral opening.

Cat catheters

Conventional catheters

These straight catheters with a Luer connection are compatible with all lubricants and are for single use. They are basically a shorter version of the dog catheter.

Jackson catheters

These catheters were designed primarily for use in male cats suffering from feline lower urinary tract disease, but they can be used in any male or female cat.

A fine metal stylet, lying in the lumen of the catheter, gives extra rigidity and provides better control for insertion into the urinary bladder. It also helps to displace any loose obstruction (e.g. protein plugs or crystals in the urethra). A normal catheter would be too flexible to achieve this. The stylet is removed once the catheter is in place.

The Jackson is much shorter than the other cat catheters. This enables the entire length of the catheter to be placed in the patient, thereby allowing the flange to be sutured to the prepuce. The circular plastic flange is present just behind the Luer fitting of the catheter. In this way the catheter becomes indwelling.

Silicone tomcat catheters

These silicone catheters with distal side holes are very similar in design to a standard Jackson cat catheter. A wire guide is supplied to assist introduction. The proximal fitting enables syringe attachment, and suture holes in the baseplate allow suturing to the prepuce.

Teflon tomcat catheters

In appearance, these are very similar to the conventional cat catheter. The very smooth catheter shaft material ensures ease of placement. The material is inert and causes no mucosal irritation. Suture holes in the silicone hub allow securing of the catheter to the prepuce. It is therefore an excellent choice for a 'blocked' cat that requires a longer-term indwelling catheter. Re-use is not recommended; these catheters are designed for single use only. All lubricants are compatible.

Care of urinary catheters
Catheter storage and checking

Catheters should be stored in a dry environment and laid flat without any pressure on top of them. Unless a suitably long drawer is available, urinary catheters are best left in their boxes and removed only when required.

All catheters have a shelf-life, after which sterility is no longer guaranteed by the manufacturer. Regular checks should be made, especially if the practice's use of catheters is infrequent.

Cleaning and sterilization

Practice policy regarding re-use of catheters is rarely the nurse's decision; however, the process of cleaning and sterilization is time-consuming and is not recommended for urinary catheters. Silicone catheters are the only variety marketed as autoclavable; however, their re-use after having been in a patient for more than 24 hours is not advised.

Cleaning urinary catheters

1. Flush, with force, copious amounts of cold water through the catheter immediately after use. This is usually done with a syringe. Cold water prevents coagulation of any protein that may be present.
2. Remove any blockages with a wire stylet and repeat step 1.
3. Wash the exterior and interior of the catheter with a mild detergent. Rinse thoroughly, as in step 1.
4. Check catheter for kinks, holes, etc. If any damage is found the catheter must be discarded.
5. Dry in a warm, dust-free atmosphere.

Sterilization

Catheters for sterilization should be packed appropriately (using autoclave bags or ethylene oxide). Autoclaving is the best method for sterilizing nylon catheters. The COSHH Regulations (see Chapter 2) have made the use of ethylene oxide in most practices difficult and expensive. There are no short cuts and it is therefore unlikely that any but the largest of veterinary establishments will continue to sterilize equipment by this method on their own premises.

Other equipment required for urinary catheterization

- **Specula:** A speculum is an instrument that assists in the viewing of cavities. Specula are used to assist catheterization of bitches by holding back the tissue in the vestibule and allowing good visualization of the urethral orifice. This is of great aid to the student nurse; digital catheterization can be difficult without a visual knowledge of the urethral position. It is preferable for all specula to be sterile. If no specula are available, bitch catheterization is still possible digitally. There are several varieties of speculum, most of which are not specifically designed for catheterization.
  - **Nasal specula:** There are many slight variations, the adult size being the most appropriate. All have two flat blades that separate when the handles are closed together (Figure 17.26a). Some have a retaining device; others have to be held open. A light source may be attached to one of the blades to illuminate the vagina. If this is not available, a pen torch held by an assistant is an effective alternative.
  - **Rectal specula:** These are used rarely, mainly due to expense. Rectal specula (Figure 17.26b) are conical in shape and, once in place, a section of the conical arm slides out to allow viewing of the urethral orifice. The main problem is to align the removable section with the urethral orifice; this is easy in theory, but difficult in practice.
- **Auriscope:** This is a normal auriscope handle and light, but the conventional aural attachment is replaced by a vaginal speculum with a section removed from its wall (Figure 17.26c).
- **Batteries and transformers:** These should be electrically tested and working correctly. Spare batteries should always be in stock. Transformers do not come into contact with the vulva and so do not require sterilization.
- **Speculum bulbs:** These are best stored separately as they break easily. They cannot be sterilized in the autoclave and therefore need gas or, more realistically, chemical sterilization.
- **Stylets:** Stylets can be made or bought. They should be long enough for easy use; they must be at least two-thirds the length of the longest Foley catheter stocked. Stylets can be packed and autoclaved or chemically sterilized. Metal guide wires are supplied for use with silicone Foleys. These are placed up the centre of the catheter and therefore need to be longer than the length of the Foley. They can be autoclaved.
- **Urine collection bags:** Manufactured varieties are pre-packed and sterile; they are designed for single use. Previously used drip-bags can be used with a giving set

attached. The end of the giving set must be thoroughly cleaned and chemically sterilized before being attached to the urinary catheter. A screw attachment bung should be attached to the end of the giving set during storage to keep it clean from dust and dirt.
- **Bungs and spigots:** Plastic bungs are supplied in multi-packs requiring sterilization, or as individually packed sterile units. Chemical sterilization is the only practical method for these bungs. Metal spigots can be autoclaved or placed in chemical sterilizing solution until needed but are rarely used in modern practice.
- **Three-way taps:** These are invaluable when draining bladders via a catheter. They avoid leakages by controlling urine flow whilst syringes are emptied.

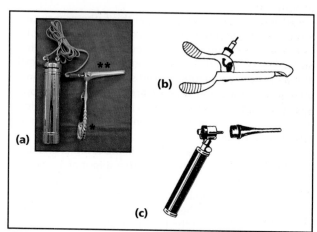

17.26 **(a)** Nasal speculum, suitable for use as a bitch vaginal speculum. Pressing together the handles causes the blades to move apart and open the vestibule. **(b)** Rectal speculum, suitable for use as a bitch speculum. The lower sliding panel is removed after insertion into the vestibule to expose the urethral opening. The lighting attachment, which is connected to a battery, provides a self-contained light source. **(c)** Catheterization speculum for attachment to an auriscope; resembles an ear speculum except that a segment of its wall is absent.

Methods for urinary catheterization

All equipment should be prepared before restraining the patient. Patient cooperation will be greater if prolonged restraint is avoided.

> **WARNING**
>
> Insertion should be stopped once urine starts to flow. Over-insertion can result in the catheter bending and re-entering the urethra or, worse, knotting in the bladder and requiring surgical removal.

Equipment preparation

Lubricants

There is some debate over the necessity for lubricants. Urinary catheterization can be carried out without lubrication; however, lubricants aid the passage of the catheter and help to avoid abrasive trauma. Their use is recommended here, especially those containing a local anaesthetic component;

this helps to desensitize tissue, aiding the catheterization procedure in conscious patients.

When using lubricants it is important to remember the following:

- The constituents of lubricants must be checked before they are used with Foley catheters; most are water-based and are compatible with commonly used catheters
- Lubricants must be sterile: small sachets (5 g) are recommended or, if only tubes are available, a new tube must be started.

Gloves

The use of gloves is recommended for the health and safety of personnel. In general, multiple packs of non-sterile gloves are adequate because the catheter will be fed from its package using a 'no touch' technique. Gloves are therefore used to prevent contamination of staff with urine, rather than protection of the patient from infection.

Sterile gloves will be required when digital catheterization is performed, as the catheter tip is inevitably guided by the finger.

Length of catheter

A dog or cat catheter should be measured against the patient before the catheter is unpacked. This measurement gives a rough estimate of the distance from the urethral orifice along the urethra to the bladder, and therefore the length of catheter to insert.

Cleaning the patient

Before a urinary catheter can be placed, the area around the prepuce or vulva must be cleaned with an antiseptic solution to remove any discharges and surface dirt. It may be necessary to clip the hair around the area, especially in longhaired breeds (although this should only be carried out with permission from the owner).

Restraint

Physical restraint

Most patients will allow urinary catheterization under gentle physical restraint without resistance. If necessary, a muzzle should be used on a dog (see Chapter 10). The patient should be placed at a comfortable working height.

Dogs and cats may be restrained in a standing position or in lateral recumbency. Bitches may be restrained in dorsal recumbency (Figure 17.27). Depending on the patient (e.g. equine) and the reason for catheterization, varying levels of manual restraint may be required.

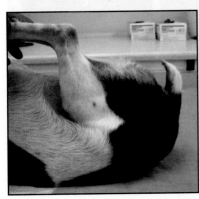

17.27 Sedated bitch in dorsal recumbency for catheterization.

Chemical restraint

Sedation

- Analgesia is appropriate for all catheterization procedures and may form part of a sedative protocol (see Chapter 23).
- Male dogs rarely require chemical sedation unless they are aggressive or very nervous.
- Most bitches will accept catheterization more readily if lightly sedated, especially if dorsal recumbency is chosen; standing catheterization is best done without sedation, otherwise the patient tends to keep sitting down (which can be tiring for the assistant).
- For cats, catheterization is generally less stressful for all concerned if the cat is sedated.
- Equine patients may require sedation depending on the patient and the reason for catheterization.

General anaesthesia

This is rarely indicated or necessary unless the patient has sustained other trauma that makes catheterization under sedation humanely unacceptable (e.g. fractured pelvis, vaginal mass). It is sensible to catheterize during general anaesthesia if this is required for other treatment (e.g. catheterizing a paraplegic patient whilst under general anaesthesia for a myelogram).

Catheterizing a male dog

Equipment:

- Catheter
- Lubricant
- Swabs for cleaning
- Syringe to assist urine drainage
- 3-way tap (if required)
- Sample pot
- Gloves
- Urine bag or a bung
- Kidney dish.

If the catheter is to be made indwelling, the following equipment is also required:

- Suture material
- Zinc oxide tape
- For silicone male Foley catheters, water sufficient to fill balloon
- Guide wire
- Syringe.

Procedure

1. Wash your hands and put on gloves.
2. Clean the prepuce.
3. Extrude the penis; if not experienced, ask an assistant to do this.

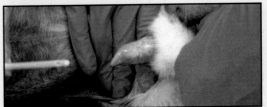

continues ▶

continued

4. Clean the prepuce again.
5. Remove the catheter from the outer wrapping and cut a feeding sleeve from the inner sterile packaging. This allows easy feeding of the catheter from the packaging into the urethra using a 'no touch' technique. For silicone male Foley catheter placement, feed the guide wire up the centre of the catheter.

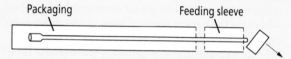

6. Lubricate the catheter and insert the tip into the urethra.
7. Advance the catheter up the urethra. Resistance may be met at the os penis, where there is a slight narrowing of the urethra, at the ischial arch and at the area of the prostate gland if enlarged. Steady but gentle pressure should overcome this resistance. If the catheter cannot be passed, re-evaluate catheter size.
8. Inflate the balloon once the tip of the catheter is in the bladder if a silicone male Foley is in use.
9. Proceed according to the reason for catheterization (e.g. drain bladder, collect sample, hydropropulsion).

To make an indwelling dog catheter from a polyamide catheter, either:

- Place zinc tape around the catheter near to the prepuce

OR

- Stitch or stick the catheter to the prepuce.

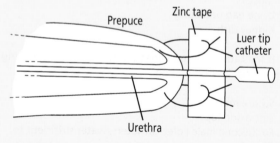

Neither of these options is ideal because dog catheters are not designed to be indwelling. It is best to use a silicone indwelling male Foley.

Catheterizing a bitch: Method 1. Urethra viewed in dorsal recumbency

Equipment:
- Speculum (with or without light source)
- Alternative light source if required
- Catheter
- Lubricant
- Swabs for cleaning
- Gloves.

If a Foley catheter is being placed, the following equipment is also needed:

- Stylet
- Sterile water/saline to inflate cuff
- Urine bag
- Syringe.

Procedure
1. Wash your hands and put on gloves.
2. Ensure the bitch is in a straight dorsal recumbent position with the hindlimbs flexed and drawn forward (see Figure 17.27). The tail must be under control too.
3. Clean the vulva.
4. Remove the catheter from its outer wrapping and expose the tip only from the inner sleeve.
5. If a Foley catheter is being used, insert the stylet.
6. Place the lubricated speculum blades between the vulval lips as caudally as possible to avoid the clitoral fossa.

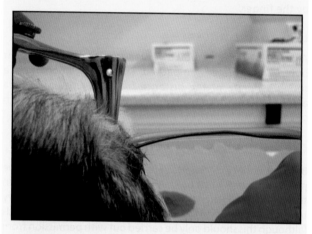

7. Insert *vertically* into the vestibule and turn the handles cranially.
8. Open the blades of the speculum. The urethral opening will be visible on the cranial side of the vertically oriented vestibule, approximately half way between the vulva and cervix.

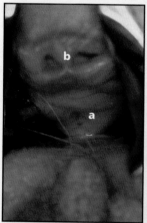
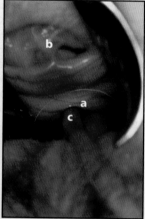

a, the urethral orifice; **b**, clitoral fossa; **c**, catheter in position

9. Insert the tip of the catheter into the urethral orifice. *Draw the hindlimbs caudally*. This straightens the

continues ▶

continued

urethra, making it easier to push the catheter into the bladder.

10. Proceed depending on the reason for catheterization. If a Foley catheter is being used, inflate the balloon, withdraw the stylet, attach the urine collecting bag and place an Elizabethan collar.

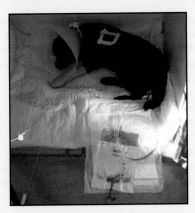

Catheterizing a bitch: Method 2. Urethra viewed standing

Equipment

The equipment required is as for Method 1. Generally only one assistant is required.

Procedure

1. Wash your hands and put on gloves.
2. Ensure the tail is well restrained.
3. Clean the vulva.
4. Place the speculum between the vulval lips and advance at a slight angle towards the spine, then horizontally.
5. Open the blades and identify the urethral orifice. This will be on the ventral floor of the vestibule.
6. Insert the catheter at a slightly ventral angle so as to follow the direction of the urethra into the bladder.
7. Proceed as for Method 1.

Catheterizing a bitch: Method 3. Digital

Equipment:

- Sterile gloves
- Catheter
- Lubricant
- Swabs for cleaning
- Collection pots.

If a Foley catheter is being placed, the additional equipment required is as for Method 1. ▶

Procedure

1. Scrub your hands and put on sterile gloves in an aseptic manner.
2. Assist to restrain the patient in the preferred position, lateral recumbency or standing (standing is generally easier).
3. Ask an assistant to clean the vulva.
4. The assistant removes the outer wrapping from the catheter and you (the scrubbed person) remove the inner package.
5. Holding the sterile part of the packaging, place the stylet if necessary.
6. Lubricate the first finger of your non-writing hand.
7. Place your finger into the vestibule and feel along the ventral surface for a raised pimple.
8. Place your finger just cranial to this raised area, which is the urethral orifice.

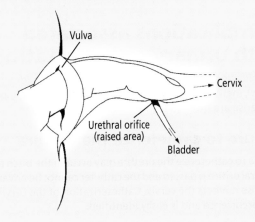

9. Raising your hand and finger dorsally, digitally guide the catheter, tipped slightly ventrally (as for Method 2) into the urethral orifice. The catheter will run past the fingertip if the orifice is missed.
10. Proceed as for Method 1.

The digital method may be difficult or even impossible in smaller breeds.

Catheterizing a tomcat

Equipment

As for dog catheterization.

Procedure

1. Wash your hands and put on gloves.
2. Restrain the patient, ensuring you have control of the tail.
3. Pull the patient's hindlimbs slightly cranially.
4. Prepare the feeding sleeve as for the dog catheter and lubricate the tip.
5. With one hand, extrude the penis by applying **gentle** pressure each side of the prepuce with two fingers.
6. Introduce the catheter into the urethra gently.
7. Collect the sample or drain the bladder.
8. If a Jackson catheter is being placed for continuous drainage, stitch the flange to the prepuce.

Catheterizing a queen

Equipment

As for dog catheterization.

Procedure

1. Wash your hands and put on gloves.
2. Restrain the patient.
3. Remove the outer wrapping and cut a feeding sleeve.
4. Lubricate the tip of the catheter.
5. Place the catheter between the vulval lips and 'blindly' introduce it into the urethra. Angle the catheter ventrally, placing gentle pressure until the catheter slips into the urethra.
6. The catheter is not designed to be indwelling.

Complications associated with urinary catheterization

Complications can arise for a number of reasons (described below); methods of prevention and actions to be taken should they arise are given in Figure 17.28.

Failure to catheterize the urethra

Failure to catheterize the urethra may occur in the bitch if the urethral orifice is passed and the catheter cannot be advanced because it meets the cervix. Catheterization of the cervix is a rare occurrence and is easily identified:

- By viewing the urethral orifice with a lighted speculum
- Because no urine flows through the catheter; although it should be noted that catheters can be placed correctly and still not produce urine, due to either an empty bladder or an obstruction to urine flow (e.g. excessive lubricant blocking the drainage holes).

Infection

Urinary tract infection (UTI) can easily be caused by catheterization if bacteria present in the urethra are pushed into the bladder by the catheter. In most circumstances the bacteria are rapidly eliminated and cause no further concern. The risk of infection is increased when:

- The bladder is traumatized
- A preputial or vaginal discharge is present
- Indwelling catheters are used, or repeated catheterization is carried out
- The patient is immunosuppressed, i.e. its immune system is compromised in some way and the body's natural defences are not operating normally.

The increase in resistance of organisms to antibiotic treatment is well documented. Prophylactic antibiotic cover for catheterization (especially where indwelling catheters are in place) is therefore less acceptable than in the past. As a result, many practices are reluctant to place indwelling catheters, preferring to use frequent visits outside or bladder expression. If catheters are placed, antibiotics are only given if a urinary tract infection is present. Monitoring for infection can be done by twice daily temperature checks and, if necessary, sending urine collected by cystocentesis for culture.

	Prevention	Action
Infection	Use only new or re-sterilized catheters. Use sterile gloves to handle catheters or employ the 'no touch' technique described for dog catheterization. Use sterile lubricants. Clean penis or vulva thoroughly before catheterization; clip surrounding hair if necessary. Catheterization should be carried out in a clean environment, not in the patient's kennel. Systemic antibiotics may be prescribed by the veterinary surgeon. Patients with indwelling catheters should receive systemic antibiotics whilst catheterized and continue the course for 5–10 days after removal	If infection becomes evident, treatment will consist of systemic antibiotics and, in some cases, soluble antibiotics flushed directly into the bladder
Cystitis after catheterization	Gentle introduction of the catheter – no force should be necessary. Use of lubricants is beneficial – they help to limit the epithelial damage to the urethral mucosa, thereby reducing inflammation. Trauma is less likely if an experienced person catheterizes debilitated patients	With indwelling catheters there is inevitably some degree of cystitis after removal of the catheter. If it is significant: • Encourage the patient to increase its fluid intake, either as water or by adding water to the food • Walk the patient frequently to allow urination; observe colour and amount of urine passed.
Patient resistance	Use desensitizing gel (e.g. lidocaine gel) on the penis tip or vestibule	Sedate or, in extreme cases, anaesthetize the patient
Blockage of indwelling catheters	General hygiene and cleaning. Encourage increased water intake (this helps to maintain a continuous flow of urine through the catheter). If bags are attached, check regularly to ensure that urine is able to drain freely	Flush with sterile saline or water
Urethral damage	Never use force. Use adequate lubrication. If an obstruction or difficulty occurs, stop and inform a senior member of staff	If trauma caused by catheterization is suspected, a veterinary surgeon will have to decide what further action is to be taken. Minor trauma may require antibiotic treatment to prevent secondary bacterial infection
Failure to catheterize the urethra in the bitch	The only prevention is to gain experience in bitch catheterization. The easiest way for the student nurse to appreciate the position of the urethral orifice is by the use of a lighted speculum to provide viewed introduction of the catheter	If catheterization of the cervix occurs, remove the catheter and begin with a new one

17.28   Complications associated with catheterization.

Other complications

- **Urethral damage.** This is most likely to occur in the male dog. Due to the ischial curve of the urethra, some epithelial damage is inevitable as the catheter is passed around the curve. This is why a small amount of blood may be present in the tip of the catheter on removal from the urethra, which should be done gently. Urethral damage in the bitch is usually due to excess force being used to advance the catheter into the bladder.
- **Cystitis after catheterization.** This is associated with indwelling catheters. It may also be seen where there has been repeated catheterization.
- **Removal of indwelling catheters by patients.** Adequate suturing (tomcat, dog) and the application of Elizabethan collars should prevent catheter removal by the patient.
- **Blockage of indwelling catheters.** Urine will cease to flow from the catheter. Flushing of catheters at regular intervals (2–3 times per day) is advisable.

Catheterizing an equine patient

Equipment

Flexible plastic equine catheters (Figure 17.29) can be used for both male and female horses. These are usually supplied with a stylet to aid placement and have an end that enables the easy attachment of a catheter tip syringe. Catheters designed specifically for stallions and geldings are longer in length and can be purchased in larger sizes if required. Metal, rigid catheters are available for catheterization of the mare, but seem to be used less commonly nowadays. For indwelling catheters, silicone catheters are recommended as they are more appropriate and less irritant, although they are more expensive. All urinary catheters must be sterile prior to use and any urine samples to be collected for urinalysis should be collected into a clean, sterile container.

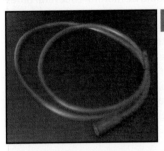

17.29 An equine urinary catheter.

Catheterizing a male horse

1. Grasp and extrude the penis and wash it thoroughly with dilute povidine–iodine.
2. Wearing gloves, and without touching the tip of a sterile flexible urinary catheter, lubricate it with a water-based lubricant (one containing local anaesthetic may be useful).
3. Gently insert the catheter into the urethral orifice and feed it in from the sterile packet (still not touching the actual catheter).
4. Slowly advance the catheter until urine is voided (this will be approximately 60 cm in a 500 kg male).
5. If no urine is voided, try moving the catheter slightly in or out, or applying syringe suction to the end using a catheter tip syringe.

Catheterizing a female horse

1. Bandage the tail and hold it to one side.
2. Wash the perineum using dilute povidine–iodine.
3. Insert a sterile gloved hand into the vagina (approximately 5–10 cm), feeling for the urethral orifice in the floor of the vagina.
4. Once the urethra has been identified, use a finger to position and guide a sterile lubricated catheter into the urethra and advance it slowly until urine is voided.

Catheter management

Appropriate catheter management is very important. Indwelling urinary catheters must be regularly plugged at the end or have a bag attached to prevent ascending infections. They must also be checked and monitored frequently, and the surrounding area kept clean and dry.

Other methods of emptying the urinary bladder

Natural micturition

This is non-invasive and usually easy to achieve with the encouragement of the nurse or owner. In most circumstances it is the preferred method for emptying the bladder; however, there are several disadvantages:

- The sample is always contaminated and therefore useless for culture and sensitivity evaluation
- If the patient is unable to urinate normally, another method has to be employed
- Patients often refuse to produce urine when convenient and required
- If not required for culture, collection of samples from the environment may be acceptable in some cases. For example, urine can be retrieved from litter trays that have been left empty or filled with non-porous beads (so-called 'washable' litter).

Manual expression of the bladder

This is probably the most common method used for cats but may also be used in dogs (especially recumbent patients) (see Figure 17.32). As long as the bladder is of a reasonable size, this task becomes easier with practice. Pressure should be applied steadily and slowly, as sudden pressure may cause trauma to the bladder. Generally, very little pressure will initiate a free flow of urine. Excessive pressure should never be required, as the bladder can become bruised or even ruptured.

Cystocentesis

This should only be carried out when the bladder is of a palpable size. The technique is fairly straightforward (see Chapter 25) and generally without complications, as long as an aseptic technique is used. It may be the only method available for urine drainage in an obstructive emergency. *As this procedure involves entering a body cavity, it must only be carried out by a veterinary surgeon.*

Nursing of common patient types

Nursing care planning for patients with particular requirements is considered in Chapter 14.

The geriatric patient

Geriatric nursing involves nursing the ageing animal in both health and disease. Geriatric patients must be treated with extra care; they are less able to adapt to change and they recover more slowly from medical or surgical interference.

The key to nursing the geriatric patient is good individual patient information (history, medication), with the provision of security, comfort (soft bedding), the correct type of food and an adequate source of water.

Changes associated with old age

Physical changes may include:

- Greying (e.g. muzzle)
- Thickening of the skin
- Coarse, thinning coat
- Loss of musculature
- Loss of stamina and strength
- Weakening of bone
- Lowered physical tolerance to change
- Loss of sight or hearing
- Poor tolerance to lack of fluid intake
- Impaired temperature regulation
- Arthritis and joint stiffness
- Raised susceptibility to infection.

Mental changes may include:

- Lowered responses to stimuli
- Less adaptable
- Increased fussiness about food
- Development of food preferences
- Less interest in activity
- Less obedient
- Disorientation.

Many of the mental alterations in old age are related to physical change; for example, disorientation is made worse when the patient is blind or deaf. Age-related changes, together with the accumulation of any injuries the patient may have sustained, result in a loss of functional reserve: the organs of the body become less capable of dealing with extra demands placed on them for repair of tissue, assimilation of substances, etc.

Changes due to disease must be carefully distinguished from those of old age, although disease can become more obvious or affect a patient more rapidly when they become old. Very few sick, elderly patients suffer from a single disease. Many conditions are subtle and multiple.

Domestic horses are increasingly surviving well into their thirties and beyond. In addition to those given above, conditions seen in geriatric equine patients include: liver disease; hormonal diseases such as Cushing's disease (pituitary tumour); and laminitis. Many conditions affecting geriatric equine patients are related to metabolic disturbance.

Diseases common in geriatric animals include:

- Cancer
- Chronic renal disease
- Cardiac disease
- Osteoarthritis (degenerative joint disease, DJD)
- Cataracts
- Dental disease
- Constipation
- Incontinence.

History

The patient's history must be known. This includes any medical conditions, current treatment and preferred food (see Chapter 15). It should be remembered that patients may be suffering from diseases other than those for which they have been admitted. Specific medical conditions of small animals are dealt with in Chapter 20.

Handling

If the patient has lost its sight or hearing, those who care for it should move slowly and talk reassuringly at all times. This will help to prevent the patient from biting, scratching (or, in horses, kicking) when suddenly touched or frightened. Discussing the pet's normal routine with the owner (see Chapter 14) will help maintain this routine where possible when hospitalized.

Bedding and accommodation

For dogs and cats, blankets and soft bedding should be provided, along with foam mattresses for those with osteoarthritis. Geriatric patients should be kept out of draughts and, if possible, somewhere not too noisy. Thermoregulation is often compromised, so additional heat sources may be required. Core temperature should be monitored several times during the day.

Some geriatric equine patients require a quieter environment, where they can rest and recover, whereas others require an environment that provides increased stimulation, e.g. the company of other patients or a companion, or background noise such as a radio. It is usually necessary for the geriatric patient to have access to a stable or shelter where they can be housed (if required) or shelter from wet or hot weather.

Feeding

Geriatric patients generally need fewer calories than younger animals, but simply feeding them less can result in a lowered intake of protein, vitamins and minerals. Suitable diets, in the absence of any disease, include a highly digestible, well balanced proprietary food such as a 'senior' dog or cat food. Various manufactured feeds are also readily available for older horses and ponies, although it is important to consider feeding in relation to the individual patient.

To avoid digestive upsets, any changes in diet should be made slowly. Hospitalized patients may need to be tempted to eat or, occasionally, hand-fed. Geriatric patients may well need prolonged periods of encouragement to eat during a convalescent period; the amount and type of food should be accurately recorded to ensure that adequate nutrition is being consumed. Dental disease should be considered as one possible medical reason for any inappetence.

Special considerations for equine patients

All feedstuffs should be of a suitable quality in order to reduce the risk of respiratory and digestive problems. Feeding may need to be increased due to reduced efficiency of digestion in the aged horse, and a more palatable and digestible diet is often required, which should include good quality roughage (see Chapter 13).

If there are problems with the horse's dentition then it is recommended to give wet or mash type feeds – usually available in the solid form of cubes or pellets that can be soaked in water prior to feeding. Soaked sugar beet can also be beneficial but the non-molassed variety is probably more appropriate, particularly for overweight patients. If a horse is suffering from laminitis then grass should be restricted and a diet of lower nutritive quality forage and minimal cereals should be given. Oil can be used as energy if required and if appropriate (providing there is no concurrent disease that contraindicates this). Some geriatric patients may require feed supplements to increase certain components of the diet, particularly if they do not have access to good quality pasture or forage.

Monitoring weight

All patients should be weighed, but it is particularly important to weigh the geriatric patient. Regular weight checks ensure that correct drug doses are given in patients where weight may change rapidly associated with ageing. Correct drug dosage and appropriate choice of medications may additionally be of concern in animals with certain age-related problems, such as liver and kidney disease.

Obesity is common in the geriatric patient and management is achieved through client education. It must be emphasized to the owner that excess weight is potentially dangerous to their pet, due to the extra strain placed on the heart, kidneys, liver and musculoskeletal system. This may help to persuade owners that their pet would be happier and healthier if it lost weight. Target weights may be suggested, but all diets should be checked with a veterinary surgeon to ensure that increased exercise (if possible) and diet changes are not contraindicated.

Exercise

Regular 'little and often' exercise is recommended for most elderly dogs, cats and horses. Frequent light exercise should be encouraged, to improve peripheral circulation and maintenance of peripheral temperature. Special care should be taken if the patient is blind or deaf.

- Elderly dogs enjoy 'pottering'. Hospitalized dogs should be given time to wander, maybe in an outside run. Frequent walks will help to exercise stiff joints and ensure plenty of opportunities to urinate. Exercise should be gentle. Physiotherapy, especially massage, may be used to improve circulation to the extremities (see Chapter 20).
- Elderly cats often sleep for long periods of time, but encouraging them to move around can be beneficial to circulation and joint health.
- Geriatric equine patients require both mental and physical stimulation. This can include physiotherapy and short walks or exercise whenever possible. Regular turn out is usually adequate for the very elderly. As a general rule, turn out and/or exercise will help prevent stiffness and promote a healthier respiratory system.

Fluid intake and output

Many elderly patients will have medical problems that result in increased thirst, such as compromised renal function. These patients may drink and urinate in excess of normal calculated volumes. If the amount of water being consumed is in doubt, it may be necessary to measure fluid intake to ensure that adequate quantities are being provided. Adequate water intake is very important; patients must be able to reach water, and water may be added to food if necessary. If there is any doubt that the patient will drink voluntarily during hospitalization then intravenous fluids should be supplied at maintenance rates (see Chapter 22). Water must never be restricted in geriatric patients. There is no requirement to withhold water for >30 minutes prior to anaesthesia (see Chapter 23). Occasionally, water may be withheld in vomiting animals and maintenance requirements replaced using intravenous fluid therapy.

Urine output can also be measured to assess adequate fluid provision. Urine should be observed for normal colour and passage (i.e. no straining). Inappropriate urination (e.g. in the house) in older dogs and cats is not always a result of urinary incontinence. Urinary incontinence arises from loss of bladder muscle or sphincter tone, and may arise as part of the ageing process or for other medical reasons. Incontinent animals typically leak urine when relaxed or asleep. Older dogs and cats that consciously urinate in the house may do so as a result of increased urine output (polyuria), often associated with increased thirst (polydipsia), or as a result of loss of learned behaviour (training) that may be associated with senility.

Defecation

Constipation is more common in elderly dogs and cats. Defecation should be observed, where possible, to enable elimination of any suspected tenesmus (difficulty in evacuation). Faecal examination should be carried out on a regular basis to detect any abnormalities.

Grooming

Elderly patients should be groomed regularly, as they are less likely to keep themselves clean. This is especially significant in longer haired breeds of dog and cat, where matting of the coat can be a source of dirt and subsequent bacterial growth. Grooming helps to give a feeling of wellbeing, encourages surface blood circulation, provides an opportunity to check the coat and skin and to clean discharges from eyes and nose. The human contact is in itself beneficial.

Dental care in horses

Older horses should have a dental examination carried out at least twice per year in order to check for problems, which may include gum disease and loose or missing teeth. As the normal grinding process is often compromised in older patients it is important that any sharp edges are checked and rasped to avoid discomfort.

Foot care in horses

Feet in all horses must be checked and picked out daily (see Chapter 16) and this is no less important in older animals. Regular visits from the farrier are also important to ensure that foot health and balance are maintained, as this can help to reduce some of the joint pain that may be caused by arthritic changes. Farrier visits should be carried out on average every 6–8 weeks, but frequency will depend on the individual horse.

Exotic pets

The geriatric phase for most small mammals is fairly short due to their lower average lifespan. Caring during this phase tends to be tailored to individual needs and conditions and there are very few generalizations that can be made. Careful attention to adequate nutrition and water intake is always the most essential of considerations; this is especially true for rabbits, where dental problems can cause greater difficulties in older age. Reptiles can live for longer in captivity than in their natural habitats and specialized advice should be sought if an aged reptile is to be nursed in the practice.

Convalescence

Recovery from illness or accident is likely to take more time in geriatric animals than in younger ones. Patience is essential and a longer period for convalescence must be allowed. If patients are discharged before they have fully recovered, the owners should be informed that it will take some time for the pet to complete its recovery.

The vomiting patient

Vomiting (emesis) is the forcible ejection of contents of the stomach through the mouth. It should not be confused with regurgitation, which is the more passive action of return of undigested food from the oesophagus. Causes of vomiting may be gastrointestinal, e.g. as a result of dietary change or indiscretion (scavenging), ingestion of foreign bodies, drug induced gastritis, or may be as a result of disease elsewhere in the body resulting in central nausea, e.g. in renal, hepatic and metabolic disorders. Nursing of the vomiting patient can therefore be either very straightforward or very complex, depending on the cause.

Care of vomiting dogs and cats

Specific medical causes of vomiting in dogs and cats and their treatment are discussed in Chapter 20.

Nausea is unpleasant for the patient and may manifest in dogs and cats as:

- Restlessness
- Salivation
- Repeated swallowing
- Retching.

These signs should be brought to the attention of the veterinary surgeon.

Considerations for nursing a vomiting patient include:

- If the first incidence of vomiting occurs in the practice or vomit has not previously been seen by the attending clinician, collect a sample for examination
- Clean away any excess vomitus and clean the mouth. If not contraindicated (see below), offer small amounts of cool fresh water (10–15 ml) to allow rinsing of the mouth.
- Handle the patient gently. Lift only if absolutely necessary, ensuring that no pressure is placed on the abdomen

  ▶

- Hand-feeding and encouragement may be required during the recovery period
- If syringe feeding of fluids is instituted at any time, remember the potential for the development of aspiration pneumonia. It is surprisingly easy to cause pneumonia, especially in smaller dogs and cats
- When patients are discharged, give the owners written instructions regarding the type of food, the amounts to be offered, its consistency and the method of feeding.

Fluids

Many patients will be able to drink small amounts of water without vomiting. Initially, small amounts should be offered frequently (50–100 ml every hour); if these are not vomited, then the amount can be increased over the next 8–12 hours. If patients have been vomiting for some time, or are unable to keep down normal volumes of water, intravenous fluid therapy will be required (see Chapter 22). Fluids will help rehydrate the patient as well as maintaining normal maintenance fluid intake until a return to normal drinking can occur. Intravenous fluids replace both water and electrolytes. In pets that can drink normally, oral electrolyte solutions may be used.

If pets are not able to drink, moist cotton wool can be wiped around the mucous membranes of the mouth; this not only freshens the mouth but also removes excess saliva that may be associated with nausea.

Reintroduction of food

Reintroduction of food can begin once oral fluids are being retained without vomiting, usually from 24 hours after the last vomiting episode. Suitable food will vary between patients but will usually consist of a bland diet offered little and often. Bland foods include boiled chicken or fish, digestible carbohydrates such as rice or pasta, and commercially prepared intestinal prescription diets. Liquidized food may be specified in some cases.

Feeding regime for a patient that has been vomiting

- Day 1: Offer small amounts of bland food 3–4 times daily. Total amount offered should equal 25–50% of the normal daily kilocalorie requirement (see Chapter 13).
- Day 2: Offer small amounts of bland food frequently, to total 50–75% of normal daily kilocalorie requirement.
- Days 3–6: Offer small amounts of bland food frequently, to total the patient's entire normal kilocalorie requirement.
- Days 7–14: Reintroduce normal diet by mixing increasing amounts with the bland diet.

  If vomiting recurs at any stage, return to the previous day's protocol.

Patients that have had a single acute vomiting episode due to scavenging will need to be starved for 24 hours before the reintroduction of food. In these cases the above regime can be followed and can also be given as advice to owners over the telephone. Veterinary attention should be sought if vomiting fails to resolve quickly.

Medical treatments

Antiemetic drugs, such as metoclopramide or maropitant, can be given via several parenteral routes: oral routes are usually avoided in vomiting patients. If given intravenously, administration as a slow continuous rate infusion may be preferred. Antiemetics may be contraindicated in some disease conditions. Other medical treatments will depend upon the underlying cause of the vomiting.

Equine patients

Horses have a strongly developed cardiac sphincter, which does not allow them to vomit. In times of crisis, however, horses will expel their stomach contents via the nasal passages; this is called nasogastric reflux. Horses with nasogastric reflux are often either in need of surgery or are recovering from it, and so need to be nursed appropriately. Nasogastric reflux is abnormal and indicates delayed gastric emptying and problems in the gastrointestinal tract; typically, reflux accompanies small-intestinal ileus (paralysis). Highly unpleasant smelling, fermented, or copious bloody reflux is usually associated with anterior enteritis, whereas reflux composed of fresh feed material and intestinal secretions is usually associated with an intestinal obstruction.

If reflux is suspected or seen, it is common practice to use a nasogastric tube to remove the stomach contents. The tube is passed into the ventral nasal meatus until it meets the pharynx and is then moved on into the oesophagus and stomach. Once the tube is in the stomach, if there is no spontaneous reflux, water should be introduced into the tube to lavage the stomach, followed by directing the end of the tube downwards into a bucket to verify the presence of reflux. The equine stomach can be a frustrating organ to decompress and the use of a siphon can be very helpful.

Following the passing of a nasogastric tube, any response to gastric decompression must be noted. Horses with functional ileus usually show relief of pain at this stage, and heart rate decreases. These horses generally require gastric decompression every 2–4 hours. If decompression is to be repeated at regular intervals then it may be appropriate to leave the tube *in situ* to reduce the risk of causing trauma to the patient by repeated introduction of the tube. This can also help to reduce stress and discomfort for the patient. However, this must be carefully considered as, for some patients, leaving the tube in place may cause added pharyngeal and laryngeal irritation and there is scientific evidence that it is contributory to delayed gastric emptying. If a tube is left *in situ* then it is important to plug the end of the tube when it is not being used. It is also imperative that patients are monitored carefully and closely, and that the area around the nasal passages and tube is kept unblocked and as clean and dry as possible in order to prevent infection and any further discomfort.

Rabbits

Rabbits, in common with many small mammals, are unable to vomit. Gastrointestinal problems are more frequently indicated by changes in appetite or defecation. Abnormal build-up of food material in or around a rabbit's mouth may be indicative of dental problems. It is very important to observe production of droppings when rabbits are inpatients and to ensure that they are eating sufficiently; critical care food is now commercially available and can be very useful for ensuring that rabbits are receiving good nutrition during recovery. Starving of small mammals is dangerous as their metabolic rates are high and they need frequent feeding for survival.

The soiled patient

Hospitalized patients may become soiled at some time during their stay. It is the nurse's responsibility to ensure that all soiling is cleaned efficiently, effectively and quickly. Animals may become soiled by urine, faeces, blood, vomit, other body fluids or food.

Reasons for soiling include:

- Confinement to a small area
- Disturbed routine
- Medical or surgical condition
- Puppies not yet house-trained
- Recumbency.

Care of soiled dogs and cats

Regular walking of inpatients may seem time-consuming but may save time that would otherwise be spent cleaning kennels and soiled patients. Cats must be supplied with litter trays; advice should be sought from the owners regarding types of litter used, as some cats are fussy.

Cleaning the soiled patient

- Clean the patient as quickly as possible.
- Choose shampoos carefully. Take into consideration the patient's coat length, the reason for its hospitalization and the area to be cleaned or bathed. Chlorhexidine gluconate and povidone–iodine are preferable if the patient has any surgical or open wounds. Dry dog shampoos are available, but they are inadequate if soiling has occurred.
- Once the area has been cleaned, dry it thoroughly. Most patients will tolerate a hair dryer after a towel rub-down. All knots in the coat should be removed as they may harbour faeces. Conditioners will make the process much less tiresome for nursing staff and for the patient (especially in longhaired breeds).
- Whilst grooming, check for any area of soreness, especially if the patient is recumbent. If necessary, clip hair away from these areas.
- It is advisable to clip heavily contaminated areas, especially if further contamination is expected (e.g. under drainage tubes). Ensure that client permission to clip has been given. White petroleum jelly can be applied around these areas after clipping, to prevent soreness and to make cleaning easier. There are also barrier film sprays that can be used to protect skin surfaces from urine and faecal scalding, and soothing gels/creams that can help prevent already challenged areas from worsening.

Cats generally keep themselves very clean. If bathing is necessary, mild shampoos should be used and products based on coal tar should be avoided (phenol is poisonous to cats). Regular grooming of hospitalized longhaired cats is essential. Cats with oral lesions or fractured jaws are unable to clean themselves and so regular cleaning of the lips, chin and paws, in addition to basic grooming, will be required.

Care of soiled equine patients

Equine patients suffering from conditions where urine and/or faecal output is increased or abnormal (e.g. salmonellosis, colitis or patent urachus in the foal) are more likely to become soiled, as are recumbent patients.

Soiling of the skin can be avoided by regular removal of droppings and urine from the bedding or mattress (foals), and regular cleaning and drying of any soiled areas. The hair surrounding soiled areas can be clipped so that adequate drying can then take place. Cleaning should be carried out using a dilute antiseptic solution (e.g. povidone–iodine); clean, dry towels should then be used to dry the area gently. Some people use hair dryers and heat lamps for drying, but care should be taken to prevent burning of the skin. Once the patient is clean and dry, protection from scalding can then be achieved by applying a suitable barrier cream. This procedure should be carried out on a daily basis, and patients should always be provided with plenty of clean, dry bedding.

The tail and surrounding areas often become heavily soiled during times when an abnormal amount of bodily fluids are produced; tail bandaging is therefore often used to prevent soiling and discomfort. Care must be taken, as bandaging can lead to pressure-related injuries that can be just as detrimental as the soiling itself, and a rectal glove rather than a tail bandage is often the safest way to cover the tail in order to keep it dry and free of faeces.

Exotic pets

Keeping these patients clean is as important as it is for dogs, cats and horses. Good husbandry and correct housing usually ensures that soiling is avoided. It is better to avoid use of antiseptics on exotic pets, as overexposure to some of the chemical contents of skin antiseptics can cause undesirable responses; use of very diluted concentrations or plain water is recommended.

The recumbent patient

An animal that is lying down and unable to rise is described as recumbent. A large number of conditions might result in recumbency; the more common conditions include:

- Fractures (e.g. pelvis, limbs)
- Spinal trauma (e.g. disc protrusion)
- Weakness due to medical disease
- Neurological injury or disease
- Shock.

Recumbency poses a serious problem in horses, particularly adult horses, because of their size and their tendency to develop muscle damage and compartmental syndrome. Once recumbent, it is difficult to move a fully grown horse. In general, horses do not cope well with recumbency, either physiologically or psychologically. In addition to those given above, a number of conditions may result in recumbency of the equine patient:

- Myopathy
- Laminitis
- Pain
- Sick/deformed foals
- Severed/traumatized tendons
- Malnourishment
- Dehydration
- Metabolic disorder/disease.

Accommodation

Size

Previously active dogs, cats and horses may attempt to drag themselves around (especially fracture and spinal cases in which pain has been relieved). The kennel or stable should therefore be large enough for patients to lie in lateral recumbency comfortably, but not so big that they have room to cause damage to themselves.

It is often necessary to house a recumbent equine patient in an area in which it can be successfully propped in sternal recumbency (Figure 17.30) to reduce the risk of hypostatic pneumonia; the area must therefore be large enough to house items that can be used as supports (e.g. hay bales, padding).

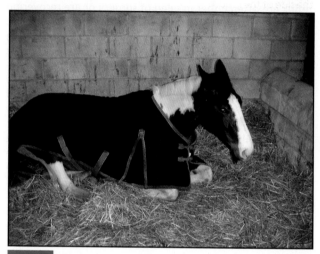

17.30 An equine patient in sternal recumbency.

Position

Most recumbent patients benefit from being housed in an area of activity; this stimulates them and relieves boredom, as nursing staff inevitably talk to them more frequently. However, this should be considered on an individual basis as some patients may require quiet in order to recover.

The kennels of recumbent dogs and cats should not be in direct sunlight, as these patients may not be able to move to a shady area.

To reduce stress levels of equine patients, neonates and foals must be kept as close as possible to their dams.

Bedding

Recumbent dogs and cats should be bedded on thick, waterproof (PVC-covered) foam mattresses, with fleece bedding on the top. If these mattresses are unavailable, thick layers of newspaper with blankets on top may be used. Beanbags, although very comfortable, become soiled very easily and are difficult to clean; they are normally impractical in the hospital situation. Use of commercial cage liners, which are absorbent with an impervious backing, can also be useful for management of urine and help keep patients dry at all times.

Neonatal and older foals should ideally be bedded on thick, waterproof, foam mattresses, with fleece veterinary bed or similar on the top. For larger equine patients, plenty of clean bedding should be supplied, and any soiled bedding must be removed and replaced on a regular basis. There are various types of equine bedding available (see Chapter 12) and the type of bedding used often depends on the individual case. As a general rule, bedding must be absorbent, warm and dust-free. Specific cases require certain types of bedding: e.g. straw would be inappropriate for patients with colic, laminitis or severe respiratory distress, while shavings would be inappropriate for a horse with an open wound or decubitus ulcers.

Food and water

Both food and water must be within easy reach or, if this is not possible for equine patients, offered at regular intervals. Patients that are recumbent due to a medical condition may be depressed, and feeding by hand may be necessary. Patients that fail to drink sufficiently can have water added to their food or be encouraged to drink by having water syringed into the side of the mouth. Recumbent equine patients may require water via a nasogastric tube; fluid therapy (see Chapter 22) and/or total parenteral nutrition (TPN, see Chapter 13) may even be necessary.

Most recumbent dogs and cats require a concentrated, highly digestible diet to meet the extra nutritional needs of stress due to kennelling or continuing tissue repair. Highly digestible diets have the added advantage of producing less faecal material. The energy requirement supplied by carbohydrates is generally lower during recumbency and the amount of carbohydrates offered may need to be reduced. Sick animals may have an increased nutrient requirement, e.g. increased protein is required for tissue repair. If the recumbent patient fails to eat, advice should be sought from the owner regarding the animal's preferences and favourite foods.

Where possible, recumbent horses should be encouraged to eat a normal diet, although highly palatable food should be offered to tempt those reluctant to eat.

Obesity may be an existing problem or weight may be gained during the period of recumbency due to less energy being used. It may be necessary to introduce reducing diets, but only in consultation with the veterinary surgeon.

Urination and defecation

Recumbent dogs and cats should, if possible, be taken outside to be given the opportunity to urinate and defecate. Natural urination and defecation are always preferable to catheterization and enemas, and the change of environment and fresh air may be beneficial to mental attitude. Patients may require help standing, as many are unwilling to urinate lying down. Towel support is useful (Figure 17.31); even tetraplegics and quadraplegics can be managed in this way, using crossed towels to support the chest. When an animal is supported, gentle manual pressure may be applied to the bladder to encourage urination (Figure 17.32).

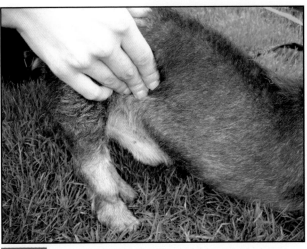

17.32 Manual bladder expression in a small dog.

A clear record of urination and defecation should be kept, as otherwise it is easy for several days of non-production to go unnoticed. If the patient becomes constipated, a laxative may be required. Any diarrhoea in the recumbent patient increases the risk of sores, infection of wounds, 'fly-strike' in the summer and discomfort to the patient. If diarrhoea develops, the veterinary surgeon should be informed. Excess hair in the perianal/anal area of dogs and cats should be clipped. Cleaning as quickly as possible after contamination occurs is extremely important.

Recumbent equine patients are at risk from colic due to changes in the motility of the digestive system. The amount, consistency, frequency and smell of urine and faeces all need to be regularly monitored and recorded. To reduce the risk of soiling, regular removal of urine and faeces is recommended.

If patients are unable to urinate normally, catheterization may be indicated (see later).

Decubital ulcers and urine scalding

It is better to prevent both decubital ulcers (Figure 17.33) and urine scalding, rather than treat them after they have occurred.

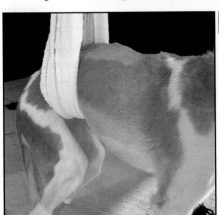

17.31 A towel is being used to assist this recumbent dog in standing.

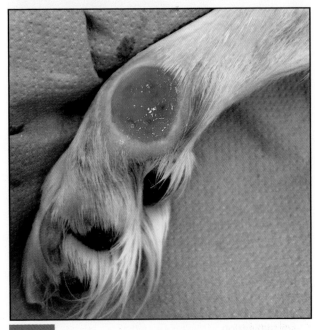

17.33 Decubital ulcer in a dog.

Preventive measures against decubital ulcers

- The use of soft bedding with absorbable blankets for dogs and cats, or adequate bedding for horses, together with regular turning of the patient (every 4 hours), will help to lessen the occurrence of sores.
- Bony prominences are most likely to suffer (e.g. in dogs and cats: elbows and ischial wings; in horses: distal limbs, elbows, hocks and tuber coxae). For dogs and cats, these areas can be padded with foam rings from the top of tablet pots (Figure 17.34) or the patient can be encouraged to lie laterally for short periods. For horses, these areas should be padded and/or lubricated.
- Massage is beneficial and can be performed while the patient is recumbent.
- Slings to raise canine and feline patients for longer periods are used in the US and at larger veterinary establishments in the UK. Slings to raise equine patients are sometimes used when appropriate; although many horses do not tolerate slings and sling-related sores can be a problem.
- Waterbeds may be useful for recumbent dogs and cats but are rarely used in the UK.

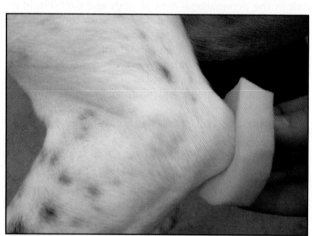

17.34   Padding of bony prominences on the elbow of a dog.

Catheterization (indwelling or repeated) enables bladder drainage without soiling. Otherwise assisted walking is essential to provide opportunities for urination.

Management of decubital ulcers

Decubital ulcers are serious and can be extremely difficult to resolve. Treatment is as follows:

1. Clip the area around the sore.
2. Clean with a mild antiseptic solution (e.g. *dilute* 1:100 povidone–iodine or chlorhexidine gluconate).
3. Dry thoroughly.
4. Apply an appropriate cream or protective barrier film.
5. If it is summer, and the position of the ulcer allows, cover with a permeable dressing (e.g. Primapore, Smith and Nephew) dressing to prevent fly-strike and contamination.
6. If on a lower limb, consider bandaging.

Management of urine scalds

Any patient that is soiled by urine should be checked for the presence of urine scalds. They begin as innocent-looking red patches and are very easily managed if treated at this stage. There is no excuse for their progressing, given proper nursing care. Urine scalding is relieved by:

- Regular washing with a mild antiseptic shampoo (e.g. dilute chlorhexidine gluconate or povidone–iodine); this must be rinsed off thoroughly
- Clipping the hair and applying soothing healing or barrier creams
- Catheterization if necessary.

Hypostatic pneumonia

Hypostatic pneumonia is caused by the pooling of blood and a consequent decrease in viability of the dependent lung. It is more likely to occur in an old, sick and debilitated animal that has been in lateral recumbency for a long period, and is a particular risk in the horse due to its size. Horses in *lateral* recumbency are at increased risk of developing hypostatic pneumonia; close monitoring and regular turning and positioning into sternal recumbency are vital, although not always easy with such large patients.

Signs of hypostatic pneumonia include:

- Rapid shallow breathing
- Increased respiratory effort
- Moist noises when breathing, possibly even gurgling
- Depressed attitude.

Serious secondary chest infections may result if hypostatic pneumonia is allowed to develop and can be life-threatening. If hypostatic pneumonia is suspected, a veterinary surgeon should be informed immediately. Auscultation of the lung fields and radiography may be required to confirm the diagnosis.

Prevention

Turning the recumbent patient at least every 4 hours, 24 hours a day, is essential. Sternal recumbency should be assisted by using sandbags, water/sand-filled containers or radiography cradles (and remembering to support the head).

For dogs and cats, regular coupage (the external impact massage of the thorax with cupped hands, see Chapter 20) 4–5 times daily for 5 minutes will improve thoracic circulation. This procedure may also be used successfully in horses. By promoting coughing it also aids removal of secretions that build up in the bronchial tree. A veterinary surgeon should be consulted before coupage is used, to ensure that there are no contraindications such as fractured ribs.

Treatment

If hypostatic pneumonia with a secondary infection is present, all of the above guidelines for prevention should be continued. In addition, treatment (e.g. with antibiotics) will probably be prescribed.

Passive physiotherapy

Physiotherapy helps to maintain and improve peripheral circulation. It is of benefit to all recumbent patients, even if only for the extra human contact and attention. This subject is covered in detail in Chapter 20 and in the *BSAVA Manual of Canine and Feline Rehabilitation, Supportive and Palliative Care*.

- **Massage:** This is particularly useful for the limbs. The patient should be massaged from the toes/foot towards the body to encourage venous return to the heart.
- **Supported exercise:** For dogs and cats, towel-walking is the most common (and inexpensive) method (see Figure 17.31). Adequate staff must be available, as both the patient and the staff member can be injured if the patient is heavy. Wheeled total support hoists for walking recumbent canine and feline patients assist mobility of heavier patients and enable effective active physical therapy with the patient in a normal walking position (Figure 17.35).
- **Hydrotherapy:** Swimming is very useful physiotherapy that can be used with dogs, cats and horses. Small dogs can be swum in large sinks and baths in the hospital; larger patients need pools. Swimming enables patients to move their limbs freely without weight-bearing forces. The temperature and the quality of the water must be checked before the patient enters. Constant support and observation are essential to prevent panic and possible drowning.
- **Passive joint movement:** Moving joints manually within their normal range helps to prevent stiffness and improves circulation.

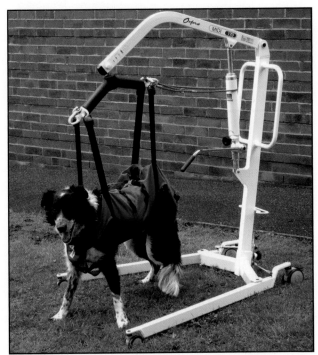

17.35 Wheeled 'total support' hoist for walking recumbent patients.

Maintenance of body temperature

Recumbent patients expend very little energy; heat production is therefore lower than normal. Body temperature may fall to a subnormal level.

Blankets to cover canine and feline patients may be sufficient; other heating methods for these patients include:

- Veterinary duvet-type covers with reflective filling
- Veterinary instant heat pads (see Figure 17.18), which should be wrapped initially; when activated, they heat to 52°C

- Hot-water bottles, which should be wrapped to prevent burning of the patient
- Heated waterbeds – these should only be used if the patient is very debilitated and will not bite or scratch; they are expensive pieces of equipment to replace if punctured
- Bubble packaging – cheap and effective
- Silver foil – good for extremities but remove if patients become active, especially if they are young, as foil may be chewed
- Silver reflective survival blankets
- Infrared lamps
- Units that blow filtered heated air through paper blankets to warm the patient gently
- Heated mats that are weight-sensitive, warming only in areas where patient weight is detected. Maximum temperature thermostats prevent inadvertent over-heating/injury
- Incubators.

> **WARNING**
>
> Standard electrically heated beds are not recommended unless the patient is under constant supervision. Some varieties have been implicated in causing serious burns when patients were placed directly on top of them. A blanket should always be placed between the heated pad and the patient.

Methods used to maintain equine body temperature include:

- Rugs (care must be taken to ensure horses do not become tangled)
- Stable bandages on limbs
- Adequate amounts of bedding
- Infrared heat lamps (care must be taken to ensure that these do not burn the skin)
- Warmed intravenous fluids (37°C).

Myopathy and neuropathy in equine patients

Muscle and nerve damage may be the cause of a horse's recumbency, but can also occur as a *result* of recumbency due to inadequate positioning (see Chapter 23). To prevent damage, careful positioning, regular turning, massage and adequate amounts of bedding are all beneficial.

Home nursing

Recumbent patients are generally managed in a hospital environment but some will be recumbent for a longer time and may then be nursed at home. Most owners are quite capable of learning how to nurse their own pet, but tasks that come automatically to a nurse must be pointed out to an owner. It is helpful to write clear instructions to which owners can refer once they are home. Assistance with provision of suitable equipment for home nursing will also help owners. Assurance should be given to the owners that they can phone the practice at any time if they are worried. Weekly checks at the surgery should be arranged to monitor for signs of decubital ulcers, urine scalding or hypostatic pneumonia.

The comatose patient

In this context, comatose is interpreted as being in a long-term coma rather than unconscious during a routine recovery from anaesthesia.

Coma may be:

- **Primary** – unconsciousness as an immediate result of an injury or accident, or after major convulsions
- **Secondary** – unconsciousness as the result of organ failure; this could be due to colic (in horses), major injury, metabolic disease, poisoning, shock, toxicity, tetanus or neurological disease.

Signs of unconsciousness and collapse include:

- Heart and pulse rate regular but slow
- Respiration regular and deep
- Eyeball in a fixed position (peripheral reflexes weakened dependent on degree of brain damage)
- Pupillary light response present (level dependent on degree of brain damage)
- Flaccid muscles.

Comatose patients are rarely nursed in general practice – they really need a critical care unit with 24-hour staffing and expert care (see Chapter 21).

The nursing of a comatose patient is essentially similar to that of a recumbent one, and many of the nursing points made above for the care of the recumbent patient can be implemented for the comatose patient. The main differences are that nutrition is best provided by total parenteral nutrition (TPN) via a jugular catheter or jejunostomy tube, and that fluid is provided intravenously.

Additional nursing requirements for a comatose patient

- Maintain a patent airway – pull the tongue forward and consider endotracheal intubation.
- Clean any secretions from the oral cavity – use suction or swabs and lower the head to encourage drainage by gravity.
- Monitor at 15-minute intervals:
  - Temperature, pulse rate and quality, respiratory rate and rhythm
  - Capillary refill time
  - Urine output (30-minute intervals if catheter is in place)
  - Drip rates
  - Drug administration.

Constant 24-hour observation is essential for the comatose patient.

When nursing the unconscious equine patient it is necessary to consider the size of the patient, safety issues, the reason(s) for the condition, the severity of symptoms, the ability to carry out normal functions, and the treatment regime in place. Prognosis is dependent on a number of factors but is generally very poor due to the patient's large size, the long-term detrimental effects of recumbency and coma, and the high costs associated with treatment and care.

Transport of the unconscious patient

The priority for these patients is maintenance of the airway. All unconscious patients should be transported from one area to another with the head and neck supported on a firm surface to enable them to be extended, thus protecting the airway. For cats this is usually in a basket (perhaps using a piece of hardboard for extra support); for dogs (and small equine patients) a trolley should be used. The unconscious patient's head should never be allowed to 'flop' towards the floor. This is similar to the transportation of anaesthetized patients (see Chapter 23).

For all patients:

- Extend the head and neck
- If possible, pull the tongue forward so that it can be seen during transport
- Monitor the colour of mucous membranes
- Observe breathing patterns
- Ensure that there are enough people to move the patient safely
- Stop transportation to readjust the position of the patient if necessary
- Transport the patient as rapidly as possible
- Cover the patient to maintain heat.

> **WARNING**
>
> As a general rule, unconscious dogs and cats should *not* be carried in the arms. Cradling the unconscious patient is bad practice and dangerous: the tongue can fall into the back of the larynx and occlude the airway.

Moving the unconscious equine patient requires an experienced team of handlers and a veterinary surgeon in order to reduce the risk of further injury to the horse and handlers involved. At least one person must be responsible for the head. In the hospital situation a headcollar, hobbles, ropes, and a hoist or winch may be used. The areas of the horse that will come into contact with this apparatus (most commonly the head and legs (pastern area)) should be padded. In the field situation it may be necessary to use ropes or a drag mat, although smaller equine patients (<100 kg) can usually be moved on a stretcher or trolley.

Small pre-warmed containers should be used for transporting unconscious small mammals, as they lose heat rapidly and hypothermia may delay recovery.

The critically ill patient

Critically ill patients must be nursed in a designated area. This should be:

- Quiet
- Well ventilated
- Well lit
- Well served with electrical points for monitors.

There must be adequate:

- Monitoring equipment for nursing staff to use effectively
- Staff members (for 24-hour care)
- On-site laboratory facilities.

Nursing care of critically ill patients is time-consuming and demanding. All care advice given for nursing of the recumbent patient and the soiled patient (above) should be applied, with any appropriate adaptations with regard to the individual patient's needs or condition.

Nurses must also remember that every patient is different and should always consider factors such as the patient's temperament and normal routine. Consideration of any other conditions that the patient may have must also be taken into account; these could be as a result of the current condition or could be a pre-existing condition such as respiratory disease.

Intensive care charts and a nursing plan (see Chapter 14) should be made up at the beginning of the day, with timed intervals for any given activity. In this way the patient's care is documented and it is easy for any member of staff to take over and assess recent progress and protocols. Checks, monitoring, drugs and nutrition are less likely to be missed accidentally if there is clear and accurately timed record keeping. In particular, vital parameters, comfort, behaviour and demeanour should all be monitored on a regular basis to ensure that the patient is receiving pain medication at accurate time intervals, especially when the patient may be unable to exhibit discomfort. In addition, the areas of intravenous and urinary catheter management, temperature control and tube management must have the highest consideration.

Intravenous catheter management

This must be exemplary, as many critically ill patients are immunosuppressed and likely to contract infections easily. Washing of hands is mandatory and wearing of gloves advisable. Any spilt blood from around the catheter should be cleaned with antiseptic solution and checks should be made to ensure that all tapes securing catheters and dressings are clean.

Catheter patency is maintained by flushing with heparinized saline (4 units of heparin per 1 ml of 0.9% saline) every 4–6 hours. Regular changing of peripheral catheters (usually every 3–5 days) should be done in line with instructions from the veterinary surgeon in charge. Jugular lines are rarely changed if they are functioning well. The skin insertion site of jugular catheters demands particular care and should be inspected at least daily, preferably twice daily, with gloved hands, and sterile dressing replaced at the site as appropriate.

For more information on intravenous fluid therapy of small animals see Chapter 22.

Intravenous fluid therapy for equine patients

It is highly likely that critically ill equine patients will at some stage require fluid therapy. Various types of fluid may be administered, including colloids, blood (Figure 17.36) and blood products, plasma and, most commonly, crystalloids.

Intravenous administration is the most common route used for fluid therapy in the equine patient. Other routes that may be used include oral, intraperitoneal and intraosseous. The preferred sites for catheter placement in the horse are the jugular vein, the cephalic vein (medial forelimb), the lateral thoracic vein and the saphenous vein (medial hindlimb). If there are no specific reasons why the jugular vein cannot be used, it is normally the preferred site.

Intravenous catheter management in horses is an important clinical skill for veterinary nurses. Not only must they become skilled at inserting catheters in a totally aseptic manner, but they must also understand and recognize potential complications of intravenous catheter use. Correct

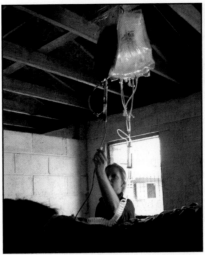

17.36

An equine patient undergoing a blood transfusion.

management of both the catheterized patient and the catheter itself is vital if complications are to be prevented.

Before inserting an intravenous catheter the area should be aseptically prepared with antiseptic solution and surgical spirit. Thought must be given as to whether a catheter should be inserted 'upstream', where loss of a catheter cap can result in significant haemorrhage, or 'downstream' where there is a risk of air embolization and cardiac arrest if a catheter cap is lost. This is a well recognized complication, although fatal air embolus is very rare. It is more common to use a 'downstream' technique.

Long-term catheters are more reliable for avoiding complications such as septic thrombophlebitis, particularly if multiple injections of potentially irritant drugs or large volumes of electrolyte solutions are to be administered. Additional caution must be observed when catheters are used in horses with endotoxaemia, where thrombosis is very common.

Regular catheter lavage with heparinized saline is essential to maintain patency. A regime of monitoring may involve the catheter and relevant vein being checked at least every 6 hours for the following:

- Firmness or swelling of the vein
- Discharge or bleeding from the catheter site
- Heat and/or pain of the vein.

In the event of any of the above conditions occurring, the catheter should be removed and a portion of it kept for culture in the laboratory.

Other checks involve:

- Vein patency
- Catheter patency
- Leaks
- Clots
- Missing stay sutures
- Damage to the catheter
- Contamination of extension sets, 3-way taps and intravenous bungs
- Managing the intravenous drip.

All giving sets must be sterile prior to use. The management of an intravenous drip requires:

- Observation of the catheter and surrounding areas
- Checking that the drip is running and there are no kinks or blockages
- Monitoring pulse rate

- Monitoring respiration rate
- Monitoring urine output
- Monitoring mucous membrane colour and capillary refill time (CRT)
- Checking for any signs of noisy breathing – fluids pooling in lung (particularly in small ponies and foals) which may indicate over-infusion.

Complications can include:

- Infection
- Transfusion reactions (e.g. increased heart rate, increased respiration rate, trembling, restlessness, urticaria and collapse)
- Over-transfusion (indicated by oedema of soft tissues, fluid within the lungs (crackling will be heard), coughing, and excessive urination).

With correct management complications should be avoided.

Urinary catheter management

Placement of urinary catheters holds a high risk of urinary tract infection (UTI). Ensuring that catheters are placed using sterile gloves and equipment will help to reduce this risk, as will keeping housing clean. The patient must be monitored for signs of infection, as UTIs can initiate a systemic response. Urinary catheterization is discussed in detail earlier in the chapter.

Temperature control

Regular monitoring of the patient's temperature is paramount. Core temperature should be monitored at least every 30 minutes. The aim is to keep the temperature at a constant level. Warming patients gradually usually prevents inadvertent overheating.

Management of tubes

These may be chest drainage tubes, active drainage tubes from wounds, feeding tubes or nasal oxygen provision tubes (see also Chapters 13, 23 and 25). The same basic rules apply to all:

- Wash hands and wear gloves on handling
- Check insertion sites (for some hourly; others daily)
- Dress sites that involve breaches in the skin with sterile dressings; change the dressings as appropriate but at least daily
- Bandage so that the tubes are protected but also in a manner that provides patient comfort; ensure that no clamps, etc., rub or press into the skin surface
- Ensure that feeding tubes are flushed thoroughly to prevent blockage.

Patients' mental attitude

Critically ill patients often respond to stimuli in a very delayed fashion, or may be unconscious. This does not necessarily mean that they are unaware. Stress, whether exhibited by the patient (e.g. by aggression or panic) or not (e.g. in the case of some neurological conditions), will actively delay recovery times. Having a radio in the background may help to calm patients, and taking time simply to sit and stroke or talk to the patient is an essential area of good nursing care for these individuals.

For horses, mental stimulation may also include grooming, physiotherapy, short walks and hand grazing (if appropriate/ possible).

Nutrition

Intake of food and water by critical patients will depend upon: whether or not the patient can or cannot physically eat and drink; whether or not it is allowed to eat and drink; the positioning of food and water; whether any adjustments to diet according to condition and impairment are required (e.g. supplements, probiotics, or electrolytes); and whether total parenteral nutrition (TPN) or fluid therapy is required. There are implications for the level of required nursing care associated with these considerations.

Critically ill patients should never be starved. They have an increased basic energy requirement (see Chapter 13) due to the stresses to which they are exposed. In the seemingly unconscious or mentally 'dull' animal, the smell of food can produce a marked response, which can be a good indicator of improvement.

Tube feeding or total parenteral nutrition must be started immediately if patients are unable to (or will not) eat for themselves (see Chapter 13). In many circumstances, fresh food should be offered to tube-fed patients regularly, as it is preferable for them to eat normally and for tube feeding to be stopped as soon as possible.

Environment

As critically ill patients begin to recover, a change in environment can be beneficial, especially if the patient has been distressed during the more critical period. The patient may be moved into a different area, or outside if monitoring equipment allows. A change of environment and different sources of stimulation can promote a more rapid recovery.

Depending on its condition, the patient may need to be housed away from other patients, in an isolation facility.

More information on the emergency intensive care of small animals is given in Chapter 21.

The neonatal patient

The care of neonates, including those that are critically ill, is considered in detail in Chapter 26.

Special considerations for neonates

- Use antiseptics and spirit carefully – they encourage heat loss. *Careless use can be the difference between survival and demise.*
- Reduce clipping of fur/hair as much as possible, to preserve body heat.
- Ensure accurate dosing of drugs – this is essential. Use of 1 ml or 100 IU syringes is advisable when drawing up small quantities. Drugs must be diluted *with care*; they must be water-miscible and thoroughly mixed.
- Move neonates around gently and do not change their orientation rapidly – the sudden need for redistribution of circulating blood volume can cause shock that they may not be able to survive.
- Keep the neonate's head slightly below the rest of the body whenever possible, to allow drainage of saliva. This is particularly important if the neonate is semi-conscious.
- Meconium impaction in foals may require an enema to be administered (see earlier).

Neonates can become critically ill very rapidly as a result of almost any insult, whether physiological or mechanical.

First aid for critical neonates

- Maintain environmental temperature at 30–33°C for the first 24 hours and then at 26–30°C for 4–5 days. Neonates need particular care in relation to temperature regulation due to their poor ability to thermoregulate.
- Begin intravenous, intraosseous or intraperitoneal fluid administration (see Chapter 22). Neonates dehydrate quickly.
- Feed as soon as possible, or at least supply some glucose in fluids.
- Encourage movement.
- If the patient is reluctant to move, massage from the periphery towards the heart to encourage better perfusion and distribution of fluids and heat.

Once these basic actions have been performed, the cause of the crisis can be investigated and treated. Even healthy neonates have a very reduced capacity for sudden changes of any kind and can deteriorate very quickly; this is even more so in the critically ill neonate and therefore *constant* monitoring is usually required.

References and further reading

Coumbe KM (2001) *Equine Veterinary Nursing Manual*. Blackwell Science, Oxford

Houlton JEF and Taylor PM (1987) *Trauma Management in the Dog and Cat*. Blackwell Science, Oxford

King L and Boag A (2007) *BSAVA Manual of Canine and Feline Emergency and Critical Care, 2nd edition*. BSAVA Publications, Gloucester

Knottenbelt DC (2003) *Handbook of Equine Wound Management*. Elsevier Science, UK

Mullineaux E and Jones M (2007) *BSAVA Manual of Practical Veterinary Nursing*. BSAVA Publications, Gloucester

Self-assessment questions

1. Explain the difference between first intention and second intention healing.
2. Name the layers of a bandage in the correct order of application and give an example of each.
3. What is the aim of an Ehmer sling?
4. List six physical changes and three mental changes commonly seen in the geriatric dog.
5. What is the difference between vomiting and regurgitation?
6. How would you feed a dog suffering from megaoesophagus?
7. List eight nursing considerations for the recumbent patient.
8. List the three methods of catheterizing a bitch and describe one in detail.
9. When might a pressure bandage be indicated and what are its benefits?
10. Identify the different types of enema that may be used for a foal with meconium impaction.
11. What factors should be taken into account when feeding a geriatric equine patient?
12. What are the problems associated with a recumbent horse? What special nursing conditions should apply?
13. List the checks that will be made when nursing an equine patient receiving intravenous fluid therapy.
14. How can hypostatic pneumonia be prevented in the foal?

Chapter 18

Diagnostic imaging

Ruth Dennis, Susan Northwood, Philip Lhermette, Simon Girling and Jan Butler

Learning objectives

After studying this chapter, students should be able to:

- **Understand the physical principles of diagnostic radiography, using both conventional film/screen systems and digital radiography**
- **Have a sound working knowledge of radiographic equipment, procedures and safety**
- **Know how to perform basic radiographic studies in dogs, cats and horses, and how to prepare for and assist in more complex investigations**
- **Identify faults in radiography and know how to correct them**
- **Understand the principles of diagnostic ultrasonography and know how to assist in ultrasound examinations in dogs, cats and horses**
- **Understand the basic principles of MRI, CT, scintigraphy and endoscopy**
- **Understand specific considerations for imaging exotic pets**

Introduction

Radiography is a fundamental part of veterinary practice and is a procedure in which most nurses become actively involved. The production of diagnostic films requires skill in the use of radiographic equipment, in patient positioning and in the processing of the films. A variety of faults may occur at each stage during the procedure and the nurse should be able to recognize and correct these problems. At the same time the procedure must be carried out safely, without hazard to the handlers or patient.

Basic principles of radiography

X-rays are produced by X-ray machines when electricity from the mains is transformed into a high-voltage current, converting some of the energy in the current to X-ray energy. The intensity and penetrating power of the emergent X-ray beam varies with the size and complexity of the apparatus and the exposure settings used; portable X-ray machines are capable of only a relatively low output, whereas larger machines are far more powerful.

X-rays travel in straight lines and can be focused into an area called the **primary beam**, which is directed at the patient. Within the patient's tissues some of the X-rays are absorbed; the remainder pass through and are detected either by photographic X-ray film or by a digital recording system, producing a hidden image. When X-ray film is processed chemically, a permanent picture or **radiograph** is produced and the image may be viewed. With digital radiography, the image is produced electronically and viewed on a computer screen.

Production and properties of X-rays

X-rays are members of the **electromagnetic spectrum**, a group of types of radiation that have some similar properties but which differ from each other in their **wavelength** and **frequency** (Figure 18.1).

The energy in a given type of radiation is *directly* proportional to the frequency of the radiation and *inversely* proportional to its wavelength. X-rays and gamma-rays are

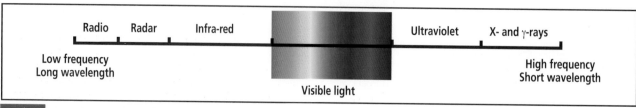

| Radio | Radar | Infra-red | | Ultraviolet | X- and γ-rays |

Low frequency
Long wavelength

Visible light

High frequency
Short wavelength

18.1 The electromagnetic spectrum.

similar types of electromagnetic radiation that have high frequency, short wavelength and therefore high energy. X-rays are produced by X-ray machines and gamma-rays by the decay of radioactive materials.

Members of the electromagnetic spectrum have the following common features:

- They do not require a medium for transmission and can pass through a vacuum
- They travel in straight lines
- They travel at the same speed: 3×10^8 m/s in a vacuum
- They interact with matter by being absorbed or scattered.

X-rays have some additional properties that mean they can be used to produce images of the internal structures of people and animals. They are also used in engineering for detecting flaws in pipes and construction materials.

- **Penetration:** Because of their high energy, X-rays can penetrate substances that are opaque to visible ('white') light. The X-ray photons are absorbed to varying degrees, depending on the nature of the substance penetrated and the energy of the photons themselves, and some may pass right through the patient, emerging at the other side. The shorter its wavelength, the higher is the energy of the X-ray photon and the greater the penetrating ability.
- **Effect on photographic film:** X-rays have the ability to produce a hidden or latent image on photographic film, which can be rendered visible by processing (film in cameras is damaged by exposure to X-radiation).
- **Fluorescence:** X-rays cause crystals of certain substances to fluoresce (emit visible light) and this property is utilized in the composition of intensifying screens, which are used in the recording of the image.
- **Energy storage:** With digital radiography systems, the energy of the emergent photons is captured and converted electronically to a digital image in several different ways, depending on the type of digital system used.

X-rays also produce biological changes in living tissues by altering the structure of atoms or molecules or by causing chemical reactions. Some of these effects can be used beneficially in the radiotherapy of tumours, but they are harmful to normal tissues and constitute a safety hazard. Aspects of radiation safety are considered later.

Production of X-rays

X-ray photons, or quanta, are tiny packets of energy that are released whenever rapidly moving electrons are slowed down or stopped. Electrons are present in the atoms of all elements and, in order to grasp the fundamentals of simple radiation physics, it is necessary to understand the structure of an atom (Figure 18.2). Atoms contain the following particles:

- **Protons** – positively charged particles contained in the centre or nucleus of the atom
- **Neutrons** – particles of similar size to protons that are also found in the nucleus but carry no electrical charge
- **Electrons** – smaller, negatively charged particles that orbit around the nucleus in different planes or 'shells'.

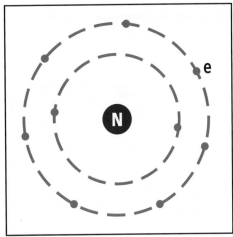

18.2 Structure of an atom. N = nucleus (protons and neutrons); e = electron (dotted lines represent electron 'shells'.)

The number of electrons normally equals the number of protons and so the atom as a whole is electrically neutral. The number of protons and electrons is unique to the atoms of each element and is called the **atomic number**. If an atom loses one or more electrons it becomes positively charged and may be written as X^+ (where X is the symbol for that element). If an atom gains electrons it becomes negatively charged (X^-). Atoms with charges are called ions or are said to be **ionized**; a positively charged ion is a **cation** and a negatively charged ion is an **anion**. Compounds are combinations of two or more elements and usually consist of positive ions of one element in combination with negative ions of another; for example, silver bromide (in X-ray film emulsion) consists of silver (Ag^+) and bromide (Br^-) ions.

In an X-ray tube head, X-ray photons are produced by collisions between fast-moving electrons and the atoms of a 'target' element. Electrons that are completely halted by the target atoms give up all of their energy to form an X-ray photon, whereas those that are merely decelerated give up smaller and variable amounts of energy, producing lower-energy X-ray photons. The X-ray beam produced therefore contains photons of a range of energies and is said to be **polychromatic**. If the number of incident electrons is increased, more X-ray photons are produced and the **intensity** of the X-ray beam increases. If the incident electrons are faster-moving, they have more energy to lose and so the X-ray photons produced are more energetic; the X-ray beam's **quality** is therefore increased and it has greater penetrating power. The intensity and quality of an X-ray beam can be altered by adjusting the settings on the machine, and the practical effect of this will be discussed in greater detail later.

The X-ray tube head

The X-ray tube head is the part of the machine where the X-ray photons are generated. A diagram of the simplest type of X-ray tube, a **stationary** or **fixed anode** tube, is shown in Figure 18.3.

The X-ray tube head contains two electrodes: the negatively charged **cathode** and the positively charged **anode**. Electrons are produced at the cathode, which is a coiled wire filament. When a small electrical current is passed through the filament it becomes hot and releases a cloud of electrons by a process called **thermionic emission**. Tungsten is used as the filament material because:

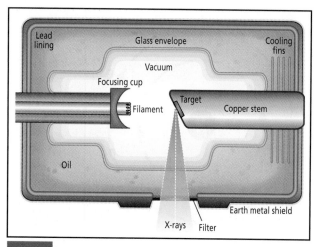

18.3 A stationary or fixed anode X-ray tube.

- It has a high atomic number, 74, and therefore has many electrons
- It has a very high melting point, 3380°C, and so can safely be heated
- It has helpful mechanical properties which mean that fine, coiled filaments can be made.

The electric current required to heat the filament is small and so the mains current to the filament is reduced by a **step-down** or **filament transformer**, which is wired into the X-ray machine (a transformer is a device for increasing or decreasing an electric current). Next, the cloud of electrons must be made to travel at high speed across the short distance to the target. This is done by applying a high electrical potential difference between the filament and the target so that the filament becomes negative (and therefore repels the electrons) and the target becomes positive (and attracts them). The filament therefore becomes a cathode and the target an anode.

The filament sits in a nickel or molybdenum focusing cup, which is also at a negative potential and so repels the electrons, causing them to form a narrow beam. The electron beam constitutes a weak electric current across the tube, which is measured in **milliamperes or 'milliamps' (mA)**. Multiplying the mA by the duration (in seconds) of the exposure reflects the total quantity of X-ray photons emitted in **milliampere seconds** or **mAs.**

The potential difference applied between the filament and the target needs to be very high and many times the voltage of the mains supply of 240 volts. In fact it is measured in thousands of volts, or **kilovolts (kV)**, and is created from the mains in a second electrical circuit using a **step-up** or **high-tension transformer**, which is also part of the electrical circuitry of the X-ray machine. The stream of electrons strikes the target, or anode, at very high speed. Tungsten or rhenium–tungsten alloy is also used as the target material because its high atomic number renders it a relatively efficient producer of X-rays. Unfortunately, the process is still very inefficient and >99% of the energy lost by the electrons is converted to heat, so the anode must be able to withstand very high temperatures without melting or cracking. Tungsten's high melting point is therefore useful in the target as well as in the filament.

In a simple type of X-ray tube (see Figure 18.3) the target is a small rectangle of tungsten about 3 mm thick set in a copper block. Copper is a good conductor of heat and so the heat is removed from the target by conduction along the

copper stem to cooling fins radiating into the surrounding oil bath, which can absorb much heat.

The target is set at an angle of about 20 degrees to the vertical (Figure 18.4). This is so that the area of the target which the electrons strike (and therefore the area over which heat is produced) is as large as possible. This area is called the **actual focal spot**. At the same time, the angulation of the target means that the X-ray beam appears to originate from a much smaller area and this is called the **effective focal spot**. The importance of having a small effective focal spot – ideally a point source – is discussed later in the chapter with regard to image definition. The design of the target to maximize actual focal spot size whilst minimizing the effective focal spot is known as the **line focus principle.**

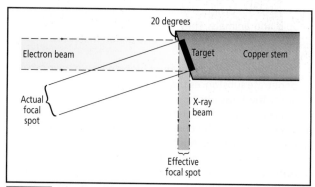

18.4 The line focus principle: how angulation of the target produces a large actual focal spot and a small effective focal spot.

Some X-ray machines allow a choice of focal spot size using two different-sized filaments at the cathode:

- The smaller filament produces an electron beam with a smaller cross-sectional area and hence smaller effective and actual focal spots. This is known as **fine focus**. The emergent X-ray beam arises from a tiny area and will produce very fine radiographic definition. However, the heat generated is concentrated over a very small area of the target and so the exposure factors that can be used are limited
- The larger filament produces a wider electron beam with larger effective and actual focal spot sizes – the **coarse** or **broad focus**. Higher exposures can be used but the image definition will be slightly less sharp due to the **penumbra effect**, a blurring of margins related to the geometry of the beam (Figure 18.5). X-ray photons produced at different points on the focal spot will travel along slightly different pathways and therefore hit the film in slightly different locations, even though they outline the same anatomical feature. 'Penumbra' is derived from Latin and means 'partial shadow'.

In practice, fine focus is selected for small parts where fine definition is required (e.g. the limbs), and coarse focus when thicker areas are to be radiographed (e.g. the chest and abdomen); the thicker areas require higher exposure factors and so the heat generated at the target is higher. The cathode, anode and part of the copper stem are enclosed in a glass envelope (Figure 18.3). Within the envelope is a vacuum, which prevents the moving electrons from colliding with air molecules and losing speed. The glass envelope is bathed in oil, which acts both as a heat sink and as an electrical insulator,

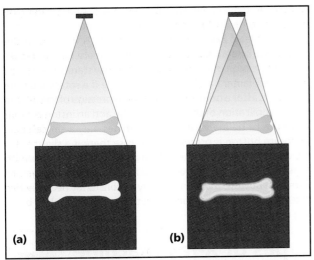

18.5 Effect of focal spot size. **(a)** The spot is a pinpoint and the projected image is sharp. **(b)** The rays from a focal spot of larger dimensions cause a penumbra effect, which blurs the projected image.

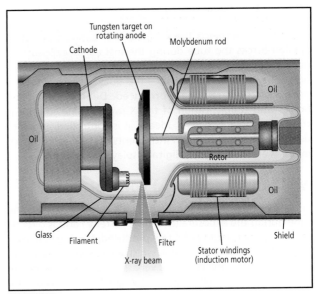

18.6 A rotating anode X-ray tube.

and the whole is encased in an earthed, lead-lined metal casing. X-rays are produced in all directions by the target but only one narrow beam of X-rays is required. This emerges through a window in the casing, placed beneath the angled target, and is used for making a radiographic image. It is called the **primary beam**. X-rays produced in other directions are absorbed by the casing.

Within the X-ray beam are some low-energy or 'soft' X-ray photons, which are not powerful enough to pass through the patient but may be absorbed or scattered by the patient and therefore represent a safety hazard. They are removed from the beam by an aluminium filter placed across the tube window; *these filters are legally required as a safety precaution and must not be removed.*

In stationary anode X-ray tubes, the X-ray output is limited by the amount of heat generated at the target. Overheating the target would produce melting and surface irregularity, which would reduce the efficiency of the tube; in modern machines, automatic overload devices prevent such high exposures from being used. Stationary anode X-ray tubes are found in low-powered, portable X-ray machines. These have limited ability to produce short exposure times for thoracic radiography or high output for large patients. More powerful machines require a more efficient way of removing the heat and this is accomplished using a **rotating anode** (Figure 18.6). In such tubes the target area is the bevelled rim of a metal disc of about 10 cm diameter whose rim is set at about 20 degrees, as in a stationary anode X-ray tube. The target area is again tungsten or rhenium–tungsten. During the exposure, the disc rotates rapidly so that the target area upon which the electrons impinge is constantly changing. The actual focal spot is therefore the whole circumference of the disc and so is many times greater than in a stationary anode X-ray tube. The heat generated is spread over a much bigger area, allowing larger exposures to be made, whilst the effective focal spot remains the same. The disc is mounted on a molybdenum rod and is rotated at speeds of up to 10,000 rpm by an induction motor at the other end of the rod. Molybdenum is used because it is a poor conductor of heat and therefore prevents the motor from overheating. Heat generated in the anode is lost by radiation through the vacuum and the glass envelope into the oil bath.

The size of the emerging X-ray beam must be controlled for safety reasons, otherwise it will spread out over a very large area. This is achieved using a **collimation device**, preferably a light beam diaphragm. Methods of collimation are described later.

The X-ray control panel

X-ray machine control panels vary in their complexity, but some or all of the following controls will be present.

On/off switch

As well as switching the machine on at the mains socket, there will be an on/off switch or key on the control panel. Sometimes the line voltage compensator (see below) is incorporated into the on/off switch, which therefore performs both functions. When the machine is switched on, a warning light on the control panel will indicate that it is ready to produce X-rays or, in the case of panels with digital displays, the numbers will be illuminated. With larger systems there may also be a link to a warning sign outside the X-ray room, which is illuminated whenever the X-ray machine is switched on. In some old machines the filament is heated continually whilst the machine is on and may burn out. Such machines should always be turned off when the exposure is terminated. X-ray machines must always be switched off when not in use, so that accidental exposure cannot occur when unprotected people are in the room.

Line voltage compensator

Fluctuations in the normal mains electricity output may occur, resulting in an inconsistent output of X-rays. The images produced may appear under- or overexposed, despite using normal exposure factors. In some machines these fluctuations are automatically corrected by an auto-transformer wired into the circuit, but in others it is controlled manually. A voltmeter dial on the control panel will indicate the incoming voltage, which can be adjusted until it is satisfactory. In such machines the line voltage should be checked before each session of radiography.

Kilovoltage (kV) control

The kV control selects the kV (potential difference) that is applied across the tube during the instant of exposure. It determines the speed and energy with which the electrons bombard the target and hence the quality or penetrating power of the X-ray beam produced. Depending on the power and sophistication of the X-ray machine, the kV is controlled in various ways. Ideally, it is controlled independently of the mA, often in increments of 1 kV, and the kV meter is either a dial or a digital display.

Milliamperage (mA) control

The mA is a measure of the quantity of electrons crossing the tube during the exposure (the 'tube current') and is directly related to the quantity of X-rays produced. Moving electrons constitute an electrical current, which is measured in amperes (amps), but the tube current is very small and is measured in 1/1000 amperes or milliamps (mA). Adjusting the mA control alters the degree of heating of the filament and hence the number of electrons released by thermionic emission, the tube current and the intensity of the X-ray beam.

In smaller machines the kV is linked to the mA, so that if a higher mA is selected only lower kVs can be used. Often there is a single control knob for both kV and mA and as the kV is increased the mA available drops. This is not ideal since, for larger patients, a high kV and high mA may be required at the same time, meaning that long exposure times are needed. In very basic machines the kV and mA are fixed, and only the time can be altered.

Timer

The quantity of X-rays produced depends not only on the mA but also on the length of the exposure, and so a composite term, the **milliamp seconds** or **mAs**, is often used. A given rate of mAs may be obtained using a high mA with a short time, or *vice versa*. The two numbers are multiplied together, for example 30 mAs = 300 mA for 0.1 s or 30 mA for 1.0 s. The effect on the film is the same except that the longer the exposure, the more likely it is that movement blur will occur. One should always, therefore, use the largest mA allowed by the machine for that kV setting, in order to minimize the exposure time. It should now be clear why machines in which kV and mA are automatically inversely linked are less than ideal.

The timer is usually electronic and is commonly another dial on the control panel, giving the choice of a wide range of exposure times up to several seconds long. Release of the exposure button terminates the exposure, even when long times have been selected. In larger machines, an automatic display of the resulting mAs is also present. At one time, X-ray machines relied on clockwork timers in hand-sets that also incorporated the exposure button. A dial was 'wound up' to an appropriate time setting and ran back to zero whilst the exposure button was depressed. The time had to be reset between exposures. These timers were not only inaccurate and noisy but also did not allow the exposure to be aborted if necessary. Some modern machines with a digital display have a single control for mAs, which automatically selects the shortest exposure time for the selected mAs.

Exposure button

The exposure button must be at the end of a cable that can stretch to >2 m, to enable radiographers to distance themselves from the primary beam during the exposure. Alternatively, the button may be on the control panel itself, provided that the panel is at least 2 m from the tube head or is separated from it by a lead screen. Most exposure buttons are two-stage devices: depression of the button to a halfway stage ('prepping') heats the filament and rotates the anode if a rotating anode is present; after a brief pause, further depression of the button causes application of the kV to the tube and an instantaneous exposure to be made. In some machines only a single-stage exposure button is present; in this case there is a slight delay between depression of the button and exposure, during which time the patient may move. In old machines with single-stage exposure buttons the filament may be constantly heated while the machine is switched on and in these there is a risk of burning out the filament.

Types of X-ray machine

X-ray machines can conveniently be divided into three broad types: portable, mobile and fixed.

Portable machines

These are the commonest type of machine found in general practice. As their name suggests, they are relatively easy to move from site to site for large animal radiography and many come with a special carrying case. The largest ones weigh about 20 kg. The electrical transformers are located in the tube head, which is usually supported on a wheeled metal stand (Figure 18.7), though some may be wall-mounted. *The tube head must never be held for radiography*, as this is very hazardous to the person holding the tube head. The controls may be either on a separate panel or on the head itself. Portable machines are low powered, producing only about 20–60 mA and often less. In most, the kV and mA are inversely linked. Although portable machines are widely used, their relatively low output means that longer exposure times are needed, and chest and abdomen radiographs of larger dogs are often degraded by the effects of movement blur.

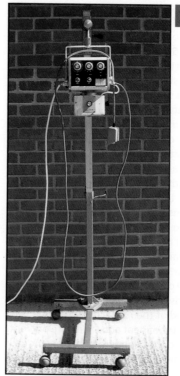

18.7   Portable X-ray machine.

Mobile machines

These are larger and more powerful than portable machines but can still be moved from room to room on wheels (Figure 18.8), some having battery-operated motors. The transformers are bulkier and encased in a large box, which is an integral part of the tube stand.

Mobile machines usually have outputs of up to 300 mA and are likely to produce good radiographs of most small animal patients. Although they are more expensive to buy new, they can sometimes be obtained second-hand from human hospitals, where they will have had relatively little use yet been well cared for, having been used mainly for bedridden patients. They are not usually suitable for equine radiography, since the tube head will not reach to the floor, but special tube arm adaptors can be fitted. If used for equine radiography, the horse should be restrained in stocks since the X-ray machine cannot be moved away quickly if the patient moves.

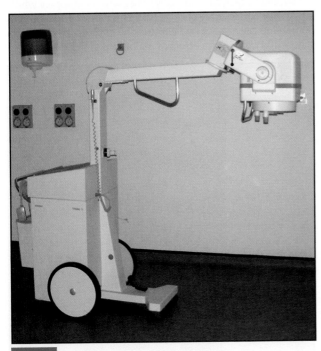

18.8   Mobile X-ray machine.

Fixed machines

The most powerful X-ray machines are built into the X-ray room and are either screwed to the floor or mounted on rails or overhead gantries (Figure 18.9). The tube head is usually quite mobile on its mounting and can be moved in several directions, which is especially valuable for equine radiography. The transformers are situated in cabinets some distance from the machine itself, and connected to it by high-tension cables.

The largest fixed machines can produce up to 1250 mA and generate excellent radiographs of all patients but, because of the high cost of purchase, installation and maintenance, they are rarely found outside veterinary institutions and large equine practices. However, several companies are now producing smaller, fixed X-ray machines especially for the veterinary market, which are much more affordable. Fixed X-ray machines are often linked electronically to a floating table top and moving grid.

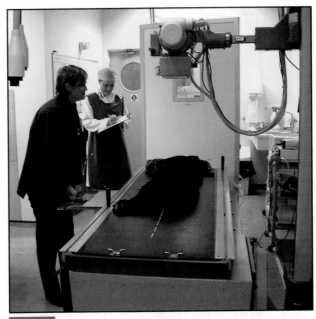

18.9   Fixed X-ray machine.

High-frequency machines

Many older X-ray machines, in particular portable machines, generate X-rays from a pulsating voltage supply. Most modern machines, including modern portable machines, use high-frequency generators to produce a stable high voltage supply to the X-ray tube. They do this by increasing the frequency of the waveform of the standard mains supply from 50 cycles per second (Hz) up to thousands of cycles per second (kHz). The advantage of this is that machines are capable of shorter exposure times, higher exposures, and improved efficiency.

Maintenance of X-ray machines

X-ray machines require little maintenance, but should be serviced annually by a qualified X-ray engineer, who will check both safety issues and calibration of the control buttons.

Formation of the X-ray image

The X-ray picture is essentially a 'shadowgraph', or a picture in black, white and varying shades of grey, caused by differences in the amount of absorption of the beam by different tissues and hence in differences in the amount of radiation reaching the X-ray film or digital detector system (Figure 18.10).

The degree of absorption by a given tissue depends on three factors:

- The **atomic number** (Z) of the tissue, or the average of the different atomic numbers present (the 'effective' atomic number)
- The **specific gravity** of the tissue
- The **thickness** of the tissue.

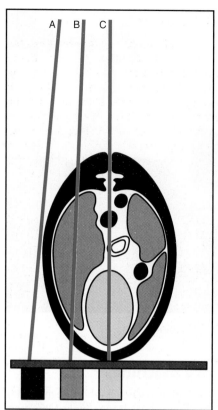

18.10 Cross-section through a thorax to illustrate formation of an X-ray 'shadowgraph'. X-ray photons passing along path C are largely absorbed, resulting in white areas on the radiograph. X-ray photons passing along path B are partly absorbed, producing intermediate shades of grey on the radiograph. X-ray photons passing along path A are outside the patient and so are not absorbed, producing black areas on the radiograph.

Bone has a higher effective atomic number than soft tissue and so absorbs more X-ray photons, producing paler areas on the radiograph. Similarly, soft tissue has a higher effective atomic number than fat.

Specific gravity is the density, or mass per unit volume. Bone has a high specific gravity, soft tissue a medium specific gravity and gas a very low specific gravity; hence gas-filled areas absorb few X-rays and appear nearly black on the radiograph.

The combination of effective atomic number and specific gravity produces five characteristic shades to be seen on a radiograph:

- Gas – very dark
- Fat – dark grey
- Soft tissue or fluid – mid grey
- Bone – nearly white
- Metal – white (as all X-rays absorbed).

It should be noted that solid soft tissue and fluid produce the same radiographic appearance; therefore fluid within a soft tissue viscus (e.g. urine in the bladder or blood in the heart) cannot be differentiated from the tissue that surrounds it. Fat is less radiopaque (darker) than soft tissue and fluid, so fat in the abdomen is helpful in surrounding and outlining the various organs. Overlap in the ranges of grey shades on the radiograph occurs due to the fact that thicker areas of tissue absorb more X-ray photons than thinner areas; hence a very thick area of soft tissue may actually appear more radiopaque (whiter) than a thin area of bone.

Selection of exposure factors

Kilovoltage

The kilovoltage (kV) controls the quality or **penetrating power** of the X-ray beam. A higher kV is required for tissues that have a higher atomic number or specific gravity, or are very thick. Both the nature and depth of the tissue being X-rayed must therefore be taken into consideration when selecting the appropriate kV setting. A range of about 40–100 kV is generally used in veterinary radiography. The kV affects both the **scale of contrast** on the image (the number of grey shades) and the **radiographic density** (the degree of blackening of the film).

Increasing the kV will cause greater penetration of all tissues and hence a darker film. Too high a kV will overpenetrate tissues, resulting in a dark film with few different shades; this is called a 'flat' film or is said to be 'lacking in contrast'. Too low a kV will underpenetrate tissue (especially bone), which will appear white, on a black or dark grey background. This type of appearance is sometimes called 'soot and whitewash'; its contrast is too high. Figure 18.11 shows the effect of alterations in the kV.

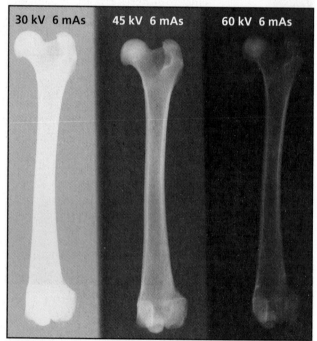

30 kV 6 mAs   45 kV 6 mAs   60 kV 6 mAs

18.11 Effect on subject penetration of altering the kV but keeping the mAs constant. With low kV there is little penetration of the subject; with high kV there is too much.

Milliamperage and time

The mA setting determines the tube current and therefore the quantity of X-rays per second in the emergent beam, also known as its intensity. Altering the mA will not affect the penetrating power of the beam (i.e. the contrast of the image) but *will* change the degree of blackening of the film under the areas that are penetrated (the radiographic density).

The product of mA and length of the exposure produces the mAs factor or total quantity of X-rays used for that particular exposure. Normally the maximum mA and shortest time possible are used for the chest, in order to reduce the effects of movement blur (times of <0.05 s are preferred). Increasing the mAs will produce more X-ray photons to blacken the film, though they have no more penetrating ability. The contrast between adjacent tissues (the difference in shades of grey) will not change, but the overall picture will be darker. Figure 18.12 shows the effect of alterations in the mAs.

Although kV and mAs can be seen to govern different parameters of the X-ray beam, in the diagnostic range of exposures they are linked, in that pictures that appear similar can be produced by raising the kV and at the same time lowering the mAs, or *vice versa*. A useful and simple rule is that for every 10 kV increase, the mAs can be halved (Figure 18.13). Conversely, if the mAs is doubled, the kV must be reduced by 10. In practice, the time factor is usually paramount and so it is normal to work with as high a kV as possible, allowing the mAs to be kept low and therefore the time short.

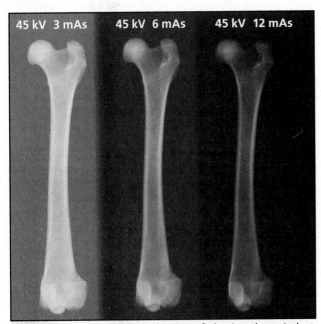

| 45 kV 3 mAs | 45 kV 6 mAs | 45 kV 12 mAs |

18.12 Effect on film blackening of altering the mAs but keeping the kV constant. The patient penetration (internal detail) is similar in each case but the image is darker with higher mAs.

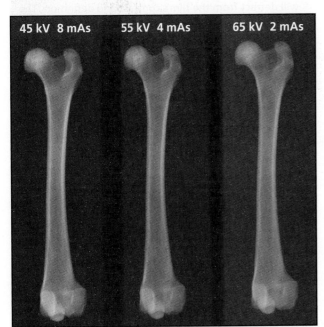

| 45 kV 8 mAs | 55 kV 4 mAs | 65 kV 2 mAs |

18.13 Interplay between kV and mAs. If the kV is increased by 10 and the mAs is halved, the effect on the film is almost identical.

Focal–film distance (FFD)

The FFD is the total distance between the focal spot and the X-ray film. It is important because, although the quality of the X-ray beam remains constant as it travels from the tube head, the intensity falls with increasing distance as the beam spreads out over a larger area. Figure 18.14 shows that if the FFD is doubled, the intensity of the beam over a given area is reduced to one-quarter and the film will appear underexposed unless the mAs is raised. Conversely, if the FFD is reduced the film will appear overexposed. The rule governing this effect is called the **inverse square law**, which states that *the intensity of the primary beam projected on to an X-ray film is reduced to one-quarter by doubling the distance from the X-ray film.* Thus a long FFD requires a higher mAs than a short FFD and the exact figure can be calculated mathematically from the equation:

$$\text{New mAs} = \text{Old mAs} \times (\text{New distance}^2/\text{Old distance}^2)$$

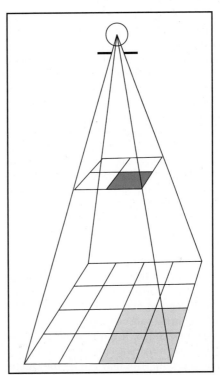

18.14 Inverse square law. The intensity of the beam falling on a given area is reduced to one-quarter by doubling the distance from the source.

Although longer FFDs require a higher mAs to be used, image definition will be improved due to a reduction in the penumbra effect as the X-ray photons are travelling more nearly parallel to each other (see Figure 18.5). It is normal practice to work always at the same FFD for a given X-ray machine; a suitable distance for a portable X-ray machine is 75 cm, whilst 100 cm is normally used for more powerful X-ray machines that produce a higher mA.

Exposure charts

In order to avoid wastage of film and time in repeating radiographs, as well as keeping the number of exposures to a minimum for health and safety reasons, it is necessary to build up an exposure chart for each machine. An exposure chart is a list of the kV and mAs required for radiography of various areas of different-sized patients. For the exposure chart to be accurate, all other parameters must be kept constant (e.g. line voltage, quality of processing, FFD) and other changeable factors should also be given on the chart (i.e. film–screen combination and use of a grid). The chart may be compiled for patients of different types (e.g. cats and small, medium, large and giant dogs) or may be made more accurate still by measuring the thickness of the part to be X-rayed using callipers. The exposure chart can be built up over a period of time by recording all exposures made in the X-ray day book, with comments. Exposure charts are not usually interchangeable between types of machine and may not even be accurate for other machines of the same make and model, because of the varying factors listed above.

Digital radiography systems are more tolerant of errors in selection of exposure factor, since the digital image can be computer-manipulated to optimize contrast and density. This means that there is less need to repeat exposures due to incorrect settings, saving time and money. The appearance of an underexposed digital image is different to that seen with a conventional X-ray film/screen system; instead of appearing pale it will have a grainy appearance as too few X-ray photons give rise to 'quantum mottle'. However, it is important not to allow the routine use of unnecessarily high exposure factors for obvious safety reasons. An additional advantage of digital radiography is that tissues of different density and thickness will usually be clearly seen using a single exposure, whereas with a conventional system two separate exposures may be needed. For example, in the thorax both the soft tissues and the spine can be demonstrated equally well with a single exposure, and an entire forelimb or hindlimb may be radiographed with one exposure, even when the difference in thickness of tissue from the proximal end to the distal is significant.

X-ray tube rating

The maximum kV and mAs produced by an X-ray tube are determined by the amount of heat production that it can withstand. If this heat production is exceeded, the tube is said to be 'overloaded' and damage may occur. The majority of X-ray machines have built-in fail-safe mechanisms that prevent these limits from being exceeded; if too high an exposure combination is selected then a warning light will come on and the machine will fail to expose. This may not be the case in old machines and so care should be taken to work within the machine's capabilities by consulting the manufacturer's details of maximum safe combinations of kV, mA and time. These details are known as **ratings charts**.

Scattered radiation

Although most of the X-ray photons entering the patient during the exposure are either completely absorbed or pass straight through, a certain proportion undergo a process known as *scattering*. Scattering occurs when incident photons interact with the tissues, losing some of their energy and 'bouncing' off in random directions as photons of lower energy (Figure 18.15). At lower kVs and when thin areas of tissue are being radiographed, the production of scattered or secondary radiation is small and most is reabsorbed within the patient. Scatter is therefore not a problem when cats, small dogs and the skull and limbs of larger dogs are

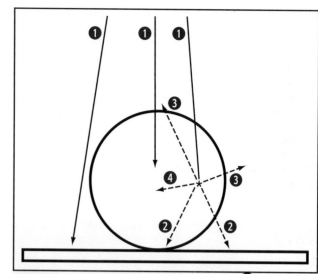

18.15 Formation of scattered radiation. **1** Photons of the primary beam. **2** Scatter in a forwards direction causing film fogging. **3** Scatter in a backwards direction, which is a safety hazard. **4** Some scatter is absorbed by the patient.

being radiographed. However, when higher kVs are required in order to penetrate thicker or denser tissues, the amount and energy of the scattered radiation increases and substantial amounts may exit from the patient's body. The problems associated with this scattered radiation are two-fold:

- Scatter is a potential hazard to the radiographers, as it travels in all directions and may also ricochet back off the tabletop or the floor or walls of the room. This remains a problem in the radiographic examination of equine limbs, but it should be less serious in small animal radiography where patients are usually artificially restrained and the radiographer stands further away
- Scattered radiation will cause a uniform blackening of the X-ray film unrelated to the radiographic image, and will detract from the film's contrast and definition. The blurring that results is called fogging.

Scatter production increases with higher kV, thicker or denser tissues, and larger field sizes of the primary beam. Digital systems are especially sensitive to the effects of scatter. The amount of scattered radiation produced may be reduced in several ways.

Reducing scattered radiation

- **Reduction of the kV** will reduce scattered radiation, so the lowest practicable kV should be selected. This is not always feasible, as in lower-powered X-ray machines the priority is usually to keep exposure time down using a low mAs factor and hence a large kV.
- **Collimation of the primary beam** (i.e. restriction in the size of the primary beam, using a device such as a light beam diaphragm) has a very large effect on the production of scatter. The primary beam should therefore cover only the area of interest, and tight collimation on to very small lesions (such as areas of bone pathology) will greatly improve the quality of the finished radiograph.

continues ▶

continued

- **Reduction of back-scatter** from the tabletop can be achieved by covering it with a 1 mm thick lead sheet.
- **Compression** of a large abdomen using a broad, radiolucent compression band will reduce the thickness of tissue being radiographed and will also reduce the amount of scattered radiation produced. Compression band devices may be attached to X-ray tables but should be used with caution in animals with abdominal pathology such as uterine or bladder distension. Compression techniques are no longer widely used in veterinary practice.

Grids

Even when the above precautions are taken, scattered radiation is still often a significant problem. The amount of scatter reaching the film can be greatly reduced by using a device known as a **grid**, which is a flat plate placed between the patient and the cassette. A grid consists of a series of thin strips of lead, alternating with strips of a material that allows X-rays through, such as plastic or aluminium, all encased in a protective aluminium cover. X-ray photons that have passed undeflected through a patient will pass through the radiolucent plastic or aluminium strips ('interspaces') but obliquely moving scattered radiation will largely be absorbed by the lead strips (Figure 18.16). Thus there will be a reduction in the degree of film fogging and an improvement in the image quality, though with coarse grids the grid lines will be visible. Significant amounts of scattered radiation are produced from depths of solid tissue >10 cm (or a 15 cm depth of chest, which contains much air) and so the use of a grid is usually recommended for areas thicker than this. Various types of grid are available, and there are two broad groups: stationary grids and moving grids.

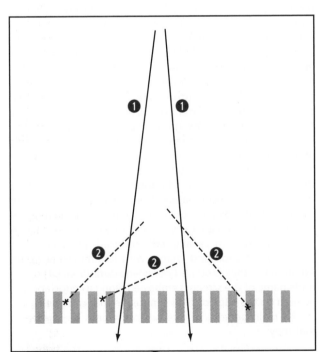

18.16 Effect of a grid. ❶ Most primary beam X-ray photons pass through the grid. ❷ Obliquely moving scattered radiation is absorbed by the strips of the grid.

Stationary grids

Stationary grids are either separate pieces of equipment or built into the front of special cassettes. Various sizes are available, but it is advisable to buy a grid large enough to cover the biggest cassette used in the practice. Grids are expensive and fragile and should be treated with care, as the strips may be broken if the grid is dropped.

Parallel grids

A parallel grid is the simplest and cheapest type of grid. The strips are vertical, and parallel to each other (Figure 18.17). This means that, since the X-ray beam is diverging from its very small source, the X-ray photons at the edge of the primary beam may also be absorbed by the lead strips, as well as scatter. There may therefore be some reduction in the quality of the film around the edges; this is called **grid cut-off**.

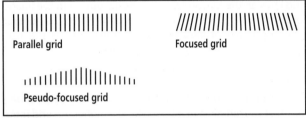

Parallel grid   Focused grid

Pseudo-focused grid

18.17 Types of stationary grid (diagrammatic cross-sections).

Focused grids

A focused grid should prevent grid cut-off, as the central strips are vertical but those on either side slope gradually, to take into account the divergence of the primary beam (Figure 18.17). A focused grid must be used at its correct focal–film distance and should not be used upside down. The X-ray beam must be centred correctly over the grid, at right angles to it.

Pseudo-focused grids

A pseudo-focused grid is intermediate between a parallel and a focused grid in efficiency and price. The strips are vertical but get progressively shorter towards the edges, so reducing the amount of primary beam absorbed (Figure 18.17). Pseudo-focused grids should also be used at the correct focal–film distance and should not be used upside down.

Crossed grids

Most grids contain strips aligned only in one direction and therefore scattered radiation travelling in line with the strips will not be absorbed. Crossed grids contain strips running in both directions and so remove much more scattered radiation. The strips may be either parallel or focused. Crossed grids are expensive and are only used in establishments routinely radiographing equine spines, chests and pelvises.

Moving grids

The use of a stationary grid results in the presence of visible parallel lines on the radiograph. These lines may be eliminated by the use of a grid that oscillates slightly during the exposure. This requires an electronic connection between the X-ray machine and the moving grid or 'Potter–Bucky diaphragm', which is built into the X-ray table. Moving grids are used in larger veterinary clinics, and moving grid tables may sometimes be available for purchase second-hand from human hospitals.

Grid parameters

Grid factor

The use of a grid means that, as well as scattered radiation, the grid will absorb some of the useful, primary beam. The mAs factor must therefore be increased when using a grid (to increase the number of X-ray photons in the beam) by an amount known as the **grid factor**. This is usually 2.5–3 times, but will be specified for each grid. In most cases a longer exposure time will be required, as it is likely that the X-ray machine will already be set at its maximum mA output. The increase in time may increase the risk of movement blur on the film, and the radiographer will have to decide whether or not this is outweighed by the advantages of using a grid.

Lines per centimetre

The greater the number of lines per centimetre, the finer the grid lines on the film and the less the disruption to the image (coarse grid lines may be very distracting). The usual number is approximately 24 lines/cm for grids used in general practice. Grids with finer lines are more expensive.

Grid ratio

The **grid ratio** is the ratio of the height of the strips to the width of the radiolucent interspace. The higher the grid ratio, the more efficient it is at absorbing scatter, but the more expensive the grid and the larger the grid factor. Practice grids usually have a ratio of between 5:1 and 10:1. Grids used with more powerful machines may have a ratio of 16:1.

Recording the X-ray image

Once the X-ray beam has passed through the subject and undergone differential absorption by the tissues, it must be recorded in order to produce a visible and permanent image. The conventional way of doing this is by using X-ray film, which has some properties in common with photographic film, including its sensitivity to white (visible) light. It must therefore be enclosed in a light-proof container, either a metal or plastic cassette or a thick paper envelope, and handled only in conditions of special subdued 'safe-lighting' until after processing. Images can also now be recorded electronically using computed or digital radiography equipment; this will be considered separately.

Structure of X-ray film

The part of the film responsible for producing the image is the emulsion, which usually coats the film base on both sides in a thin, uniform layer. The emulsion gives unexposed film an apple green, fawn or mauve colour when examined in daylight (obviously an unexposed film examined in this way will then be ruined for X-ray purposes). The emulsion consists of gelatine, in which tiny grains of silver bromide are suspended. The silver bromide molecules are sensitive to X-ray photons and visible light, both of which change their chemical structure slightly. During a radiographic exposure, X-ray photons passing through the patient will cause this invisible chemical change in the underlying film emulsion, but the picture is not visible to the naked eye and the film will still be spoilt by blackening ('fogging') if exposed to white light. The picture is therefore a hidden or **latent** image and must be rendered visible to the eye by chemical processing or development. When the film is developed, the chemical change in the emulsion continues until those silver bromide grains that were exposed lose their bromide ions and become grains of pure silver, appearing black when the film is viewed.

The emulsion layers are attached to the transparent polyester film base by a sticky 'subbing' layer and the outer surfaces are protected from damage by a supercoat (Figure 18.18).

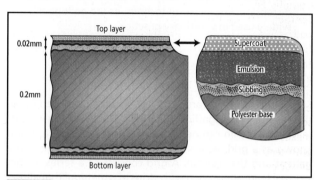

18.18 Section of X-ray film, showing emulsion coats bound to the base by subbing layers and protected by supercoats.

Intensifying screens and cassettes

Unfortunately, X-ray film used alone requires a very large exposure to produce an image and the use of film in this way is unacceptable in most circumstances. However, it was discovered many years ago that the exposure time could be greatly reduced for the same degree of blackening if some of the X-ray photons emerging from the patient were converted into visible light photons. This is achieved by coating flat sheets with crystals of phosphorescent material and holding these sheets against the X-ray film. These devices are known as **intensifying screens** (because they **intensify** the effect of the X-rays on the film) and for many years the most common phosphor used in the construction of intensifying screens was calcium tungstate, which emits blue light when stimulated by X-rays. In the 1970s a new group of phosphors was first used in intensifying screens; these were the so-called **rare-earth phosphors**, which produce blue, green or ultraviolet light. It is important that the X-ray film used is primarily sensitive to the right colour of light and for this reason some film–screen combinations are incompatible. One advantage of rare-earth screens is that they are more efficient at converting X-radiation into light than are calcium tungstate screens and so exposure factors can be markedly reduced, producing less scattered radiation and images with less movement blur. Additionally, they produce finer image definition. Often the trade name of the screen is embossed along its edge and can be seen on the edge of films exposed in that cassette.

The main benefits of intensifying screens are therefore that they:

- Allow much lower mAs settings to be used and so reduce movement blur, scatter production and patient exposure
- Prolong the life of the X-ray tube
- Increase radiographic contrast.

Screens consist of a stiff plastic base covered with a white reflecting surface and then a layer of the phosphor. Over the top is a protective supercoat layer. The screens are usually used in pairs and are enclosed in a light-proof metal, plastic or carbon fibre box known as a **cassette** (Figure 18.19) with the film sandwiched between. Occasionally a single screen is used together with single-sided emulsion film used for human mammography; such a combination produces images of higher definition but requires slightly longer exposures. These systems are especially popular for equine orthopaedic radiography. For good detail, the film and screens must be in close contact; the cassette therefore contains a thick felt or foam pad between the back plate and the back screen. Poor screen–film contact causes blurring in that part of the film as the light from the intensifying screens spreads out slightly before impacting on the film. The top of the cassette must be radiolucent (i.e. allow X-rays through), and the bottom may be lead-lined to absorb remaining X-rays and prevent backscatter, though this is uncommon with modern cassettes as it makes them very heavy. The cassette must be fully light-proof with secure fastenings and should be robust. Small flexible plastic cassettes containing one or two screens may be used for small animal intraoral radiography, since the larger sizes of non-screen film previously used are no longer manufactured and only small, dental non-screen film is available.

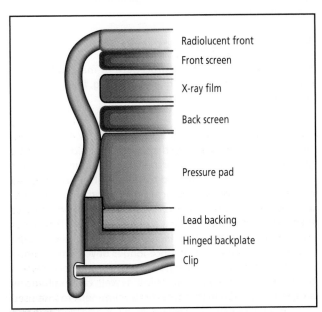

18.19 Cross-section through an X-ray cassette.

Labels:
- Radiolucent front
- Front screen
- X-ray film
- Back screen
- Pressure pad
- Lead backing
- Hinged backplate
- Clip

Care of intensifying screens and cassettes

Intensifying screens are expensive and fairly delicate and should be treated gently. Scratches or abrasions will damage the phosphor layer permanently, resulting in white (unexposed) marks on all subsequent radiographs produced in that cassette. Screens should not be splashed with chemicals or touched with dirty or greasy fingers. Any dust particles or hairs falling on the screens when the cassette is open in the darkroom will prevent light from reaching the film and will produce fine white specks or lines on the image (even minute particles will prevent the visible light from the intensifying screens from blackening the film in that area, though they will not, of course, interfere with the passage of X-rays). Screens should therefore

be cleaned periodically by wiping them gently with lint in a circular motion using a proprietary antistatic screen-cleaning liquid. The cassettes are then propped open in a dust-free environment in a vertical position to allow the screens to dry naturally. If they are reloaded whilst the screens are still damp, the film will stick to the screens and damage them.

Cassettes should be handled carefully and never dropped. They should be kept clean, as stains on the front may produce artefactual shadows on the radiograph and fluids seeping in will mark the screens. The catches must not be strained by closing the cassette when a film is trapped along the edges.

Types of X-ray film
Non-screen film

Non-screen film is film designed for use without intensifying screens, i.e. the image is solely due to X-rays. This requires a very large mAs (usually a long exposure time) but produces extremely fine image definition. The film comes wrapped in thick, light-proof paper rather than being used in a cassette. Non-screen film is now only available as small dental film, which is used for dental radiography and other intraoral views in cats and small dogs. The patient will be anaesthetized for this type of study and so the very high exposure required is not a problem, as the radiographer can retire to a safe distance, and movement blur should not occur. The 13 x 18 cm film that was previously popular for intraoral radiography of dogs and for radiography of small exotic species is no longer manufactured; it has been replaced by flexible plastic cassettes of the same size containing one or two high-detail screens that can be inserted into the mouth of an animal for intraoral radiography. Image quality is inferior to that which is obtained with non-screen film. The flexible nature of these 'cassettes' means that image blurring due to poor screen–film contact will occur if the device is bent in the mouth, but they can be reinforced by taping thick cardboard to them. Care should be taken that the patient's teeth do not damage the device and so an appropriate level of anaesthesia is needed.

Screen film

Screen film is designed for use in cassettes and is used for all other studies. The detail produced is less than with non-screen film, as the visible light produced by the phosphor crystals spreads out in all directions and will result in blackening of a larger number of silver halide grains than the initial X-ray photon would have done – an effect called **screen unsharpness** (Figure 18.20). **Monochromatic** or blue-sensitive film is for use with calcium tungstate or blue light-emitting rare-earth screens; it is sensitive only to visible light in the blue part of the spectrum. For use with green light-emitting rare-earth screens, the sensitivity of the film emulsion is extended to

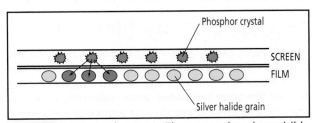

Labels: Phosphor crystal, SCREEN, FILM, Silver halide grain

18.20 Screen unsharpness. The arrows show how visible light emitted from each phosphor crystal may affect several silver halide grains, resulting in some loss of definition of the image.

include green as well as blue light; this is called **orthochromatic** film. It can therefore be appreciated that whilst green-sensitive film can be used with blue light-emitting screens as well (since it is sensitive to both colours), blue-sensitive film can only be used with blue light-emitting screens. One manufacturer produces ultraviolet light-emitting screens, which should therefore be used only with the same brand of film.

Most types of film are duplitized or double-sided, i.e. there is a layer of emulsion on both sides of the base, which doubles the efficiency of the film and the contrast and density of the image. However, this does result in some loss of definition, due to the superimposition of two slightly different images, and so single-sided emulsion film has become quite popular, especially for equine limb radiography. Human mammography film is used and gives very finely detailed images with good soft tissue and bone detail; it is used in a cassette containing a single green light-emitting screen. The main disadvantages are that the system requires about five times more exposure and the film cannot be processed in glutaraldehyde-free developer.

Film and screen speed

The speed of a film, a screen or a film–screen combination describes the exposure required for a given degree of blackening of the film. The speed is due to the silver bromide grains in the film emulsion size and the shape of the phosphor crystals in the screens, as well as to the thickness of the layers. Fast film–screen combinations require less exposure but produce poorer image definition (the image is more blurred) whereas slow film–screen combinations produce finer detail and are often called 'high definition'. In practice, a medium-speed system is usually the best compromise for keeping exposure times down and still getting reasonable quality images. Rare-earth systems give better definition at the same speed. Different manufacturers describe their various films and screens with different terms, which makes it difficult to make direct comparisons, but most produce several speeds of film and screen, e.g. slow (high detail), medium and fast. If a choice of speeds of film–screen combinations is available in the practice, then a slow high-definition combination may be used where exposure times are not a problem (e.g. for bone detail in limbs and skulls) but a faster combination should be used where it is important to keep exposure times short in order to reduce movement blur (e.g. for the chest and abdomen), especially if a grid is used.

Films, screens and cassettes come in a range of sizes from 13 x 18 cm to 35 x 43 cm. It is wise to have several different sizes available so as not to waste film by radiographing small areas on large cassettes, though multiple exposures can be made on the same film. Hangers of corresponding size must be available if the films are processed manually. Some table-top automatic processors will not accept larger sizes of film.

Storage of X-ray film

As has already been mentioned, unexposed X-ray film is sensitive to light and so must be stored in a light-proof container. This may be either the original film box or a light-proof hopper. Film boxes and loaded cassettes should be kept away from the X-ray area in case they are fogged by scattered radiation; they should be kept in lead-lined cupboards if stored near a source of radiation.

Films are also sensitive to certain chemical fumes and of course to chemical splashes, so good darkroom technique is essential. They may be damaged by pressure or folding and so should be stored upright and handled carefully without being bent or scratched. In hot climates high temperature or humidity may be a problem and so film should be refrigerated. This is not usually necessary in the UK. Film has a finite shelf-life which varies with the type of film. It is therefore wise to date the film boxes on arrival and use them in sequence, within the expiry date shown on the box.

Radiographic processing

The invisible or latent image on the exposed X-ray film is rendered visible and permanent by a series of chemical reactions known as processing. As with photographic film, this must be carried out under conditions of relative darkness, as the X-ray film is sensitive to blackening by white light (fogging) until processing is complete. Although most people now use automatic processors, an understanding of the principles of manual processing is essential since automatic processors operate on the same principles. This will also permit identification of processing faults, some of which will appear similar whether caused by problems with manual or automatic processing.

Manual processing

There are five stages in the procedure of manual film processing: development, intermediate rinsing, fixing, washing and drying.

Development

The main active ingredient in the developing solution is either phenidone-hydroquinone or metol-hydroquinone. These chemicals convert the exposed crystals of silver bromide into minute grains of black metallic silver, whilst the bromide ions are released into the solution. This process is known as **reduction** and the developer acts as a **reducing agent**. The length of time for which the film is immersed in the developer (usually 3–5 minutes) is critical, since longer development times will allow some of the unexposed silver bromide crystals to be converted to black metallic silver as well, causing uniform darkening of the film (chemical or development fog: see section on film faults). The developer must also be used at a constant and uniform temperature (usually 20°C) and ways of achieving this will be considered later. Precise times and temperatures for developing films are given in the manufacturer's instructions along with some indication of how the development time may be altered to compensate for unavoidable changes in the temperature of the solution.

Other chemicals present in the developing solution include an accelerator and a buffer, to produce and maintain the alkalinity of the solution necessary for efficient development, and a restrainer to reduce the amount of development fog (development of unexposed silver bromide crystals by fresh developer). X-ray developing solutions are purchased as concentrated liquids. Skin irritation may be observed after handling processing solutions; this may be due to an allergic reaction or due to the alkaline nature of the developer. *Gloves should be worn when the chemicals are handled.* If the problem is marked, the person's doctor should be consulted and informed of the chemicals involved.

During the development of each film a certain quantity of the developer will be absorbed into the film emulsion and so the level in the developer tank will gradually fall. On no account should the solution be topped up with water, as this will cause dilution and subsequent underdevelopment of films. The original developer solution is also unsuitable for topping up, as the proportions of the different chemical constituents of the developer change with each film that is developed and the solution becomes imbalanced. Instead, special developer replenisher solutions should be used, which take into account, and compensate for, this imbalance. Eventually, the developer will become exhausted as the active ingredients are used up and the solution becomes saturated with bromide ions.

Developer will also deteriorate with time by the process of oxidation, which will again result in underdevelopment of films. This process can be slowed by keeping the developer tank covered; in larger replenishment tanks there may also be a floating lid on the surface of the solution. Whether or not the developer is used, it is therefore unlikely to be fit for use after 3 months and so the general rule is to change the developer completely either every 3 months or when an equal volume of replenisher has been used, whichever is the sooner.

Rinsing

After the appropriate development time the film and hanger are removed from the solution and quickly transferred to the rinse water tank. Surplus developer should not be allowed to drain back into the developer tank, because it will be saturated with bromide ions and will contribute to developer exhaustion. The film should be rinsed for about 10 seconds to remove excess developer solution and prevent carryover into the fixer tank. Ideally the rinse tank will be situated between the developer and the fixer to prevent splashes of developer falling into the fixer.

Fixing

Following immersion in the developer, development is halted and the image is rendered permanent by a process known as **fixing**. The fixer is acidic and this neutralizes the developer, preventing further development of the emulsion. The fixer also removes the unexposed silver halide crystals, leaving a metallic silver image that can be viewed in normal light, a process known as **clearing**. The fixer contains sodium or ammonium thiosulphate, which dissolves the unexposed silver halide, causing the emulsion to take on a milky-white appearance until the process is complete. The time taken for the removal of all of the unexposed halide is called the 'clearing time' and depends on the thickness of the film emulsion, the temperature and concentration of the solution and the degree of exhaustion of the fixer. The fixer becomes exhausted as the amount of dissolved silver halide builds up within it, and exhaustion of fixer will occur more quickly than exhaustion of developer.

Fixer temperature is not critical but warm fixer will clear a film faster than cold fixer. However, staining may occur above 21°C and so the fixer should not be overheated. Fixing can also be speeded up by agitating the film slightly in the fixer. After 30 seconds' immersion in the fixer it is safe to switch on the darkroom light, and the film may be viewed once the milky appearance has cleared. The total fixing time should be at least twice the clearing time, a total of about 10 minutes.

A third function of the fixer bath is to harden the film emulsion (a process known as **tanning**) to prevent the film from being scratched when handled.

As well as the fixing agent (thiosulphate) and the hardener, the fixer solution contains a weak acid (to neutralize any remaining developer), a buffer (to maintain the acidity) and a preservative.

Fixing solutions are normally made up from concentrated liquids by the addition of water, according to manufacturer's instructions, as are developing solutions. They should be changed when the clearing time has doubled.

Washing

Following development and fixing, the film must be washed thoroughly to remove residual chemicals which would cause fading and yellow-brown staining of the film. Washing is best achieved by immersion of the film and hanger in a tank with a constant circulation of water, using at least 3 litres per minute so that the film is properly rinsed; static water tanks are much less satisfactory. Washing time should be 15–30 minutes.

Drying

Following adequate washing the films should be removed from their hangers for drying. Films left in hangers of the channel type will not dry adequately around the edges. The usual method is to clip the films to a taut line over a sink, taking care that they do not touch each other. The atmosphere should be dust-free with a good air circulation. Drying frames and warm-air drying cabinets are also available and are useful if film throughput is high.

Manual processing procedure

In order to ensure that no mistakes are made a strict protocol should be adhered to and all those involved in film processing must be familiar with it. The following steps should be carried out.

Preparation

1. Check that the developer and fixer are at the correct level. Check that the developer is at the required temperature and is adequately stirred.
2. Ensure that hands are clean and dry.
3. Select a suitable film hanger and check that new films for reloading the cassette are available.
4. Lock the door, switch on the safe-light (see below) and switch off the main light.

Unloading the cassette

1. Open the cassette and take hold of the film gently by one corner between finger and thumb, taking care not to damage the screen; shaking the cassette slightly first may help to dislodge the film.
2. Remove the film and close the cassette to prevent dirt falling into it.

Identifying the film

If labelling has not been performed during radiography, label the film using a light marker if available. These simple devices allow details written or typed on a thin piece of paper to be imprinted on to the corner of the film before processing, using a small flash of light. Often, cassettes contain small lead blockers in one corner to prevent that part of the film being exposed to X-rays and preserving it for the light-marking identification. The paper slips can be overprinted with the practice's name, which adds a professional touch.

Loading the hanger

Load the film into the hanger, handling it as little as possible and touching it only at the edges.

Processing the film

The processing stages are illustrated in Figure 18.21.

1. Remove the developer tank lid, insert the film and hanger and agitate gently to remove air bubbles from the film's surface
2. Close the lid and commence timing. The lid is kept on for two reasons: firstly it reduces the amount of oxidation of the developer by the atmosphere; and secondly the developing film is still sensitive to fogging by prolonged exposure to the safe-light.
3. The film may be agitated periodically during development to bring fresh developer into contact with the film surface and prevent streaking.
4. At the end of the development period, remove the film and transfer quickly to the rinse tank.
5. Immerse and agitate the film in the rinse water for about 10 seconds.
6. Transfer the film to the fixing tank. After 30 seconds the light may be switched on or the door opened. The film may be examined briefly once the milky appearance has cleared but it should be fixed for at least 10 minutes to allow hardening to take place.
7. Wash in running water for half an hour. (If running water is not available in the darkroom, the film may be washed elsewhere.)
8. Dry the film by hanging it on a taut wire in a dust-free atmosphere. Films in channel hangers must be removed first and hung by clips. Films must not touch each other during drying.

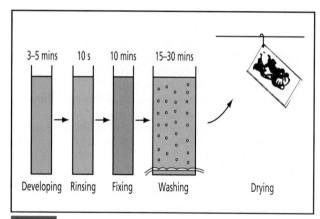

18.21 Processing routine.

Reloading the cassette

This stage may be performed whilst the film is developing.

1. Ensure hands are clean and dry.
2. Open the cassette.
3. Remove a new film from the film box or hopper. Handle carefully without excessive pressure or bending, as unprocessed films are susceptible to damage by pressure.
4. Lay the film in the cassette and, with a fingertip, ensure that it is seated correctly and will not be trapped when the cassette is closed.

Manual processing of non-screen film

As the emulsion of non-screen film is thicker than that of screen film, it takes longer for the developing and fixing chemicals to penetrate the emulsion and act on the silver halide crystals. Development time should normally be increased by about one minute and clearing time in the fixer will be several minutes longer. Since the only non-screen film currently available is the very small dental film, it is more practical to process these in small plastic cups or trays.

Automatic processing

Automatic film processing has several advantages over systems of manual film development, as it saves considerable time and effort and produces a dry radiograph that is ready to interpret in a very short time (as little as 90 seconds with some machines). In addition, the films should be processed to a consistently high standard if the processor is operated and maintained correctly. However, with poor use of the automatic processor film, faults may still arise.

Automatic processors are now widely used in general practice. A darkroom is still required to unload and reload the cassettes, but only a dry bench is necessary. The processor may be entirely within the darkroom, or the feed tray may pass through the darkroom wall to a processor that is located outside.

An alternative is a daylight processor such as may be used in a human hospital; these automatically unload and process the exposed film and then reload the cassette. Daylight processors do not require a darkroom but do require special cassettes and need regular servicing. A daylight processor found in some practices is a small automatic processor with light-proof sleeves into which the forearms are inserted, manipulating the cassette inside a dark area and feeding the film into the machine by feel.

Construction of an automatic processor

An automatic processor consists of a light-proof container enclosing a series of rollers that pass the film through developer, fixer, wash water and warm air (Figures 18.22 and 18.23). The intermediate rinse is omitted, as excess developer is removed from the films by squeegee rollers. The chemicals are used at a higher temperature (about 28°C) to speed up the process, and the solutions are pumped in afresh for each film at a predetermined rate; there is therefore no risk of poor

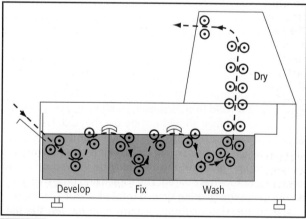

18.22 Essential features of an automatic processor.

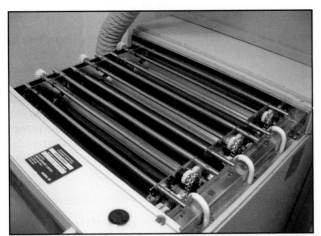

18.23 Automatic processor with lid removed, showing rollers and tanks.

processing due to the use of exhausted chemicals. A considerable amount of water needs to flow through the unit for the final rinse and so there must be an adequate water supply and adequate drainage. Finally, the films are dried by a flow of warm air. If the film throughput is high, a silver recovery unit may be attached to the processor to retrieve silver from waste chemicals.

Maintenance of the automatic processor

Automatic processors usually require a warm-up period of 10–20 minutes prior to use (longer in cold weather). Films processed before the machine has reached its operating temperature will be underdeveloped, although some machines will not accept film until they have reached the correct operating temperature. After the warm-up period a piece of unexposed film should be passed through to check the correct functioning of the processor and to remove any dried-on chemicals from the rollers by adherence to the unhardened emulsion. At least 10 films per day should be put through the processor to ensure adequate replenishment of the chemicals in the tanks. If necessary these may be old films; although new, unfixed films work better at cleaning the rollers this is more wasteful and expensive. At the end of the working day the machine should be switched off and the superficial rollers wiped or rinsed to remove any chemical scum.

Once a week the machine may be given a more thorough clean according to the manufacturer's instructions. This requires a deep sink so that the whole roller assembly for each of the three tanks can be removed and thoroughly cleaned. An old toothbrush is useful for cleaning around the cogs, especially in hard water areas in which lime scale will develop. The tanks also need to be cleaned once the chemicals have been drained out. An algicide solution such as 'Milton' can be added to the wash tank to help to remove algae from the tank walls and roller assembly, and a lime scale treatment may also be required. Care should be taken when handling chemical solutions as they contain substances that are classified as irritant and can also lead to sensitization from cumulative exposure. Cleaning and mixing tasks should therefore always be undertaken using appropriate eye protection and protective clothing. Splashes of developer reaching work surfaces, walls and floors will quickly oxidize and become brown; this may cause a permanent stain and so any splashes should be wiped off quickly.

The chemicals required are produced specifically for automatic processors and are not usually interchangeable with solutions for manual processing as they are formulated for use at higher temperatures. Since fresh chemicals are pumped in for each film and then discarded, there is no need for developer replenisher solution. The chemicals are made up by mixing concentrated solutions thoroughly with water; in the case of the developer there are three concentrates, one acting as a 'starter' solution; for the fixer there are two. The constituents must be mixed in the correct order and with the correct amount of water. The developer and fixer solutions are mixed and then stored in tanks ready to be pumped into the processor.

An alternative means of mixing chemicals for automatic processors is by automatic mixer unit. This method provides a safer and more convenient way of mixing and storing chemical solutions. Chemical concentrates for automatic processors are packaged in bottles with plastic seals and screw caps. Mixing is achieved by removing the screw cap and placing the upturned bottle on to the seal opener of the mixing unit; the seal is automatically broken and the contents flow into the tank below, where the correct amount of water is then added. The prepared chemicals can be pumped directly from the mixer unit tanks into the processor.

The automatic processor should be serviced regularly by the manufacturer's engineers as breakdowns can be very inconvenient. Most engineers will also operate an emergency service but nevertheless it may be wise to have the facility to process by hand, should the occasion arise.

Film quality with automatic processing

Although automatic processing will produce films of a consistently good standard, there is always a slight loss of contrast compared with the best that can be achieved by perfect hand processing. The latter is not often achieved and so the automatic processor is usually of great benefit to a practice with a reasonable throughput of radiographic cases.

Automatic processing of non-screen film

Non-screen film may be put through the automatic processor but will usually require subsequent manual fixing and further washing and drying to finish the clearing process in the thicker emulsion layers. A small amount of the fixer solution placed in a small plastic box is adequate for this. Depending on the nature of the processor, dental non-screen film may be too small to pass through the roller system and will need complete manual development.

Film faults

Radiographic quality is often degraded by faults arising during exposure or processing of the film. It is important to be able to recognize the cause of film faults in order to correct them. Sometimes there may be several possible causes for a given fault. Common film faults, their causes and remedies are discussed in detail in the section 'Assessing radiographic quality' below.

Disposal of waste chemicals

Spent chemical solutions should not be poured into the normal drainage system as they are environmentally damaging. Solutions should be collected and disposed of by a licensed waste disposal company. It is now a legal requirement to notify the Environment Agency when hazardous waste, such as spent developer and fixer, is produced or removed from any premises. Records of types and quantities of hazardous waste must then be kept for at least 3 years. Certain types of premises, including veterinary practice, are exempt from having to notify the Environment Agency provided that <200 kg of hazardous waste is produced per year.

Fixer solution can be collected and re-used several times in automatic processors, using dipsticks to test it for activity and to show when it is exhausted. To retrieve the silver content of waste fixer it can then be passed through a silver recovery system, though the cost-effectiveness of this depends upon the world price of silver. Another alternative may be to take fixer to a local hospital to pass through their silver recovery unit.

Darkroom design and maintenance

Requirements

The darkroom is an important part of the radiography set-up within each practice (Figure 18.24). The following factors should be considered in its construction.

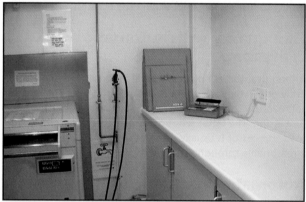

18.24   A darkroom for an automatic processor.

Size

Ideally it should be of a reasonable size to allow for satisfactory working conditions, and should not be used for any other purpose.

Light-proofing

The darkroom must be completely light-proof, and this must be checked by standing inside the darkroom for about five minutes until the eyes becomes dark-adapted, as small chinks of light entering may otherwise go unnoticed. The room must be lockable from the inside to prevent the door being opened inadvertently whilst films are being processed. Light-proof maze entrances or revolving cylindrical doors are used in busy hospital departments so that radiographers have free access to the darkroom.

Services

There usually needs to be a supply of electricity and mains water and a drain, though some tabletop processors use water in bottles rather than mains water. Access to a sink for cleaning the processor also needs to be considered when designing the room.

Ventilation

Due to the presence of chemical fumes, some form of light-proofed ventilation is essential.

Walls, floor and ceiling

The walls and ceiling should be painted white or cream (not black) so as to reflect the subdued lighting and make it easier for those working inside to see what they are doing. The walls and floor should be washable and resistant to chemical splashes; it may be wise to tile any wall areas likely to be splashed.

Safe-lighting

Since X-ray film is sensitive to white light until the fixing stage, illumination must be achieved using light of low intensity and a specific colour from safe-lights, which are boxes containing low-wattage bulbs behind brown or dark red filters. The colour of light produced must be safe for the type of film being processed, as green-sensitive films require different filters to blue-sensitive films. If the wrong filter is used, the films will become uniformly fogged whilst being handled in the darkroom. Safe-light filters must be checked carefully for flaws and damage, as even small pinpricks will allow light leakage.

The efficiency of the safe-lights may be checked by laying a pair of scissors or a bunch of keys on an unexposed film on the work bench for periods of up to 2 minutes and then processing it. If significant fogging is occurring, the metal object will be visible on the film. It should be noted that no safe-light is completely safe if the films are exposed for too long or if the safe-light is too close to the handling area. Film manufacturers will advise on the correct filter colour needed for particular types of film.

Two types of safe-light are available: *direct* safe-lights shine directly over the working area and *indirect* safe-lights produce light upwards which is reflected from the ceiling. The number of safe-lights required varies with the size of the room but should be sufficient to allow efficient film handling without fumbling.

Dry and wet areas

If manual processing is used, the darkroom should be divided into two working areas: the **dry area** and the **wet area**. If the room is large enough, these areas may be separated by being on opposite sides of the room, but where this is not possible they must be separated by a partition to prevent splashes from the wet area reaching the dry bench and damaging the films or contaminating the intensifying screens.

- In the **dry area**, the films are stored in boxes (preferably in cupboards) or in film hoppers, loaded into and out of cassettes and placed in the film hangers prior to processing. Sometimes films are also labelled at this stage. Dry film hangers should be stored on a rack above the dry bench and there may also be a storage area for cassettes.
- In the **wet area**, the processing chemicals are kept and used. There should be a viewing box with a drip tray for initial examination of the films, a wall rack for wet hangers and some arrangement for allowing films to dry without dripping over the floor or other working areas.

Usually, the processing solutions are contained in tanks. The **developer tank** should have a well fitting lid to slow down the rate of deterioration of the developer due to oxidation by the atmosphere. Ideally, the intermediate **rinse water** is held in a separate tank situated between the developer and the fixer so as to prevent splashes of developer falling into the fixer. The rinse water should be changed frequently. The final **wash tank** should contain running water if possible and should be at least four times the size of the developer tank.

In a busy radiography unit, the tanks should be housed together in a larger container filled with water and maintained at a constant temperature (usually 20°C). This **water bath** ensures that the chemicals are always at the correct, uniform temperature for processing and saves time, as well as helping to avoid underdevelopment of films. It is not essential to heat the fixer but inclusion in the water bath will prevent fixing from slowing down in very cold weather. Water bath arrangements may be purchased as special units or may be constructed, using an immersion heater and a thermostat.

If a water bath is not available, the tanks should sit in a shallow sink to prevent wetting the floor. In this case, the developer must be heated prior to use using an immersion heater with a thermostat or a thermometer (the latter requires constant checking). The solution must not be allowed to overheat and must be thoroughly mixed before the film is placed in the tank, as an uneven temperature in the solution will result in patchy development and a mottled appearance to the film.

If few radiographs are processed, the chemicals may be kept in dark, stoppered bottles and poured into shallow dishes when needed (as in photography). It may also be necessary to employ this technique should the automatic processor break down or for small dental films that cannot be put through an automatic processor. Unused cat litter trays make ideal processing dishes for radiographs, and dental film can be processed in small plastic drinking cups. The correct development temperature is achieved either by heating the solution prior to use or by placing the dish on an electric heating pad. The solutions are usually discarded after use as the developer oxidizes rapidly.

Other darkroom equipment

Film hangers are required for manual processing and are available in two types: channel hangers and clip hangers. Each type has its advantages and disadvantages. **Channel hangers** are easier to load but may result in poor development of the edges of the film. Films must be removed for drying and attached to the drying line using clips. The hangers should be washed after the films are removed, as chemicals may otherwise build up in the channels, causing staining of subsequent films. Very large films may not be held securely in channel hangers. **Clip hangers** avoid these disadvantages but are more fragile and more cumbersome to use and they may tear the films if not used correctly.

A timer with a bell should be present in the darkroom so that the period of development can be timed accurately. The timer should ideally be capable of being pre-set to a given time.

A hand towel and a waste-paper bin are also useful additions to the darkroom.

General care of the darkroom

Most film faults arise during processing and often radiographs that have been carefully taken are spoilt by careless darkroom technique. Competent handling of the films during this stage is therefore vital to the success of radiography within the practice and it is a duty usually delegated to the veterinary nurse. Film faults can also arise during automatic processing.

The darkroom should be kept tidy, clean and uncluttered, with all the equipment in its correct place. Cleanliness is particularly important, as undeveloped films handled with fingers that are dirty or contaminated with developer, fixer or water will show permanent fingerprints. Splashes of liquid falling on to undeveloped films result in black (developer), grey (water) or white (fixer) patches on the film after processing. Splashes of liquid falling on to screens result in pale areas on all subsequent films placed in that cassette, due to interference with light emission. Dust and dirt falling into open cassettes will result in small white screen marks on the radiographs.

With manual processing, attention must also be paid to the maintenance of the processing solutions, as underdevelopment is a common film fault. The tanks should be topped up when the fluid levels fall and the chemicals should be changed regularly, with a record being kept of the date on which they are changed. Developer should be renewed every 90 days or when it has been replenished by the same volume as the original solution, whichever is sooner. Whether using manual or automatic processing, separate mixing rods should be used for making up developer and fixer and should be cleaned after use. Chemicals splashing on to the walls or the floor should be wiped up, as they produce dust when dry and they may stain or corrode the surfaces. The chemical solutions may also damage clothing and so aprons should be worn while they are being mixed. The temperature of the solutions for manual processing should be checked regularly and the heater or thermostat adjusted if necessary.

Other important points are to ensure that the cassettes are always reloaded ready for use when the previous film is removed and to check that a sufficient number of film hangers are always clean and dry.

Viewing the radiograph

Although the radiograph may be examined whilst it is still wet (for technical quality, a provisional diagnosis or the need for a contrast study), the image will be somewhat blurred due to swelling of the two layers of wet emulsion. Full examination must be delayed until the film has dried, when the emulsion will have shrunk and the image is clearer. Radiographs should be examined on clean viewing boxes (not held up to a window) in a dim area to allow the eyes to pick out detail on the film without distracting glare from elsewhere. If the film is small, the rest of the viewer may be masked off with black card or other opaque objects – a simple procedure that will allow very much more detail to be appreciated. Relatively overexposed areas should be examined with a special bright light, and a magnifying glass is useful to look for fine detail.

Assessing radiographic quality

Radiographs must be of high technical quality if a radiographic examination is to produce maximum information about the patient. Errors can arise both during radiography and in the darkroom and the veterinary nurse should be able to assess the film for its quality, recognize any faults and know how to correct them (Figure 18.25). Before film faults can be recognized, it is necessary to understand the terms **density**, **contrast** and **definition**.

Fault	Cause	Remedy
Film too dark	Overexposure	Reduce exposure factors; check thickness of patient; check correct film/screen combination used
	Overdevelopment	Check developer temperature; time development accurately; check automatic processor cycle and thermostat
	FFD too short	Increase FFD
	Fogging	See below for causes and remedies
Film too pale	Underexposure (background black but image too light	Increase exposure factors; check thickness of patient; check correct film/screen combination used
	Underdevelopment (background pale only)	Check developer temperature; time development accurately; check automatic processor cycle and thermostat; change developer
	FFD too long	Decrease FFD
Patchy film density	Developer not stirred; film not agitated in developer	Correct the development technique
Contrast too high ('soot and whitewash film')	kV too low	Increase kV
Contrast too low ('flat film')	Overexposure	Reduce exposure factors
	Underdevelopment	Correct the development technique
	Overdevelopment	Correct the development technique
	Fogging	See below for causes and remedies
Fogging	Scattered radiation from patient	Collimate the beam; use a grid
	Scattered radiation from elsewhere	Change storage area for films and cassettes
	Exposure to white light before fixing stage	Check darkroom and safe-lights, film hoppers, lids on film boxes, keep lid on developer whilst film in the tank
	Storage fog	Use films before expiry date
	Chemical or development fog	Avoid overdevelopment
Image blurring	Patient movement Tube head movement Cassette movement Scattered radiation Fogging Poor film–screen contact Large object–film distance (OFD) Double exposure	Depends on the cause
Extraneous marks:		
Small, bright marks	Dirt on the intensifying screens	Clean the screens
Black patches	Developer splashes on film	Careful processing
White patches	Fixer splashes on film	Careful processing
Grey patches	Water splashes on film	Careful processing
	Chemical splashes on intensifying screens	Careful processing
Scratches	Careless handling of unprocessed film	Clean the screens
	Guideshoes of automatic processor malaligned	Handle unprocessed film carefully
Crescentic black crimp marks	Bending of unprocessed film	Handle unprocessed film carefully
Fingerprints	Handling of unprocessed film with dirty hands	Wash and dry hands before processing
Branching black marks	Static electricity	Handle unprocessed film carefully; use antistatic screen cleaner
Parallel marks on film	Roller marks	Check seating and cleanliness of rollers
Scum on surface	Scale or algae in processor	Clean processor; use water softener or anti-algal agents
Chemical stains:		
Yellowing/browning on storage	Insufficient fixing or washing	Correct fixing/washing
Areas of film supposed to be clear are grey and opaque	Insufficient fixing	Increase fixing time; change fixer
Borders around films	Dirty channel hangers	Clean the hangers
Grid lines too coarse	X-ray beam not perpendicular to grid; focused or pseudo-focused grid used upside down	Correct alignment of beam and grid
Damp films for automatic processor	Thermostat malfunction	Call service engineer
	Dryer temperature too low	Call service engineer
	Insufficient fixing	Change fixer

18.25 Common faults and their remedies.

Density

Radiographic density is the degree of blackening of the film and is determined by two factors: the exposure used and the processing technique.

Exposure

Film blackening is affected by the quantity of X-rays passing through the patient and reaching the film. It is influenced by the kV, the mAs and the FFD. If the patient's image is generally too dark, then the film is overexposed and the exposure factors should be reduced or the FFD increased; conversely, if it is too light, then it is underexposed and the exposure factors should be increased or the FFD reduced. Usually, corrections are made to the exposure factors; the FFD should remain constant unless it has been inadvertently altered.

Processing

Radiographic density can also be affected by processing. Underdevelopment, due to the use of diluted, exhausted or cold developer or development for too short a time, will cause all areas of the film to be too light, including the background outside the area covered by the primary beam. Development can be tested by performing the finger test, i.e. putting a finger between the film and the light viewer in an area where the film was not covered by the patient and which should therefore be completely black. If the finger is visible, the film is underdeveloped. Underdevelopment is the most common film fault arising with manual processing, and should be corrected by topping up the developer with replenisher (not water), by changing the solution regularly and by ensuring that it is used at the correct temperature and for the correct length of time. Underdevelopment may also occur with automatic processing, if the machine is not working at the correct temperature. Overdevelopment may occur if the developer is too hot or if the film is inadvertently left in the solution for too long. In this case, some of the *un*exposed silver halide crystals will be converted to black metallic silver, leading to uniform darkening of the film or 'development fog'.

Overexposure and overdevelopment may be hard to differentiate, as both will cause an increased radiographic density. However, areas covered by metal markers during the exposure will remain white if the fault is overexposure but will darken if the film is overdeveloped.

Underexposure and underdevelopment can usually be easily differentiated. Underdevelopment will produce a grey background using the finger test; with underexposure the background should still be black but the area covered by the patient will be too pale as the tissues have not been adequately penetrated by the X-ray beam.

In general, films that are too dark are to be preferred to those that are too light, as they may still yield adequate information when examined under a bright light.

Contrast

Contrast is the difference between various radiographic densities (shades of grey) seen on the radiograph. A medium contrast film with a reasonable number of grey shades as well as white and black on the image is desirable, as it will yield most information. A film that shows a white image on a black background with few intermediate grey shades has too high a contrast ('soot and whitewash') and is due to the use of too low a kV with insufficient penetrating power. A film without extremes of density, showing mainly grey shades, has a very low contrast and is called a 'flat' film. Poor contrast is usually due to underdevelopment, in which case the background will be grey (use the finger test). Overexposure, overdevelopment and various types of fogging including scattered radiation will also produce a flat film but in this case the background density will be black and the remainder of the film will also be very dark.

Definition

Definition refers to the sharpness and clarity of the structures visible on a radiograph. Good definition is usually essential if the film is to be diagnostic. Definition may be affected by a number of factors, as follows:

Movement blur

This is the most common cause of poor definition on chest and abdomen radiographs and is usually due to respiratory movement or struggling by the patient. It may also occur if the tube stand is unstable or if the cassette moves during the exposure (the latter is applicable only to equine radiography when a cassette holder may be supported by hand). Patient movement is minimized by the use of sedation or general anaesthesia and by adequate artificial restraint using sandbags, etc. The exposure time should be kept as low as possible as this will minimize the effect of motion.

Scattered radiation

Scattered radiation produced when thick or dense areas of tissue are X-rayed will produce random darkening of the film, resulting in loss of both definition and contrast. Its effects may be reduced significantly by collimating the beam and by using a grid.

Fog

Fogging is darkening of the film unrelated to the image and has a number of causes. These include the following: scattered radiation, accidental exposure of the film to radiation or white light prior to or during processing, poor light-proofing of the darkroom, the use of an unsuitable safe-light filter, prolonged or incorrect storage of film and overdevelopment. The result is a loss of definition and contrast.

Poor film–screen contact

Poor contact between the intensifying screen and the film within the cassette due to shrinkage of the felt or foam pad will cause blurring of the image in the affected area as light produced by the intensifying screens spreads out slightly before contacting the film. It will be present in the same place on all films taken in that cassette. Poor film–screen contact may also occur if the edge of the film is trapped in the side of the cassette, preventing it from closing snugly.

Film and screen speed

Fast film–screen combinations require a lower exposure for a given degree of film blackening than do slower combinations, but the definition of the image is poorer due to the larger size of the phosphor crystals in the intensifying screens and to the characteristics of the film emulsion.

Focal spot size

Some machines allow a choice of focal spot size. Fine focus produces finer radiographic detail but the exposure factors available are limited. Coarse focus allows higher exposure factors but, since the effective focal spot is larger, some detail is lost by the penumbra effect (see Figure 18.5). The penumbra effect is reduced in two ways: firstly by keeping the object–film distance as small as possible to reduce the amount of divergence between the photons, and secondly by using a reasonably long focus–film distance, which means that the photons are travelling more nearly parallel to each other.

Magnification and object–film distance (OFD)

As the X-ray beam diverges from the focal spot, the geometry of the X-ray beam results in some degree of magnification of the image. Magnified images will usually also be blurred, because the penumbra effect increases with increasing OFD. In order to reduce this effect, the part being radiographed should always be positioned as close as possible to the film, with the focal–film distance as long as is practicable for that machine (Figure 18.26).

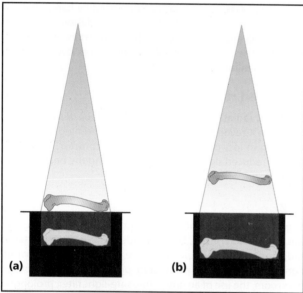

18.26 Magnification and object–film distance (OFD). **(a)** Object close to film, so reproduced accurately on radiograph. **(b)** Object not close to film, so image is magnified.

Labelling, storage and filing of radiographic films

Labelling

All radiographic films should be permanently labelled with the case identification (name or number), the date, a right or left marker if appropriate and any other relevant details (e.g. time after administration of a contrast medium). Labelling of the paper sleeve or film envelope only is inadequate and liable to cause mix-ups, especially on busy days. Films can be labelled at one of three stages: during exposure, in the darkroom or on dry film after processing.

Labelling during exposure

Films can be identified during radiography by placing lead letters on the cassette or by writing details on special graphite tape, which is then stuck to the cassette. Care should be taken to ensure that the whole of the information appears on the film after processing and is neither lost on the edge of the film nor overexposed. Right or left markers should be used at this stage (and not substituted for by the use of personal codes such as scissors or keys).

Labelling in the darkroom

Films may also be identified by labelling in the darkroom prior to processing. The most efficient method is to use a light marker, which is a small device that prints information, written or typed on paper, on to the corner of the film, using white light. A small rectangular area in the corner of the film must therefore be protected from exposure to X-rays by the incorporation of a piece of lead in the cassette to act as a blocker and leave a space on the film on which these details may be printed. There are also special cassettes available with a movable window, which can be inserted into a light-marking camera for imprinting the details; this can be done in daylight outside the darkroom.

Labelling of the dry film

Information may be written on the film after processing using a white 'Chinagraph' pencil, white ink or a black felt-tip pen. Such identification may not be acceptable for films used in legal cases, and so labelling after processing is not good practice.

Identification of radiographs for the BVA/KC scoring schemes

The requirement for submission of films to the BVA/KC Hip and Elbow Dysplasia Scoring Schemes is that they must be identified with the dog's Kennel Club and microchip numbers, the date and right or left markers *during* radiography, i.e. using lead letters or tape (or by a light marker before processing if using conventional film/screen systems). If the dog is not registered with the Kennel Club or other breed club, another form of identification may be used. Labelling after processing and computer-generated labelling with digital systems are not acceptable.

Storing and filing radiographic films

Radiographs may be required for retrospective study or as legal documents and so radiographs on film ('hard copies', as opposed to digital images) should be clearly labelled and carefully filed. Many films can accumulate within a short space of time in a busy practice and the filing system must be simple and foolproof.

Films processed manually must be completely dry before filing, otherwise they will be damaged by sticking to paper. Films may be stored in their original paper folders or in special X-ray envelopes, with case details (e.g. owner's name, patient information and date) marked clearly on the outside. These may then be kept in film boxes, filing cabinets or on shelving depending on the number of films involved. Films may be stored either chronologically or in alphabetical order of owner's surname, with films from each year usually being kept separately. Films of special interest and good examples of normal anatomy should be noted for future reference.

Digital radiography

With modern technological advances, new methods of acquiring and viewing radiographic images have become available. These methods are based on digital acquisition of the image; the radiographer is still required to position the animal and collimate accurately and to select the appropriate exposure factors but the acquired image is viewed on a computer monitor (Figure 18.27). Advantages include:

- Greater tolerance to suboptimal exposure factors, reducing the need for repeat exposures
- The ability to see a wide range of tissues on the same image
- The ability to computer-manipulate images
- Savings in processing and storage space
- Important radiographs should never go missing.

Image quality, however, is not inherently better than with high-standard conventional film/screen radiographs.

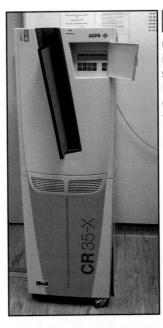

18.28 Digitizer for computed radiography. The cassette is inserted into the vertical slot, the image is 'read' by laser, and the cassette cleared and ejected ready for its next use.

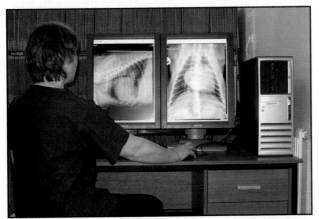

18.27 Digital radiographs are viewed on a computer screen.

There are two types of digital radiography: computed radiography and direct digital radiography.

Computed radiography

Computed radiography (CR) replaces the conventional film and cassette with a CR cassette containing an **imaging plate (IP)**, which can be used in conjunction with a conventional X-ray machine. IPs look very similar to conventional intensifying screens and are available in the same sizes. The IP absorbs X-rays and stores this as energy. The stored energy is released as visible light after stimulation of the atoms on the phosphor plates with a laser beam, and is converted into a digital signal. The patient's details are entered into the CR system and the type of examination selected (e.g. thorax, abdomen, spine) so the system can apply the correct **algorithm** or reconstruction for that body part. CR systems can be set up with small animal, equine or mixed examination selections, depending on the needs of the practice.

Following exposure, the cassette is inserted into the reader or 'digitizer' (Figure 18.28) and the IP is stimulated to release the image by the laser beam; the image then appears on the workstation monitor within about a minute. The IP is then usually automatically erased and inserted back into the cassette for re-use.

IPs are more sensitive to radiation than are conventional intensifying screens and should be erased, prior to use, if they have not been used for a few days. They should be used in rotation and periodically cleaned with the appropriate CR manufacturer's IP plate cleaner. CR systems allow greater flexibility with exposures than do conventional film/screen radiography but the optimum quality image is still achieved with the correct exposure and radiographic technique, including accurate collimation.

Most systems have an exposure range displayed, to indicate whether an image is under- or overexposed. Under- and overexposure appear differently to the same faults on conventional images: an underexposed CR image may have a higher degree of 'noise', creating a grainy appearance, whereas an overexposed image is less easily detected and may appear lacking in density. As an overexposed image can be adjusted on the workstation and a repeat avoided (unless extremely overexposed), it is important that the system exposure range is checked frequently to ensure that the minimum radiation dose is used consistently by all staff.

Direct digital radiography

Direct digital radiography (DR) may be of two types:

- **Flat panel systems** use a detector panel synchronized with the X-ray equipment. In the veterinary market, the flat panel first converts the X-ray energy to light and then to a digital signal to be interpreted by computer to produce an image file
- **Charged coupled device systems** rely on a fluorescent screen positioned directly under the X-ray table and the screen is linked to a charged coupled device via a lens and/or mirrors.

The resultant radiograph from either DR system is displayed on the workstation screen almost immediately, within 2–10 seconds.

As with CR, the animal's details are entered on the system and the examination selected. When the exposure is made, the image is sent directly to the workstation without the DR panel or screen being moved. The DR workstation software allows images to be manipulated as with CR. DR systems can be integrated with the X-ray equipment, especially in small animal use, but there are also many portable equine systems available which are ideally suited to mobile work for pre-purchase and yearling radiography due to the short image acquisition and display time.

Viewing digital images

Images acquired using CR or DR systems are normally viewed on the CR/DR LCD monitor (see Figure 18.27) and can be manipulated using the various viewing tools available. The computer image can be manipulated in several ways:

- Rotation
- Flipping
- Magnification
- Adjustment of density/contrast
- Inversion of black and white
- Annotation (e.g. adding a L/R marker or time after contrast study)
- Measurement of line distance or angles.

Images can also be enhanced by adjusting the density and contrast ('window levelling') to improve the diagnostic value depending on the tissue of interest.

It is usually possible to compare different images of the same study on the same screen on the CR/DR monitor.

LCD monitors can vary in size and resolution and if the CR/DR monitor is the only screen where images will be viewed, it is important that this monitor is of a high specification. The larger veterinary establishments may have a dry laser printer, which allows the images to be printed on to thermal film from the CR/DR if required. Images may also be printed on photographic paper, although this often results in very inferior reproduction.

Storage and distribution of digital images

Storage

There is normally limited storage on the CR/DR system without internal disc back-up, so it is important that an additional storage method is used. The storage of digital images acquired from CR/DR systems can be either off-line or on-line. Off-line storage can be on a CD/DVD, whereas on-line storage will typically be on a central archive. An on-line archive system allows the automatic saving of images from the CR/DR or other digital imaging system to a secure location without the manual task of copying to CD/DVD by veterinary staff.

The central archive will have a server with hard discs that would normally have built-in disc back-up and will store a minimum of 30,000 images. A mini-archive will connect to a single modality such as CR; and a small archive could connect to additional modalities such as a DR system and ultrasound scanner (assuming they have a DICOM (Digital Imaging and Communications in Medicine) output). Archive systems are specified for small, medium, referral or university veterinary establishments and can connect to multiple modalities for larger sites with storage of >250,000 images. It may be possible to import DICOM or JPEG images or digital photographs acquired elsewhere into the archive from CD/DVD/memory stick, such as images from a mobile MRI scanner or from equine pre-purchase examinations taken by another veterinary practice. The archive system may need to be expanded in the future, with the procurement of a new modality such as an MRI or CT

scanner or scintigraphy. A branch practice may add a CR/DR system, and storage at the main practice archive server may be preferred – a routing device can be added that encrypts and compresses the images and sends them on to the main practice archive server for storage and distribution across all sites.

Images can be copied to a CD or DVD in DICOM or JPEG format. Images copied in DICOM format will normally include a DICOM viewer which will allow the CD to be read on a normal PC with the DICOM viewing tools available as above. DICOM 3.0 is an industry standard for the viewing and storage of X-ray images which secures the patient details, and the image is stored in full resolution on the CD/DVD. The CD/DVD may be used to store images at a practice, given to a referring vet or sent away for second opinion, etc. Images copied into JPEG format are compressed, of lower resolution, and may not contain the patient details. They are used where e-mailing of images is required, e.g. for an urgent second opinion at a referral centre, or for lecture presentations.

Image distribution

Images can be viewed on the archive server but even in a small veterinary practice it is very useful to be able to access images in consulting rooms, theatre, offices, etc. An image archive can be supplied with a web browser to enable PCs within the practice to access the archive server. The browser may be restricted to three users at the same time, or up to 25+ at larger establishments. Veterinary surgeons and nurses can search for the patient's images using the animal's or owner's name, the animal's ID number, date of examination, etc., and view and manipulate images in the full-resolution DICOM format. Images from different dates and imaging modalities can be compared on the same screen for diagnosis or discussion with clients (Figure 18.29). The image archive system may also have complete integration with the practice management system (PMS), enabling users to query X-ray images from the PMS software.

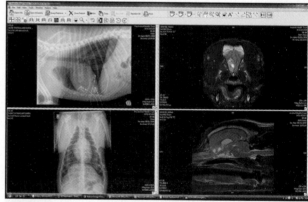

18.29   MRI scans (right) of a dog's brain showing a brain tumour, and thoracic radiographs (left) obtained to look for lung metastases, demonstrated simultaneously using digital technology.

Although DICOM images can be viewed in full resolution throughout the practice, PC monitors may not be of ideal resolution. If not using the dedicated CR/DR monitor, one practice PC could be upgraded to a DICOM-calibrated monitor (available in a selection of sizes and resolutions). For more in-depth radiology reporting of CR/DR, ultrasound, MRI and CT images, a dedicated PACS (picture archiving and communication system) workstation with DICOM calibrated or diagnostic monitors would be recommended. However, monitor resolution is reflected in the price.

Teleradiology

Teleradiology is the ability to transmit digital imaging files, normally in DICOM format, from one location to another for a veterinary or medical radiologist to interpret, and is a more efficient system than sending CDs or DVDs. Subsequently a report is transmitted back to the practice. This means that expert advice may be obtained very quickly from off-site professionals, even working on different continents. Images are normally sent electronically from the practice PACS system to the radiologist using a broadband Internet connection.

Radiation protection

Dangers associated with radiography

Exposure of the human or animal body to radiation is not without hazard, because of the biological effects that X-rays have on living tissues via cellular chemical reactions. X-rays have four properties that mean that the danger from them may be seriously underestimated:

- They are invisible
- They are painless
- The effects are latent, i.e. they are not evident immediately and may not manifest until some time later – even several decades in some cases
- Their effects are cumulative and so repeated very low doses may be as hazardous as a single large exposure.

Large doses are unlikely to occur in human or veterinary radiography but may be seen after nuclear accidents. It is the danger arising from *repeated* exposure to small amounts of radiation that concerns people working with radiation. Despite these hazards, it is possible to perform radiography in veterinary practice with no significant risk to any of the people involved, provided that adequate precautions are taken.

The adverse effects of radiation on the body may be divided into three groups: **somatic**, **carcinogenic** and **genetic**. They may also be classified as **stochastic** and **non-stochastic** or **deterministic**. Stochastic effects are those which occur by chance and which have no threshold, so could be caused by any size of dose, for example neoplasia and genetic mutations. Deterministic, or non-stochastic, effects have a dose-specific threshold after which acute radiation burns can occur.

Somatic effects

These are direct changes in body tissues that usually occur soon after exposure. They include skin reddening and cracking, blood disorders, baldness, cataract formation and digestive upsets. Gastrointestinal side effects cause severe dehydration, which is the usual cause of death following nuclear accidents or bombs. Different tissues vary in their susceptibility to this type of damage, with the developing fetus being particularly susceptible. The somatic effect is used to advantage in the radiotherapy of tumours, since tumour cells are often more sensitive to radiation damage than are normal cells.

Carcinogenic effects

These concern the induction of cancer in tissues that have been exposed to radiation. There may be a considerable time lag before tumours arise; this may be as long as 20–30 years in the case of leukaemia.

Genetic effects

These occur when gonads (ovaries and testes) are irradiated and mutations are induced in the chromosomes of germ cells. The mutations may give rise to inherited abnormalities in the offspring.

Sources of radiation hazard

During an exposure, there are three potential sources of X-rays that may be hazardous to the radiographers: the tube head, the primary beam, and secondary or scattered radiation (Figure 18.30).

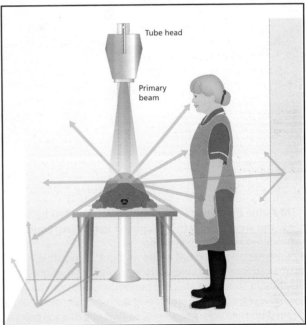

18.30 Spread of scattered radiation. The radiographer is too close to the X-ray beam and should ideally be 2 m away from it and behind a lead screen.

Tube head

Although the tube head is lead-lined (except at the window where the primary beam emerges), older machines may have suffered cracks in the casing that allow X-rays to escape in other directions. For this reason, the tube head should never be held or touched during an exposure. Checks on the efficiency of the casing can be made by taping envelope-wrapped non-screen film to the tube head, leaving it for a few exposures and then processing it. Any cracks in the casing will cause black lines to appear on the film, where it has been exposed. The integrity of the tube head should be checked by an engineer during the machine's annual service, as well as testing for electrical safety. The tube window must be covered by an aluminium filter, which removes low-energy X-ray photons from the primary beam. These photons do not contribute to the useful X-ray beam but are still a potential source of radiation hazard.

Primary beam

The beam of X-rays produced at the anode is directed out of the tube head through the window. This primary beam constitutes the greatest safety hazard, since it consists of high-energy X-rays. It may be delineated using a **light beam diaphragm**, a device attached to the tube head that produces visible light over the area covered by the X-ray beam (Figure 18.31). The light beam diaphragm usually contains crossed wires that produce a shadow in the illuminated area, showing the position of the centre of the beam (the central ray).

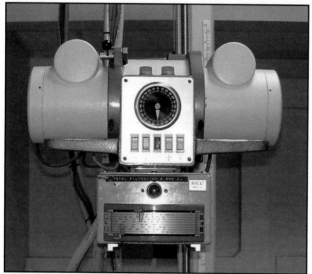

18.31 A light beam diaphragm attached to an X-ray tube head.

Movable metal plates or diaphragms operated by knobs allow the area covered to be adjusted to the size required, a procedure known as **collimation**.

Collimation should always be as 'tight' as possible (i.e. to as small an area as possible) and the accuracy of the light beam diaphragm should be checked periodically. This can be done by arranging pairs of coins along each margin of the light beam with their edges touching, so that one of each pair lies inside and one outside the light beam, and making an exposure. After processing, the image should show four coins inside the black area and the other four coins outside, if the light beam diaphragm is accurate. Good collimation is especially important in equine radiography when flexed 'skyline' views are obtained, as there is often an assistant restraining the limb in flexion.

An alternative, but now uncommon, method of collimation is to use conical or cylindrical devices or cones attached to the tube window to produce a circular primary beam of varying diameter. Cones are much less satisfactory than light beam diaphragms, since the area covered by the primary beam is not seen. Whichever method of collimation is used, the area covered by the primary beam should be no larger than the size of the cassette, and so the borders of the beam should be visible on the processed radiograph.

No part of any handler should come within the primary beam, even if protected by lead rubber clothing. In the rare cases where small animals have to be held for radiography, a light beam diaphragm *must* be used to ensure that the primary beam is safely collimated. Manual restraint is usual in equine radiography; *however, safety must still be observed at all times.* To prevent the primary beam from passing through the table and scattering off the floor or irradiating the feet of any handlers, the tabletop should be covered with lead or else a lead sheet should be placed underneath the cassette; in the case of a table with a grid cassette holder beneath the table top, the lead may be below this. In equine radiography, a lead sheet can be incorporated into the back of the cassette holder.

The use of a horizontal X-ray beam is especially hazardous, as the primary beam will pass, with little attenuation, through doors, windows and thin walls. This procedure should only be performed with great care, with the primary beam directed only towards a thick wall. The procedure for the use of horizontal beam radiography should be described in the practice's Local Rules (see below). Although the use of a horizontal beam is mainly employed for large animal radiography, there are occasions when it may be necessary for dogs and cats, for example for animals that are too dyspnoeic to lie in lateral recumbency.

Secondary or scattered radiation

Scattered radiation is produced in all directions when the primary beam strikes a solid object (see Figure 18.30), and so it arises from the patient and the cassette. It is produced by the table or floor if the tabletop is not lead-lined; it can also bounce off walls and ceilings and travel in random directions. It is, however, of much lower energy than the primary beam and is absorbed by lead rubber protective clothing. Its intensity falls off rapidly with distance from the source, as described by the inverse square law. The best protection against scatter is to stand as far from the X-ray machine and patient as possible – a minimum of 2 m, and better still behind a lead-lined screen.

Ways of reducing the amount of scatter produced (see above) include tight collimation of the primary beam, compression of large areas of soft tissue, reduction in the kV where possible, and the use of a lead-topped table or lead-backed cassettes. Protection against scatter is also afforded by radiographic protective clothing. The rotation of staff involved in large-animal radiography is advisable, since personnel may of necessity stand closer to the primary beam, although this should not be the main method of dose restriction. With small-animal radiography and non-manual restraint, rotation of staff is less important.

Legislation

In 1985 the law governing the use of radiation and radioactive materials was revised and updated with the publication of The Ionising Radiations Regulations (IRR) 1985, since updated as The Ionising Radiations Regulations 1999. This legal document covers all uses of radiation and radioactive materials, including veterinary radiography. As it is written in legal terms and is somewhat lengthy, a second booklet was published at the same time which attempted to explain the Regulations and is called the Approved Code of Practice for the Protection of Persons against Ionising Radiation arising from any Work Activity. The Code of Practice does contain some specific references to veterinary radiography but is also rather long and complex and so guidance notes explaining the law as it applies to veterinary radiography were published by the BVA in 2002 (Guidance Notes for the Safe Use of Ionising Radiations in Veterinary Practice). These cover premises, equipment, personnel and procedures and aim to minimize radiation doses received by veterinary staff. A summary of the legislation is given in the following paragraphs.

Principles of radiation protection

Protection follows three basic principles:

- Radiography should only be undertaken if there is definite clinical justification for the use of the procedure
- Any exposure of personnel should be kept to a minimum. The three words to remember are: Time, Distance, Shielding (i.e. reduce the need for repeat exposures, stand well back, and wear protective clothing or stand behind a lead screen)
- No dose limit should be exceeded.

The aim is to avoid exposure at all times, but failing this a high standard of protection will exist if the advice contained in the Guidance Notes is followed.

Local Rules and written arrangements

The Local Rules are a set of instructions drawn up by the practice's Radiation Protection Adviser (RPA), which set down details of equipment, procedures and restriction of access to the controlled area for that practice. The written arrangements are part of the Local Rules and include the sequence of actions to be followed for each exposure, including the method of restraint of patients for radiography and the precautions to be taken should manual restraint be necessary. A copy of the Local Rules should be given to anyone involved in radiography (veterinary surgeons and veterinary nurses) and should also be displayed in the X-ray room.

Radiation Protection Supervisor (RPS)

An RPS must be appointed within the practice and will usually be the principal or a senior partner, although may be the Head Nurse in some practices. The RPS is responsible for ensuring that radiography is carried out safely and in accordance with the Regulations, and that the Local Rules are obeyed, but the person need not be present at every radiographic examination.

Radiation Protection Adviser (RPA)

Most practices will also need to appoint an external RPA. RPAs must hold a certificate of competence issued by an appropriate body, stating that they have the knowledge, experience and competence required to act as a veterinary RPA. They are usually medical physicists, although holders of the RCVS Diploma in Veterinary Radiology who have undertaken appropriate further training may also be eligible. The RPA will give advice on all aspects of radiation protection and the demarcation of the controlled area, and will advise on drawing up the Local Rules and instructions for safe working.

The controlled area

A specific room should be identified for small animal radiography and should have walls of sufficient thickness that no part of the controlled area extends outside the room (single brick is usually adequate; thin walls may be reinforced with lead ply or barium plaster). The room should be large enough to allow people remaining in the room to stand at least 2 m from the primary beam. If this is not possible, a protective lead screen should be provided, unless the radiographer can routinely step outside the room and stand behind a brick wall during the exposure. Unshielded doors and windows may be acceptable if the workload is low and the room is large enough. Special recommendations are made for flooring in cases where there may be an occupied area below or above the radiography room.

Technically, the controlled area is the area around the primary beam within which the average dose rate of exposure exceeds a given limit (laid down in the Regulations). The controlled area for a typical practice is within a 2 m radius from the beam but usually needs to be defined by the RPA. Since the controlled area must be physically demarcated and clearly labelled, it is usually simpler to designate the whole X-ray room as a controlled area and to place warning notices on its doors to exclude people not involved in radiography. When the radiographic examination is completed, the X-ray machine must be disconnected from the power supply; the room then ceases to be a controlled area and may be entered freely.

A **warning sign** should be placed at the entrance to the X-ray room, consisting of the radiation warning symbol and a simple legend (see Chapter 2). For permanently installed equipment there should also be an automatic signal at the room entrance indicating when the X-ray machine is in a state of readiness to produce X-rays. This signal usually takes the form of a red light or an illuminated sign. Whilst not a legal requirement for portable and mobile X-ray machines (which comprise the majority of practice X-ray machines), many practices have installed red lights outside their radiography rooms to warn when radiography is in progress and prevent accidental entry, and this is to be recommended.

In addition, all X-ray machines should have lights visible from the control panel indicating (a) when they are switched on at the mains and (b) when exposure is taking place; sometimes exposure is indicated by a noise such as a beep or buzz. Illuminated signs outside the X-ray room may also have two different legends, for example one showing in yellow light when the X-ray machine is switched on and the other in red light when an exposure is taking place (Figure 18.32).

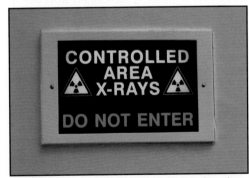

18.32 Two-stage illuminated warning sign outside an X-ray room.

For equine radiography at a practice there is usually a specific room, with the same control measures warning of a radiographic procedure and restricting access. Because much of the work with horses is with a horizontal beam, the walls should be of adequate construction and the doors and windows shielded. When radiography is carried out away from the practice, a temporary controlled area must be established. This will be defined by the RPA and the area must be clearly demarcated with cones, ropes and portable warning signs. The whole of the controlled area should be visible to the radiographer.

X-ray equipment

Radiation safety features of the X-ray machine should be checked annually by a qualified engineer.

- Leakage of radiation from the tube housing must not exceed a certain level and the beam filtration must be equivalent to at least 2.5 mm aluminium.
- All machines must be fitted with a collimation device, preferably a light beam diaphragm.
- The exposure button must allow the radiographer to stand at least 2 m from the primary beam, which means either that it must be at the end of a sufficiently long cable or else that it should be on the control panel, which is placed well away from the tube head.
- The timer should be electronic rather than clockwork, as exposures cannot be aborted with the latter, should the patient move.

Suppliers of X-ray machines have a responsibility to ensure that they are safe and functioning correctly, and they should provide a report to this effect when installing the equipment. *Servicing of X-ray machines is a legal requirement and should be carried out at least once a year.*

The X-ray table must be lead-lined, or else a sheet of lead 1 mm thick and larger than the maximum size of the beam should be placed on or below the table to absorb the residual primary beam and reduce scatter. Many practices now use purpose-built X-ray tables that are not only lead-lined but are also fitted with hooks to aid in patient positioning.

Practices performing equine radiography also require cassette holders with long handles for supporting cassettes during limb radiography, and various types of wooden blocks for positioning the lower limbs with the minimum of manual restraint.

Film and film processing

The Regulations recommend the use of fast film–screen combinations in order to reduce exposure times. They stress the importance of correct processing techniques in order to minimize the number of non-diagnostic films and avoid the need for repeat exposures. Digital radiography has important safety benefits as the number of repeat exposures required is reduced, since exposure factors chosen are less critical, and since bone and soft tissues can be seen on the same exposure of a given area.

Recording exposures

It is necessary to record each radiographic exposure made and this is done using a daybook for radiography including the following details for each exposure: date; patient identity and description; exposure factors used; quality of image; and means of restraint. If the animal has had to be held during radiography, the name(s) of the person(s) doing so must be recorded.

Protective clothing

Protective clothing consists of aprons, gloves, sleeves and neck (thyroid) protectors and is usually made of rubber impregnated with lead. The thickness and efficiency of the garment is described in millimetres of lead equivalent (LE), i.e. the thickness of pure lead that would afford the same protection. It is important to remember that *protective clothing is only effective against scatter and does not protect against the primary beam.* Fixed or mobile lead screens with lead glass windows are also useful as the radiographer can stand behind them during the exposure and still see the patient. Unfortunately they are very expensive.

Lead rubber aprons should be worn by any person who needs to be present in the X-ray room during the exposure unless they are behind a protective lead screen. They are designed to cover the trunk (especially the gonads) and should reach at least to mid-thigh level. Their thickness should be at least 0.25 mm LE; many are 0.35 or even 0.5 mm LE, though the latter are rather heavy to wear. Single-sided aprons covering the front of the body but with straps at the back are cheaper but provide less protection than double-sided aprons covering both front and back and are also less comfortable to wear for long periods. Aprons are expensive items and should be handled carefully; when not in use they should be stored on coat hangers or on rails (Figure 18.33). They must never be folded as this can lead to undetected cracking of the material.

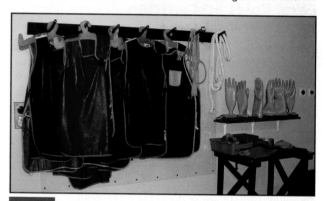

18.33   Correct storage of lead aprons and gloves.

Lead rubber gloves, open-palm mitts and hand shields must be available for use in those cases where manual restraint of the patient is unavoidable. They are also required for equine radiography when a limb or a cassette holder may need to be held. Lead sleeves are tubes of lead rubber into which the hands and forearms may be inserted as an alternative to gloves. Single sheets of lead rubber draped over the hands are not adequate, as they do not protect against back-scatter.

Gloves, hand shields and sleeves should be at least 0.35 mm LE and must never appear in the primary beam, since they offer inadequate protection against high-energy primary beam X-rays. It is important to remember that, although a lead glove may appear completely opaque on a radiograph, the film is being protected by two layers of lead rubber but the hand by only one (Figure 18.34).

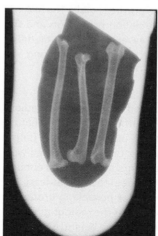

18.34   Radiograph of bones covered by a single thickness of lead rubber: compare with the edge, where there are two layers of lead rubber and all of the primary beam appears to have been absorbed.

Cassettes are occasionally hand-held in equine radiography; gloves worn should be 0.5 mm LE for maximum protection. Lead rubber neck guards for protection of the thyroid gland may also be used and are held in place using Velcro. Thyroid collars should be used in equine radiography where personnel are in close proximity to the source of radiation. Their use should be defined in the Local Rules.

All items of protective clothing should be checked frequently for signs of cracking. A small defect may not allow many X-rays through but will always be over the same area of skin. If in doubt, the garment may be X-rayed or examined with fluoroscopy and image intensification (a moving X-ray image obtained with low energy photons, which is electronically enhanced) to check for cracks (Figure 18.35).

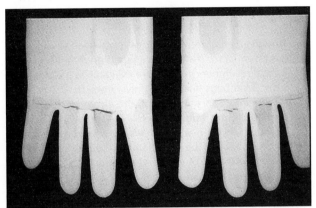

18.35 Radiograph of gloves showing cracking of the lead rubber at the usual site – the base of the fingers. These gloves should now be discarded.

Dosimetry

All persons who are involved in radiography should wear small monitoring devices or **dosemeters** to record any radiation to which they are exposed. The main dosemeter should be worn on the trunk beneath the lead apron, but an extra dosemeter may be worn on the collar or sleeve to monitor the levels of radiation received by unprotected parts of the body. Extremity ring or fingerstall dosemeters are available for wearing on the hands beneath lead gloves and are used for large animal radiography and for work with radioactive materials (e.g. during scintigraphy). Each dosemeter should be worn only by the person to whom it is issued and it must neither be left in the X-ray room whilst not being worn nor exposed to heat or sunlight. Dosemeters should only be worn on the veterinary premises (or when performing off-site large animal radiography) as it is important that they reflect accurately any radiation dose acquired at work and not false readings due to other factors.

Two types of dosemeter are available:

- **Film badges** contain small pieces of X-ray film and are usually blue. They contain small metal filters that allow assessment of the type of radiation to which the badge has been exposed
- **Thermoluminescent dosemeters** (TLDs) contain radiation-sensitive lithium fluoride crystals and are usually orange. On exposure to radiation the electrons in the crystals are rearranged, thus storing energy. During the reading process the crystals are heated and give off light in proportion to the amount of energy that they have stored – this gives a quantitative reading.

Dosemeters are obtained from dosimetry services such as the National Radiological Protection Board (NRPB; now part of the Health Protection Agency, HPA), or local hospital. They should be sent off for reading every 1–3 months, depending on the radiographic caseload. Dosemeters may also be used to monitor radiation levels in the X-ray room or in adjacent rooms by mounting them on the wall. They can be used to check the adequacy of protection offered by internal walls and doors. The exact arrangement for dosimetry in the practice will be made in consultation with the RPA, and the records must be filed for easy retrieval or available for new employers if a staff member leaves. Anyone whose badge reveals a reading should be informed, so that the cause can be identified if possible and working practices adjusted accordingly.

Dose limits

Dose limits are amounts of radiation that are thought not to constitute a greater risk to health than those encountered in everyday life. Legal limits have been laid down for various categories of person and for different parts of the body. Maximum permitted doses (MPDs) are laid down for the whole body, for individual organs, for the lens of the eye and for pregnancy. 'Classified' persons are those working with radiation who are likely to receive >30% of any relevant MPD. However, in veterinary practice these levels should not be reached and so veterinary workers rarely need to be designated as classified persons, provided they are working under formal written arrangements drawn up by the practice's RPA.

Staff involved in radiography

The Local Rules will include a list of names of designated persons authorized to carry out exposures. It should be remembered that nurses and other lay staff aged 16 or 17 have a lower MPD than do adults aged 18 or over, and therefore their involvement in radiography should be limited. *Young people under 16 years of age should not be present during radiography under any circumstances.* Owners should not routinely be present as they are members of the general public and are neither trained in radiography nor wearing dosemeters, although their presence may be necessary in emergency situations or during equine radiography. The Local Rules should ensure that doses to pregnant women are well within the legal limit, but nevertheless it is wise to avoid the involvement of pregnant women in radiography whenever possible.

The general rule is that the minimum number of people should be present during radiography. When, as is usual, the patient is artificially restrained, only the person making the exposure need be present and this should be the case in the majority of radiographic studies. Usually the radiographer will be able to stand behind a protective screen or outside the room during the exposure.

Radiographic procedures and restraint

Whenever possible, the beam should be directed vertically downwards on to an X-ray table. The minimum number of people should remain in the room and they should either stand behind lead screens or wear protective clothing. All those present must obey the instructions given by the person operating the X-ray machine. The beam must be collimated to the smallest size practicable and must be entirely within the borders of the film. Grids should only be used when the part being X-rayed is >10 cm thick, as their use necessitates an increase in the exposure.

The method of restraint of the patient is of paramount importance. The Approved Code of Practice states that 'only in exceptional circumstances should a patient or animal undergoing a diagnostic examination be supported or manipulated by hand'. These *exceptional circumstances* may include severely ill or injured animals for whom a diagnosis requires radiography but for whom sedation, anaesthesia or restraint with sandbags is dangerous (e.g. very young puppies and kittens, congestive heart failure, ruptured diaphragm or other severe traumatic injuries). In these cases the animal may be held, provided that those restraining it are fully protected and provided that no part of their hands (even in gloves) enters the primary beam. A light beam diaphragm is essential for manual restraint. The majority of patients may be positioned and restrained artificially using positioning aids under varying degrees of sedation or general anaesthesia, and sometimes with no chemical restraint at all.

Positioning

In order to produce radiographs of maximum diagnostic value it is necessary to position the patient carefully and to centre and collimate the beam accurately. Poor positioning, with rotation or obliquity of the area being radiographed, will result in a film that is hard to interpret or misleading or that fails to demonstrate the lesion. There are several general rules that should be adhered to when positioning the patient.

Patient positioning

- Use a large enough cassette to cover the whole area of interest, such as the chest or abdomen in a large dog – it is very difficult to interpret images that are made up of a mosaic of smaller radiographs.
- Place the area of interest as close to the film as possible in order to minimize magnification and blurring and to produce an accurate image.
- Centre over the area of interest, especially if it is a joint or a disc space.
- Ensure that the central ray of the primary beam is perpendicular to the film; otherwise distortion and non-uniform exposure of the structures will result. If a grid is being used, accurate alignment of the primary beam is essential to prevent grid faults.
- Collimate the beam to as small an area as possible, to reduce the amount of scattered radiation produced.
- Since a radiograph is a two-dimensional image of a three-dimensional structure, it is usually necessary to take two radiographs at right angles to each other in order to visualize the area fully. Oblique views may then be taken to highlight lesions seen on the initial films if appropriate.

Restraint

Small animals should be held for radiography *only in exceptional circumstances* (see above), when a radiograph is essential for a diagnosis but their condition renders other means of restraint unsafe. In practice, patients rarely need to be held and most views may be achieved using a combination of chemical restraint and positioning aids.

Simple lateral views of chest, abdomen and limbs may be possible in placid animals without any form of sedation. Other views require varying degrees of sedation or general anaesthesia; the positioning requirements and the temperament of the patient must be taken into consideration when assessing the depth of sedation required. It is also important to handle patients gently, calmly and firmly during radiography, and to reassure them with touch and voice. The room should be quiet, and subdued lighting will not only help to settle the patient but is also necessary for use of the light beam diaphragm.

Positioning aids

With the skilful use of positioning aids and the correct degree of chemical restraint, almost any radiographic view may be achieved without the need to hold the animal. The following positioning aids should be present in the practice.

Positioning aids

- **Troughs:** Radiolucent plastic or foam-filled troughs are essential for restraining animals on their backs (dorsal recumbency). They are available in a variety of sizes. Bean-bags filled with polystyrene beads are also helpful in supporting the patient, although they may be very slightly radiopaque.
- **Foam pads:** When lateral views are required, wedge-shaped pads may be placed under the chest, skull or spine to prevent rotation and to ensure that a true lateral view is achieved. They are also useful for accurate limb positioning. They are radiolucent and may therefore be used in the primary beam. It is useful to have several, in different shapes and sizes, and to cover them with plastic for easy cleaning.
- **Sandbags:** Long, thin sandbags of various sizes may be wrapped around limbs or placed over the neck for restraint. They should only be loosely filled with sand, so that they can be bent and twisted. As they are radiopaque they should not be used in the primary beam. They should be plastic-covered for easy cleaning.
- **Tapes:** Cotton tapes are looped around limbs and may then be tied to hooks on the edge of the table or wrapped around sandbags, for positioning of the limbs. Medical sticky tape may also be useful at times. Ties should only be attached to hooks in anaesthetized patients, in case of unexpected patient movement, which might lead to injury.
- **Velcro bands:** Fabric bands with Velcro fastenings are especially useful for VD hip radiographs, as they can be placed around the stifles to align the femora correctly. Non-stick elasticated bandage can also be used.
- **Wooden blocks:** These are used to raise the cassette to the area of interest for certain views (e.g. DV skull). They are radiopaque and so should not be placed between the patient and the film.

Nomenclature

Each radiographic projection is named with a composite term describing first the point of entry and then the point of exit of the beam. For example, a DV view of the chest involves the X-ray beam entering through the spine (dorsally) and emerging through the sternum (ventrally). An exception is the lateromedial (LM) or mediolateral (ML) view, which is commonly just called the lateral view. A standardized nomenclature has been devised for veterinary radiology (the naming of the various body regions is illustrated in Chapter 3). The correct terminology will be used throughout this section.

Note that the terms anterior and posterior are no longer used in veterinary radiography as they are not appropriate to four-legged creatures. Instead, anteroposterior (AP) and posteroanterior (PA) views of the limbs are called:

- Craniocaudal (CrCd) or caudocranial (CdCr) above the radiocarpal and tibiotarsal joints
- Dorsopalmar (DPa)/palmarodorsal (PaD) below the radiocarpal joint in the forelimb and dorsoplantar (DPl)/plantarodorsal (PlD) below the tibiotarsal joint in the hindlimb.

Dorsal recumbency (supine) describes an animal lying on its back and sternal recumbency (prone) describes the crouching position.

Positioning for common views in dogs and cats

The following notes describe in brief the positioning for the more common views performed in veterinary practice in small animals. The resultant images of various views can be found in BSAVA Manuals on diagnostic imaging.

Thorax

The right lateral recumbent position is usually preferred to the left lateral for a single screening film, as the heart outline is more consistent in shape. However, when assessing the lungs it is useful to perform the left lateral recumbent view too, as the uppermost lung field is better aerated in lateral recumbency and is therefore more likely to show pathology. Therefore when investigating known or suspected lung disease (such as a search for metastases) both right and left lateral radiographs with or without a DV or VD view should always be obtained. For cardiac examination a right lateral and DV are recommended for consistency of cardiac shape.

If performing radiography under general anaesthesia, the animal should be radiographed as soon as possible after induction, as collapse of the dependent lung area occurs quickly and can mimic pathology. Ideally, the patient should be kept in sternal recumbency until the lateral radiograph is to be taken. Manual inflation of the chest (taking all necessary safety precautions for the person doing this) will be of great benefit in aerating the lungs and improving the image. The kV should be reduced slightly, by about 2–5 kV, for manually inflated lungs.

Lateral view

1. Place the patient in right or left lateral recumbency.
2. Place a radiolucent foam wedge under the sternum to raise it to the same height above the tabletop as the spine (Figure 18.36), thus ensuring that there is no lateral rotation of the chest.
3. Place a sandbag carefully over the neck for restraint if the patient is not anaesthetized.
4. Draw the forelimbs forwards and fix them in place with tapes or sandbags to prevent them from overlying the cranial thorax.
5. Restrain the hindlimbs with a sandbag, extending them slightly caudally.
6. Centre by palpation on the middle of the fifth rib and level with the caudal border of the scapula (slightly caudal to this if manual lung inflation is to be used).
7. Collimate to include lung fields and expose on inspiration for maximum aeration of the lungs.

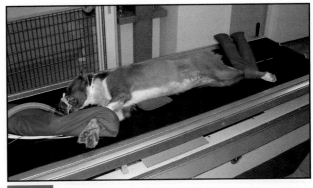

18.36 Positioning for lateral view of thorax/abdomen.

The trachea, heart, aorta, caudal vena cava, diaphragm, bronchovascular lung markings and skeletal structures can be identified on a lateral view. The oesophagus is not normally visible on plain radiographs.

In a very dyspnoeic patient, a lateral view may be obtained with the patient standing or crouching and using a horizontal X-ray beam. This is safer for the patient than being placed in lateral recumbency. Cats and small dogs may be restrained in narrow cardboard boxes instead of being held; larger dogs can usually be held on the end of a lead with the handler standing well back. Care should be taken with the direction of the primary beam, which should only be directed towards a substantial wall. Although the resulting image will be poor, with the elbow area overlying and obscuring the cranioventral thorax, in such dyspnoeic patients there is usually major thoracic pathology which is still easily visible.

Dorsoventral view

The DV and not the VD view must be used for assessment of the heart, because in the latter position the heart may tip to one side and appear distorted. Animals that are dyspnoeic or may have significant thoracic pathology must not be placed on their backs, and so the DV and not the VD view is required.

1. Position the patient in sternal recumbency, crouching symmetrically (Figure 18.37). This may be difficult in conscious animals that have arthritis of the elbows, hips or stifles.
2. Push the elbows laterally to 'prop' up the dog or cat symmetrically.
3. Drape a sandbag carefully over the neck to keep the head down, shaking the sand into either end to produce a sparsely filled area in the middle of the sandbag. It may be useful to rest the patient's chin on a foam pad or wooden block.
4. Centre in the midline between the tips of the scapulae.
5. Collimate to include the lung fields and expose on inspiration.

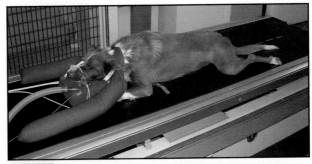

18.37 Positioning for dorsoventral view of the thorax.

The trachea, heart, aorta, caudal vena cava, diaphragm, bronchovascular lung markings and skeletal structures can be identified on a DV view. The oesophagus is not normally visible on plain films.

Ventrodorsal view

> **WARNING**
>
> Patients must never be placed on their backs if pleural fluid, pneumothorax or a ruptured diaphragm is suspected, as this may cause respiratory embarrassment.

1. Position the patient in dorsal recumbency using a radiolucent trough or sandbags around the hind end (Figure 18.38). The hindlimbs may be flexed or 'frog-legged' and supported on foam wedges or sandbags.
2. Ensure that the patient is lying straight and not tipped to one side.
3. Draw the forelimbs forwards with tapes or by placing a sandbag gently over them. Secure the hindlimbs too if necessary.
4. Centre on the mid-point of the sternum, collimate to the lung field and expose on inspiration.

The trachea, heart, aorta, caudal vena cava, diaphragm, bronchovascular lung markings and skeletal structures can be identified on a VD view. The oesophagus is not normally visible on plain films.

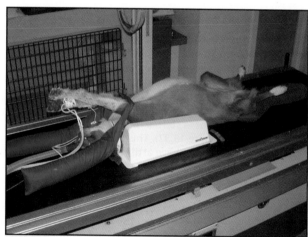

18.38 Positioning for ventrodorsal view of thorax/abdomen.

Abdomen

Lateral view

Positioning is similar to that for the thorax.

1. Position the patient in lateral recumbency and pad up the sternum if necessary (see Figure 18.36).
2. Place a sandbag carefully over the neck if the patient is not anaesthetized.
3. Restrain the fore- and hindlimbs with sandbags or ties, ensuring that the hindlimbs are pulled back so that they do not obscure the caudal abdomen.
4. Centre over the area of interest and collimate as necessary. In large dogs two radiographs may be

required to cover the entire abdomen, one for the cranial area and one for the caudal area.

5. Expose on expiration to give a more 'spread out' view of the abdominal viscera.

The liver, spleen, kidneys, bladder, stomach, small and large intestine, and skeletal structures can usually be identified on a lateral view.

Ventrodorsal view

Positioning is similar to that for the thorax.

1. Position in dorsal recumbency using a trough, or by placing sandbags on either side of the chest (see Figure 18.38).
2. Sandbag or tie the fore- and hindlimbs if necessary.
3. Centre and collimate as required and expose on expiration.

The liver, spleen, kidneys, bladder, stomach, small and large intestine, and skeletal structures can usually be identified on a VD view.

DV views of the abdomen are rarely taken, as the viscera are usually compressed and distorted, but they may be all that is possible if the patient is dyspnoeic, or very large and conscious, and cannot be placed on its back.

Skull

Skull views generally require general anaesthesia, as accurate positioning cannot otherwise be achieved.

Lateral view

1. Position the animal in lateral recumbency, using small foam wedges under the nose and mandible to ensure that the line between the eyes is vertical and that the midline is horizontal and parallel to the table (Figure 18.39). The degree of padding depends on the shape of the patient's skull.
2. It may also be necessary to place a pad under the middle of the neck and under the sternum.
3. Centre and collimate as required, according to the shape of the head and the area of interest.

The cranium, frontal sinuses, nasal cavity, teeth, maxillae, mandibles, temporomandibular joints and tympanic bullae can be identified on a lateral view.

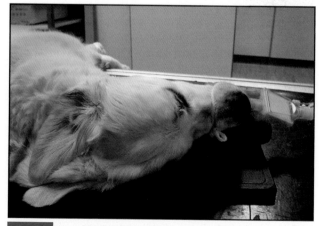

18.39 Positioning for lateral view of the skull.

Dorsoventral view

1. Place the animal in a symmetrical crouching position, with the chin resting on a wooden or foam block, on which is placed the cassette (Figure 18.40).
2. Secure the head with a sandbag draped loosely over the neck if necessary. Ensure that the line between the eyes is horizontal.
3. Centre and collimate as required.
4. If an endotracheal tube is being used, it may require removal before exposure so as not to obscure any structures in the midline.

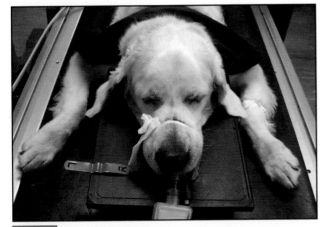

18.40 Positioning for DV view of the skull.

Ventrodorsal view

Symmetrical positioning is more difficult than for the DV view, as facial landmarks are not visible. The DV view is therefore usually preferred, and there is little benefit to a VD.

1. Place the animal in dorsal recumbency in a trough, with the head and neck extended (Figure 18.41).
2. Put foam pads under the neck and nose.
3. Fix the nose down using a tape placed over the chin, or using sticky tape.

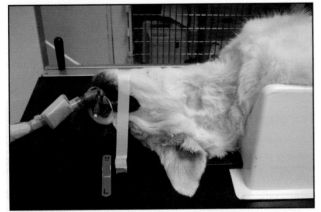

18.41 Positioning for VD view of the skull.

Lateral oblique view for tympanic bullae

1. Place the animal in lateral recumbency with the side to be radiographed down.
2. Using foam pads, rotate the skull about 20 degrees around its long axis, towards the VD position (this will skyline the tympanic bulla nearer the table) (Figure 18.42).

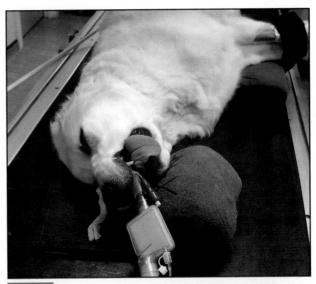

18.42 Positioning for oblique tympanic bullae view.

3. Centre and collimate by palpation of the bulla, which will now lie ventral to the main part of the skull.
4. It is usually necessary to repeat the procedure for the other bulla, either to give a normal for comparison or to check whether it is also affected. Care should be taken to ensure that the positioning is the same for the two sides.

Intraoral DV (occlusal) view for nasal chambers

This view always requires general anaesthesia.

1. Place the animal in sternal recumbency with the chin resting on a wooden or foam block.
2. Insert a small dental non-screen film (cats and small dogs) or flexible plastic cassette (medium and larger dogs) into the mouth above the tongue, placing it corner first so as to get it as far back in the mouth as possible (Figure 18.43).
3. Ensure that the head is level and not laterally tilted by looking for facial landmarks such as the eyes.
4. Centre and collimate over the nasal cavity, bearing in mind the size of the film.

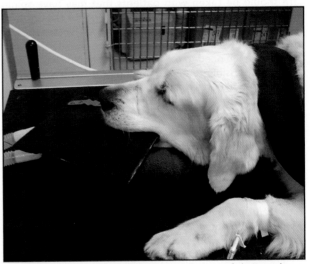

18.43 Positioning for DV intraoral view of the nasal cavity.

Intraoral VD (occlusal) view of the mandible

This view always requires general anaesthesia.

1. Place the animal in dorsal recumbency in a trough.
2. Insert a small dental non-screen film (cats and small dogs) or flexible plastic cassette (medium and larger dogs) into the mouth, placing it corner first so as to get it as far back in the mouth as possible (Figure 18.44). The tongue can be moved so as not to obscure the main area of interest.
3. Ensure that the head is level and not laterally tilted by looking for symmetry of the mandibles.
4. Centre and collimate over the area of interest, bearing in mind the size of the film.

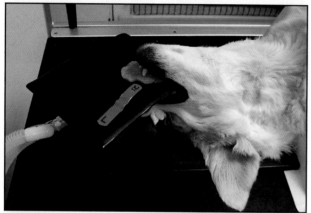

18.44 Positioning for VD intraoral view of the mandible.

Other views

A number of other views of the skull are possible but their detailed description is beyond the scope of this chapter. They include special obliques for temporomandibular joints, obliques for dental arcades and the frontal sinuses, skyline views of the frontal sinuses and cranium and the open-mouth rostrocaudal view for tympanic bullae (see Further Reading).

Vertebral column

Spinal pathology is often undramatic using radiography and therefore requires particularly careful positioning, especially if disc spaces are under scrutiny. General anaesthesia is usually required in order to obtain diagnostic radiographs. Great care should be taken with patients that may have spinal fractures or dislocations in case positioning for radiography causes displacement of the fragments; in such cases the use of a horizontal beam for VD views could be considered as this will remove the need to roll the patient on to its back.

It is not possible to get an accurate picture of the entire spine on one film, since the X-ray beam is diverging and will not pass equally through all disc spaces, and so it is usually necessary to take several radiographs of smaller areas. In medium and large dogs, up to six films may be required for a spinal survey, as follows: cervical C1–C6; cervicothoracic C6–T3; thoracic T3–T11; thoracolumbar T11–L3; lumbar L1–L7; sacral and caudal (coccygeal) L6–Cd4. Once a lesion is suspected, tightly collimated views taken over the area of interest should be made. For disc disease, only the few disc spaces in the centre of the film are fully assessable (Figure 18.45). It is important to note that many spinal diseases produce minimal or no radiographic changes, and that some apparent radiographic lesions, such as lumbosacral spondylosis, are clinically silent. Magnetic resonance imaging (MRI, see below) is a far superior technique for spinal imaging.

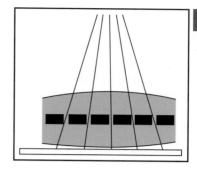

18.45 Radiography of disc spaces.

Lateral view

Judicious use of foam pads is required to prevent the spine sagging or rotating (Figure 18.46) and to ensure that it forms a straight line parallel to the tabletop. Otherwise, the positioning is similar to that for lateral chest and abdomen views (see Figure 18.36). It is necessary to centre and collimate to the area of interest by the palpation of relevant bony landmarks (in obese animals the spine may be some distance below the skin surface).

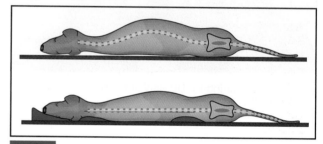

18.46 Use of foam pads for spinal radiography.

Ventrodorsal view

1. Place the animal in symmetrical dorsal recumbency, using a trough or sandbags (similar to positioning for VD chest and abdomen radiographs, see Figure 18.38)
2. Secure the limbs as appropriate.
3. Centre and collimate over the area of interest.
4. For VD views of the caudal cervical spine and cervicothoracic junction, the X-ray beam must be angled 15–20 degrees towards the patient's head in order to pass through the disc spaces, which lie obliquely at this level.

The DV view of the spine is rarely obtained, as the unavoidably large OFD results in magnification and blurring of the image.

Forelimbs

Although many diagnoses may be possible from a single view (usually the mediolateral) it is often necessary to obtain the orthogonal view as well (i.e. the view at right-angles to this), and sometimes flexed views or obliques are also required. For investigation of suspected joint disease, centre over the joint of interest. Some joint diseases, such as osteochondrosis (OCD), are commonly bilateral and so the opposite limb should be radiographed as well. For long bones, the beam should be centred over the middle of the bone but including the joints above and below, with the long bone parallel to the film. If there is doubt about the significance of a lesion or if the normal length of a bone must be known for a fracture repair, then the opposite limb may be used as a useful control. Note that, except for the scapula and shoulder in giant dogs, a grid is not necessary for forelimb radiography.

Mediolateral (ML) scapula

The scapula is a difficult bone to radiograph, as it is very thin. The distal part of the scapula can be seen on shoulder radiographs, but the following special ML and CdCr views may occasionally be required for the proximal scapula.

1. With the animal lying on the side to be radiographed, pull the lower limb caudally and the upper limb cranially, flexing it towards the head and securing it with a tape. It may also be pushed slightly dorsally so that it lies above the level of the spine.
2. Centre and collimate to the dependent scapula by palpation.

Caudocranial (CdCr) scapula

1. Place the animal on its back in a trough, tipping it slightly over to the side that is not under investigation.
2. Draw the limb cranially and secure in maximum extension with a tape.
3. Centre and collimate to the scapula by palpation.

Mediolateral shoulder

1. With the animal lying on the side to be radiographed, draw the lower limb cranially and secure it with a tie or sandbag (Figures 18.47 and 18.48); pull the upper limb so that it is well back out of the way and secured.
2. Extend the head and neck to reduce the amount of soft tissue overlying the shoulder of interest.
3. Centre and collimate to the dependent shoulder joint by palpation.

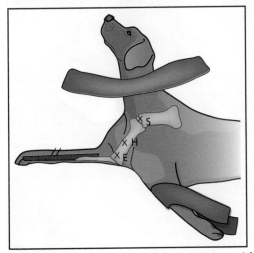

18.47 Positioning for mediolateral forelimb view.

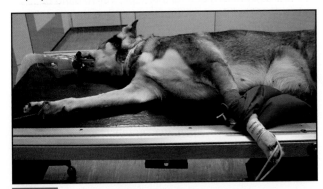

18.48 Centring points (X) for mediolateral forelimb views: S = shoulder, H = humerus; E = elbow.

Caudocranial shoulder

As for caudocranial scapula but centred on the shoulder joint.

Cranioproximal-craniodistal (CrPr-CrDi) shoulder

This special oblique view is used to skyline the bicipital groove of the humerus in cases of suspected shoulder tenosynovitis, and is obtained with the shoulder flexed.

1. Place the patient in sternal recumbency (as for a DV chest) and flex the forelimb to be radiographed at the shoulder and elbow, the opposite side of the body being raised on a sandbag and the head displaced away from the shoulder under investigation.
2. Support the cassette above the forearm but beneath the shoulder joint, pushed back to contact the front of the elbow.
3. Centre and collimate to the humeral head by palpation.

Mediolateral humerus

As for the lateral shoulder (see Figures 18.47 and 18.48) but centred on the mid-humerus. Collimate to include both the elbow and shoulder joints.

Caudocranial humerus

As for the caudocranial scapula but centred on the mid humerus. Collimate to include both the elbow and shoulder.

Craniocaudal humerus

An alternative view. The animal is placed on its back and the limb to be radiographed is pulled caudally, securing with a tape. The humerus should lie parallel to the film. It may not be possible to use a trough for this view.

Mediolateral elbow

Extended view: as for mediolateral shoulder (see Figures 18.47 and 18.48) but centred on the elbow by palpation and collimated to include the distal humerus and proximal radius and ulna.

Flexed view (more useful for assessing degenerative joint disease): as for mediolateral shoulder but with the lower limb flexed at the elbow so that the paw comes up towards the patient's chin. Secure with a tape or sandbag (Figure 18.49). Overflexion should be avoided, as this may also cause rotation of the limb and distortion of the image. For the BVA/KC Elbow Dysplasia Scheme, both views are required (see relevant Procedure Notes published by the BVA). Details of image labelling are given below, under Pelvis and Hips.

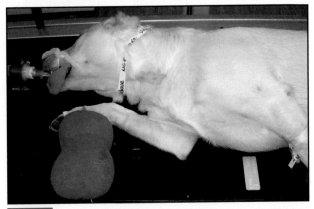

18.49 Positioning for flexed mediolateral elbow view.

Craniocaudal elbow

1. Position the animal in sternal recumbency with the forelimb to be radiographed extended and pulled cranially, and secured with a sandbag and/or tie. The other forelimb may be allowed to remain more flexed.
2. Turn the head and neck to the side which is not being radiographed and restrain by draping a sandbag over the neck. Take care that the elbow to be radiographed does not slide sideways (further sandbags and ties may be required) (Figure 18.50).
3. Centre on the elbow joint by palpation, angling the beam about 10 degrees towards the patient's tail in order to demonstrate the joint space. Collimate to include the distal humerus and proximal radius and ulna.

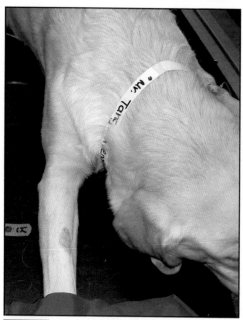

18.50   Positioning for craniocaudal elbow view.

Caudocranial elbow

An alternative view: as for caudocranial shoulder but centred on the elbow joint. However, the large OFD results in some magnification and blurring of the image.

Mediolateral forearm (radius and ulna), carpus and paw

1. With the animal lying on the side to be radiographed, draw the lower limb cranially and the upper limb caudally out of the way (see Figures 18.47 and 18.48).
2. Ensure that a lateral position is achieved, using foam pads or sticky tape.
3. Centre and collimate to the appropriate area.
4. For individual toes, it may be useful to separate them by drawing the affected one forwards and the others backwards with tapes.

Craniocaudal forearm and dorsopalmar (DPa) carpus and paw

As for craniocaudal elbow (see Figure 18.50), but centred and collimated to the appropriate area and using a vertical beam. The limb may be extended using a tie rather than a sandbag, as the latter is radiopaque.

Hindlimbs

Lateral pelvis and hips

The animal is positioned on its side, using foam pads under the spine and sternum to achieve a true lateral position. The beam is centred on the hip joints by palpation of the greater trochanter of the uppermost femur. For medium and large dogs a grid is required, although no grid is required for more distal parts of the limb.

VD pelvis and hips: extended hip position

This position is described in some detail as it is required for official assessment of hip dysplasia in dogs under the BVA/KC Hip Dysplasia Scheme (see also the relevant Procedure Notes published by the BVA). This position requires general anaesthesia or a reasonable degree of sedation, and perfect positioning may be achieved without the need for manual restraint. For medium and large dogs a grid is required.

1. Place the animal on its back in a trough, ensuring that the thorax is perfectly upright and not tipped to either side.
2. Extend the forelimbs cranially and secure them with tapes; a sandbag may also be draped over the sternum, taking care not to impair respiration.
3. Extend the hindlimbs caudally, using tapes looped just above the hocks and tied to hooks on the edge of the table. The femora should be parallel to each other and to the tabletop, and the stifles should be rotated inwards by means of a further tape, Velcro band or bandage tied firmly around them so that they are also parallel (Figure 18.51).
4. Centre on the pubic symphysis at the level of the greater trochanter of the femur, by palpation of these bony landmarks. Generally the whole pelvis is included in the image but note that it is not necessary to include the stifles in the radiograph; this is a common misconception, but in order to centre over the hips and still include the stifles an unacceptably large area would need to be irradiated.

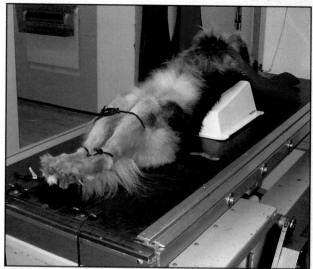

18.51   Positioning for assessment of hip dysplasia: extended ventrodorsal pelvic view.

For submission to the BVA/KC Hip Dysplasia Scoring Scheme, the radiograph must be permanently identified with the patient's Kennel Club number (or other identification if the dog is unregistered), microchip number, the date and a right or left marker *before* processing. Radiographs labelled after processing or, in the case of digital images, labelled by computer at printing, will not be accepted by the scheme. In the case of digital images, therefore, the use of graphite tape or lead letters placed within the primary beam is still necessary. Submission of digital images in DICOM format is now possible and further information about this procedure may be obtained from the BVA Canine Health Schemes office.

The various anatomical areas of the hip joint assessed under the scoring scheme should all be identifiable; if the image is under- or overexposed certain important features may not be seen and the radiograph may be rejected. Lateral tilting of the pelvis results in the hip joint which has moved up and away from the table appearing falsely deeper (better) than it really is and the hip joint which has moved towards the table appearing shallower (poorer); therefore the hip score will not accurately reflect the true hip status. This may also result in rejection of the radiograph, especially if the hips are very good and the scrutineers feel that the score on the tilted radiograph will be artificially high (i.e. poor). If the hips are dysplastic, lateral tilting is less important as the score is unlikely to be significantly affected.

VD pelvis and hips: flexed or frog-legged view

This view allows some assessment of the hips but is not as satisfactory as the extended view for assessment of subluxation or mild degrees of arthrosis. The hindlimbs are flexed and allowed to fall to either side. Sandbags may be used to steady the hindpaws (Figure 18.52).

VD pelvis and hips: dorsal acetabular rim (DAR) view

This is used to provide measurements prior to triple pelvic osteotomy surgery. The exposure needs to be increased by about 5–10 kV from that used for the extended VD projection.

1. Position the dog in sternal recumbency with a trough under its chest.
2. Pull the hindlimbs forwards so that the pelvis is rotated towards a more vertical position and raise the hocks on sandbags.
3. Palpate the pelvis to ensure that it is symmetrical and extend the tail caudally.
4. Centre at the base of the tail.

Mediolateral femur

Two methods are used, both requiring the animal to lie on the side to be radiographed. In the first method the uppermost limb is pulled upwards so that it is roughly vertical, and is secured with tapes or sandbags. It may be difficult to prevent superimposition of part of this limb over the femur under investigation and so an alternative is to pull the lower hindlimb cranially and the upper hindlimb back. In this case the lower femur is radiographed through the soft tissues of the abdomen.

Craniocaudal femur

1. Position the animal in dorsal recumbency in a trough and extend and restrain the limb that is to be radiographed (Figure 18.53).
2. The other hindlimb may be left free.
3. It may be useful to tilt the animal slightly away from the side which is being radiographed to ensure a true craniocaudal view.
4. Centre on the mid-femur by palpation, and collimate to include the hip and stifle.

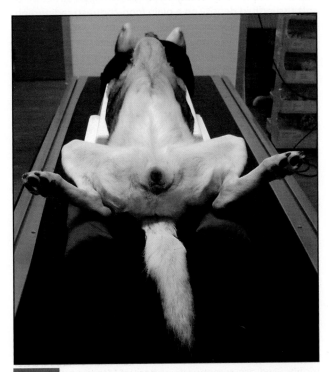

18.52 Positioning for flexed ventrodorsal pelvic view.

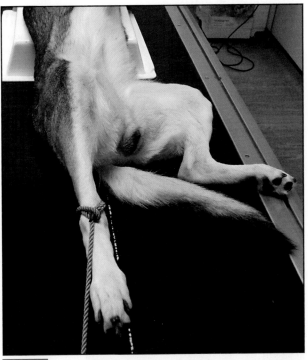

18.53 Positioning for craniocaudal hindlimb views.

Mediolateral stifle

1. Position the animal so it is lying on the side to be radiographed (Figure 18.54).
2. Move the other hindlimb upwards or caudally so that it is not superimposed over the lower stifle.
3. Ensure that a true lateral projection is obtained by placing a small pad under the hock.
4. In obese animals, the mammary tissue or sheath may obscure the stifle joint; this may be prevented by tying a tape around the caudal abdomen to act like a corset.
5. Centre on the stifle by palpation, and collimate to include the distal femur and proximal tibia.

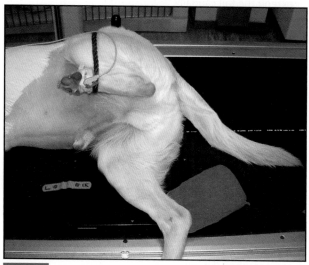

18.54 Positioning for mediolateral stifle view.

Craniocaudal stifle

This is identical to the extended CrCd femur view (see Figure 18.53), but centring and collimating to the stifle by palpation.

Caudocranial stifle

An alternative view (Figure 18.55), with the animal positioned in sternal recumbency and with the affected limb extended caudally. The opposite side of the animal may need to be raised on sandbags to obtain a true CdCr position. This position results in less magnification and sharper definition of the stifle than with the CrCd view as the stifle is closer to the film, but the joint space may be slightly distorted.

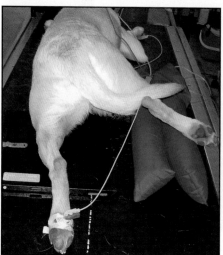

18.55

Positioning for caudocranial stifle view.

Mediolateral tibia, hock and paw

1. The patient lies on the side to be radiographed; the uppermost limb is drawn cranially or caudally to prevent superimposition.
2. Use foam wedges to achieve a true lateral position if necessary.
3. Centre and collimate to the required area by palpation.

Craniocaudal tibia and dorsoplantar hock

As for CrCd stifle, but centred and collimated to the appropriate area (see Figure 18.53). For the hock, the tape is looped around the paw. To reduce the object–film distance for the hock view, it may be necessary to raise the cassette from the table with a wooden block or rectangular foam wedge. The X-ray tube head should be raised by the same amount in order to keep the focal–film distance the same.

Dorsoplantar paw

Two methods are available. The patient may be positioned as above, but with the paw held down to the cassette with strong radiolucent tape. Alternatively, the animal may crouch, with the affected paw pulled slightly outwards and resting on the cassette; this results in a slightly oblique view.

Radiographic contrast studies

Although much information about soft tissues can be gained from good-quality radiographs, certain structures may be unclear either because they are of the same radiographic opacity as surrounding tissue or because they are masked by other structures. In addition, the inner lining (the mucosal surface) of hollow, fluid-filled organs cannot be assessed, because it is of the same radiographic density as the fluid contained within the organ. A good example is the urinary bladder, which appears simply as a homogeneous pear-shaped structure of soft tissue/fluid density on a plain (non-contrast) radiograph.

Contrast studies aim to render these structures and organs more visible and to outline the mucosal surface where appropriate, either by changing the radiopacity of the structure itself or by altering that of the surrounding tissue. Both methods increase the contrast (difference in grey shade) between the structure of interest and the surrounding tissues, allowing assessment of its position, size, shape and internal architecture. If serial films are taken over a period, it may also be possible to gain some idea of the function of the organ, for example the rate of stomach emptying or small intestinal transit time.

Many contrast techniques are possible, but only those of most relevance to veterinary radiography will be discussed.

Types of contrast media

Two broad groups of contrast media exist: positive and negative.

Positive contrast agents

Positive contrast agents contain elements of high atomic number that absorb a large proportion of the X-ray beam and are therefore relatively radiopaque, appearing whiter on radiographs than do normal tissues. They are said to provide *positive contrast* with soft tissues. The agents most commonly used are compounds of barium (atomic number 56) and iodine (atomic number 53).

Barium sulphate preparations

Barium sulphate is a white, chalky material, which may be mixed with water to produce a fine, colloidal suspension. It is available as a liquid, a paste or a powder that is made up to the desired consistency by the addition of water. It is used for gastrointestinal studies and is not suitable for injection into blood vessels. Being inert, it is non-toxic and well tolerated by the patient and it produces excellent contrast with clear delineation of the lumen of the gut. Its inert nature means that it does not become diluted by body fluids and so it maintains its contrast along the length of the gut. Its main disadvantages are that if it is inadvertently aspirated it may cause pneumonia and if it leaks through a perforated area of gut into the thoracic or abdominal cavities it may provoke the formation of granulomas or adhesions by causing a foreign body reaction. Barium should not be given to constipated patients as it will exacerbate the condition, although it is otherwise somewhat soothing to an inflamed gastrointestinal tract.

Water-soluble iodine preparations

The iodine compounds are water-soluble and may therefore be injected into the bloodstream. However, anaphylaxis is a possibility (although it is extremely rare) and so an emergency protocol for such an eventuality should be in place. Most of the iodine compounds are excreted by the kidney and they therefore outline the upper urinary tract (kidneys and ureters). They are also safe to use in many other parts of the body, for example the bladder, gut and sinus tracts. Despite being radiopaque, they appear as clear solutions to the eye (unlike barium). Iodine compounds fall into two categories: ionic media, which dissociate in solution; and non-ionic media, which remain as single molecules in solution. The ionic media have a higher osmotic pressure, several times that of normal body fluids. Intravascular injection of ionic media may cause nausea and retching and so the patient must be heavily sedated or anaesthetized. Ionic media must not be used for myelography as they can cause seizures and even death. The non-ionic media were developed in the 1970s for myelography, as their lower osmotic pressure means that they have much less effect on sensitive nervous tissues. They are also suitable for use in all the studies for which the ionic media can be used, although they are more expensive.

Being water-soluble, the iodine preparations are absorbed by the body and so should be used in the gut in preference to barium if there is a possibility of perforation. However, due to their high osmotic pressure the ionic media absorb fluid during their passage through the gut, with the result that they become progressively diluted and so the pictures they produce have much less contrast than those obtained using barium; there is also a risk of collapse in a dehydrated patient. They are therefore not routinely used for gut studies. Non-ionic iodinated media can be used for gastrointestinal studies and produce an image quality intermediate between that of barium and the ionic iodinated media; non-ionic media should be used if gut perforation is a possibility. Many different water-soluble iodine preparations are available but most ionic media contain diatrizoate, metrizoate or iothalamate as the active ingredients. Non-ionic iodinated media include iohexol and iopamidol.

Negative contrast agents

These are gases, which because of their low density appear relatively radiolucent or black on radiographs, providing negative contrast with soft tissues. Room air is usually used in veterinary radiography although N_2O, CO_2 or O_2 from cylinders may also be used.

Double-contrast studies

Studies on hollow organs may utilize both a positive and a negative agent in a *double-contrast* study. In these cases a small amount of positive contrast agent is used to coat the inner lining of the organ, which is then distended with gas. This provides excellent mucosal detail and prevents the obscuring of small filling defects, such as calculi, by large volumes of positive contrast. Examples of commonly performed studies are double-contrast cystography (bladder) and double-contrast gastrography (stomach).

Patient preparation

Adequate patient preparation is essential before many of the contrast studies, which are usually performed as elective procedures. Prior to a barium study of the stomach or small intestine, the animal must be fasted for at least 24 hours to empty the gut of residual ingesta. If food remains in the gut it will mix with the barium, mimicking pathology. Patients should also be fasted prior to studies on the kidneys, as a full stomach may obscure the renal shadows. However, most patients are anaesthetized for these studies and so will have been fasted anyway.

The presence of faeces in the colon will also obscure much abdominal detail and so an enema is often required prior to the contrast study. This is particularly important before investigations of the urinary tract as faeces may obscure or distort the kidneys, ureters, bladder or urethra. The colon must be completely empty of faeces if a barium enema is to be performed as even a small amount of faecal material will produce filling defects, giving the appearance of severe pathology. The patient should therefore be fasted for 24 hours and the colon must be thoroughly washed out with tepid saline or water.

Plain radiographs must *always* be taken and examined before the contrast study commences. They are assessed for the following factors:

- Any pathology previously overlooked
- Correct exposure factors, to avoid the need to repeat films after the contrast study has begun
- Adequacy of patient preparation
- Assessment of the amount of contrast medium required
- Comparison with subsequent radiographs (to show whether any shadows on the images are due to contrast media or were already present).

Techniques for contrast radiography in dogs and cats
Oesophagus (barium swallow)

Indications

Regurgitation, retching, dysphagia (difficulty in swallowing).

Preparation

No patient preparation required; plain radiographs must be obtained first.

Equipment

- Barium paste is usually preferred as it is sticky and adheres to the oesophageal mucosa for several minutes.
- Barium liquid may be used if paste is not available (5–50 ml, depending on patient size).
- Oral water-soluble iodine preparations should be used if a perforation is suspected.
- Liquid barium mixed with tinned pet food should be used if a megaoesophagus is suspected clinically or on plain radiographs, as paste or liquid alone may fail to fill a dilated oesophagus.

Restraint

Moderate sedation sufficient to allow non-manual restraint is required. Heavy sedation or general anaesthesia is contraindicated because of the possibility of regurgitation and aspiration; in addition both procedures may induce a transient megaoesophagus.

Technique

Barium paste is deposited on the back of the tongue. Barium or iodine liquids should be given slowly by syringe into the buccal pouch, allowing the patient to swallow a small amount at a time to avoid aspiration. Barium/tinned pet food mixture is often eaten voluntarily, as animals with megaoesophagus tend to be hungry; if not, then the patient may be hand-fed.

Radiographs are taken immediately after administration of the contrast medium. Lateral views are usually sufficient but VD views may also occasionally be indicated. In medium and large dogs two separate radiographs may be needed to cover the cervical and thoracic areas of the oesophagus due to the differences in exposure factors required and the length of the area of interest.

Stomach (gastrogram)

Three techniques are used: air alone (pneumogastrogram), barium alone (positive gastrogram), or barium and air (double-contrast gastrogram). The latter gives better mucosal detail. Gastrography is less often performed now due to the increasing use of endoscopy.

Indications

Persistent vomiting, haematemesis, displacement of stomach, assessment of liver size.

Preparation

24 hours of fasting; enema if necessary; plain radiographs.

Equipment

- Barium liquid (20–100 ml, depending on patient size) unless the study is a simple pneumogastrogram. Note: barium paste and barium/tinned pet food mixtures are not suitable, and oral water-soluble iodine preparations should be used if a perforation is suspected.
- Syringe or stomach tube plus three-way tap.

Restraint

Moderate sedation (to allow positioning and non-manual restraint); acepromazine has least effect on gut.

Technique

Pneumogastrogram

This technique may be used to show position and distensibility of the stomach and large gastric masses or foreign bodies, but will not show mucosal detail.

1. Administer the required dose of room air by stomach tube.
2. Take four radiographs: DV, VD, left and right lateral recumbency; each will highlight a different area of the stomach.

Barium gastrogram

This technique will show position of the stomach and the thickness of its wall and may be followed by a small intestinal examination. However, smaller foreign bodies may be 'drowned' by the barium, and mucosal detail will not be shown.

1. Administer the required dose of barium liquid by syringe or stomach tube.
2. Roll the patient to coat the gastric mucosa.
3. Take four radiographs: DV, VD, left and right lateral recumbency; each will highlight a different area of the stomach with barium lying in the lowest part of the stomach and any gas which was present rising to the highest area.
4. Take further radiographs as indicated, e.g. to follow stomach emptying.

Double-contrast gastrogram (DCG)

This technique will give better distension of the stomach than a barium gastrogram, and will show mucosal detail. Small, radiolucent foreign bodies are more likely to be visible as 'filling defects' in the barium or else coated with residual barium after stomach emptying. A DCG is preferred if a definite gastric lesion is suspected, but follow-up radiographs of the small intestine may be hard to interpret because of the presence of the air creating bubbles in the barium.

1. Stomach tube the patient.
2. Give liquid barium, using the syringe and three-way tap, roll the patient (with the stomach tube still in place) and then distend the stomach with room air.
3. Remove the stomach tube and immediately take four views of the stomach as above.

Small intestine (barium series)

Indications

Persistent vomiting, haematemesis, abdominal masses, weight loss, malabsorption, intestinal dilatation (usually unrewarding in cases of chronic diarrhoea).

Preparation, equipment and restraint

As for stomach.

Technique

Liquid barium is administered by syringe or stomach tube. Serial lateral and VD radiographs are taken to follow the passage of barium through the small intestine (usually at intervals of 15–60 minutes, plus a 24-hour radiograph) depending on rate of transit and any pathology seen.

Large intestine

Three techniques are used: air only (pneumocolon), barium only (barium enema), and barium and air (double-contrast enema). A pneumocolon will outline soft tissue masses within the colon and the use of barium alone will demonstrate displacement or compression of the colon, but for most purposes a double-contrast enema is indicated, as it yields maximum information about the colonic mucosa. Large intestinal contrast studies are less often performed now due to the increasing use of endoscopy.

Indications

Tenesmus, melaena, colitis, identification of certain abdominal masses.

Preparation

Fasting for 24 hours; thorough enema, using tepid water or saline until no faecal matter returns; plain radiographs.

Equipment

- Cuffed rectal catheter or Foley catheter.
- For pneumocolon: three-way tap and large syringe.
- For barium and double-contrast enemas: gravity feed can and hose or a proprietary barium enema bag; barium sulphate liquid diluted 1:1 with warm water.

Restraint

Moderate to deep sedation or general anaesthesia is required, to allow positioning with non-manual restraint. With anaesthesia a purse-string suture may be used to hold the rectal catheter in place.

Technique

Pneumocolon

The rectal catheter is positioned and the colon is inflated with room air, using the syringe and three-way tap, until air leaks out around the catheter. Lateral and VD radiographs are taken without removing the catheter.

Barium enema

The rectal catheter is positioned and barium allowed to flow into the colon under gravity, until it just begins to leak out around the catheter (usually 10–20 ml/kg is required). Lateral and VD radiographs are taken without removing the catheter.

Double-contrast enema (DCE)

The barium technique is followed for initial radiographs. Then, excess barium is allowed to drain out and the colon is re-inflated with air. This can be a very messy procedure unless a special barium enema bag is used; when the bag is lowered to the floor the barium drains back down the tube from the colon into the bag. If the bag is then compressed, the air within it will inflate the colon (Figure 18.56).

Kidneys and ureters: intravenous urography (IVU), excretion urography

Contrast radiography of the upper urinary tract involves the intravenous injection of a water-soluble iodine preparation, which is subsequently excreted by, and opacifies, the kidneys and ureters. Two methods are used: rapid injection of a small

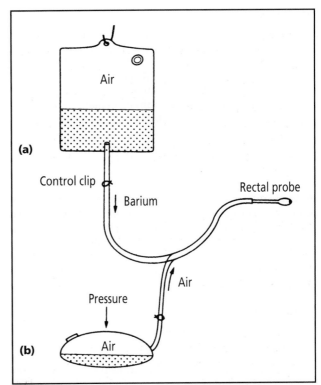

18.56 Barium enema bag. **(a)** In this position barium flows down into the colon due to gravity. **(b)** In this position, barium empties from the colon into the bag. Applying pressure to the bag will distend the colon with air to produce the double-contrast effect.

volume of a very concentrated solution (bolus intravenous urogram) and a slow infusion of a large volume of a weaker solution (infusion intravenous urogram). The bolus IVU produces excellent opacification of the kidneys. The infusion IVU is preferred for investigation of the ureters, as it produces more ureteric distension by inducing a greater degree of osmotic diuresis.

Indications

Identification of kidney size, shape and position, haematuria, urinary incontinence.

Preparation

Fasting for 24 hours; enema; plain radiographs.

Equipment

- Intravenous catheter (perivascular leakage of contrast medium is irritant).
- **For bolus IVU:** syringe and three-way tap; concentrated contrast medium (300–400 mg iodine/ml) at a dose of up to 850 mg iodine/kg bodyweight, i.e. about 50 ml for a 25 kg dog (if there is poor renal function, the dose may be increased by up to 50% more).
- **For infusion IVU:** drip giving set; less concentrated contrast medium (150–200 mg iodine/ml) at a dose rate of up to 1200 mg iodine/kg bodyweight, i.e. about 200 ml for a 25 kg dog. Concentrated solutions may be diluted with saline for this study if necessary.

Restraint

General anaesthesia is required to prevent patient nausea and to allow positioning with non-manual restraint.

Technique

Bolus IVU

1. Warm the contrast medium to body temperature to reduce its viscosity and make it easier to inject.
2. Inject the whole amount as quickly as possible.
3. Take VD and lateral radiographs immediately and at 2, 5, 10 minutes and so on as indicated by the initial images. The VD view is generally more helpful, as the two kidneys are seen without superimposition.

Infusion IVU

If the patient has urinary incontinence and the position of the ureteric endings is being assessed, a pneumocystogram should be performed first to produce a radiolucent background against which the location of the ureters can be seen.

1. Infuse the total dose over 10–15 minutes.
2. Take VD and lateral radiographs once most of the contrast medium has run in.
3. Oblique radiographs are also useful for ureteric endings.

Bladder (cystography)

Direct or retrograde cystography may be performed in three ways: using negative contrast alone (pneumocystogram), positive contrast alone (positive contrast cystogram) or a combination of the two (double-contrast cystogram). Non-ionic iodine media are preferred for the positive and double-contrast studies, as they are less irritant to inflamed bladder mucosa than the ionic media. Pneumocystography is quick and easy but gives poor mucosal detail and will fail to demonstrate small bladder tears, as air leaking out will resemble intestinal gas. Positive contrast cystography is ideal for the detection of bladder ruptures but will mask small lesions and calculi. Double-contrast cystography is usually the method of choice, as it produces excellent mucosal detail and will demonstrate all types of calculi as filling defects in the 'contrast puddle'. A positive contrast cystogram will also be seen following an IVU, if the patient cannot be catheterized for any reason. Excreted contrast should be mixed with urine already present in the bladder by rolling the animal. This type of cystogram is not ideal, as adequate bladder distension cannot be ensured.

Indications

Haematuria, dysuria, urinary incontinence, urinary retention, suspected bladder rupture, identification of the bladder if not visible on the plain radiograph, assessment of prostatic size.

Preparation

Enema, if faeces are present; plain radiographs.

Equipment

- Appropriate urinary catheter
- Syringe and three-way tap
- Dilute water-soluble iodine contrast medium for positive and double-contrast cystogram.

Restraint

Sedation or general anaesthesia is required to allow catheterization and positioning using non-manual restraint.

Technique

The bladder is first catheterized and drained completely of urine, obtaining a sterile urine sample if required.

Pneumocystogram

The drained bladder is inflated slowly with room air, using a syringe and three-way tap. The bladder should be inflated until it is felt to be moderately firm by abdominal palpation (usually requires 30–300 ml air, depending on patient size). It is important to avoid overdistension, especially if the bladder may be fragile or in cats with cystitis in which mucosal sloughing may occur.

Positive contrast cystogram

Procedure as for pneumocystogram but using diluted iodine contrast medium instead of air. However, for detection of bladder rupture, a much smaller quantity is required.

Double-contrast cystogram (DCC)

1. Inject 2–15 ml iodine contrast medium (depending on patient size) at a concentration of approximately 150 mg iodine/ml into the empty bladder via the catheter.
2. Palpate the abdomen or roll the patient to coat the bladder mucosa.
3. Inflate with air until the bladder feels turgid.
4. The bladder wall will be lightly coated with positive contrast, and residual contrast will pool in the centre of the bladder shadow, highlighting calculi and other filling defects.

Lateral radiographs are usually more informative, but VD and oblique views may be taken if required.

Urethra: retrograde urethrography (males); retrograde vagino-urethrography (females)

These studies are less frequently performed in cats than in dogs, but may be carried out using simple cat catheters.

Indications

Haematuria, dysuria, urinary incontinence, urinary retention, prostatic disease, vaginal disease.

Preparation

Enema, if faeces are likely to obscure the urethra on either view; plain radiographs.

Equipment

- Appropriate urinary catheter.
- Syringe.
- Dilute iodine contrast medium (150 mg iodine/ml) (may be mixed with an equal amount of K-Y jelly for studies on male dogs, to increase urethral distension).
- Gentle bowel clamp (for bitches).

Restraint

Sedation (dogs) or general anaesthesia (bitches, cats).

Techniques

Retrograde urethrography (males)

1. Insert the urinary catheter into the penile urethra.

2. Occlude the urethral opening manually, to prevent leakage of contrast.
3. Inject 1 ml/kg bodyweight contrast or contrast/K-Y jelly mixture slowly.
4. Release the urethral occlusion and stand back prior to exposure (or make the injection via an extension tube wearing lead mittens and an apron, and ensuring tight collimation to exclude the hands).

Lateral views are most useful and should be taken with the hindlimbs pulled forwards for the ischial arch and backwards for the penile urethra.

Retrograde vaginourethrography (females)

1. Snip off the tip of a Foley catheter, distal to the bulb.
2. Insert the catheter just inside the vulval lips, inflate the bulb and clamp the vulval lips together with the bowel clamp to hold the catheter in place. In cats a non-cuffed catheter is used.
3. Carefully inject up to 1 ml iodine contrast medium/kg bodyweight (vaginal rupture has been reported).

Lateral views are most informative, and demonstrate filling of the vagina and urethra.

Spine (myelography)

A narrow gap surrounds the spinal cord as it runs along the vertebral column; this is called the **subarachnoid space** and it contains cerebrospinal fluid (CSF). It may be opacified by the injection of positive contrast medium and will then demonstrate the spinal cord, showing areas of cord swelling (e.g. tumours) or cord compression (e.g. prolapsed intervertebral discs) not evident on plain radiographs. This technique, which is called **myelography**, requires the use of non-ionic water-soluble iodine preparations, which have lower osmotic pressures than do the ionic iodine media and which are therefore less irritant to nervous tissue. The two low osmolar contrast media currently used in veterinary myelography are iohexol and iopamidol.

Two approaches may be made to the subarachnoid space. The one most commonly used in veterinary radiology is the cisternal puncture, where the needle is inserted into the cisterna magna – the wide cranial end of the subarachnoid space just behind the skull. Myelography may also be performed by injection in the lumbar area via a lumbar puncture, which is more commonly used in humans. Lumbar myelography involves passing the needle through the cauda equina (the termination of the spinal cord) and injecting into the ventral subarachnoid space. Both techniques involve practice and skill and the patient must be anaesthetized to prevent movement during needle placement or injection.

Myelography has been largely replaced by MRI, when available, as the latter is safer and gives much more information about the different spinal tissues.

Indications

Spinal pain, spinal neurological signs (ataxia, paresis or paralysis), identification of location of prolapsed intervertebral discs prior to surgery.

Preparation

Clip relevant area, i.e. caudal to skull or over lumbar spine.

Equipment

- Spinal needle of suitable length, depending on patient size.
- Contrast medium, warmed to body temperature to reduce viscosity and ease injection (dose rate 0.25–0.45 ml/kg of 200–350 mg iodine/ml solution – dose administered depends on size of patient and expected site of lesion but no more than a maximum of 15 ml).
- Syringe
- Sample bottles for CSF if required for analysis.
- Some means of elevating the head end of the table for cisternal punctures, to aid flow of contrast along the spine.

Restraint

General anaesthesia is essential.

Cisternal puncture

1. Elevate the table to about 10 degrees of tilt, with the animal's head at the raised end.
2. Clip and surgically cleanse the injection site.
3. The veterinary surgeon will flex the head to an angle of 90 degrees to the neck. It is then held by an assistant, e.g. the VN.
4. The veterinary surgeon will insert the needle carefully between the skull and atlas vertebra (Figure 18.57), advancing the needle slowly until CSF drips out of the hub when the needle is in the cisterna magna.
5. Several millilitres of CSF will be collected. The veterinary surgeon will then slowly inject warmed contrast medium. The syringe plunger should be withdrawn very slightly at intervals to check that CSF flows back into the syringe, confirming that the tip of the needle is still in the correct place.
6. The needle is removed by the veterinary surgeon and the head is extended again.
7. Several lateral radiographs are taken, either until contrast medium reaches the lesion or until the whole spine is shown well. VD and oblique views may also be taken, especially if a lesion is found. Improved filling of the subarachnoid space in the lower neck area can be ensured by obtaining DV rather than VD views of this area. When the animal is on its back for the VD view, this area is furthest from the table and contrast medium runs cranially and caudally away from the area of interest; with the dog in sternal recumbency, this area is closest to the table and therefore contrast medium pools here.

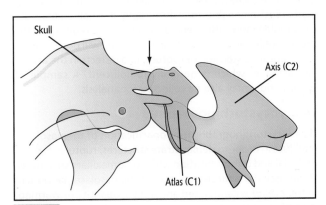

18.57 Myelography: site for cisternal puncture (arrowed).

Lumbar puncture

1. Clip and surgically cleanse the injection site in the caudal lumbar area.
2. Flex the vertebral column by pulling the hindlimbs forwards; the animal may be in lateral or sternal recumbency depending on preference.
3. The veterinary surgeon will insert the needle carefully (usually at L5–6); as it passes through the cauda equina, the animal's hindlimbs and anus will usually twitch slightly. Little or no CSF may appear from this site and if this is the case a small test injection is required to check needle placement.
4. The veterinary surgeon injects contrast medium.
5. The needle is removed and the spine is extended again.
6. Radiographs are taken as above.

> ### WARNING
>
> It is important that the VN keeps the animal's head raised during the recovery period after cisternal or lumbar myelography, since contrast medium entering the brain may precipitate fits.

Other contrast techniques

Some other contrast techniques occasionally performed in small animals are described briefly.

Portal venography

Portal venography is used to diagnose certain types of liver disease (e.g. congenital portosystemic shunts, cirrhosis and acquired shunts) by demonstration of the vascular system within the liver parenchyma. Under general anaesthesia a laparotomy is performed and a splenic or mesenteric vein is catheterized. A small quantity of concentrated iodine contrast medium is injected as a bolus and a single radiograph, either lateral or VD depending on preference, is taken at the end of the injection. The contrast medium enters the liver via the hepatic portal vein and in the normal animal shows branching and tapering portal vessels throughout the liver. In the case of a congenital shunt the liver is bypassed by an anomalous vessel, which connects to the caudal vena cava or azygos vein; with acquired shunts numerous small and tortuous vessels are seen between the hepatic portal vein and the caudal vena cava.

Arthrography

Arthrography is the demonstration of a joint space using negative contrast (air), positive contrast (iodine) or double-contrast techniques injected under sterile conditions. The joints most amenable to arthrography in small animals are the shoulder and stifle. General anaesthesia is required as the procedure is uncomfortable. Arthrography will demonstrate joint capsule distension or rupture, and defects in the articular cartilage, which is normally radiolucent. A sample of synovial fluid may also be collected for analysis.

Dacryocystorhinography

Dacryocystorhinography uses opacification of the nasolacrimal duct in order to demonstrate strictures, rupture, foreign material and communication with cystic maxillary structures. Under general anaesthesia, one of the nasolacrimal puncta in the eyelids is cannulated and a small quantity of warmed, non-ionic iodine contrast medium is instilled. Lateral views are usually most helpful.

Fistulography/sinography

Fistulography and sinography use the opacification of fistulae and sinus tracts by water-soluble iodine contrast media injected via cuffed catheters. They demonstrate the extent and course of these lesions and may outline radiolucent foreign bodies such as pieces of wood. These techniques have largely been superseded by MRI, which gives much more information about the soft tissues.

Angiography

Angiography comprises the opacification of blood vessels by injected iodine contrast medium and a rapid series of radiographic exposures made immediately after injection. It demonstrates the location and size of arteries (arteriography) or veins (venography), depending on the site of deposition of the contrast medium. Although still used in humans for the investigation of cerebral aneurysms and varicose veins, its applications in veterinary patients are extremely limited, with the exception of portal venography (described above). It has been largely superseded in both medical and veterinary diagnosis by ultrasonography, CT and MRI.

Equine radiography

Restraint

The horse should be restrained manually by an experienced handler. There is often a second or even a third person involved supporting the plate holder and positioning the limb. In addition to radiographic PPE, a hard hat, gloves, etc. may be required by handlers, depending on the appropriate risk assessment.

Very few radiographic examinations are carried out on the anaesthetized horse but most horses will require some form of chemical restraint to restrict movement and reduce the risk of the handlers being kicked. The temperament of the patient should be considered when assessing the amount and type of sedation required. It is also necessary to consider whether a limb will need to be lifted for views of the foot, or if flexed views are required. A nose twitch (see Chapter 10) can be useful, although some horses resent these. Lifting another limb can also be useful to restrict movement.

Positioning

Some general points of small animal positioning apply. Additional points to note in equine radiography include:

- Four views are usually acquired to fully visualize the equine limb: lateral, dorsopalmar (dorsoplantar, craniocaudal) and two oblique views
- For fractures, or suspected fractures, several views at slightly different obliquity may be required to visualize the full extent and configuration of the fracture
- On occasion, specific views, e.g. 'skyline' (i.e. DPr-DD or PaP-PaD or even CrPr-CrDi), are essential to demonstrate a lesion
- For distal limb radiography, use a large enough cassette for the region; all four margins of collimation must be visible on the radiograph
- Areas such as the cervical and thoracic vertebrae will require several overlapping images to visualize the whole length of the spine.

Safety considerations

Special consideration should be given to equine radiography using a horizontal beam.

- The investigation may need to be undertaken outside an X-ray room, when it should preferably take place in a walled or fenced area with the primary beam directed at a wall of double brick.
- The extent of the controlled area should be identified using portable warning signs, in order to prevent people not involved from being accidentally irradiated.
- The patient must be adequately restrained by an experienced handler, for its own physical safety as well as that of personnel and equipment.
- Everyone taking part in radiography must wear radiographic protective clothing and dosemeters.
- The extra hazards posed by the use of a horizontal beam must be remembered and care must be taken not to irradiate the legs of anyone assisting in the procedure.
- Collimation must be tight and accurate, especially if a limb or cassette holder is being held by a gloved hand close to the primary beam.

Positioning aids and cassette holders

A selection of 'blocks' of differing heights are useful for positioning limbs, either for weight-bearing or flexed views. Cassette holders are essential to distance the assistant from the source of radiation. These are available commercially, or can be made 'in-house'.

- Foot blocks should include flat blocks for weight-bearing views. These ideally should have slots to support the cassette.
- A 'navicular' block (Figure 18.58) is essentially a block of wood with a groove along the top, in which to rest the toe of the foot. These can also be useful to support the limb for flexed views.
- A cassette tunnel is essential to protect the cassette when the horse is required to stand on the cassette, i.e. the 'skyline' for view of the navicular bone (Figure 18.59). The tunnel should be made of material that is radiolucent, but strong enough to protect the cassette.
- A support for the head for skull radiography is useful (e.g. a small table or a bale of straw)
- A long-handled cassette holder is required for limb radiography (see Figure 18.72).
- A floor-standing cassette holder (Figure 18.60) is required for upper limb, skull, thorax and spine radiography.
- An adjustable stand for holding a large cassette is invaluable for radiography of the head, neck, back and chest.

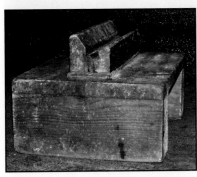

18.58 The navicular block is used to support the foot to obtain the DPr-PaDiO (upright) view (see also Figure 18.70) It can also be used to support the limb for some flexed views.

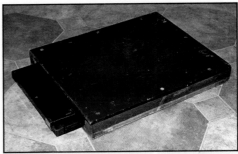

18.59 A cassette tunnel is used to protect the cassette when the horse is required to stand on it. It should be made of a radiolucent material that will not interfere with the quality of the image (see also Figures 18.69 and 18.71).

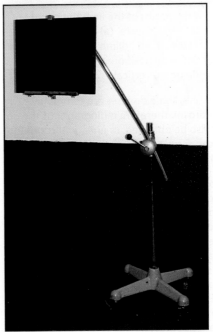

18.60 A method of supporting the cassette, such as this floor-standing cassette holder, is essential for radiation safety when obtaining radiographs of upper limbs, the skull, neck and back.

Positioning for common equine views

These notes describe in brief the technique for the more common views required in equine practice. Radiological atlases should be consulted for identification of normal anatomical structures.

There are some general points to follow when obtaining radiographs of the equine limb:

- Brush the limb to remove dried dirt and mud from the coat
- The horse should be standing square with the metacarpus/metatarsus vertical (Figure 18.61).
- Four projections are usually required for complete evaluation of the region or joint.
- For flexed projections, avoid abduction or adduction of the distal limb; the foot should be vertically under the upper limb (see Figure 18.64).

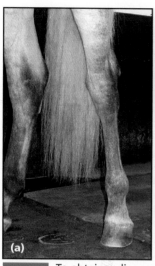
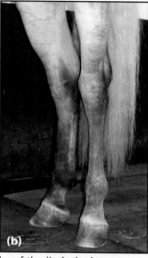

18.61 To obtain radiographs of the limb the horse should be standing square. **(a)** This horse is positioned incorrectly, with the hindlimb placed out to the side (abduction). **(b)** Correctly positioned hindlimbs, with the metatarsus (cannon bone) vertical.

As with small animals, some diseases are commonly bilateral (e.g. osteochondrosis); therefore radiographs of the opposite limb should also be obtained. In unilateral conditions the opposite limb can serve as a 'control' (this is particularly valuable in foals when physeal complexity can be confusing).

- The cassette should be positioned parallel to the tube head, perpendicular to the X-ray beam.
- Labelling should be placed on the cassette so that it lies within the primary beam.
- Left/right markers should be placed on the cassette within the primary beam.
- Lateral markers should be place on the cassette on dorsopalmar (dorsoplantar, craniocaudal) views to identify the lateral aspect of the limb.
- When acquiring radiographs of the hindlimb, because of the 'toe-out' stance of most horses, it is important to align the X-ray beam to the limb and not to the long axis of the spine (Figure 18.62).
- Select the appropriate size cassette and cassette holder.

- Ensure the handler and assistant are wearing suitable PPE and dosemeters.
- A grid is not normally required.

Carpus

For the lateral, oblique and dorsopalmar views of the carpus, collimate to include the distal aspect of the radius and proximal aspect of the metacarpus.

Lateromedial (LM)

1. Position the cassette in the holder on the medial side of the joint.
2. The assistant should stand in front of the horse.
3. Centre on the middle carpal joint, lateral to the limbs.
4. Position the X-ray beam *horizontally*

Dorsolateral-palmaromedial oblique (DL-PaMO)

1. Position the cassette in the holder on the palmaromedial aspect of the joint.
2. The assistant should stand to the lateral side of the horse.
3. Centre on the middle carpal joint; angle 45 degrees from dorsal towards lateral.
4. Position the X-ray beam *horizontally.*

Dorsomedial-palmarolateral oblique (DM-PaLO)

1. Position the cassette in the holder on the palmarolateral aspect of the joint.
2. The assistant should stand to the lateral side of the horse.
3. Centre on the middle carpal joint; angle 45 degrees from dorsal towards medial.
4. Position the X-ray beam *horizontally..*

Dorsopalmar (DPa)

1. Position the cassette in the holder to the palmar aspect of the horse (Figure 18.63).
2. The assistant should stand to the side of the horse.

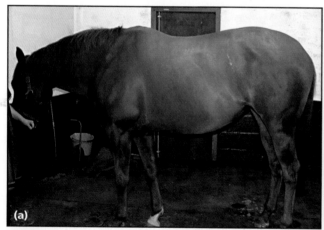
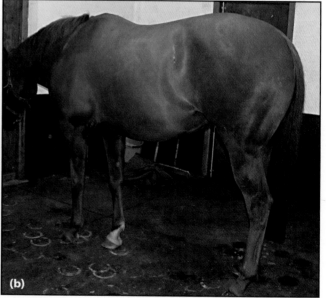

18.62 For a lateral view, the hindlimb should be perpendicular to the X-ray beam. **(a)** With the horse square-on to the beam, it is aligned incorrectly for the hindlimb. **(b)** Aligned correctly to the hindlimb. The beam is now perpendicular to the limb.

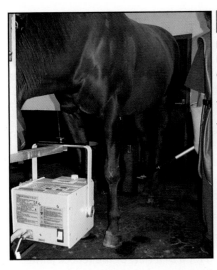

18.63

Positioning for a DPa view of the carpus. The X-ray beam is centred on the middle carpal joint. The assistant stands to the side of the horse.

3. Centre on the middle carpal joint; align dorsopalmar to the limb.
4. Position the X-ray beam *horizontally*.

Dorsoproximal-dorsodistal oblique views (DPr-DDiO)

These views are not standard for every examination of the carpus, but are commonly used to highlight the dorsal aspect of the distal and proximal rows of carpal bones, and the cranial margin of the distal radius.

1. Flex the limb and ease it slightly forward of the other limb. If possible rest the carpus on a suitable support with the metacarpus horizontal, restraining the limb at the toe (Figure 18.64).
2. Place the cassette horizontally under the carpus on the support.
3. The assistant should wear gloves and a thyroid collar.
4. Centre in the midline of the carpus in the dorsopalmar plane.
5. Collimate carefully to avoid the assistant restraining the foot.
6. For the distal row, angle the beam 35 degrees downward from horizontal. For the middle row, angle the beam 55 degrees downward from horizontal. For the distal radius, angle the beam 85 degrees downward from horizontal.

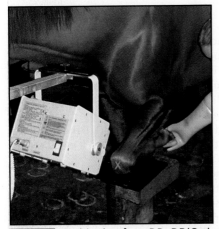

18.64 Positioning for a DPr-DDiO view of the carpus. Centre in the middle of the joint (**X**). The foot is placed vertically under the upper limb and restrained at the toe. The assistant stands to the side.

Lateromedial (flexed)

1. A flexed lateral view may be obtained instead of, or as well as, a weight-bearing lateral.
2. Flex the joint, supporting the foot vertically under the elbow.
3. Place the cassette in a holder on the medial side of the joint.
4. The assistant should stand in front of the horse.
5. Centre on the middle carpal joint, at right angles to the limb.
6. Position the X-ray beam *horizontally*.

Metacarpus (metatarsus)

A horizontal X-ray beam is used for the lateromedial, oblique and dorsopalmar views.

The centre of the X-ray beam and collimation varies according to the region of interest.

1. Place a lateral marker on dorsopalmar views.
2. The assistant should stand in front of the limb for the lateral view, and to the lateral side of the horse for the oblique and dorsopalmar views.

Third metacarpus (metatarsus)

1. Centre halfway between the distal carpus (tarsus) and fetlock.
2. Collimate so that the proximal and distal margins of the primary beam are visible on the radiograph.

Second and fourth metacarpal (metatarsal) bones ('splint' bones)

1. Centre just above halfway between the distal carpus (tarsus) and fetlock (Figure 18.65).
2. Collimate proximally to include the carpometacarpal (tarsometatarsal) joint and distally to include the distal margin of the splint bones.
3. For the second metacarpal (metatarsal) bone, angle 45 degrees from dorsal towards medial. For the fourth metacarpal (metatarsal) bone, angle 45 degrees from dorsal towards lateral.

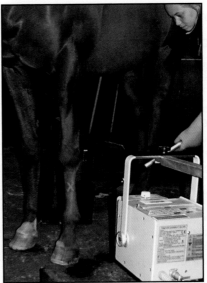

18.65 Positioning for a DL-PaMO of the metacarpus to highlight the lateral splint bone (fourth metacarpus). The X-ray beam is centred just above the middle of the metacarpus.

Proximal half of the metacarpus (metatarsus)

1. Centre between the distal carpus (tarsus) and the mid third of the metacarpus (metatarsus).
2. Collimate to include the distal row of carpal (tarsal) bones and distally to half way down the third metacarpus (metatarsus).

Metacarpophalangeal/metatarso-phalangeal joint (fetlock)

For views of the metacarpophalangeal (metatarsophalangeal) joint, collimate to include the distal aspect of the third metacarpus (metatarsus) and proximal aspect of the middle phalanx (short pastern bone/P2).

The technique for the forelimb is described; for the hindlimb it is plantar instead of palmar.

Lateromedial (LM)

1. Position the cassette in holder on medial side of joint.
2. The assistant should stand in front of the limb.
3. Centre on the joint, perpendicular to it.
4. Position the X-ray beam horizontally.

Dorsolateral-palmaromedial oblique (DL-PaMO)

1. Position the cassette in the holder on the palmaromedial aspect of the joint.
2. The assistant should stand to the lateral side of the horse.
3. Centre on the joint; angle 45 degrees from dorsal towards lateral.
4. Position the X-ray beam *horizontally*.

Dorsomedial-palmarolateral oblique (DM-PaLO)

1. Position the cassette in the holder on the palmarolateral aspect of the joint.
2. The assistant should stand to lateral side of the horse.
3. Centre on the joint; angle 45 degrees from dorsal towards medial.
4. Position the X-ray beam *horizontally*.

Dorsopalmar (DPa)

1. Place the lateral marker on the cassette.
2. Position the cassette in the holder to the palmar aspect of the joint.
3. Angle the cassette so it is perpendicular to the X-ray beam (Figure 18.66).
4. The assistant should stand to lateral side of the horse.
5. Centre on the joint; align dorsopalmar to the joint.
6. Angle the X-ray beam 10–15 degrees downwards.

Lateromedial (flexed)

A flexed lateral view may be obtained instead of, or as well as, a weight-bearing lateral view. The flexed view highlights a greater extent of the sagittal ridge of the third metacarpus and the articular margins of the proximal sesamoid bones.

1. Flex the joint and rest the toe of the foot on a navicular block.
2. Ensure the metacarpus is vertical in a lateral/medial plane.

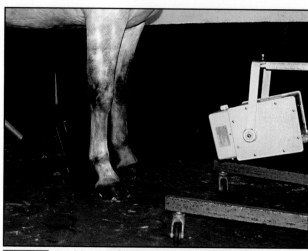

18.66 Positioning for a DPa view of the fetlock joint. The X-ray beam is angled 15 degrees down from the horizontal. The cassette is aligned parallel to the front of the X-ray machine, perpendicular to the primary beam.

3. Place the cassette in a holder on the medial side of the joint.
4. The assistant should stand in front of the horse.
5. Centre on the middle of the joint, at right angles to the limb.
6. Position the X-ray beam *horizontally*.

Other views

There are a number of special oblique and flexed views of the metacarpophalangeal (metatarsophalangeal) joint that are beyond the scope of this chapter (see Further reading).

Pastern

The four standard views are a lateromedial, two 45 degree obliques and a dorsopalmar (dorsoplantar).

1. Centre halfway between the fetlock joint and the coronary band.
2. Collimate to include the proximal aspect of the proximal phalanx and the distal interphalangeal joint.
3. For the dorsopalmar (-plantar) view angle 5–10 degrees downwards.

Foot

Before obtaining radiographs of the foot, the shoe should be removed and the hoof wall and sole cleaned of mud and dirt. In some cases (e.g. in acute laminitis), shoe removal may be contraindicated, and in other horses demonstrating poor shoeing dorsopalmar foot balance is best (and most dramatically) achieved by radiography with the shoes on. The sole and frog should be trimmed, particularly if the frog clefts are deep. Packing the sole (Figure 18.67) will eliminate air shadows, especially for navicular views.

The frog clefts must be packed evenly; loose packing may mask or mimic fractures, whereas radiopaque artefacts may be created by excessive packing. Packing the sole and sulci of the frog with a material such as Play-doh decreases gas artefacts from the trapped air. This packing is especially important for the navicular and P3 examinations. Although acceptable views can be obtained without the use of a grid, they should normally be used for lateral and dorsopalmar views.

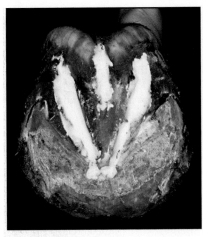

18.67 The foot should be thoroughly cleaned before radiography, and the frog trimmed if necessary. The frog clefts and central sulcus are packed to eliminate air shadows.

A minimum of four views are required for complete evaluation of the foot: lateromedial; dorsoproximal-palmarodistal oblique for the distal phalanx; dorsoproximal-palmarodistal oblique for the navicular bone; and a palmaroproximal-palmarodistal oblique for the navicular bone.

In the case of laminitis or suspected fractures it may be preferable to leave the shoe on for initial survey radiographs. In cases of laminitis lateral views may be sufficient. It is useful to place a radiopaque marker on the dorsal hoof wall, with the proximal edge of the marker placed on the coronary band. A radiopaque marker should also be placed on the point of the frog.

The technique for the forefoot is described below. For the hindfoot it may be easier to obtain some views in a plantarodorsal direction.

Lateromedial (LM)

1. Place the foot on a block so the horse is standing square and a horizontal X-ray beam can be centred below the coronary band.
2. Place the cassette to the medial side of the foot. The bottom of the cassette must be lower than the solar surface of the foot so that it appears on the radiograph.
3. Centre 1 cm below the coronary band, halfway between the heel and the toe of the foot (Figure 18.68).
4. With a horizontal X-ray beam, align parallel with an imaginary line drawn across the bulbs of the heel.
5. Collimate to include the proximal interphalangeal joint, the solar surface of the foot, the toe and the heel.

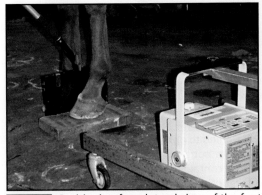

18.68 Positioning for a lateral view of the foot. The foot is placed on a block so that the X-ray beam can be centred below the coronary band (**X**). The bottom of the cassette should be below the level of the sole of the foot.

Dorsoproximal-palmarodistal oblique (DPr-PaDiO) – 'high-coronary' technique

This is the recommended technique to obtain the DPr-PaDiO views for radiation safety reasons, as there is no manual restraint of the limb or cassette. It can also be easier to acquire in difficult horses. However, because the X-ray beam is not perpendicular to the image plane, there is some distortion of the image. It is sometimes referred to as the 'high coronary' view. Two radiographs are taken, one exposed for the distal phalanx, the second exposed and collimated for the navicular bone. The distal phalanx requires less exposure than the navicular bone. To avoid grid cut-off, this technique is best used without a grid.

1. Place the cassette in a protective tunnel on the floor.
2. Place the foot of the horse on the tunnel.
3. Angle the X-ray beam 65 degrees downwards (Figure 18.69).
4. Align the X-ray beam in the dorsopalmar plane.
5. For the distal phalanx, centre on the coronary band and collimate for the whole of the foot. For the navicular bone, centre 1–2 cm above the coronary band and collimate to halfway up the pastern, halfway down the hoof wall, and within the lateral and medial margins of the foot.

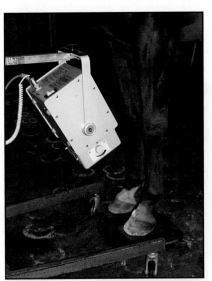

18.69 Positioning for the DPr-PaDiO view of the distal phalanx and navicular bone using the 'high coronary' technique. This technique is recommended for radiation safety reasons as it does not require manual restraint of the limb or cassette (compare with Figure 18.70).

Dorsoproximal-palmarodistal oblique (DPr-PaDiO) – 'upright' technique

The advantage of this technique is that the X-ray beam is perpendicular to the cassette, resulting in no distortion of the image.

> **WARNING**
>
> This technique is not recommended for radiation safety reasons, as the limb is restrained manually. If this technique is used, the assistant should wear protective gloves and a thyroid collar.

Distal phalanx

1. Place the foot in an upright position with the toe resting on a block with the sole vertical.
2. Avoid the fetlock 'knuckling' forward too far.
3. Place the cassette in a holder against the solar surface of the foot with the lower edge below the toe.
4. Centre on the coronary band.
5. With a horizontal X-ray beam align dorsopalmar to the foot.
6. Collimate to include the whole of the foot.

A grid is not required.

Navicular bone

This requires a higher exposure than the distal phalanx for adequate visualization of the navicular bone. A grid is preferable.

1. Position the foot in an upright position with the toe resting on a navicular block.
2. The dorsal wall of the hoof should be just forward (5 degrees) of vertical (Figure 18.70).
3. Place the cassette in a holder against the solar surface of the foot in an upright position.
4. Centre 1–2 cm above the coronary band.
5. With a horizontal X-ray beam align dorsopalmar to the foot.
6. Collimate to halfway up the pastern, halfway down the hoof wall, and within the lateral and medial margins of the foot.

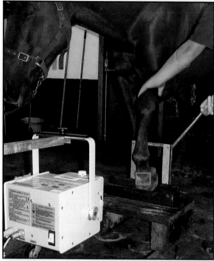

18.70 Positioning for the DPr-PaDiO view of the distal phalanx and navicular bone using the 'upright' technique. Collimation for the navicular bone is shown.

Palmaroproximal-palmarodistal oblique (PaPr-PaDiO)

Two techniques have been described to obtain this view of the navicular bone:

1. Place the cassette in a protective tunnel on the floor.
2. The foot to be imaged is placed on the tunnel caudal to the opposite forelimb (Figure 18.71a). The heels of the foot should be on the ground but the weight of the horse forward on the other limb.

3. Angle the X-ray beam 45 degrees downwards from horizontal.
4. Position the X-ray machine ventral to the abdomen of the horse.
5. Centre between the bulbs of the heel at the base of the pastern.
6. Collimate to include the palmar processes of the distal phalanx and the bulbs of the heel.

Alternatively:

1. Place the cassette in a protective tunnel on a wedge-shaped block with a slope of approximately 10 degrees on the floor.
2. Stand the horse square on the tunnel so that the toe is raised (Figure 18.71b).
3. The opposite limb can be raised if necessary to restrict movement.
4. Angle the X-ray beam 30 degrees downwards from horizontal.
5. Position the X-ray machine ventral to the abdomen of the horse.
6. Centre between the bulbs of the heel at the base of the pastern.
7. Collimate to include the palmar processes of the distal phalanx and to the bulbs of the heel.

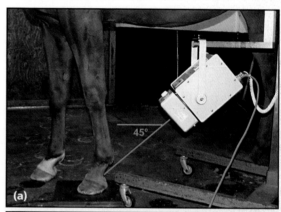

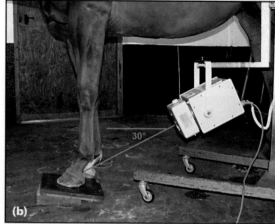

18.71 Positioning to obtain the PaPr-PaDiO view of the navicular bone. **(a)** The foot is placed on a protective tunnel containing the cassette, caudal to the contralateral limb. The X-ray beam is angled 45 degrees down from horizontal. **(b)** Alternatively, the horse is placed on the tunnel standing square. A wedge under the tunnel raises the toe of the foot and the X-ray beam is angled down 30 degrees from horizontal.

Other views

There are a number of additional oblique views of the foot that are beyond the scope of this chapter (see Further reading).

Tarsus (hock)

For views of the tarsus, collimate to include the point of the hock and distal tibia proximally, and the proximal aspect of the metatarsus distally. It is important to align the X-ray beam to the limb, not the long axis of the spine.

Lateromedial (LM)

1. Position the cassette in a holder on the medial side of the joint.
2. The assistant should stand at the side of the horse in front of the limb (Figure 18.72).
3. Centre on the intertarsal joints, lateral to the limb.
4. Use a horizontal X-ray beam, or angle 5–10 degrees downwards, and align perpendicular to the tarsus.

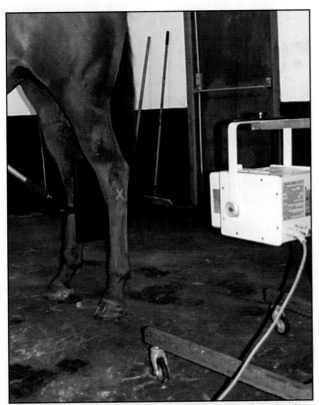

18.72 Positioning for a lateromedial view of the hock. The beam is aligned lateral to the limb, centred on the intertarsal joints (X). The assistant stands on the same side of the horse, in front of the limb to be imaged.

Dorsolateral-plantaromedial oblique (DL-PlMO)

1. Position the cassette in a holder on the plantaromedial aspect of the joint.
2. The assistant should stand to the lateral side of the horse.
3. Centre on the intertarsal joints; angle 45 degrees from dorsal towards lateral.
4. Position the X-ray beam *horizontally.*

Dorsomedial-plantarolateral oblique (DM-PlLO)

1. Position the cassette in a holder on the plantarolateral aspect of the joint.
2. The assistant should stand to the lateral side of the horse.
3. Centre on the intertarsal joints; angle 45 degrees from dorsal towards medial.
4. The X-ray machine will be on the other side of the horse, and the X-ray beam is directed under the abdomen.
5. Position the X-ray beam *horizontally.*

This oblique view can be acquired as a plantarolateral-dorsomedial oblique.

Dorsoplantar (DPl)

1. Position the cassette in a holder to the plantar aspect of the tarsus.
2. The assistant should stand to the lateral side of the horse.
3. Centre on the intertarsal joints; align dorsoplantar to the limb.
4. Position the X-ray beam *horizontally.*

Other views

There are additional views for the malleoli of the tibia and flexed views (e.g. skyline of sustentaculum tali) that are beyond the scope of this chapter (see Further reading).

Stifle

Radiography of the stifle in the conscious horse should be carried out with caution. In almost all situations, sedation is a prerequisite but not such heavy sedation as to cause movement artefact. Horses often resent a cassette being placed in the groin and may cause serious injury to personnel and damage to equipment. The horse should be familiarized to the feel of the cassette before attempting the procedure. Cassette holders should be used if possible, but are often too bulky for placement inside the limb; therefore large cassettes (35 x 43 cm) may be hand-held. Because of the difficulty in alignment of the primary beam with the cassette in the conscious horse, it is advisable not to use a grid. Two views of the stifle are commonly acquired.

> **WARNING**
>
> The X-ray beam must be well collimated with gloved hands well out of the primary beam. The assistant should also wear a thyroid collar.

Lateromedial (LM)

1. The limb should be placed caudal to the contralateral limb, fully weight-bearing.
2. Position the cassette on the medial aspect of the stifle, as high in the groin as possible.
3. Centre on the femorotibial joint, 10 cm caudal to the cranial skin margin (Figure 18.73).
4. Horizontal X-ray beam, perpendicular to the limb.
5. Collimate to include the proximal margin of the patella, and the proximal aspect of the tibia.

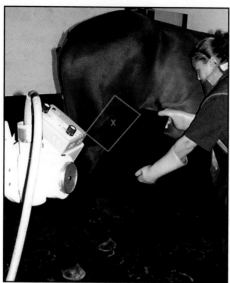

18.73 Positioning for a lateromedial view of the stifle. The beam is centred on the femorotibial joint (**X**) and the area of the primary beam is outlined. The assistant is wearing gloves and a thyroid collar. Careful collimation is essential for radiation safety.

Caudocranial (CdCr)

1. The limb should be placed caudal to the contralateral limb, fully weight-bearing.
2. Ensure the heels of the foot are on the ground.
3. Position the cassette against the cranial aspect of the joint, taking care not to touch the sheath of male horses.
4. Centre the X-ray beam in the midline on the caudal aspect of the limb.
5. The beam should exit on the cranial aspect at the level of the tibial tuberosity.
6. Angle the beam 15 degrees downwards from the horizontal (Figure 18.74).
7. Collimate proximally to include the distal aspect of the femur and distally to include the proximal tibia.
8. Collimate carefully lateral and medial to just inside the skin.

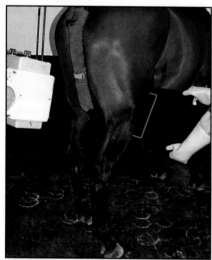

18.74 Positioning for a caudocranial view of the stifle. The beam is centred on the femorotibial joint (**X**). The lateral margin of the primary beam is outlined. The assistant is wearing gloves and a thyroid collar. Careful collimation is essential for radiation safety.

Non-routine views of the stifle include a flexed lateromedial and a cranioproximal–craniodistal oblique (flexed) view of the patella. Oblique views may also be taken and can be very useful for imaging osteochondral lesions of the trochlear ridges.

The head

Radiography of the head in the conscious horse is difficult because it is very mobile and high off the ground. Sedation is essential to lower the head and reduce movement. Providing a solid support for the head, e.g. a small table or trolley or a proprietary head stand, will avoid the need for manual support. *The handler is potentially close to the source of radiation and should wear gloves and a thyroid collar.* To avoid the head collar and its buckles being superimposed over an area of interest, a lightweight rope halter may be used. Lateral and oblique views can be obtained in the conscious horse. It is very difficult to obtain good alignment for DV views (but with care and practice this can be done); anaesthesia should be considered. In cases of nasal discharge or facial swelling, the cassette should be placed on the affected side of the head. In the anaesthetized horse, the head will need to be supported to position it in lateral or VD alignment.

Lateral sinus

1. Support the head in an upright, neutral position.
2. Place a large cassette in a holder next to the side of the head, parallel with the midline of the head.
3. Centre between the orbit and the distal aspect of the facial crest, just dorsal to the facial crest.
4. With a horizontal beam, align at right angles to the midline of the head and the cassette (Figure 18.75).
5. Collimate to include the frontal sinus that lies proximal and dorsal to the orbit, and distally to between the facial crest and the nostril.

A grid is not necessary for the sinus.

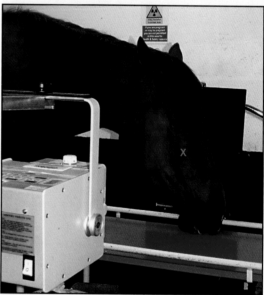

18.75 Positioning for a lateral view of the sinus. The horse has been adequately sedated with the head resting on a support. The cassette is in a floor-standing cassette holder. The beam is centred dorsal to the facial crest (**X**). The head collar has been removed to avoid superimposition of buckles.

Lateral teeth

1. Support the head in an upright, neutral position.
2. Place a large cassette in a holder next to the side of the head, parallel with the midline of the head.
3. Centre 2 cm ventral to the distal margin of the facial crest.
4. With a horizontal beam, align at right angles to the midline of the head and the cassette
5. Collimate to the orbit proximally and to the nostrils distally.

A grid is useful.

Oblique view of teeth to visualize tooth roots

1. Support the head in an upright, neutral position.
2. Place the cassette in a holder adjacent to the tooth arcade of interest, perpendicular to the X-ray beam.
3. For maxillary teeth: angle the beam 30 degrees downwards from the horizontal, align 60 degrees from dorsal towards lateral, and centre at the distal margin of the facial crest on the side of interest. For mandibular teeth: angle the beam 30 degrees upwards from horizontal, align 60 degrees from ventral towards lateral, and centre on the region of interest.
4. Careful collimation is essential for safety because of the obliquity of the X-ray beam.

Other regions of the head can be obtained, the beam being centred on the point of interest and collimated appropriately (see Further reading).

There are also a variety of specialized oblique views, e.g. for the temporomandibular joint and petrous temporal bone.

Spine, thorax and pelvis

Radiography of the equine spine, thorax, upper forelimb and pelvis can be carried out. It may be possible to radiograph some of these regions in the foal with portable equipment but in the adult horse high-output equipment is required. In the adult horse a series of overlapping views of the spine, thorax and pelvis is required to image each region fully. In the foal, one or two views may be sufficient .

Radiographs of the cervical, thoracolumbar and sacral spine are taken in the standing horse in the lateral plane. The cranial cervical area is relatively easy to image but care should be maintained to avoid rotation of the neck, as this can cause confusion in interpretation of cervical vertebral stenosis. Oblique views are taken of the facet joints of the thoracic spine, and have been described for the cervical spine. A technique for obtaining standing VD views of the pelvis has been described, but these are best acquired in dorsal recumbency. VD views of the pelvis may be obtained in the sedated recumbent foal. Left and right lateral views of the thorax should be taken to compensate for magnification; detail of the lung next to the cassette is sharper. The location of a lesion can be identified using the sharpness and magnification factors. VD views of the thorax may be possible in foals; otherwise radiography of the equine thorax is limited to lateral views. Radiography of the abdomen can be useful in foals, usually in the case of acute abdominal discomfort. Equine radiographic texts should be consulted for a more detailed description of these regions (see Further reading).

Contrast radiography in the horse

Although the size of equine patients limits some of the radiographic contrast studies undertaken, the contrast media described above can be used to some extent in horses. As with small animal contrast radiography, plain radiographs should be obtained before the contrast medium is introduced. It should be noted, however, that ultrasonography has replaced most of the gastrointestinal and urinary indications for radiography.

Barium swallow

Indications are a history of dysphagia, oesophageal obstruction or recurrent oesophageal disease. Barium paste is used to evaluate the oesophageal mucosa. Barium sulphate suspension is suitable where mega-oesophagus or diverticuli are suspected. In the conscious horse, barium paste is less likely to be aspirated than barium suspension. Barium-coated food such as horse nuts may also be used to identify some strictures. Contrast medium is introduced into the mouth using a 50 ml catheter tip syringe, or into the cranial oesophagus by stomach tube, and the horse encouraged to swallow. Lateral views of the pharynx and cervical oesophagus can be obtained with portable equipment but higher output equipment is required for thoracic and abdominal regions. Note that sedation can significantly delay passage of contrast material down the oesophagus and artefactual mega-oesophagus can be created by sedation with nasogastric intubation.

Gastrointestinal tract

Positive, negative or double-contrast studies can be performed in the standing horse. They are most commonly carried out in the foal. Starvation prior to a contrast study in the foal should be limited in order to maintain fluid and electrolyte balance. A neonate foal should have fluids withdrawn for no more than 2 hours. For a foal on a solid diet, solids may be withdrawn for up to 8 hours, but fluids for 4 hours at most. Contrast medium is administered by nasogastric tube. A double-contrast technique (**air and barium**) is best for evaluation of the stomach. The cassette should be on the left side of the horse. Although standing views are preferable for the abdomen, left and right recumbent views in the foal can be taken. VD views can also be obtained in the foal.

Cystography

Positive or double-contrast studies can be useful in foals and give information in cases of rupture of the bladder, cystitis and patent urachus. The contrast medium is introduced via a flexible catheter positioned in the urinary bladder.

Arthrography and bursography

Indications are possible rupture or penetration, or to outline cartilaginous or osseous 'joint mice'. The most common use may be navicular bursography in foot penetration injuries, and the next most common use is probably for tendon sheaths. Contraindications to this technique would be possible infection of the joint or adjacent tissue, or inflammation.

Under sterile conditions, a volume of synovial fluid is withdrawn before injection of the contrast agent, with the horse sedated. Flexion and extension of the joint helps to distribute the contrast medium evenly.

Myelography

This is used in the horse to identify the site, or sites, of cervical spinal cord compression. It is carried out in the anaesthetized horse. With the head raised, cerebrospinal fluid is withdrawn under sterile conditions, then 50 ml of a non-ionic water-soluble contrast agent is injected slowly over 5 minutes. Five minutes after injection the head is lowered and lateral views are obtained with the neck in a normal position. Some lesions are dynamic in nature. If a lesion is not identified with the neck in the normal position, radiographs with the neck flexed and extended are obtained. VD views can also be taken to identify lateral compression, although these are difficult to align correctly.

Fistulography

This technique is used to outline sinus tracts or to identify foreign bodies. Depending on the size and position of the sinus, the contrast medium may be introduced via a Foley catheter or a flexible catheter. Contrast medium often leaks from the sinus; therefore the skin should be cleaned before radiography is carried out. False negative results are a possibility, as the sinus tract often does not fill completely.

Other contrast studies in the horse have been used: angiography, venography, intravenous pyelography, dacryocystorhinography.

Radiography of exotic species

Most of the exotic species seen in general practice are smaller than the more commonly seen cats and dogs. The smaller size of the species means lower voltages (kV) are generally used, particularly in small mammals and birds. In chelonians, however, the kV may need to be disproportionately *greater* per kilogram of bodyweight, due to the density of the bony shell. Grids are rarely, if ever, used in commonly seen exotic species as few patients are >10 cm in depth. Due to the smaller size of these patients, non-screen films may be more helpful in demonstrating the finer details of their anatomy. These types of film require higher amperage (mAs) in general. Alternatively, rare-earth intensifying screens and so-called 'detail' films (high-definition fine-grain films) are used.

For most small exotic pets, particularly birds, mammals, snakes and lizards, a radiography unit capable of a range of 40–70 kV with a rapid exposure time of 0.008–0.016 seconds is helpful. The rapid exposure time is important, as many small mammals in particular have rapid respiration rates and therefore longer exposures can lead to blurring of the image produced.

It may also be useful to have a radiography unit that has the facility to alter the focal–film distance, as reducing the distance can allow some magnification of the image produced, which may be of help when imaging very small patients.

Smaller radiographic units, such as human dental machines, are beneficial. They generally operate on a fixed voltage and amperage, the only variable being the exposure time, which may be varied from 0.1 to 3 seconds on modern digital machines. This will allow the fine detail imaging of distal limbs and the head, and, if combined with non-screen dental film,

can provide superior imaging to standard veterinary radiography. Because of longer exposure times patients generally have to be restrained chemically to avoid motion blurring of the image.

Positioning and restraint
Small mammals

The usual two views (a lateral and a VD or DV view; Figure 18.76 a,b) for small mammals are advisable in order to build up a three-dimensional picture. In addition, further specialist views may be useful. For example, in rabbits and chinchillas particularly, where dental disease is a common problem, oblique lateral views (Figure 18.76c) with contrast medium injected into the lacrimal ducts may help to highlight dental and nasolacrimal disease (see Chapter 26).

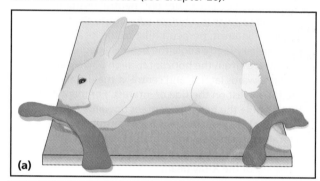

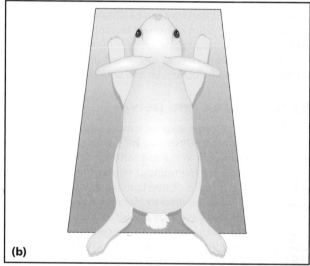

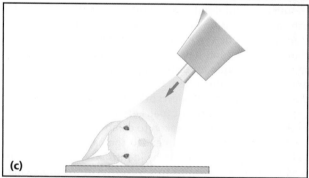

18.76 Positioning a rabbit for radiography. **(a)** Right lateral view: the limbs are drawn away from the body. **(b)** Standard dorsoventral whole body view. **(c)** Oblique lateral dental arcade and head view. (Reproduced from the *BSAVA Manual of Rabbit Medicine and Surgery, 2nd edition*)

Rabbits also commonly suffer from otitis media, and DV views specifically focusing on the auditary bullae are necessary to confirm the presence of disease. Skyline views of the frontal sinuses and craniocaudal views of the skull may also be used where disease is suspected in sinuses or in the temporomandibular joints.

Dental disease is also common in ferrets, and bisecting angle radiographs as used in cat and dog dental radiography are helpful to obtain an accurate image of the roots of affected teeth.

Birds

As with small mammals, two views are essential and these usually comprise a lateral (generally a right lateral) and a VD view (Figure 18.77). For the lateral view the wings are pulled dorsally away from the body to prevent superimposition. It is advisable to anaesthetize the patient to prevent struggling and minimize stress.

These two views are suitable for imaging the body cavity, but they actually result in exactly the same view for the wings, i.e. a VD view. To obtain a caudocranial view of the wing, it is necessary to position the patient vertically. This is achieved by positioning the anaesthetized and intubated bird head downwards and extending the wing over the radiographic cassette, which can be challenging.

It may also be necessary from time to time to perform skyline views of the skull when examining the sinuses for signs of disease.

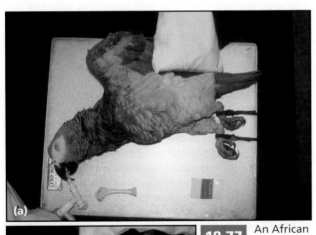

(a)

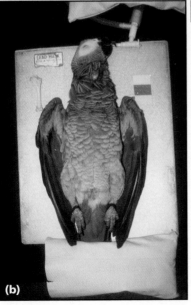

(b)

18.77 An African Grey parrot positioned for **(a)** lateral and **(b)** ventrodorsal views. (Reproduced from the *BSAVA Manual of Psittacine Birds, 2nd edition.* © Nigel Harcourt-Brown)

Reptiles

Chelonians may be immobilized by propping up the centre of the plastron, for example with tin cans or upturned feeding bowls, so that the legs cannot reach the ground (Figure 18.78). Snakes can be encouraged to enter a clear plastic tube to restrain them for such procedures, but the tube itself will reduce the clarity of the image produced. Lizards, and some snakes, may be placed into a hypotonic immobility by using the vagovagal response. This is where pressure applied gently to the eyes stimulates the vagal nerve and results in a slowing of respiration, heart rates and a semi-sedated state. Pressure may be maintained by placing cotton-wool balls over the closed eyes and wrapping them in place with bandage material. Chemical restraint should be used for fractious animals or dangerous species.

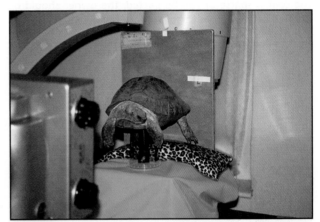

18.78 Tortoises can be propped up by the plastron to keep them immobile during radiography. (Courtesy of Mike Jessop)

Due to the absence of a diaphragm in reptiles, the lungs are fully collapsible (unlike birds, where the lungs are relatively rigid in structure). It is therefore advisable to use horizontal beam radiography when performing lateral radiography, to avoid the viscera obscuring the lung fields. This allows the assessment of the lung fields and viscera in their normal positions without superimposition.

A DV view is also necessary, to provide a three-dimensional picture, and in chelonians a third view, the craniocaudal view (again using horizontal beam radiography), is helpful. This is because the chelonian lungs sit in the most dorsal part of the carapace. Lateral horizontal beam radiographs will allow the lungs to be examined, but the right and left lung fields are superimposed on each other. The DV view in chelonians provides little information on the lungs due to their superimposition on the ventrally situated viscera. Therefore to compare left and right lung fields a craniocaudal horizontal beam radiograph (with the X-ray beam centred on the nuchal scute just behind the head) can be performed.

In snakes, it is not advisable to allow the snake to coil up on the cassette, as this distorts the anatomy and makes interpretation difficult. The snake should instead be stretched out; if necessary, sequential sections of body can be radiographed. It is helpful to place radiodense markers on the dorsal body wall when performing lateral radiographs, and on the lateral body wall when performing DV radiographs to help with the accurate localization of any abnormalities found.

Other imaging techniques

Ultrasonography

Diagnostic ultrasonography is common in small animal practice as a complementary imaging tool to radiography. Ultrasound imaging can be performed on the conscious patient using manual restraint without the need for sedation or anaesthesia (Figure 18.79), although nervous or tense animals may be more easily scanned under some form of chemical restraint, especially for abdominal ultrasonography when a better image is usually obtained in a more relaxed patient. Ultrasonography requires clipping of the hair, unless the coat is sparse or can be parted; the owner should be warned of this before the procedure is undertaken.

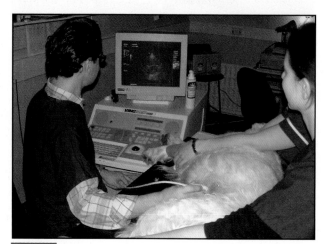

18.79 Ultrasonography of a conscious patient.

Ultrasonography can differentiate soft tissue from fluid, which radiography cannot, and shows the internal architecture of soft tissues that appear homogeneous on radiography. Unlike a conventional radiograph, the ultrasound image is a 'real-time' or moving picture, which is invaluable in the assessment of cardiac function and of peristalsis, and it therefore gives information about the function of certain organs. The applications of ultrasonography are continually advancing, and very small structures such as the adrenal glands, pancreas and lymph nodes, which were once thought to be beyond detection with ultrasonography, are now routinely examined. Furthermore, ultrasonography allows guided biopsy or fine-needle aspiration of very small lesions deep within the patient, and often avoids the need for a more invasive diagnostic procedure.

The main disadvantage is that ultrasound does not penetrate bone or air so it cannot usually be used for investigations of the skeletal system or lungs, with the exception of examination of superficial lesions. Bone reflects all of the incident ultrasound, resulting in 'acoustic shadows' or radiating black streaks in deeper tissues (Figure 18.80), whereas air in normal aerated lungs creates reverberations.

Ultrasonography is a difficult technique to master, since experience is required both to obtain and to interpret the images. Unlike radiographs, MRI and CT images, ultrasound scans are not suitable for remote interpretation, since frozen images lose much of their value and much of the interpretation depends on hand–eye coordination of the operator.

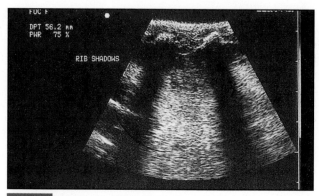

18.80 Acoustic shadows created by ribs.

However, some simple interpretations, such as pregnancy, pericardial effusion, large abdominal masses or ascites, may be made even by relatively inexperienced operators. A range of normal and abnormal ultrasound images are presented in the *BSAVA Manual of Canine and Feline Ultrasonography*.

Principles of ultrasonography

Ultrasound is sound energy at a higher frequency than can be detected by the human ear. In the diagnostic range, the frequencies used range from about 2.5 to 15 megahertz (MHz). Ultrasound of higher frequency produces better image resolution but cannot penetrate as far into the body as lower frequencies, and so the highest frequency compatible with the type of study and patient is selected. For abdominal ultrasonography of larger dogs, a 5 MHz transducer is used. For cats and smaller dogs, 7.5 MHz may be preferred; and for very superficial examinations, such as of the eye or tendons, transducers of 10 MHz or higher are needed.

In an ultrasound machine the sound waves are created by the vibrations of special crystals in the probe or transducer that alter their shape when an electrical current is applied to them. This is known as the piezoelectric effect. When the transducer is applied to the patient's skin, the sound waves are passed through the patient's soft tissues as pressure waves, and at interfaces between tissues or between clusters of different cells within an organ a certain percentage of the sound waves are reflected and may return to the transducer (Figure 18.81). Returning sound waves in turn create a vibration of

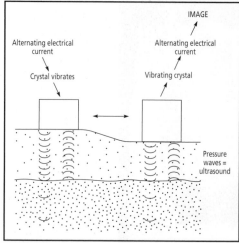

18.81 Ultrasound waves are produced by the transducer and pass into the tissues. Reflected waves are detected by the same transducer and an image created.

the tissues and of the crystals in the probe and this is converted back into electrical impulses, which are almost instantly converted by a computer into an image. The image is basically built up from many tiny dots of different brightness, depending on the strength of the returning pulses of ultrasound and the location in the body from which they have been reflected. It is a cross-sectional picture of the internal architecture of the tissues under investigation.

Equipment

Ultrasound equipment consists of one or more transducers, a TV monitor and a control panel (Figure 18.82). There is also likely to be some sort of printer for recording the images and a computer to record the studies.

Ultrasound transducers are of two main types: linear array and sector scanner (Figure 18.83). In linear array transducers, the piezoelectric crystals are arranged in a line and the image is rectangular. Although a wide image of the tissues close to the transducer is obtained, linear array transducers need a long contact area with the patient, which is hard to achieve

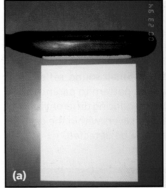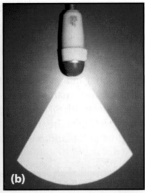

18.83 Transducers. **(a)** Linear array transducer and image field. **(b)** Sector scanner transducer and image field.

in small animals (note: ultrasound does not pass through air). Linear array transducers are mainly used for rectal investigations in large animals. Sector scanning transducers are much more suitable for small animal work, since the crystals are arranged close together so that only a small area of contact with the patient is required. The ultrasound beam fans out to produce a triangular image that shows as much of the deeper tissues as possible. The image can be altered in depth, size, brightness and contrast, using the ultrasound machine's controls, and measurements and annotations can be made on a frozen image.

Care of the ultrasound machine

- Schedule regular machine maintenance visits by a service engineer.
- Check the ultrasound equipment regularly.
- Make sure that all connections are plugged in properly.
- Check the integrity of the wiring, cables and transducers.
- Wipe down the transducers and cables that monitor the heart rate after each patient examination, using a special cleaner.
- Follow any recommended cleaning protocols, such as sterilization for certain types of transducers used for specific procedures.
- Wipe down the machine thoroughly at the end of each use.
- Report any problems to the service representative.

Technique

Usually for dogs and cats, the fur must be clipped to allow good contact between the transducer and the skin, as small air bubbles trapped in hair will greatly degrade the image. A special coupling gel is then applied to improve contact further. In long-haired animals it may be possible simply to part the hair and hold it aside using gel, but this means that only a small area can be examined.

Most ultrasound examinations are performed with the animal in lateral or dorsal recumbency, scanning from the ventral surface of the body or through the uppermost body wall. However, echocardiography (ultrasonography of the heart) is best performed from beneath, through a cut-out in a special tabletop. In lateral recumbency, the heart sinks

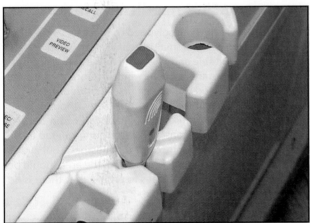

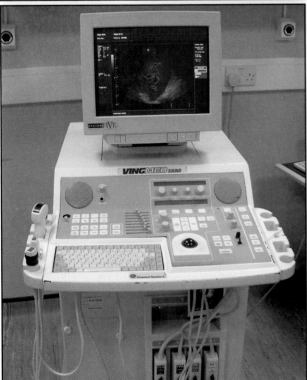

18.82 Ultrasound transducer, TV monitor and control panel.

towards the dependent chest wall, compressing the lung between it and the chest wall, and therefore the best 'acoustic window' (the least intervening lung) is on the underside.

Most ultrasonography performed uses B-mode ('brightness' mode ultrasound, described above) to create a two-dimensional image of the tissues. Small sound reflections within tissues create a fine granular pattern to parenchymatous organs, with different organs producing different brightnesses on the image (Figure 18.84). Layers within the gastrointestinal and bladder walls can also be detected.

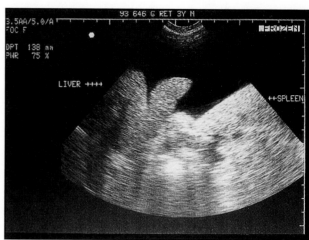

18.86 Ultrasound image of free abdominal fluid, seen as a black area outlining abdominal organs.

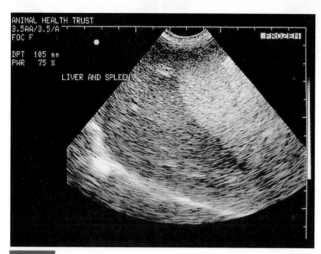

18.84 Ultrasound image of normal liver and spleen.

Pathology within an organ can often be recognized as a change in the overall brightness or **echogenicity** of the organ, or a mottled appearance disrupting normal architecture (Figure 18.85). Areas of altered echogenicity are said to be **anechoic** (black), **hypoechoic** (dark) or **hyperechoic** (bright). An area of mixed echogenicity is described as **complex**.

Fluid is usually seen as an anechoic area, because it gives rise to very few ultrasound reflections. Thus, free abdominal fluid can be seen as a black background surrounding abdominal organs (Figure 18.86). One of the main advantages of ultrasonography is that it allows examination of the abdominal structures when free fluid renders radiography unhelpful by obscuring the organs.

Special applications

Biopsy and fine-needle aspiration

Ultrasonography is increasingly used to assist biopsy or fine-needle aspiration (FNA) of small diseased areas within organs, provided that a suitable and safe route to the area of interest exists via an appropriate acoustic window. Since the internal organ architecture and the needle tip can both be seen, the needle can be guided into the affected area without damaging other structures (Figure 18.87). FNA can often be performed with the patient conscious; ultrasound-guided tissue biopsy is more likely to require general anaesthesia but avoids the need for surgery. Following sampling, the area should be scanned for several more minutes to ensure that there is no after-effect such as haemorrhage.

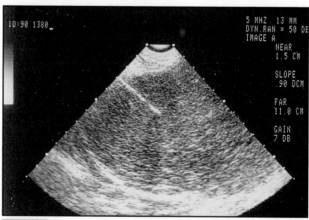

18.87 Fine-needle aspiration of an abdominal mass. The needle is seen as a bright line entering the mass.

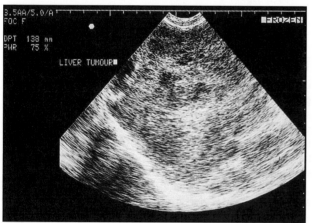

18.85 Ultrasound image of a liver tumour in a dog, giving rise to a mottled, irregular pattern to the liver.

Ultrasound-guided cystocentesis is a very useful and quick procedure when the bladder is small and cannot be palpated for cystocentesis.

Heart motion

A further refinement of ultrasonography is the use of M-mode ('movement' mode) to quantify heart motion. First, a B-mode image is obtained and a cursor (line of dots) is placed on it and moved right or left until it passes through the heart in the required position. At the touch of a button, the ultrasound beam produced by the transducer is converted into a thin line that produces a vertical band of dots, indicating reflections at tissue interfaces along that fixed line. This is rapidly updated with the movement of the heart and the image is scrolled along a horizontal axis with time. The resultant image shows the degree of heart motion and can be frozen to allow measurements of the heart chambers and walls in systole and diastole. Figure 18.88 shows a combined B-mode and M-mode image of a heart.

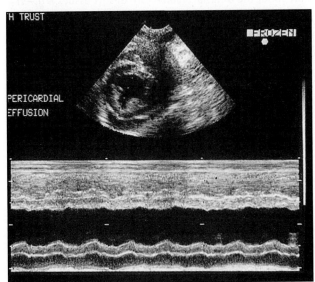

18.88 Ultrasound image from a dog with a pericardial effusion. Top: B-mode image of the heart; the line of dots indicates the position of the linear ultrasound beam. Bottom: M-mode image, with time along the horizontal axis. Blood in the left ventricle and the pericardial fluid are seen as black areas on both images.

Doppler ultrasonography

Doppler ultrasonography is the use of ultrasound waves to detect movement, usually blood flow. It is based on the principle that echoes returning from moving reflective surfaces will be of shorter wavelength if the movement is towards the transducer and longer wavelength if it is away. Spectral Doppler displays flow quantitatively and graphically against a baseline, whilst colour-flow Doppler assigns a colour according to speed and direction of flow and this colour mapping is superimposed over a B-mode or M-mode image. Doppler ultrasonography is used mostly in cardiac investigations (echocardiography) but can also be used to show the vascularity of structures, which is helpful prior to biopsy and to detect portosystemic shunts.

Contrast ultrasonography

There is increasing interest in contrast ultrasonography, in which small quantities of microbubbles of sulphur hexafluoride gas within phospholipid capsules suspended in liquid are injected into the blood stream. The microbubbles reflect ultrasound, producing increased echogenicity of the tissues in proportion to their vascularity. This allows vascular and non-vascular structures to be differentiated (for example, tumour masses from blood clots), and the time scale of 'wash in' and 'wash out' of the contrast medium may suggest whether a lesion is benign or malignant, especially in the liver.

Equine diagnostic ultrasonography

Diagnostic ultrasonography has a wide range of applications in equine practice: ligaments and tendons, joints and bursae, cardiac, abdominal, guided biopsy and injections, location of non-radiopaque foreign bodies and reproduction. As with small animals, the hair should be clipped and the skin cleaned before applying ultrasound gel. Some horses will tolerate ultrasonography without restraint but many will require sedation. Some will not tolerate clipping without sedation.

Ultrasonography is frequently used to assess ligaments and tendons of the distal limb (Figure 18.89). A high frequency linear array transducer is used. A stand-off (Figure 18.90) may be used to aid visualization of superficial structures.

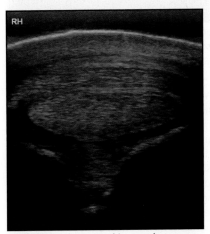

18.89 Ultrasound image (transverse plane) of the tendons of the plantar aspect of the hindlimb at the level of the proximal sesamoid bones of the fetlock joint.

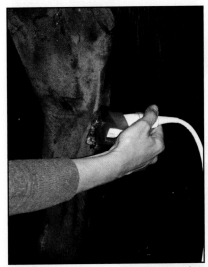

18.90 Performing an ultrasound scan of the tendons of the hindlimb. A stand-off has been placed over the probe to obtain images of superficial structures.

Ultrasonography is also used in other areas, such as the supraspinous ligament of the back, and the dorsal sacroiliac ligaments, and can identify muscle tears. Imaging joint capsules also yields important information (Figure 18.91). In particular, joints such as the femorotibial joint can be imaged to evaluate the menisci and this may be more useful than other techniques in some instances.

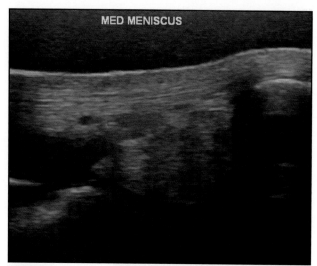

18.91 Ultrasound image of the stifle joint highlighting the meniscus, which is not normally seen on radiographs. Proximal is to the right.

Ultrasonography can also provide information on superficial bone lesions. Periosteal bone formation can be detected earlier on ultrasonography than on radiography. Fractures of the ilium of the pelvis have been detected on ultrasonography by identifying an incongruity in the surface of the bone. Ultrasound guidance is also used for intra-articular treatment of facet joints of the cervical and thoracic spine, or for injecting subchondral bone cysts.

Low-frequency sector scanners are used for cardiac and abdominal ultrasonography. Rectal linear array probes (Figure 18.92) are used for reproduction scanning in mares to assess the stage of ovulation and for pregnancy confirmation.

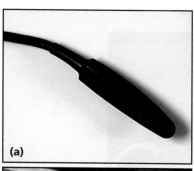

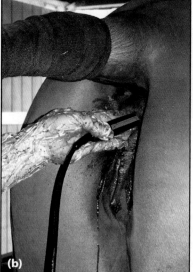

18.92 Pregnancy diagnosis. **(a)** A rectal probe used for scanning mares. **(b)** The probe is introduced per rectum to scan the ovaries and to confirm pregnancy. Some pelvic structures can also be imaged in this way.

Computed tomography (CT scanning)

Principles and equipment

CT involves using X-rays to produce a highly detailed cross-sectional radiograph of the patient's tissues. Tissue contrast is much greater than with conventional radiography, and so fluid and solid tissue can be distinguished and some information about the internal architecture of soft tissues is given.

The CT scanner is a large piece of apparatus shaped like a ring doughnut with a central orifice within which is the patient table (Figure 18.93). The X-ray tube head moves rapidly around the circumference of the ring during the exposure, and radiation emerging from the patient is detected electronically and digitized, producing image information that can be manipulated by computer. The table moves forward slowly or in very small increments, and this movement results in the production of many cross-sectional, slice-like images of the area under investigation.

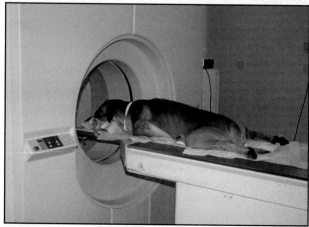

18.93 CT scanner and patient.

Differences in mathematical reconstruction of the emerging radiation, or 'algorithms', are used to emphasize different types of tissue and the grey scale of the final image can be altered further according to the tissue of interest. Thus, settings such as 'bone', 'lung' and 'soft tissue' can be selected. The **grey scale** of CT is described in terms of 'Hounsfield units' (HU), named after the engineer who invented CT, Sir Godfrey Hounsfield. The Hounsfield scale extends from approximately +3000 to –1000, with water being 0, bone being up to nearly 3000 and air being –1000 HU. Within the **grey scale** of the image, a range of Hounsfield units can be selected for viewing; all values higher and lower than these are displayed as white and black, respectively, and the values between are spread out over a range of grey shades that are discernible by the human eye. The centre of the range of Hounsfield units selected for viewing is known as the **window level** and the range is the **window width**. For examination of bone a window level of about +200 to +600 and window width of about +1000 to +2000 are used; for lung, the values are about –500 to –800 and +1000 to +2000, respectively.

Technique

Veterinary patients must be anaesthetized or heavily sedated for CT scanning because the very high doses of radiation involved preclude manual restraint, but conventional anaesthetic and monitoring equipment can be used. Each exposure takes between a few seconds and one minute, depending on the study.

With older CT machines, images are always obtained transverse to the patient as it passes through the gantry. Images in other planes must be reformatted, which results in considerable loss of detail. The newer 'spiral' or 'helical' CT scanners are capable of producing images in any plane in very short scan times. Images can also be displayed in three dimensions and with different layers of tissue 'stripped away', allowing surgical planning. Advanced applications such as angiography and 'virtual endoscopy' are also possible.

Applications

Although this is essentially a radiographic technique, CT images have much more tissue definition than radiography and can differentiate between different types of soft tissue and between fluid and soft tissue. CT is especially valuable for imaging the skeletal system, as it is very sensitive to areas of osteolysis and new bone formation, and can therefore detect bony lesions that are invisible on radiography (Figure 18.94).

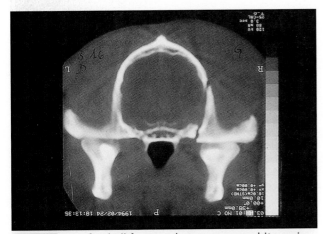

18.94 CT of a skull fracture: bone appears white, as in radiography. This image has been 'windowed' by the computer to 'flatten' the soft tissues into a single grey shade to give better emphasis to bone.

CT is also useful for imaging thoracic and abdominal masses, as it is less susceptible to movement artefacts than is MRI (see below). CT is especially valuable for imaging the lung, due to the very fine definition produced (Figure 18.95), and is the technique of choice for detection of lung metastases.

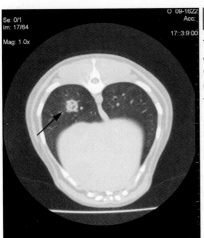

18.95 CT of a bronchial foreign body, seen as a white (hyperdense) area (arrowed) within a thickened bronchus.

CT can be used for the brain, although the images are greatly inferior to those obtained with MRI. For the spine, excellent bone detail is obtained but changes in the spinal cord are not likely to be visible. Iodine radiographic contrast media can be given intravenously or into the spinal subarachnoid space to enhance the images further, demonstrating the vascularity of a lesion or damage to the blood–brain barrier and permitting myelography to be performed. CT-guided biopsy may be performed with the needle trajectory planned by computer from the CT images.

There is currently limited availability for CT scanning of the horse in the UK. The horse is generally anaesthetized for the procedure; however, a system has been devised to obtain CT scans of the skull in the standing horse and is arguably one of the greatest uses for the technique in equine patients. Scanning is limited to the skull, cervical spine and distal limb (or to any part of the horse that can be inserted into the 'doughnut').

Magnetic resonance imaging (MRI scanning)

Principles and equipment

MRI involves completely different physical principles to radiography and CT, combining magnetism and radio waves. The scanner itself is a very powerful magnet, which may be cylindrical in the case of medium- and high-field magnets (Figure 18.96) or open in the case of low-field (weaker) systems. The tissues within the magnetic field become magnetized, which has the effect of aligning the protons of the hydrogen atoms in the body. The patient is then subjected to a series of radio waves emitted by a radiofrequency aerial, or RF coil, each lasting for several minutes; these disorientate the protons so that they emit tiny radio signals themselves. The emitted signals are detected by the same RF coil and are converted to an image by a computer using very complex mathematical procedures.

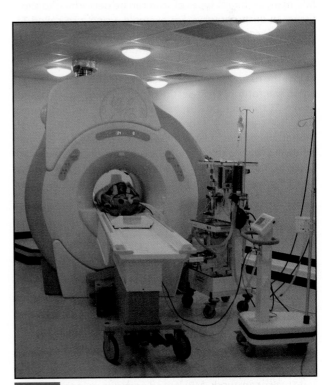

18.96 MRI scanner and anaesthetized patient.

Because MRI does not use ionizing radiation, unlike radiography and CT, it is thought to be completely safe, but veterinary patients must be anaesthetized to keep them still during the scanning time, as any movement will render the images non-diagnostic. This may sometimes be for up to an hour or more in complex cases or when using low-field systems, in which scan times are longer. The main danger to patients and handlers lies in the fact that ferrous metal objects taken near the magnet may become dangerous missiles, and serious injuries and even deaths have occurred in medical MRI as a result. Fortunately, however, pet microchips remain unaffected by the powerful magnetic field and retain their data.

The presence of a strong magnetic field means that conventional anaesthetic and monitoring equipment cannot be used. In the case of low-field magnets, placing the anaesthetic machine at a distance from the magnet and using a long circuit may be sufficient to overcome this problem. With higher-field systems, dedicated non-ferrous machines may be required and this of course adds to the expense of MRI. Although total intravenous anaesthesia may be possible, patients with severe disease, especially of the CNS, are often at high risk from anaesthesia, especially if they cannot be monitored adequately.

Technique

During scanning, the patient lies on the table in the magnetic field with the part to be imaged in an RF coil. The RF coils are of varying size and shape depending on the part of the body for which they are designed. There are now some MRI scanners and RF coils that are manufactured especially for veterinary patients (including a low-field unit for scanning the lower limbs of standing horses), but most are designed for human patients; nevertheless, the equipment is well suited to scanning veterinary patients.

Unlike CT, in which there is a single image acquisition, with MRI many different types of scan can be performed to show tissues in different ways. For example, using a so-called T1-weighted scan, fluid such as CSF and ascites is dark, whereas with a T2-weighted scan it is bright. Other types of scan or 'pulse sequences' such as fat suppression can be employed to detect the nature of a tissue or lesion. As with CT, the images are in the form of cross-sectional 'slices' of the patient, but unlike CT they can be acquired in any plane. Studies usually comprise transverse, sagittal and dorsal plane images, although sometimes oblique slices are helpful too, for example following the orbital structures. Since many more studies are possible than with CT and since each set of image acquisitions takes a number of minutes, overall scan times are much longer than with CT.

Applications

The soft tissue information produced by MRI is much better than with CT, provided the tissue is still during scanning. Moving areas, such as the heart and lungs, require more complex '**gating**' techniques during which the application of the RF pulses is synchronized with heartbeat or respiration. Although slightly less sensitive for bony structures and calcification than CT, MRI provides excellent orthopaedic images by showing articular cartilage, joint fluid, subchondral bone and so on.

In veterinary work, MRI is used particularly in the diagnosis of brain (Figure 18.97) and spinal (Figure 18.98) conditions

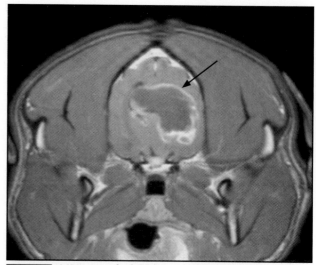

18.97   MRI scan of a brain tumour (arrowed) in a dog. On this contrast-enhanced, T1-weighted transverse brain image, the vascularized part of the brain tumour appears white and the necrotic part is dark.

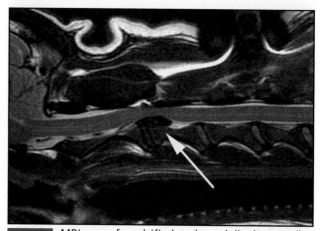

18.98   MRI scan of a calcified prolapsed disc (arrowed) causing spinal cord compression. Calcified material is black on MRI.

in small animals in which it is by far the technique of choice. Conditions such as brain and spinal cord tumours, inflammatory CNS disease, congenital deformities, disc disease and trauma can all be readily diagnosed, improving the diagnosis and treatment of the patients and allowing a more accurate prognosis to be given.

MRI can also be used to investigate many other disease processes, such as neoplasia, soft tissue foreign bodies and other space-occupying lesions and inflammation. Intravenous MRI contrast medium is given in many cases. MRI contrast media are complex molecules that usually contain the element gadolinium, which has 'paramagnetic' properties. Use of contrast medium will show damage to the blood–brain barrier and vascularity of lesions, due to 'enhancement' of the tissues absorbing the contrast medium. As with CT, angiography can be performed to show blood vessels in three-dimensional detail.

The use of MRI, and to a lesser extent CT, has meant that surgery and radiotherapy of brain tumours in cats and dogs can now be performed successfully. The two techniques are also very helpful in planning surgery or radiotherapy for diseases elsewhere in the body, as the full extent of a disease process is often not evident on radiographs. MRI and CT are becoming increasingly used in veterinary diagnostic imaging as referral centres gain access to human scanners or mobile MRI systems or even obtain their own machines, and as owner expectations and the number of insured animals continue to rise. MRI and CT are, however, open to misuse. As with other imaging techniques, appropriate patient selection is required, together with expert acquisition and interpretation of images.

MRI is widely used in horses. There is limited availability of equipment to carry out an MRI scan on the anaesthetized horse but equipment has been developed to obtain MRI scans of the limb in the standing horse. All horses are sedated for MRI scanning to limit movement and allow the coils to be placed on the horse's foot or limb. The horse's shoes must be removed before entering the scanning room, even for scanning regions other than the foot. A thorough check must be made to ensure that nail clenches have not been left in the hoof wall. In the standing horse the main use of MRI is imaging the distal limb, especially the foot (Figure 18.99). Damage to the distal aspect of the deep digital flexor tendon and the collateral ligaments within the hoof capsule that are difficult to visualize with other imaging techniques can be shown by MRI. Osseous changes are also identified that are not visible on radiographs. At some equine centres the limb can be examined as far proximally as the carpus and tarsus.

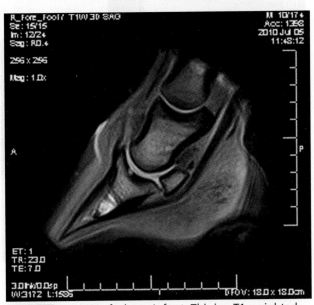

18.99 An MRI of a horse's foot. This is a T1-weighted image in the sagittal plane, outlining anatomy as on a lateral radiograph. Soft tissue as well as bone can be identified.

Nuclear medicine (scintigraphy)

Scintigraphic studies involve the use of radioactive isotopes and are defined as 'open sources'. Use of these isotopes is governed by the Radioactive Substances Act 1993. Licences must be obtained from the Environment Agency for activities involving radioactive isotopes. One is for keeping and using isotopes (the Registration), and the second governs the accumulation and disposal of radioactive waste (the Authorization). As with radiography, safe working procedures should be defined in the Local Rules.

Use in small animals

Scintigraphy is occasionally used in small animals. Figure 18.100 shows a sedated cat positioned on a gamma camera for scintigraphy of the thyroid gland. Radioactive iodine is injected intravenously and is taken up by the thyroid gland. The activity of the thyroid is compared with that of the zygomatic salivary glands in the head, and the relative activity of the two areas will show whether hyperthyroidism is present, in which gland (or both) the abnormality is, and whether or not there is any ectopic thyroid tissue elsewhere. Figure 18.101 shows the location of abnormal thyroid tissue in a hyperthyroid cat, allowing surgical planning if thyroidectomy is to be performed. Scintigraphy is occasionally used for other purposes such as detection of a portosystemic shunt and comparison of ventilation and perfusion in the lungs. However this is a very specialized technique, which is performed in relatively few veterinary institutes. Following scintigraphy, small animals must be isolated, usually for 24 hours.

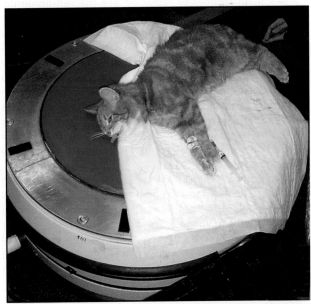

18.100 A sedated cat lying on a gamma camera during scintigraphy.

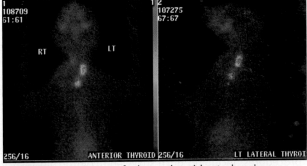

18.101 Scintigram of a hyperthyroid cat, showing abnormal tissue in the caudal neck.

Use in horses

In the veterinary field scintigraphy is used mainly in horses, for the diagnosis of bony orthopaedic problems. A gamma ray-emitting radioactive substance attached to a molecule that will be taken up by the tissue under investigation (usually bone) is injected into the bloodstream under conditions that protect the handler from irradiation. The horse is then returned to an isolation stable. Several hours later the radioactivity will have become concentrated in areas of increased bone turnover, creating 'hot spots' that are emitting more gamma-radiation than are the surrounding tissues. The emitted photons can be detected either by a hand-held radioactivity counter or by a large detector known as a gamma camera. A pattern of emitted radioactivity is produced that allows the source of the lameness to be diagnosed. Although the 'image' itself is rather crude, since it reflects metabolism rather than anatomical detail, the technique is very sensitive to early bone changes that cannot be seen with radiography and is used to localize the source of lameness. It can also confirm whether a lesion seen on radiography is currently active.

Scintigraphy has enabled the reliable identification of stress fractures for which rest provides 100% cure. Prior to this, a significant proportion of such cases suffered catastrophic long bone fracture and were euthanased.

The main sources of radiation are the radiopharmaceutical, the injection, the horse, urine, bedding and waste material. Following scintigraphy, the horse must be confined to an isolation stable with minimal handling until readings obtained with a Geiger counter show that it is no longer emitting significant amounts of radiation. The stable is designated as a Controlled Area with appropriate signs on the door, and access restricted. The bedding must also be checked with a Geiger counter to ascertain when the levels of radioactivity are no longer significant. All areas where the radiopharmaceutical is prepared and used must also be routinely monitored.

Ideally there should be a delay of 7 days after performing multiple perineural local analgesic techniques before nuclear scintigraphy is carried out. Diuretics can be used to encourage urination prior to imaging. The horse should be lunged for 10–15 minutes before injection of the isotope to increase peripheral perfusion. An intravenous jugular catheter can aid in safe injection of the isotope, and also in the administration of diuretics and sedatives.

Diagnostic endoscopy

Endoscopy is the use of optical devices that give visual access to the inside of the body and provide high-quality magnified images of tissues and organ systems (Figure 18.102). Foreign bodies can be removed and tissue samples taken, often without the need for open surgery (Figure 18.103). Where surgery is required, the clear magnified image gives greater precision and access to otherwise inaccessible places. Procedures are carried out through natural orifices or tiny incisions (keyhole surgery), resulting in less tissue trauma, reduced intraoperative and postoperative pain, quicker recovery and reduced infection rates. For this reason, these procedures are termed minimally invasive. An increasing number of routine procedures, including bitch spays and cryptorchid testicle removal, are being carried out using these techniques (see Chapter 25), and this trend is likely to continue as it has in human surgery.

Flexible endoscopy

Flexible endoscopes comprise an umbilical cord connected to a light source and suction/irrigation pump, a handpiece and a long flexible insertion tube, the tip of which can be manipulated in two directions (bronchoscopes) or four

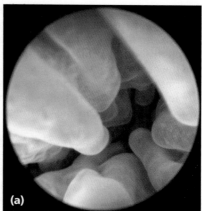
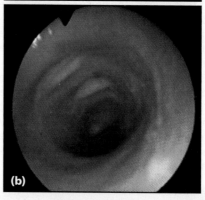

18.102 Endoscopic images of **(a)** normal nasal turbinates and **(b)** normal duodenum in a dog.

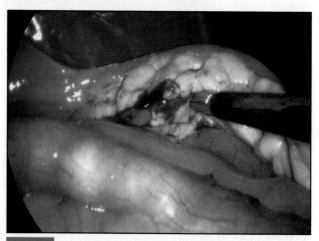

18.103 Laparoscopic biopsy of the pancreas.

directions (gastroscopes). These endoscopes are used for examination of the respiratory tract and gastrointestinal tract, respectively, where they can be directed deep within the body to remove foreign bodies, visualize lesions and take fluid or tissue samples. Images are observed either through the eyepiece or preferably on a television monitor by means of an attached camera or dedicated video-endoscope. Patients are examined under general anaesthesia and a suitable mouth gag must always be used to prevent inadvertent reflex biting and damage to the endoscope.

Instrumentation

Instruments used in flexible endoscopy must be chosen to suit the diameter and length of the endoscope's instrument channel. Biopsy forceps (oval cupped with serrated edges are preferred) and a variety of grasping forceps are routinely used. Instruments are necessarily small and fragile and limit the size of biopsy specimen that can be obtained. Guarded brushes can also be obtained for retrieving samples for cytology and culture from the bronchial or intestinal mucosa. Sterile sample tubing may also be used through the instrument channel when performing bronchoalveolar lavage (BAL).

Routine positioning for flexible endoscopy

- Upper GI tract (**gastroduodenoscopy**) – left lateral recumbency.
- Lower GI tract (**colonoscopy**) – left lateral recumbency.
- Lungs (**tracheobronchoscopy**) – sternal recumbency.
- Nose/pharynx (**rhinoscopy**) – sternal recumbency.
- Urethra (especially male dogs) (**urethroscopy**) – lateral recumbency.

Special considerations

Insufflation (filling with air) of the stomach in upper GI tract endoscopy may reduce diaphragmatic excursion and venous return. Air should always be removed by suction at the end of the procedure. Any fluid in the oesophagus should also be removed to prevent oesophagitis and possible stricture formation. Airways will be partially occluded during bronchoscopy. Careful attention to the pulse oximeter is essential. Patients should be maintained on oxygen for 10 minutes before and after the procedure.

Rigid endoscopy

Rigid endoscopes are relatively simple steel tubes containing rod lenses, with an eyepiece at one end, and a connection for a light guide cable. They are extremely delicate and require careful handling and care during cleaning. These endoscopes are used for a wide variety of diagnostic and surgical procedures, including:

- **Otoscopy** (examination of the ear)
- **Rhinoscopy** (examination of the nose)
- **Tracheoscopy** (examination of the trachea)
- **Colonoscopy** (examination of the colon)
- **Vaginoscopy** and **urethrocystoscopy** (examination of the vagina and urogenital tract/bladder)
- **Laparoscopy** (examination of the abdomen)
- **Thoracoscopy** (examination of the thorax)
- **Arthroscopy** (examination of the joints).

Instrumentation

Smaller endoscopes are always placed in a specially designed rigid sheath with instrument and irrigation channels to protect the endoscope and allow biopsy samples to be taken in restricted spaces such as the nose and bladder. Grasping forceps or laser fibres can also be passed down the channel for foreign body removal or surgical resection, respectively. Arthroscopic sheaths are used to protect the endoscope in joints. These have no instrument channels, but have a tap with a luer fitting for instillation of saline under pressure from a pump or pressure bag. Instruments are introduced through separate cannulae.

Larger endoscopes, usually 5 mm diameter, are used in the abdomen or thorax through specially designed cannulae, which have gas-tight valves and are inserted through the body wall. A variety of endoscopic instruments may be passed through separate cannulae to perform surgical procedures or take tissue samples. Most instrumentation used in veterinary laparoscopy and thoracoscopy is of 5 mm diameter for use in 6 mm laparoscopic cannulae. A wide variety of instrumentation is available but most commonly used are biopsy forceps, Babcock's forceps, curved scissors, Maryland forceps and a palpation probe – a blunt metal rod used for manipulating tissues. A detachable camera clipped to the eyepiece enables procedures to be observed on a television monitor.

In addition to the basic instrumentation, a light source is required; this is often shared with a flexible endoscope, though older halogen light sources may give insufficient light for laparoscopy. A xenon or metal halide light source is preferred. For laparoscopy an electronic carbon dioxide insufflator is used and connected to the tap on a cannula via a filter and some sterile insufflation tubing. This maintains intra-abdominal pressure at a pre-set level, providing a space in which the surgeon can work.

Electrosurgery is the preferred method of haemostasis for routine minimally invasive procedures, and a radiosurgery generator is therefore essential. Many instruments are electrically shielded and have electrodes for attachment of monopolar leads. Bipolar instruments are also widely used, especially for operative surgery. Note that the generator should always be set on the 'cutting' current, even when coagulating vessels, as this has a lower voltage and is less likely to cause sparking to other instruments and cannulae, resulting in tissue damage.

Routine positioning and preparation for rigid endoscopy

Vaginoscopy and otoscopy may be carried out on conscious patients, but all other procedures require general anaesthesia. Positioning will depend on the site being examined, and the procedure being undertaken.

- **Rhinoscopy** and **urethrocystoscopy** – sternal recumbency (some prefer lateral), with nose or abdomen propped up on a rolled-up towel.
- **Laparoscopy** – dorsal recumbency (sometimes dorsolateral).
- **Thoracoscopy** – dorsal recumbency (sometimes lateral).
- **Arthroscopy** – usually lateral but depends on the joint being examined.

Rhinoscopy and urethrocystoscopy are best carried out on a wet table as they require considerable amounts of saline flushing. Alternatively, a deep tray covered with a wire grid may suffice.

Special considerations

Copious saline flushing may also result in the induction of hypothermia, especially in small patients. Careful monitoring of core body temperature is advisable and small patients should be maintained on heat mats or warm air circulation blankets.

It should be noted that laparoscopy requires insufflation of the abdomen with an inert gas (usually carbon dioxide). This increases abdominal pressure on the diaphragm and can restrict respiration, which requires careful monitoring during anaesthesia. Thoracoscopy is an open chest procedure, resulting in collapse of the lungs. All patients will require positive pressure ventilation throughout the operation and careful monitoring using pulse oximetry and capnography if available. A chest tube will be placed at the end of the procedure to allow re-inflation of the lungs through intermittent or continuous suction. It is not unusual for the surgeon to change the position of the patient during laparoscopy or thoracoscopy in order to allow gravity to move viscera out of the surgical field. For this reason, rigid ties should not be used, and movable cradles may be substituted. Alternatively an adjustable operating table that can tilt in four directions is ideal.

Patients should be clipped widely to allow optimal positioning of cannulae and also to enable conversion to an open procedure if it should become necessary. A suitable surgical kit should always be immediately available.

Equine endoscopy

Endoscopic examination of the respiratory tract is carried out in the conscious standing horse. The handler stands to one side of the horse. On the other side an assistant passes the endoscope along the ventral meatus of one of the nasal passages. Many horses can be examined without significant restraint, although a nose twitch may be helpful in some circumstances. Some horses will become dangerous and can 'strike out' when twitched, and sedation is often a useful tool to facilitate endoscopic examination, except when laryngeal function is to be assessed. Sedation may also be contraindicated if the horse is due to compete, because of 'doping' considerations. Endoscopy is usually carried out with the horse standing still, but may be performed during exercise (i.e. on a treadmill or using remote dynamic endoscopic equipment) to assess dynamic upper respiratory tract disorders.

In the adult horse, a 100–110 cm endoscope is sufficient to examine the upper respiratory tract (Figure 18.104). For bronchoscopy, or for broncho-alveolar lavage a longer endoscope of >160 cm is required. For gastroscopy (Figure 18.105) an endoscope with a working length of 250–300 cm is required.

There are many indications for endoscopic examination of the respiratory tract, including nasal discharge, epistaxis, dysphagia, coughing, exercise intolerance, respiratory noise and loss of appetite. Examination of the nasal meatuses, guttural pouches and airways of foals and small ponies is carried out with an endoscope with a smaller diameter (7–9 mm). Using a narrow diameter endoscope of 8 or 9 mm facilitates the examination of the upper airway in horses and ponies of all ages. Epistaxis occasionally occurs, as the turbinates are very vascular and inadvertent injury can happen, usually because the endoscope is in the narrower middle meatus or traumatizes the ethmoid region or because a fractious horse moves its head when the endoscope is being withdrawn.

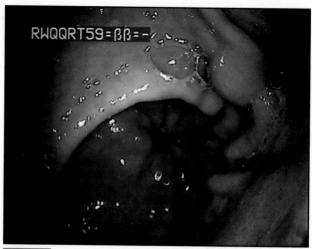

18.105 Gastroscopic image of the stomach of a horse.

Care and cleaning of endoscopic equipment

All endoscopes require meticulous care and attention to cleaning protocols if they are not to suffer irreversible damage. Delay may make cleaning very difficult or impossible. Most endoscope suppliers will provide in-house training in care and maintenance, and it is advisable to ensure all cleaning is done by trained personnel.

Both rigid and flexible endoscopes may be gas-sterilized or soaked in a suitable cold sterilizer solution. Some rigid endoscopes are autoclaveable, although this is not recommended as the majority of veterinary autoclaves cycle too quickly and may shorten the life of the instrument. Most instruments, cannulae and trocars can be cleaned in an ultrasonic bath.

- Rinse immediately after use to remove gross contamination.
- Flexible endoscopes should be pressurized with a pressure tester before immersion.
- Soak in an approved enzymatic cleaner.
- Brush all channels in flexible endoscopes and rigid cannulae.
- Rinse in clean water.
- Soak in an approved cold sterilizer for a further 15 minutes – never soak any endoscope for longer than one hour as this may result in damage to the seals.
- **Never attempt to clean an endoscope or light guide cable in an ultrasonic bath as this will cause irreparable damage.**
- Rinse in deionized water and dry carefully.
- Hang flexible endoscopes vertically with the umbilicus and insertion tube straight and all taps removed to allow drainage.
- Store rigid endoscopes in a protective sheath in a suitable container or drawer.

Single-use bipolar instruments designed for human surgery may be re-used if carefully cleaned and re-sterilized. These instruments cannot be autoclaved or cold-sterilized. Care must be taken not to allow fluids to run up the shaft towards the handle, which houses the electronic circuitry. The tip of the instrument is cleaned carefully with enzymatic cleaner, rinsed and dried. The instrument can then be gas-sterilized.

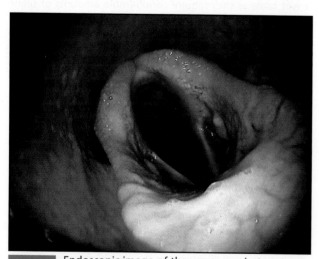

18.104 Endoscopic image of the upper respiratory tract of a horse, showing the epiglottis in the foreground and the arytenoid cartilages behind.

Further reading

Baines E (2005) Practical contrast radiography 3. Urogenital studies. *In Practice* **27**, 466–473

Barr F and Gaschen L (2011) *BSAVA Manual of Canine and Feline Ultrasonography*. BSAVA Publications, Gloucester

Barr F and Kirberger R (2006) *BSAVA Manual of Canine and Feline Musculoskeletal Imaging*. BSAVA Publications, Gloucester

Barrett E (2007) Practice radiography: time to go digital? *In Practice* **29**, 616–619

Bradley K (2005) Practical contrast radiography 2. Gastrointestinal studies. *In Practice* **27**, 412–417

Bradley K (2006) Digital radiography – considerations for general practice. *UK Vet* **11**, 81–84

Butler JA, Colles CM, Dyson SJ *et al.* (2008) *Clinical Radiology of the Horse, 3rd edn*. Wiley-Blackwell, Oxford

Caine A (2009) Practical approach to digital radiography. *In Practice* **31**, 334–339

Crane L and Barrett E (2008) Advanced imaging. In: *BSAVA Manual of Canine and Feline Advanced Veterinary Nursing, 2nd edn*, ed. A Hotston Moore and S Rudd, pp.220–249. BSAVA Publications, Gloucester

Dennis R, Kirberger RM, Barr FJ and Wrigley RH (2010) *Handbook of Small Animal Radiology and Ultrasound: Techniques and Differential Diagnoses, 2nd edn*. Elsevier, Oxford

Latham C (2005) Practical contrast radiography 1. Contrast agents. *In Practice* **27**, 348–352

Lhermette P and Sobel D (2009) *BSAVA Manual of Canine and Feline Endoscopy and Endosurgery*. BSAVA Publications, Gloucester

Llabres Diaz F (2005) Practical contrast radiography 4. Myelography. *In Practice* **27**, 502–510

Llabres Diaz F (2006) Practical contrast radiography 5. Other techniques. *In Practice* **28**, 32–40

O'Brien R and Barr F (2009) *BSAVA Manual of Canine and Feline Abdominal Imaging*. BSAVA Publications, Gloucester

Rudorf H, Taeymans O and Johnson V (2008) Basics of thoracic radiography and radiology. In: *BSAVA Manual of Canine and Feline Thoracic Imaging*, ed. T Schwarz and V Johnson, pp. 1–19. BSAVA Publications, Gloucester

Wallack ST (2003) *The Handbook of Veterinary Contrast Radiography*. San Diego Veterinary Imaging Inc.

Ward A and Prior J (2007) Diagnostic imaging techniques. In: *BSAVA Manual of Practical Veterinary Nursing*, ed. E Mullineaux and M Jones, pp. 229–267. BSAVA Publications, Gloucester

Weaver M and Barakzai S (2009) *Handbook of Equine Radiography*. Saunders, Philadelphia

Self-assessment questions

1. Draw simple diagrams of the construction of stationary (fixed) anode and rotating anode tube heads. Describe the design features which permit the production of higher exposures in rotating anode tubes.
2. What is scattered radiation and how is it produced? What steps may be taken to minimize the effect of scatter on radiographs?
3. Describe the stages of processing a radiographic film by the manual method. How does automatic processing differ?
4. Define the terms 'density', 'contrast' and 'definition', as applied to radiographic images.
5. What sources of radiation hazard exist in veterinary radiography? How may the potential risk to personnel involved be minimized?
6. Describe the restraint, positioning and views required for submission of hip and elbow radiographs to the BVA/KC Hip and Elbow Dysplasia Schemes.
7. What preparations are required prior to radiographing a horse's foot?
8. Describe the positioning required for obtaining a lateromedial radiograph of the stifle in a horse. What special safety measures are required?
9. Describe the techniques used for myelography in small animal practice.
10. What is the difference between linear array and sector scanning ultrasound transducers?
11. Define 'Hounsfield unit', 'window level' and 'window width', as applied to CT scan images.
12. What are the advantages and disadvantages of MRI scanning compared with CT?
13. What is the main use for scintigraphy in horses?
14. Describe the cleaning and care of endoscopic equipment following its use. How should flexible and rigid endoscopes be stored?

Chapter 19

Laboratory diagnostic aids

Gemma Irwin-Porter

Learning objectives

After studying this chapter, students should be able to:

- **Identify the requirements of a veterinary practice laboratory**
- **Demonstrate an understanding of laboratory equipment and safe working practices**
- **Explain and describe the preparation, collection, preservation and processing of laboratory samples from dogs, cats, equine species and exotic pets**
- **Explain the requirements for packaging and despatching samples to external laboratories**
- **Record the results of laboratory analysis and understand the interpretation of common findings**

Diagnostic testing and the in-house laboratory

The need for fast and accurate test results has meant that most veterinary practices are now equipped with their own laboratory with up-to-date equipment allowing staff within the practice to carry out laboratory analysis on samples immediately so that a clinical diagnosis can be made. Laboratory diagnostics carried out by the veterinary nurse allow the veterinary surgeon to make an accurate diagnosis, assess the degree of the problem and monitor the condition or treatment effectively.

The reliability of test results ultimately depends on the following factors:

- **Knowledge**: For example, have the staff been shown how to perform the diagnostic tests correctly?
- **Collection**: Was the correct gauge needle used for blood collection?
- **Preservation**: Was the correct anticoagulant used for the blood sample? Was the correct preservative used for other fluids or tissues collected for histological examination?

- **Equipment**: Has the weekly quality control been carried out on the biochemistry analyser?

Before a diagnostic test is performed:

- Check with the veterinary surgeon to confirm which test is to be carried out
- Check the patient ID and clinical history
- Check that all equipment required is present and in full working order
- Check that a safe area is available in which to perform the test
- Check that another person is available in order to assist with collection if required.

The following samples may need to be collected:

- Blood
- Urine
- Faeces
- Other bodily fluids, such as cerebrospinal fluid
- Tissue, including cells for cytology
- Skin and hair samples.

Details for each of these are given later.

After the diagnostic test has been performed:

- Label all samples with the patient ID, date and sample type
- Record that the diagnostic test has been carried out
- Record the results of the test
- Inform other members of staff of the results.

Some samples will need to be sent to external laboratories for further investigation or for more detailed procedures, requiring practice staff to package and despatch pathological samples safely (see end of chapter).

Health and safety

The veterinary practice laboratory houses many potential hazards and is therefore subject to strict health and safety protocols in line with current legislation (see also Chapter 2).

508

Relevant legislation includes:

- Health and Safety at Work etc. Act 1974
- The Control of Substances Hazardous to Health Regulations 2002 (COSHH)
- Environmental Protection Act 1990
- The Control of Pollution (Special Waste) (Amendment) Regulations 1988
- The Collection and Disposal of Waste Regulations 1988
- The Hazardous Waste (England and Wales) Regulations 2005 (amended 2009)
- The Reporting of Injuries, Diseases and Dangerous Occurrences Regulations 1995 (RIDDOR)
- Health and Safety (First Aid) Regulations 1981
- The Electrical Equipment (Safety) Regulations 1994.

In order to ensure safe working practice in the laboratory, risks and hazards must be identified and protocols developed and reviewed. Potential hazards and risks include:

- Chemicals that may have harmful effects (Figure 19.1)
- Equipment, such as electrical items
- Biological agents, including zoonoses (see Chapters 5, 6 and 7)
- Waste, including sharps
- Fumes and aerosols
- Fire/explosion
- Slips/trips/falls.

Symbol and classification	Precautions
Toxic	Wear PPE, including eye protection Rinse immediately if in contact with skin or eyes Dispose of safely
Explosive	Use only as directed Keep tightly closed, cool and in a well ventilated area Keep away from heat or ignition Dispose of safely
Flammable	Keep away from heat or ignition Keep container tightly closed away from sunlight Do not breathe vapours
Oxidizing	Use only as directed Keep tightly closed, cool and in a well ventilated area Keep away from heat or ignition Dispose of safely
Corrosive	Wear PPE, including eye protection Rinse immediately if in contact with skin or eyes Dispose of safely
Harmful	Avoid contact with skin and eyes Do not inhale vapour, dust or spray Rinse immediately if in contact with skin or eyes
Dangerous for the environment	Dispose of safely – do not empty into drains or water sources The container must also be disposed of safely

19.1 'Dangerous substances': common health hazards in the laboratory.

Staff who may be pregnant or who are immunosuppressed may be at greater risk. In order to minimize the risk to staff, risk assessments should be carried out in accordance with current legislation (see Chapter 2). A general code of conduct must be followed when working within the laboratory.

Laboratory code of conduct

- All staff must have read and understood the practice health and safety policy and specific protocols for the laboratory area.
- Entry must be restricted to authorized persons only.
- Authorized members of staff should be fully trained and supervised wherever necessary.
- Jewellery must be removed and long hair tied back.
- Personal protective equipment (PPE) (e.g. laboratory coat) must be worn whilst in the laboratory. Additional PPE should be available and worn wherever necessary, e.g. gloves, mask, goggles.
- No eating, smoking or drinking should take place within the laboratory.
- The laboratory must be kept well organized, tidy and clean.
- All hazardous items should be clearly labelled and kept secured.
- Cupboards should not be above eye level.
- A sink should be provided in the laboratory.
- Containers, chemicals and other material should all be fully labelled and datasheets available.
- All waste should be disposed of correctly.
- A well stocked and in-date first aid box must be available, including eye wash. A First Aider must also be available within the practice.
- Firefighting equipment must be available and appropriate for the area.
- Records of diagnostic tests carried out should be kept within the laboratory.
- Any accidents, spillages, etc., must be reported to a senior member of staff immediately.
- All staff should be aware of potential zoonotic risks, such as from faeces.

Disposal of laboratory waste

The disposal of waste within the laboratory is regulated by the legislation discussed in detail in Chapter 2. It is important that correct segregation, storage, removal and destruction of waste are carried out in accordance with these regulations and in line with the practice's waste collection service.

Laboratory equipment

A range of laboratory equipment may be used within the veterinary practice. In order that equipment is used safely, reliably and accurately, correct management is required.

Glassware

Glassware, such as flasks and beakers, should be thoroughly cleaned before use to avoid contamination.

Cleaning and care of laboratory glassware

1. Wear suitable PPE – this must include gloves.
2. Remove organic material/contaminants from the glassware. Appropriate soaking may be required in order to remove dried substances. A soft-bristled brush may be used to assist the removal.
3. Wash the glassware in a detergent to remove remaining organic material, grease, etc.
4. Disinfect using an approved solution for the required contact time.
5. Rinse in distilled or deionized water.
6. Allow to drain.
7. Dry in a drying cabinet or oven.
8. Ensure the glassware is thoroughly clean, free from cracks/chips and suitable for use before storage.
9. Store in a clean, dry and dust-free environment.

Microscopes

A microscope is one of the most commonly used pieces of equipment within a laboratory. A binocular microscope with a built-in light source (Figure 19.2) is the most suitable. Figure 19.3 explains the functions of the various components.

Using a binocular light microscope

1. Use PPE if necessary.
2. Remove the dust cover and ensure the microscope is plugged into an electrical socket.
3. Lower the stage to its lowest point.

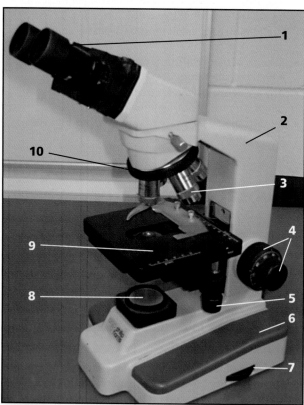

19.2 Binocular microscope with a built-in light source. **(1)** Eyepiece containing ocular lenses. **(2)** Limb. **(3)** Objective lens. **(4)** Focus knobs. **(5)** Stage control. **(6)** Base. **(7)** Rheostat. **(8)** Light source. **(9)** Stage. **(10)** Rotating nosepiece.

Component	Function
Eyepiece	The eyepiece, through which the operator views the specimen, contains ocular lenses that magnify the primary image formed by the objective lens. Typically X10
Nosepiece	The rotating nosepiece holds the objective lens
Objective lenses	There are normally four objective lenses, each with a different magnification. Typically X4, X10, X40 and X100 (oil immersion)
Stage	A flat platform that holds the microscope slide. The hole in the centre of the platform allows light to illuminate the specimen. The stage can then be moved up and down using the focus control knobs. The stage houses the mechanical stage, which allows the slide to be moved left, right, horizontally and vertically
Vernier scale	A horizontal and vertical Vernier scale allows the position of specific points of the specimen to be recorded and relocated
Substage condenser	Condenses light from the light source on to the specimen. The position of the substage condenser and the amount of light passing through it can be adjusted
Iris diaphragm	By adjusting the iris diaphragm, the amount of light passing through the condenser can be increased or decreased
Focus knobs	Coarse (larger knob) and fine focus (smaller knob) raise and lower the stage to allow the image to be focused
Rheostat	Alters the level of light produced by the light source

19.3 The main components of a microscope.

4. Adjust the substage condenser so that it is a few millimetres below the stage.
5. Move the rheostat to ensure that it is turned down low.
6. Switch on the light and turn the rheostat to allow a medium light.
7. Place the microscope slide on to the stage, using clips to hold it in position if required.
8. Move the lowest objective lens (X4) into position, ensuring it clicks firmly in place.
9. *Without looking down the eyepiece*, move the stage up until it almost touches the objective lens. Ensure that the lens does not touch the slide.
10. Look down the eyepieces and adjust the distance between them so that the two fields can be viewed as one.
11. Slowly move the stage downwards using the coarse focus control, whilst looking down the eyepiece until the image comes into view.
12. Once an image can be seen, use the fine focus control to sharpen the image.
13. In order to move to the X10 objective lens, take your eyes away from the eyepiece and slowly move the X10 objective lens into place, checking that it does not come into contact with the slide. Use the fine focus control to focus the image.
14. In order to move to the X40 objective lens take your eyes away from the eyepiece and slowly move the X40 objective lens into place, checking that it does not come into contact with the slide. Use the fine focus control to focus the image.

Using oil immersion

First, carry out steps 1 to 14 above.

1. Fully open the iris diaphragm.
2. Move the stage down and place a drop of oil on the specimen. NB Remove the coverslip first if one is in place.
3. Rotate the oil immersion lens (X100) into place.
4. *Without looking down the eyepiece*, move the stage upwards slowly until the objective lens comes into contact with the oil on the slide.
5. Look down the eyepiece and slowly focus the image using the fine focus control.

Viewing the slide

Once an image is in view, the slide/specimen must be viewed in a methodical manner. Use the 'battlement technique' to scan the slide (Figure 19.4).

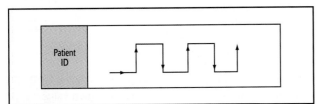

19.4 When viewing a slide, start on the left hand side. Move 3–5 fields to the right and view again; then move 3–5 fields up the slide vertically (i.e. away from you) and view again; then move 3–5 fields to the right and view again; then 3–5 fields downwards (i.e. towards you) and view again. This is continued across the slide, forming a 'battlement' pattern.

Vernier scales

The Vernier scales can be used to record the location of a particular part of an image or specimen, e.g. an ectoparasite on a skin scraping or a blood cell in a blood smear, so that it can be relocated easily on a subsequent viewing. There are two scales: the horizontal Vernier and the vertical Vernier. Both must be read and recorded, stating which is horizontal and which vertical.

Using a Vernier scale

- The stage can be lowered if needed to enable the scale to be read accurately but should not be touched again.
- For each direction, there is a main scale (marked on the stage) and a smaller, Vernier, scale located next to the main stage.
- For the main scale reading, the number on the main scale opposite the Vernier scale zero is read, i.e. 28 in the diagram below.
- For the Vernier scale reading, the point at which a line on the Vernier scale matches one on the main scale is located. Readings are taken from the Vernier scale, e.g. 4 in the diagram below.
- This will give the complete reading as 28.4 mm.

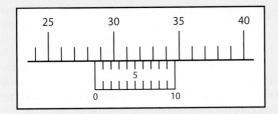

After viewing the specimen:

1. Work out the magnification factor of the image by multiplying the eyepiece lens magnification by the objective lens magnification (e.g. X10 times X40 = X400).
2. Turn down the light.
3. Lower the stage completely.
4. Remove the slide.
5. Rotate the nosepiece to the lowest objective lens.
6. Move the stage up but do not touch any of the lenses.
7. Switch off the light.
8. Remove the plug from the electrical socket.
9. Clean the microscope, including the lenses.
10. Replace the dust cover.

Microscope care and cleaning

- The microscope must be stored in a safe position away from water, moisture and excessive heat.
- The base must be supported during lifting of the microscope.
- The microscope must never be pulled or pushed along a surface; it should instead be lifted and placed where required.
- The microscope must be cleaned regularly, using a suitable disinfectant.
- Lenses should be wiped with lens tissue.
- Safety checks must be carried out regularly, including electrical testing.
- The light must never be left on for long periods of time.

Centrifuges

A centrifuge uses centrifugal force to separate substances of varying densities. Dense particles such as solids will settle to the bottom of the sample; this is known as the **sediment**. The less dense liquid portion will remain at the surface; this is known as the **supernatant**. There are two types of centrifuge:

- **Angle-head**: This is the most common type of centrifuge. Tubes are held in a fixed position, usually at 40 degrees from vertical (Figure 19.5a). Care must be taken when removing the sample from the fixed angle position.
- **Swing-out head**: The specimen starts in the vertical position. As the rotor turns the head, the specimen buckets swing out (Figure 19.5b). Once the centrifuge slows and eventually stops, the buckets revert to the vertical position.

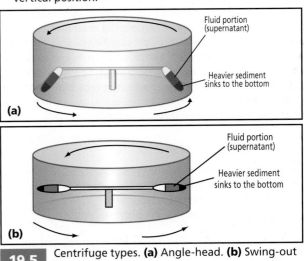

19.5 Centrifuge types. **(a)** Angle-head. **(b)** Swing-out head.

A microhaematocrit centrifuge has a special type of rotor consisting of individual slots on a horizontal surface for holding capillary tubes (Figure 19.6).

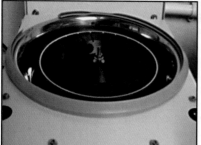

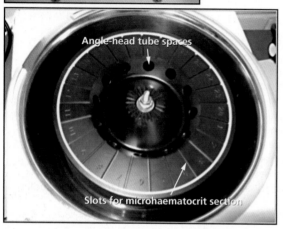

19.6 Angle-head centrifuge with a section for microhaematocrit tubes.

Using a centrifuge

- Always use the centrifuge on a flat surface.
- Make sure the safety plate in the lid is secure before turning on.
- Always balance the samples around the machine.
- Select the most appropriate speed for the sample and the centrifuge. As a guide:
  - Urine: 2000 rpm for 5 minutes
  - Blood: 10,000 rpm for 5 minutes
- Never lift the lid whilst the centrifuge is still rotating.
- Clean the whole centrifuge after each use.
- The centrifuge must be serviced regularly.

Analysers

Biochemistry, haematology, electrolyte and hormone analysers are the types found most commonly in veterinary practices. There are a variety of commercial machines available and most manufacturers provide specific training for staff. Analysers can provide quick and reliable results and avoid the delay of sending to external laboratories. This is particularly important in urgent cases, such as severe haemorrhage (packed cell volume (PCV) can be measured quickly in house), severe metabolic disturbances, or organ failure.

All analysers should:

- Be kept in a safe and secure position
- Be used in accordance with manufacturer's instructions by trained personnel
- Be serviced regularly by the provider, including electrical testing
- Have quality control performed regularly for reliable results.

Quality control and quality assurance

Quality control and quality assurance procedures must be carried out on any analyser used within the in-house laboratory.

- **Quality control** (QC) refers to the measures that must be included during each assay run, in order to verify that the test is working properly.
- **Quality assurance** (QA) is defined as the overall programme which ensures that the final results reported by the laboratory are correct. QA includes ensuring that the right test is carried out on the right specimen, and that the right result and right interpretation is delivered to the right person at the right time.

Analyser quality control should ideally be carried out:

- At the beginning of each shift or day
- After an analyser is serviced
- When reagent lots are changed
- After calibration
- When patient results seem inappropriate
- As indicated by the manufacturer.

Manufacturers produce QC products for each of their analysers. These consist of samples with known values, e.g. biochemical ranges, which can then be compared to the results formulated by the in-house analyser. Any inconsistencies in the results produced from the machine should be reported to the manufacturer.

In addition to internal QC procedures, QA through referral of internal samples to external laboratories, or internal analysis of external samples, should be routinely undertaken and results documented. The frequency of external QA testing should be related to the number of tests undertaken. This is likely to be at least quarterly.

Biochemistry analysers

These measure levels of biochemical substances (e.g. calcium, glucose) contained within a patient's blood. There are two types of machine.

- **Dry chemistry analysers:** These use slides impregnated with chemicals. The machine drops the sample on to the slides and then reads and interprets the colour change. The colour change reflects the level of the substance in the patient sample.
- **Wet chemistry analysers:** These use containers of wet fluids. The machine uses chemical reactions to determine the levels in the sample.

Some biochemical analysers have additional functions such as hormone analysis, e.g. T4 (thyroxine) levels.

Haematology analysers

These quickly determine the quantities and types of red and white blood cells within a blood sample (see below).

Electrolyte analysers

These can vary from large in-house laboratory analysers to hand-held portable analysers. They are able to give rapid results on the levels of electrolytes (e.g. Na^+, K^+, Cl^-) in a sample. Some machines can be used for additional tests, such as measuring blood gas levels, which can be extremely important in critical care patients and during general anaesthesia.

Blood

Sample collection

Preparation and equipment

Preparation is important prior to blood collection in order to obtain accurate results. Before the patient is restrained, all equipment should be prepared. The following is required for venepuncture:

- Syringe of appropriate size (smallest size possible to reduce the pressure and avoid rupturing red blood cells)
- Needle of appropriate size (largest gauge possible to avoid rupturing red blood cells)
- Materials for skin preparation (chlorhexidine and surgical spirit)
- Cotton wool or swab to assist in skin preparation
- Clippers or scissors to remove hair
- Receptacle, e.g. blood tube, vacutainer (see Figure 19.10 for colour coding)
- Dry swab for applying pressure after venepuncture
- Gloves.

Venepuncture

Sites for venepuncture are given in Figure 19.7. Restraint of the patient is described in Chapters 8 and 10.

Species/group	Veins used for blood sample collection
Dog	Cephalic, jugular, lateral saphenous
Cat	Jugular, cephalic, lateral saphenous
Rabbit	Jugular, cephalic, lateral saphenous, marginal ear
Horse	Jugular, lateral saphenous, cephalic, lateral thoracic (rarely), transverse facial (small volume only)
Birds	Jugular, medial metatarsal, alar
Tortoises	Subcarapacial, jugular, dorsal tail
Lizards	Jugular, cephalic, ventral tail (only in larger species)
Snakes	Jugular, ventral tail

19.7 Common sites for venepuncture in a range of species.

Technique for needle venepuncture

1. Assemble the equipment required. Ensure equipment such as the needle and syringe are sterile and assembled aseptically. Ensure the plunger is pre-released on the syringe. It is also useful to pre-label blood collection tubes.
2. Ensure correct identification of patient.
3. Confirm the tests/sample required from the patient.
4. Request assistance from a colleague to restrain the patient. The restraint technique will vary depending on the species and site used for venepuncture (Figure 19.8).
5. Put gloves on.
6. Prepare the venepuncture site aseptically. This may involve clipping in mammalian species.
7. Depending on the venepuncture site, ask the assistant to occlude the vein if required. ▶

8. Once the vein is visible, insert the needle into the vein at a slight angle from the skin surface.
9. Once in the vein, pull back gently on the syringe plunger, allowing blood to fill the syringe barrel.
10. Once the required volume has been collected, remove the needle slowly from the vein. The assistant should then use the dry swab to apply pressure on the collection site.
11. Remove the needle from the syringe and dispose of it as hazardous sharps waste.
12. Transfer the sample to the desired collection tube. If the sample tube contains an anticoagulant, the blood tube filled with blood should be gently inverted to ensure mixing.
13. Label the blood tube with the patient ID and date of sample collection if this has not already been done.
14. Dispose of the used syringe and pressure swab as hazardous waste.
15. Monitor the patient for signs of haemorrhage.

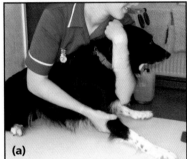 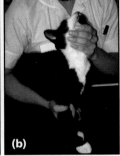

(a) (b)

19.8 (a) Restraint of a dog for cephalic venepuncture. (b) Restraint of a cat for jugular venepuncture.

Collecting a blood sample from a horse

Blood can be collected using either a hypodermic needle and syringe or a vacutainer.

1. The horse must be appropriately restrained.
2. Raise the jugular vein by applying pressure to the neck.
3. Clip the hair over the site.
4. Clean the site with surgical spirit.
5. If using a vacutainer, connect the vacutainer to the needle and holder without breaking the vacuum, i.e. with the needle partially within the bung.
6. Gently insert the needle, bevel uppermost and parallel to the vein, through the skin and into the vein.
7. If using a vacutainer, advance the tube into the holder, so the needle fully penetrates the bung. Hold whilst blood enters the chamber (Figure 19.9).
8. Remove the needle from the vein and apply pressure. Separate any vacutainer from its needle and holder.
9. Invert tube or vacutainer gently if it contains anticoagulant.
10. Dispose of the needle as hazardous waste.
11. Label the blood tube or vacutainer with the patient's ID and date of sample collection, if this has not already been done.

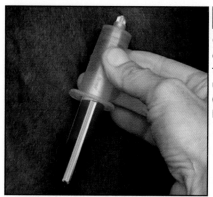

19.9

Collection of equine blood from the jugular vein using a vacutainer. (Courtesy of B&W Equine Group)

The sample will settle if allowed to stand, so it is important that the sample is mixed gently before it is used.

Sample preservation

The preservation method chosen is dependent upon the required diagnostic test. In order to preserve a sample, the following can be used:

- A receptacle containing an anticoagulant
- A receptacle containing no anticoagulant, allowing the sample to clot so that the serum can be removed (see Figure 19.11)
- Preparation of a blood smear that can be viewed with a microscope.

Anticoagulants

Anticoagulants prevent blood clotting (see Figure 19.11). A collection tube with the appropriate anticoagulant for the diagnostic test to be carried out must be selected (Figure 19.10). Incorrect selection can result in inaccurate results.

- For routine haematology EDTA (ethylenediamine tetra-acetic acid) is used. The benefit of this anticoagulant is that it causes minimal changes in the morphology of the blood cells, thus making it useful for blood smears and cell counts. It is not suitable, however, for avian or reptile blood samples.
- Samples for glucose estimation are collected into a tube containing fluoride/oxalate or into a vacutainer that inhibits the oxidation of glucose.
- Heparin salts may be used for blood samples to undergo other biochemical tests where plasma is required.

Heparin salts (sodium, ammonium and lithium) bind and inhibit thrombin, thus preventing the formation of clots. Samples with heparin may also be used for various hormone tests.

Serum samples

Serum is obtained from a clotted sample (without anticoagulant; Figure 19.11). Serum does not contain clotting factors, such as fibrinogen, as they have been used in forming the blood clot. Serum may be extracted from a clotted sample and used in house or sent to an external laboratory. Separated serum can be stored in a refrigerator for a few days and in some cases the separated serum may be frozen and then thawed to room temperature before use. The appearance of serum and plasma can be affected by various factors (Figure 19.12).

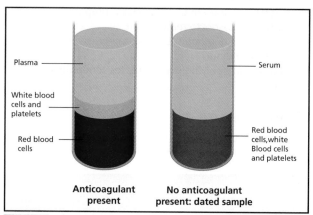

19.11 The individual components of a blood sample can be seen once it has been centrifuged. Plasma is obtained from samples collected into tubes containing anticoagulant. Serum is obtained from a clotted sample (no anticoagulant).

Colour	Reason for change
Pink/red	Haemolysed sample – red blood cells have been damaged due to incorrect sampling or preservation
Yellow	Icteric sample – the colour change is caused by the presence of bilirubin, which indicates liver damage
Milky white	Lipaemic sample – due to the presence of fat in unstarved animals or evidence of liver disease

19.12 The colour of a serum or plasma sample may vary, for a number of reasons.

Anticoagulant	Tube cap colour	Vacutainer cap colour	Used for
Lithium heparin	orange	green	Biochemistry
Ethylenediamine tetra-acetic acid (EDTA)	pink	mauve	Haematology
Fluoride/oxalate	yellow	grey	Glucose
Sodium/lithium citrate	blue	blue	Coagulation profiles
No anticoagulant	white brown	red	Serum collection

19.10 Common anticoagulants used in blood collection containers.

Blood smears

A blood smear, or blood film as it is sometimes known, is a method by which blood is spread across a glass slide. The method is used to produce a sample that may be sent to an external laboratory or used in house to be examined for a differential white blood cell count or cellular abnormalities. Blood smears are an important tool, even in practices with haematology analysers, as they can detect cell abnormalities and inclusions not detected by an automatic analyser.

Preparation of a blood smear

1. Put on gloves.
2. Select a microscope slide and clean it using ethanol or absolute alcohol (methanol) and dry with lint-free tissue.
3. Select a blood sample containing EDTA.
4. Gently mix the sample.
5. Insert a plain capillary tube into the blood sample and draw up a small amount of blood into the tube.
6. Place a finger over the top of the tube or keep the tube horizontal to prevent leakage of blood.
7. Remove the tube and place a dot of blood near one end of the slide.
8. Discard the capillary tube as hazardous waste.
9. Select a spreader slide.
10. Holding the blood sample slide firmly on the work surface, place the spreader on the opposite end of the slide to the blood.

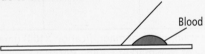

11. Draw the spreader back into the drop of blood at an angle of 45 degrees and allow blood to spread along the edge of the spreader.

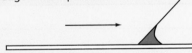

12. Push the spreader away from the blood drop using a single, smooth motion.

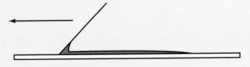

13. Rapidly air-dry the slide.
14. Label the slide.
15. Check and comment on the quality of the smear.

The final blood smear should look like a thumbprint with a feathered edge (Figure 19.13) and should be of equal thickness. Common faults include hesitation bands, grease spots, thick/thin smears and uneven smears. Faults can be avoided through correct preparation and technique.

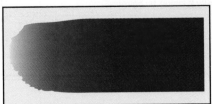

19.13

Correct appearance of a blood smear.

Staining

Smears are then stained prior to examination to distinguish individual cells and to identify cellular abnormalities. There are two common types of stain used for blood smears in veterinary practice:

*   **Romanowsky stain** – e.g. Leishman's, Giemsa, Diff-Quik. These stains can be used when performing a differential white blood cell count. They will also detect the presence of blood parasites such as *Babesia*.
*   **Supravital stain** – e.g. methylene blue. Supravital stains can be used for smears that are to be used to perform a reticulocyte count. They will also detect Heinz bodies.

Staining procedures

Leishman's

1. Put on gloves.
2. Place slide on staining rack with smear uppermost.
3. Cover with Leishman's stain and leave for 2 minutes.
4. Add twice the stain's volume of buffered distilled water pH 6.8 and gently mix using a Pasteur pipette.
5. Leave for 10–15 minutes.
6. Wash the slide with buffered distilled water pH 6.8.
7. Allow slide to dry.

Giemsa

1. Put on gloves.
2. Fix the slide by dipping in methanol for 1 minute.
3. Flood the slide with diluted Giemsa stain and leave for 30 minutes.
4. Rinse the slide with distilled water.
5. Allow slide to dry.

Diff-Quik

1. Put on gloves.
2. Dip slide into the fixative (methanol) solution (pale blue) five times. Allow excess fluid to drip back into the jar.
3. Dip slide into stain (eosin) solution (red) five times. Allow excess fluid to drip back into the jar.
4. Dip slide into stain (methylene blue) solution 2 (purple) five times. Allow excess fluid to drip back into the jar.
5. Rinse slide with distilled water.
6. Place slide vertically and leave to dry.

Once the slide has been correctly stained and is dry, examination can be carried out. The smear should be examined under X10, X40 and X100 (with oil immersion) objectives.

Blood smear examination
Blood cell morphology

Qualitative examination should be carried out first. This involves examination of red blood cells (RBCs, erythrocytes), white blood cells (WBCs, leucocytes) and thrombocytes (platelets) for morphological abnormalities. Normal blood cell morphology is shown in Figure 19.14 and in Chapter 3. Erythrocyte abnormalities are described and illustrated in Figures 19.15 to 19.17.

Cell type	Normal appearance	Description	Role/ Significance	Reference values (number of cells per litre of blood or percentage of white blood cells)		
				Cat	Dog	Horse
Erythrocyte		Pink, biconcave disc with no nucleus	Transport of blood gases	$5–10 \times 10^{12}$/l	$5.5–8.5 \times 10^{12}$/l	$6–11 \times 10^{12}$/l
Mature neutrophil		Multi-lobed nucleus, pale granules in cytoplasm	Phagocytosis	60%	70%	45–65%
Immature neutrophil		Horseshoe-shaped nucleus	Phagocytosis	Variable	Variable	No data
Eosinophil		Pink granules with bilobed or segmented nucleus	Increased in parasitic conditions	4%	$0.1–1.25 \times 10^9$/l	0–3%
Basophil		Irregular nucleus with blue granular cytoplasm	Increased in allergic reactions	Rare	Rare	Rare
Lymphocyte		Larger cells, nucleus occupies majority of cell	Immune response: B cells and T cells	30%	20%	36–49%
Monocyte		Horseshoe-shaped nucleus. Larger cells. No granules in cytoplasm	Phagocytosis	3%	5%	0–6%
Thrombocyte (platelet)		Very small cells	Clotting	200×10^9/l	200×10^9/l	120–220 $\times 10^9$/l

19.14   Normal blood cell morphology and numbers. (Modified Wright's stain, original magnification X100) (Images courtesy of Axiom Laboratories. Equine reference ranges courtesy of Newmarket Equine Hospital.)

Abnormality		Description
Size	Macrocyte	Larger than normal
	Microcyte	Smaller than normal
	Anisocytosis	Great variation in size of cells
Shape	Crenation (crenellation)	Distortion giving a spiky appearance (Figure 19.16a). Caused by damage to the cell. Seen in patients with autoimmune haemolytic anaemia
	Schistocyte	Red blood cell fragment (Figure 19.16b)
	Spherocyte	Spherical (Figure 19.16c)
	Rouleaux (normal in the equine patient)	Individual cells are of normal shape but cells are stacked and formed into chains (Figure 19.16d)
Colour	Hypochromasia	Reduced cellular haemoglobin, giving paler appearance
	Polychromasia	Larger bluer cells (Romanowsky stain). Often seen in regenerative anaemia
Inclusions	Heinz bodies	Blue (Supravital stain) and granular in appearance; formed from denatured haemoglobin
	Howell–Jolly bodies	Basophilic nuclear remnants seen in young red blood cells (Figure 19.17a). Seen in regenerative anaemia and after splenectomy
	Babesia	Parasite transmitted by ticks. Detected using Romanowsky staining techniques
	Mycoplasma haemofelis	Parasite causing feline infectious anaemia
Immaturity	Reticulocyte	Immature red blood cells (anuclear) with stainable cytoplasmic RNA (blue cytoplasm, Supravital stain) (Figure 19.17b)

19.15   Abnormalities of red blood cells.

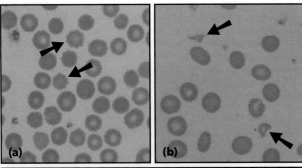

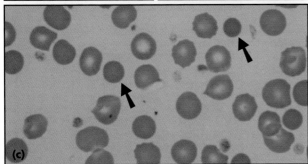

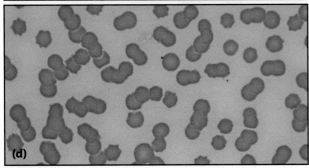

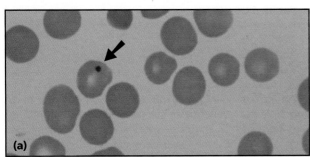

19.16 Abnormally shaped erythrocytes:
(a) crenated; **(b)** schistocytes; **(c)** spherocytes;
(d) rouleaux. (Modified Wright's stain; a, b and c, original
magnification X100; d, original magnification X50)
(Courtesy of Axiom Laboratories)

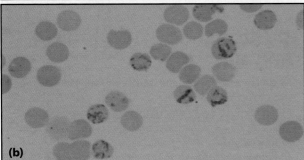

19.17 Erythrocytes with inclusions: **(a)** Howell–Jolly
body (Wright's stain); **(b)** canine reticulocytes
(new methylene blue) (original magnifications X100).
(Courtesy of Axiom Laboratories)

Common abnormalities in white blood cells include:

- **Toxic neutrophils:** Blue/pink cytoplasm with blue cell inclusions
- **Left shift:** Increase in the number of immature neutrophils. Indicates the presence of an inflammatory condition.

White blood cell counts

A differential white blood cell count is performed to determine the relative proportions of the different cell types (see Figure 19.14 for normal values). The procedure is time-consuming but can be a crucial aid to diagnosis in practices that do not have a haematology analyser.

- The main body of the smear is examined under oil immersion.
- Cells are counted and recorded using a standard manual laboratory counter or using an electronic tabulator. If these are not available a tally chart can be used.
- Usually 100 cells are counted, so that the number of each cell counted can be expressed as a percentage.

Once the quantitative analysis of the smear has been carried out, the results must be correctly recorded and passed to the veterinary surgeon who will interpret the results (Figure 19.18).

Cells counted	Increase and possible causes	Decrease and possible causes
All white blood cells	**Leucocytosis:** Presence of infection, neoplasia, haemorrhage	**Leucopenia:** Severe bacterial infection/sepsis, some viral disease, Cushing's disease, bone marrow suppression
Neutrophils	**Neutrophilia:** Bacterial infection, inflammation, stress, neoplasia	**Neutropenia:** Severe bacterial infections, some viral infections, cytotoxic medications, bone marrow disorders
Eosinophils	**Eosinophilia:** Allergic reactions, parasitism	**Eosinopenia:** Cushing's disease, corticosteroid therapy
Basophils	**Basophilia:** Rare, sometimes seen with allergy, parasitism or neoplasia	**Basopenia:** Basophils rare in all common domestic animals. Therefore basopenia difficult to document and of no diagnostic significance
Lymphocytes	**Lymphocytosis:** Chronic disease, exercise/ excitement, stress, lymphoproliferative disease	**Lymphopenia:** Cushing's disease, corticosteroid therapy, acute viral or bacterial infection
Monocytes	**Monocytosis:** Infection/ inflammation, steroids/ stress, immune-mediated conditions	**Monopenia:** Rare

19.18 Interpretation of quantitative analysis of white blood cells.

Packed cell volume

Packed cell volume (PCV) (also known as the **haematocrit**) is the percentage of the total blood volume that is occupied by red blood cells. This quick and easy test rapidly gives information on hydration status, level of blood loss in haemorrhaging patients, or degree of anaemia.

Preparing a PCV sample

1. Put on gloves.
2. Select a blood sample with EDTA.
3. Mix the sample gently.
4. Insert a plain microhaematocrit tube into the sample (holding the sample tube at an angle) and fill the tube to at least three-quarters full by capillary action.
5. Place a finger over the top end of the tube or keep the tube horizontal.
6. Remove the tube from the sample.
7. Wipe the outside of the tube with a tissue.
8. Plug one end of the tube with soft clay sealant.
9. Place the tube into the microhaematocrit centrifuge with the clay plug against the rim.
10. Screw the inner safety lid down over the samples.
11. Close and lock the main lid.
12. Set at 10,000 rpm (or fast setting, depending on make of centrifuge) for 5 minutes.
13. Dispose of any used capillary tubes and other used materials as hazardous waste.

Once the microhaematocrit tube has been centrifuged the blood will have separated into three layers (Figure 19.19).

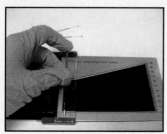

19.19 Layers of a centrifuged sample in a microhaematocrit tube for PCV evaluation. The buffy coat layer contains the white blood cells and platelets. (Reproduced from *BSAVA Manual of Canine and Feline Clinical Pathology, 2nd edn*)

Ideally, the PCV should be read using a Hawksley microhaematocrit reader. If one is not available a ruler can be used along with the following calculation:

PCV (%) = (height of red blood cells/total column height) × 100

Using a Hawksley reader

1. Place the tube into the slot in the reader, with the sealed end downwards.
2. Align the top of the seal, i.e. the bottom of the red blood cell layer, with the zero line on the reader.

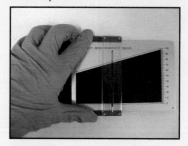

3. Move the tube holder across until the top of the plasma is lined up with the 100% line on the reader.

4. Move the adjustable PCV reading line to intersect the top of the RBC layer.

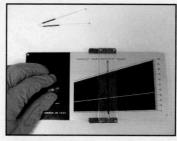

5. Record the PCV reading correctly as a percentage.

Reference ranges for dogs, cats and horses are given in Figure 19.20. It is important to note that in all species, and especially in horses, PCV readings vary significantly with breed, age and fitness. Equine neonates have a normal PCV range of 40–52%, which will decrease with age. Greyhounds have significantly higher numbers of red blood cells than other breeds of dog, which is one reason why they are often popular as blood donors. Reference ranges for some exotic pets are as follows:

- Mouse 39–49 %
- Rat 36–54%
- Hamster 40–61%
- Guinea pig 37–48%
- Birds 35–55%
- Reptiles 20–40%.

An *increase* in PCV may indicate dehydration due to reduced plasma levels, but an increase is also present in other conditions such as endotoxic shock and splenic contraction. A *decrease* in PCV may indicate anaemia or haemorrhage, due to a decrease in the number of red blood cells.

Additional haematological analysis

- **Mean corpuscular volume (MCV)** indicates the average size of the red blood cells.
- **Mean corpuscular haemoglobin concentration (MCHC)** indicates the average haemoglobin concentration per red blood cell.
- **Haemoglobin (Hb)** estimations indicate the level of haemoglobin found in the red blood cells.

All these parameters are provided by automated haematology analysers. Reference ranges are shown in Figure 19.20.

Species	RBC count (10¹²/l)	WBC count (10⁹/l)	PCV (%)	Hb (g/dl)	MCV (fl)	MCHC (g/dl)
Dog	5.5–8.5	6–17	37–55	12—18	60–70	32—36
Cat	5–10	5.5–19.5	24–45	9—17	39–55	30—36
Horse	6–11	5.5–10	30–49	12–16	37–50	34–37

19.20 Reference ranges of haematological values for dogs, cats and horses. For values in exotic pets please refer to relevant BSAVA Manuals. (Equine data courtesy of Newmarket Equine Hospital)

Blood clotting (coagulation) tests

Thrombocytes assist in haemostasis through the coagulation of blood. Blood clotting analysis can be a vital test in the diagnosis and treatment of many conditions, such as von Willebrand's disease and warfarin poisoning. The normal clotting time of blood is usually 1–2 minutes. Buccal mucosal bleeding time, activated clotting time and thrombocyte counts can all be used to determine the animal's coagulation profile.

- **Buccal mucosal bleeding time** (BMBT; Figure 19.21): A commercially available kit is available to create a small incision in the mucosa – normally in the patient's inner lip. Blotting paper or tissue is held against the incision and a timer used to calculate the length of time taken for it to stop bleeding.
- **Activated clotting time** (ACT): This is measured by placing 1 ml of whole blood into a small glass tube or ACT tube. The tube should be kept at 37°C. The time is recorded from aspiration to the formation of the first clot.
- **Thrombocyte counts** are performed by haematology analysers.

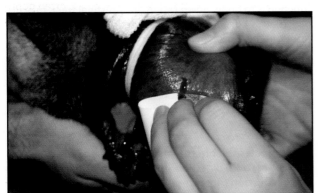

19.21 A veterinary nurse performing a buccal mucosal bleeding time test. Note the upper lip is everted by a bandage; filter paper is used to absorb excess blood without disturbing the primary clot. (Reproduced from *BSAVA Manual of Advanced Veterinary Nursing, 2nd edn.*)

Blood biochemistry

Biochemical parameters are used in the diagnosis of many conditions (see Figure 19.10 re blood sample containers and anticoagulants required for different tests). A variety of methods can be used to measure biochemical parameters:

- In-house biochemistry analyser
- External laboratory
- Commercial test strips
- Hand-held analyser.

It is important to note that precise reference ranges for biochemical parameters vary for each laboratory and also that regular quality assurance tests must be carried out on biochemistry analysers to ensure that reliable results are produced (see above). Figure 19.22 provides some common biochemical reference ranges for the cat and dog. Figure 19.23 provides these for the horse.

Biochemical parameter	Dogs	Cats
Albumin (g/l)	25–40	25–40
Alanine aminotransferase (ALT) (IU/l)	10–75	35–134
Alkaline phosphatase (ALP) (IU/l)	0–80	15–96
Blood urea nitrogen (mmol/l)	2.5–7	5–11
Calcium (mmol/l)	2–3	1.8–3
Cholesterol (mmol/l)	2.5–8	2–6.5
Creatinine (µmol/l)	40–130	40–130
Glucose (mmol/l)	3.3–6	3.3–6
Pancreatic amylase (IU/l)	350–1200	515–2210
Phosphate (mmol/l)	0.8–1.6	1.3–2.6
Total bilirubin (µmol/l)	1.7–10	2–5
Total protein (g/l)	54–71	54–78

19.22 Representative reference ranges for common biochemical tests in dogs and cats. Note that precise reference ranges vary from laboratory to laboratory.

Biochemical parameter	Equine reference range
Albumin (g/l)	25–35
Alkaline phosphatase (ALP) (IU/l)	250–400
Aspartate aminotransferase (AST) (IU/l)	150–600
Bilirubin (µmol/l)	20–50
Calcium (mmol/l)	1.3–1.7
Creatine phosphate kinase (CPK) (IU/l)	100–300
Creatinine (µmol/l)	80–150
Gamma-glutamyl transferase (GGT) (IU/l)	20–60
Globulin (g/l)	25–35
Intestinal alkaline phosphatase (IU/l)	70–100
Potassium (mmol/l)	3–4.5
Sodium (mmol/l)	128–142
Total protein (g/l)	55–70
Urea (mmol/l)	3–8

19.23 Representative reference ranges for common biochemical tests in horses. Note that precise reference ranges vary from laboratory to laboratory. (Data courtesy of Newmarket Equine Hospital)

Ammonia

Ammonia is a result of the metabolism of protein and should be excreted. Elevated levels in blood may be associated with portosystemic shunts. High concentrations of ammonium can cause neurological problems.

Blood urea nitrogen

Blood urea nitrogen (**BUN**) is a waste product formed by the liver and excreted by the kidneys as a result of amino acid metabolism. Elevated BUN can occur as a result of infection, necrosis, metabolic disease, high-protein diet, chronic heart failure, urethral obstruction, renal failure, ruptured bladder, or corticosteroid therapy. Decreases in BUN can occur as a result of low-protein diet, anabolic steroids, liver failure or portosystemic shunts.

Normal BUN levels are as follows:

* Dogs: 2.5–7 mmol/l
* Cats: 5–11 mmol/l
* Horses: 3–8 mmol/l.

Calcium

The majority of calcium is found in bone and it is also involved in the maintenance of neuromuscular function. Calcium concentrations are usually related to phosphorus concentrations. Increased levels of calcium may occur in parathyroid gland disease, renal disease and some types of neoplasia. It is important to note that EDTA or citrate anticoagulants will affect the calcium result produced by the analyser.

Cholesterol

Cholesterol is a plasma lipoprotein that is produced primarily in the liver, but is also obtained from food. An increase in cholesterol may be seen in patients with diabetes mellitus, hypothyroidism, hyperadrenocorticism, liver disease and renal disease and also in post-feeding samples. Decreases may be seen in patients with maldigestion, malabsorption and severe hepatic insufficiency.

Creatinine

Creatinine is formed from creatine, which is found in skeletal muscle. Creatinine diffuses out of the muscle cell and into most body fluids, including blood. In normal conditions the creatinine is filtered through the glomeruli in the kidney and is eliminated in urine. Creatinine is not an accurate indicator of early kidney function compromise because approximately 75% of the kidney tissue must be non-functional before elevated blood creatinine levels are seen.

Creatine phosphokinase (CPK)

The highest levels of CPK are found in skeletal and cardiac muscle and brain tissue. When muscle cells become damaged CPK is excreted into the blood. The most common cause of a rise in blood CPK in small animals are muscle disorders such as exertional hyperthermia. Hypothyroidism, heart disease, recent exercise prior to a blood test, selenium/vitamin E deficiencies and trauma to the muscles may also contribute to a rise in the CPK value.

In horses, CPK testing is used in association with aspartate aminotransferase (AST, see above) as a useful indicator of muscle cell damage in conditions such as exertional rhabdomyolysis or post-anaesthetic myopathy. When monitoring muscle damage, a peak of plasma CPK is typically seen within 6 hours, which then rapidly decreases in concentration. AST serum concentrations will typically peak at 24 hours but will then continue to remain high for at least 7 days.

Glucose and fructosamine

Glucose is the main source of energy for cells in the body and its concentration is controlled by the hormones insulin and glucagon. Elevated levels may be seen in diabetes mellitus, hyperadrenocorticism, corticosteroid therapy, stress and pancreatitis and in post-feeding samples. Decreased levels may be seen in hepatic insufficiency, hypoadrenocorticism, neoplasia, malabsorption, starvation or insulin treatment.

Animals with diabetes mellitus may have a disturbance in the oxidation and use of glucose for energy production. This may be secondary to decreased production or release of insulin by beta-cells in the pancreatic islets of Langerhans, or due to an abnormal tissue response to the presence of insulin.

Fructosamine is formed by the glycosylation of circulating proteins and is related to circulating glucose concentration. Fructosamine measurement can aid in the diagnosis of diabetes mellitus and in the ongoing assessment of blood glucose in diabetic patients. Fructosamine results must be evaluated in the context of the patient's total clinical findings. Falsely low fructosamine results may be seen with decreased blood total protein and/or albumin levels, with conditions associated with increased protein loss, or with changes in the type of protein produced by the body. In this case, a discrepancy between the results obtained from daily glucose monitoring and fructosamine testing may be noticed.

Lipase

Lipase is a water-soluble enzyme secreted by the pancreas. Its function is to break down fats in the intestinal tract. In acute pancreatitis (see Chapter 20), destruction of pancreatic tissue results in the escape of pancreatic enzymes into the pancreas and peritoneal cavity. The enzymes enter the blood by way of lymphatics or capillaries with subsequent elevation of serum levels. Lipase levels may also be increased by kidney disease and corticosteroid drugs.

Pancreatic amylase

This is a water-soluble enzyme secreted by the pancreas. It is involved in starch digestion. In acute pancreatitis (see Chapter 20), destruction of pancreatic tissue results in the escape of pancreatic enzymes into the pancreas and peritoneal cavity. The enzymes enter the blood by way of lymphatics or capillaries with subsequent elevation of serum levels. Pancreatic amylase levels may also be increased in intestinal disease.

Phosphate

Phosphate levels are very closely linked with calcium levels (see above). Increased levels are seen in renal insufficiency in cats and dogs.

Total bilirubin

Bilirubin is formed from the breakdown of haemoglobin and is a component of bile. Elevated levels may be seen in haemolytic anaemia, liver disease and biliary obstruction. An animal with an elevated bilirubin level may appear icteric (jaundiced; see Chapter 20).

Liver enzymes and liver function tests

- **Alanine aminotransferase (ALT)** is found within the cytoplasm of the hepatocyte, as well as in renal cells, cardiac muscle, skeletal muscle and pancreas. Alterations in ALT levels can be indicative of damage/disease of the aforementioned areas, as the enzyme escapes from damaged cells. Administration of corticosteroids and anticonvulsants may also lead to increases in ALT.
- **Alkaline phosphatase (ALP)** is widely distributed in the body, including liver, intestines and bone. Younger animals have naturally higher levels due to the growth and development of bone. Elevated levels of ALP may indicate liver disease or hyperadrenocorticism. Corticosteroids can also cause elevated levels in dogs and cats.
- **Aspartate aminotransferase (AST)** is found in the liver, red blood cells and in muscle tissue. Increases in blood levels can reflect muscle damage or liver disease.
- **Gamma-glutamyl transferase (GGT):** Alterations in levels may indicate liver disease/cholestasis. Particularly useful in horses.
- **Glutamate dehydrogenase (GLDH):** A liver-specific enzyme that can indicate acute liver damage. Particularly useful in horses.
- **Lactate dehydrogenase (LDH):** Not liver-specific, but can be useful when measured with other liver enzymes.
- **Sorbitol dehydrogenase (SDH):** A liver-specific enzyme that can indicate acute and current liver damage in horses (and cattle).

The biochemical assays described above may indicate liver cell damage and bile stasis (cholestasis) but they are not necessarily good measures of liver function. Albumin and ammonia levels (see below) may reflect abnormalities in liver function, as may measurement of blood clotting factors. The most commonly used liver function test is the measurement of bile acids, often as part of a bile acid stimulation test (see below). Liver biopsy (see later) is, however, often the only definitive way to diagnose liver disease.

Following a fatty meal the normal gall bladder contracts and releases bile acids into the duodenum, to allow emulsification and absorption of fats. Bile acids are then reabsorbed from the small intestine, via the portal blood stream and into the hepatocytes. In normal animals this process is very efficient, with only low levels of bile acids being present in the bloodstream after a meal. Liver dysfunction or shunting of blood away from the liver can result in high post-feeding bile acid levels.

Bile acid stimulation test

1. Fast the animal for 12 hours.
2. Collect about 1–2 ml of blood into a plain (serum) tube.
3. Feed a fatty meal – puppy or kitten food is good. If the pet is not eating, give it vegetable oil carefully by syringe.
4. Take a second sample of blood into a plain (serum) tube 2 hours after eating.

Plasma proteins

Total protein

Total *plasma* protein measurements include fibrinogen, whereas total *serum* protein levels do not as it is used in the clotting process. Elevated TP levels may occur as a result of dehydration, immune-mediated disease, lactation, infection or neoplasia. Decreased levels may occur as a result of renal disease, haemorrhage, malnutrition, malabsorption, hepatic insufficiency or pancreatic insufficiency.

Albumin

Albumin is one of the most important proteins in plasma or serum, making up 35–50% of the total plasma protein in most animals. Hepatocytes synthesize albumin, and levels may therefore be influenced by liver disease. In addition, intestinal disease and kidney disease can lead to loss of albumin from the blood.

Globulins

Globulin concentration is usually calculated by subtracting albumin from total protein. Specific measurements of specific immunoglobulins are useful in determining the immune status of the patient. IgG test kits are routinely used to assess the immunity of neonatal foals following antibody transfer in the mare's colostrum.

Electrolytes and acid–base balance

Electrolytes are the negative ions and positive ions found in body fluids. Their functions (Figure 19.24) include water balance in the body. Serious consequences can follow even relatively small changes in their absolute or relative levels (acid–base balance, see Chapter 22). Measurements of electrolyte concentrations are used in the diagnosis and management of many conditions, including renal, endocrine and metabolic disorders. Electrolytes commonly measured are sodium (Na^+), potassium (K^+), chloride (Cl^-) and bicarbonate HCO_3^-.

Electrolyte	Importance	Causes of increase	Causes of decrease
Sodium (Na^+)	Water distribution; osmotic pressure maintenance; temperature control	Intestinal disease Kidney disease	Hypoadrenocorticism Intestinal disease
Potassium (K^+)	Muscular function; respiration; cardiac function; nerve impulse transmission; carbohydrate metabolism	Hypoadrenocorticism Renal disease	Intestinal disease
Chloride (Cl^-)	Water distribution; osmotic pressure; normal anion/cation ratio	Renal disease	Renal disease

19.24 Importance of common electrolytes and causes of abnormal concentrations.

Electrolytes are measured by a process known as potentiometry. This measures the potential difference (voltage) that develops between the inner and outer surfaces of an electrode that is selectively permeable to the ion being measured. This is then compared to that of a reference electrode. Electrolyte tests can be performed on whole blood, plasma or serum.

Sodium

Sodium is required for many vital functions in the body, including the regulation of blood pressure and volume, and the transmission of nerve impulses. **Hypernatraemia** (increased levels of sodium in the blood) may be seen where there has been an abundant loss of water through the gastrointestinal tract along with sodium intake, perhaps caused by excessive sodium replacement in fluid therapy or low water intake (dehydration). **Hyponatraemia** (decreased levels) may arise as a result of excessive loss of sodium, which may be seen in renal failure, intestinal obstruction or urinary tract problems.

Normal sodium levels in blood serum are:

- Dogs: 140–153 mmol/l
- Cats: 142–155 mmol/l
- Horses: 132–146 mmol/l.

Chloride

Chloride plays an important role in helping to maintain a normal balance of fluids. Significant increases (**hyperchloraemia**) may be associated with diarrhoea, kidney disease and overactivity of the parathyroid glands. Vomiting or excessive sweating may be associated with a decrease in chloride (**hypochloraemia**).

Potassium

Potassium has a key role in maintaining the electrical potential of the cell membrane (see Chapter 22 for details). Normal potassium levels in blood are:

- Dogs: 3.5–5.8 mmol/l
- Cats: 3.4–5.6 mmol/l
- Horses: 145–150 mmol/l.

Hormones
Thyroid disease

Measurement of thyroxine (T4) is used to assess thyroid function (triiodothyronine, T3, is also sometimes considered). Increased T4 may be seen in hyperthyroidism (cats), oestrus, pregnancy and young age. Decreased levels may be seen in hypothyroidism (dogs), hyperadrenocorticism, chronic illness, advanced age and iodine deficiency. Many factors, including illness and drug therapy, can affect levels of T4 in the blood and so testing can be unreliable. Additional tests (e.g. thyroid stimulating hormone, TSH) are used to confirm conditions such as hypothyroidism.

Adrenal disease

The most common conditions affecting the adrenal cortex are hyperadrenocorticism (Cushing's disease) and hypoadrenocorticism (Addison's disease), where levels of cortisol are affected. A basal cortisol test is unreliable in the diagnosis of these and so adrenocorticotrophic hormone (ACTH) stimulation or dexamethasone suppression tests are performed. The diagnosis of equine Cushing's disease is complex and may require a thyroid-releasing hormone (TRH) stimulation test and a dexamethasone suppression test to be carried out; it is likely that this will involve an external laboratory.

- **ACTH stimulation test:** Basal cortisol level is first measured in a sample of the patient's blood. The patient is then given an intravenous injection of synthetic ACTH, which will stimulate the release of cortisol. A second blood sample is taken 2 hours later (depending upon specific laboratory preferences) and the cortisol level is measured. Elevated post-injection levels of cortisol indicate Cushing's disease, whereas a reduced level indicates Addison's disease, although clinical interpretation of the test results may be influenced by other clinical factors.
- **Low-dose dexamethasone suppression test:** Basal cortisol level is first measured in a sample of the patient's blood. The patient is then given an intravenous injection of a low dose of dexamethasone. A second blood sample is taken 8 hours later, to assess the response. Cortisol levels should normally decrease significantly, and a high post-injection cortisol level may be indicative of hyperadrenocorticism. An overnight dexamethasone suppression test is performed in horses with suspected Cushing's disease.
- **High-dose dexamethasone suppression test:** This is used to distinguish between pituitary-dependent and non-pituitary-dependent hyperadrenocorticism in dogs. Basal cortisol level is first measured in a sample of the patient's blood. The patient is then given an intravenous injection of a high dose of dexamethasone. A second sample is taken 3 hours later and a third at 8 hours, to assess the response. Patients with pituitary-dependent Cushing's disease commonly have a post-injection cortisol level *below* the base level, whereas those with non-pituitary-dependent Cushing's will have a post-injection cortisol level *above* the base level.

In-house test kits

Manufacturers have developed a number of in-house test kits that are quick and reliable. ELISA (enzyme-linked immunosorbent assay) is one of the most sensitive and reproducible diagnostic technologies available. Kits are available for the detection of diseases in small animals and equine species, as well as ruminants and poultry. Blood tests for feline leukaemia and feline immunodeficiency detect exposure to, or infection with, FeLV or FIV. They can be run individually but are most commonly run together.

In-house test kits are available for:
- FeLV/FIV
- *Giardia*
- Heartworm
- *Leishmania*
- Parvovirus
- cPLI (canine pancreatic lipase immunoreactivity)
- Foal IgG
- Thyroxine
- Cortisol
- Bile acids.

Urine

Analysis of urine samples can be a non-invasive, simple and quick method of determining the health status of a patient and can assist the veterinary surgeon in the diagnosis of many conditions of the urinary system and other body systems.

On average, a cat, dog or horse will produce 1–2 ml/kg of urine per hour. Alterations to normal production may occur (see Chapter 15). In order to assess water intake and urine output fully, a thorough 12-hour or 24-hour measurement is required.

Collection

A variety of methods are available for collecting urine (see below). Ideally a morning sample should be collected, as the urine tends to be of a higher concentration at this time. Any urine sample should be examined within 1 hour of collection. The chemistry of urine alters when it is left standing and this may cause inaccurate test results. Urine samples can be stored in the refrigerator for up to 6 hours, although the sample must be allowed to warm to room temperature before analysis. Samples for bacteriology should not be refrigerated and should be examined immediately if performing the task in house.

Urine samples are of significant diagnostic value in birds, although collecting urine presents some obvious problems, such as collecting a large enough volume to analyse, and separating urine from urates and faeces in the droppings.

Containers

Depending on the method of collection, urine should ideally be collected straight into a sterile universal container. Urine for microbial examination should be collected directly into a container with boric acid (red-topped container). Boric acid will preserve the existing bacteria and prevent the growth of further microorganisms. Thymol (1 mg/ml) is an alternative.

If the primary collection receptacle is not a sterile pot (e.g. jam jar, ice cream tub, kidney dish) then it must be thoroughly cleaned and dried before use. All containers must be adequately labelled.

Collection methods

For all collection methods, personal protective equipment (PPE) such as gloves should be worn. If the sample is being collected by the owner then the practice should provide the client with a pair of disposable gloves.

Collection methods include:

- **Mid-stream free collection:** This method is ideal for owners to collect samples at home, although it can be challenging, particularly in some species. Commercial sterile collection kits are available, consisting of a funnel with a universal container attached (Figure 19.25). Urine from cats can be collected using non-absorbable cat litter, which can then be transferred to a universal container. These methods are relatively easy to perform in both cats and dogs, although the sample is not sterile.
- **Manual expression:** This is relatively easy to perform on cats, dogs and small mammals, although the bladder must contain sufficient urine in order to be palpated and expressed. Care must be taken to avoid rupturing the

bladder or causing other trauma. The method is classed as non-sterile and the urine collected is therefore not suitable for microbial examination.
- **Catheterization:** This method involves passing a urinary catheter directly into the bladder via the urethra (see Chapter 17). The procedure is relatively easy to perform, although sedation or general anaesthesia may be required. Catheterization provides a sterile sample, although the process may cause trauma or infection. The urinary catheter, once in place, can be used for contrast imaging or left *in situ* to monitor urine output and maintain urethral patency.
- **Cystocentesis:** This method involves the passage of a sterile needle through the abdominal wall and into the bladder (see Chapter 17). Strict asepsis is required. It can be a relatively quick method of obtaining a sterile sample, although rarely the patient may require sedation or general anaesthesia. The method is reliant upon there being sufficient urine in the bladder. Cystocentesis may result in blood contamination of the sample.

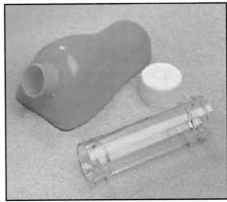

19.25   Commercial urine collection funnel with container.

Analysis
Physical appearance

Before tests are performed on the urine, it is important to record the physical characteristics of the sample.

- **Colour:** Urine should be pale yellow in colour. The pigment urochrome is responsible for this colour. The depth of colour may change according to the concentration of the urine. Rabbit urine can range in colour from clear to yellow, red, rust or orange. This colour variation is normal and is not a cause for concern unless it is accompanied by other signs such as straining to urinate, elevated temperature, sudden changes in drinking, polyuria or anuria, or loss of litter tray habits.
- **Turbidity:** Dog and cat urine is usually clear, although, if the urine is left to stand precipitation of phosphate can occur and cause turbidity. Rabbit urine and horse urine appear naturally turbid due to the presence of calcium carbonate crystals. Urine from birds and reptiles is also cloudy due to the presence of uric acid crystals.
- **Odour:** Normal urine has a slight sour smell. The urine of entire male cats can have a distinct putrid smell, which is used for scent marking.

Alterations in the physical appearance can be fundamental for diagnosis (Figure 19.26).

Characteristic	Abnormality	Causes
Colour	Pale/clear	Polyuria/polydipsia
	Dark yellow/orange/brown	Dehydration
	Red, brown or black	Presence of blood Certain drugs
	Green/yellow	Biliverdin (oxidization of bilirubin)
	Blue/green-tinged	Certain drugs
Turbidity	Cloudy	Contamination, e.g. pus, semen Presence of mucus Phosphate precipitation
Odour	Sweet/fruity	Presence of ketones (ketonuria), e.g. in diabetes mellitus
	Ammonia	Fresh samples – bacteria present Old samples – stale
	Foul	Excess protein

19.26 Abnormalities in the physical characteristics of canine urine.

Specific gravity

Specific gravity (SG) is the relative density (mass per unit volume) of a known volume of fluid compared to an equal volume of distilled water. Distilled water has an SG of 1.000 and is used in the calibration of SG measuring devices. Elevated levels can be caused by dehydration, acute renal failure, shock, diabetes mellitus or fluid loss, or by sediment such as crystals (see below). Decreased levels can be seen with chronic renal failure, diabetes insipidus, polydipsia, fluid therapy and corticosteroid therapy.

Normal values (depending on hydration status and water intake) are given as:

- Dogs: 1.015–1.045
- Cats: 1.035–1.060
- Horses: 1.020–1.050.

A refractometer is used for accurate measurement.

Using a refractometer

1. Put on gloves.
2. Place 2–3 drops of distilled water on the prism surface of the refractometer.
3. Hold the refractometer up to a light source and look down the eyepiece.
4. Calibrate the refractometer to 1.000 on the USG (or W) scale.
5. Lift the cover and dry the prism surface using a dry tissue.
6. Invert the tube to mix the urine sample gently.
7. Pipette 1–2 drops of urine on to the prism surface.
8. Close the cover.

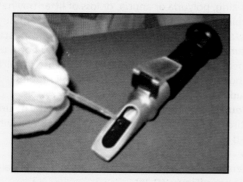

9. Hold up to the light source and look down the eyepiece.
10. Read and record the actual urine specific gravity reading.
11. Rinse the prism with water.
12. Dry the prism.
13. Dispose of used materials as hazardous waste.

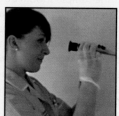

Chemical tests

Commercial dipsticks are available for the quick and inexpensive chemical analysis of urine in house.

For accurate results, ensure that:

- The test strips come in an airtight container
- The test strips are in date before using
- The sticks are not damp or discoloured
- The lid is closed immediately after removing the strip
- Urine less than 1 hour old is used
- The urine has been kept at room temperature, away from sunlight, in a closed container.

Dipstick analysis

1. List the chemicals on a piece of paper before starting, to enable results to be recorded efficiently.
2. Put on gloves.
3. Select urine dipstick test strips; remove one test strip and replace the lid immediately.
4. Invert the fresh urine sample to mix.
5. Cover the test strip pads with urine (ideally using a 1 ml syringe; alternatively the test strip can be immersed in the urine sample).
6. Immediately note the time.
7. Wait for the appropriate length of time and then read and record the dipstick measurements correctly.
8. Dispose of used dipsticks as hazardous waste.

Dipsticks measure pH, proteins, glucose, ketones, bilirubin, urobilinogen, nitrite and blood in urine. Causes of abnormal levels are noted in Figure 19.27.

It should be noted that some dipsticks available are designed for measuring human parameters. Although some dipsticks measure specific gravity (SG), these are not reliable and SG should be measured using a refractometer (see above).

Chemical test	Normal value	Possible causes of increase	Possible causes of decrease
pH	Dogs: 5–7 Cats: 7–9 Horses: 7–9	Bacterial infection, cystitis, alkalosis, certain drugs	Fever, starvation, diabetes mellitus, chronic renal failure, acidosis
Proteins	Trace	Renal failure, haemorrhage, inflammatory disease	Rare
Glucose	None	Stress, excitement, diabetes mellitus, Cushing's disease, hyperthyroidism	Not applicable
Blood	None	Oestrus, cystitis, urolithiasis, acute nephritis	Not applicable
Ketones	None	Diabetes mellitus, starvation, liver damage	Not applicable
Bilirubin	Trace	Liver disease, haemolytic or obstructive jaundice	Rare
Nitrite	None	Bacterial infection	Not applicable
Urobilinogen	Trace/small amount	Liver dysfunction	Liver dysfunction

19.27 Chemical analysis of urine.

Microscopic analysis of urine

Centrifugation of the urine allows the sediment to be separated from supernatant and examined microscopically. The procedure is inexpensive and can be carried out within the practice laboratory relatively quickly. Normal urine may contain a small amount of sediment, consisting of:

- Epithelial cells
- Mucus
- Blood cells
- Bacteria.

Method for microscopic analysis of urine

1. Wear gloves.
2. Mix the urine sample gently, and pipette urine into the centrifuge tube.
3. Centrifuge the sample at 1500 rpm for 5 minutes.
4. Remove the supernatant, leaving a few drops in which to re-suspend the sediment.
5. Re-suspend the sediment by 'flicking' the base of the tube.
6. Add a stain to the sediment if required. New methylene blue or Sedi-Stain can be added to facilitate examination.
7. Pipette a drop of the suspension on to a clean, labelled microscope slide.
8. Carefully place a coverslip on top of the sediment. Avoid creating air bubbles by lowering the coverslip at an angle of 45 degrees.
9. Dispose of the used pipette, urine and used materials as hazardous waste.
10. Examine the slide using the battlement technique under low power, X10 then X40.
11. Record any findings. The Vernier scale reading can be used to relocate items.

Sediment analysis: cells

The following cells may be found:

- **Epithelial cells** (Figure 19.28):
  - Transitional cells from the bladder – these are small round polyhedral cells and indicate cystitis or pyelonephritis
  - Squamous cells from the lower urethra, vagina and prepuce – these are large granular cells with nuclei

- Renal tubular cells – these are cuboidal to columnar cells; a large number would indicate active renal tubule disease.
- **Blood cells:**
  - Erythrocytes – these indicate trauma, oestrus and infection/inflammation
  - Leucocytes (Figure 19.28) – these indicate inflammation and infection
- **Spermatozoa:**
  - These may be seen in entire male animals
- **Yeast cells:**
  - These are non-nucleated round or oval cells
- **Bacterial cells:**
  - A small number of bacterial cells is always present
  - Further staining, culture and sensitivity may be required.

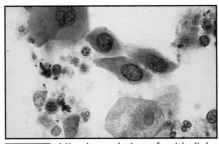

19.28 Mixed population of epithelial cells and leucocytes in canine urine sediment. (Sedi-Stain; original magnification X400) (Reproduced from *BSAVA Manual of Canine and Feline Nephrology and Urology, 2nd edn*)

Sediment analysis: casts

Casts are formed in the distal convoluted tubules and collecting ducts of the kidney, where the concentration and acidity of urine are greatest. Secreted protein is precipitated in acidic conditions. Casts are composed of a matrix of protein and mucoprotein. Mucus threads can be differentiated from casts by their irregularly spaced, twisting sides and pointed, wispy ends.

- **Hyaline casts** (Figure 19.29a):
  - Clear, colourless, composed only of protein
  - More easily identified in stained samples
  - Present in patients with poor renal perfusion and fever, and those that have recently undertaken strenuous exercise
- **Granular casts** (Figure 19.29b):
  - The most common type seen in animal urine

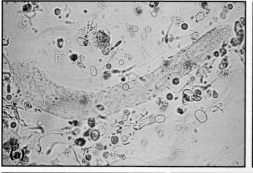
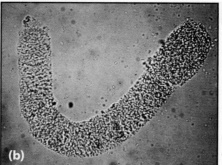

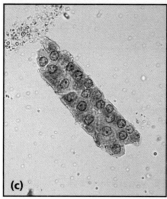
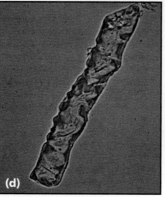
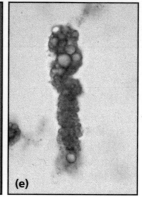

19.29 Casts found in urine. **(a)** Curved hyaline renal tubular cast. (Unstained; original magnification X400) **(b)** Granular cast. (Unstained; original magnification X400) **(c)** Epithelial cast from a dog with acute renal failure. (New methylene blue; original magnification X400) **(d)** Waxy cast with characteristic broken, blunt ends. (Unstained; original magnification X400) **(e)** Fatty cast in feline urine; note the lipid droplets. (New methylene blue; original magnification X100) (Reproduced from *BSAVA Manual of Canine and Feline Nephrology and Urology, 2nd edn*)

- Appear granular due to the degeneration of other cells, such as red blood cells
- Seen in patients with acute nephritis and chronic renal failure
- **Epithelial casts** (Figure 19.29c):
  - Consist of epithelial cells from the renal tubules in a hyaline matrix
  - Seen in patients with acute nephritis
- **Leucocyte casts**:
  - Contain white blood cells (normally neutrophils)
  - Indicate inflammation in the renal tubules
- **Erythrocyte casts**:
  - Formed from red blood cells
  - Indicate renal haemorrhage
- **Waxy casts** (Figure 19.29d):
  - Similar to hyaline casts but have a square end
  - Indicate extensive renal damage
- **Fatty casts** (Figure 19.29e):
  - Contain small droplets of fat
  - Mainly seen in cats with renal disease and dogs with diabetes mellitus.

Cellular casts are rarely seen in equine urine, while hyaline casts can occasionally be seen.

Sediment analysis: crystals

The presence of crystals may or may not be of clinical significance. Some crystals form through normal renal activity; others form as a result of metabolic disturbances. Crystals may aggregate to form large uroliths (also called calculi). The damage these cause to the urinary tract is known as urolithiasis (see Chapter 20). It is important to note that the appearance of crystals can vary greatly depending on the position in which they are sitting and if they are incomplete or complete.

- **Struvite (magnesium ammonium phosphate or triple phosphate) crystals** (Figure 19.30a):

- Typically resemble the shape of coffin lids, although their shape may vary
- Found in alkaline urine
- **Cystine crystals** (Figure 19.30b):
  - Flat and thin with hexagonal outline
  - Found in acidic urine and associated with renal tubular dysfunction
  - Not seen in equine samples
- **Calcium oxalate crystals** (Figure 19.30c):
  - Dihydrate crystals appear as small square crystals with an 'X' in the centre
  - Found in acidic or neutral urine
  - Commonly seen in urine from certain breeds that are genetically predisposed (e.g. Yorkshire Terrier, Miniature Poodle, Lhaso Apso, Miniature Schnauzer and Burmese, Himalayan and Persian cats)
  - Also found in animals that have ingested ethylene glycol (antifreeze)
  - Rarely seen in equine samples
- **Ammonium urate crystals** (Figure 19.30d):
  - Appear as spindles, thorn apple-shaped or rosettes
  - Found in acidic and neutral urine
  - Seen in clinically normal Dalmatians due to the way they metabolize and excrete protein
  - In other dog breeds and in cats their presence can indicate liver disease or portosystemic shunts
  - Not seen in equine samples
- **Uric acid crystals** (Figure 19.30e) :
  - Vary in shape but usually diamond-shaped or rhomboid
  - Occur in acidic urine, although they are rare
- **Calcium phosphate crystals**:
  - Long and flat with a rectangular outline
  - Typically form in alkaline urine but are rare
- **Calcium carbonate crystals** (Figure 19.31):
  - Commonly seen in urine from clinically normal equine species and rabbits
  - Cause urine to appear turbid and cloudy, which is normal in these species.

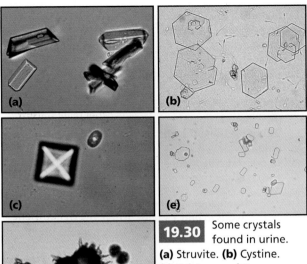

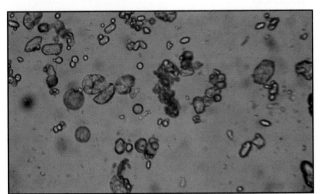

19.30 Some crystals found in urine. **(a)** Struvite. **(b)** Cystine. **(c)** Calcium oxalate dihydrate. **(d)** Ammonium urate. **(e)** Uric acid. (Original magnifications: (a) X500, (b-e) X100)

19.31 Calcium carbonate crystals in equine urine. (Courtesy of Newmarket Equine Hospital)

Faeces

Faecal samples can be very useful as an aid to the diagnosis of endoparasites, viral diseases and gastrointestinal disease. Although the collection of faeces may be simple, it is important that strict hygiene is employed to avoid contamination and exposure to potential zoonoses. Depending on the diagnostic test to be performed, it may be necessary to withdraw medication, such as antibiotics or antidiarrhoeal preparations, or to withhold red meat from the diet, prior to sampling.

Collection

Samples can be collected directly from the rectum or from passed faeces. It is important to consider contamination if faeces have been collected from the animal's enclosure or from the ground and also the date on which they were passed.

- **Collection from the rectum** can be carried out using gloved fingers. Once the sample has been collected, the glove can be turned inside out and the faeces kept within it, secured and labelled, or the sample transferred to a universal container. Direct collection is particularly useful in animals that are generally housed with others, such as horses.
- **Collection from the ground** involves transferring the faeces into a universal container using gloves, and a spatula if required.

Specimens that cannot be examined within a few hours should be refrigerated or mixed with an equal part of 10% formalin to preserve the sample. NB Formalin should not be used if the sample is to be used for culture and sensitivity testing.

Examination of faecal samples

All faecal samples should be handled with care, as they may contain bacteria, viruses and parasites that may be potentially zoonotic or harmful to humans. Special attention must be paid to hygiene and personal protective clothing, not only during collection but also during examination of the sample.

Normal contents of faeces of carnivorous animals include:

- Water
- Undigested food (small amounts only)
- Enzymes such as trypsin
- Bile products (biliverdin)
- Small amounts of mucus
- Bacteria
- Small numbers of epithelial cells
- Small amounts of blood from prey
- Small amounts of hair from prey.

Equine faeces contain large amounts of cellulose (fibre) plus undigested seeds, water and electrolytes.

Gross/macroscopic examination

Consistency

This will depend on the species of the animal. The faeces should be formed, and any variations such as hard dry faeces (constipation) or liquid faeces (diarrhoea) should be noted. If someone observed the animal passing faeces they may be able to comment further, e.g. did they observe tenesmus (straining)? Some veterinary practices have developed a faecal consistency scoring chart to standardize reporting.

Odour

This will depend on the species, as well as the diet the animal receives. Increased fat levels in the diet can result in rancid smells. Some conditions cause distinct odours, e.g. with haematochezia in parvovirus infection.

Colour

This will depend on the species of the animal and the food that it eats. Colour will also change as the age of the specimen increases, hence the need to examine fresh samples. Blood may appear in faeces as fresh blood (bright red) or older blood (darker red/brown); it is important to note the colour, as this is indicative of the origin. Variations in colour for canine faeces are described in Figure 19.32.

Colour	Possible causes
White	Increased fat in the diet Feeding of bones Digestive problems such as exocrine pancreatic insufficiency (EPI; see Chapter 20)
Yellow	Increased bile pigments due to liver disease
Pink	Hepatic dysfunction such as biliary obstruction
Bright red	Fresh blood (normally seen on top/coating the faeces) Haemorrhage from the lower part of the gastrointestinal tract
Dark red/brown/black	Older blood Diet high in red meat Haemorrhage from the upper part of the gastrointestinal tract

19.32   Colour abnormalities in canine faeces.

Mucus

Any presence of mucus should be noted. In some cases it can indicate the presence of digestive disorders (in particular colitis) and parasitic conditions.

Parasites

Some parasites, such as adult worms or tapeworm segments, may be found in the sample. Parasites should be identified (see below and Chapter 7).

Microscopic examination

Microscopic examinations are required to detect parasites, impaired digestion and bacterial/yeast infections.

A direct smear can be made by spreading a small amount of fresh faeces (collected from the rectum or off a rectal thermometer) on to a microscope slide. The faeces are gently mixed on the slide with saline or water, using a toothpick, and a coverslip applied. The smear should be examined using the X10 objective and X40 objectives. This is a quick method, requiring minimal equipment. However, the small sample used may not be sufficient to detect low parasite burdens. The Modified McMaster technique (for eggs) and the Baermann technique (for larvae) may be employed for better detection of parasites in faecal samples.

Modified McMaster technique

1. Measure 3 g of faeces and place in a glass beaker.
2. Add 42 ml of water to the beaker and mix with the faeces.
3. Pour the mixture through a tea strainer or sieve, collecting the filtrate in a separate bowl.
4. Discard the debris in the sieve as hazardous waste.
5. Add 15 ml of the filtrate to a test tube and centrifuge at 1500 rpm for 5 minutes.
6. Remove the supernatant and discard.
7. Add a few millilitres of saturated salt solution to the sediment and resuspend. Once suspended, add further amounts of saturated salt solution until 15 ml of fluid is present.

▶

8. Remove a small amount with a Pasteur pipette and fill one side of a McMaster chamber.
9. Repeat step 8, filling the other side of the McMaster slide.
10. Examine the McMaster slide under X40 magnification.
11. Using the grid on the McMaster slide examine each section, recording the eggs present. Repeat this technique using the grid on the other side of the slide.
12. To calculate the number of eggs per gram of faeces, add the total together and multiply by 50.

**Number of eggs per gram of faeces =
(eggs in grid 1 + eggs in grid 2) x 50**

Baermann technique

Equipment:

- Baermann apparatus (funnel, metal clamp stand, short section of rubber tube, clip)
- Gauze/muslin
- Centrifuge tube
- Microscope slides
- Glass coverslips
- Lugol's iodine.

Method

1. Attach the rubber tubing to the end of the funnel. Place the clip over the end of the rubber tubing to seal.
2. Clamp the funnel in the metal clamp stand.
3. Fill the funnel with warm water, up to about 1 cm from the rim.
4. Place the gauze/muslin (twice the diameter of the funnel) on top of the funnel.
5. Place 5–15 g of faeces on to the gauze/muslin, ensuring it is covered with water.
6. Allow the apparatus to stand overnight.
7. In the morning unclip the clip from the tubing and fill a centrifuge tube with the filtrate.
8. Centrifuge the tube for 1 minute at 1500 rpm.
9. Remove the supernatant and place the sediment on a microscope slide using a pipette.
10. Add a drop of Lugol's iodine and examine under the microscope.
11. Record any findings.

Skin and hair

The testing of skin and hair is invaluable in the diagnosis of ectoparasites and conditions such as ringworm (dermatophytosis). It is important that the correct technique is used for sample collection, and knowledge of the potential condition is also required.

Sampling techniques

Whilst sampling it is important to be aware of potential zoonoses and cross-contamination. Personal protective equipment should be worn at all times and, if necessary, the procedure should be performed in an isolation unit away from other patients. Various methods are used to collect skin and hair. The clinical signs, along with differential diagnoses, should be considered to ensure that the correct sampling technique and area of sampling are used. See Chapter 7 for identification of parasites.

Skin scrapes

Skin scraping is one of the most common diagnostic procedures used for evaluating patients with dermatological conditions. The area selected is usually one that contains lesions or is most likely to harbour the particular parasite, e.g. ear margins for *Sarcoptes scabiei*.

Skin scrape procedure

1. Assemble equipment required: clippers, size 10 scalpel blade (blunt), liquid paraffin or 10% potassium hydroxide, microscope slide, glass coverslip, chinagraph pen/permanent marker and microscope.
2. Select the area to be scraped.
3. Clip the area using clippers with a size 40 blade. This will allow more accurate scraping and will remove hair that may obscure findings. Clipping is not necessary where surface-dwelling parasites are suspected.
4. Dip the scalpel blade into liquid paraffin or potassium hydroxide and moisten the surface of the skin.
5. Hold the blade between the thumb and forefinger.
6. Stretch the skin to be scraped with the other hand and then gently scrape the area (usually a 3 cm by 3 cm area). The depth of scraping will vary according to the parasite in question, although most scraping should result in capillary ooze.

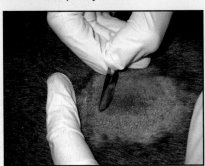

7. Transfer the collected material from the forward surface of the blade on to a glass slide. A drop of liquid paraffin or 10% potassium hydroxide can be added to the slide.
8. Place a coverslip over the top of the sample and label the slide.
9. Set up the microscope and examine the slide using the lowest power first. Vernier scale readings can be used to relocate parasites, although live parasites may move.
10. Slides should be viewed immediately after the sample has been collected to avoid parasites leaving the slide.
11. Once the slide has been examined and results recorded, dispose of correctly.

Adhesive tape impressions

This method can be used to detect superficial parasites (e.g. *Cheyletiella*), bacteria, fungi and yeasts (e.g. *Malassezia*). Clear adhesive tape is applied to the skin to collect epidermal debris. The adhesive side of the tape is then placed on a glass slide, which is labelled with the patient's details. The slide is then viewed with a microscope, starting with the lowest power.

Hair plucks

Hair plucks may be used to identify the presence of fungal spores, superficial mites (including *Demodex*, which lives in the hair follicle) and parasitic eggs such as those from *Cheyletiella*. A small number of hairs (including the roots) are plucked from the affected area using artery forceps. The hairs are placed on a glass slide with a drop of liquid paraffin. A glass coverslip is placed on top and the slide labelled. The slide can then be examined using a microscope.

Hair brushings

Hair brushings can be used to identify superficial parasites and eggs. This method is also used to identify the faeces of fleas where the fleas cannot be seen on the coat by the naked eye.

The animal should be placed near a white background, e.g. white paper. The coat is then brushed by hand or using a comb and the debris collected. The debris can then be transferred to a labelled microscope slide with liquid paraffin and a coverslip placed on top. This can then be examined using the microscope.

A wet paper test can also be performed by dabbing the collected debris with wet cotton wool. Flea faeces will dissolve with the wet cotton wool and appear as red/brown tinged marks.

Impression smear

Impression smears can be used to detect bacterial, fungal or yeast skin conditions. The hair is first clipped and then a microscope slide pressed directly on to the skin. The slide can then be stained and viewed with a microscope.

Swab samples

Skin swabs can be used to identify bacterial, fungal and yeast skin conditions. The swab is rolled over the surface of the affected area, e.g. skin, inside the ear canal. The swab can then be labelled and sent to an external laboratory. Alternatively, the swab can be rolled/smeared on a microscope slide, stained and viewed with a microscope.

In cases where *Otodectes* ear mites are suspected, small amounts of wax can be collected from the ear canal and then transferred to a microscope slide with liquid paraffin. A glass coverslip should then be placed over the top before the slide is labelled and examined with a microscope.

Analysis of skin and hair samples

Ectoparasites (see Chapter 7), bacteria, fungi and yeasts may be detected. Methods for bacterial detection are outlined later in the chapter.

Tissue samples for cytology

Cytology uses microscopic examination of tissue or fluid samples to differentiate normal from abnormal cells to aid diagnosis. The samples may be obtained from a variety of areas, such as the ear canal, skin, abdominal cavity and subarachnoid space. Various techniques are used for sampling each area, and testing can be carried out in house or via an external laboratory.

Samples for cytological examination include:

- Tracheal washes
- Nasal flushes
- Vaginal swabs
- Ear swabs
- Semen
- Cerebrospinal fluid
- Abdominal fluid
- Synovial fluid
- Thoracic fluid.

Sample collection

Swabs

Swabs are generally used to collect samples from mucous membranes such as those lining the nasal cavity, vagina (see Chapter 26) or eyes (Figure 19.33). The swab should be gently placed into the cavity and rolled/stroked on the lining. Once removed from the cavity, the swab should be gently stroked down the length of a clean microscope slide. The slide should be air-dried or heat-fixed. The slide can be stained (e.g. with Diff-Quik) before microscopic examination. The cells seen should be identified and recorded. Bacterial cells are identified using Gram staining (see Bacteriology, below).

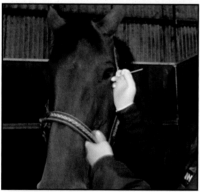

19.33 Swabs can be used to obtain cytology samples from the eye. (Courtesy of B&W Equine Group)

Scrapings

Scraping (see Skin, above) has the advantage of collecting many cells from the area being sampled; however, such samples only provide details of the superficial layer.

Direct smears

Inflammatory exudate from ulcerated surface lesions can be sampled by direct application of a microscope slide to the lesion. This may be of limited value, however, as deeper tissues are not included.

Impression smears may also be made of biopsy specimens (see later) to give an immediate indication of the type of lesion before sending a sample for histopathological interpretation. The cut surface of the sample is blotted to remove surface blood and serum. The dried surface is then applied to a clean dry slide, using gentle pressure. Several areas can be sampled on a single slide. The preparations are quickly air-dried and then stained as for a fluid sample.

Fine-needle aspiration

Specimens for cytology may be collected from organs, lymph nodes and masses. The most common method used in practice is fine-needle biopsy, commonly known as fine-needle aspiration (FNA). Ultrasound guidance may be helpful (see Chapter 18). The procedure will be carried out by a veterinary surgeon but may require assistance from a veterinary nurse.

- The mass is stabilized using the hand and a sterile 21–25G needle inserted. Negative pressure may be created by attaching a syringe and drawing back on the plunger. The needle is redirected several times while still in the mass.
- The needle is then removed from the mass and the syringe, if used, removed.
- A syringe is then filled with air and attached to the needle. Pushing down on the plunger forces the sample on to a clean microscope slide, which is then air-dried.
- The sample may be stained and examined in house (Figure 19.34) or sent to an external laboratory.

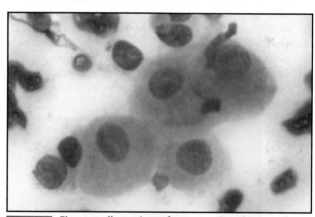

19.34 Fine-needle aspirate from a perianal mass on a dog, showing a cluster of epithelial cells with round nuclei and grainy cytoplasm. (Wright's stain; original magnification X1000) (Courtesy of Elizabeth Villiers; reproduced from *BSAVA Manual of Canine and Feline Clinical Pathology*, 2nd edn.)

Tissue biopsy

Tissue biopsy can be used to obtain samples for cytological and histopathological examination. Biopsy can be performed for most organs and tissues, including the skin, liver and lymph nodes, depending on location and accessibility; some samples may be taken using endoscopy (see Chapter 18). The procedure will be carried out by a veterinary surgeon where it requires entry into a body cavity.

- **Wedge biopsy**: Commonly performed using a surgical scalpel. Specific lesions can be included within the sample and a good cross-section of the mass/area can be obtained.

- **Punch biopsy**: Normally much easier and quicker to perform than wedge biopsy. Specialized punch biopsy instruments are available, e.g. skin punches and Tru-cut needles.

Sample handling

All tissue samples should be preserved (unless required for bacteriology). There are a variety of preservatives available (Figure 19.35).

Preservative	Details
10% formalin	This contains 40% formaldehyde gas
10% formal saline	Most common solution used. It is made by diluting formalin with saline solution
10% neutral buffered formalin	This is a 10% solution of formalin with added buffers. The buffers prevent any changes in pH, which may affect cells
Alcohol	This may be used but causes unwanted shrinkage of tissue and hardness

19.35 Tissue preservatives.

Considerations for tissue samples

- Be aware of health and safety (see Chapter 2). The sample is a pathological hazardous specimen and formalin is toxic and irritant. PPE should be worn at all times.
- A wide-necked container should be used so that samples can be removed easily after they have been fixed.
- Sample containers should be robust, leak-proof and tightly secured.
- Every container/microscope slide should be labelled.
- Tissue samples should be of a small size, to allow penetration of formalin for preservation of the cells.
- Enough formalin should be used for preserving. All tissue samples should be immersed in formalin, ideally at 10 times volume of fixative to the tissue volume.
- Samples should not be frozen, as this damages the cells.
- Only representative samples should be collected and sent to external laboratories. Whole organs should not be sent.
- Correct paperwork should accompany the tissue sample. This must include the details of the submitting veterinary surgery, the patient's details, and details of the area sampled, including the margins.

Centesis

Centesis involves placing a needle into a body cavity or organ in order to remove fluid. This procedure will be carried out by a veterinary surgeon but may require assistance from a veterinary nurse.

Cerebrospinal fluid

Examination of CSF is often required in the diagnosis of neurological conditions such as meningitis. The technique is very specialized and should only be carried out by experienced personnel due to the location of sampling.

- The area for needle insertion must be aseptically prepared by clipping the hair and using skin disinfectants. Personnel must also adhere to aseptic techniques by wearing sterile surgical gloves and using sterile equipment and consumables.
- In dogs and cats, the patient is anaesthetized and placed in lateral recumbency. The head and neck are flexed and held securely in position. The veterinary surgeon inserts a 20–22G spinal needle carefully into the subarachnoid space.
- In equine patients, CSF can be collected from the atlanto-occipital space in recumbent patients or from the lumbosacral space in standing patients.
- The CSF is collected by allowing the fluid to drip into the collecting tubes. A maximum of 1 ml per 5 kg of bodyweight should be collected, using only EDTA and plain tubes.
- The veterinary surgeon then slowly removes the needle.
- The point of insertion is covered with a sterile adhesive dressing.

Normal CSF should be clear, colourless and slightly viscous. Alterations in the visual appearance should be noted. Cytological analysis must be performed on CSF in order to assess the fluid accurately. This should be carried out immediately after collecting the sample. The sample is examined for the presence of red blood cells and nucleated white blood cells. Other tests performed on CSF include: protein analysis; bacteriology; antibody titres; electrolyte concentrations.

Thoracic fluid

Thoracocentesis can be undertaken in order to obtain fluid from the thoracic cavity. Fluid should be collected into EDTA and plain collection tubes and examined under the microscope. Visual inspection of the fluid should also be carried out, noting any differences in colour and turbidity such as pus (pyothorax), blood (haemothorax) or chyle (chylothorax) (see Chapter 20).

Abdominal fluid

Abdominocentesis may be undertaken to obtain abdominal fluid. Fluid should be collected into EDTA and plain collection tubes and examined microscopically. Visual inspection should also be carried out, noting differences in colour and turbidity. Additional testing for protein levels and bacteriology can also be carried out.

In equine patients, collection of peritoneal fluid is vital for the diagnosis of abdominal disease and emergency conditions such as colic. Fluid can be collected from a standing horse from the ventral midline, 15 cm from the xiphisternum. Suitable patient restraint and aseptic preparation of the site is required prior to sampling. Once prepared, an 18G 1.5-inch needle is usually inserted into the linea alba and advanced until peritoneal fluid can be collected into an EDTA and plain tube. This can then be analysed.

Synovial fluid

Synovial fluid is collected from a joint via arthrocentesis. This can be very useful in assisting the diagnosis of joint conditions such as septic arthritis. Small amounts of fluid should be collected into a plain tube and examined microscopically.

Normal synovial fluid is clear to straw yellow in colour, and non-turbid. Turbidity can indicate the presence of cells, protein or cartilage.

The collection of synovial fluid in the horse is commonly carried out in joint conditions and in lameness investigations.

The anatomical site will vary according to the patient and condition. The patient should be adequately restrained and the site of collection aseptically prepared. Local anaesthetic may be used by the veterinary surgeon at the sample site to reduce the possibility of movement. A suitable needle and syringe should be selected and synovial fluid collected into an EDTA and plain tube. The fluid can then be sent to an external laboratory for cytology or bacteriology, or stained and examined in house (Figure 19.36).

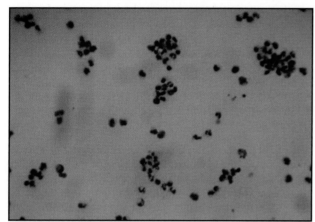

| 19.36 | Arthrocentesis sample from a horse, showing a high number of white blood cells. Modified Wright's stain; original magnification X25) (Courtesy of Newmarket Equine Hospital) |

Airway washes

Tracheal wash or bronchoalveolar lavage (BAL) can be particularly useful for the diagnosis of respiratory disease. An endoscope is used to visualize the area to be investigated. Saline is then flushed into the area via the port on the endoscope and drawn back up with a syringe or suction device on the endoscope. The collected fluid should be placed in a sterile container and examined in house or preserved and sent to an external laboratory for examination.

Bacteriology

When infection is suspected bacteriological samples may be investigated. The type of bacteria (see Chapter 6) can be identified and further testing, such as drug sensitivity testing, can be undertaken to aid treatment of the condition. A range of samples may be collected, e.g. blood, skin, CSF, faeces. A variety of sampling techniques may be used, as discussed earlier in the chapter.

Considerations for bacteriological samples

- A generous sample, or multiple samples, should be submitted.
- Samples should be collected using aseptic techniques and sterile equipment.
- Samples should be collected and transported in appropriate media and containers.
- The collection/transport container should be sealed as soon as possible to avoid contamination. ▸

- All containers should be labelled, to avoid confusion.
- Sampled should be examined as soon as possible after collection.
- Samples should be delivered as soon as possible to the laboratory, if sending externally.

Bacterial culture

Bacteria are specialized microorganisms that will only grow in a suitable environment. The correct environment for growth should include:

- Water
- Essential nutrients
- Correct pH
- Correct temperature (most bacteria are normothermic and therefore require body temperatures of 37–40°C)
- Correct gaseous environment.

Culture media

Bacteria are grown on or within a culture medium. Culture media provide the essential nutrients the bacteria require in order to reproduce. There are two types of medium:

- Liquid (also known as broth)
- Solid.

For bacteriology, culture media may be purchased as dehydrated powder or as prepared agar plates in Petri dishes or liquid media jars. Solidifying agents used in solid media include gelatine and agar (dried extract of sea algae). Unused agar plates should be kept refrigerated at 5°C.

Simple media

Simple agar or nutrient agar media provide the basic nutrients for undemanding species such as *Escherichia coli*.

Enriched media

These media are used to culture bacteria that require additional nutrients. Examples include:

- **Blood agar**: This contains 5–10% blood, and is used to support the growth of most mammalian pathogens. It may also be used to detect haemolysis
- **Chocolate agar**: This contains blood that has been heated to 80°C. By heating the blood, the red blood cells rupture and release haemoglobin, which adds nutrition to the agar.

Enrichment broths are also used. This liquid medium is selective for a particular bacterium. Enrichment broth has no inhibitory agent preventing growth of other organisms. It allows the growth of the target species and allows it to outgrow other species that may be present. An example of an enrichment broth includes selenite broth used for the growth of *Salmonella*.

Selective media

This type of medium allows a particular bacterium or group of bacteria to grow whilst inhibiting the growth of unwanted species. Some of these media change colour with microbial growth; these are known as indicator media. Examples include:

- **MacConkey's agar**: This contains crystal violet (which suppresses the growth of Gram-positive bacteria) and bile salts (selective for lactose-fermenting enteric bacteria and other bile salt-tolerant Gram-negative bacteria)
- **Deoxycholate–citrate agar**: This inhibits non-enteric bacteria and is used for growing *Salmonella*.

Media for fungal culture

Selective media may also be used for **fungal** culture. **Sabouraud's agar** has a high glucose content and low pH, which is ideal for fungal growth. It is used as an indicator medium, changing from yellow to red in the presence of fungal growth.

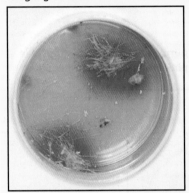

Colour change from yellow to red indicates growth of a ringworm fungus on this 'dermatophyte test medium'.

Transport agar

Transport agar is used for the temporary storage and transport of a specimen, by acting as a maintenance agar. It merely supports the survival of the organism rather than aiding growth.

Producing a bacterial culture

In order to culture bacteria, a sample is transferred to an appropriate culture medium. The aim is to obtain single bacterial colonies in order to observe colonial morphology, antibiotic sensitivity and biochemical identification. The quadrant streak method is the preferred method of inoculating an agar plate.

The quadrant streak method

1. Put on PPE.
2. Label the Petri dish.
3. Heat a wire inoculation loop by passing it through the flame of a Bunsen burner. Cool the loop in the air for a few seconds or by touching it gently on to the surface of the agar at the edge of the plate.
4. Dip the loop into the sample.
5. Pick up the Petri dish and smear the loop over one quarter of the agar surface. Be sure to keep the loop almost parallel to the agar surface to avoid digging into it.

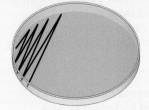

6. Pass the inoculating loop through the Bunsen burner flame again and allow it to cool.
7. Place the inoculating loop on the edge of the first set of streaks and create further streaks at right angles to them.

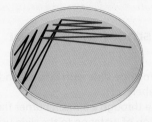

8. Pass the inoculating loop through the Bunsen burner flame again and allow it to cool.
9. Place the inoculating loop on the edge of the second set of streaks and create further streaks at right angles.

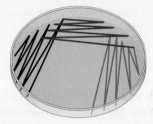

10. Pass the inoculating loop through the Bunsen burner flame again and allow it to cool.
11. Place the inoculating loop on the edge of the third set of streaks and create a final set, again at right angles.

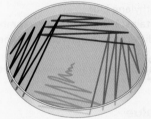

12. Place the lid on the dish and place in the incubator at 37°C.
13. Remove the plate after 18–24 hours and examine for colony growth. Re-incubate if necessary.

Examining the colony

An experienced microbiologist can recognize several bacteria on gross examination of cultured colonies. When looking at the colonies, the following examination and recordings should take place:

- Size (either measured or described as pinpoint, medium, large)
- Pigment/colour
- Density (opaque, transparent)
- Elevation (raised, flat, convex, drop-like)
- Shape (circular, irregular)
- Texture (smooth, sticky)
- Odour, if appropriate (sweet, pungent)
- Haemolysis.

Once gross examination has occurred, individual colonies can be isolated and grown on if required. An inoculation loop is used to remove an individual part of the bacterial culture and a new agar plate inoculated as described above. Culture samples may be transferred to a microscope slide, stained and examined with a microscope.

Bacterial smear preparation

1. Put on PPE.
2. Clean a microscope slide with ethanol and lint-free tissue and label it.
3. Pass the slide through a Bunsen burner flame.
4. Place one drop of water on to the slide using a sterile inoculating loop.
5. Using the sterile inoculating loop, remove a portion of the bacterial culture and place it on to the slide.
6. Mix the sample on the slide and spread evenly.
7. Allow the smear to dry thoroughly.
8. Fix the slide by passing through the Bunsen burner flame three times.

Staining

Once the smear is prepared and fixed, a stain may be used to aid identification. Taking into consideration the colour, size, shape and arrangement, common types of bacteria may be identified.

There are three types of stain that can be used:

- **Simple stains**: These colour the cell or the background so that the size, shape and arrangement of the cells can be seen, e.g. methylene blue
- **Differential stains**: These stains use a combination of two dyes to differentiate between cell types, e.g. Gram stain
- **Structural stains**: These stains only dye part of the cell structure.

Methylene blue

This is a simple stain, which can be used to identify size, shape and arrangement. Methylene blue is relatively cheap and easy to use.

Methylene blue staining

1. Put on PPE.
2. Place the microscope slide on a staining rack.
3. Flood the slide with 1% methylene blue stain.
4. Leave for 2 minutes.
5. Wash off with distilled water.
6. Stand vertically and allow to dry.
7. Examine under the microscope, using X100 with oil immersion.

Gram stain

The Gram stain is the most common differential stain used, as it divides bacteria into two groups: Gram-positive and Gram-negative (see Chapter 6).

Gram staining procedure

1. Put on PPE.
2. Place the microscope slide on a staining rack.
3. Flood the slide with crystal violet for 30 seconds.
4. Gently rinse in tap water.
5. Flood slide with Gram's iodine for 30 seconds.
6. Gently rinse in tap water.
7. Wash slide with decolorizer (acetone) for 5 seconds.
8. Gently rinse in tap water.
9. Flood slide with carbol fuchsin or safranin for 30 seconds.
10. Gently rinse in tap water.
11. Air-dry smear or gently blot with paper towel.
12. Examine under the microscope, using X100 and oil immersion.

Results:

- Bacteria that stain **purple** are termed **Gram-positive**
- Bacteria that stain **pink** are termed **Gram-negative**

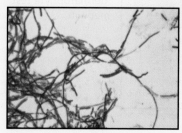
Gram-positive bacilli

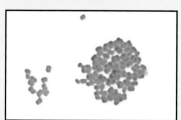
Gram-negative cocci

Ziehl–Neelsen/acid-fast staining

This stain is used to identify acid-fast bacteria such as *Mycobacterium* spp.

Ziehl–Neelsen staining procedure

1. Put on PPE.
2. Place the microscope slide on a staining rack.
3. Flood the slide with Ziehl–Neelsen carbol fuchsin solution and apply gentle heat until steam rises.
4. Leave for 5 minutes.
5. Rinse gently with tap water.
6. Decolorize with acid alcohol for at least 1 minute.
7. Rinse gently in tap water and repeat decolorization until the smear is pale pink.
8. Flood with Loeffler's alkaline methylene blue.
9. Leave for 2–3 minutes.
10. Rinse gently with tap water.
11. Blot dry with paper towel and examine.

Results:

- **Acid-fast** bacteria stain **bright red**
- **Non-acid-fast** bacteria stain **blue**

Antimicrobial sensitivity testing

In order to establish the best treatment for a bacterial infection, antimicrobial sensitivity testing can be carried out using agar Petri dish cultures. Specialized discs impregnated with antibiotics are placed on the surface of the agar, which has been previously inoculated with a pure bacterial culture. After incubation of 18–24 hours the plate is removed and examined. Where bacteria are sensitive to a particular antibiotic, there will be a clear zone of growth inhibition around that disc (Figure 19.37).

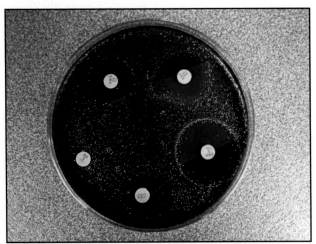

19.37 Antibacterial sensitivity plate: the organism was sensitive to three of the antibiotics (no growth zone around the disc) but resistant to the other two (no zone of inhibition).

Toxicology

Toxicological testing is carried out by specialist laboratories. Veterinary practices should check with the laboratory which are the most appropriate samples and/or tests available before sampling. Samples can be taken from both living and dead animals and they include blood, organs, stomach contents and vomit.

Virology

Testing for some viruses can be carried out in the practice using simple in-house testing kits (see above). For other viruses samples will need to be sent to external laboratories.

Considerations for toxicological and virological samples

- Check the laboratory's requirements before sampling.
- Wear PPE, to avoid contamination and potential zoonoses.
- The container used should be appropriate, robust and leak-proof.
- Separate containers should be used for each sample, to avoid cross-contamination. ▶

- If samples are not being examined for histopathology, they may be frozen to preserve them.
- All containers should be labelled, and accurate and detailed paperwork submitted.
- Copies of documentation and samples sent must be kept, as these may be required for legal reasons in some cases, e.g. poisoning.

Package and despatch of samples

It may be necessary to send samples to specialized external laboratories. If this situation arises, it is important that the external laboratory receives the sample in excellent condition.

Considerations for packaging

- Ensure the correct preservative is used for the sample.
- Ensure the correct collection container is used. These must be robust and leak-proof.
- Ensure accurate labelling of containers/samples.
- Ensure detailed paperwork is sent with the sample.
- Ensure national postal regulations are followed.
- If possible, blood samples should be submitted as either serum or plasma samples (see above) to avoid haemolysis.
- Ensure the correct packaging is used, i.e. to absorb spillages, prevent damage to containers.
- Ensure samples are kept at the correct temperature and humidity prior to dispatch.
- Be aware of postal strikes, bank holidays and weekends, which will delay delivery and affect sample quality.

External laboratories often supply their own containers and packaging to be used for submitting laboratory samples. These normally consist of:

- Containers, e.g. blood collection tubes, universal containers
- Forms/paperwork
- Absorbent material
- Secondary layer, e.g. plastic biohazard bag, polystyrene box
- Tertiary layer, e.g. padded bag-type envelope, cardboard box.

Packing and posting samples

1. Put on PPE, to avoid contamination and potential zoonoses.
2. Check that the sample is preserved correctly, i.e. is there adequate formalin?
3. Ensure the container is labelled with the animal's name, species, breed, age, sex, owner's name and date.
4. Ensure the container is airtight, moisture-proof and robust.
5. Ensure the total volume/mass of the sample in one package does not exceed 50 ml or 50 g.
6. Wrap the container in sufficient absorbent material to absorb the total volume of fluid in the sample, should the container leak or break. ▶

7. Place the sample in a secondary layer, e.g. plastic biohazard bag.
8. Ensure the laboratory paperwork/form has been completed and place this in a plastic bag separate from the sample.
9. Place all the items into the tertiary layer, e.g. a prepaid padded bag supplied by the laboratory.
10. Ensure the outer packaging contains the sender's name and address.
11. Ensure the outer packaging states the nature of the sample and any special instructions, e.g. handle with care, fragile, pathological specimen.
12. Ensure the sample is sent by first class post or via a courier.

Further details on the correct packaging and posting of samples can be checked through the Royal Mail or courier service.

Acknowledgement

The author would like to thank Alistair Foote for providing the information on horses.

Further reading

Bexfield N and Lee K (2010) *BSAVA Guide to Procedures in Small Animal Practice*. BSAVA Publications, Gloucester
Knottenbelt C (2007) Practical laboratory techniques. In: *BSAVA Manual of Practical Veterinary Nursing*, ed. E Mullineaux and M Jones, pp. 205–228. BSAVA Publications, Gloucester
Villiers E and Blackwood L (2005) *BSAVA Manual of Canine and Feline Clinical Pathology, 2nd edn*. BSAVA Publications, Gloucester

---

Self-assessment questions

1. List five pieces of legislation concerned with laboratory diagnostics.
2. What is the difference between plasma and serum?
3. List three types of urinary crystals.
4. What does a macroscopic examination of faeces involve?
5. List three types of media for bacterial culture.
6. What is a Gram stain?
7. List three types of bodily fluids that may be obtained via centesis.
8. What factors may alter the specific gravity of urine in the dog, cat and horse?
9. Define diagnostic cytology.
10. How should samples be packaged if sending to an external laboratory?

Chapter 20

Medical disorders of dogs and cats and their nursing

Robyn Gear and Helen Mathie

Learning objectives

After studying this chapter, students should be able to:

- **List the common medical disorders**
- **List the presenting signs, initial treatment and nursing care for a range of common medical conditions**
- **Describe the effects of the pathophysiological states and common pathologies on the animal body**
- **Explain the nurse's role when dealing with a range of medical conditions**
- **List the more commonly recognized complementary therapies and their uses**

Upper respiratory tract disease

The upper respiratory tract comprises the nasal cavity, pharynx, larynx and trachea.

Definitions

- **Sinusitis** – inflammation of one or more sinuses.
- **Rhinitis** – inflammation of the nasal lining.
- **Epistaxis** – bleeding from the nose.
- **Laryngitis** – inflammation of the larynx.
- **Tracheitis** – inflammation of the trachea.

Nasal disease

Clinical signs

- Sneezing.
- Snorting.
- Facial swelling.
- Facial rubbing.
- Dyspnoea.
- Nasal discharge.

Nasal discharge

Nasal discharge can be either bilateral or unilateral, depending on the causal factor. A good indicator as to the causal factor can be the type of discharge:

- Serous
- Mucoid
- Mucopurulent (Figure 20.1)
- Bloody.

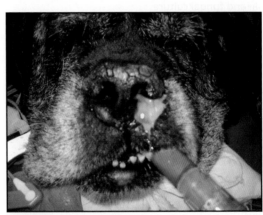

20.1 Mucopurulent nasal discharge from a dog with a nasal tumour.

Causes of nasal discharge (Figure 20.2) include viral, bacterial and fungal infections, allergies, neoplasia and foreign bodies. Trauma, tumours and coagulopathies can cause epistaxis (Figure 20.3).

Dogs
<ul><li>Distemper</li><li>Kennel cough complex</li><li>*Aspergillus* spp.</li><li>Foreign bodies, e.g. grass seeds</li><li>Neoplasia</li></ul>
Cats
<ul><li>Feline upper respiratory disease</li><li>*Chlamydophila*</li><li>Foreign bodies, e.g. blades of grass</li><li>Neoplasia</li><li>Trauma</li></ul>

20.2 Causes of nasal discharge and respiratory disease in various species.

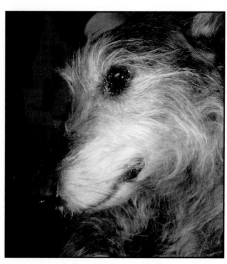

20.3

Epistaxis in a dog with a nasal tumour.

Diagnostics

- History and clinical examination.
- Blood tests: haematology, biochemistry, clotting profile and serology if pathogens suspected.
- Radiography of the nasal chambers and thorax.
- Rhinoscopy.
- Magnetic resonance imaging (MRI), computed tomography (CT).
- Bacterial and fungal culture.
- Nasal flush for cytology examination.
- Nasal biopsy and histopathology.

Treatment

The correct treatment will depend on the causal factor (e.g. supportive treatment for viral infections; antibiotics for primary and secondary infections; antifungal treatment for aspergillosis; removal of foreign bodies; surgery or radio-therapy for neoplasia).

Nursing care

- Isolate and barrier nurse the patient if it is thought to be infectious.
- Monitor vital signs.
- Keep the patient clean, bathe away discharge and groom as necessary. Prevent excoriation around orifices by the use of petroleum jelly.
- Encourage the patient to eat by feeding highly palatable, strong-smelling food, warming the food, hand-feeding, etc.
- Humidify the air.

Laryngeal disease

This can include conditions such as laryngitis, laryngeal paralysis, oedema and trauma. Causes of laryngitis include persistent barking in dogs and respiratory tract infections in dogs and cats.

Clinical signs

- Change in vocal ability (dysphonia).
- Coughing or gagging when attempting to bark or purr.
- Exercise intolerance or dyspnoea in the case of laryngeal paralysis; commonly, ageing medium to large breeds.

Diagnostics

- History and clinical examination.
- Examine larynx when patient is being anaesthetized.

Treatment

Treatment depends on the cause:

- Severe laryngeal paralysis – surgery often indicated
- Laryngitis – supportive treatment and possibly use of anti-inflammatory drugs and antibiotics.

Nursing care

- Use a head collar or harness to prevent pressure around the neck.
- Provide rest and avoidance of excitement.
- Keep patient cool.
- Administer oxygen if necessary.
- Veterinary surgeon to anaesthetize and intubate for severe laryngeal paralysis.

Tracheal disease

This can include conditions such as tracheitis and tracheal collapse and trauma. Clinical signs may include:

- Honking noise (tracheal collapse) – middle-aged obese dogs, especially Yorkshire Terriers
- Dry hacking cough
- Exercise intolerance or dyspnoea in tracheal collapse.

Diagnosis

- History and clinical examination.
- Radiography, tracheoscopy, tracheal wash.

Treatment

- Treatment depends on the cause.

Nursing care

- Use a head collar or harness to prevent pressure around the neck.
- Restrict exercise.
- Revise diet if the patient is obese (especially in the case of tracheal collapse).
- Avoid dry, dusty or smoky atmospheres.

Lower respiratory tract disease

The lower respiratory tract comprises the bronchi, bronchioles and alveoli.

Definitions

- **Dyspnoea** – difficulty in breathing.
- **Apnoea** – cessation of breathing.
- **Tachypnoea** – increased breathing rate.
- **Orthopnoea** – dyspnoea in lateral recumbency (usually improved in sternal recumbency).

Acute respiratory disease

Acute respiratory disease will occur when any part of normal respiration is interrupted or fails to function adequately. This will lead to the failure of oxygen being transferred to the circulation and of carbon dioxide being eliminated, resulting in hypoxia and hypercapnia. Causes can include the following:

- Ruptured diaphragm
- Pneumothorax, haemothorax, pyothorax, chylothorax
- Airway obstruction (e.g. foreign body, tracheal collapse)
- Neoplasia
- Infections
- Pulmonary oedema
- Pulmonary haemorrhage
- Paraquat poisoning
- Gastric torsion.

Clinical signs

- Tachypnoea, orthopnoea, dyspnoea.
- Mouth breathing.
- Cyanosis.
- Tachycardia.
- Collapse.

Nursing care

Acute respiratory disease is an immediate life-threatening emergency. When the patient arrives at the surgery the veterinary nurse should inform the veterinary surgeon and begin to set up and administer oxygen therapy. It is vital that the patient should not be stressed, as this will increase the patient's demand for oxygen. The method by which oxygen therapy is given should be chosen carefully to suit the patient (see Chapter 21). Minimal restraint should be used for any procedure to avoid the patient struggling. Tight-fitting collars and leads should be removed or loosened.

The patient may have to be supported in sternal recumbency to allow maximum lung inflation. If the patient is collapsed, the head and neck should be extended and the airways kept as clear as possible, without causing further stress.

Equipment should be prepared in case the patient deteriorates further. This equipment might include:

- Various sizes of endotracheal tube (local anaesthetic spray for cats) and bandage for securing the tube in place
- Oxygen supply and suitable anaesthetic circuit to provide intermittent positive pressure ventilation (IPPV)
- Laryngoscope
- Tracheostomy tube and surgical kit or large-gauge needle
- Thoracocentesis equipment
- 'Crash' box.

The patient should be monitored continually for any changes in its respiratory rate and character, heart rate, blood pressure and oxygenation if equipment available. The veterinary surgeon should be informed of such changes. See also Chapter 21.

Chronic pulmonary disease

Causes of chronic pulmonary disease (CPD) include:

- Bronchitis
- Pneumonia
- Pulmonary oedema (e.g. in cardiac failure)
- Feline asthma
- Lungworm
- Neoplasia
- Pulmonary haemorrhage.

Clinical signs

- Coughing.
- Wheezing.
- Tachypnoea.
- Exercise intolerance.
- Debility.

Diagnostics

- History and clinical examination.
- Blood tests for haematology and biochemistry.
- Thoracic radiographs.
- Bronchoscopy.
- Faecal analysis for lungworm larvae.
- Bronchoalveolar lavage to obtain a sample for culture and cytology.

Treatment

Treatment depends on the cause, but may include:

- Anti-inflammatory medication – to reduce inflammation
- Bronchodilators – to treat narrowing of the airways (e.g. in the case of feline asthma)
- Mucolytics – to reduce mucous viscosity to aid removal
- Expectorants – to aid removal of secretions
- Antibiotics – for primary or secondary bacterial infections
- Anthelmintics – for lungworm infections
- Antitussives – to suppress coughing if indicated, when coughing is persistent and unproductive
- Diuretics – for pulmonary oedema.

Nursing care

- Monitor vital signs.
- Provide rest and avoid stress.
- Provide oxygen therapy with or without nebulized medication.
- Ensure adequate fluid intake (dyspnoea increases fluid loss).
- Give coupage if indicated (check with veterinary surgeon).

Extrapulmonary disease

Clinical signs

The lungs are unable to inflate adequately as a result of air, fluid, abdominal organs or neoplasia in the thoracic cavity (Figure 20.4). The clinical signs are directly attributable to this.

The signs depend on the severity of the underlying condition but may include:

- Tachypnoea, shallow respiration, orthopnoea, dyspnoea
- Cyanosis
- Severe respiratory distress
- Shock
- Collapse.

Condition	Description	Cause	Other information
Diaphragmatic rupture	Abdominal organs in the thoracic cavity	Rupture of the diaphragm due to blunt trauma (e.g. road traffic accident, being kicked)	Heart can sound muffled, depending on extent of condition Size of rupture can determine how many of the abdominal organs are present in the chest cavity Patient should be handled carefully as viscera can move around, making the condition worse
Pneumothorax	Accumulation of air in thoracic cavity	Trauma to chest wall either blunt or penetrating (e.g. often seen following road traffic accidents)	Can be classified as **open** (e.g. when thoracic wall is penetrated, air is sucked into thorax from outside) or **closed** (e.g. following rupture to lungs, allowing air to leak from lungs into thoracic cavity) Chest percussion will produce increased resonance
Haemothorax	Accumulation of blood in thoracic cavity	Trauma or disease affecting pulmonary veins, arteries or other blood vessels in chest cavity	Heart can sound muffled depending on the extent of the condition Chest percussion will show decreased resonance in ventral thorax when patient in sternal recumbency
Hydrothorax	Accumulation of fluid (pure or modified transudate) in thoracic cavity	Hypoproteinaemia causing fluid to leak from blood vessels (pure transudate) Congestive heart failure or neoplasia (modified transudate)	Appearance of fluid (pure = clear and colourless; modified = straw coloured, pink, slightly opaque) Laboratory test will reveal: nucleated cell count <7 (1 x 10^9/l), specific gravity 1.018 or less with pure transudate, protein content <35 g/l Chest percussion as above
Pyothorax	Accumulation of pus (or exudates) in thoracic cavity	Bacterial infection (pyothorax) Feline infectious peritonitis (wet) Neoplasia	Appearance of fluid – often thick, yellow-brown and foul smelling Laboratory test will reveal: nucleated cell count 5–300 (1 x 10^9/l), specific gravity >1.018, protein content >30 g/l Chest percussion as above These patients are often pyrexic
Chylothorax	Accumulation of chyle in thoracic	Trauma or rupture of thoracic duct Congenital abnormalities of thoracic duct	Appearance of fluid – milky, fails to clear when centrifuged Triglyceride levels of the fluid should be tested to confirm that it is chyle Chest percussion as above
Neoplasia	Development of neoplasia involving thymus, mediastinal and sternal lymph nodes	Lymphosarcoma – common in ferrets FeLV infection Cysts	Neoplasia if large enough will interfere with normal lung expansion, but usually it is the pleural effusion generated that produces the clinical signs A non-compressible cranial mediastinum may be present with dull heart and lung sounds on auscultation
Ascites	In avian and reptile patients that do not possess diaphragm, development of ascites places pressure on air sacs (birds) or lungs directly (reptiles), causing dyspnoea	Usual causes of ascites (e.g. congestive heart failure, liver disease etc.)	Radiographically, loss of detail in coelomic cavity; ultrasonography will demonstrate hypoechoic fluid in normally air-filled spaces

20.4 Extrapulmonary disease.

Diagnosis

- Clinical examination.
- Blood tests.
- Thoracic radiographs.

Treatment

- Thoracocentesis.
- Indwelling chest drain (indicated for pyothorax and chylothorax).
- Specific treatment depending on the cause of the condition (e.g. surgery to repair ruptured diaphragm).

Nursing care

- Monitor vital signs.
- Decrease stress and provide a warm quiet environment.
- Provide oxygen therapy.
- Provide intravenous access and administer fluid therapy under veterinary surgeon's direction.
- Set up for and assist with thoracocentesis.

Nursing assistance with a thoracocentesis procedure

Equipment:

- Clippers
- Cotton wool swabs and skin disinfectant
- Local anaesthetic
- Sterile gloves
- Intravenous catheter – suitable size for patient; extension set and three-way tap, suitable size syringe
- Bowl for collection of any fluid
- Sterile sample pots (plain and EDTA).

Procedure

1. Place patient in sternal recumbency.
2. Clip thorax over 7th/8th intercostal space.
3. Veterinary surgeon will inject local anaesthetic and wait for it to take effect.
4. Surgically prepare thoracocentesis site.

continues ▶

continued
5. Veterinary surgeon will put on sterile gloves.
6. Hand equipment to surgeon in a sterile manner.
7. Veterinary surgeon will hand syringe to nurse.
8. Veterinary surgeon will insert catheter into thoracic cavity.
9. Attach syringe to catheter.
10. Gently withdraw plunger.
11. Once syringe is full, turn the three-way tap and empty of fluid or air.
12. Repeat procedure until no further air or fluid can be aspirated.
13. Repeat on other side of chest if required.
14. Fill sample pots and send for analysis.

Circulatory system disease

Definitions

- **Myocarditis** – inflammation of the muscular walls of the heart.
- **Endocarditis** – inflammation of the endocardium (endothelial membrane lining the cavities of the heart), most commonly involving a heart valve.
- **Endocardiosis** – chronic fibrosis and thickening of the atrioventricular valves.
- **Tachycardia** – rapid heart rate.
- **Bradycardia** – slow heart rate.
- **Pericarditis** – inflammation of the pericardium (sac around the heart).
- **Cardiomyopathy** – primary disease of the heart muscle.
- **Cardiac tamponade** – compression of the heart due to fluid accumulation in the pericardial sac.

Congenital heart disease

Congenital heart disease is present at birth. Many breeds have a predisposition to a specific defect or defects. Often it is detected at the first vaccination, when a heart murmur is auscultated. Clinical signs depend on the severity of the defect and include poor growth and those of heart failure: exercise intolerance, lethargy, dyspnoea and coughing. The diagnosis is made from the signalment of the patient, history, clinical examination, thoracic radiographs (including contrast studies), echocardiography and electrocardiography (ECG). Congenital conditions include: patent ductus arteriosus, valvular defects, septal defects and persistent right aortic arch.

Patent ductus arteriosus (PDA)

This is the most common congenital defect in dogs. In the fetus a vessel (ductus arteriosus) connects the pulmonary artery to the aorta, allowing blood to bypass the lungs. At birth this vessel normally closes but in a PDA it fails to do so and blood is shunted from the aorta into the pulmonary artery, thereby overloading the lungs. This causes left-sided heart failure and ultimately death if not treated.

Clinical signs

- A PDA is usually detected at first vaccination when a loud machinery-type murmur is auscultated.
- The patient may be poorly grown, asymptomatic or in heart failure.

Treatment

Treatment is via closure of the vessel with either surgery or implantation of a coil (both carried out by cardiac specialists). The prognosis is excellent with treatment.

Aortic and pulmonic stenosis

Stenosis is a narrowing of the aortic or pulmonic valves, obstructing the blood flow leaving the ventricles. This requires the heart muscle to work harder and there is compensatory hypertrophy of the muscle.

Clinical signs

- A heart murmur is auscultated, which may or may not be accompanied by clinical signs.
- Patients can present with syncope or signs of heart failure.

Treatment

Pulmonic stenosis can be treated with dilation of the area with a balloon (balloon valvuloplasty). Aortic stenosis is treated symptomatically. The narrower the outflow, the worse the prognosis.

Mitral/tricuspid valve dysplasia

This is a malformation of the mitral or tricuspid valves. Blood regurgitates into the atria, increasing their workload, and they enlarge. This leads to congestion and right- (tricuspid) or left-sided (mitral) heart failure. In some cases both valves will be affected. The condition is less common than PDA or aortic/pulmonary stenosis.

Clinical signs

- A heart murmur is auscultated, which may or may not be accompanied by clinical signs.
- Patients can present with heart failure.

Treatment

Treatment is symptomatic treatment for heart failure (see below).

Ventricular/atrial septal defects

These defects are known as 'holes in the heart'. A hole connects either the atria or the ventricles. Blood flows through the heart abnormally, leading to heart failure. Ventricular septal defects are the most common congenital defects in cats.

Clinical signs

- A heart murmur may be auscultated.
- The patient may be asymptomatic or have congestive heart failure.

Treatment

Symptomatic treatment of heart failure. Animals with small defects can live normal lives. The larger the lesion, the more guarded the prognosis.

Combined defects – tetralogy of Fallot

Some patients can present with a combination of defects. The most common is tetralogy of Fallot, which is a combination of a ventricular septal defect, pulmonic stenosis, compensatory right-sided hypertrophy and an overriding aorta. These patients present with cyanosis, as the blood bypasses the lungs. The prognosis is guarded.

Persistent right aortic arch (vascular ring anomaly)

This is a congenital malformation of the major arteries of the heart which traps the oesophagus, obstructing boluses of food from reaching the stomach.

Clinical signs

- Regurgitation and failure to thrive are usually evident when the animal is weaned.
- Aspiration pneumonia can be a complication.

Treatment

Treatment is surgery to ligate and cut the remnant. If there is permanent oesophageal dysfunction and megaoesophagus, the patient needs to be managed with feeding from a height and monitoring for aspiration pneumonia (see 'Regurgitation'). The prognosis is excellent as long as no permanent damage has been done to the oesophagus.

Acquired heart disease

Endocardial disease: endocardiosis

Disease of the heart valves is most commonly due to chronic fibrosis (endocardiosis). Endocardiosis is the most frequently encountered heart disease in dogs, but is very rare in cats. The mitral value is most commonly affected, although the tricuspid valve can be affected. It is a progressive condition. Endocardiosis prevents the valves from functioning correctly and blood regurgitates into the atria, increasing their workload, causing congestion and heart failure. Infection of the heart valves (endocarditis) is less common.

Clinical signs

Clinical signs of mitral valve endocardiosis include a murmur. Other signs are those of left-sided heart failure (see later). Clinical signs of tricuspid valve endocardiosis are those of right-sided heart failure (see later).

Treatment

Endocarditis is inflammation of the inside lining of the heart chambers and heart valves (endocardium).
Clinical signs of endocarditis include:

- Pyrexia
- Lethargy
- Shifting lameness
- Anorexia
- Heart murmur.

Diagnostics

A presumptive diagnosis can be made on history and clinical examination:

- Thoracic radiographs: right lateral and dorsoventral views
- Echocardiography
- ECG
- Blood culture.

Treatment

- Patients with endocardiosis are treated when heart failure has developed (see below).
- Endocarditis is treated with broad-spectrum antibiotics pending blood culture results.

Recording an electrocardiogram

This should be carried out with minimal stress to the patient and without sedation.

- The animal is placed in right lateral recumbency and gently restrained.
- ECG pads can be placed on the main pads of the paws. Alligator forceps can be traumatic and painful and should if possible be reserved for emergency situations; they can be attached on the upper part of the leg, where there is some loose skin.
- Good contact is made by using ECG gel or spirit. The latter should not be used if there is a chance that the animal may be defibrillated.
- The electrodes are attached as follows:
  - Red – right forelimb
  - Yellow – left forelimb
  - Green – left hindlimb
  - Black – right hindlimb.
- A standard six-lead ECG is recorded (leads I, II, III, aVL, aVR, aVF), usually at settings of 10 mV and 25 mm/s.
- The ECG should be labelled with the animal's details, date, settings and leads used.
- Ensure that it is of diagnostic quality, with minimal interference.

The electrode placement can be remembered as 'Red = Right' (both begin with R) and then work in an anti-clockwise direction in the order of traffic lights – yellow, green. Black is placed on the remaining limb, i.e. right hindlimb.

Myocardial disease

Cardiomyopathies are diseases of the myocardium associated with cardiac dysfunction. Cardiomyopathy is the most frequently recognized cardiac condition in cats (commonly hypertrophic cardiomyopathy). It is also seen in large and giant breeds of dog (commonly dilated cardiomyopathy).

Hypertrophic cardiomyopathy

Thickening of the heart muscle interferes with relaxation of the heart, preventing normal filling, leading to poor diastolic function, decreases in cardiac output and heart failure. In cats the condition is not uncommon and may be secondary to hyperthyroidism.

Clinical signs

Many cases in cats are clinically 'silent', but if congestive heart failure is present signs include:

- Dyspnoea, tachypnoea
- Tachycardia
- Heart murmur.

A common complication in cats is aortic thromboembolism, where a thrombus (blood clot) leaves the heart and lodges in the caudal aorta (most commonly), obstructing blood flow to the hindlimbs. Clinical signs include:

- Acute onset of unilateral/bilateral paresis/paralysis of the hindlimbs
- Lack of arterial pulse in the affected leg(s)
- Pain
- Hindlimb(s) cool to the touch
- Dyspnoea, tachypnoea.

Diagnostics

- Echocardiography.
- Thoracic radiographs: right lateral and dorsoventral views.
- ECG.
- Blood pressure measurement.
- Blood tests: T4 (for hyperthyroidism), renal function.
- Additional tests if a clot is suspected include blood tests: haematology and biochemistry, clotting profile and abdominal ultrasonography.

Treatment

Treatment of hypertrophic cardiomyopathy is aimed at improving cardiac relaxation and slowing the heart rate: calcium channel blockers (e.g. diltiazem) and beta blockers (e.g. atenalol, propranalol). Blood clots are treated with pain relief, antithrombotics and vasodilators.

Dilated cardiomyopathy

This is characterized by dilatation of the heart chambers and poor systolic function and heart failure. In dogs, dilated cardiomyopathies are seen most frequently in large breeds and there is a familial predisposition in Dobermanns, Irish Wolfhounds, Great Danes, Newfoundlands, Boxers and other breeds. The heart enlarges and there is reduced cardiac contractility, decreasing forward flow of blood and causing congestion and heart failure. In cats, the cause may be idiopathic or due to taurine deficiency, though the latter is now rare because of good commercial diets.

Clinical signs

- Apparently acute onset.
- Anorexia, weight loss, reduced exercise tolerance, lethargy.
- Usually present with signs of left-sided heart failure (coughing, dyspnoea, tachypnoea) and sometimes concomitant right-sided heart failure.
- Ascites.
- Heart murmur, tachycardia.
- Arrhythmias.
- Sudden death.

Diagnostics

- Echocardiography.
- Thoracic radiographs: right lateral and dorsoventral views.
- ECG.

Treatment

Each patient is assessed and treated based on the severity of the disease but general guidelines are as per management of heart failure (see below).

Arrhythmias

Arrhythmias occur as a result of a disturbance of the electrical activity in the heart. This can be due to primary heart disease, or secondary to another systemic disease. Arrhythmias can be broadly categorized into bradycardic (slow) arrhythmias and tachycardic (fast) arrhythmias (Figure 20.5). They are further divided according to where the arrhythmia arises, either in the ventricles or above the ventricles.

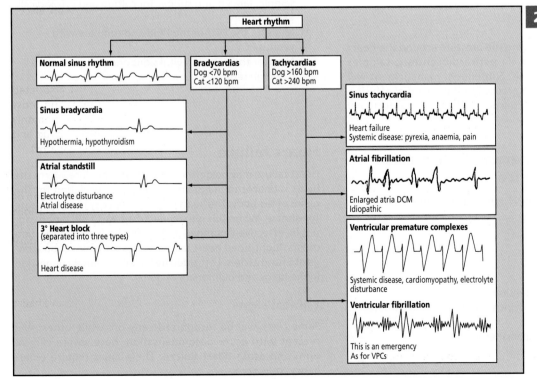

20.5 Arrhythmias.

Clinical signs

- May be asymptomatic.
- Collapse.
- Exercise intolerance, weakness.

Diagnostics

- Blood tests: electrolytes.
- ECG to document type of arrhythmia.
- Thoracic radiographs, echocardiography for underlying cause.

Treatment

Treatment depends on the type of arrhythmia and whether or not the patient is symptomatic. If possible, the underlying cause should be treated. Tachycardia is treated with antiarrhythmic drugs. Bradycardia can be treated with a pacemaker.

Pericardial disease

An effusion accumulates in the pericardial sac and restricts filling of the right side of the heart, leading to right-sided heart failure. A pericardial effusion is usually either idiopathic or secondary to a tumour of the heart.

Clinical signs

- Collapse.
- Exercise intolerance.
- Pale mucous membranes.
- Muffled heart sounds, tachycardia.
- Distended abdomen.
- Variable pulse quality.

Diagnostics

- Echocardiography.
- Thoracic radiographs: right lateral and dorsoventral views.
- ECG.

Treatment

Treatment involves relieving the pressure around the heart and removing the fluid via pericardiocentesis; samples should be sent for analysis. Subsequent management will depend on the underlying cause but if pericardial effusion recurs, surgical removal of the pericardium (pericardectomy) is indicated.

Procedure for pericardiocentesis: nursing assistance

The following is one of various pericardiocentesis techniques.

Equipment:

- 60 ml syringe
- Three-way stopcock
- Intravenous fluid extension line
- 16 gauge $3\frac{1}{4}$-inch or 5-inch over-the-needle catheter
- Sterile gloves
- Lidocaine for local anaesthesia
- Scalpel blade.

  ▶

Technique

This is a sterile procedure. It may be carried out with the patient standing or in sternal or left lateral recumbency.

If sedation is required, it should be administered according to the veterinary surgeon's instructions. The patient should have constant monitoring throughout the procedure. The patient should be monitored with ECG if available.

1. Surgically clip the ventral third of the right hemithorax from the 3rd to the 8th intercostal space.
2. The veterinary surgeon will infiltrate the areas with lidocaine.
3. Surgically prepare the clipped area.
4. Pass the equipment to the surgically scrubbed and gloved veterinary surgeon in a sterile manner.
5. The veterinary surgeon will pass the syringe, 3-way stopcock and one end of the extension set to the veterinary nurse. Connect the syringe to the 3-way stopcock and intravenous extension tubing.
6. The veterinary surgeon will make a small cutaneous incision with the scalpel blade and advance the catheter into the pericardial space. The veterinary surgeon's end of the intravenous extension is then attached to the catheter.
7. The veterinary nurse will then be instructed to aspirate the fluid slowly. A small volume is removed first to check it does not clot. If it does this may indicate incorrect placement of the needle within a vessel.
8. During the procedure the catheter may block and the veterinary surgeon will need to reposition it.
9. Ventricular premature complexes may be seen during the procedure. These usually resolve once the procedure is completed. The ECG may need to be monitored intermittently for abnormal rhythms once the procedure is complete.
10. The fluid is usually very bloody. Collect a sterile sample, label it and submit for culture and cytological examination.
11. Measure the PCV of the fluid and compare with venous PCV.
12. Monitor the patient's vital signs once the procedure is completed.

Heart failure

Heart failure may be defined as circulatory failure where the heart is unable to maintain an adequate circulation for the needs of the body. The heart has some capacity to compensate for disease. When this is exceeded the heart fails; blood cannot be effectively pumped around the body and congestion occurs. Right-sided heart failure causes systemic venous congestion and ascites. Left-sided heart failure causes congestion in the lungs and pulmonary oedema.

Clinical signs

Some cases will be recognized early on, while others will present with acute decompensation, have severe clinical signs and acute heart failure. These cases require emergency treatment.

Acute heart failure

- Collapse.
- Pale mucous membranes.
- Slow capillary refill time.
- Weak pulse.

This is an emergency and requires immediate treatment (see Chapter 21).

Left-sided heart failure

- Pulmonary oedema.
- Cough.
- Dyspnoea, tachypnoea.
- Tachycardia, weak pulses.
- Murmurs, dysrhythmias (in many cases).
- Exercise intolerance, fatigue, lethargy.
- Cyanosis in severe cases.

Right-sided heart failure

- Ascites, abdominal distension.
- Hepatomegaly, splenomegaly.
- Exercise intolerance, fatigue, lethargy.
- Pale mucous membranes, tachycardia, weak pulses.
- Dyspnoea, tachypnoea, cyanosis.
- Murmurs, dysrhythmias (in many cases).

Diagnostics

In a patient with heart disease the first indication of failure can be an increased breathing rate and heart rate. Therefore, these need to be monitored at home by the owners.

- Thoracic radiographs: right lateral and dorsoventral views.
- Echocardiography.
- ECG.
- Blood tests: biochemistry, especially urea, creatinine and electrolytes.

Treatment

Acute heart failure

- Strict cage rest.
- Oxygen supplementation.
- Glyceryl trinitrate (applied topically to inside of ear; wear gloves).
- Diuretics.

Chronic heart failure (left-sided, right-sided, congestive)

- Reduce exercise.
- Reduce obesity if present.
- Low salt diet (see below).
- Diuretics to relieve pulmonary oedema, ascites.
- Cardiac drugs – ACE inhibitors (decreases upregulation of fluid retention), pimobendan (improves contractility).
- Anti-arrhythmic drugs if required.

Nursing care

Acute heart failure

- Do not stress.
- Provide oxygen.
- Provide cage rest.
- Keep warm.

- Monitor vital signs; the resting respiratory rate is a good indication of response to treatment.

Chronic cases

- Decrease stress and exercise.
- Manage for weight loss if the patient is overweight.
- Monitor vital signs – particularly resting respiratory rate.
- Blood tests to monitor for dehydration and electrolyte imbalances secondary to diuretic treatment.

Nutrition

Animals with heart failure can be anorexic; therefore it is important that the diet is palatable. Various formulated diets are available. These have added nutrients and usually increased potassium and magnesium but decreased sodium (salt restriction) (see Chapter 13). As treats are often high in salt, low-salt alternatives need to be used (e.g. formulated treats or a slice of apple or orange). Overweight patients must be given a weight-control diet.

It should be noted that new cardiac drugs may alter the electrolyte balance of the patient and so these need to be monitored and the diet adjusted as necessary.

Haemopoietic system disease

Definitions

- **Anaemia** – reduced number of red blood cells or reduced quantity of haemoglobin.
- **Erythrocytosis** – increased number of red blood cells.
- **Leucocytosis** – increased number of white blood cells.
- **Leucopenia** – reduced number of white blood cells.
- **Thrombocytopenia** – reduction in number of platelets.
- **Lymphocytosis** – increase in number of lymphocytes.
- **Leukaemias** – distorted proliferation and development of leucocytes and their precursors in the blood and bone marrow.

Anaemia

Anaemia is a clinical sign rather than a diagnosis. It may have many causes (Figure 20.6).

- In regenerative anaemias, the bone marrow is capable of making an appropriate response to the anaemia: it increases the production of red blood cells and releases immature red blood cells (reticulocytes) into the circulation. Regenerative anaemias are distinguished by the presence of these reticulocytes in the blood.
- In non-regenerative anaemias the bone marrow is not capable of making an appropriate response to the anaemia: there is no increase in red blood cell production.

Clinical signs

In acute anaemias the clinical signs can be severe and require emergency treatment. Conversely, mild and chronic anaemias can have very few apparent clinical signs.

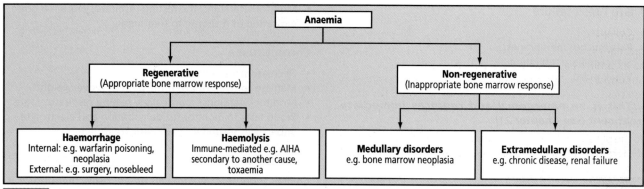

```
                              ┌──────────────┐
                              │   Anaemia    │
                              └──────┬───────┘
                      ┌──────────────┴───────────────┐
```

| **Regenerative** (Appropriate bone marrow response) | **Non-regenerative** (Inappropriate bone marrow response) |

| **Haemorrhage** Internal: e.g. warfarin poisoning, neoplasia External: e.g. surgery, nosebleed | **Haemolysis** Immune-mediated e.g. AIHA secondary to another cause, toxaemia | **Medullary disorders** e.g. bone marrow neoplasia | **Extramedullary disorders** e.g. chronic disease, renal failure |

20.6   Types and causes of anaemia.

- Collapse.
- Lethargy.
- Inappetence.
- Exercise intolerance.
- Pale mucous membranes.
- Dyspnoea, tachypnoea.
- Tachycardia sometimes with an anaemia induced (haemic) murmur.

Diagnostics

- Blood tests: haematology – full blood count and fresh blood smear; morphology of the cells is important as it can help with determining the cause, including presence of reticulocytes.
- Biochemistry (disease in other organs may result in secondary anaemia).
- In-saline agglutination (slide agglutination test) and Coombs' test for autoimmune haemolytic anaemia.
- Serology, especially if travel history.
- FeLV/FIV tests in cats.
- *Mycoplasma* – fresh blood smear needed (see 'Feline infectious anaemia').
- Faecal occult blood (red-meat-free diet for 3 days).
- Non-regenerative anaemias: bone marrow aspiration (see Chapter 19).

  Other tests that may be indicated include:

- Coagulation profile
- Radiographs – chest, abdomen (e.g. evidence of bleeding or neoplasia)
- Ultrasonography – chest, abdomen (e.g. evidence of bleeding or neoplasia).

Treatment

The animal may need a blood transfusion (Figure 20.7) if the anaemia is severe or if there are severe clinical signs. The underlying cause needs to be treated (e.g. immunosuppresion for immune-mediated disease; chemotherapy for neoplasia; tetracyclines for *Mycoplasma*).

Nursing care

- Monitor vital signs.
- Restrict exercise, keep quiet and avoid stress.
- Monitor blood transfusion.
- Take blood samples to monitor progress.

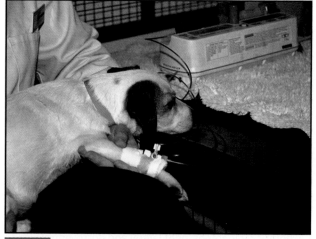

20.7   Blood transfusion in an anaemic dog.

Clotting disorders

The normal blood clotting mechanism (haemostasis) is described in Chapter 3. Clotting defects can result in haemorrhage and thus give rise to anaemia. Clotting disorders may result from primary or secondary defects:

- Primary haemostatic defect:
  - Vessel defect
  - Platelets (decreased number or increased consumption)
  - von Willebrand factor deficiency (rarely seen in cats but commonly seen in certain breeds of dog, e.g. Dobermann, Rottweiler, poodles and Golden Retriever)
  - Often presents with no clinical signs until the dog begins bleeding for some reason, e.g. after surgery or a bitch in oestrus
  - Signs may include nose bleeds, vaginal or penile bleeding and petechiae.
- Secondary haemostatic defect:
  - Decreased levels of clotting factors
    o Decreased production (e.g. liver disease, warfarin toxicity)
    o Increased consumption (e.g. disseminated intravascular coagulation, DIC).

Clinical signs

A primary abnormality in haemostasis usually leads to haemorrhages in the skin or mucous membranes. These are referred to as **petechial** (pinpoint) or **ecchymotic** (Figure 20.8). An abnormality in clotting factors can lead to bleeding into body cavities such as the pleural or peritoneal space. If the blood loss is severe, the patient will have clinical signs of anaemia. Other clinical signs will be related to the underlying cause and to the physical effect of accumulation of blood (e.g. dyspnoea if there is bleeding in the pleural space).

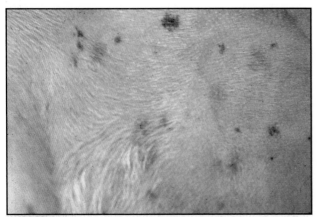

20.8 Ecchymotic haemorrhages in the skin as a result of a primary haemostatic disorder.

Diagnostics

Caution is required when nursing, as the patient can bleed. It is important to have a confident and careful approach to taking blood and to ensure that there is adequate pressure applied to the venepuncture site afterwards to prevent haemorrhage. For clotting factors, fresh blood should be collected into a tube containing sodium citrate anticoagulant and tested within 2 hours.

- Haematology and biochemistry.
- Clotting profile: prothrombin time, activated partial thromboplastin time.
- Activated clotting time.
- Buccal mucosal bleeding time (This is performed if the above tests are normal; it assesses primary haemostasis).
- von Willebrand factor.
- Clotting factor assays.
- Platelet function tests.
- Fibrin degradation products, D-dimers.

Buccal mucosal bleeding time (BMBT)

1. Restrain the patient in lateral recumbency (cats usually require light sedation).
2. Fold back the upper lip and tie a strip of gauze around the maxilla, enough to cause moderate mucosal engorgement.
3. Make an incision on the upper lip by gently holding the buccal mucosal bleeding spring-loaded blade on the lip and firing it.
4. Start the timer. ▶

5. Gently blot away bleeding with filter paper, taking care not to disturb the incision and the formation of the clot.
6. When bleeding ceases, stop the timer.

The normal bleeding time for dogs is <4.2 minutes and for cats <2.4 minutes.

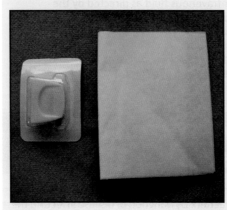

Spring-loaded buccal mucosal bleeding device and filter paper

Treatment

The underlying cause needs to be treated (e.g. immunosuppression for immune-mediated disease; vitamin K for warfarin poisoning). If the bleeding is severe, the patient may require whole blood or plasma to replace clotting factors. Desmopressin can be used to increase von Willebrand factor and can be used prior to surgery in affected animals.

Nursing care

- Handle very gently, padded beds, minimal manual handling.
- Blood samples should be taken from a peripheral vein to ensure that adequate pressure can be applied to the site.
- Avoid intramuscular injections.
- Monitor vital signs.

Lymphoma

This is a cancer of the lymphoid tissue.

Clinical signs

- Enlarged lymph nodes.
- Weight loss.
- Anorexia, inappetence.
- Vomiting, diarrhoea.
- Clinical signs associated with other organs affected.

Diagnostic tests

- Haematology.
- Biochemistry.
- Fine-needle aspiration (FNA) of an enlarged peripheral lymph node (ideally unassociated with the head).
- Biopsy of the lymph node if FNA cytology non-diagnostic.
- Radiography, ultrasonography.

Treatment

- Chemotherapy.
- Intravenous fluids.

Nursing care

- Monitor vital signs.
- Assist the veterinary surgeon when administering chemotherapy.
- Practise safe handling of chemotherapeutic drugs and excreted waste and fluid from the patient (see Chapters 2 and 8).
- Administer intravenous fluid as directed by the veterinary surgeon.
- Administer medication as directed.
- Offer palatable food.
- Provide water.
- Keep the patient clean and comfortable.

Gastrointestinal tract disease

The GI tract comprises the oesophagus, stomach, small intestine, colon and rectum. Dysfunction or disease affecting these organs can lead to regurgitation, vomiting and diarrhoea.

Definitions

- **Dysphagia** – difficulty in swallowing.
- **Coprophagia** – eating of faeces.
- **Anorexia** – absence of appetite.
- **Pica** – depraved appetite (e.g. eating of unusual foodstuff).
- **Inappetence** – reduced appetite.
- **Polyphagia** – increased appetite.
- **Megaoesophagus** – flaccid dilatation of oesophagus.
- **Regurgitation** – passive process of returning ingesta, usually from oesophagus.
- **Vomiting** – active process of expelling stomach contents.
- **Diarrhoea** – increased passage of abnormally softer liquid faeces.
- **Tenesmus** – straining to pass faeces.
- **Dyschezia** – pain on defecation.
- **Melaena** – dark tar-like faeces containing digested blood.
- **Constipation** – failure to pass faeces of normal frequency or consistency.

Regurgitation

It is important to be able to differentiate between regurgitation and vomiting. Regurgitation is a *passive* process: there is no contraction of the abdominal muscles; the head is lowered and undigested food is ejected from the mouth. The severity of the condition can vary from the regurgitation of all solid food to regurgitation of some ingested matter and saliva. Malnutrition and aspiration pneumonia can result, depending on the severity of the condition. If there is any doubt as to the origin of the undigested food matter (i.e. whether it is from the oesophagus or from the stomach) a dipstick can be used to check the pH, as it can sometimes be difficult to determine (true stomach contents will be acidic).

Causes of regurgitation can include:

- Megaoesophagus
- Oesophagitis

- Oesophageal foreign bodies
- Oesophageal strictures
- Persistent right aortic arch.

Diagnostics

- Blood samples for haematology and biochemistry; other specific tests to detect myasthenia gravis, and hypoadrenocorticism (Addison's disease).
- Plain and barium swallow radiographs.
- Oesophagoscopy.

Treatment

The treatment will vary depending on the underlying cause of the problem:

- Medical management to treat any underlying disease that causes megaeosophagus
- Anti-inflammatories and histamine H_2 blockers for oesophagitis
- Endoscopic or surgical removal of oesophageal foreign bodies
- Ballooning for oesophageal strictures
- Surgery for animals with persistent right aortic arch.

Further management can include feeding animals from a height (see Chapter 13). Gravity-assisted feeding can help to control the clinical signs if the problem is not too severe. Keeping the patient's head and forelimbs elevated for 10 minutes after a meal will allow the food to enter the stomach. In other cases liquid food can be fed to pass a stricture, or balls of food may be given for megaoesophagus if some peristaltic activity is present.

Nursing care

- Monitor patient's vital signs and hydration status.
- Monitor and record patient's weight.
- Observe for regurgitation and record frequency and consistency.
- Observe for signs of aspiration pneumonia (coughing, depression, pyrexia).
- Offer food and water from a height.
- Groom and clean patient as necessary.
- Administer medication and fluid therapy as directed by the veterinary surgeon.

Vomiting

Vomiting is an *active* process, where the stomach contents are forcefully ejected out of the mouth by the contraction of the abdominal muscles. It is a common clinical sign of many conditions, as it is a protective mechanism that helps to eliminate toxic substances from the body. Receptors in the brain are triggered by the presence of certain toxins or when normal levels of substances found in the body are exceeded (e.g. urea). Causes of vomiting are shown in Figure 20.9.

Prior to vomiting the animal may show signs of restlessness, abdominal pain, salivating or licking of the lips. An episode of vomiting may occur many hours after the animal has eaten and the vomitus may contain partially digested food, bile or a mixture of both.

Vomiting can be classified as **acute** or **chronic**, depending on the speed of onset and its duration. Depending on the frequency of vomiting and the volumes involved, there can

Gastrointestinal disease
• Dietary indiscretion • Infectious agents: viral (e.g. parvovirus); bacterial (e.g. *Salmonella*); parasitic (e.g. roundworms) • Gastric foreign bodies • Intestinal foreign bodies • Intussusception • Gastrointestinal ulceration • Pyloric stenosis • Gastrointestinal neoplasia

Systemic disease
• Uraemia – due to either renal disease or urinary tract obstruction • Hepatic failure • Pyometra • Pancreatitis • Peritonitis

Metabolic/endocrine disorders
• Diabetic ketoacidosis • Hypercalcaemia • Hypoadrenocorticism

Drugs/toxins
• NSAIDs • Chemotherapy drugs • Heavy metal toxicity • Insecticide toxicity (e.g. organophosphates) • Herbicide toxicity (e.g. chlorates) • Molluscicide toxicity (e.g. metaldehyde)

20.9   Causes of vomiting.

be a significant loss of water from the body and dehydration if the animal is unable to replace these losses. Electrolytes (sodium, chloride and potassium) are also lost, along with hydrogen ions, and this can result in electrolyte imbalances and metabolic alkalosis (see Chapter 22).

Diagnostics

It can sometimes be difficult to discover the cause of vomiting in a patient. Obtaining a detailed history is an important part of the diagnostic approach. It is equally important that close observations of a patient are made if an animal is hospitalized.

- History (see below).
- Clinical examination – abdominal palpation important.
- Blood samples for haematology and biochemistry to confirm or rule out systemic disease.
- Abdominal radiography and/or ultrasonography.
- Barium meal.
- Gastroscopy.
- Exploratory laparotomy.
- Biopsy (via endoscopy or laparotomy).

Assessing the vomiting patient

- **Body condition:** A depressed or lethargic patient is more likely to have systemic disease, dehydration or electrolyte imbalances. Weight loss and general body condition can also provide important information about the cause of vomiting.
- **Age:** Older animals are more likely to have neoplasia. Younger animals are more likely to have infections or have eaten foreign bodies. ▶

- **Other clinical signs:** Clinical signs such as polyuria and polydipsia can indicate the presence of systemic disease.
- **Vaccination history:** Up-to-date vaccination status can help to rule out some infectious agents.
- **Dietary changes:** Changes in feeding can help to confirm or rule out uncomplicated gastroenteritis. A history of scavenging (or opportunity to scavenge) should also be ascertained.
- **Frequency of vomiting:** Can provide important information about the causal factor. For example, infectious agents such as parvovirus or *Salmonella* are often associated with acute bouts of frequent vomiting.
- **Type of vomit:** Vomit containing blood can indicate ulceration or severe inflammation of the GI tract. Vomition of undigested food long after a meal can suggest gastric motility problems.
- **Faeces:** Lack of faeces can indicate obstruction. Diarrhoea indicates intestinal involvement. Melaena (blackened by digested blood) indicates ulceration and bleeding from the upper GI tract. Fresh (undigested) blood indicates bleeding from the lower GI tract.

Treatment

Uncomplicated **acute** vomiting is managed by starving the patient for 24 hours, whilst providing oral fluid and electrolyte replacement. If the animal responds successfully, an investigation of the cause is often not undertaken. Further symptomatic treatment may also be required.

Treatment for **chronic** vomiting is aimed at treating the underlying disease, controlling the clinical signs and correcting the dehydration. Drug therapy may include:

- Specific drugs acting on the GI tract (see Chapter 8)
- Fluid therapy – important to correct dehydration, electrolyte and acid–base imbalances (see Chapter 22)
- Analgesia – to make the patient more comfortable (NSAIDs should be avoided).

Surgery may be indicated for correction of pyloric stenosis, intussusception or removal of foreign bodies and tumours.

Nursing care

- Isolate and barrier nurse if an infectious agent is suspected (see Chapter 12).
- Starve the patient for 24 hours and then feed small frequent meals.
- Feed a bland easy-to-digest single-source protein diet.
- Keep the patient clean and groom as necessary.
- Monitor clinical signs, weight and hydration status and record findings.
- Observe and record vomiting type and frequency.
- Administer medication and fluid therapy, as directed by the veterinary surgeon.

Diarrhoea

Diarrhoea can be classified as either acute or chronic and can originate from the small intestine, the large intestine or both (Figure 20.10). It results in a loss of water from the body, leading to dehydration, electrolyte imbalances and metabolic acidosis.

Clinical sign	Origin: small intestine	Origin: large intestine
Vomiting	Commonly seen	Occasional
Weight	Loss common	Maintained
Appetite	Often increased	Normal
Faecal volume	Increased	Normal
Faecal type	Watery	Varies with cause
Faecal frequency	3–4 times daily	Up to 10 times daily
Faecal mucus	None	Often present
Blood in faeces	Melaena	Haematochezia
Urgency to pass faeces	Not present	Present; straining on defecation
Flatulence	Minimal	Common

20.10   Clinical signs suggesting the origin of diarrhoea.

Causes

Acute diarrhoea

- Sudden change of diet or scavenging.
- Dietary intolerance or hypersensitivity.
- Colitis and other GI disturbances.
- Viral infections (e.g. parvovirus, FIV, FeLV).
- Bacterial infections (e.g. *Salmonella*, *Campylobacter*, *Escherichia coli*).
- Intestinal parasites (e.g. *Toxocara*, *Giardia*, *Cryptosporidium*).
- Intussusception.
- Neoplasia.
- Foreign bodies.

Chronic diarrhoea

- Long-term dietary intolerance or hypersensitivity.
- Chronic infections (e.g. *Giardia*, *Campylobacter*).
- Antibiotic-responsive diarrhoea.
- Malabsorption (e.g. inflammatory bowel disease (IBD)).
- Maldigestion (e.g. exocrine pancreatic insufficiency (EPI)).
- Colitis and other GI disturbances.
- Intussusception.
- Neoplasia.
- Foreign bodies.
- Liver disease, due to lack of bile salts being produced.
- Endocrine disease (e.g. hyperthyroidism, hypoadrenocorticism).

Clinical signs

- **Acute** diarrhoea can be mild or severe. In mild cases the animal appears bright and alert with no signs of dehydration. In severe cases the animal is dull, depressed and dehydrated, especially if accompanied by vomiting.
- In **chronic** diarrhoea clinical signs are more commonly weight loss and loss of bodily condition, as the causes result in the animal receiving inadequate nutrition over a period of time.

Diagnostics

A thorough history can provide important information as to the cause of the diarrhoea. Also observation of the frequency and the consistency of the diarrhoea (e.g. steatorrhoea) can indicate exocrine pancreatic insufficiency (EPI).

- Clinical examination.
- Routine biochemistry and haematology to rule out systemic disease.
- Specific blood tests: trypsin-like immunoreactivity (TLI); to confirm or rule out EPI, cobalamin (vitamin B12) is checked as it can be low in gastrointestinal disease.
- Faecal analysis – for parasites, undigested food, culture; ELISA for parvovirus antigen.
- Abdominal radiography and/or ultrasonography.
- Contrast radiography.
- Endoscopy of upper or lower GI tract.
- Exploratory laparotomy.
- Biopsy (via endoscopy or laparotomy).

Treatment

Acute diarrhoea

In cases of acute diarrhoea, fasting for 24–48 hours is usually sufficient as long as during this period of time the animal is not vomiting, and fluid and electrolytes are supplemented. In severe acute cases, intravenous fluid therapy is indicated to prevent dehydration and electrolyte imbalance. Fasting for longer periods should be avoided, as the intestine absorbs the majority of its nutrition from the digested food that passes through it. Long periods of starvation can therefore result in reduced functioning capabilities of the intestine.

Treatment of any underlying cause is also important.

When food is reintroduced it should be a bland, easy-to-digest, low-fat and single-source protein diet. This should be fed for a number of days before gradually reintroducing normal food.

Chronic diarrhoea

In cases with chronic diarrhoea, investigation of the underlying cause is important for successful treatment. Treatments can include:

- In cases of hypersensitivity, feeding a protein that the animal has never eaten before
- Anthelmintics and antiparasitic drugs
- Antibacterials for antibiotic responsive diarrhoea
- Corticosteroids for inflammatory bowel disease
- Enzyme supplementation in cases with EPI
- Surgery for intussusception, neoplasia and foreign bodies
- Treatment of underlying systemic disease.

Nursing care

- Isolate and barrier nurse if an infectious agent is suspected (see Chapter 12).
- Feed a diet that contains high-quality protein and is low in fat (see Chapter 13).
- Feed small frequent meals.
- Keep the patient clean and groom as necessary. It may be necessary to bandage the tail, clip the hair and apply barrier cream to the skin if diarrhoea is severe.
- Monitor clinical signs, weight and hydration status and record findings.
- Observe and record passing of any diarrhoea.
- Allow frequent visits outside to defecate (if not thought to be infectious).
- Administer medication and fluid therapy, according to veterinary surgeon's instructions.

Colitis

The cause of colitis is often not determined. Many cases of acute colitis are associated with dietary indiscretion, resulting in a secondary bacterial infection. Causes of chronic colitis can include: inappropriate immune response to antigens in the colon (e.g. eosinophilic colitis); infections – *Campylobacter*, *Salmonella*; neoplasia or polyps; motility disorders and food hypersensitivity reactions. Treatment includes: hypoallergenic diet; change of diet; increase or reduce fibre, sulfasalazine – as anti-inflammatory; metronidazole – anti-bacterial but also has anti-inflammatory effect; corticosteroids – used in cases not responding to other treatment.

Constipation

Constipation is the failure to pass faeces either in normal quantity or at normal frequency, resulting in impaction of the colon and rectum with faecal material. There are many causes of constipation (Figure 20.11). It is seen more commonly in elderly patients taking less exercise.

Dietary
• Fibre content of diet too low • Eating bones
Colonic
• Rectal strictures • Rectal foreign bodies • Rectal tumours • Perineal ruptures • Megacolon (dysautonomia) • Anal sac disease
Orthopaedic
• Pelvic fractures causing narrowing of pelvic canal
Other
• Dehydration • Neurological dysfunction (Key–Gaskell syndrome; spinal damage) • Prostatic hyperplasia

20.11 Causes of constipation.

Clinical signs

- Failure to pass faeces.
- Tenesmus.
- Passing of very hard faeces (often with fresh blood).
- Vomiting.
- Dyschezia (pain on passing faeces).

Diagnostics

- Physical examination/rectal examination.
- Radiography.
- Proctoscopy.

Treatment

It is important to find the underlying cause to provide the best treatment, but treatment may include:

- Enemas – various types (use most suitable) (see Chapter 17)
- Changes to diet
- Stool-softening agents (lactulose, pumpkin)
- Bulking agents
- Surgical correction of obstruction.

Nursing care

- Administer enema under veterinary surgeon's instructions.
- Administer fluid therapy.
- Monitor vital signs.
- Keep the patient clean.
- Encourage the patient to eat a suitable diet.

Hepatic disease

Definitions

- **Hepatitis** – inflammation of the liver.
- **Cirrhosis** – a degenerative change, causing fibrosis of the organ, resulting in a loss of functional cells and therefore loss in normal function.
- **Ascites** – accumulation of fluid in the abdominal cavity.
- **Jaundice** – elevated levels of bilirubin in the tissues and circulation, resulting in a yellowing of the skin and mucous membranes.

Causes

Liver disease may be congenital or acquired, and acute or chronic. There are many causes which are often not identified, including:

- Acute:
  - Drug-induced (e.g. paracetamol, phenobarbital)
  - Toxins (e.g. bacterial endotoxin, blue-green algae)
  - Bacterial infection (e.g. *Leptospira*, *Salmonella*)
  - Viral infection (e.g. adenovirus I (ICH), canine herpes)
  - Parasitosis (e.g. toxoplasmosis)
  - Acute pancreatitis
  - Surgical hypotension or hypoxia
  - Trauma (e.g. bruising or rupture).
- Chronic:
  - Drug-induced (e.g. phenobarbital)
  - Neoplasia (e.g. haemangioma, haemangiosarcoma)
  - Metabolic (e.g. diabetes mellitus, hyperadrenocorticism)
  - Copper toxicity (in Bedlington Terrier and West Highland White Terrier)
  - Immune-mediated (e.g. cholangiohepatitis, chronic progressive hepatitis)
  - Congenital (e.g. portosystemic shunts).

Portosystemic shunt

The hepatic portal system enables the products of digestion that are absorbed by the gut to be transported directly to the liver for storage or use (see Chapter 3). In a normal animal the blood flows:

- From the heart to the capillary beds of the stomach and intestines

- From here to the liver via the hepatic portal vein, where it enters the capillary bed of the liver
- From the liver via the hepatic vein to the posterior vena cava.

With a portosystemic shunt the blood bypasses the liver and deposits blood directly back into the systemic circulation. Clinical signs are frequently seen post feeding, and blood ammonia levels are elevated. Shunts can be a developmental abnormality or they can be due to advanced cirrhosis. Ultrasonography is used to identify the location and extent of shunting and possible treatment options. Some congenital shunts can be surgically ligated, others can only be treated medically. In cirrhosis multiple shunting vessels develop which cannot be ligated.

Clinical signs of liver disease

The liver has enormous regenerative capabilities and chronic clinical signs will not be noticed until 70–80% of the liver cells have been lost due to damage.

Non-specific signs include:

- Vomiting
- Diarrhoea
- Weight loss
- Polydipsia
- Polyuria
- Anorexia.

Specific signs include:

- Anterior abdominal pain
- Jaundice
- Ascites
- Hepatomegaly
- Hepatoencephalopathy
- Pale fatty faeces – due to decreased bile production
- Dark urine – due to bilirubin from red cell breakdown
- Bleeding disorders – due to clotting factor deficiency.

Jaundice (icterus)

Jaundice of the skin (Figure 20.12) and mucous membranes will occur if the capacity of the liver to excrete bilirubin in the bile becomes unbalanced:

- Prehepatic (e.g. excessive haemolysis)
- Intrahepatic (e.g. degenerative liver function)
- Posthepatic (e.g. bile flow obstruction).

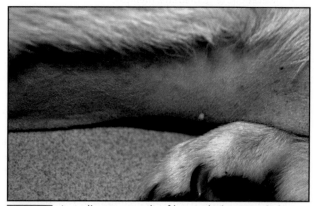

20.12 Jaundice as a result of haemolytic anaemia in a 6-year-old Labrador Retriever.

Hepatic encephalopathy

This occurs when >70% of hepatic tissue is lost and neurotoxic substances build up, causing toxaemias and neurological signs. The toxins are mainly from the gastrointestinal tract (e.g. ammonia is a by-product of protein breakdown).

Diagnostics

- Biochemistry:
    - Albumin
    - Globulin
    - Alanine aminotransferase (ALT)
    - Alkaline phosphatase (ALP)
    - Gamma glutamyltransferase (GGT) (cats).
- Bile acid stimulation test (liver function test).
- Haematology:
    - Full blood count
    - Coagulation screen.
- Radiography – can provide information about the size of the liver.
- Ultrasound scan – can give a more useful indication of internal structure of the liver and can identify focal or diffuse lesions.
- Fine needle aspirate of the liver – can give indication as to cause or nature of the disease.
- Liver biopsy – will most likely provide definitive diagnosis, but coagulation screen should be run first.

Treatment

- Intravenous fluids (acute cases).
- Antibiotics (to reduce bacterial load).
- Anti-inflammatories.
- Water-soluble bile acids.
- Lactulose (helps to bind ammonia).
- Special diet and supplements (see Chapter 13).

Nursing care

- Isolate and barrier nurse the patient if cause is infectious.
- Monitor vital signs.
- Administer medication and therapy.
- Provide comfort and TLC.
- Provide nutritional support (see Chapter 13).

Pancreatic disease

The pancreas is composed of two types of tissue:

- Exocrine – produces digestive enzymes
- Endocrine – produces hormones (insulin, glucagon).

Diseases of the exocrine pancreas can be divided into:

- Pancreatitis – acute and chronic
- Exocrine pancreatic insufficiency
- Exocrine tumours.

Pancreatitis

Pancreatitis, inflammation of the pancreas, is caused by self-digestion (**autolysis**) of the pancreas by the digestive enzymes that are stored inside specialized storage pockets. It can be acute or chronic.

Acute pancreatitis

This can be life-threatening, as complications such as peritonitis can develop. Predispositions include:

- Obesity
- High-fat diet
- Pancreatic duct occlusion
- Hypotension.

Clinical signs

- Vomiting (not seen as often in cats).
- Pyrexia.
- Anorexia.
- Acute abdominal pain.
- Dehydration.
- Shock.
- Collapse.

Diagnostics

- Blood tests (elevated levels of canine specific pancreatic lipase or feline specific pancreatic lipase).
- Radiography.
- Ultrasonography.

Treatment

- Nothing by mouth (*nil per os*, NPO) until vomiting stops.
- Intravenous fluid therapy.
- Analgesics.
- Low-fat diet.
- Antiemetics if vomiting persists.

Nursing care

- Monitor vital signs (this is important, as disease can quickly progress to a life-threatening state).
- Withhold food if instructed by the veterinary surgeon.
- Keep the patient away from the sight and smell of other patients' food.
- Groom and keep the patient clean (it is often necessary to clean the gums and mucous membranes, as the animal is unable to drink oral fluids).
- Administer fluid therapy and other medications, as instructed by the veterinary surgeon.
- After clinical signs have resolved, and on the instruction of the veterinary surgeon, introduce small amounts of water and observe the patient's vital signs closely.
- If the patient tolerates water, introduce small frequent low-fat meals (see Chapter 14) and observe the patient's vital signs closely.

Chronic pancreatitis

This is a low-grade but continual inflammation of the pancreas, leading to functional destruction. The causes include:

- Idiopathic
- Infection
- Cholangiohepatitis (especially in cats)
- Ascending infection (especially in cats)
- Bile duct obstruction (especially in cats).

Clinical signs

- Recurrent vomiting and discomfort.
- Weight loss.
- Reduced appetite.
- Abdominal pain.

Diagnostics

Diagnostic tests are as for acute pancreatitis, with the addition of testing for trypsin-like immunoreactivity (TLI) and vitamin B12 levels.

Treatment

- Long-term dietary management (low/reduced fat) use low fat for acute then reduced fat.
- Fluid and electrolyte support.
- Enzyme supplementation if EPI occurs.

Exocrine pancreatic insufficiency (EPI)

This condition is caused by insufficient production of pancreatic enzymes, resulting in maldigestion and malabsorption of food. Pancreatic atrophy occurs. It can be congenital and may be hereditary in German Shepherd Dogs. It can also occur following a severe case of pancreatitis if the cells of the pancreas are damaged. The condition is relatively common in dogs but rare in cats.

Clinical signs

- Diarrhoea.
- Steatorrhoea.
- Ravenous appetite.
- Coprophagia (eating faeces) – due to presence of undigested food.
- Weight loss.

Diagnostics

- Blood test for haematology and biochemistry, to include trypsin-like immunoreactivity (TLI).
- Faecal analysis for undigested food.

Treatment

- Supplementation of food with pancreatic enzymes – amylase, lipase, and protease; dietary management still required.

Nursing care

- Feed small frequent meals of low/reduced-fat diet.
- Mix enzyme supplement with food.
- Monitor faecal output – colour, consistency and frequency.
- Groom and keep the patient clean.
- Check and record weight.

Renal disease

Definitions

- **Nephritis** – inflammation of the kidney.
- **Glomerulonephritis** – inflammation of the glomerulus.
- **Pyelonephritis** – inflammation of the kidney and renal pelvis.
- **Interstitial nephritis** – inflammation of the renal interstitium.

Acute renal failure

Acute renal failure may occur as a consequence of:

- Decreased blood flow to the kidneys (e.g. hypovolaemic shock)
- Direct effect on the cells of the kidneys (e.g. toxins: ethylene glycol toxicity (antifreeze); infectious causes: leptospirosis)
- Post-renal obstruction (e.g. urethral stone causing obstruction, blocked bladder or rupture of the urinary tract)
- Acute exacerbation of chronic renal failure.

Clinical signs

- Sudden-onset anorexia, lethargy, depression.
- Oliguria and anuria, followed by polyuria.
- Vomiting, diarrhoea.
- Polydipsia.
- Dehydration.
- Uraemic breath.

Diagnostics

- Blood tests: haematology and biochemistry (urea, creatinine, electrolytes – specifically potassium, phosphate).
- Urinalysis: specific gravity, dipstick and sediment examination.
- Abdominal radiography: right lateral and ventrodorsal views.
- Abdominal ultrasonography.

Treatment

Treatment involves removing the inciting cause and if possible treating the underlying cause. It is usually supportive.

- Intravenous fluid therapy is very important for several reasons: to decrease potassium (which is the initial life-threatening complication); to dilute the built-up waste products; and to rehydrate the animal. It is also the first line in establishing urine output.
- If oliguria persists, drugs such as furosemide, dopamine and mannitol may be administered to improve urine output.
- Antiemetics can be used to manage persistent vomiting.
- Peritoneal dialysis is used to remove nitrogenous waste products when urine output has failed to be re-established with the above treatment.

The condition is often reversible if the patient comes through the acute crisis.

Nursing care

- Barrier nurse the patient if an infectious cause is suspected.
- Administer fluid therapy, as directed by the veterinary surgeon.
- Monitor vital signs, respiratory rate and sounds – especially for signs of volume overload.
- Monitor urine output. If normal output (1–2 ml/kg/h) is not re-established, discuss with the veterinary surgeon; a urinary catheter may need to be placed (this must be managed aseptically).
- Monitor hydration status.
- Monitor bodyweight.
- Administer drugs as directed by the veterinary surgeon.
- Encourage the patient to eat, and feed a renal diet (see Chapter 13).
- Monitor vomiting.
- Keep animal clean, grooming and bathing as necessary.

Chronic renal failure

This slowly progressive loss of renal function over an unidentified period of time results in **azotaemia** (uraemia). The onset of the clinical signs is gradual and may only become noticeable when 75% of the nephrons have already been lost. It is most often seen in animals over 7 years of age (Figure 20.13) but this can depend on the causal factor, as younger animals can be affected.

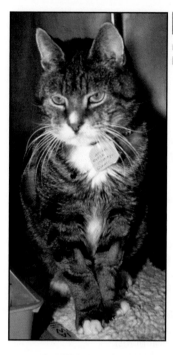

20.13 A 13-year-old cat with chronic renal failure showing poor body condition.

Causes of chronic renal failure include:

- Idiopathic
- Acute renal failure
- Nephrotoxins
- Pyelonephritis
- Glomerulonephritis
- Ischaemic damage
- Hypercalcaemia
- Congenital/hereditary disease (e.g. polycystic kidney disease).

Clinical signs

- Polyuria/nocturia (as the kidney loses its ability to concentrate the urine).
- Polydipsia.
- Uraemia – anorexia, vomiting, lethargy, depression.
- Weight loss.
- Dehydration.
- Oral ulceration and halitosis.
- Non-regenerative anaemia (due to lack of erythropoietin production by the kidney).

- Hypertension.
- Rubber jaw (renal hyperparathyroidism) – kidneys fail to excrete phosphorus, effectively causing phosphorus levels in blood to become elevated (hyperphosphataemia); parathyroid responds by triggering release of parathyroid hormone (PTH), resulting in demineralization of calcium from bones to correct imbalance in blood.
- Seizures – end-stage of disease.

Diagnostics

- Biochemistry – high levels of urea, creatinine and phosphorus.
- Hypokalaemia often evident.
- Haematology: non-regenerative anaemia.
- Urinalysis: lower than normal specific gravity often evident.
- Abdominal radiography and/or ultrasonography.
- Blood pressure frequently increased.

Treatment

Chronic renal failure is not reversible. Treatment is aimed at preventing further damage and reducing the workload of the remaining nephron.

- Treatment of any underlying cause.
- Intravenous fluid therapy if required (allow water to drink, unless vomiting). Subcutaneous fluid if the patient is treated as an outpatient.
- Antiemetics if vomiting.
- Electrolyte supplementation, if required due to increased losses.
- Dietary management (see Chapter 13).
- ACE inhibitors such as benazepril to help treat systemic and glomerularhypertension.
- Vitamin B supplementation.
- Erythropoietin by injection.

Nursing care

- Monitor vital signs and urine output.
- Administer fluid therapy and any other medication.
- Provide water *ad libitum*.
- Take patient outside regularly or keep litter tray clean.
- Feed special diet (see Chapter 13).
- Encourage patient to eat if inappetent.

If the animal is anorexic it should be offered other more palatable foods; for example, a recovery diet can be used initially until the patient's appetite improves. If the patient does not eat it will become catabolic, as it is metabolizing protein (its own body mass), and byproducts of protein metabolism can still contribute to azotaemia. However, in this case the animal will also be losing weight and body condition.

Nephrotic syndrome

This is caused by either immune-mediated damage to the glomerular basement membrane or amyloidosis.

Clinical signs

- Ascites.
- Subcutaneous oedema.
- Hydrothorax (dyspnoea).
- Weight loss.
- Exercise intolerance.

May initially be bright until chronic renal failure develops; then additional signs of CRF (see above).

Diagnostics

- Biochemistry – hypoproteinaemia.
- Urinalysis – severe proteinuria.
- Urine protein-to-creatinine ratio.
- As for chronic renal failure.

Treatment

- Diet – high biological value protein, low phosphate, high B vitamins.
- Diuretics.
- As for chronic renal failure.

Lower urinary tract disease

The lower urinary tract comprises the ureters, bladder and urethra. Disease of these organs results from inflammation, obstruction or dysfunction.

Definitions

- **Cystitis** – inflammation of the urinary bladder.
- **Urinary incontinence** – involuntary passing of urine.
- **Urinary tenesmus** – straining to pass urine.
- **Haematuria** – the presence of blood in the urine.
- **Polyuria** – passing of increased volumes of urine.
- **Dysuria** – difficulty and pain passing urine.
- **Oliguria** – reduced urine production.
- **Anuria** – absence of urine production.
- **Pollakiuria** – abnormal frequency of urination (used in paediatrics, where it is a benign condition), passing very small amounts of urine.

Diagnostic tests

- Blood tests for biochemistry and haematology.
- Urinalysis: specific gravity, dipsticks, sedimentation examination, culture and sensitivity (urine for this test must be obtained via cystocentesis).
- Ultrasonography.
- Radiography: contrast studies such as pneumocystograms and double-contrast cystograms.
- Intravenous excretory urography (IVU).
- Retrograde urethrography.
- Histology.

Cystitis

Causes of cystitis include:

- Idiopathic
- Trauma
- Urolithiasis (urinary calculi)
- Neoplasia

- Primary bacterial infection – often ascending, common in females
- Bacterial infection secondary to other diseases (e.g. diabetes mellitus, hyperadrenocorticism (Cushing's disease), immunosuppressive infections – FIV, FeLV).

Clinical signs

- Pollakiuria.
- Urinary tenesmus.
- Haematuria.
- Incontinence.
- Dysuria.

Treatment

- Identification and treatment of any underlying cause.
- Appropriate antibiotic therapy if a bacterial Infection has been diagnosed – bacteria such as *Escherichia coli*, *Staphylococcus*, *Streptococcus* and *Pseudomonas* have all been identified as causal agents.

Nursing care

- Monitor vital signs.
- Ensure that water is freely available.
- Take patient outside frequently.
- Monitor urine output (note volume and frequency, and whether straining or haematuria is present).
- Administer medications, as directed by veterinary surgeon.

Urolithiasis (urinary calculi)

Urinary calculi or uroliths (see Chapter 19) can form within the urinary tract in the renal pelvis, ureters, bladder or urethra. Causes include:

- Urinary tract infection
- High dietary intake of certain minerals
- Systemic disease (e.g. liver disease)
- Genetic predisposition (e.g. high incidence of urate calculi in Dalmatians).

See also FLUTD below.

Clinical signs

- Pollakiuria.
- Urinary tenesmus.
- Haematuria.
- Dysuria.
- Distended bladder.

Treatment

Diet plays a major role in the control and management of some types of urinary calculi (i.e. struvite, urate and cystine) (see Chapter 13). Dietary dissolution of calculi is possible for certain uroliths, but surgical removal is required for some calculi such as those composed of calcium oxalate or calcium phosphate. Diet is used to prevent the recurrence of calculi after removal. These diets change the urinary pH, make the urine more dilute, and contain lower dietary levels of the minerals that contribute to calculi formation.

If urinary obstruction occurs, the same steps should be followed as for obstructed feline lower urinary tract disease (see below).

Nursing care

- Monitor vital signs.
- Ensure that water is freely available.
- Take outside frequently.
- Monitor urine output (note volume and frequency, and whether straining or haematuria is present).
- Administer medications as directed by the veterinary surgeon.

Urinary incontinence

Urinary incontinence is the involuntary passing of urine. Leakage of urine may be continuous or intermittent and may occur when the animal is recumbent or standing. Causes include:

- Urethral sphincter mechanism incontinence
- Ectopic ureters (congenital; more common in females; ureter often ends in vagina)
- Bladder-neck tumour (transitional cell carcinoma)
- Prostatic disease
- Neurological disease
- Cystitis.

Clinical signs

- Passing of urine when lying down or walking.
- Urine around perineum.
- Urine scalding of the skin around the perineum.

Treatment

Treatment will be specific to the cause, but can include:

- Phenylpropanolamine or oestrogen for sphincter mechanism incontinence
- Surgery for ectopic ureters
- Surgery with or without chemotherapy for tumours
- Castration or hormone treatments for prostatic hyperplasia
- Antibiotic therapy for cystitis.

Nursing care

- Clip and clean the perineum.
- Apply barrier creams to prevent urine scalding.
- Provide suitable bedding to draw urine away from the patient, change bedding often.
- Administer medication as directed by the veterinary surgeon.
- Monitor for signs of secondary urinary tract infections.

Feline lower urinary tract disease (FLUTD)

FLUTD may be obstructive or non-obstructive. In many cases the cause is unclear, but FLUTD is commonly seen in overweight, young to middle-aged, indoor cats fed on dry food in multi-cat households. It is thought that these cats have a tendency to urinate less frequently than outdoor cats, resulting in stale urine remaining in the bladder for longer periods, which gives rise to increased levels of bacteria in the urine and precipitation of crystals. Stress is also thought to be a contributing factor. Research has found that cats with cystitis have reduced levels of glycosaminoglycan (GAG), a component of the bladder membrane.

FLUTD affects both male and female cats, but male cats tend to be affected by obstructive disease due to the narrow size of the urethra in comparison with females. The distal end of the urethra becomes blocked with calculi or clumps of crystals and mucus (urethral plugs).

Causes of FLUTD include:

- Idiopathic (up to 65% of cases)
- Urethral plugs
- Uroliths
- Bacterial infection.

Clinical signs

Clinical signs for both non-obstructive and obstructive FLUTD are as for cystitis (see above). With obstructive FLUTD these signs may lead to:

- Distress
- Anuria
- Distended bladder
- Renal damage.

Treatment of obstructive FLUTD

Urethral obstruction is a serious life-threatening condition, which requires urgent medical attention.

- Blood tests should be performed to assess the patient's metabolic state (urea and creatinine often elevated due to postrenal azotaemia; potassium levels elevated; analysis of blood gases if available).
- Cystocentesis should be performed to empty the bladder or at least alleviate the pressure. A sample can be taken at this time for analysis and culture.
- Intravenous fluid therapy should be initiated (a fluid type that does not contain potassium).
- Once the cat is stable he should be anaesthetized.
- The blockage can then be dislodged; massage of the penis tip or retrograde flushing is often required to pass a urinary catheter, and the bladder should then be flushed with saline.
- The veterinary surgeon will decide whether or not an indwelling catheter should be left in place, as this can increase the urethral inflammation already present.
- If a urinary catheter is fitted, it should be sutured in place and either plugged or a closed collection system fitted, to prevent ascending infection. The patient should also be fitted with an Elizabethan collar to prevent interference.
- Antibacterial, analgesic and anti-inflammatory drugs are given (avoid NSAIDs in cases with possible renal involvement).

Nursing care of obstructive FLUTD

- Monitor vital signs.
- Perform regular blood test as described by the veterinary surgeon to monitor azotaemia and potassium levels.
- Administer and maintain fluid therapy.
- Monitor urine output and aseptically maintain urinary catheter if in place; apply barrier creams to prevent scalding.
- Groom and keep patient clean, especially if fitted with an Elizabethan collar.
- Administer any other medications as per veterinary

surgeon's instructions.
- Encourage eating of a suitable urinary diet; if inappetent, tempt patient with other food initially.

Treatment of non-obstructive FLUTD

This usually involves long-term management by the owners at home.

- Dietary management: feeding a diet that has low levels of magnesium and phosphorus. Wet foods are preferable as this increases the urine output. Weight loss is to be encouraged if the cat is overweight.
- Increase water consumption: ensure that the cat always has access to clean water. Cats prefer large shallow bowls. Commercial water fountains are available that provide filtered running water; these are often successful, as cats tend to prefer to drink running water.
- Provide glycosaminoglycan (GAG) supplementation to promote the health of the bladder lining.
- Reduce stress levels; use pheromones or, in severe cases, amitriptyline.
- Make regular biochemistry and urinalysis checks.

Prostatic disease

The prostate can be affected by:

- Benign prostatic hyperplasia (BPH)
- Prostatitis
- Prostatic abscessation
- Prostatic cysts
- Prostatic neoplasia (rare; may occur in young and old dogs).

Clinical signs

- Haematuria.
- Dysuria.
- Urinary incontinence.
- Urinary and faecal tenesmus.
- Constipation.

Diagnostics

- Ultrasonography.
- Radiography.
- Urinalysis.
- Prostatic massage/flushing/biopsy.

Treatment

- BPH is treated with castration or hormone treatment.
- Prostatitis is treated as for BPH and with antibiotics.
- Surgical intervention is required for cysts and abcessation.
- Palliative treatment for neoplasia.

Reproductive system disease

Diseases of the reproductive system are discussed in detail in Chapter 26.

Endocrine and metabolic disorders

The hormones are manufactured and secreted by various endocrine glands and the functions of those hormones are described in Chapter 3.

Diabetes mellitus

Diabetes mellitus is caused by the lack of insulin, or a relative lack of insulin. Insulin is required to regulate glucose in the body. In the absence of insulin the animal will become hyperglycaemic. Clinical signs are attributable to this.

In the majority of dogs the condition is caused by immune destruction of the insulin-producing cells in the pancreas. Dogs generally require insulin therapy for treatment. In cats diabetes is often a result of insulin resistance due to obesity. These cats may produce insulin but the cells do not respond adequately. The cat may only be temporarily diabetic and can sometimes be managed with oral hypoglycaemic drugs. Insulin resistance can also be seen in entire bitches, in hyperadrenocorticism (Cushing's disease) and pancreatitis.

If diabetes is left untreated, fats are broken down, leading to a build-up of ketones. These patients quickly become dehydrated, are acidotic and have electrolyte abnormalities. This condition is called **diabetic ketoacidosis** (DKA).

Clinical signs

The majority of cases present with a history of:

- Polyuria/polydipsia
- Increased appetite (polyphagia) with weight loss.

More serious clinical signs that may indicate that the animal has developed DKA include:

- Vomiting
- Diarrhoea
- Anorexia
- Depression
- Collapse.

Other clinical signs include:

- Cataracts in dogs
- Plantigrade posture in cats.

Diagnostics

- Blood: haematology, biochemistry and fructosamine levels.
- Urinalysis: dipstick, especially for presence of glucose and ketones in the urine, culture and sensitivity.

Treatment

Treatment involves subcutaneous administration of insulin.

The only insulin with a veterinary authorization is Caninsulin (Intervet/Schering-Plough), which is a porcine lente insulin (40 IU/ml) and is generally used twice daily. Where this is ineffective, other insulins authorized for human use, such as human protamine zinc insulin (PZI) or glargine insulin (both usually 100 IU/ml) may also be prescribed.

Patients undergoing anaesthesia should have their glucose measured on the morning of surgery and the insulin given as directed by the veterinary surgeon. Blood glucose levels should be monitored during anaesthesia, and dextrose saline administered intravenously as necessary.

If there is insulin resistance, the underlying cause needs to be treated (e.g. treat hyperadrenocorticism; spay a diabetic bitch).

The 'well' diabetic dog

It is very important that patients follow a routine in their insulin administration, diet and exercise. Routine should be adapted to the owner's lifestyle and can be flexible, to a small degree.

- Insulin therapy: intermediate-acting insulin lente or protamine zinc insulin (PZI) administered once or twice daily or as per the veterinary surgeon's instructions (note that insulin preparations authorized for veterinary use are usually 100 IU/ml or 40 IU/ml).
- Diet: high-fibre, medium-protein, low-fat diet for dogs and low-carbohydrate, high-protein diet for cats (see Chapter 13)
  - If receiving once-daily insulin, feed once when insulin administered and the second meal 6–8 hours later to coincide with lowest glucose point
  - If receiving twice-daily insulin, meals are given at the time of insulin administration, usually every 12 hours.
- Exercise – same time every day.

The 'well' diabetic cat

- Insulin therapy:
  - Intermediate-acting insulin or PZI once or twice daily as per veterinary surgeon's instructions
  - Insulin therapy can be discontinued in some cats with non-insulin-dependent diabetes
  - Glucose needs to be monitored closely.
- Diet: high-protein or high fibre/low carbohydrate, ad libitum (see Chapter 13) or twice daily to coincide with insulin.
- Exercise: as per usual.

The diabetic ketoacidotic patient

DKA is a life-threatening condition and needs intensive treatment.

- Fluid therapy to rehydrate the patient and correct acidosis and electrolyte imbalances.
- A short-acting human neutral (soluble) insulin is given intravenously or intramuscularly to lower blood glucose slowly.
- Glucose, electrolytes and phosphate need to be monitored frequently and treatment adjusted as directed by the veterinary surgeon.

Long-term monitoring

The diabetic patient is monitored by owner observations (appetite, water consumption, urine output, weight control) and blood tests. The insulin is adjusted on the basis of a combination of these findings.

- Fructosamine: indication of blood glucose control over 2–3 weeks.

- Serial blood glucose curves: give indication of how long the insulin is effective for and the time the lowest glucose level occurs. Blood is usually taken every 2 hours over a 24-hour period and the glucose level plotted on a graph. This needs to follow as normal a routine as possible, with minimal stress to the patient, as stress causes hyperglycaemia (this is especially important in cats).
- Urinalysis to monitor for ketones, glucose and developing urinary tract infections.

Urine glucose monitoring and subsequent adjustment of insulin by the owner is *not* recommended, as urine glucose can be misleading. The presence of glucose in the urine can be a result of underdosing with insulin but can also be as a result of *over*dosing in the case of insulin-induced hyperglycaemia (see below).

Hyperglycaemia

Hyperglycaemia in diabetic patients most commonly results from underdosing with insulin or poor control of diabetes due to other medical conditions (e.g. hyperadrenocorticism, infections). Hyperglycaemia can also confusingly arise as a result of overdosing with insulin. The reason for the latter is a compensatory mechanism called the Somogyi overswing. An overdose of insulin will make the patient hypoglycaemic; hormones are then released to increase the glucose in the blood; there is a compensatory overswing and the patient becomes hyperglycaemic. Therefore if a patient is found to have an unexpected increase in blood or urine glucose prior to the administration of the morning insulin, it may be an indication to perform a serial blood glucose curve or other diagnostic tests.

Hypoglycaemia

Hypoglycaemia is a complication that occurs as a result of an insulin overdose. Clinical signs include:

- Lethargy
- Ataxia
- Muscle twitching
- Severe seizures.

It is most likely to occur at the time of peak activity of the insulin. Immediate action must be taken, which may involve feeding, rubbing honey or glucose on the gums, or administering intravenous dextrose (as directed by veterinary surgeon). If left untreated, coma and death will ensue.

Nursing care

Uncomplicated diabetes mellitus

- Assist the veterinary surgeon with diagnostic tests.
- Administer insulin, as directed by the veterinary surgeon.
- Feed appropriate diet at times requested (see Chapter 13).
- Ensure that water is freely available.
- Take the patient outside frequently.
- Monitor blood glucose levels.
- Monitor urine for glucose and ketones.
- Monitor vital signs.
- Clean and groom the patient as necessary.
- Administer fluid therapy, as directed by the veterinary surgeon.

- Administer any other medication.
- Provide outpatient support to clients (diabetic clinics): weight; urine sample; blood sample (fructosamine); discuss progress, appetite, water intake, urination, vision (diabetic cataracts), exercise tolerance.

Diabetic ketoacidosis

- Monitor vital signs.
- Monitor glucose and electrolyte levels, as directed by veterinary surgeon.
- Administer intravenous fluid therapy, as directed by veterinary surgeon.
- Administer insulin injections, as directed by veterinary surgeon. Take particular note of the type of insulin to be administered and the route of administration.
- Administer intravenous glucose if blood levels fall, as directed by veterinary surgeon.
- Supplement intravenous fluids as directed by veterinary surgeon (or with electrolytes and phosphate).
- Encourage the patient to eat suitable food, or *any* food if anorexic.
- Clean and groom as necessary.
- Monitor animal's response to treatment.

Nutrition

Successful management of a diabetic patient involves an appropriate dietary regime as well as insulin therapy (see Chapter 13).

Hyperadrenocorticism (HAC) (Cushing's disease)

Hyperadrenocorticism is common in the dog but rare in the cat. It occurs as a result of excessive cortisol in the body. This may be due to excessive administration of steroid or an overproduction of cortisol by the adrenal glands. The latter is a result of either a tumour in the pituitary gland (pituitary-dependent HAC), which overstimulates the adrenal glands to produce cortisol, or a tumour of the adrenal gland (adrenal-dependent HAC). Pituitary-dependent HAC is the most common form.

Clinical signs

- Polyuria/polydipsia.
- Polyphagia.
- Pot-belly (Figure 20.14).
- Panting.
- Bilateral alopecia and skin changes (thin inelastic skin).
- Muscle atrophy and weakness.

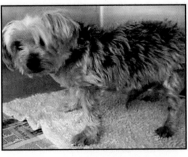

20.14 A dog with hyperadrenocorticism. Note the pot-bellied appearance.

Diagnosis

- Blood tests: haematology and biochemistry.
- ACTH stimulation test.
- Low-dose dexamethasone suppression test (LDDST).
- High-dose dexamethasone suppression test (HDDST).
- Endogenous ACTH assay.
- Abdominal ultrasonography.
- Abdominal radiography.
- MRI or CT (pituitary and adrenal areas).

The ACTH stimulation and LDDST are confirmatory tests. The HDDST and endogenous ACTH assay are used to differentiate between pituitary-dependent and adrenal-dependent HAC (see Chapter 19).

Treatment

Pituitary-dependent HAC is treated medically. Trilostane (veterinary licensed product) is the first-line medication. Mitotane (human-licensed product) may be administered if there are complications with trilostane. Adrenal tumours can be treated with drugs or by surgical removal.

Nursing care

- Monitor vital and clinical signs.
- Assist veterinary surgeon with diagnostic tests.
- Observe the patient after blood sampling for haematoma formation and handle carefully for other procedures, as bruising can occur easily in patients with HAC.
- Ensure that water is freely available.
- Take patient outside frequently.
- Clean and groom patient as necessary.
- Administer medications, as directed by the veterinary surgeon.

Hypoadrenocorticism (Addison's disease)

Hypoadrenocorticism is a reduction in, or failure of, steroid production by the adrenals. This usually occurs as a result of immune destruction of the adrenal gland, but may also be a consequence of treating *hyper*adrenocorticism. Hypoadrenocorticism causes electrolyte imbalances, hyponatraemia (low sodium), hyperkalaemia (high potassium) and dehydration. The hyperkalaemia can be life-threatening and needs to be treated promptly.

Clinical signs

Clinical signs are often initially vague and wax and wane; they include lethargy and inappetence. In the untreated patient this will progress to:

- Anorexia
- Vomiting
- Haemorrhagic diarrhoea
- Hypotension
- Weakness
- Bradycardia
- Collapse.

Diagnostics

- Blood tests: haematology and biochemistry (sodium:potassium ratio).
- ACTH stimulation test (protocol as for hyperadrenocorticism).
- ECG (Figure 20.15).

Treatment

An acute crisis is an emergency. Treatment involves fluid therapy at shock rates to reduce the potassium level and re-hydrate the patient (see Chapter 22). Intravenous corticosteroids are administered. In the stable patient, glucocorticoids (prednisolone) and mineralocorticoids (fludrocortisone acetate) are administered. Treatment is monitored by measuring the sodium:potassium ratio.

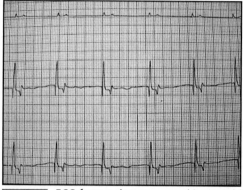

20.15   ECG from a dog presented in an Addisonian crisis. There is bradycardia, and no P waves are evident.

Nursing care

- Monitor vital signs (especially heart rate, if patient is in a crisis) and clinical signs.
- Assist veterinary surgeon with diagnostic tests.
- Administer medication, as directed by the veterinary surgeon.
- Administer fluid therapy (high in saline/low potassium) if patient is in a crisis, as directed by the veterinary surgeon.
- Encourage patient to eat.
- Ensure that water is freely available.
- Clean and groom patient as necessary.
- Take patient outside frequently.
- ECG when heart rate is low.

Hyperthyroidism

Patients with hyperthyroidism have an overactive thyroid gland usually as a result of benign neoplasia. There is overproduction of thyroxine (T4) that increases the metabolic rate. This is a common condition in the older cat but rare in dogs.

Clinical signs

- Polyphagia with weight loss.
- Emaciation.
- Aggression and hyperactivity.
- Heart murmur and tachycardia.
- Polyuria/polydipsia.
- Vomiting and diarrhoea.

Diagnostics

- Blood tests: haematology and biochemistry, total T4.

Treatment

Treatment involves administration of methimazole or carbimazole, radioactive iodine, or thyroidectomy. Treatment is monitored by measuring T4 levels.

Nursing care

- Monitor vital and clinical signs.
- Assist veterinary surgeon with diagnostic tests.
- Reduce patient stress as much as possible.
- Feed patient a suitable diet.
- Ensure that water is freely available.
- Clean and groom patient as necessary.
- Administer medication, as directed by veterinary surgeon.
- Provide postoperative nursing and observation for hypocalcaemic complications following thyroidectomy.
- Follow protocol for nursing patients after radioactive iodine treatment.

Hypothyroidism

Patients with hypothyroidism have an underactive thyroid gland. There is decreased production of thyroxine (T4) as a result of atrophy or lymphocytic infiltration of the thyroid gland. This results in a decreased metabolic rate. It is most common in middle-aged dogs and rare in the cat. It is occasionally seen in cats after thyroidectomy.

Clinical signs

- Lethargy, exercise intolerance.
- Obesity.
- Bradycardia.
- Dermatological abnormalities: alopecia, seborrhoea, hyperpigmentation, pyoderma.

Diagnostics

- Blood tests: haematology and biochemistry.
- Total T4, free T4 and thyroid stimulating hormone (TSH) assay treatment trial.

Treatment

Supplement thyroxine (levothyroxine). Treatment is monitored by measuring T4 levels and observing clinical signs.

Nursing care

- Monitor vital and clinical signs.
- Assist veterinary surgeon with diagnostic tests.
- Feed patient a suitable diet.
- Ensure that water is freely available.
- Clean and groom patient as necessary.
- Administer medication, as directed by veterinary surgeon.

Hypercalcaemia

Calcium is required for many functions in the body. It is regulated in the body by vitamin D, which is ingested and metabolized in the kidneys, and parathyroid hormone (PTH) produced in the parathyroid gland (Figure 20.16). Increased vitamin D and PTH will increase the calcium in the body. There are other substances that are able to increase calcium in the body and they are released in certain disease states. In excess, calcium can cause renal failure and death.

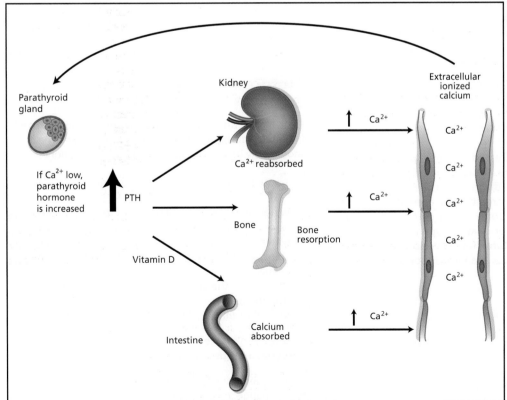

20.16 Calcium regulation in the body. Low calcium: PTH production rises; calcium absorbed by intestine and kidney. High calcium: PTH production decreases; calcium lost in urine and taken up by bones.

Differential diagnoses

- Neoplasia (e.g. lymphoma, Figure 20.17).
- Primary hyperparathyroidism.
- Vitamin D toxicity (e.g. some toxic rat baits).
- Renal failure (see 'Chronic renal failure').

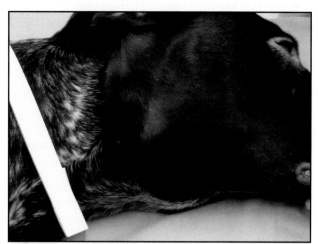

20.17 This dog was presented with hypercalcaemia. It has enlarged submandibular lymph nodes and was diagnosed with lymphoma.

Clinical signs

- Polyuria, polydipsia.
- Anorexia, lethargy, weakness.
- Vomiting, diarrhoea.
- Tremors.

Diagnostics

- Blood tests: haematology and biochemistry (total calcium and ionized calcium).
- Urinalysis: specific gravity, dipstick and sediment.
- Fine-needle aspiration of a lymph node to rule out lymphoma.
- Radiography.
- Ultrasonography.
- PTH assay and parathyroid-related protein assay to diagnose occult tumours.

Treatment

Hypercalcaemia should be treated promptly to decrease risk of permanent renal damage. Patients should be placed on intravenous fluids. Once a diagnosis has been made, the underlying cause should be treated (e.g. chemotherapy for lymphoma; parathyroidectomy for primary hyperparathyroidism). After surgery for primary hyperparathyroidism the patient should be monitored for hypocalcaemia. Clinical signs include tremors, seizures and facial rubbing.

Nursing care

- Monitor vital and clinical signs.
- Monitor urinary output.
- Assist veterinary surgeon with diagnostic tests.
- Monitor blood calcium and electrolyte levels.
- Feed patient a suitable diet.
- Ensure that water is freely available.
- Clean and groom patient as necessary.

- Administer medication, as directed by veterinary surgeon.
- Administer intravenous fluids, as directed by veterinary surgeon.

Diabetes insipidus (DI)

This disease is caused by an impairment in the production of ADH (antidiuretic hormone/vasopressin) or a failure in response. The animal produces large quantities of dilute urine with a compensatory polydipsia. The condition may be referred to as water diabetes. Animals are normally well in all other aspects.

There are two forms of diabetes insipidus:

- **Central DI** – a deficiency in ADH produced by the pituitary, thought to be either congenital or as a result of trauma to the hypothalamus (e.g. tumours, head trauma)
- **Nephrogenic DI** – failure of the collecting tubules in the nephrons to respond to ADH. A primary problem is very rare.

Normally ADH controls the water balance within the body by concentrating the urine. If the animal's water intake is decreased, the body will respond by producing more ADH and this will then stimulate the collecting tubules to retain water, preserving the body's water balance.

Clinical signs

- Marked polyuria.
- Marked polydipsia.
- Vomiting after drinking large amounts.
- Weight loss due to poor appetite, due to constant thirst.

Diagnostics

- Haematology and biochemistry – normal.
- Urinalysis (SG <1.009).
- Water deprivation test.
- Trial of ADH.

Protocols for water deprivation test and ADH trial

Prior to starting this test, the patient should be well hydrated and have a normal blood urea level. The test should only be performed under close observation.

1. Empty the bladder and measure urine specific gravity (SG).
2. Weigh animal and calculate 5% of its bodyweight.
3. Place animal in a kennel with no access to food or water.
4. Empty bladder every hour, check SG and weigh the animal.
5. Once 5% of the animal's bodyweight has been lost, stop the test.
6. Normal result: SG >1.025. If SG is <1.020, suspect DI.

Once rehydrated, repeat as above but give ADH injection or drops.

- Increased urine SG = central DI
- No change in SG = nephrogenic DI

Treatment

Central DI

Desmopressin acetate (DDAVP) nasal/eye drops, synthetic vasopressin.

Nursing care

- Monitor vital and clinical signs.
- Monitor for dehydration.
- Assist veterinary surgeon with diagnostic tests.
- Ensure that water is freely available (except during water deprivation test).
- Take patient outside frequently.
- Clean and groom patient as necessary.
- Administer medication, as directed by veterinary surgeon.

Nervous system disease

Definitions

- **Convulsions** – a series of involuntary contractions of the muscles.
- **Seizures** – clinical manifestation of a paroxysmal cerebral disorder resulting from a transitory disturbance of brain function due to abnormal electrical activity.
- **Epilepsy** – an intracranial disorder that produces recurrent seizures.
- **Status epilepticus** – life-threatening series of epileptic spasms without intervals of consciousness.
- **Paresis** – weakness of one or more limbs.
- **Hemiplegia** – paralysis of one side of the body.
- **Paraplegia** – paralysis of the caudal limbs.
- **Tetraplegia** – paralysis of all four limbs.

Clinical signs of nervous system disease include:

- Cerebral:
  - Behaviour changes
  - Ataxia
  - Circling
  - Pacing
  - Seizures
  - Weakness.
- Cerebellar:
  - Ataxia
  - Tremors
  - Dysmetria
  - Hypermetria
  - Head tilt
  - Nystagmus.
- Spinal:
  - Abnormal spinal reflexes
  - Weakness
  - Paresis/paralysis
  - Faecal/urinary incontinence.

Seizures

Differential diagnoses

Seizures can result from abnormalities within or outside the brain.
Causes within the brain include:

- Idiopathic epilepsy
- Brain tumours
- Head trauma
- Infections (e.g. canine distemper)
- Congenital abnormalities (e.g. hydrocephalus).

Causes outside the brain include:

- Metabolic (e.g. hypoglycaemia, hypocalcaemia, hepatic encephalopathy, uraemia)
- Toxins (e.g. ethylene glycol (antifreeze)).

Idiopathic epilepsy is more likely to occur in dogs under 3 years of age. Most brain tumours are more common in the older animal.

Clinical signs

Signs can vary from animal to animal, but usually take the form of three phases.

- **Preictal** – just before the fit the animal will usually be asleep or resting; it will then appear restless or anxious.
- **Ictal** – this period describes the actual fit, varying degrees of collapse, clonic and tonic activity. Unconsciousness, vocalization, jaw champing, hypersalivation, involuntary urination or defecation may also be present.
- **Postictal** – this is the period following the fit: the animal may be exhausted, disorientated or anxious.

Seizures may be single, multiple (**cluster seizures**) or continuous (**status epilepticus**). They also need to be distinguished from **syncopal episodes** (fainting).

Diagnosis

- History and neurological examination.
- Blood test for haematology and biochemistry.
- Cerebral spinal fluid (CSF) tap.
- Magnetic resonance imaging (MRI) scan.
- Computed tomography (CT) scan.
- Electroencephalography (EEG).

Treatment

Any underlying cause should be treated. To control cluster seizures or status epilepticus, initial treatment involves:

- Diazepam initially, can be repeated (intravenously or per rectum) if unsuccessful. This should be used with care for cats and under the direction of the veterinary surgeon
- Phenobarbital or propofol infusion
- Status epilepticus should be dealt with as an emergency
- If idiopathic epilepsy is diagnosed, anticonvulsant therapy should be started.

Phenobarbital is used to control seizures; this can also be used in conjunction with potassium bromide.

Nursing care

- Observe and record seizure activity. Contact the veterinary surgeon when this occurs.
- Monitor vital signs, especially temperature and breathing.
- Dim the lighting or partially cover the kennel.
- Pad the kennel to prevent trauma.
- Keep the room as quiet as possible.
- Place and maintain intravenous access.
- Administer medication, as directed by the veterinary surgeon.
- Administer fluid therapy, as directed by the veterinary surgeon.
- Keep airway clear.
- Administer oxygen if required.
- Cool the patient if hyperthermic, keep warm if hypothermic.

Spinal injuries

Differential diagnoses

- Intervertebral disc disease.
- Fibrocartilaginous embolism.
- Discospondylitis.
- Wobbler syndrome.
- Cauda equina syndrome.
- Tumour.
- Fracture.

Clinical signs

- Ataxia.
- Paresis of one or more limbs.
- Paralysis of one or more limbs (paraplegia, tetraplegia, hemiplegia).
- Urinary or faecal incontinence.
- Lack of panniculus reflex.
- Lack of tail function.
- Pain.

Diagnosis

Neurological assessment

- Localization of pain.
- Examination of gait.
- Detection of proprioceptive deficits.
- Assessment of muscle atrophy/tone.
- Assessment of limb, tail, anal and panniculus reflexes.
- Assessment of deep pain.
- Assessment of bladder function.

Other diagnostic tests

- Radiography.
- Myelography.
- MRI/CT scan.
- CSF analysis.

Treatment

Surgical correction of some conditions is possible. Other conditions cannot be corrected surgically, or surgical repair is precluded by financial constraints. These patients are then managed by medical treatment, which includes:

- Analgesia
- Restricted or supported exercise (depending on condition)
- Urinary and faecal management – use of catheters and enemas
- Physiotherapy (depending on condition).

Nursing care

- Monitor patient's vital signs.
- Assess for progression of neurological clinical signs.
- Assist veterinary surgeon with examination and other diagnostic procedures.
- Prevent pressure sores (suitable padded bedding) and turn patient frequently.
- Avoid excessive movement with spinal fractures.
- Assist with emptying bladder and rectum.
- Keep patient clean and groom as necessary (this also helps to prevent patient boredom).
- Provide adequate nutrition – make sure that the animal can reach its bowls. Hand feeding or other methods of assisted feeding may be required.
- Carry out physiotherapy, as directed by veterinary surgeon (see below).
- Administer medication, as directed by veterinary surgeon.

Musculoskeletal system disease

Definitions

- **Myositis** – inflammation of a voluntary muscle.
- **Tendonitis** – inflammation of a tendon.
- **Arthritis** – inflammation of a joint.

Bone disease

Rickets

This disease is seen in young growing animals that are fed a diet deficient in vitamin D. The affected animal is unable to absorb calcium from the intestines, leading to reduced bone mineralization around the growth plates. Clinical signs include lameness, bowing of limbs and swollen joints. Radiographic examination shows enlargement of growth plates. Treatment involves feeding an appropriate balanced diet for a young growing dog.

Nursing care

- Feed a balanced diet suitable for a growing puppy.
- Administer analgesics as necessary.
- Provide soft comfortable bedding.

Metaphyseal osteopathy

This is also known as hypertrophic osteodystrophy and Möller Barlow's disease. Metaphyseal osteopathy occurs in young growing dogs, particularly giant breeds. It is associated with abnormal metaphyseal bone formation, usually affecting long bones of the distal limbs. Clinical signs include swollen and painful growth plate regions on all limbs, severe lameness, pyrexia, depression and anorexia. The cause of metaphyseal osteopathy is unknown. Treatment consists of pain relief and feeding an appropriate diet for a young growing dog.

Nursing care

- Feed a balanced diet suitable for a growing puppy.
- Administer analgesics as necessary.
- Provide soft comfortable bedding.
- Ensure urination and defecation are possible.

Hypertrophic osteopathy

This is also known as pulmonary osteopathy and Marie's disease. It is associated with a thoracic mass. There is periosteal proliferation, particularly of the metacarpals and metatarsals. There is no joint involvement. Clinical signs include lameness, bilateral soft tissue swelling of the lower limbs and pain. These changes are usually seen before thoracic signs develop. Treatment depends on the underlying condition but the prognosis is usually poor unless the thoracic mass is operable.

Nursing care

- Monitor vital signs.
- Provide soft, comfortable bedding.
- Administer analgesics as necessary.
- Administer medications as per the veterinary surgeon's instructions.

Secondary nutritional hyperparathyroidism

This is caused by a diet grossly deficient in calcium or containing an excess of phosphorus. It is most commonly associated with feeding all-meat diets. Calcium is resorbed from bone, giving rise to lameness, pain, reluctance to stand or walk, and pathological fractures of long bones. Treatment consists of feeding a balanced diet, cage rest to allow fractures to heal, and analgesics.

Nursing care

- Feed a balanced diet.
- Administer analgesics as required.
- Provide soft comfortable bedding.
- Ensure urination and defecation are possible.

Osteomyelitis

Osteomyelitis is inflammation, most commonly due to infection, of bone. Clinical signs include pain, swelling, lameness, loss of function, pyrexia, depression and inappetence. A draining sinus tract may develop. Causes include bacterial or fungal infection (the latter is uncommon in the UK) and corrosion of surgical implants. Radiography reveals destruction of existing bone and new bone formation. Treatment includes administration of antibiotics (based on culture and sensitivity results), antifungals and removal of surgical implants or necrotic bone fragments (sequestra) that may be associated with the osteomyelitis.

Nursing care

- Monitor vital signs.
- Provide soft, comfortable bedding.
- Administer analgesia as necessary.
- Administer antibiotics as per the veterinary surgeon's instructions.
- Provide postoperative care.
- Manage and change dressings as necessary.

Arthritis

Joint disease can be categorized as immune-mediated (e.g. idiopathic polyarthritis, systemic lupus erythematosus, rheumatoid arthritis), inflammatory (infectious or non-infectious) or degenerative (Figure 20.18).

Clinical signs

Patients with arthritis have a variable degree of lameness, pain in the affected joint or joints, and exercise intolerance. A specific clinical sign of degenerative joint disease is that the condition improves with exercise.

- Degenerative:
  - Gradual onset
  - Improvement with exercise
  - Crepitus on extension/flexion.
- Immune-mediated:
  - Pyrexia
  - Inappetence
  - Usually multiple joints involved
  - Other signs of systemic disease.

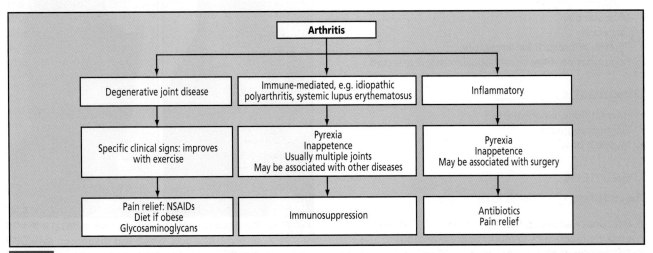

20.18   Classification of arthritis.

- Inflammatory:
  - Joint pain
  - Pyrexia
  - Recent history of surgery or medication.

Diagnostics

- Blood tests for haematology, biochemistry, rheumatoid factor and antinuclear antibody.
- Radiography.
- Joint tap (arthrocentesis) for cytology and culture.

Treatment

Treatment is aimed at the underlying cause, or managing the pain associated with degenerative changes:

- Immune-mediated: immunosuppressive drugs
- Infectious: antibacterials, pain relief
- Degenerative: pain relief (NSAIDs), diet, glycosaminoglycans.

Nursing care and nutrition

- Monitor vital signs.
- Provide soft, comfortable bedding.
- Encourage frequent short walks.
- Administer medication, as directed by the veterinary surgeon.
- Adjust diet if obese (see Chapter 13).

Muscle disease

Myopathies can be classified as inflammatory and non-inflammatory:

- **Inflammatory:**
  - Infectious (e.g. *Toxoplasma gondii*, *Neospora caninum*)
  - Immune-mediated.
- **Non-inflammatory:**
  - Endocrinopathies (e.g. hyperadrenocorticism, hypothyroidism)
  - Congenital (e.g. 'floppy Labrador').

Clinical signs

- Muscle weakness and loss of function.
- Muscle atrophy.
- Muscular pain.
- Lameness.
- Pyrexia, anorexia if inflammatory.
- Regurgitation if the oesophageal muscle is affected.

Diagnostics

- Haematology, biochemistry.
- Electromyography.
- Muscle biopsy.

Treatment

The underlying cause needs to be treated:

- Infectious – antibacterials
- Immune-mediated – immunosuppressive drugs
- Endocrinopathies – treat underlying disease
- Congenital – usually no treatment available.

Nursing care

- Monitor vital signs.
- Assist walking if required (see Chapter 17).
- Provide soft comfortable bedding.
- Turn patient every 4 hours if recumbent.
- Carry out physiotherapy (see later).
- Assist feeding if dysphagic.
- Feed from a height if regurgitating.
- Administer medication, as directed by veterinary surgeon.
- Monitor progress.

Tumours of the musculoskeletal system

- Bone tumours – most commonly osteosarcoma (malignant) and osteoma (benign); other tumours include fibrosarcomas, haemangiosarcomas and chrondrosarcomas.
- Soft tissue tumours – fibrosarcoma, haemangiosarcomas.

Clinical signs

- **Osteosarcomas** most commonly affect the long bones. Patients may present with only a swelling (Figure 20.19) but these are usually very painful and the patient will be lame and often unable to bear its weight on the affected leg.
- **Chondrosarcomas** affect bones such as ribs and the nasal cavity.
- **Fibrosarcomas** usually affect the bones of the axial skeleton, including the skull and mandible.

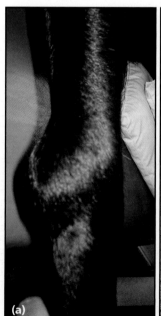
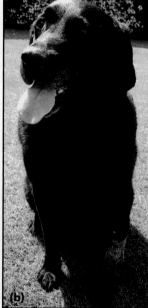

20.19 Bone tumour. **(a)** A swelling on the distal left forelimb of a dog, which was diagnosed as osteosarcoma. **(b)** The dog underwent a course of radiotherapy, as evidenced by the white square.

Diagnostics

- Haematology, biochemistry.
- Radiography – local area, thorax (metastasis).
- Ultrasonography – abdomen (metastasis).
- Biopsy.

Treatment

Treatment of osteosarcomas involves amputating the affected leg to relieve pain and/or cure. The best results are achieved by combining this with chemotherapy to slow the development of any metastases. Radiotherapy will also relieve the pain of the tumour.

Soft tissue tumours are best treated by surgical excision.

Nursing care

- Monitor vital signs.
- Provide soft comfortable bedding.
- Help with walking – sling walk if necessary.
- Administer analgesia and other medications, as directed by the veterinary surgeon.
- Provide postoperative care.
- Assist veterinary surgeon with chemotherapy.
- Ensure adequate nutrition.

Nutrition

- Convalescent diets should be used for patients following surgery and initial chemotherapy.
- Specially formulated diets that help to reduce tumour growth may be fed.
- Excess weight should be avoided or managed if limbs are amputated.

Diseases of the skin and coat

Definitions

- **Alopecia** – the absence of hair from areas of the skin where it is normally present; can be partial or complete, symmetrical or patchy, diffuse or focal.
- **Erythema** – reddening of the skin.
- **Pyoderma** – a pyogenic (pus-forming, e.g. infected) condition of the skin.
- **Pruritus** – sensation within the skin that provokes the desire to scratch (animal may persistently lick, chew, or rub itself to alleviate the irritation; this can lead to self-trauma).
- **Seborrhoea** – excessive secretion of sebum by the sebaceous glands within the skin, giving the coat and skin an oily appearance.

Parasitic and fungal skin disease

These are discussed in Chapters 6 and 7.

Pyoderma

This condition is more common in the dog than the cat and there is usually an underlying cause for its development. The severity of the condition is determined by the depth of the tissue affected (Figure 20.20). *Staphylococcus intermedius* is the most commonly involved bacterium, but other secondary opportunist bacteria such as *Pseudomonas* may also be present.

Tissue depth	Condition	Presentation	Treatment
Surface	Acute moist dermatitis	Often occurs where skin has become damaged due to self-trauma Can occur anywhere but especially over face, feet and tail base Erythema often present and area is often moist or crusty due to serum exudates	Treatment of underlying cause (e.g. ear infection) Clip hair from site – patient may require sedation as area can be very painful Clean area with chlorhexidine Elizabethan collar to prevent further self-trauma Topical or systemic antibiotics and anti-inflammatories may be required
	Skin fold dermatitis	Commonly found around lip folds, vulval folds and tail folds Common in breeds with excessive skin folds	Treat as above Surgical correction or cosmetic surgery may be required to correct anatomy of skin in severe cases that recur
Superficial	Impetigo	Often known as juvenile pustular dermatitis or puppy pyoderma Multiple pustules and yellow scabs commonly found along ventral abdomen	Antibacterial shampoo with additional systemic antibiotic and anti-inflammatory therapy if condition extensive
	Folliculitis	Formation of pustules with hair protruding Sometimes the lesions in ring-like formation, especially ventral abdomen As a result of underlying disease	Treatment of underlying disease Appropriate antibiotic medication
Deep	Interdigital pyoderma (pododermatitis)	Often seen in short-haired dogs – paws become painful and swollen and may discharge pus Area of alopecia seen with ulceration and fistulas in severe cases	Surgical drainage of infected material Treatment of underlying cause Long-term antibiotic therapy
	Furunculosis	Often associated with underlying disease such as demodicosis, dermatophytosis or hypothyroidism Clinical signs include pustules, discharging pus, fistulas, alopecia, pain Lesions often found on muzzle, flanks and anal regions but can occur anywhere on body	Treatment of any underlying disease Long-term antibiotic therapy In severe cases, surgical resection of fistulas may be required if problem recurs

20.20 Classification of pyoderma.

Feline pyoderma is associated with cat bites. Bacteria such as *Pasteurella, Staphylococcus* and *Fusiformis,* which are routinely found in the cat's mouth, cause cellulitis when bite wounds penetrate deep within the skin. Other clinical signs include pyrexia, anorexia, depression, pain and swelling at the site of the bite wound. This condition is usually successfully treated with antibiotics and drainage of pus from the site of infection.

Allergic skin disease

This is caused by an inappropriate immune response to an antigen, which in cases of allergic skin disease can include many factors. Figure 20.21 outlines the causes, presentation, diagnoses and treatments of various allergic skin diseases.

Hormonal alopecia

This is usually associated with one of the following:

- Hypothyroidism
- Hyperadrenocorticism (Cushing's disease)
- Sertoli cell tumour
- Canine ovarian imbalance.

In conjunction with clinical signs of the underlying condition, it usually presents as a bilateral alopecia, often on the flanks. It is usually non-pruritic and the skin is not inflamed. Treatment is based on identifying and treating the underlying cause.

Diseases of the eye
Conditions that affect the eyelids

- **Entropion** – inturning of the upper or lower eyelid, towards the eyeball (often hereditary).
- **Ectropion** – eversion of the lower eyelid, away from the eyeball, with exposure of the conjunctiva; less common than entropion.
- **Distichiasis** – extra row of eyelashes behind the normal row; most common hereditary eye abnormality in the dog.

All of these abnormalities can result in irritation, inflammation, infection or damage to the cornea and conjunctiva, depending on the severity.

Clinical signs

As well as visible evidence of one of the above conditions, clinical signs may include:

- Blepharospasm (constant blinking)
- Squinting
- Increased lacrimation (tear production)
- Ocular discharge.

Condition	Cause	Presentation	Diagnosis	Treatment
Urticaria	Induced by drugs, vaccines and insect stings	Sudden development of multiple oedematous swellings or wheals on skin, with hair becoming erect; they are pruritic and can remain for hours or days	Based on clinical signs and accurate history	Removal of cause Treatment with corticosteroids Future avoidance of causal agent
Atopic dermatitis	Large numbers of unknown antigens, including house dust mites, pollens, danders	Usually affects dogs 1–3 years old Intense pruritus and alopecia, especially around eyes, feet, axilla and ventral abdomen Secondary infection common, due to self-trauma Otitis externa and ocular discharges may also be present Cats may present with miliary eczema and eosinophilic granuloma complex	Intradermal skin testing with multiple allergens to determine cause Serum testing for specific antigens	Allergies usually lifelong Depending on causal factors, changes to environment may be required Treatment may include corticosteroids, antihistamines, essential fatty acid supplementation, desensitizing vaccinations
Food hypersensitivity	Causes individual to each animal but can include beef, milk, gluten	Pruritic skin disease and/or gastrointestinal symptoms	Clinical signs and exclusion diet food trial (see Chapter 13)	Avoidance of specific allergens identified by food trial Long-term feeding of novelty diet fed during exclusion trial
Contact dermatitis	Commonly caused by soaps, detergents or chemicals of any kind	Pruritic erythematous lesions mainly on feet, ventral abdomen, neck and face Often secondary bacterial infection due to self-trauma Intolerance generally develops 4–6 weeks after initial exposure	Patch testing: suspected allergen applied to clipped area of skin and kept in contact 48 hours then examined for reaction Contact elimination: hospitalize animal from usual environment to see if clinical signs resolve; suspected items or substances then reintroduced and patient observed for reaction	Avoid contact with identified allergens

20.21 Causes, diagnosis and treatment of allergic skin diseases.

Treatment

- Anti-inflammatory eyedrops.
- Antibacterial eyedrops.
- Surgical correction of condition.

Conjunctivitis

Inflammation of the conjunctiva can be unilateral or bilateral, depending on the cause.

Causes include bacterial infections (sometimes primary but usually secondary), viral infections (e.g. distemper, herpesvirus) or allergies. It may also be associated with foreign bodies, strong winds, trauma and ectropion.

Clinical signs

- Blepharospasm.
- Increased lacrimation.
- Chemosis (oedema and swelling of the conjunctiva).
- Conjunctival hyperaemia.
- Ocular discharge ranging from serous to mucopurulent.

Treatment

This will vary depending on the causal factor, but may include:

- Surgical correction of eyelid deformities, removal of foreign bodies
- Antibiotic eyedrops
- Anti-inflammatory eyedrops
- Antiviral eyedrops
- Antihistamine eyedrops.

Nursing care

- Prevent patient self-trauma and interference (e.g. Elizabethan collar).
- Bathe eyes to remove any discharge.
- Apply medication, following veterinary surgeon's instructions.

Keratoconjunctivitis sicca

KCS ('dry eye') is due to a reduction in aqueous tear production from the lacrimal and third eyelid gland. This often results in an overproduction of mucus as an attempt to keep the cornea moist. Most commonly the condition is immune-mediated but it may also be caused by drug toxicity (e.g. sulfasalazine), trauma or surgery (e.g. following removal of the third eyelid gland in dogs with 'cherry eye'). There is considerable variation in the degree of severity.

Clinical signs

- Vascularization, ulceration, opacity of the cornea.
- Recurrent conjunctivitis.
- Mucoid or mucopurulent discharge on and around the surface of the eye.

Diagnostics

A Schirmer tear test (Figure 20.22) will show insufficient tear production. Readings of <10 mm in a minute will confirm the diagnosis, but the test should be repeated for monitoring purposes.

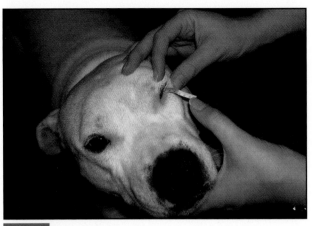

20.22 Schirmer tear test.

Treatment and nursing care

- Ciclosporin to treat immune-mediated destruction of the lacrimal gland.
- Tear substitutes.
- Antibiotic drops if infected.
- Anti-inflammatory eye drops.
- Good ocular hygiene and frequent cleaning to remove discharge from around the eyes.

Corneal ulceration

This common condition can vary in severity depending on depth. Deep ulcers may result in corneal rupture. Causes include:

- Eyelash/eyelid disorders
- Trauma (e.g. cat scratch)
- Keratoconjunctivitis sicca
- Bacteria (primary trauma due to any of the above often allows bacterial overgrowth)
- Melting ulcers – these occur due to bacterial infections (e.g. *Pseudomonas*) resulting in enzymes being released to aid removal of devitalized cells and debris. These enzymes also contribute to the melting of the cornea.

Clinical signs

- Ocular pain.
- Ocular discharge.
- Blepharospasm.
- Increased lacrimation.

Diagnostics

- Visual inspection of the cornea.
- Fluorescein dye – this dye is taken up by any exposed stroma so that epithelial erosions can be detected.

Treatment

This will vary depending on the severity of the ulcer but may include:

- Antibiotic eyedrops
- Analgesia
- Fitting of contact lenses
- Surgical procedures (e.g. debridement of damaged cornea, grid keratotomy, conjunctival grafts).

Nursing care

- Monitor carefully to check for deterioration – infected ulcers can progress rapidly (melting ulcers).
- Prevent patient self-trauma. As well as using correctly fitting Elizabethan collars, prevent the patient from rubbing on cage bars, etc.
- Carefully follow medication regimes.

Uveitis

Uveitis is inflammation of the iris, ciliary body and/or choroid. It can be caused by trauma, neoplasia, infection or immune-mediated disease, lens-induced, or associated with corneal insult.

Clinical signs

Clinical signs vary according to duration of the condition, the cause of the inflammation and the extent of the uveal tract involvement. Bilateral uveitis usually indicates systemic involvement. Secondary complications include glaucoma and cataracts.

- Pain.
- Blepharospasm.
- Miotic pupil.
- Red eye.
- Photophobia.
- Lacrimation.
- Reduced intraocular pressure.

Diagnostics

Underlying cause must be determined.

- Haematology, biochemistry, specific diagnostic tests (e.g. FeLV, FIV, FIP).
- Serology.
- Ophthalmoscopy.
- Tonometry.
- Fluorescein staining.
- Diagnostic imaging.

Treatment

- Treat underlying cause.
- Topical atropine (contraindicated if glaucoma present).
- Topical corticosteroids (avoid in corneal ulceration, with caution in viral/fungal infections) or topical NSAIDs.
- Systemic corticosteroids.
- Systemic NSAIDs if systemic corticosteroids contraindicated.
- Evaluate response to treatment at regular intervals.

Nursing care

- Keep patient away from bright light if photophobic.
- Follow treatment regimes carefully.

Glaucoma

This is a condition in which there in an elevation in intraocular pressure due to inadequate drainage of aqueous humour within the globe. This eventually affects the vision and health of the eye, and the condition can be very painful. In acute cases permanent blindness can result if untreated. The condition may be idiopathic: many breeds have a predisposition (including many terrier and spaniel breeds as well as the Great Dane and Flat-coated Retriever). There is a list of breeds that are tested for this condition on the KC/BVA eye testing scheme (see Chapter 4). Other causes include:

- Uveitis
- Cataracts
- Lens luxation
- Neoplasia.

Clinical signs

- Painful red eye(s).
- Corneal oedema.
- Swelling of the globe.
- Dilated pupil.
- Retinal damage.

Diagnostics

- Examination of the eye with an ophthalmoscope.
- Measuring the intraocular pressure with a tonometer (this is also monitored to check the response to treatment) (Figure 20.23).
- Gonioscopy to measure the iridocorneal drainage angle.

Treatment

- Emergency treatment: intravenous mannitol, to help to draw fluid from the aqueous and vitreous humours and therefore decrease intraocular pressure.
- Carbonic anhydrase inhibitors reduce formation of aqueous humour.

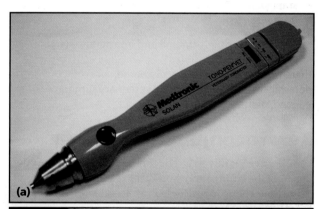

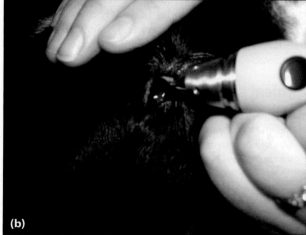

20.23 (a) Tonometer. (b) Using a tonometer to measure intraocular pressure.

- Miotics to increase aqueous outflow.
- Analgesia.
- Surgical treatment in specialist centres.
- Enucleation.

Nursing care

- Prevent patient self-trauma (patient may rub eye when uncomfortable).
- Carefully follow medication regimes.

Conditions affecting the lens

These include cataract formation and lens luxation, both of which require surgical correction (see Chapter 25). Cataract formation is a common finding in dogs with diabetes mellitus. Visual inspection of the eye reveals a clouding of the lens. Poor night vision leading to progressive blindness is the common progression of the disease.

Conditions affecting the retina

Collie eye anomaly

This is a disorder of the deep structures of the eye that affects collie breeds. It is a congenital disorder and can be detected with an ophthalmoscope in puppies. It can affect the eye in the following ways:

- Choroid hypoplasia – inadequate development of the choroids
- Coloboma – a cleft or defect in the optic disc
- Staphyloma – an area of thinning in the sclera, adjacent to the choroids
- Retinal detachment, with or without haemorrhage.

The severity of the condition varies. In its mildest form there is little effect on sight. In a severe form, total retinal detachment will cause blindness. Affected animals should not be used for breeding (see Chapter 4 for details of BVA/Kennel Club/International Sheep Dog Society Eye Scheme).

Progressive retinal atrophy (PRA)

This is a hereditary disease of the eye that causes blindness. The retina is composed of two types of photoreceptor cells: rods and cones. The rods function in dim light and the cones in bright light. A dog affected with PRA begins to have difficulty seeing in dim light and then gradually looses the ability to see in bright light, eventually becoming completely blind. Although most common in dogs, some forms can occur in cats. Age at onset and rate of progression vary. Generalized retinal thinning occurs, manifest as tapetal hyper-reflectivity and attenuation of the superficial retinal vessels. There is no available treatment. Genetic testing is now available to identify carrier animals that are unaffected (see Chapter 4).

Nursing animals with poor vision

If a patient's sight is badly affected, it is important that the patient is aware of the nurse's presence before trying to handle them or apply any medication. Talking to them and stroking should reassure them. Otherwise the patient may be aggressive due to fear. To transport such patients around unfamiliar areas, it is often easier to carry smaller dogs; larger dogs need to be led slowly.

When these animals are nursed as inpatients, food and water bowls should always be located in the same position.

Infectious diseases – canine

Figure 20.24 summarizes information on common canine infectious diseases. Two important features in the care of patients with infectious diseases are barrier nursing and the provision of isolation facilities, which are described in Chapter 12. The subject of vaccination is discussed in principle in Chapter 5.

Disease/ infection	Type of infectious agent	Incubation period	Major organs affected	Main method of transmission	Zoonotic	Diagnostics	Major nursing needs	Control/ prevention
Canine distemper	Virus	7–21 days	Respiratory, gastrointestinal systems	Inhalation	No	History, clinical signs Blood analysis Post-mortem examination	Fluid therapy Symptomatic	Vaccination Client education
Infectious canine hepatitis	Virus	5–10 days	Liver	Inhalation/ ingestion	No	History, clinical signs Blood analysis	Pain management Fluid therapy	Vaccination Client education
Canine parvovirus	Virus	3–5 days	Gastrointestinal system, bone marrow, heart	Ingestion of faecally contaminated material	No	History, clinical signs CITE faecal test	Fluid therapy Symptomatic Antibiotics	Vaccination Isolation Avoid risk
Leptospirosis	Bacterium	5–7 days	Kidneys, liver	Through mucous membranes and skin abrasions	Yes	History, clinical signs Urinalysis Blood analysis	Antibiotics Fluid therapy	Vaccination Avoid risk

20.24 Common canine infectious diseases.

continues ▶

Disease/ infection	Type of infectious agent	Incubation period	Major organs affected	Main method of transmission	Zoonotic	Diagnostics	Major nursing needs	Control/ prevention
Kennel cough complex	Mixed – bacteria/ virus	5–7 days	Respiratory system	Inhalation	No	History, clinical signs	Antibiotics Symptomatic	Vaccination Isolation
Rabies	Virus	1 week to 1+ years, normally 3–8 weeks	Nervous system	Saliva to skin wound	Yes – fatal	History, clinical signs Post-mortem examination	N/A	Stray dog control Vaccination Pet Travel Scheme
Salmonellosis	Bacterium	2–3 days following a stressful experience	Gastrointestinal system	Ingestion of faecally contaminated material	Yes	History, clinical signs Culture	Fluid therapy, +/– antibiotics	Hygiene, disinfection

20.24 *continued* Common canine infectious diseases.

Canine distemper

Canine distemper is caused by canine distemper virus, a morbillivirus related to measles virus in humans and rinderpest virus in cattle. Both dogs and ferrets are susceptible. In warm climates the virus persists for 1–2 days in the environment. It is susceptible to routine disinfection.

The disease is most commonly seen in unvaccinated 3–6-month-old puppies. This time coincides with the waning of maternal antibodies (see Chapter 5). In susceptible populations a dog of any age may be affected. Outbreaks occur where there is a high density of dogs, such as rescue centres, housing estates and cities generally.

The virus is shed most commonly in respiratory exudates as well as in urine, faeces, saliva, vomitus and ocular discharges, up to 60–90 days post-infection. The incubation period is 7–21 days and infection is via inhalation. The aerosol droplets, when inhaled, come into contact with the upper respiratory epithelium of the susceptible animal and spread through the body from this point. The respiratory, gastrointestinal and central nervous systems, nose, footpads and conjunctiva can be affected. The severity of the disease depends on the efficacy of the immune response that is mounted and ranges from no clinical signs to death. Secondary bacterial infections can complicate the infection.

Clinical signs (generalized distemper)

- Depression.
- Pyrexia.
- Anorexia.
- Lymphadenopathy.
- Conjunctivitis giving ocular discharge (initially serous but rapidly becoming mucopurulent with secondary bacterial infection).
- Rhinitis giving nasal discharge (initially serous but rapidly becoming mucopurulent with secondary bacterial infection).
- Cough (initially dry, may become moist and productive).
- Exudative pneumonia – complicated by a secondary bacterial infection – leading to tachypnoea, dyspnoea.
- Vomiting, diarrhoea, dehydration, loss of body condition.
- Hyperkeratosis of nose and footpads; footpads become thickened and fissures appear ('hard pad').
- Enamel hypoplasia – permanent damage to tooth enamel in puppies under 6 months old.
- Neurological signs (see below).
- Skin rash – pustules, thought to be associated with an immune response (animals that develop rashes often recover).

Neurological signs

Some animals, including those with subclinical infection, can develop neurological signs 2–3 weeks after infection. Clinical signs are usually acute in onset and progressive and are associated with a poor prognosis. Clinical signs depend on the part of the nervous system that is affected and include seizures, paresis/paralysis of one or more limbs, and optic neuritis. Involuntary twitching of muscles (myoclonus) may also occur and is said to be a classic sign.

Diagnostics

A presumptive diagnosis is usually based on the history and classical clinical signs in an at-risk patient.

- Blood tests: haematology and biochemistry.
- Thoracic radiography: right lateral and ventrodorsal views.
- CSF sample.
- Specific tests:
  - Epithelial cells with eosinophilic bodies
  - Antibody titre rising at least four-fold
  - Immunofluorescence for virus in lymphoid tissue
  - Detection of antibody in CSF.
- Post-mortem examination.

Treatment

Prevention is by vaccination. Specific treatment is not available and the patient is treated symptomatically:

- Isolation and barrier nursing – of particular importance
- Antitussives for *dry* cough
- Broad-spectrum antibiotics for secondary bacterial infections
- Intravenous fluids for dehydration and electrolyte losses
- Anticonvulsants for seizures
- Antiemetics for vomiting.

Nursing care

The nursing care of a patient with CDV is centred on managing the clinical signs.

- Barrier nurse the patient to prevent transmission.
- Monitor vital signs.
- Administer medication, as directed by the veterinary surgeon.
- Administer and maintain fluid therapy.
- Provide general nursing of the clinical signs, cleaning of nasal and ocular discharges, and application of petroleum jelly to prevent skin excoriation.
- Ensure adequate nutrition of the patient; use of convalescing diets and assisted feeding may be required.
- Disinfect the environment.
- Provide the owner with advice on vaccination protocols for any other dogs in the household.

Infectious canine hepatitis (ICH)

Infectious canine hepatitis is caused by canine adenovirus type I (CAV-1), similar to the CAV-2 adenovirus that causes respiratory disease (see 'Kennel cough complex', below). It is a resistant virus and can survive for days on fomites in the environment. It survives disinfection with various chemicals but is inactivated at temperatures >50°C.

The incubation period is 5–10 days. During the initial infection, virus is shed in all bodily secretions. From around 10 days post-infection, the virus is shed in the urine for at least 6 months. Animals become infected through the oronasal route. The virus localizes in the tonsils and regional lymph nodes before disseminating to other parts of the body and localizing in the liver and vascular endothelial cells. If an appropriate immune response is not made, acute or chronic hepatitis can occur. Immune complexes (antibody and viral antigen complexes) can lodge in the uveal tract and glomerulus and cause a severe uveitis and corneal oedema, or glomerulonephritis.

Dogs younger than 1 year are usually affected, but unvaccinated dogs of any age can be affected. Mortality rate can be high in unweaned puppies. Disease can progress rapidly and the puppies may die within a few hours of developing clinical signs. Infection in older animals is less severe.

Clinical signs

Clinical signs in acute infections may include:

- Pyrexia, depression, anorexia
- Lymphadenopathy
- Vomiting, diarrhoea
- Shock
- Hepatomegaly and anterior abdominal pain
- Jaundice (in a third of cases)
- Petechial haemorrhages
- Corneal oedema (blue eye)
- Neurological signs (in terminal stages)
- Severely affected dogs may die suddenly, without the owner noticing other clinical signs.

In subacute infections, clinical signs include depression, anorexia and mild pyrexia.

Diagnostics

- History and clinical signs.
- Blood tests: haematology and biochemistry (especially liver enzymes), clotting profile.
- Serological tests – rising antibody titre.
- Intranuclear inclusion bodies found within hepatocytes.
- Virus isolation from affected organs.
- Post-mortem examination.

Treatment

Prevention is by vaccination (CAV2 cross-protective).
ICH patients are treated symptomatically:

- Intravenous fluids to rehydrate the animal
- Analgesics to control abdominal pain
- Topical steroids should only be used with caution; topical NSAIDs may be preferred.

The corneal changes may remain as a complication leading to permanent visual impairment, but in the majority of cases these are temporary.

Nursing care

- Barrier nurse the patient to prevent transmission.
- Monitor vital signs.
- Administer medication, as directed by the veterinary surgeon.
- Administer and maintain fluid therapy.
- Provide general nursing of the clinical signs.
- Ensure adequate nutrition of the patient; use of convalescing diets and assisted feeding may be required.
- Disinfect the environment.
- Provide the owner with advice on vaccination protocols for any other dogs in the household, as after recovery dogs can become convalescent carriers for up to 6 months.

Canine parvovirus

Canine parvovirus (related to feline panleucopenia virus) is very resistant and can survive in the environment from months to years. It is not killed by normal routine disinfection and a parvocidal disinfectant needs to be used.

It is a common infection and is highly contagious with a high mortality rate. Young puppies are most susceptible between the waning of maternal antibodies and efficacy of a vaccination programme. However, an unvaccinated dog of any age can be affected. Black and tan dogs are at increased risk.

Parvovirus is shed in the faeces. It is spread by direct or indirect contact with infected dogs or their faeces. Infection occurs through ingestion. The incubation period is 3–5 days. The severity of the disease depends on the age, immune/antibody status of the animal, stress and concurrent infections. The virus targets rapidly dividing cells, i.e. the gastrointestinal tract, cardiac tissue and bone marrow. In the gastrointestinal tract there is generalized inflammation, causing the gastrointestinal signs. The virus causes flattening of the villi, which causes malabsorption. Destruction of the bone marrow causes immunosuppression and susceptibility to secondary bacterial infections. In puppies under 4 weeks of age, the myocardium is rapidly dividing and will also be targeted by parvovirus, causing heart failure. The infection is often complicated by secondary bacterial infections.

Clinical signs

- Anorexia, depression, lethargy.
- Vomiting and foul-smelling haemorrhagic diarrhoea.
- Pyrexia.
- Shock, dehydration, hypothermia.
- Sudden death.

Diagnostics

A presumptive diagnosis is based on history (general and vaccination) and clinical signs.

- Blood tests: haematology (leucopenia) and biochemistry.
- Faecal sample: antigen tests – CPV antigen ELISA test.
- Serology.
- Post-mortem examination – histopathology.

Treatment

Prevention is by vaccination and reducing the exposure of at-risk animals.
Treatment involves:

- Isolation and barrier nursing
- Supportive – intravenous fluid therapy to correct dehydration and electrolyte imbalance; whole blood or colloids may be indicated
- Interferon
- Antiemetic if vomiting is intractable
- Nutrition (microenteral nutrition has been shown to decrease the time for which a patient is hospitalized)
- Antibiotics to treat secondary bacterial infections.

Once vomiting has ceased, water can be introduced. If this is kept down, small highly digestible low-fibre low-fat meals need to be offered to the patient. The amounts are gradually increased over the following few days. Sometimes parvovirus causes permanent damage to the gastrointestinal tract and malabsorption may then occur; these patients will need to be maintained on a special diet. Antibiotics are important in treating the secondary bacterial infections.

Nursing care

- Barrier nurse the patient to prevent transmission.
- Potential zoonoses (parvoviruses are able to cause cross-species infections).
- Monitor vital signs.
- Administer medication as directed by the veterinary surgeon.
- Administer and maintain fluid therapy.
- Provide general nursing of the clinical signs.
- Keep patient clean from vomitus, clip hindquarters, bathe and apply barrier creams to prevent scalding from diarrhoea.
- Offer small amount of electrolyte fluid when vomiting stops; then offer small meals as described above.
- Disinfect the environment using a suitable parvocide.
- Provide the owner with advice on vaccination protocols for any other dogs in the household.

Leptospirosis

This is a zoonotic disease. It is important that effective precautions are taken when nursing these cases.

Leptospirosis is caused by the Gram-negative bacterium *Leptospira canicola* or *L. icterohaemorrhagiae*. Other serovars may also be involved. Leptospires can survive in a suitable environment and contaminate water supplies. They are destroyed by desiccation, disinfection and ultraviolet light.

Transmission occurs through contact with infected urine and contaminated water sources, food, soil or bedding. Recovered dogs can excrete organisms, through urine, intermittently for months. Some species of animal can be carriers without exhibiting signs. Rats can be carrier animals of *L. icterohaemorrhagiae* and the source of contamination.

The organism penetrates through mucous membranes or damaged skin, spreads through the body and infects many tissues. The incubation period is approximately 7 days. The extent of damage to organs depends on the serovar. *L. icterohaemorrhagiae* predominantly causes hepatocellular damage, giving rise to hepatitis, whereas *L. canicola* predominantly causes renal dysfunction, leading to an acute interstitial nephritis.

Young animals are usually more severely affected. *L. canicola* infection has a low incidence of clinical disease and is more common in urban areas. *L. icterohaemorrhagiae* causes very severe illness and is more common in rural areas. Peracute cases may die before clinical signs develop. The acute form is the most frequently recognized, as the subacute form often only manifests very mild clinical signs. Mortality rates can be high, with sudden death or rapid deterioration within a few hours.

Clinical signs

- Anorexia, pyrexia, depression, dehydration.
- Vomiting, diarrhoea.
- Anterior abdominal pain, jaundice, petechiae, bleeding from gum margins (*L. icterohaemorrhagiae*).
- Renal enlargement and pain, polyuria/polydipsia or oliguria (*L. canicola*).

Diagnostics

A presumptive diagnosis is usually made based on history and clinical signs.

- Blood tests: haematology and biochemistry, clotting profile.
- Urinalysis: specific gravity, dipstick, sediment and dark field microscopy and culture for leptospires.
- Serological testing: demonstration of a fourfold increase in antibody titre.
- Post-mortem examination.

Treatment

Prevention is through pest control and vaccination.

Antibiotics are used specifically to treat the infection. Penicillins are effective against the bacteraemic state but other antibiotics are required to eliminate the carrier state. Some antibiotics can be nephrotoxic and need to be avoided (e.g. tetracyclines). Doxycycline is not eliminated via the kidneys and therefore can be used.

Supportive treatment is aimed at restoring fluid and electrolyte balance. If acute renal failure has occurred, urine output needs to be restored. Blood transfusions may be required if the patient is anaemic.

Nursing care

- *This is a zoonotic disease* – care must be taken when nursing.
- Barrier nurse the patient to prevent transmission.
- Monitor vital signs.
- Administer medication, as directed by the veterinary surgeon.
- Administer and maintain fluid therapy.
- Provide general nursing of the clinical signs.
- Ensure adequate nutrition of the patient.
- Monitor urine output and dispose of urine-soaked bedding carefully.
- Disinfect the environment.
- Provide the owner with advice on vaccination protocols for any other dogs in the household.

Canine contagious respiratory disease ('kennel cough complex')

A complex of microorganisms can cause the clinical signs of kennel cough. The organisms include canine parainfluenza virus 5 (PI-5), canine herpesvirus, canine reovirus, canine adenovirus 2 (CAV-2), *Bordetella bronchiseptica* and *Mycoplasma*. *B. bronchiseptica* can cause the most severe form of kennel cough when involved in an outbreak. Parainfluenza virus does not last long away from the host. CAV-2, like CAV-1, is relatively resistant but is susceptible to heat. Quaternary ammonium disinfectants are effective against these viruses. *Bordetella* can be shed for months.

Kennel cough is highly infectious but mortality rate is low. Spread usually occurs in areas of high density by direct dog-to-dog contact, hence the name kennel cough. Transmission occurs through aerosol droplets that localize in the respiratory system and cause a tracheobronchitis. The incubation period is 5–7 days and the clinical signs tend to resolve after 3–7 days. Damage to the respiratory epithelium can predispose to secondary bacterial infections.

Clinical signs

These are usually restricted to a goose-honking cough that is dry and unproductive, and may be associated with retching.

Gentle pressure on the trachea will elicit this cough. The animal will remain bright and alert unless the condition is complicated by bronchopneumonia, in which case anorexia, pyrexia, depression, tachypnoea and dyspnoea will be present.

Diagnostics

A presumptive diagnosis is usually made on history and clinical signs.

Treatment and prevention

Vaccination is available against *B. bronchiseptica* (intra-nasal vaccine), CAV-2 and PI-5, the latter as part of combination vaccines including canine distemper virus and canine parvovirus.

The disease is usually self-limiting, but antibiotics can be used to reduce the time of clinical signs and risk of secondary bacterial infections. Antitussives can be used to reduce the persistent cough, but should not be used if there is bronchopneumonia.

Nursing care

- Barrier nurse the patient (aerosol transmission is an important mode of transmission).
- Monitor vital signs.
- Administer medication, as directed by the veterinary surgeon.
- Provide general nursing of the clinical signs, cleaning of nasal discharge.
- Ensure adequate nutrition of the patient.
- Disinfect the environment.
- Provide the owner with advice on vaccination protocols for any other dogs in the household.

Infectious diseases – feline

Common feline infectious diseases are summarized in Figure 20.25.

Disease/ infection	Type of infectious agent	Incubation period	Major organs affected	Transmission	Zoonotic	Diagnostic methods	Major nursing needs	Control/ prevention
Feline panleucopenia	Virus	2–10 days	Gastrointestinal system Bone marrow	Body excretions	No	History, clinical signs Faecal analysis	Fluid therapy Symptomatic Antibiotics	Vaccination
Feline upper respiratory disease	Virus Bacteria	1–10 days	Upper respiratory tract	Saliva Ocular and nasal discharges	No	History, clinical signs Swabs	Symptomatic Antibiotics for secondary bacterial infections	Vaccination Isolation
Feline leukaemia	Virus	Months/years	Immune system Neoplasia	Saliva	No	Blood analysis	Symptomatic	Vaccination
Feline immuno-deficiency	Virus	Variable – may not show clinical signs for many years	Immune system	Cat bites – saliva	No	Blood analysis	Symptomatic	Restrict cat's movements

20.25 Common feline infectious diseases.

continues ▶

Disease/ infection	Type of infectious agent	Incubation period	Major organs affected	Transmission	Zoonotic	Diagnostic methods	Major nursing needs	Control/ prevention
Feline infectious peritonitis	Virus	Variable	Severe inflammation of body tissues	Ingestion	No	Combination of history, clinical signs, blood tests, tissue biopsy	Symptomatic	Unknown
Feline infectious anaemia	Bacterium		Red blood cells	Unknown Fighting/fleas?	No	Blood analysis	Antibiotics, immunosuppression Symptomatic	Flea control, cat fight control
Toxoplasmosis	Coccidian	3–10 days	Intestinal tract Systemic	Ingestion faeces, meat	Yes	Tissue biopsy Serology	Antibiotics	

20.25 *continued* Common feline infectious diseases.

Feline panleucopenia (feline infectious enteritis, FIE)

Feline panleucopenia is caused by a feline parvovirus and infects domestic and wild cats. It is very similar to the canine parvovirus, with similar properties. It survives for long periods in the environment and is very resistant to heating and routine disinfectants. Parvocidal products are required for disinfection.

The disease is usually seen in unvaccinated kittens living in close proximity (e.g. in rescue shelters). Maternal antibodies protect the kittens in the first 3 months of life.

The virus is shed in faeces, vomit, saliva and urine up to 6 weeks after infection. Transmission occurs via the oral route or transplacentally. Fomites play an important role in transmitting the virus. The incubation period is 2–10 days.

As a parvovirus, feline panleucopenia targets rapidly dividing cells: the lymphoid tissue, bone marrow and intestinal mucosal crypts. Destruction of the lymphoid tissue and bone marrow results in immunosuppression. Damage to the gastrointestinal system leads to gastroenteritis. In the late prenatal and early neonatal stages the lymphoid tissue, bone marrow and central nervous system can be affected. Early *in utero* infection can cause abortion and infertility. The cat recovers when an adequate immune response is mounted.

Damage to the bone marrow (panleucopenia results in low white blood cell counts) and enteritis increase susceptibility to bacterial infections.

Clinical signs

Many cats will have mild or subclinical infection and the disease is unlikely to be recognized. In peracute cases there will be sudden death. In acute cases the clinical signs include:

- Pyrexia, depression, anorexia
- Vomiting
- Diarrhoea (less frequent)
- Dehydration, hypothermia
- CNS signs: ataxia, tremors, incoordination. Cerebellar hypoplasia if fetus infected in second half of pregnancy
- Retinal lesions
- Queens: abortion, infertility.

Diagnostics

A presumptive diagnosis is usually made on history, clinical signs and demonstration of leucopenia on haematology.

- Blood tests: haematology and biochemistry.
- ELISA test: faecal sample.

Treatment

Prevention is by vaccination.

Supportive and symptomatic treatment includes interferon, intravenous fluid therapy, antibiotics for secondary bacterial infections and antiemetics for intractable vomiting.

Nursing care

- Barrier nurse the patient to prevent transmission.
- Monitor vital signs.
- Administer medication, as directed by the veterinary surgeon.
- Administer and maintain fluid therapy.
- Provide general nursing of the clinical signs.
- Keep patient clean from vomit and diarrhoea.
- Offer small amount of electrolyte fluid when vomiting stops, then offer small meals of a low-fat highly digestible diet.
- Advise the owner regarding other cats in the household. As the virus can persist in the environment, advise owners that new cats/kittens are fully vaccinated before entering the household.
- Advise owners re disinfection of the environment.

Feline upper respiratory disease (FURD, 'cat 'flu')

FURD is a common syndrome involving several primary infectious agents. It usually causes high morbidity but low mortality. The main infectious agents are:

- Feline herpesvirus type 1 (FHV-1)
- Feline calicivirus (FCV)
- *Bordetella bronchiseptica*
- *Chlamydophila felis*.

FHV-1 and FCV account for 80% of cases.

FURD is a highly infectious disease and the infectious organisms are shed in nasal and ocular discharges and saliva from cats exhibiting clinical signs or from asymptomatic carriers. Aerosolized droplets and contaminated fomites transmit the viruses to susceptible individuals. The virus can remain in the environment for a week following the presence of an infected cat.

Purebred cats, especially Siamese, are prone to a more severe infection. Cats of all ages are susceptible but the disease may be more severe in kittens, elderly cats and immunocompromised cats.

After inhalation, the virus replicates in the local lymph nodes before targeting the epithelial cells of the respiratory tract and conjunctiva. Most cats will become carriers after the clinical signs are no longer evident.

Infectious agents and clinical signs

Feline herpesvirus type 1

FHV-1 survives in the environment for hours only and is killed by routine disinfection. The incubation period is 2–10 days and infection usually lasts for 10–14 days. After infection >80% of animals become carriers, shedding the virus when stressed. Cats remain carriers for life. Severe illness and fatalities can occur in young and old cats. Some cats develop chronic rhinitis or sinusitis ('chronic snufflers').

Clinical signs

- Depression.
- Inappetence/anorexia.
- Paroxysmal sneezing.
- Pyrexia.
- Conjunctivitis.
- Rhinitis (serous ocular/nasal discharges rapidly become mucopurulent with secondary bacterial infection).
- Salivation.
- Dyspnoea and cough if pneumonia develops.

Feline calicivirus

The incubation period is 1–7 days and infection usually lasts for 7–14 days. Disease is usually not as severe as with FHV-1. Carriers of FCV shed the virus continuously, some for a short period and some for years.

Clinical signs

- Mild ocular/nasal discharge (becoming mucopurulent with secondary bacterial infection).
- Sneezing.
- Inappetence.
- Depression.
- Pyrexia.
- Ulceration of hard and soft palates, tongue and cheeks.
- Chronic ulcerative stomatitis and gingivitis in some individuals.

Bordetella bronchiseptica

Infection with this bacterium causes mild upper respiratory tract disease in cats. Coughing is less prominent than in infected dogs. Bronchopneumonia may develop and can cause death, especially in kittens. Recovered cats may remain infectious for several months. Infections are more prevalent in multi-cat households, in rescue catteries and in cats in contact with dogs with respiratory disease, suggesting interspecies transmission.

Clinical signs

- Sneezing.
- Nasal discharge.
- Coughing.
- Submandibular lymphadenopathy.

Chlamydophila felis

Chlamydophila felis (formerly *Chlamydia psittaci* var. *felis*) is an intracellular parasite. Strains are species-specific. It is present on the ocular, respiratory, gastrointestinal and genitourinary mucosa of infected cats. The organism is very short lived off the host and transmission is likely to occur through direct contact with infected ocular and nasal discharges. All ages can be affected but kittens the most severely. The incubation period is 4–10 days. Infection may be unapparent to overt. The most common illnesses are acute, chronic and relapsing conjunctivitis. Improvement is normally seen after 2–3 weeks. The organism is responsible for about 30% of conjunctival cases and can cause nasal and lower respiratory infections. Abortions or infertility may also be caused by *Chlamydophila felis* but this remains to be proved clinically.

Clinical signs

- Conjunctivitis, hyperaemia, blepharospasm.
- Serous to mucopurulent ocular discharge.
- Mild upper respiratory tract disease (less common).

Diagnostics

A presumptive diagnosis is usually made on history and clinical signs.

- Oropharyngeal swab in viral transport medium for isolation of FHV-1 or FCV.
- Oropharyngeal or nasal swab in charcoal Amies transport medium for culture of *Bordetella*.
- Ocular swab in chlamydial transport medium for detection of *Chlamydophila* antigen.

Treatment

Prevention is by vaccination.

Treatment is symptomatic and supportive. Nursing care is particularly important.

- Antibiotics if viral infection complicated by secondary bacterial infection.
- Chlamydophilosis: topical or systemic tetracyclines. In multi-cat households the whole cat population should be treated at the same time. Treatment should continue for 2 weeks after clinical signs have abated.
- Bordetellosis: antibiotics (tetracyclines, enrofloxacin).
- Intravenous fluid therapy if cat dehydrated and anorexic.
- Interferon.

Nursing care

- Barrier nurse the patient (aerosol transmission is an important mode of transmission).
- Monitor vital signs.
- Monitor weight and hydration status if the patient is anorexic.
- Provide general nursing care, with attention given to cleaning of nasal discharges and grooming.
- Provision of a steamy room with added decongestant can help if nasal discharge is severe.
- Attention to nutrition is important, as these patients often need assisted feeding due to anorexia.
- Administer fluid therapy and medication, as directed by veterinary surgeon.
- Advise the owner about contamination, especially in multi-cat households.
- Advise the owner regarding vaccination protocols for other cats in the household.
- Advise the owner regarding the carrier state of the patient once recovered.

Preventive measures in a cattery

- Ensure that all animals are vaccinated before entering the premises.
- Cats should not be able to gain access to other cats. Ideally runs should have Perspex walls to provide a sneeze barrier.
- Use of disposable feeding bowls to reduce fomite transmission.
- Maintain correct disinfection protocols.
- Isolate any cats showing clinical signs.

Feline leukaemia (FeLV infection)

Feline leukaemia virus is a retrovirus. It is host species-specific and affects both domestic and wild cats around the world. It is an important cause of death in young adult cats. It is associated with leukaemia and other lymphoproliferative diseases and non-neoplastic disease.

The virus is shed constantly in saliva; therefore, close contact and mutual grooming are required for spread. Cats in close contact or living in the same household are most likely to become infected. Vertical transmission from dam to offspring via the placenta and milk also occurs. The main source of infection is the persistently viraemic cat that is either a healthy carrier or has FeLV-related disease. Kittens are more susceptible than adults and are more likely to become persistently viraemic.

Although the virus is shed in other bodily fluids (e.g. mucus and faeces), it is unlikely to be spread via this route; it is readily inactivated in the environment. Iatrogenic spread could occur through blood transfusions and contaminated needles or instruments.

After initial oronasal infection the animal may exhibit mild, vague clinical signs of lethargy and inappetence and a corresponding lymphadenopathy. At this point most cats mount an appropriate immune response, recover and do not become carriers. In a minority of cases the cat becomes permanently viraemic. The most important factors that determine whether a cat recovers or is permanently infected are its age at infection and the dose of virus to which it is exposed. Cats with persistent viraemia have a high risk of developing FeLV-related disease.

The diseases caused by FeLV can be divided into two categories: neoplastic and non-neoplastic. Malignancy may be caused by the virus being inserted into the genome and causing changes in the expression of the oncogene, which results in abnormal 'growth' and control of some cell lines. The transformation is usually of lymphoid and myeloid cells, causing lymphoma, leukaemias and myelodysplastic disorders. Anaemias may occur as a result of interference with normal maturation of the red blood cell line in the bone marrow or due to anaemia of chronic disease. Thrombocytopenia and leucopenia are a result of decreased production caused by suppressed or infiltrated bone marrow. The virus also interferes with a normal immune response; therefore these cases are more prone to infections. Circulating immune complexes may cause immune-mediated disease (e.g. glomerulonephritis, polyarthritis). Reproductive disorders include infertility and abortions.

Latent infections may revert to overt viraemia in times of stress, such as pregnancy and glucocorticoid treatment, but this is unusual and latent infection is most likely to be eliminated over time.

The prevalence of FeLV has declined over the years with effective routine testing of kittens in shelters and use of early vaccination.

Clinical signs

Neoplastic FeLV

Lymphoma can be categorized by the site of origin. FeLV may be associated with some sites, including mediastinal lymphoma. Clinical signs for the latter include:

- Tachypnoea
- Dyspnoea
- Regurgitation
- Horner's syndrome
- Non-specific signs of disease.

Alimentary lymphoma is usually FeLV-negative even though other lymphomas can be associated with FeLV. It affects the lymph nodes surrounding the alimentary tract
Clinical signs include:

- Vomiting
- Diarrhoea
- Weight loss
- May only present with anorexia.

Clinical signs for leukaemia include:

- Lethargy
- Bleeding
- Sepsis
- Splenomegaly.

Non-neoplastic FeLV

- Anaemia (see above).
- Platelet abnormalities:
  - Bleeding tendencies (see clotting section).
- Leucocyte abnormalities:
  - Increased incidence of bacterial infections
  - Gingivitis.
- Immunosuppression:
  - Increased incidence of infections, e.g. toxoplasmosis, cat 'flu, gingivitis.
- Reproductive disorders:
  - Infertility
  - Abortions.

If kittens are infected *in utero* they often die at an early age of 'fading kitten' syndrome (see Chapter 25). They fail to nurse and become dehydrated and hypothermic within the first 2 weeks of life.

Diagnostics

Before diagnosis in an apparently healthy cat, a definitive test using virus isolation or immunofluorescence is recommended.

- Specific blood tests: ELISA for FeLV.
- Other blood tests: haematology for haemopoietic cell lines.
- FIV test as may occur concurrently.
- Bone marrow cytology.
- Fine-needle aspiration/biopsy of lymph nodes.
- Radiography and/or ultrasonography.

Treatment

Prevention is by vaccination of at-risk cats. Treatment is supportive: although the underlying virus cannot be treated, the secondary disease should be treated as for an FeLV-negative cat.

Good routine management of disease needs to be maintained to avoid stress to the immune system. For example, good flea and worm control and routine vaccinations need to be continued.

FeLV-positive cats should be removed from multi-cat households if the other cats are found to be negative, using 'test and remove' schemes.

Nursing care

- Barrier nurse the patient away from other cats.
- Ensure feed bowls, anaesthetic equipment, dental equipment, etc. are sterilized after use.
- Monitor vital signs.
- Administer medication, as directed by the veterinary surgeon.
- Administer and maintain fluid therapy if required.
- Provide general nursing of the clinical signs.
- Ensure adequate nutrition of the patient. Advise the owner *not* to feed raw meat (due to increased risk of infection by *Toxoplasma gondii*).
- Advise the owner regarding preventive vaccination, worming and flea control to protect the patient from contracting other diseases.
- Advise the owner to neuter the cat and keep it indoors to prevent transmission to other cats.

Feline immunodeficiency (FIV infection)

Feline immunodeficiency virus is a retrovirus. It is related to human immunodeficiency virus (HIV) but is host species-specific, i.e. it only infects cats, both wild and domestic. It is labile and does not survive in the environment.

The virus is transmitted predominantly via bite wounds. The virus is found in large quantities in the saliva. Kittens can also be infected via the placenta and milk. Transmission to other cats in a multi-cat household is infrequent. Intact male cats are at increased risk as they are most likely to roam and fight. The average age of infected cats is around 6 years.

After infection, replication of the virus occurs in the salivary glands and lymphoid tissue. At this point there may be mild and vague clinical signs or infection may be subclinical. An immune response can be mounted that decreases the circulating virus and the cats generally become asymptomatic for a period of time. The virus, however, continues to replicate and over time there is destruction of the cat's immune system. This leaves the cat susceptible to infections and developing various tumours. The brain and kidneys can also be affected, leading to neurological signs and renal failure, respectively.

There are no vaccines for FIV and the virus cannot be eliminated by a normal immune response elicited by infection. The cat will produce antibodies but these are largely ineffective.

Clinical signs

Clinical signs are non-specific. After the initial infection the cats may have mild lethargy, inappetence and pyrexia. In the later stage of infection, clinical signs are associated with opportunistic infections, neoplasia or other syndromes, such as wasting, and include:

- Weight loss, emaciation
- Lethargy
- Inappetence
- Lymphadenopathy
- Pyrexia
- Gingivitis/stomatitis
- Chronic diarrhoea
- Chronic nasal discharge
- Chronic ocular discharge
- Anterior uveitis (directly FIV-related or as a result of toxoplasmosis)
- Chronic renal failure
- Chronic respiratory infection
- Abscesses
- Neurological signs (behaviour changes, seizures, paresis).

Diagnostics

- Blood tests: haematology, biochemistry.
- FIV-specific ELISA for antibodies.
- Confirmatory tests: virus isolation from the lymphocytes, PCR.
- FeLV test as can be concurrent.

ELISA-based tests

Some FIV-positive cats produce different antibodies to those detected on the test, leading to a false-negative result. Negative tests should be repeated after 8–12 weeks (anti-FIV antibodies are not produced in the first 8 weeks of infection).

Queens transfer antibodies to their newborn kittens via milk. These maternally derived antibodies (MDA) are then detected when the kittens are tested. FIV is usually only passed on to about one-third of the litter, but all the kittens will have MDA at the time of sampling as they may remain in the kitten's immune system for up to 4 months. Kittens that have been infected with the virus do not usually produce their own antibodies to the virus for a further 2 months. Therefore, to avoid false-positive results, kittens born to FIV-positive queens should not be tested until 6 months old or should be tested repeatedly until at least 6 months old.

Treatment

At this time there is no specific treatment with proven long-term efficacy, although antiviral drugs may be used. Treatment is aimed at the complications of FIV infection, i.e. opportunistic infections and neoplasia. Infections should be treated with appropriate antimicrobials. Dental hygiene is important to reduce stomatitis.

Routine inactivated vaccines can be given to asymptomatic FIV-positive cats living in a high-risk population to reduce the effects of stress that these diseases could have on the cat. The PCR test needs to be used to test these cats for FIV following vaccination. Other measures include:

- Routine flea and worming prevention
- Neutering
- Removal of kittens from FIV-positive queens from birth
- Keeping FIV-positive cats indoors and away from FIV-negative cats.

Nursing care

The nursing of a patient with FIV is based on generalized symptomatic care. Clinical signs can vary from patient to patient, but in addition to general nursing care the following measures should be taken.

- Barrier nurse away from other cats.
- Ensure feed bowls, anaesthetic equipment, dental equipment, etc. are sterilized after use.
- Administer fluid therapy and other medications, as directed by the veterinary surgeon.
- Keep the patient clean and groomed.
- Ensure adequate nutrition of the patient.
- Advise the owner not to feed raw meat (due to increased risk of infection by *Toxoplasma gondii*).
- Advise the owner regarding preventive vaccination, worming and flea control.
- Advise the owner to neuter the cat and keep it indoors to prevent transmission to other cats.

Feline infectious peritonitis (FIP)

Feline infectious peritonitis is caused by a coronavirus. Although the incidence is low, the disease is usually fatal. It is a disease of multi-cat households and there is an increased risk in pedigree households. Clinical disease is seen most frequently in cats under 2 years of age, stressed or with concurrent disease.

The virus is shed via the faeces. Cats are usually infected via the oronasal route by direct contact with infected individuals or indirectly through contaminated fomites. Although the virus may survive in the environment, it is readily destroyed by routine disinfection.

Coronavirus infection is common. In the majority of cases the cats are asymptomatic or develop mild signs of diarrhoea and eliminate the virus. Less commonly the virus causes FIP. The reason why these cats develop FIP is not fully understood but it is thought likely to be associated with an inappropriate immune response.

The coronavirus infects macrophages, which are then dispersed around the body via the circulation, targeting the vascular beds of the peritoneum, pleura, eyes, meninges or kidneys. Antibodies produced against the coronavirus form complexes with the antigen that lodge in the vasculature and cause a vasculitis.

- If this occurs in the peritoneum or pleura, it causes protein-rich fluid leakage and accumulation in the cavities. This is referred to as wet effusive FIP and is generally seen in cats under 2 years old.
- The dry form of FIP is seen in older cats, often after stress. There is inflammation and development of pyogranulomatous lesions throughout the body, without fluid accumulation.

Both forms are difficult to treat and, as the immune response is not appropriate, the disease is invariably fatal. Therefore the prognosis is poor.

Clinical signs

FIP cats have clinical signs of systemic disease – anorexia, lethargy and depression. The signs may be variable depending on the affected organs.

Wet effusive FIP

- Pleural effusion: dyspnoea and tachypnoea.
- Ascites: pot-bellied appearance.
- Weight loss.

Dry FIP

Common presenting signs include:

- Weight loss
- Inappetence.

Other signs depend on the organs affected:

- Neurological signs
- Eye disease
- GI disease
- Renal disease.

Diagnostics

Diagnosis can be difficult, as the majority of cats are seropositive for coronavirus but do not have FIP. A combination of criteria is therefore used to make a diagnosis of FIP:

- History and clinical signs
- Blood tests: haematology and biochemistry (especially looking for increased globulins)
- FeLV and FIV test as may occur concurrently
- Fluid analysis: exudates with increased proteins
- Biopsy of enlarged organs
- Post-mortem examination.

Treatment

The prognosis is poor and treatment is palliative. Corticosteroids may target the inflammation and slow the deterioration of the cat's condition, but may also result in immunosupression. Supportive treatment involves thoracocentesis to relieve dyspnoea associated with a pleural effusion.

Prevention is aimed at managing the multi-cat households by reducing faecal contamination, keeping cat numbers low, and isolation and early weaning of the kittens.

Nursing care

- Monitor vital signs.
- Provide general nursing of clinical signs presented.
- Provide assisted feeding of the anorexic patient.
- Advise the owner regarding other cats in the household.

Feline infectious anaemia (FIA)

The organism causing feline infectious anaemia was previously known as *Haemobartonella felis* but it has recently been reclassified as *Mycoplasma felis* and *M. haemominutum*. It is a parasite of feline red blood cells and lives on the cell surface.

The route of transmission is not completely understood. It is potentially spread by cat bites, fleas and blood transfusions. Kittens can be infected transplacentally and via the milk. There is an increased incidence in cats that are FeLV-positive, unvaccinated, roaming or involved in frequent cat fights.

The organism causes damage to the red blood cell surface. This is recognized by the immune system and the red blood cells are destroyed. This results in anaemia, which can be severe, especially if there is a concurrent FeLV infection.

Once infected, there is cyclical parasitaemia resulting in a cyclical anaemia. Some cats will be asymptomatic for infection and others will have severe disease. Infected cats will remain carriers for life.

Clinical signs

Clinical signs may be acute or chronic. The chronic form is the more common. Because cats can adapt their lifestyle they are often very anaemic when first presented.

- Acute:
  - Collapse
  - Dyspnoea
  - Pale mucous membranes.
- Chronic:
  - Lethargy, anorexia
  - Tachypnoea, tachycardia
  - Pale mucous membranes
  - Splenic enlargement
  - Enlarged lymph nodes
  - Pyrexia.

Diagnostics

The diagnostic plan is the same as for anaemia:

- Blood tests: haematology (including reticulocytes) and biochemistry (the anaemia is regenerative)
- Fresh blood smears to stain for *Mycoplasma* – Wright–Giemsa stain. The parasites are visible on the surface of the red blood cells. Due to the cyclical nature, multiple smears over time may need to be examined.
- FeLV and FIV testing.

Treatment

The infection is treated with doxycycline for 2–3 weeks. As there is an immune component to the red blood cell destruction, the patient is also given immunosuppressive drugs. Supportive care includes blood transfusions for severe anaemia.

Nursing care

- Monitor vital signs.
- Administer medication, as directed by veterinary surgeon – especially flea treatment to prevent disease transmission.
- Administer fluid therapy with or without blood transfusion, as directed by veterinary surgeon.
- Ensure adequate nutrition; assisted feeding may be required.
- Reduce environmental stress.
- Advise the owner regarding flea control.

Toxoplasmosis

This is an important zoonotic disease, especially for pregnant women. Toxoplasma gondii is an intracellular proto-zoan parasite (see Chapter 7). It infects all warm-blooded animals but cats are the only species in which the parasite can complete its life cycle (the definitive host) and the only species that sheds oocysts. The other species act as

intermediate hosts. The organism has a predilection for placental tissue, especially in ewes and in women. It is a multisystemic infection. Neurological signs are seen in 10% of affected animals.

Clinical signs

Most infections are subclinical. Most adult cats are immune to infection as a result of previous exposure. If infection occurs in a previously uninfected queen during pregnancy, the parasite can multiply in the placenta and spread to the fetuses. Affected kittens may be stillborn or may die before weaning.

Clinical signs depend on the organs affected:

- Pyrexia
- Anorexia
- Lethargy
- Weight loss
- Ophthalmitis (especially uveitis)
- Pneumonia
- Hepatitis
- Myositis
- Pancreatitis
- Myocarditis
- Skin lesions (rare)
- Diarrhoea
- Vomiting
- Muscle hyperaesthesia
- Lameness
- Ascites
- Neurological signs
- Sudden death.

Diagnostics

- Blood tests: haematology and biochemistry.
- FeLV and FIV testing as may occur concurrently.
- Cerebrospinal fluid (CSF) sample if neurological signs are present.
- Faecal examination.
- Serology.
- Biopsy.

Treatment

Systemic disease should be treated with clindamycin. Corticosteroids are contraindicated.

Nursing care

- *This is a zoonotic disease.* Appropriate care and use of disinfectants are important when handling faeces or cleaning litter trays.
- Administer drugs, as directed by the veterinary surgeon.

Advice for clients on avoiding toxoplasmosis

- Prepare animal food in a separate area, using separate utensils and feeding bowls.
- Do not allow pets to lick bowls, utensils or cooking items that will be used by people.
- Empty cat litter trays daily and clean with boiling water and disinfectant.
- Regular and prompt cleaning of litter trays will

continues ▶

continued

prevent oocysts from sporulating and becoming infectious.

- Pregnant women should wear waterproof protective gloves when gardening to avoid contact with buried or decomposed cat faeces, as the oocysts in the environment will have sporulated and become infectious. Hands should be washed thoroughly prior to contact with cups, food, etc.
- Wash all vegetables thoroughly for the same reason.
- Cook meat thoroughly.
- Cover children's sand pits to prevent cats using as litter trays.
- Ensure regular worming of cats to prevent infection.

Infectious diseases – canine/feline

Rabies

This is a zoonotic disease.

Rabies is caused by a lyssavirus. It is quite labile and does not survive in the environment. Rabies is an important fatal zoonotic disease and is widely spread through the rest of the world except Australasia and Antarctica; the UK is currently rabies-free. Control of stray dogs and rabies vaccinations have been important in reducing the number of rabies cases in pet dog and human populations. Dogs that travel abroad as part of the Pet Travel Scheme are required to be vaccinated against rabies.

Rabies is transmitted directly via saliva in bite wounds or abrasions from infected animals. All warm-blooded animals are variably susceptible to infection. Wild animals can act as a reservoir of infection.

The incubation period can be prolonged, with an average of around 2 months. The length of time to clinical signs is related to the infective dose and the distance the virus has to travel to the central nervous system: after the animal is bitten, the virus replicates locally before spreading up the nerves to the central nervous system. It replicates in the central nervous system before spreading along nerves to other parts of the body and into the salivary glands, where it is secreted in the saliva and capable of infecting another animal. Clinical signs of abnormal behaviour and paralysis are caused by direct damage to the central nervous system. The disease is considered fatal.

Clinical signs

The clinical signs of rabies have classically been divided into two major types: excitative ('furious') and paralytic ('dumb'). However, atypical signs are commonly seen. From the onset of clinical signs in pets, death usually occurs within 2–7 days.

Excitative

These animals become irritable, restless and vicious. They usually develop other neurological signs of incoordination, disorientation and generalized grand mal seizures. Wild animals may be less fearful of humans.

Paralytic

Incoordination is one of the first signs of the paralytic form. The motor neurons are damaged, resulting in hindlimb ataxia progressing to paralysis. Progressive laryngeal and pharyngeal paralysis occurs, giving difficulty in swallowing and profuse salivation and drooling. Facial expression is affected, resulting in drooping eyelids, sagging jaw and squinting. Progressive paralysis ensues, leading to respiratory arrest and death.

The distinction between the two forms is often not clear-cut and both forms progress toward paralysis, coma and death. The paralytic form is very uncommon in cats.

Diagnostics

There are no reliable ante-mortem tests for diagnosis of rabies; therefore, a presumptive diagnosis needs to be based on history and clinical signs. As rabies is a fatal zoonotic disease, suspected cases are euthanased and the diagnosis is made on post-mortem examination of the brain. Rabies is a **notifiable** disease. Suspect cases should be isolated and Defra contacted immediately.

Any animal that has potentially been exposed should be handled with great care. Transmission routes should be borne in mind and any abrasions, especially to the hands and face, should be covered. Masks with visors should be worn to avoid infection via mucous membranes.

Treatment

- Dogs are vaccinated in areas where there is a risk of rabies and in those taking part in the Pet Travel Scheme (see Defra website and Chapters 5 and 10).
- Humans are vaccinated if they are deemed at risk (e.g. staff working in quarantine kennels or handling certain wildlife species such as bats).
- Dogs with clinical signs should be placed in strict isolation and Defra contacted immediately. These cases are not treated.
- If bitten, the wound should be washed immediately with detergent and then 40–70% alcohol. Medical attention should be sought urgently.

Salmonellosis

This is a zoonotic disease.

Salmonellosis is caused by *Salmonella*, of which there are many serotypes. The bacterium is not host species-specific and occurs commonly in the intestinal tract of healthy mammals, birds and reptiles. Under certain circumstances it can cause systemic disease. It can survive for relatively long periods in the environment.

It is shed in the faeces, and transmission occurs through ingestion of faecally contaminated food, water or fomites. The bacteria multiply rapidly in foodstuffs stored at room temperature and in food that is inadequately cooked. Shedding can be intermittent and is usually increased when the animal is stressed. Younger animals are more susceptible to infection and illness. Overcrowding, stress and immunosuppression increase the risk of salmonellosis in dogs and cats.

After ingestion, the bacteria localize in the intestinal epithelium. Acute gastroenteritis is the most common clinical manifestation, but septicaemia can occur and the infection may become established in other tissues (placenta, conjunctiva, joints, meninges). Carrier animals may exhibit GI signs when subject to stress.

Clinical signs

- Anorexia, depression.
- Diarrhoea – haemorrhagic in severe cases.
- Vomiting, abdominal pain.
- Dehydration.
- Weight loss.
- Pyrexia.
- If severely affected and has a bacteraemia, will present in shock.
- *In utero* infections result in abortions, stillbirths and the birth of weak puppies.

Diagnostics

The diagnosis may be suspected from history and clinical signs.

- Blood tests: haematology/biochemistry are non-specific.
- Faecal culture: may be supportive but bear in mind that *Salmonella* can be isolated from healthy individuals.

Treatment

- Barrier nursing and isolation.
- Antibiotics are only used if the disease is systemic, as they (except fluoroquinolones) may increase risk of shedding once the animal has recovered. The disease is usually self-limiting.
- Fluid therapy and other supportive care for acute diarrhoea.

Nursing care

- *This is a zoonotic disease* – care must be taken when nursing.
- Barrier nurse the patient to prevent transmission.
- Monitor vital signs.
- Administer medication, as directed by the veterinary surgeon.
- Administer and maintain fluid therapy if required.
- Provide general nursing of the clinical signs.
- Ensure adequate nutrition of the patient.
- Dispose of faeces carefully.
- Advise owner regarding contamination.

Campylobacteriosis

This is a zoonotic disease.

The bacterium *Campylobacter* is an opportunistic organism whose role as a primary pathogen is not fully known. *Campylobacter* species probably act synergistically with other infections. Spread is through ingestion of undercooked raw food, contaminated water or faeces from infected animals, or via food/water bowls. Clinical infection is more common in animals under 6 months of age.

Clinical signs

- Watery or mucoid diarrhoea.
- Faecal tenesmus.
- Dullness, inappetence.

Diagnostics

- Culture of organisms from fresh (<24h old) faeces, using selective media.
- Detection of *Campylobacter* – not always diagnostic on its own because of carrier state.

Treatment

- The disease is self-limiting.
- Antibiotics may be given to reduce duration and severity of diarrhoea, minimizing risk of infection to humans and other animals.
- Fluid therapy.

Nursing care

- *This is a zoonotic disease* – care must be taken when nursing.
- Barrier nurse the patient to prevent transmission.
- Monitor vital signs.
- Administer medication, as directed by the veterinary surgeon.
- Administer and maintain fluid therapy if required.
- Provide general nursing of the clinical signs.
- Ensure adequate nutrition of the patient.
- Dispose of faeces carefully.
- Advise owner regarding contamination.

Complementary therapies – an overview

Complementary therapies incorporate a range of treatment approaches designed to facilitate and promote healing alongside conventional veterinary medicine. There is growing evidence from the medical literature that they can aid recovery and promote restoration of health in human patients when used appropriately following an accurate diagnosis. These techniques have since been extrapolated and applied with success to the field of veterinary medicine, although there is a paucity of randomized, controlled clinical trials. Further research is warranted to compile an evidence base and help inform best practice for use of these techniques in animals.

The complementary therapies and treatment approaches discussed in this chapter are by no means an exhaustive list. There are other alternative treatment approaches, such as Shiatsu, Bowen therapy, Rolfing and Reiki, all of which need further research and evidence into their effectiveness in the treatment of animals.

The practice of complementary therapies is restricted to registered members of the Royal College of Veterinary Surgeons (RCVS) with the exemptions of listed or Registered Veterinary Nurses and qualified physiotherapists (which includes osteopaths and chiropractors). This is currently under consultation review, following which paraprofessionals working with animals will be more closely regulated in conjunction with their respective governing bodies.

Acupuncture

Acupuncture has gained considerable popularity and credibility within the fields of human and veterinary medicine as a method of pain control. It is a treatment technique that originated in China and has been used in the Far East for the past 2000 years. It involves the insertion of fine metal needles at varying depths into the skin at localized points within the body to treat pain or disease (Figure 20.26). Research suggests that the needles activate naturally occurring pain-relieving

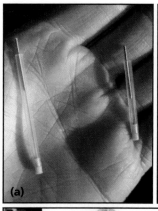 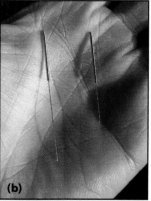

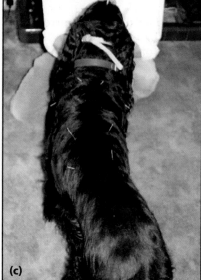

20.26

Acupuncture needles: **(a)** within and **(b)** removed from their plastic casings; **(c)** in use in a dog. (Courtesy of N Thompson)

Physiotherapy

Physiotherapy or physical therapy is the treatment of illness and injury by physical means. It encompasses manual therapies (stretches, massage, joint mobilizations), exercises, hydrotherapy (see later), thermal modalities (heat and cold), electrotherapeutic modalities (ultrasound, laser, TENS, NMES) and respiratory physiotherapy techniques.

In the UK there are currently three subgroups of physiotherapists treating animals:

- ACPAT (Association of Chartered Physiotherapists in Animal Therapy) members – dually qualified healthcare professionals that train extensively with human patients to degree level before embarking upon further postgraduate degree programmes (MSc/PGDip) to enable them to treat animals
- IRVAP (Institute of Registered Veterinary and Animal Physiotherapists) members – comprising veterinary surgeons, veterinary nurses and chartered physiotherapists
- NAVP (National Association of Veterinary Physiotherapists) members – who train solely with animals.

Physiotherapists can only treat an animal legally in the UK following permission from the referring veterinary surgeon in accordance with the Veterinary Surgeons Act 1966. Veterinary nurses can treat animals using physiotherapy techniques provided the referring veterinary surgeon feels they are competent to do so.

Manual therapies

These include techniques such as massage, limb stretches and joint mobilizations, as well as specialized positioning methods used to treat respiratory patients, such as postural drainage. Additional details of these techniques and their applications can be found in the *BSAVA Manual of Canine and Feline Advanced Veterinary Nursing, 2nd edition* and the *BSAVA Manual of Canine and Feline Rehabilitation, Supportive and Palliative Care: Case Studies in Patient Management*.

Massage

This involves the manipulation of the muscles and associated soft tissue structures of the body through rhythmical motions of the therapist's hands. There are various different massage techniques designed to influence the tissues in different ways.

- **Stroking** (Figure 20.27) involves gentle sweeping movements across the muscles and is generally used as a relaxation and preparatory phase of massage treatment prior to working the tissues using the deeper techniques. It allows the animal to become accustomed to the therapist's touch, thus enabling trust and patient compliance.
- **Effleurage** is similar to stroking but requires more pressure and is therefore only appropriate to use once the animal has become accustomed to the therapist and the muscles have been warmed up by stroking. The therapist should allow his/her hands to follow the contours of the animal's musculature, taking care not to put pressure over bony areas such as the spine.
- **Tapotement** (percussion) (Figure 20.28) and **petrissage** are more vigorous, stimulating techniques that need to be introduced gradually to prevent the animal becoming alarmed.

chemicals in the brain (endogenous opiates and endorphins) by sending messages via the spinal cord from the sensory nerves in the skin.

The Chinese Medicine theory believes that acupuncture works by stimulating the body's natural energy known as 'Chi' via energy channels known as 'meridians' but the scientific literature to date has difficulty proving the existence of these meridians, as they cannot be measured or quantified. Nevertheless, acupuncture is a popular method of achieving natural pain relief in human patients and has since been applied successfully to animals. It can be a useful adjunctive treatment in postoperative or chronic pain cases (see *BSAVA Manual of Canine and Feline Rehabilitation, Supportive and Palliative Care: Case Studies in Patient Management*).

Acupuncture needle insertion may be slightly uncomfortable initially but seems to be tolerated well by most animals if performed correctly and sympathetically. The needles are left *in situ* for anything up to 30 minutes during which they may be 'stimulated' by being gently rotated several times. The number of needles used during a treatment session varies depending on the condition being treated. Frequency of treatment also depends on the chronicity and nature of the presenting condition; an animal may start off with two treatments per week initially.

Under the Veterinary Surgeons Act 1966 acupuncture is classified as minor surgery. It may be performed by a veterinary surgeon who has received specialist training or by a listed or Registered Veterinary Nurse under the direct supervision of a veterinary surgeon, but by no other individual, even if they are qualified to use acupuncture in human medicine.

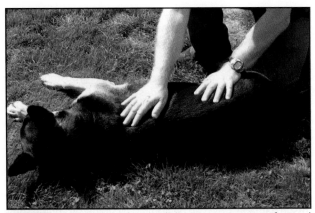

20.27 Stroking involves a gliding movement performed in any direction on the surface of the body, although it usually starts proximally and ends distally. (Courtesy of Brian Sharp; reproduced from *BSAVA Manual of Canine and Feline Rehabilitation, Supportive and Palliative Care: Case Studies in Patient Management*)

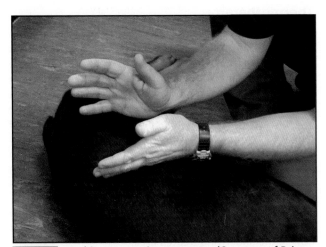

20.28 Hacking percussion massage. (Courtesy of Brian Sharp; reproduced from *BSAVA Manual of Canine and Feline Advanced Veterinary Nursing, 2nd edition*)

Research suggests that massage, when applied appropriately, can effectively promote blood and lymph circulation and is therefore an effective adjunct in oedema control. In addition it helps to mobilize the tissues, promoting collagen extensibility and elasticity as well as providing relaxation and pain relief (due to stimulation of pressure receptors in the skin that interact with the nervous system, involving the brain). Animals seem to enjoy massage if performed in an appropriate, timely manner by a trained professional, and evidence from human medicine suggests that it promotes psychological and emotional wellbeing. It must be noted that massage may be contraindicated in certain cases, e.g. around unstable fracture sites, around unstable joints, over bony prominences in general, and around neoplastic or infected tissue (as it will promote blood supply). A thorough working knowledge of veterinary anatomy is an absolute prerequisite before treating any animal with massage techniques, to ensure appropriate application.

Limb stretches

Limb stretches involve gently taking a muscle to a lengthened position without causing pain. Again, a thorough working knowledge of animal anatomy is an absolute necessity prior to attempting these techniques to prevent damage to the soft tissue structures. When executed appropriately, stretches can help maintain muscle/tendon length and health, thereby facilitating normal joint range of movement. This can help with restoration of movement and therefore ultimately function. Stretches can help prevent painful contractures and improve as well as maintain extensibility of collagen fibres within the connective tissue matrix, thus promoting flexibility and suppleness.

Joint mobilizations

This technique involves gently moving the joints through their normal physiological range of motion (ROM). Joint mobilizations may be performed passively or actively.

- **Passive joint mobilizations** involve the therapist gently taking the animal's joints from flexion through to extension and back again (Figure 20.29). They are particularly useful in recumbent animals that are not actively able to move the joints themselves, e.g. tetraplegics and paraplegics.
- **Active joint mobilizations** involve the animal taking the joints from flexion to extension and back again itself, e.g. asking a dog to sit and then stand for a treat will result in hip, stifle and tarsus flexion followed by hip, stifle, tarsus extension.

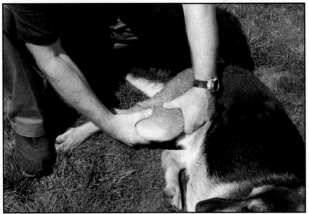

20.29 Flexion and extension passive movements performed on the stifle. The joint is moved into flexion to the first point of resistance (or animal reaction), and then similarly into extension. This is repeated in a rhythmic manner 15–20 times, and should be performed several times daily. (Courtesy of Brian Sharp; reproduced from *BSAVA Manual of Canine and Feline Rehabilitation, Supportive and Palliative Care: Case Studies in Patient Management*)

Joint mobilizations, whether active or passive, are necessary for normal joint nutrition and, ultimately, cartilage health. Articular cartilage lines the surface of all synovial joints and obtains its nutrition via the synovial fluid present within the joint cavity. The synovial fluid is moved around the joint surface thus 'feeding' the articular cartilage with nutrients in response to flexion/extension movements of the limbs. Joints that haven't been moved for some time or have only been moved in a restricted manner will become stiff, dysfunctional and at more risk of degeneration. A thorough knowledge of anatomy, especially normal joint angle ranges, is essential before performing these techniques to ensure patient safety.

Therapeutic exercises

Therapeutic exercises consist of a multitude of planned, repetitive series of events designed to facilitate muscle hypertrophy, activate joint range of movement(ROM) and stimulate balance and co-ordination, as well as influencing cardiovascular/respiratory endurance and fitness. They are intended to prepare condition and restore function to the neuromusculosketetal, cardiovascular and respiratory systems after injury, surgery or disease. These exercises may include (Figure 20.30):

- Harness-controlled lead-walking up or down slopes, over different surfaces (e.g. sand, gravel, grass) or through weave poles
- Using apparatus to challenge the animal's balance, proprioception and core stability, e.g. stepping over poles, balancing on wobble cushions, working over a 'physio-roll' and performing sit-to-stand exercises.

Such exercise programmes must be designed with clear goals in mind, which are ultimately influenced by the clinical diagnosis. They must be progressively incremental in design, thus allowing for training and subsequent recovery effect. This should aim for controlled stresses on the muscles, joints, ligaments, tendons and nervous system, which ultimately facilitate restoration of function without increasing pain or lameness. During the rehabilitation process it is important for the animal to receive suitable pain management; this will enable it to participate in the programme without being caused unnecessary discomfort or suffering. Analgesia should be discussed with the referring veterinary surgeon.

Thermal modalities

These involve the application of cold (cryotherapy) or heat (thermotherapy) to the muscles and associated soft tissues of the body to promote pain relief and facilitate healing after injury.

Cryotherapy

The application of cold can help reduce swelling postoperatively or following trauma, and provides a natural form of pain relief to inflamed/injured structures. Initially the application of cold causes the blood vessels to constrict (vasoconstriction), which reduces blood flow to the area. This is then followed by a period where the blood vessels expand again (vasodilatation), therefore enabling an increase in blood flow to the area. These changes in blood flow can help control inflammation and are useful in the acute stage, helping to limit further tissue damage. Cold can be applied by simply wrapping some ice in a damp towel or using special gel packs that can be kept in the freezer. Care must be taken not to expose the treated area to the cold for too long, otherwise an ice burn and further tissue damage may be caused (10–15 minutes is usually adequate per treatment).

Thermotherapy

This involves the application of heat to the tissues, which can help with pain relief, promotion of blood flow (causes vasodilatation) and tissue elasticity/extensibility. This can make it a useful treatment adjunct prior to massage or stretching in certain cases. Heat can be applied by special gel or wheat bag packs that can be warmed to a comfortable temperature in a microwave oven before being applied directly over the muscles. As with ice application, precautions must be taken to avoid skin burns to the animal. Hot packs can be left in place for 20–30 minutes, as they tend to cool down during this time; however, the animal must be supervised at all times to ensure safety. It is important to note that neoplastic, infected or haemorrhaging tissue must *not* be exposed to thermotherapy treatments, as heat causes an increased blood flow to the underlying treated area.

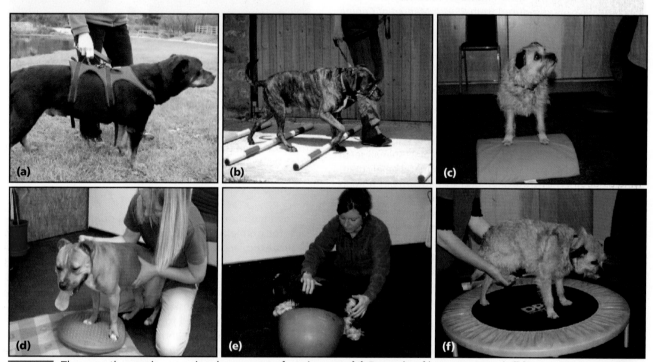

20.30   Therapeutic exercises may involve a range of equipment. **(a)** Example of harness control. **(b)** Stepping over poles. **(c)** Balancing on a wedge. **(d)** Balancing on a wobble cushion. **(e)** Core stability/strengthening work uisng a physio roll. **(f)** Limb lifts on a trampette. © Linhay Veterinary Rehabilitation Centre

Electrotherapy

This involves treating soft tissue structures with specific machines that produce electrical energy in a variety of different waveforms, which can help promote healing and repair at a cellular level. Electrotherapy includes modalities such as ultrasound, laser, and electrical nerve stimulation (NMES, TENS). These machines can cause significant damage if used inappropriately at the wrong dosages and it is important that those administering such treatments have received appropriate training. In addition, there are specific precautions and contraindications to using these treatment modalities which once again highlight the need for specialized training prior to use in animals. A thorough anatomical and physiological knowledge base is therefore paramount for their safe use in animal treatments.

Ultrasound therapy

Ultrasound machines use mechanical vibrations to generate sound waves of a frequency too high for the human ear to detect. The waveform can produce both thermal and non-thermal effects within body tissues, depending on how much energy the tissue absorbs. Ultrasound therapy is useful for increasing tissue extensibility, and promotes normal collagen fibril alignment. It is therefore advocated in managing contractures and scar tissue, as well as for tendon and ligament injuries. A coupling medium such as gel is needed to transmit the ultrasound waves to the underlying tissues (Figure 20.31).

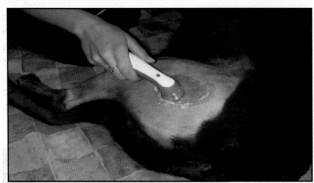

20.31 Ultrasound therapy being used on a dog. Note the clipped area and use of a gel to enable more effective transmission of the ultrasound waves). © Linhay Veterinary Rehabilitation Centre

Lasers

Laser is an acronym of light amplification by stimulated emission of radiation. Lasers deliver light energy into the underlying tissue structures, thus creating an optimum environment for healing to occur. Studies in animal and human models have found that laser energy can help reduce the inflammatory chemicals that have an adverse effect on normal tissue homeostasis and function. Laser light is therefore beneficial for wound healing and, in addition, can help provide pain relief. As with all electrotherapy modalities, it is important that it is used only by trained personnel; otherwise significant tissue damage can occur.

Neuromuscular electrical nerve stimulation (NMES)

This involves stimulation of nerve fibres on the skin surface by a series of gel-covered electrodes attached to a small hand-held unit. TENS (transcutaneous electrical nerve stimulation) machines are one type of electrical stimulation unit. They can be used in pain relief, and work by stimulating the nervous system to release naturally produced pain-relieving chemicals from the brain. Depending on the electric current frequency and intensity used, they can cause a muscle to contract by stimulating its motor unit. This can help promote blood and lymph circulation (thus reducing swelling), optimize muscle health and strength, and assist in healthy nerve functioning at a cellular level, depending on the machine type and frequency/intensity of current used.

Hydrotherapy

Hydrotherapy involves swimming or walking in a body of water such as a pool or water treadmill. Submerging an animal in water has a number of physiological effects that can help provide a therapeutic treatment if performed correctly by qualified physiotherapists or veterinary nurses who have received further specialist training. These therapeutic effects involve the principles of buoyancy, hydrostatic pressure and viscosity.

- **Buoyancy** is based on Archimedes' principle that pushing an object into water will cause an upthrust on the object equal to the weight of the water it has displaced. From a clinical perspective, the effect of buoyancy means that weak patients or those with joint pain are able to move more freely in water, with less pain, and therefore to build muscle. By building up the relevant muscle groups and gently mobilizing the associated joints, the animal becomes stronger and therefore better able to cope with exercise on land.
- **Hydrostatic pressure** works on the principle that the deeper an object is immersed, the more pressure is exerted on it by the surrounding water. Clinically, this means that submerging an animal's limbs in water can help control swelling, as the pressure exerted by the water will help push the venous blood back to the heart. As a result, the limb may be less swollen after hydrotherapy, which will be more comfortable for the animal.
- **Viscosity** measures the degree of resistance to movement created by the water molecules; this decreases as temperature increases. Clinically, this is advantageous as it will enable weak muscles to move bones and joints in water more easily than on land. This is particularly useful in some orthopaedic postoperative or neurological cases. Treatment times need to be closely monitored and increased gradually, depending on the patient's problem. The skill lies in knowing when to challenge the musculoskeletal structures without causing a concomitant increase in pain and lameness.

Hydrotherapy can thus help strengthen muscles (due to water resistance) without placing extra weight-bearing forces on the joints (due to the effect of buoyancy). It also has a place in cardiovascular/respiratory conditioning and oedema control. Psychological benefits may also be gained from the animal being able to exercise and expend energy in a controlled environment.

Care must be taken with geriatric animals and those with heart or lung conditions as the water will place extra pressure on the heart and lungs when the animal is submerged; each animal should be examined by a veterinary surgeon prior to undertaking any form of hydrotherapy.

Practical considerations

Ideally, animals should receive hydrotherapy in a veterinary-run establishment (usually run in conjunction with a qualified physiotherapist) or in one that has received approval from the Canine Hydrotherapy Association (CHA). Sometimes natural bodies of water such as lakes or ponds can be utilized; however, the water temperature is usually too cold and therefore will not have a thermal therapeutic effect on the joints and tissues. In addition, there is the issue of safety when swimming an animal in an open body of water, due to external influences such as current, water depth and hidden reeds or weeds.

Water temperature and quality should be strictly controlled to ensure patient safety and satisfy hygiene/infection control regulations. Water temperature should be between 26 and 30°C to enable a therapeutic effect on the musculoskeletal system. In addition, it is important that the animal is adequately dried afterwards to prevent chills, especially in colder weather.

Good control and handling of the animal is imperative to ensure an appropriate, effective and safe treatment. When using a pool, the therapist must be present in the pool with the animal at all times and use appropriate buoyancy aids or harnesses to aid control, thus ensuring animal/handler safety (Figure 20.32). Dogs on treadmills should be secured centrally on the treadmill belt via a harness and bungee system (Figure 20.33) to facilitate a safe, therapeutic treatment, and should be supervised at all times. In addition, all dogs must be introduced to the aquatic environment in a controlled, sympathetic manner, ideally via a shallow, non-slip ramp. In some cases it may be appropriate to hoist the animal into the pool environment; this must be undertaken by experienced personnel.

Swimming in a pool often encourages the patient to take its joints through a large active range of motion (ROM), which may not always be appropriate immediately after surgery. For this reason, the hydrotherapy treadmill may be a more suitable treatment option, but the water height and belt speed must be carefully controlled to prevent worsening of the condition. It is also easier to control the amount of work performed by the patient in a treadmill compared to a pool.

Both pools and treadmills can be useful rehabilitation tools if used sensibly but it must be noted that in certain

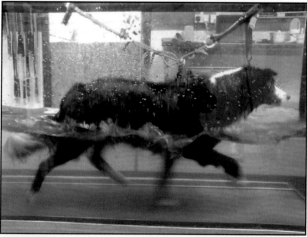

20.33 A dog undergoing treatment on a hydrotherapy treadmill. Note the harness and bungee control system. © Linhay Veterinary Rehabilitation Centre

cases/conditions they can make the animal lame, increase pain and, in the case of postoperative orthopaedic cases, cause surgery to fail.

It is paramount that the physiotherapist/veterinary nurse collaborate closely with the referring veterinary surgeon so as not to adversely affect treatment outcome. Knowledge of normal healing timescales for both soft tissue and bone/fractures, alongside a thorough working knowledge of animal anatomy, are very important.

Other forms of complementary therapy

Aromatherapy

Aromatherapy involves the use of aromatic plant extracts in oil form to promote health and wellbeing. Certain plant materials are believed to possess therapeutic properties, which may prevent illness and disease. The oils may be administered to the animal by massaging them into the skin or via direct inhalation. Treatment of animals (other than one's own) using aromatherapy is restricted to members of the RCVS who have undergone further training in these areas.

Homeopathy

Homeopathy is the oral administration of diluted plant or mineral extracts designed to boost the body's natural energy and promote a state of health. The treatment can be given in tablet or liquid form and relies on the theory 'treat like with like', i.e. the substance given is meant to cause a similar effect to the clinical signs of dysfunction presented. Homeopathy can only be administered (other than by the owner) to animals by a member of the RCVS who has received further specialist training in this field of naturopathic medicine.

Chiropractics

Chiropractic treatment involves the identification and subsequent treatment of musculoskeletal dysfunction within the body. Particular emphasis and treatment is focused on the spine and its associated bony and soft tissue structures by performing a manipulation or 'adjustment' to correct areas of 'subluxation'. Chiropractors use the term 'subluxation' to

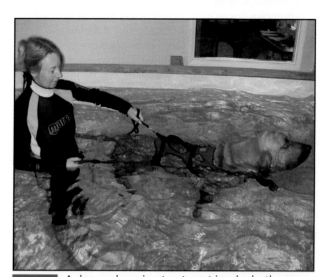

20.32 A dog undergoing treatment in a hydrotherapy pool. Note the harness control and use of a buoyancy aid. © Linhay Veterinary Rehabilitation Centre

describe a loss of function in an area of the spine and associated spinal nerves due to a reduction in normal movement or alignment. Chiropractors undergo specialized training before they can treat humans and animals and are regulated by the General Chiropractic Council in the UK. The chiropractic treatment of animals must be approved by a qualified veterinary surgeon in accordance with the Veterinary Surgeons Act 1966.

Osteopathy

Osteopathy involves the identification and subsequent treatment of imbalances and dysfunction within the skeleton involving the bones, joints, muscles, ligaments, tendons and nerves. Osteopaths use a variety of treatment techniques including manipulation, massage and stretches to create a state of balance within the body. They are required to undergo 4–5 years' specialist training at degree level with human patients prior to further postgraduate study which enables them to treat animals following veterinary permission. The osteopathic treatment of animals must be approved by a qualified veterinary surgeon in accordance with the Veterinary Surgeons Act 1966.

Further reading

Bowden C and Masters J (2003) *Textbook of Veterinary Medical Nursing*. Butterworth Heinemann, London

Hall EH, Simpson JW and Williams DA (2005) *BSAVA Manual of Canine and Feline Gastroenterology, 2nd edn.* BSAVA Publications, Gloucester

Klide AM and Kung SH (2002) *Veterinary Acupuncture.* University of Pennsylvania Press, Philadelphia

McGowan C, Goff L and Stubbs N (2007) *Animal Physiotherapy – Assessment, Treatment and Rehabilitation of Animals.* Blackwell Publishing, Oxford

Millis DL and Levin D (2004) *Canine Rehabilitation and Physical Therapy.* Saunders, St. Louis

Mooney CT and Peterson ME (2004) *BSAVA Manual of Canine and Feline Endocrinology, 3rd edn.* BSAVA Publications, Gloucester

Ramey DW and Rollin BE (2004) *Complementary and Alternative Veterinary Medicine Considered.* Iowa State Press, Ames

Ramsey IK and Tennant B (2001) *BSAVA Manual of Canine and Feline Infectious Diseases.* BSAVA Publications, Gloucester

Rew K (2007) Rehabilitation offers effective way to restore form and function. *Veterinary Times*, October 22nd pp. 16–18

Rew K, Davies L and Sharples R (2009) Don't drown the dog: practical and safe approaches to rehabilitation. *Veterinary Times* February 2nd pp. 16–19

Sharp BJ (2008) Physiotherapy and rehabilitation. In: *BSAVA Manual of Canine and Feline Advanced Veterinary Nursing, 2nd edn*, ed. A Hotson Moore and S Rudd, pp. 72—102. BSAVA Publications, Gloucester

Watson P and Lindley S (2010) *BSAVA Manual of Canine and Feline Rehabilitation, Supportive and Palliative Care: Case Studies in Patient Management.* BSAVA Publications, Gloucester

Useful websites

www.linhayvet.co.uk
www.acpat.org
www.navp.co.uk
www.abva.co.uk

Self-assessment questions

1. Describe the clinical signs of acute heart failure, how this is initially treated and how these patients are nursed.
2. Cats and dogs both get pancreatitis. How do the clinical signs, treatment and nursing differ between the two species?
3. What are the clinical signs of acute and chronic renal failure and how are these patients treated and nursed?
4. What are the clinical signs of diabetes mellitus? How is it treated and how are these patients nursed and monitored long term?
5. What are the causes of arthritis and how are these conditions treated and nursed?
6. How is parvovirus shed and what age group is most susceptible to infection? Describe how to nurse these patients.
7. Describe how to nurse a patient with cat 'flu.
8. Advise a client on how to avoid contracting toxoplasmosis.
9. What is the difference between regurgitation and vomiting? How would nursing differ between the two conditions?
10. What are the clinical signs of a bleeding disorder and how is it diagnosed and nursed?
11. When might the following therapies be used and why:
    a. Effleurage
    b. Petrissage
    c. Cryotherapy
    d. Hydrotherapy?
12. How can ultrasound benefit an injured tendon?
13. What role do the following professionals carry out when working alongside the veterinary team in providing alternative treatments to promote health:
    a. The chiropractor
    b. The osteopath
    c. The acupuncturist
    d. The physiotherapist?

Chapter 21

Small animal first aid and emergencies

Amanda Boag and Kate Nichols

Learning objectives

After studying this chapter, students should be able to:

- **Define a veterinary emergency and provide advice on emergency care over the telephone**
- **Recognize the severity of an emergency and perform appropriate triage**
- **Describe the approach to the assessment of the emergency patient**
- **List the major body systems and understand their importance in the evaluation of the emergency patient**
- **Describe the procedure to follow if a patient undergoes cardiopulmonary arrest**
- **Explain the veterinary nurse's role when evaluating emergency patients and understand professional limitations**
- **List common veterinary emergencies, their presenting signs and their initial stabilization and treatment**

Introduction

Veterinary emergency medicine is a rapidly developing area of the profession. In general, an emergency is classified as any illness or injury where the animal's owner or guardian perceives that urgent veterinary attention is needed. Once the animal has been examined by a trained veterinary professional (veterinary surgeon or veterinary nurse), emergencies may be further categorized as those that are **unstable** where immediate/urgent diagnostics and treatment are required and those that are **stable** where further diagnostics and treatment may be delayed safely.

The Royal College of Veterinary Surgeons (RCVS) requires that all veterinary surgeons take steps to provide 24-hour emergency cover for their patients. Emergency cover is defined in the *RCVS Guide to Professional Conduct* as 'the provision of immediate first aid and pain relief to deal promptly with emergencies'. Historically, most practices have provided their own cover. Increasingly, practices are working together to provide out-of-hours care or are using one of the dedicated emergency service clinics that have opened in the last few years.

While veterinary surgeons and nurses are able to develop a special interest in this field, it is vital that *all* members of nursing staff are confident and competent in dealing with emergencies. These can present at any time, including during routine daily clinics, and some practices (especially in rural areas) will continue to provide their own out-of-hours cover. Although practices may focus on treating only certain species, on an emergency basis 'a veterinary surgeon must not unreasonably refuse to provide first aid, and facilitate the provision of pain relief for all other species until such time as a more appropriate emergency veterinary service accepts responsibility for the animal'.

This chapter will outline the general approach to the veterinary emergency patient and the role of the nurse, and will summarize some of the common clinical conditions seen in an emergency practice. Emergency work is *always* a team effort and the emergency nurse is a vital part of the veterinary team.

A successful outcome for the patient depends on:

- Early **recognition** of the severity and nature of the problem
- Good **communication** with the owner and with other members of the team
- **Implementation** of appropriate treatment
- Careful and diligent **monitoring**.

Although a veterinary surgeon will ultimately examine every patient, the experienced emergency nurse should be able to assess the severity of illness of each animal. This allows cases to be prioritized on the basis of clinical need and determines the optimal order in which they should be treated. The goal is to ensure a successful outcome for as many patients as possible, although the decision to euthanase an individual patient will sometimes need to be made.

Rules for emergency practice

- Remain calm.
- Be prepared.
- Do not put yourself, the owner or other staff members at risk.
- Ensure that the animal is at no further risk.
- Assess severity of injury/illness.
- Contact the veterinary surgeon as soon as possible.

Types of emergency

Veterinary emergencies comprise a wide range of clinical problems, ranging from those that are imminently life-threatening to minor injuries and ailments.

Triage is the process of rapidly classifying patients on the basis of their clinical priority, allowing identification of those patients that need urgent life-saving help and ensuring that this occurs immediately and before patients with less severe problems are dealt with.

In emergency practice, one of the nurse's major roles is to perform triage so that the veterinary surgeon can focus his/her attention on the patients that need them the most. The process of triage involves assessing information from the patient's history and initial clinical examination, in particular an assessment of their major body systems.

- Severe life-threatening emergencies are those that involve significant disturbances in the major body systems, where there is the potential for rapid deterioration and death.
- The list of minor emergencies is long but includes problems such as minor wounds, mild vomiting or diarrhoea, polydipsia, skin lesions/scratching and lameness. Although these animals may be dealt with on an emergency basis, their full evaluation and treatment can be delayed until after the needs of those patients with life-threatening emergencies have been addressed.

Telephone calls

This form of communication is often the first contact the practice will have with a client and their pet during an emergency. Understandably, clients may be very distressed and concerned at this time. It is vital that the veterinary nurse or receptionist remains sympathetic, calm and patient, and shows that they are aware that the client is distressed. Owners may not understand why certain questions are being asked and may become upset. They need to be reassured that the questions are being asked in order to ensure that the best advice and help are provided

The immediate aim of the telephone conversation is to establish whether the pet has a life-threatening problem. If this is the case, the owner should be advised that the pet should be brought to the practice as soon as possible. Further questioning at this point will only delay the pet's arrival at the practice and may have a negative impact on its chances of survival.

Emergencies for which examination at a veterinary practice should be advised without delay

- Respiratory distress.
- Severe bleeding, either from wounds or from body orifices.
- Collapse or unconsciousness.
- Rapid and progressive abdominal distension.
- Inability to urinate.
- Sudden onset of severe neurological abnormalities.
- Protracted vomiting, especially if animal is also depressed.
- Severe diarrhoea, especially if haemorrhagic.
- Witnessed ingestion of toxin.
- Severe weakness or inability to stand.
- Extreme pain.
- Fracture with bone ends visible or wounds in close . proximity to fracture site.
- Dystocia.

In other situations, further questioning may be needed to determine whether the animal needs to be seen immediately or whether an appointment can be made. Examples of this include:

- Mild to moderate vomiting
- Non-haemorrhagic diarrhoea
- Small wounds with minimal blood loss
- Discomfort on urinating but urine is being passed
- Polyuria/polydipsia
- Weight-bearing lameness.

Questions to be asked if the emergency is *not* life-threatening

- What is the breed, age and sex of the pet?
- Is it on any medication? If so, what medication is this and when was it last given?
- What is the exact nature of the problem?
- When did the problem start and has it been progressive?
- Has the animal ever had this problem before? If so, when? Was it treated?
- Does the animal seem depressed or lethargic?
- Does the animal have any other signs?

In general, questions should be asked about the nature of the problem before asking for owner details such as name and address. It can be frustrating for a distressed owner to be asked administrative questions before being asked about their pet's problem. To gain maximum information, questions should be specific and concise. To avoid misunderstanding, it is preferable to speak directly to the owner rather than to a third party.

Occasionally telephone advice is sought when the pet seems relatively normal but a serious incident has occurred recently. It is recommended that the following advice is given.

- **Recent trauma** (e.g. glancing blow from a car, fall from a height) has occurred and the animal appears to have recovered.
  - In this situation a full clinical examination by a veterinary surgeon should be recommended. It is possible that the animal has internal injuries. A

veterinary surgeon may be able to identify these injuries, allowing early treatment. If the owners are unwilling to bring the pet to the practice, they should be asked to observe the pet closely and call back immediately if any unusual signs (especially respiratory distress, weakness and pale mucous membranes) are observed.

- The animal has suffered a **seizure** but it has stopped by the time the owner contacts the veterinary practice.
  - It is recommended that the animal be seen as soon as possible. Although many seizures are single incidents, an underlying medical problem may be identified.

Owners will often ask if there is any treatment or first aid they can give at home. Any advice should be given with caution. Very few owners have medical training and their interpretation of clinical signs may be misleading. If in doubt, it is always advisable to recommend that a pet is seen at the practice in order that it may be examined by a trained professional.

In some situations, first aid provided by the owner before reaching the practice may be helpful:

- With haemorrhage, owners should be advised to apply pressure directly over an area of profuse bleeding, using a clean towel or cloth, whilst the animal is transported to the clinic
- In rare cases where a foreign object is present in the wound, the owner should be instructed *not* to remove it but to transport the animal to the practice with the object in place. It may be possible to apply pressure around the foreign object. Removing the object can potentially make any bleeding much worse
- On rare occasions, either as a result of trauma or if a surgical wound has broken down, owners may report being able to see internal organs (often fat or intestines) protruding through the wound. The owners should be advised to cover the pet's abdomen lightly (not tightly) with a clean towel for transportation and prevent the animal from licking the area.

The owner's personal safety is paramount and it may not be possible for first aid measures to be carried out on animals with painful wounds.

Rules for telephone conversations

- Always answer the phone by introducing yourself and your practice. A panicking owner needs to know that they have contacted their vet.
- Always be polite.
- Ascertain as quickly as possible whether the problem is life-threatening.
- Be able to provide clear directions to the practice.
- Be able to offer alternative means of transport (local pet ambulances, taxi firms) in case the owner has transport difficulties.
- Obtain an estimated time of arrival.
- Obtain the owner's contact details, including a mobile telephone number if possible. Repeat this information back to the caller to ensure that it is correct.
- Give the owner a financial quote for an emergency consultation.
- Check whether the pet regularly attends a veterinary surgery and, if so, which one.

Practices should consider having a telephone logbook where details of emergency telephone calls can be recorded. This book can also contain useful information such as pet ambulance numbers.

When an emergency call is taken, the veterinary nurse or receptionist should inform the rest of the team about the nature of the emergency and its expected arrival time. The surgery should be prepared to receive the patient. This may include preparing equipment for oxygen administration, intravenous fluid administration or wound dressings.

Handling and transport of emergency patients

Emergency patients generally have the same considerations regarding handling and transportation as other patients (see Chapter 10). Importantly, emergency patients may be shocked and in pain. Dogs and cats that are normally considered to be friendly and placid may become aggressive when injured and in pain. Veterinary staff should be cautious when approaching these animals and should use a muzzle or other restraint if concerned. Analgesia, under veterinary direction, should be given at the earliest possible opportunity; this will facilitate further handling. Owners should also be reminded that they should be cautious even when handling their own pet.

The dyspnoeic patient, especially the dyspnoeic cat, warrants special consideration. These patients may already be stressed due to their underlying disease and the journey to the practice. Further handling of these patients on arrival, especially if they struggle, may precipitate cardiopulmonary arrest. Dyspnoeic animals should be placed in an oxygen-enriched environment and given time to settle after arrival before a full examination or further procedures (e.g. catheter placement, radiography) are carried out.

Consideration should also be given to location when handling small mammal and exotic emergencies; many of these species are natural prey species and can find the presence and even odour of dogs and cats very distressing.

Arrival at the surgery

The key to treating emergencies successfully is to be prepared. As much paperwork as possible, including a consent form, should be prepared in advance. All practices, including both general practices and those that predominantly carry out emergency or out-of-hours work, should have a designated area for dealing with emergency patients. This emergency area or room should be easily accessible from as many other areas of the building as possible, including the client entry area/consulting rooms and areas with diagnostic equipment such as the laboratory and radiography room. Oxygen and anaesthetic equipment should be readily available. In most practices, the preparation area or induction room is best suited, as it is usually fitted with most of the emergency equipment required. Figure 21.1 gives a suggested list of equipment and drugs that should be readily available.

Emergency equipment

- Endotracheal tubes (varying sizes)
- Laryngoscope
- Oxygen supply
- Anaesthetic circuits
- Intravenous catheters (varying sizes)
- Tape for tying in ET tube
- Tape for securing IV catheters
- ECG machine
- Assortment of syringes and needles
- Suction machine/bulb syringe
- Dog urinary catheter (for difficult intubations)
- Good light source
- Drug dosage chart
- Fluid administration equipment
- Scalpel blades/suture material

Emergency drugs

- Adrenaline (epinephrine)
- Atropine
- Lidocaine
- Diazepam
- Calcium gluconate (10%)
- Dextrose solution (50%)
- Furosemide
- Dexamethasone
- Propofol
- Glyceryl trinitrate paste
- Opioid analgesics
- Intravenous fluids – replacement crystalloid
- Intravenous fluids – colloid
- Mannitol

21.1 Emergency equipment and drugs that should be readily available in the designated emergency area.

All staff (veterinary surgeons, veterinary nurses, other patient care staff and reception staff) should know that this area is where emergencies should be taken. The area should be well lit and spacious, with items and equipment stored tidily.

There should be a mobile crash box or trolley that is fully stocked and ready for use at all times (Figure 21.2). It should be the responsibility of one person in the practice (usually a veterinary nurse) to ensure that it is checked after every use and at least once weekly.

Any patient with a potentially life-threatening condition should be taken immediately to the designated emergency area on arrival at the practice for a primary survey.

Primary survey

This starts with an assessment of whether the animal has just undergone, or is likely to undergo, imminent cardiopulmonary arrest. The mnemonic **ABC** should be followed:

- **A**irway – does the patient have a patent airway?
- **B**reathing – is the patient making useful breathing efforts?
- **C**irculation – does the patient have evidence of spontaneous circulation (heartbeat, pulses)?

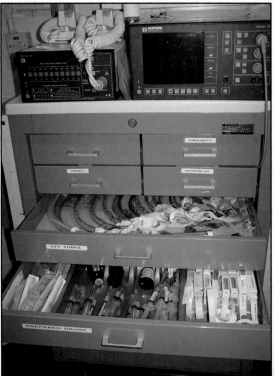

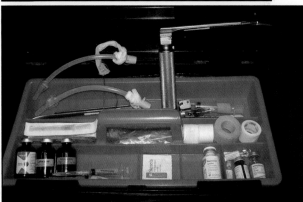

21.2 Example of a crash trolley from a large veterinary hospital and a crash box from a smaller practice. A variety of endotracheal tubes, intravenous catheters, drugs and monitoring equipment is present.

It should also be determined whether the patient is conscious or unconscious.

The primary survey should take approximately 30 seconds to perform. Once this assessment has been carried out and it is established that the patient is unlikely to undergo cardiorespiratory arrest, the triage nurse should carry out a major body systems assessment.

If the nurse has any concerns at all that the patient has arrested, the veterinary surgeon should be called and cardiopulmonary resuscitation should be started.

Major body system assessment

The three major body systems are considered to be:

- Cardiovascular
- Respiratory
- Neurological.

When triaging a patient, these systems should always be examined first, regardless of any other injuries. Dysfunction in any of these systems is potentially life-threatening. If a patient dies, it is always the result of failure of one of these systems.

Although other injuries may be more obvious, they are unlikely to kill the patient unless they have a secondary effect on one of the major body systems. For example, in a dog that has been hit by a car and has a fracture of the femur with a large open wound, although that injury may appear dramatic it will not on its own lead to the dog's death. However, the haemorrhage from the fracture site may lead to hypovolaemic shock, cardiovascular system compromise and death. Shock is detected by examination of the cardiovascular system.

The major body system assessment provides a means of assessing whether the patient's injuries are life-threatening. All parameters should be recorded at the time they are measured.

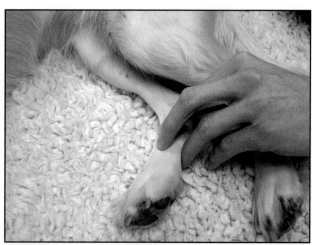

21.3   Locating the metatarsal pulse. Palpation of this pulse is especially useful in patients with pelvic or femoral fractures.

A pulse deficit occurs when a heart beat is heard but there is no corresponding pulse. Thus, the pulse rate measured will be lower than the heart rate. Pulse deficits are a sign of arrhythmia.

Mucous membrane colour

The normal colour is pale pink (paler in cats than dogs), though it should be remembered that some breeds (e.g. Chow-Chow) have pigmented dark mucous membranes. Some disease states cause abnormalities in mucous membrane colour; for example, pale or white in hypovolaemic shock or anaemia, bright red in distributive shock, or blue with hypoxia.

The capillary refill time (CRT) is checked by applying firm pressure with the thumb on the gingival mucosa to blanche the mucous membranes and timing how quickly the colour returns (see Chapter 15). A normal refill time is 1–2 seconds. The CRT may be rapid (<1 second) in early shock or slow (>2.5 seconds) in late shock.

Respiratory system

Respiratory system assessment involves evaluation of the animal's respiratory rate and effort. It is useful to record whether there are any audible noises associated with the respiratory effort and, if possible, whether the greater effort is associated with inspiration (breathing in) or expiration (breathing out). This information can assist the veterinary surgeon in diagnosing the cause of the breathing difficulty.

> ## Findings that suggest severe respiratory distress
>
> - Cyanotic (blue) mucous membranes.
> - Open-mouth breathing (especially in cats).
> - Abducted elbows.
> - Extended neck.
> - Paradoxical abdominal movement (abdomen moves in while chest moves out).
> - Dilated pupils.
> - Anxious facial expression.

Oxygen should always be supplied while a dyspnoeic animal is being examined (Figures 21.4, 21.5 and 21.6). Care should be taken that the method of oxygen supplementation does not distress the patient further.

> ## Parameters that should be recorded during a primary survey
>
> - Heart rate.
> - Pulse quality.
> - Mucous membrane colour.
> - Capillary refill time.
> - Respiratory rate.
> - Respiratory effort.
> - Gait.
> - Mentation.
> - Temperature.

Cardiovascular system

Information from the cardiovascular system examination is the best way the veterinary team has of quickly assessing the degree and type of shock. Repeat cardiovascular system examination, as the animal receives treatment for shock, is the simplest and most cost-effective way of monitoring the animal's response to treatment. The information provided by the nurse has a vitally important role in the outcome of the case.

The cardiovascular system examination involves assessment of a patient's heart rate, pulse quality, mucous membrane colour and capillary refill time.

Heart rate

Heart rate should be measured while auscultating the patient's heart with a stethoscope (see Chapter 15) and should be compared with the patient's pulse rate. The heart and pulse rates should be the same. If they are not, the veterinary surgeon should be alerted.

Pulse

The easiest pulse to feel is the femoral pulse. It is felt by sliding the fingers gently into the inguinal region (see Chapter 15). In some patients (e.g. those with femoral or pelvic fractures, heavily muscled or obese animals) this pulse can be difficult to feel and palpation of a metatarsal pulse on the dorsomedial aspect of the metatarsus may be easier (Figure 21.3).

With practice, pulse quality can be assessed. Pulse quality can be classified as: normal; tall and narrow (bounding or hyper-kinetic); or weak (thready). Information on the quality of the pulse should be recorded each time it is felt.

Method of oxygen supplementation	Advantages	Disadvantages
Flow-by (hold oxygen source close to patient's nose or mouth)	Cheap. Easy. Well tolerated	Does not allow high inspired concentration of oxygen
Mask	Cheap. Easy	Not tolerated by some patients. Does not allow high inspired concentration of oxygen
Nasal prongs	Cheap	Not tolerated by some patients. Tend to fall out frequently (designed for human noses). May cause sneezing
Nasal catheter (Figure 21.5)	Cheap. Catheter easy to place with practice	May require sedation for placement of catheter. Catheter irritates some patients. May cause sneezing
Transtracheal catheter	May be useful in patients with upper airway problems	Difficult to maintain and use in conscious patient. Not tolerated by some patients
Improvised oxygen cage (e.g. Elizabethan collar with cling-film)	Cheap. Widely available	Patients rapidly become hot. Can get CO_2 build-up
Oxygen cage/incubator (Figure 21.6)	Allows delivery of up to 90% oxygen. Minimal stress. May allow temperature and humidity control	Not widely available. Expensive
Intubation and ventilation	Allows 100% oxygen delivery. Allows control of breathing	Requires anaesthesia. Not possible long term except in specialist institutions

21.4 Methods of oxygen supplementation.

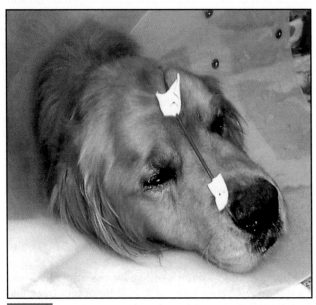

21.5 Nasal oxygen catheter in place.

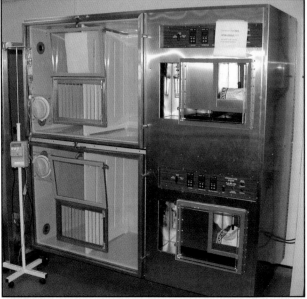

21.6 Oxygen cage allowing supplementation of up to 90% oxygen, with temperature and humidity control.

Nervous system

Initial evaluation of the nervous system involves an assessment of the patient's gait and mentation.

Gait

During assessment of gait, the following terms are used:

- **Paresis** – weakness
- **Plegia** – paralysis (unable to move)
- **Quadriplegia** – paralysis of all four limbs
- **Paraplegia** – paralysis of any two limbs
- **Hemiplegia** – paralysis of one side of the body
- **Hypermetria** – exaggerated limb movements.

In a paralysed animal it is important to note whether the animal can feel its limbs (e.g. turns its head toward the handler when its toes are squeezed) even though it may be unable to move them.

Mentation

The animal's mentation may be classified as:

- **Alert**
- **Obtunded** (mentally dull)
- **Stuporous** (semi-conscious, able to be roused only by a painful stimulus)
- **Coma** (unconscious and unable to be roused).

Other neurological features to note include:

- Pupil size and symmetry
- Presence or absence of pupillary light reflexes
- Presence or absence of palpebral reflex
- Facial asymmetry and any head tilt
- Nystagmus (abnormal flicking eye movements)
- Presence of gag reflex (in stuporous or comatose patients only)
- Anal tone (may be assessed when taking the temperature).

Body temperature

Once the major body system assessment has been completed, the animal's temperature can be taken and recorded. These points should be noted:

- Any faecal staining of the perineum
- Any blood or melaena on the thermometer
- Whether normal anal tone was present.

After the primary survey has been completed, any major body system conditions can be prioritized, and stabilization started as soon as possible.

Secondary survey

A secondary survey to establish other abnormalities can be performed once the primary survey is complete and treatment for any major body system abnormalities has been started. A **head-to-tail approach** is recommended to ensure that a systematic examination is performed.

Nose

Note any discharge (serous, purulent, haemorrhagic) and whether it is unilateral or bilateral. Note any swellings or asymmetry that may suggest nasal fractures or tumours.

Mouth

Note the colour of the mucous membranes. Initial examination of mucous membrane colour and capillary refill time (CRT) should have been performed as part of the major body systems assessment (see above). Normal mucous membranes are pale to medium pink in colour.

Abnormal mucous membrane colours

- **Pale** – suggestive of anaemia or hypovolaemic shock.
- **Red** – suggestive of distributive shock or localized inflammation (gingivitis).
- **Cyanotic** (blue) – suggestive of severe hypoxia.
- **Jaundiced** (yellow) – suggestive of liver disease or haemolytic anaemia.
- **Cherry red** – suggestive of carbon monoxide poisoning. (This is rare. Red mucous membranes are much more likely to be seen with distributive shock).

The oral cavity should be examined for any signs of haemorrhage, including both gross haemorrhage and petechial (pinprick) haemorrhages in the mucosa. The moistness of the mucous membranes can be assessed. Dry mucous membranes are suggestive of dehydration. Any ulcers on either the mucosa or the tongue should be noted. The hard palate should be assessed to see if it is split (a common injury in cats with head trauma). The mouth should be closed and an assessment made of whether the jaw closes properly or whether there is any asymmetry that may suggest a fracture. Excessive salivation should be noted.

Eyes

The eyes should be assessed for any discharge (serous or purulent) and whether it is unilateral or bilateral. The symmetry of the eyes should be assessed and any blepharospasm (indicative of ocular pain) noted. If there is no obvious ocular injury, the conjunctival mucous membranes should be assessed for their colour and the presence of haemorrhage. The position of the eyeball should be noted. An abnormal position is known as **strabismus** ('squint') and the direction of the strabismus should be noted. Abnormal ocular movements (**nystagmus**) should be noted and the direction of the fast component of the movement should be recorded. The pupil size and symmetry should be noted. The presence of asymmetrical pupils is known as **anisocoria** and it should be noted which pupil is larger. The palpebral reflex and pupillary light response should be checked.

Ears

Both ears should be checked for any discharge and the nature of the discharge noted. The pinnae should be observed for any petechial haemorrhages.

Limbs

Any obvious wounds should be noted. The limbs should be gently palpated and any swellings, pain or crepitus (abnormal cracking or grinding sound or sensation) should be recorded. If a limb is clearly being held at an abnormal angle and a fracture is suspected, this limb should not be palpated but the veterinary surgeon should be alerted. The animal should be prevented from using this limb until the veterinary surgeon has examined it. If the animal is ambulatory, it should be noted if it is lame and if so on which limb(s) it is lame and how severe the lameness is.

It is important to note whether the neurological function of each limb is intact. If the animal is moving the limb voluntarily, there must be some functioning nerve supply. If there are concerns that an animal cannot move or feel a limb, the toes on that foot should be pinched. Withdrawal of the limb implies that local nerve reflexes are intact but does not necessarily mean that the spinal cord is functioning normally. The animal should be closely observed to see whether there is pain sensation accompanying the reflex. This may involve vocalizing, turning its head towards the limb or attempting to bite. Loss of conscious pain perception in a limb indicates a poor prognosis.

Thorax

Any external wounds or swellings should be noted. If there is any evidence of a penetrating chest wound (e.g. a piece of skin sucked in and out as the animal breathes, sometimes accompanied by a gentle hissing sound) the wound should be covered with a sterile adherent dressing until it can be examined by the veterinary surgeon.

Thoracic auscultation is a useful skill for the emergency nurse to develop. When auscultating the chest, the nurse should listen to whether the lung sounds are abnormally quiet or loud. The distribution (e.g. left *versus* right, dorsal *versus* ventral) of any abnormal sounds should be recorded.

Abdomen

The hands should be run gently over the abdomen. Any wounds, swellings or bruising should be noted. Deep abdominal palpation is a skill that can take years to develop. The ability to palpate the bladder in the caudal abdomen is a useful skill for the emergency nurse to master. An obstructed bladder or urethra is a common emergency. Obstructed bladders feel firm, hard and enlarged. If this condition is suspected, the nurse should *not* attempt to express the bladder as there is a chance it may rupture.

External genitalia

In both sexes, the external genitalia should be checked for any discharge and for discoloration of the mucous membranes. Any evidence of urine scalding should be noted, as this could be suggestive of a more chronic urinary problem.

Tail

Any wounds should be noted. It should also be noted whether the animal can move its tail. Neurological injuries to the tail are common in cats following trauma and may be accompanied by neurological injury to the bladder and anus.

Capsule history

A 'capsule history' should be obtained from the owners of all emergency patients. This history focuses on the essential information that could alter the early management of the patient. A more detailed history may be taken once the patient is more stable.

Important questions to ask for a capsule history

- What is the age, sex and neutering status of the animal?
- If an entire female, when was her last season or litter?
- Is the animal on any medications?
- Has the animal been diagnosed with any long-term medical problems?
- Does the animal have any known allergies?
- Has the animal had access to any known toxins?
- When was the last time the animal ate and drank?
- When was the last time the animal passed faeces and urinated, and was it normal?
- How long has the animal been showing signs of its current problem?
- Has this problem got better, worse or stayed the same since it was first noticed?

Intravenous access

Vascular access is required in most emergency and critically ill patients, and the placement of intravenous catheters (see Chapter 25) is a key skill for nurses working in emergency and critical care to master. Intravenous access is required for the administration of fluid and drug therapy and can provide a means of atraumatic serial blood sampling. Vascular access should be obtained early in the management of many emergency patients and sometimes before the secondary survey is complete.

In dogs and cats, the most common vein used is the cephalic vein; patients can generally be restrained in sternal recumbency during placement and the vein is easily identified with practice. If the cephalic vein cannot be used (e.g. injuries to both forelimbs), the saphenous vein is a useful alternative. In very collapsed or very small patients, the peripheral veins may be difficult to identify. In this situation, options include placement of a catheter directly into the jugular vein or placement of an intraosseous catheter into the bone marrow. Intraosseous access is usually obtained via the femur, although the tibia, humerus and ilium may all be used.

In rabbits, the ear vein is the most easily catheterized vessel, although the cephalic vein can be used. Obtaining vascular access in smaller mammals is challenging, and jugular or intraosseous access is usually required.

In avian emergencies, options for venous access include the right jugular vein (larger than the left in all avian species), the ulnar vein running on the ventral aspect of the wing or the medial metatarsal vein. Intraosseous access can also be used in avian species, although bones that contain air sacs must be avoided. Suitable bones include the distal ulna and proximal tibiotarsus.

Regardless of the site used, the catheter chosen should be the largest that will fit into the vessel; this facilitates rapid fluid administration and reduces the risk of thrombophlebitis. Aseptic technique should always be used during catheter placement, and the catheter should be carefully secured immediately following placement.

General nursing care

The stabilization of life-threatening medical conditions must take priority but, having addressed these, the patient's general physical comfort and level of psychological stress should be considered (see Chapter 14).

Mental welfare

Many emergency patients are distressed, in pain or confused. Being in the unfamiliar environment of the veterinary practice surrounded by strangers can serve to make this worse.

- Be kind and gentle with the patient. Talk softly and use the patient's name as much as possible.
- Be aware if the patient has any physical disabilities, such as being blind, deaf or recumbent, that may make the situation more unsettling.
- Always approach the patient slowly and perform any procedures with the minimum handling necessary. Some patients may benefit from a period in a kennel or basket without being handled whilst they become accustomed to the environment.
- Emergency patients should *never* be covered from view.
- Be aware that some patients (especially prey species, e.g. rabbits) may find the presence of other animals stressful; organize kennelling to reduce this if possible.

Physical comfort

The patient should be given a warm and comfortable bed. If the patient is recumbent, it should be turned regularly and at least every 4 hours. Environmental temperature should allow maintenance of a normal body temperature. Hypothermia is a common problem in small critically ill patients (cats and other small mammals).

If the patient is able to stand and walk, then it should be allowed to do this. Critically ill patients should not walk long distances, but the benefit of standing and walking around the room should not be underestimated, especially in older patients who may have concurrent chronic orthopaedic disease (e.g. arthritis). Patients that are able to walk outside will benefit from the fresh air and sunshine.

Toileting needs

The necessity for the patient to urinate and defecate should be considered. Although it may not be possible or advisable for critically sick dogs to be walked outside, they should be allowed to leave their kennel regularly for toileting purposes. If they are recumbent, a urinary catheter should be considered.

If a patient soils itself or its bedding, it should be cleaned immediately. In patients with diarrhoea, clipping the perineal and caudal thigh region should be considered and a barrier cream applied. A tail bandage may be beneficial, and should be replaced regularly. Cats should be provided with a litter tray, containing a familiar type of litter if possible.

Dressings, catheter sites and tube sites

All dressings and catheter or tube insertion sites should be checked regularly. Any dressings that become soiled or displaced should be changed as soon as possible. All catheter sites should be unwrapped and checked at least once daily, and more frequently if the site appears to cause discomfort. Other tubes (e.g. oesophagostomy tubes, gastrostomy tubes) should be checked and rewrapped on the advice of the veterinary surgeon.

A record should be made each time dressings are replaced; the necessity for frequent dressing changes, especially if this represents an increase on previous needs, may indicate a problem, e.g. local infection.

Oral food and water

The decision to offer food and water should be made by the veterinary surgeon and is dependent on the underlying disease process. The nurse should be proactive in ascertaining when food and water can be offered.

If food can be offered, small amounts of fresh food should be placed in the patient's kennel. If the patient does not want to eat, the food should be removed after 1 hour and more fresh food offered at a later time. The presence of stale food in the patient's kennel may act as an adverse stimulus and decrease the patient's appetite. Some patients may have trouble moving to their water or food bowl and may benefit from hand-feeding.

Monitoring

The nurse is responsible for monitoring the patient. Although many advanced monitoring techniques are now available in veterinary practice, the most important monitoring tool is the serial clinical examination.

The following parameters should be recorded at regular intervals (up to every 15 minutes in unstable patients; every 6–8 hours in stable patients).

Regular monitoring

- Pulse rate.
- Pulse quality.
- Mucous membrane colour.
- Capillary refill time.
- Respiratory rate.
- Respiratory effort.
- Temperature.
- Demeanour.
- Bodyweight (every 12 hours).

Other monitoring techniques that can be considered include:

- Urine output
- Urine specific gravity
- Blood pressure
- Pulse oximetry
- ECG
- Central venous pressure
- Serial electrolyte and blood gas parameters.

It is vital that any parameter monitored is recorded accurately. Successful management of emergency patients often involves several members of staff and it is essential that the patient's status is communicated accurately between staff members. Emergency patients often require a great deal of effort but can be some of the most rewarding patients to nurse.

Cardiopulmonary arrest, resuscitation and death

Early recognition of cardiopulmonary arrest or impending cardiopulmonary arrest is vital.

Signs of impending or actual cardiac arrest

- Agonal (gasping) breathing pattern *or* absence of useful respiratory movements.
- Absence of a heartbeat and pulse, *or* weak and rapid pulses that will usually slow rapidly and dramatically shortly prior to arrest.
- Loss of consciousness.
- Fixed dilated pupils and lack of a palpebral and corneal reflex.

Patients that have suffered cardiopulmonary arrest shortly before arrival at the practice will be identified during the primary survey and resuscitation attempts should be started immediately. The longer the time from arrest to return of spontaneous circulation, the worse the prognosis is likely to be. If in doubt, resuscitation procedures should always be started. It may be necessary to do this before the veterinary surgeon arrives and before speaking to the owner.

Mucous membrane colour and capillary refill time may remain normal for a brief period after cessation of effective circulation. If the patient is being monitored by an ECG, this may also remain relatively normal for several minutes after cessation of cardiac contractions.

Cardiopulmonary–cerebral resuscitation

Cardiopulmonary–cerebral resuscitation (**CPCR**) is the provision of artificial support of ventilation and circulation (**basic life support**) until spontaneous circulation and breathing are restored and sustained. Basic life support (see below) is based around the familiar 'ABC' mnemonic (Airway, Breathing, Circulation).

Advanced life support (see below) refers to the administration of drugs or other treatments to restart and maintain spontaneous circulation.

Cardiopulmonary–cerebral resuscitation procedure

All members of staff should be trained in basic CPCR, including student veterinary nurses, animal nursing assistants and receptionists. They can all be trained to carry out one or more tasks. Successful CPCR requires a team approach. Planning and practice is the key. The minimum number of people required for CPCR is three, but more (four to six) is ideal.

Following recognition that a patient has undergone cardiopulmonary arrest, the following tasks should be carried out as quickly and smoothly as possible:

- Placement and securing (tying in) of an endotracheal tube
- Provision of oxygen and ventilation
- Provision of external cardiac compressions
- Placement and securing of an intravenous catheter
- Placement of an ECG to assist the veterinary surgeon in making decisions on appropriate medication.

These tasks are usually carried out in the order listed above, but this may change depending both on the patient and the number and experience of staff present. The patient is typically placed in right lateral recumbency.

It is vital that a person is nominated to 'run the crash' as soon as possible. This person would usually be a veterinary surgeon but an experienced nurse may need to fulfil this role until a veterinary surgeon arrives. It is this person's responsibility to direct the other members of the team and ensure all tasks are being carried out.

Depending on the number and training of staff present, the following roles are usually assigned:

- One person to provide adequate ventilation
- One person to undertake chest compressions
- One person to monitor the patient, including palpating for the presence of pulses
- One person to draw up drugs as requested and record all medications given, as well as any other interventions.

All practices should have regular CPCR training sessions where all can practise their responsibilities. Various veterinary CPCR models are available but even stuffed toys of various sizes can be used to represent patients. Different scenarios should be considered. After the practice session, or after a real CPCR, there should be a review and evaluation to encourage and facilitate ongoing improvements.

Basic life support

Airway

An airway is best provided by an endotracheal tube that is tied securely in place. On rare occasions an animal will have undergone cardiopulmonary arrest because of an obstructed airway. If airway obstruction is suspected, a variety of endotracheal tubes should be available, including some much smaller than would normally be chosen for the size of patient. A stiff male dog urinary catheter is also useful as it can be placed through the larynx and passed beyond the obstruction. It can then be used to deliver oxygen while the obstruction is addressed.

Very rarely, an endotracheal tube cannot be placed and an emergency tracheotomy must be carried out. The patient should be rolled into dorsal recumbency with hyperextension of the neck. An area over the trachea in the mid-cervical region is rapidly clipped and a brief surgical preparation is performed. The veterinary surgeon will rapidly make an incision through the subcutaneous tissues of the neck and then between the tracheal rings. Ideally, a specially designed tracheostomy tube (see Chapter 25) is placed through the tracheal incision into the airway, but if this is not available a standard endotracheal tube can be used.

Breathing

Ventilation is usually provided by connecting the endotracheal tube to an anaesthetic circuit (preferably a Bain) or an Ambu bag (Figure 21.7). The respiration rate should be 6–12 breaths per minute. The volume of air per breath should be judged so that the chest wall can be seen to rise only a small amount. In an arrest situation it is very easy either to ventilate too quickly or to overinflate on each breath. This has the potential to damage the lungs by causing barotrauma and so caution must be exercised.

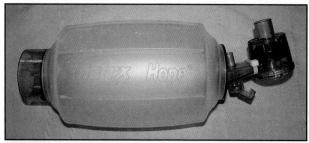

21.7 Ambu bag, designed to be attached to an endotracheal tube and used to ventilate patients.

Circulation

Circulation is maintained by chest compressions. In dogs and cats, effective chest compression is best accomplished with the animal in right lateral recumbency. In cats and small dogs, pressure should be applied using the heel of the hand directly over the heart (rib spaces 4 to 6). In cats and other small mammals it may be most effective to hold the thorax within the hand so pressure can be applied directly across the heart. In larger dogs, pressure should be applied, again using the heel of the hand, at the highest point on the thoracic wall (Figure 21.8). Chest compressions should be given at a rate of approximately 100 per minute, with an equal time for compression and relaxation. If chest compressions are successful, a palpable femoral pulse is generated.

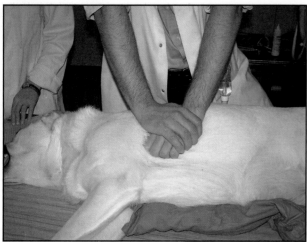

21.8   Position for administering external cardiac compression to a large dog.

Abdominal counter-pressure

If there are a large number of people (more than four) present for CPCR, it may be helpful for someone to perform abdominal counter-pressure. This involves pressing down firmly on the abdomen between chest compressions. It acts to increase venous return to the chest and improves blood pressure and cerebral and myocardial perfusion.

Advanced life support

Once ECG monitoring has started, the veterinary surgeon may wish to administer drugs to return the heart to a normal rhythm. Although a veterinary nurse does not need to understand fully the mechanism of action of each drug, having an understanding of which drug is appropriate and why can make both the veterinary nurse's and the veterinary surgeon's job quicker and easier. An experienced nurse can start to prepare drugs that are likely to be necessary, so that they can be administered as soon as they are requested.

The three common cardiac arrest rhythms in dogs and cats (Figure 21.9) are:

- Pulseless electrical activity (PEA)
- Asystole
- Ventricular fibrillation.

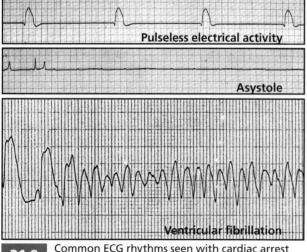

21.9   Common ECG rhythms seen with cardiac arrest in dogs and cats. (Courtesy of V Luis Fuentes)

The three drugs used most commonly during resuscitation are:

- **Adrenaline** (epinephrine), a peripheral vasoconstrictor that acts to increase blood flow to the heart and brain. It is used in asystole and PEA
- **Atropine,** an anticholinergic drug used to reduce vagal tone. It is used to control severe bradycardia, which may lead to asystole or PEA
- **Lidocaine**, an antiarrhythmic drug. It is used for the treatment of ventricular arrhythmias such as fast ventricular tachycardia. It may be used as a chemical defibrillator but is rarely successful in this situation.

Electrical defibrillation

Electrical defibrillation is occasionally used to shock the heart from chaotic non-pulse-producing electrical activity (commonly ventricular fibrillation) to normal sinus rhythm. A large electrical charge is passed through the heart, with the aim of causing the cardiac cells to depolarize and then repolarize synchronously.

Defibrillation is only useful in cases where arrest has been caused by ventricular fibrillation or rapid ventricular tachycardia. The most common arrhythmia in human cardiopulmonary arrest is ventricular fibrillation and this is why defibrillators are so readily available and commonly used in human medicine. It is, however, a rare cause of arrest in dogs and cats. The earlier a heart is defibrillated, the better chance the patient will have of survival. The energy necessary for external defibrillation is approximately 5 joules/kg. Excessive energy levels and repeated defibrillation can cause myocardial damage; therefore it is advisable to start at the lower energy levels and increase as needed.

Extreme caution must be exercised whenever a defibrillator is being used. One person who is trained to operate the machine should be in charge and should instruct all other personnel to 'Clear!' before discharging the defibrillator. To prevent risk of serious injury, all personnel must be clear of the patient *and* the table on which the patient is lying before the defibrillator is discharged. Defibrillators should never be used by untrained personnel. Alcohol-based solvents should never be used in the proximity of the defibrillator.

Collapse and unconsciousness

Many emergency patients will present because of collapse. The term collapse is used when an animal is unable or unwilling to stand and walk but remains aware of its surroundings. During the initial major body systems assessment, it should be ascertained whether an animal is:

- An **alert** collapsed animal with normal mentation
- A **depressed** collapsed animal that is quiet but will respond to stimuli such as calling its name or clapping hands behind its head
- An **obtunded** collapsed animal with a decreased level of consciousness that will only respond to painful stimuli such as squeezing hard on its toes or touching a painful area

- An **unconscious** (comatose) collapsed animal that does not respond to stimuli but has a palpable pulse and heart rate.

If the animal does not respond to stimuli and has no heart beat on thoracic auscultation, then it is considered to be dead. However, if it is still making breathing movements, death may only just have occurred and resuscitation efforts should be started.

In an unconscious collapsed patient the airway may become blocked or narrowed due to the position of the neck and the tongue. The patient's muscles will tend to relax and can occlude the pharyngeal region, especially in breeds with a large amount of soft tissue in this area, such as Bulldogs. If this occurs, it can lead to respiratory and then cardiac arrest. It is vital that the airway is clear and open to allow adequate ventilation and oxygen delivery to the lungs.

Unconscious patients should be placed in lateral recumbency with their heads tilted dorsally (up), their mouths held gently open and the tongue gently pulled out. The airway should be examined to ensure that it is clear, but caution should be exercised and the safety of veterinary personnel must not be compromised.

There are many potential causes of collapse. The most common groups are summarized in Figure 21.10.

Presentation	Possible causes of collapse
Alert collapsed animal	Orthopaedic disease Peripheral neurological disease
Depressed collapsed animal	Mild to moderate shock Pain
Obtunded collapsed animal	Moderate to severe shock Neurological disease Metabolic disease
Unconscious collapsed animal with very fast or slow heart rate	Severe shock – cardiopulmonary arrest imminent
Unconscious collapsed animal with normal heart rate	Neurological disease Metabolic disease (e.g. hypoglycaemia)

21.10 Groups of differential diagnoses to be considered in a collapsed animal.

Shock

Shock is defined as a state of acute circulatory collapse where the circulation is unable to transport sufficient oxygen to meet the tissues' needs. The consequences of untreated shock are severe, as a lack of oxygen supply to the tissues will have significant effects on all organs, especially the brain, heart and kidneys. If the state of shock is prolonged, it may lead to organ failure and death.

The lack of tissue oxygen supply may be secondary to a number of circulatory system problems. Four major types of shock are recognized and are described in Figure 21.11. The distinction between the types of shock is important, as the treatment strategy varies. In most situations, the different types of shock can be distinguished by a careful and thorough physical examination focusing on the cardiovascular system and, most importantly, the perfusion parameters (heart rate, pulse quality, mucous membrane colour and capillary refill time).

Type of shock	Description	Common causes
Hypovolaemic	Decreased circulating blood volume	Haemorrhage Severe vomiting and diarrhoea Third spacing (loss of fluid into body cavities, e.g. abdomen)
Distributive (includes anaphylactic, toxic and septic shock)	Abnormal distribution of body fluids secondary to body-wide dilation of all blood vessels	Sepsis Systemic inflammatory response syndrome (e.g. severe pancreatitis) Severe allergic reaction
Cardiogenic	Failure of the heart to act as an effective pump	Dilated cardiomyopathy Severe arrhythmias
Obstructive	Physical obstruction to blood flow within the vascular system	Pulmonary thromboembolism Pericardial effusion

21.11 Different forms of shock.

Types of shock
Hypovolaemic shock

Hypovolaemic shock is the most common form of shock seen in veterinary patients. It occurs secondary to significant loss of circulating fluid volume that may happen following haemorrhage or rapid fluid loss through other sites, such as the gastrointestinal tract, urinary system or into third spaces, e.g. peritoneal cavity.

Physical examination findings of severe hypovolaemic shock

- Tachycardia (up to 220 beats per minute (bpm) in dogs and 250 bpm in cats).
- Prolonged capillary refill time.
- Pale mucous membranes
- Poor pulse quality.
- Low blood pressure.

Fluid replacement

As hypovolaemic shock occurs due to reduced circulating blood volume, treatment revolves around replacing the fluid deficit. The fluid used to restore the deficit is dependent on the type of fluid loss (e.g. haemorrhage, vomiting, diarrhoea). The commonest fluids used are isotonic replacement crystalloid fluids, such as Hartmann's solution, but occasionally it is necessary to use colloids or whole blood.

When treating shock, the fluid is given intravenously (or, rarely, via the intraosseous route). Initially the fluid is given at a fast rate over a relatively short period. The dose (or bolus) of fluid used varies, with a full shock dose of crystalloid being 60–90 ml/kg bodyweight in the dog and 40–60 ml/kg in the cat. As cats are susceptible to volume overload, it is recommended that this is given in 10–20 ml/kg increments. Depending on the severity of the shock, this dose may be given over a period as short as 30 minutes (see Chapter 22). The principles of treating hypovolaemic shock with a large fluid bolus delivered over a short time frame should also be used when treating small mammals and exotic species.

Arrest of haemorrhage

Haemorrhage is one possible cause of hypovolaemic shock. The haemorrhage may be external or internal. When dealing with very small patients, it should be remembered that shock can result from only small blood losses; for example, a budgerigar can show signs of shock with the loss of only 20 drops of blood. If there is an obvious site of haemorrhage, efforts should be made to arrest it. However, external haemorrhage is a rare cause of severe hypovolaemic shock in dogs and cats.

Methods of arresting haemorrhage

- **Direct digital pressure** – ensure that gloves are worn and apply pressure for at least 5 minutes.
- **Artery forceps** (haemostats) – if a bleeding vessel can be seen it may be possible to clamp it directly with artery forceps.
- **Pressure dressing** – apply direct pressure over the bleeding area using an absorbent pad and cohesive bandage. If blood seeps through, reapply another layer. Do not remove the initial layer as a clot may be dislodged. If a pressure dressing is used on a limb, the toes should be monitored carefully for both swelling and colour; if the toes become markedly swollen or lose their pink colour the pressure being applied should be carefully reduced.

Haemorrhage into the peritoneal cavity is a common cause of hypovolaemic shock in dogs. If this is suspected, the veterinary surgeon may suggest placement of an abdominal pressure (belly) wrap (Figure 21.12). The aim is to increase pressure within the abdominal cavity to promote the formation of a clot at the site of bleeding. As this increase in pressure can lead to decreases in blood flow to intra-abdominal organs, the wrap should only be left in place for relatively short periods of time and certainly no longer than 12 hours.

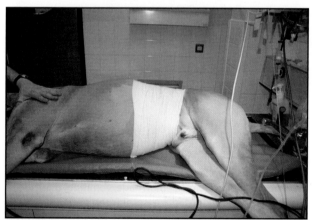

21.12   Abdominal pressure wrap for a patient with haemoabdomen. (Courtesy of D Hughes)

Distributive shock

This type of shock occurs when the body suffers an insult (often severe infection or inflammation) that causes the generalized release of inflammatory mediators (cytokines) that promote peripheral vasodilation. The body can no longer properly control where the blood volume is distributed. The peripheral tissues may have an increased blood supply to the detriment of the more important internal organs. Anaphylactic, toxic and septic are all forms of distributive shock.

Physical examination findings of distributive shock

- Tachycardia.
- Poor pulse quality.
- *Red* mucous membranes.
- Capillary refill time initially rapid, progressing to slow.

As the body is unable to constrict its blood vessels normally, the mucous membranes appear abnormally red. It is the presence of these inappropriately red mucous membranes that should alert the nurse to the presence of distributive shock.

The successful treatment of distributive shock involves rapidly identifying and treating the underlying cause. This may involve medical therapy (e.g. anaphylactic shock, pneumonia) or surgical therapy (e.g. ruptured pyometra). Fluid therapy is important but complications of fluid therapy (development of oedema or effusions) are more common in these patients, as they frequently have inflamed and leaky blood vessels. Peripheral oedema is common if a large volume of crystalloid fluid is used.

In anaphylactic shock (e.g. insect stings) the patient can be treated with adrenaline, corticosteroids, antihistamines and fluid therapy if seen soon after exposure to the allergen.

Cardiogenic shock

This is seen in conditions where the heart can no longer pump effectively. It is most commonly seen in degenerative conditions of the heart muscle, such as dilated cardiomyopathy, or in severe arrhythmias. The findings on physical examination depend on the nature of the heart disease but may include heart murmurs, irregular pulses (especially if pulse deficits are present) and either very fast (>240 bpm) or very slow heart rates. Treatment depends on the underlying heart disease and is covered in the cardiovascular emergencies section. Fluid therapy is generally contraindicated in this form of shock.

Obstructive shock

This is the rarest form of shock in veterinary medicine. It may be seen in pericardial effusion and pulmonary thromboembolism. These conditions are covered under the cardiovascular and respiratory emergencies sections, respectively.

General treatments for shock

Patients with shock are likely to benefit from oxygen supplementation and being hospitalized in a comfortable stress-free environment. They may have a reduced body temperature and should be rewarmed slowly, but only after fluid therapy has started. Patients with shock require careful and close monitoring, especially in the first few hours after presentation.

Other markers of shock
Blood pressure

A drop in blood pressure is a late change in shock, as the body has a number of mechanisms to maintain blood pressure. A mean arterial blood pressure of <60 mmHg is of serious concern, as there may be damage to vital organs such as the brain, heart and kidneys.

Urine output

When monitoring a patient in shock, measurement of urine output (in ml per kg bodyweight per hour) is useful as it is a non-invasive method of evaluating blood supply (perfusion) to the kidneys. If the animal is producing plenty of urine (>2 ml/kg/h) the kidneys are likely to be well perfused. Normal urine production is 1–2 ml/kg/h. Serial measurements of urine output are a useful and cheap monitoring tool that can be used in most practice situations.

Lactate

Lactate is generated secondary to anaerobic respiration in the tissues and is the best objective marker of shock. Until recently it could not easily be measured in veterinary patients but there are now several machines available to veterinary practices allowing in-house measurement of lactate. Normal lactate values are <2.5 mmol/l and values >6 mmol/l imply severe shock. Lactate values should return rapidly to normal if the shock is treated successfully.

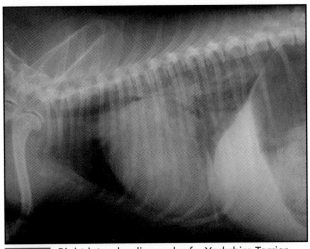

21.13   Right lateral radiograph of a Yorkshire Terrier with congestive heart failure. Note the enlarged cardiac silhouette and the increased opacity in the perihilar and caudal lung fields.

Cardiovascular emergencies

Many emergency patients present with cardiovascular system abnormalities on examination (e.g. tachycardia, poor pulse quality). In many cases these abnormalities represent the cardiovascular response to shock and are not indicative of primary cardiovascular system disease. This section focuses on those emergencies that are primarily cardiovascular in nature.

Acute congestive heart failure (CHF)

CHF may occur secondary to a number of heart conditions. The most common are:

- Chronic mitral valve disease in small-breed dogs
- Dilated cardiomyopathy (weakness of the heart muscle) in large-breed dogs and older rabbits
- Hypertrophic cardiomyopathy (thickening and stiffening of the heart muscle) in cats.

CHF is usually seen in older patients but can occur in younger animals. Whatever the underlying cause, the clinical signs and emergency stabilization procedures are the same.

Clinical signs

- Cough, especially at night.
- Dyspnoea/tachypnoea.
- Reluctance to exercise.
- Tachycardia.
- Poor pulse quality.
- Pale mucous membranes.
- Cyanosis.
- Heart murmur or gallop rhythm on cardiac auscultation.

Diagnostic aids

If the patient is stable:

- Thoracic radiography (Figure 21.13)
- ECG
- Echocardiography (ultrasonography of the heart).

Treatment

- Do not stress.
- Oxygen therapy.
- Medical intervention, including:
  - Thoracocentesis if pleural effusion (commoner in cats)
  - Loop diuretic, e.g. furosemide intravenously or intramuscularly
  - Glyceryl trinitrate paste has been used topically (on skin in ear or groin) in these patients. Use non-latex gloves to apply.
- Once stabilized, medical therapy including ACE (angiotensin-converting enzyme) inhibitors, diuretics, pimobendan, digoxin, calcium-channel blockers may be used depending on the nature of the underlying disease.

Pericardial effusion

This condition is principally seen in older large-breed dogs where the pericardial sac becomes full of fluid. This puts pressure on the heart so that it cannot fill properly and leads to signs of right-sided congestive heart failure.

Clinical signs

- Exercise intolerance.
- Dyspnoea/tachypnoea
- Ascites (fluid in the abdomen).
- Muffled heart sounds on cardiac auscultation.
- Tachycardia.
- Poor pulse quality.

Diagnostic aids

- Echocardiography (ultrasonography of the heart).
- Thoracic radiography.
- ECG – electrical alternans (height of QRS complex alters from beat to beat) due to fluid in the pericardial sac.

Treatment

- Pericardiocentesis (a needle is used to drain the fluid from the pericardial sac) (Figure 21.14).

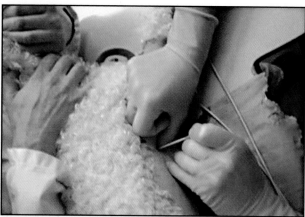

21.14 Placement of a large-bore intravenous catheter into the pericardial sac during pericardiocentesis in a Bichon Frise. Note the ECG leads running to the patient's feet, allowing essential monitoring of the patient.

- Placement of intravenous catheter in case emergency treatment with lidocaine is necessary due to arrhythmias during pericardiocentesis.
- In recurrent cases, surgery to remove the pericardial sac may be necessary.
- Medical therapy is not effective.

Aortic thromboembolism

This is a relatively common condition in cats but a rare condition in dogs. A thrombus (clot) blocks the aorta, disrupting blood flow to the hindlimbs. In cats it usually occurs secondary to underlying heart disease, whereas in dogs it usually occurs secondary to abnormal blood clotting. Rarely, thrombi can occur at other sites.

Clinical signs

- Unilateral or bilateral paresis or paralysis of the hindlimb(s); forelimbs can be affected, but much less commonly.
- Cold hindlimb(s) with non-palpable pulse(s).
- Extreme pain (vocalizing) – less common in dogs.
- In the cat, dyspnoea or tachypnoea (signs of underlying cardiomyopathy).
- History of heart disease.

Diagnostic aids

Diagnosis is usually based on a physical examination; supportive tests may be useful, especially in dogs, where an underlying medical disease is often the precipitating factor:

- Haematology and biochemistry
- Urinalysis
- Abdominal ultrasonography
- Echocardiography
- Thoracic radiography
- Blood pressure
- Endocrine testing.

Treatment

- Prognosis poor.
- Oxygen therapy.

- Analgesia.
- Environmental comfort.
- Treatment of underlying disease.
- Thrombolytic drugs – for example tissue plasminogen activator. There is limited experience of their use in veterinary medicine. They are very expensive and associated with a number of side effects. If used, they are likely to be more effective within hours of the clot first forming.
- Antithrombotic drugs (e.g. aspirin, heparin) – these may help to reduce the risk of further clots forming but will not break down clots that are already present.

Arrhythmia – tachycardia

Animals present with an abnormal heart rhythm that is so fast that the heart does not have time to fill properly with blood between beats. This is a rare emergency but needs to be identified quickly or heart failure can follow.

Clinical signs

- Collapse or syncope.
- Exercise intolerance.
- Severe tachycardia (>240 bpm).
- Poor or intermittent pulses.

Diagnostic aids

- ECG (Figure 21.15).

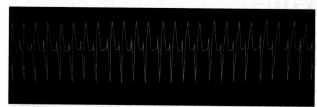

21.15 Ventricular tachycardia in a German Shepherd Dog that presented with gastric dilatation–volvulus.

Treatment

- Medical therapy with antiarrhythmic drugs.
- Therapy is challenging as the drugs used have side effects, including the potential to worsen the arrhythmia.

Arrhythmia – bradycardia

Animals present with an abnormally slow heart rate, leading to collapse. This is rare. Medical causes such as hyperkalaemia should be ruled out at an early stage.

Clinical signs

- Collapse or syncope.
- Exercise intolerance.
- Marked bradycardia (usually <60 bpm).

Diagnostic aids

- ECG (Figure 21.16).
- Serum potassium level.
- Other medical tests dependent on potassium level.

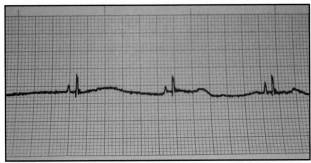

21.16 Sinus bradycardia in a Miniature Poodle that presented with severe head trauma and raised intracranial pressure.

Treatment

- If serum potassium level high, this should be treated urgently (see 'Metabolic emergencies').
- Cage rest.
- Medical therapy unlikely to be effective unless patient is hyperkalaemic.
- Pacemaker implantation may be necessary.

Respiratory emergencies

Respiratory emergencies are very common and can be challenging to treat successfully. Several treatment strategies can be used irrespective of the cause of the dyspnoea, notably:

- Oxygen therapy
- Stress-free cool (but not cold) environment
- Maintain in sternal recumbency.

Upper airway disease

Upper airway problems generally present as dyspnoea associated with an audible noise (stridor or stertor). The emergency treatment of upper airway disease involves oxygen therapy and calming and cooling the patient. If the patient is in severe distress, it may be necessary to bypass the upper airway temporarily by anaesthetizing and intubating the patient. Emergency tracheotomies need to be performed rarely.

Common causes of upper airway dyspnoea are discussed in more detail below. Rarer causes include laryngeal masses, severe trauma to the upper airway and airway foreign bodies.

Laryngeal paralysis

This is a common cause of dyspnoea in older large-breed dogs. The muscles that hold the larynx open during inspiration become paralysed and the larynx collapses as the dog tries to breathe in.

Clinical signs

- Marked dyspnoea, often with paradoxical abdominal movement.
- Stridor (audible whistling noise) on inspiration.

- Exercise intolerance.
- History of change in bark.
- Cyanosis.
- Hyperthermia.

Diagnostic aids

The diagnosis is often suspected on the basis of the history and physical examination.

- Laryngoscopy under a light plane of anaesthesia is confirmatory.

Treatment

- Oxygen therapy.
- Sedation (commonly low doses of acepromazine) to reduce stress and inspiratory effort.
- Cooling.
- If severe, the patient may need to be anaesthetized and intubated. The patient can then be cooled and allowed to recover slowly from the anaesthetic. Rarely, a tracheostomy needs to be performed.
- Long-term treatment requires surgery (usually a 'tie-back' procedure) but this is not commonly done on an emergency basis.

Brachycephalic obstructive airway syndrome (BOAS)

This is a common disease in brachycephalic breeds such as Bulldogs and Pugs. It can be seen in brachycephalic cats such as Persians, but is less severe in this species. The dyspnoea is caused by airway obstruction secondary to the abnormal anatomy of these breeds. It is considered to include several components:

- Stenotic nares
- Long soft palate
- Everted laryngeal saccules
- Hypoplastic (narrow) trachea.

Clinical signs

- Dyspnoea.
- Exercise intolerance.
- Stertorous (snoring) breathing sounds.
- Collapse/syncope.
- Cyanosis.

Diagnostic aids

Diagnosis is usually made on the basis of compatible clinical signs, breed and physical examination. Anaesthesia and examination of the upper airway confirms the diagnosis.

Treatment

- Oxygen therapy.
- Sedation (commonly acepromazine).
- Cooling.
- If severe, the patient may need to be anaesthetized and intubated. The patient can then be cooled and allowed to recover slowly from the anaesthetic. Rarely, a tracheostomy needs to be performed.
- If severe, surgery may be needed to correct the anatomical abnormality, but this surgery is not commonly done on an emergency basis.

Tracheal collapse

This condition typically occurs in small-breed dogs where the cartilaginous tracheal rings are abnormal or degenerate and the trachea collapses as the animal breathes in and out.

Clinical signs

- Cough (goose-honk) and dyspnoea commonly occur with stress or excitement.
- Cyanosis.
- Collapse/syncope.

Diagnostic aids

Diagnosis is usually made on history, clinical signs and examination. Thoracic radiography and/or tracheal endoscopy may be used to confirm the diagnosis.

Treatment

- Oxygen therapy.
- Stress-free environment and strict rest.
- Sedation if necessary.
- If severe, the patient may need to be anaesthetized and intubated. This should be avoided if possible as the endotracheal tube will cause further irritation to the trachea and the patient may be worse following an anaesthetic.
- Long-term medical management includes weight loss and drug therapy but is rarely curative.
- Invasive treatment options are available (e.g. placement of a tracheal stent, surgery) but these have a variable success rate and are only available at specialist institutions.

Pleural space disease

Animals with dyspnoea secondary to pleural space disease commonly present with short shallow respiration and dull lung sounds on thoracic auscultation.

Pleural effusion

This occurs when fluid accumulates in the pleural space. There are a number of types of fluid but the emergency treatment is the same.

Types of fluid

- **Transudate** – secondary to severe hypoalbuminaemia (low blood protein).
- **Modified transudate** – secondary to heart failure.
- **Neoplastic exudate** – secondary to neoplasia within the chest, commonly lymphoma in cats.
- **Pyothorax** – infected purulent fluid in the chest.
- **Haemothorax** – blood in the chest secondary to trauma or a clotting disorder.
- **Chylothorax** – a milky fluid that builds up due to problems with lymphatic drainage in the chest or rupture of the thoracic duct.

Clinical signs

- Dyspnoea and tachypnoea.
- Dull lung sounds on auscultation.
- Inappetence.
- Weight loss.

Diagnostic aids

- Thoracocentesis – this is therapeutic as well as diagnostic. The fluid obtained should be analysed.
- Thoracic radiography.
- In dyspnoeic patients, radiographs should not be taken until after thoracocentesis has been performed.
- In non-traumatic cases, advanced imaging (computed tomography, CT) may be useful.
- Thoracic ultrasonography.

Treatment

- Oxygen therapy.
- Thoracocentesis.
- Treatment of the underlying cause – this may be medical or surgical.
- Occasionally it is necessary to place thoracostomy (chest) tubes to allow frequent drainage.

Pneumothorax

This occurs when air accumulates in the pleural space. Causes include:

- Trauma – most common cause
- Inhaled foreign body
- Idiopathic (especially in large-breed dogs)
- External penetrating wound (open pneumothorax).

Clinical signs

- Dyspnoea with short shallow respirations.
- Dull lung sounds on auscultation.
- External wound (open pneumothorax).
- Cyanosis.

Diagnostic aids

- Oxygen therapy.
- Thoracocentesis – this is therapeutic as well as diagnostic.
- Thoracic radiography.
- In non-traumatic cases, advanced imaging (computed tomography, CT) may be useful.

Treatment

- Thoracocentesis – in most cases of traumatic pneumothorax, thoracocentesis is the only treatment required as the leak will heal itself.
- In non-traumatic cases, surgical exploration of the chest may be necessary.
- Thoracostomy tubes may need to be placed if large volumes of air produced quickly.
- Open pneumothorax requires surgical treatment; a sterile adherent dressing should be placed over the wound until the patient is stable for surgery.

Feline asthma

This is the only lower airway disease of importance in veterinary emergency patients.

Clinical signs

- Dyspnoea principally on expiration.
- Wheezes on auscultation.
- Abdominal effort on expiration.

Diagnostic aids

- Physical examination.
- Thoracic radiography.
- Cytology on wash samples taken from the airways.

Treatment

- Oxygen therapy.
- Medical treatment:
  - Corticosteroids
  - Bronchodilators
  - Inhaled medications (Figure 21.17).

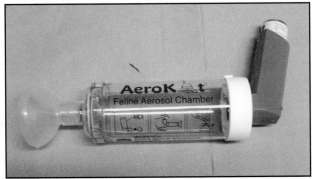

21.17 An inhaler used for administration of inhaled medications.

Parenchymal disease

Parenchymal disease develops when the alveoli become filled with either fluid or tissue.
Common causes include:

- Heart failure (pulmonary oedema)
- Pneumonia (bacterial or parasitic) (Figure 21.18)
- Neoplasia
- Non-cardiogenic oedema (e.g. secondary to head trauma, airway obstructions, severe systemic illness)
- Pulmonary contusions (bleeding into lung following trauma)
- Pulmonary thromboembolism.

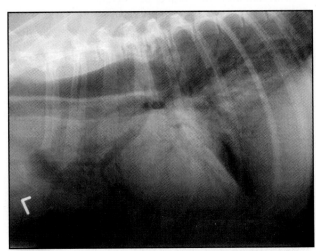

21.18 Left lateral thoracic radiograph of a dog with megaoesophagus and aspiration pneumonia. Note the branching air bronchogram in the cranial lung field.

Clinical signs

- Dyspnoea.
- Cyanosis.
- Crackles on auscultation of the lungs.
- Inappetence.

Diagnostic aids

- Thoracic radiography.
- Haematology and biochemistry.
- Urinalysis.
- Bronchoscopy with airway washes in some patients.
- Echocardiography (heart ultrasonography).

Treatment

- Oxygen therapy.
- Medical treatment of the underlying disease may include:
  - Diuretics (e.g. furosemide)
  - Antibiotics
  - Anthelmintics.

Neurological emergencies

Head trauma

Head trauma is a common emergency in both dogs and cats. It can occur secondary to road traffic accidents, falling from a height or being attacked by other animals (bitten by a dog or cat, kicked by a large animal). Head trauma may or may not be associated with traumatic brain injury. Clinical signs are variable, depending on whether the brain has been damaged and, if so, which part.

Clinical signs

- Depression.*
- Anisocoria (variation in pupil size).*
- Nystagmus.*
- Strabismus.*
- Cranial nerve deficits.*
- Epistaxis.
- Bruising or swelling of face.
- Asymmetry of face or jaw.
- Inability to close mouth properly (mandibular or maxillary fractures).
- Ocular haemorrhage (scleral or within eye).
- Bradycardia.*
- Abnormal breathing pattern.*
- Seizures.*
- Coma.*
- Signs of trauma in other body areas (especially thorax or limb fractures).

(Those marked * indicate brain injury.)

Diagnostic aids

- Frequent neurological examination – these should be recorded using a standard system such as the modified Glasgow Coma Scale. This scale is an objective way of

recording the severity of neurological injury by assigning a point value (1–6) to the patient's level of consciousness, motor activity and brainstem reflexes. A low score indicates more severe injury.
- Haematology and biochemistry.
- Blood pressure.
- Skull radiographs.
- Advanced imaging techniques (CT, MRI).

Treatment

- Ensuring patent airway.
- Supplementing oxygen (take care that this does not cause stress).
- Intravenous fluid therapy to maintain blood pressure.
- Head elevated at 30 degrees to reduce intracranial pressure.
- Avoidance of any techniques that may increase intracranial pressure, such as jugular venepuncture
- Monitoring and maintaining body temperature.
- If recumbent, turning every 4 hours.
- Monitoring bladder size and catheterization or expression if necessary.
- Medical therapies to reduce intracranial pressure (e.g. hypertonic saline, mannitol).
- Analgesia.
- Treat concurrent injuries.
- Corticosteroids are now considered to be **contraindicated** in patients with head trauma.

Seizures

Seizures occur relatively commonly in dogs and rarely in cats. They represent an acute and usually brief disturbance of normal electrical activity in the brain and can be very distressing for both the patient and the owner. Most seizures are short (<2 minutes) and owners often only manage to telephone for veterinary advice once the seizure is over. As seizures can sometimes occur close together, it is always best to advise that the animal is examined by a veterinary surgeon as soon as practical even if the seizure has stopped. This is particularly important in very young (< 6 months old) and older animals where there is more likely to be a medical cause for the seizures.

Seizures are often described as having a **pre-ictal**, **ictal** and **post-ictal phase**. During the pre-ictal phase the animal may show mild behaviour changes, though these are not always recognized by owners. The ictal phase represents the seizure itself and the post-ictal phase a period after the seizure where the animal displays abnormal neurological signs.

Status epilepticus is a condition where seizures are prolonged (>5 minutes) or where there are multiple seizures in a short space of time (e.g. 30 minutes) and the animal does not recover completely between them. Animals with status epilepticus should be seen immediately, as prolonged or very frequent seizures may cause permanent brain damage.

Clinical signs

Ictal phase

- Loss of motor coordination with paddling of the limbs.
- Rigid collapse.
- Loss of consciousness.
- Hypersalivation and abnormal chewing movements.
- Defecation.

- Urination.
- Signs are usually generalized but, rarely, partial seizures are seen where the animal does not lose consciousness totally but becomes less aware, with focal twitching of the face or a single limb.

Post-ictal phase

- Confusion.
- Depression/listlessness.
- Ataxia.
- Visual disturbances, including blindness.

The post-ictal phase may last for several hours after a seizure episode.

Causes

- Idiopathic epilepsy.
- Brain tumour (neoplasia).
- Trauma.
- Infection.
- Inflammation.
- Toxin.
- Metabolic problems (hypoglycaemia, hepatic encephalopathy).

Diagnostic tests

- Blood glucose level (especially in young animals).
- Haematology and biochemistry.
- Full neurological examination.
- Cerebrospinal fluid (CSF) tap.
- Brain imaging (CT, MRI) if available.

Treatment

If the animal is having a seizure when it arrives at the practice, or starts to do so whilst hospitalized, medications should be given to control the seizure. Although most seizures are short, longer seizures (especially if lasting >5 minutes) can lead to further brain damage. Drugs used to treat seizures include:

- Diazepam (valium) – intravenous or per rectum
- Phenobarbital – intravenous or oral
- Potassium bromide – oral or per rectum.

The drug of choice for acute control of seizures is diazepam given by the intravenous route, but the rectal route can be used if intravenous access cannot be obtained. If diazepam does not work for the acute control of seizures, other intravenous drug therapy such as propofol infusions may need to be considered. Phenobarbital and potassium bromide are more commonly used as oral medications for the longer-term control of seizures.

If a seizuring animal develops respiratory distress or cyanosis, it is important to secure an airway. However, drugs (sedative or anaesthetic) must be given to allow this to happen safely. ***Never* put your hand in the mouth of a seizuring animal.**

Nursing care

- Monitor body temperature and cool if hyperthermic.
- Monitor heart rate and respiratory rate.
- Ensure patent intravenous access in case further seizures occur.
- Turn patient every 4 hours.

- Monitor bladder size and catheterize or express if necessary.
- Lubricate eyes.
- Maintain a calm environment. However, it is *not* necessary to maintain a dark room and this can in fact be detrimental, as it can compromise the ability to monitor the patient.

Spinal cord disease

Causes

- Intervertebral disc disease.
- Direct trauma (e.g. road traffic accident, inadequate restraint (rabbit)).
- Anatomical abnormalities (e.g. 'wobbler' dogs).
- Vascular disease (e.g. fibrocartilaginous emboli).
- Spinal cord haemorrhage.
- Spinal cord neoplasia.
- Infection.
- Degenerative spinal cord disease (e.g. degenerative myelopathy).

Clinical signs

These will be variable depending on the site and severity of the spinal cord injury. In general, cervical spinal cord disease has signs involving all four limbs, whereas thoracolumbar spinal cord disease has signs involving the hindlimbs only. It is very important to assess whether the animal can feel pain in each of its legs, which is usually done by squeezing firmly on one of the animal's toes. It should be remembered that the animal simply withdrawing its leg when the toe is squeezed is a local reflex arc and does not necessarily mean that the animal is aware and feeling the sensation. Signs that the animal can feel the sensation include vocalization, turning the head to look at the leg or pupillary dilation at the time the toe is squeezed. If deep pain sensation is lost, the animal's prognosis, in terms of the likelihood of it walking again, is much worse.

Clinical signs may include:

- Limb weakness (paresis) and proprioceptive deficits (mild disease)
- Ataxia (mild disease)
- Paralysis (severe disease)
- Recumbency/inability to walk (severe disease)
- Pain on palpation of spine
- Urinary incontinence
- Lack of anal tone
- Loss of deep pain sensation (severe disease)
- Change (either decrease or increase dependent on location of lesion) of the strength of the local reflexes (e.g. patellar reflex)
- Normal mentation and cranial nerve examination.

Rarely, severe thoracolumbar spinal cord disease will cause the Schiff–Sherrington phenomenon, where the forelimbs are rigid and the hindlimbs flaccid. This is most often seen following trauma and has a poor prognosis.

Treatment

- Analgesia.
- Cage rest.

- Monitoring bladder size and expression or catheterization if necessary.
- Maintaining warm and comfortable environment.
- Turning regularly (every 4 hours) if recumbent.
- Surgical treatment required for most causes of acute spinal cord disease.
- Use of corticosteroids (e.g. methylprednisolone, dexamethasone) is no longer recommended.
- Intravenous fluids only required if the animal shows concurrent signs of hypovolaemia or dehydration, or if the animal is not eating and drinking.

If a spinal fracture is suspected, great care must be taken when moving the patient. If possible, the animal should be strapped to something rigid during transport to the practice. A specially designed animal stretcher is ideal but other rigid objects may be used in an emergency.

Vestibular disease

The vestibular system controls balance and the animal's awareness of its body position in space. Vestibular disease may occur at the level of the inner ear, where the sense organs of balance are located (known as peripheral vestibular disease), or within the brain (known as central vestibular disease). Vestibular signs are not uncommon in rabbits where infection with *Pasteurella* spp. or *Encephalitozoon cuniculi* are common causes.

Causes

- Infection (e.g. otitis media).
- Inflammation.
- Neoplasia.
- Benign polyps (especially in young cats).
- Idiopathic ('old dog' vestibular disease).
- Trauma.
- Toxic (including drugs, e.g. high doses of metronidazole).
- Postsurgical (e.g. following ear surgery).

Clinical signs

- Nystagmus (abnormal eye movements).
- Strabismus.
- Ataxia.
- Mental depression.
- Other neurological signs.
- Horner's syndrome (constricted pupil, flaccid eyelids, enophthalmos, third eyelid protrusion).
- Nausea.
- Signs of external ear disease.

Figure 21.19 summarizes the clinical signs that can help to distinguish peripheral from central vestibular disease.

Clinical sign	Peripheral	Central
Nystagmus	Usually horizontal	Can be vertical or rotatory
Horner's syndrome	May be present	Absent
Mentation	Normal	May be depressed
Hemiparesis	Absent	Possible

21.19 Clinical findings that can help to differentiate between peripheral and central vestibular disease.

Treatment

- Treatment of underlying cause (medical or surgical).
- Maintaining in a comfortable padded environment.
- May need intravenous fluids and/or nutritional support as may be unable to eat or drink.
- Time.

Reproductive emergencies

Dystocia

Dystocia refers to problems during the parturition (birthing) process (see also Chapter 26). There are a large number of causes of dystocia but some of the more common ones are:

- Primary uterine inertia (i.e. failure of uterus to contract)
- Secondary uterine inertia after prolonged straining
- Fetal malpresentation
- Maternal–fetal disproportion (common in breeds such as Bulldogs)
- Maternal pelvic abnormalities (e.g. previous fractured pelvis)
- Fetal death.

Clinical signs

If the bitch is showing any of the following signs, veterinary advice should be urgently sought:

- She has been straining unproductively for more than 1 hour from the onset of stage II labour without producing a puppy
- She has been straining unproductively for more than 30 minutes without producing subsequent puppies
- She has a green/black vulval discharge or fetal fluids are seen and 2 hours have elapsed without producing a puppy
- She rests for more than 2 hours between puppies without straining
- She appears unwell or depressed
- A puppy can be seen stuck in the birth canal.

For queens, the interval between kittens may be much longer and the entire parturition process may take up to 24 hours. If concerned, it is better to err on the side of caution and recommend that the pet is examined for signs of fetal or maternal distress.

The occurrence of dystocia in exotic pets is very variable between the species. Egg binding in birds and reptiles may also occur. Reasons for dystocia in small mammals may include those factors listed above. Other factors may be related to husbandry, such as lack of suitable substrate or nesting material, or to hormonal or metabolic imbalances. A clinical history should therefore include how the pet is managed and all relevant husbandry information. Veterinary advice should be sought if there is unproductive straining or an abnormal vulval or cloacal discharge. The reader is referred to exotic pet texts for specific information on individual species.

Diagnostic aids

- Digital vaginal examination.
- Abdominal radiography.
- Abdominal ultrasonography.

Treatment

- Keep the bitch/queen in a warm and comfortable environment.
- If a puppy/kitten is visible in the birth canal, manually assisted delivery may be attempted.
- Medical therapy (e.g. oxytocin).
- Surgical delivery (caesarean operation).

Nursing care for caesarean operation

For a successful outcome, the time taken for the anaesthesia and surgical procedure should be minimized. The bitch may be clipped and an initial surgical preparation carried out prior to anaesthesia. All instruments for the surgery and for neonatal resuscitation and care should be prepared before the procedure.

Neonatal resuscitation

Equipment that should be prepared prior to delivery includes:

- A warm environment (incubator) or box with heat lamp
- Plenty of soft, dry, warm towels
- Haemostats for clamping the umbilical cord
- Suture material
- Suction bulb syringe for clearing oral secretions
- Emergency drugs (adrenaline, naloxone).

The following procedures should start once the neonate has been handed over to the nurse:

- Clean the fetal membranes from the puppy's mouth and gently suction the oral cavity (check for cleft palate when doing this)
- Clamp and cut the umbilical cord approximately 3 cm from the puppy's abdomen
- Stimulate and dry the neonate by rubbing with a warm towel
- Check that the puppy is breathing and has a heartbeat (using digital palpation).

If a puppy is not breathing or does not have a heartbeat, supply oxygen via a tight-fitting face mask or endotracheal tube and continue vigorously rubbing the puppy to stimulate respiration. 'Swinging' puppies is no longer recommended, due to the potential for causing brain damage. If there is no heartbeat, start gentle external compressions and administer adrenaline.

Pyometra

This is an infection of the uterus that is common in older entire female dogs and occasionally cats. It occurs secondary to hormonally induced changes and is commonest about 5–6 weeks after a season.

Clinical signs

- Vomiting.
- Polyuria/polydipsia.

- Weakness and lethargy.
- Purulent vaginal discharge (not always present).
- Abdominal pain.
- Shock.

Diagnostic aids

- Haematology and biochemistry.
- Urinalysis.
- Vaginal swab.
- Abdominal radiography.
- Abdominal ultrasonography.

Treatment

- Intravenous fluid therapy.
- Antibiotic therapy.
- Surgery to remove the infected uterus.

Eclampsia

This is hypocalcaemia secondary to pregnancy or more commonly lactation. It is most often seen in small-breed dogs within 2 weeks of parturition.

Clinical signs

- Restlessness and anxiety.
- Panting.
- Hypersalivation.
- Twitching/muscle spasms.
- Hyperthermia.
- Tachycardia.
- Collapse.

Diagnostic aids

- Blood calcium level.

Treatment

- Slow intravenous infusion of 10% calcium gluconate (monitor heart rate while doing this).
- Oral calcium supplementation.
- Wean the puppies.

Paraphimosis

This is an inability to retract the penis into the prepuce. It commonly occurs in entire male small-breed dogs following an episode of sexual excitement.

Clinical signs

- Engorged protruding penis, often dry and may be necrotic.
- Dysuria.
- Pain and excessive licking associated with penile region.

Treatment

- Analgesia.
- Gentle cleaning of penis with warm water or saline solution.
- Topical hyperosmolar solution to reduce swelling.
- Manual replacement of penis within prepuce (commonly requires heavy sedation or anaesthesia).
- Surgical correction, especially if situation recurs.

Paediatric emergencies

Young puppies, kittens and neonates of other species may present in a collapsed state. It is often challenging to achieve a specific diagnosis but the two most common problems are:

- Hypoglycaemia
- Hypothermia.

Clinical signs

- Weakness or collapse.
- Persistent crying.
- Decreased feeding.
- Decreased movement.

Treatment

Due to patient size, diagnostic tests and treatment are challenging but the following guidelines should be used:

- Monitor body temperature and warm if hypothermic
- Measure blood glucose
- Supplement glucose:
  - Intravenous – a standard intravenous catheter may be used in the jugular vein in paediatric patients
  - Intraosseous – easy to place in paediatric patients and can be life saving
  - Oral – much less effective.
    (NB if a blood sample to measure glucose cannot be obtained, it is recommended that treatment with glucose is started, as hypoglycaemia is so common)
- Supplement fluids.
- Once normothermic, initiate oral feeding regime.

Nursing the paediatric patient

- Ensure warm and comfortable environment.
- Feed regularly by bottle or stomach tube:
  - Every 2 hours in puppies and kittens up to 5 days old
  - Every 4 hours in puppies and kittens >5 days old.
- Use a commercial hand-rearing formula to supply the patient's needs.
- After feeding, stimulate the patient to defecate by gently rubbing the perineum with a damp cotton bud (this function is usually undertaken by the mother).

For further information on neonatal care, see Chapter 26.

Urological emergencies

Urethral obstruction

This occurs when there is a blockage in the urethra and therefore the animal cannot pass urine. As urine cannot be voided from the body, waste products (especially potassium, urea and creatinine) build up rapidly in the bloodstream and can cause life-threatening signs within 24 hours of the obstruction occurring. It occurs most commonly in overweight male neutered cats, but some dog breeds (e.g. Dalmatians) and rabbits are also predisposed. It is very rare in female animals, as they have a much shorter wider urethra.

Causes

- Urethral calculi (stones).
- Urethral plug (consists of crystals and a mucoid material).
- Urethral neoplasia (cancer) (rare).
- Urethral stricture (may occur secondary to previous obstruction with stones or a plug).

Clinical signs

- Stranguria (straining to urinate without passing any urine).
- Frequent visits to litter tray with no urine produced.
- Vocalization (pain) when attempting to urinate.
- Licking at urethra.
- Depression (dependent on duration of blockage, but most animals are markedly depressed by 24–36 hours after the blockage occurs).
- Anorexia.
- Bradycardia (secondary to potassium build-up in bloodstream).
- Distended painful bladder on palpation of the abdomen.
- Vomiting.
- Collapse.

Urethral blockage must be distinguished from cystitis, where the bladder is inflamed but not blocked. Animals with cystitis may also strain to urinate, urinate frequently and show pain when urinating, but they will pass small amounts of urine. Cystitis is more common in female animals. Cystitis is an uncomfortable condition but, as the animal can still void urine, it is not life-threatening.

Diagnostic aids

- Palpation and gentle attempts at expression of the bladder.
- Blood tests, especially blood potassium level.
- ECG – can help to identify signs of hyperkalaemia (high blood potassium).

Once the patient has had the obstruction relieved (been 'unblocked'), the following tests can be carried out:

- Urinalysis and culture
- Ultrasonography of the bladder
- Radiography, including retrograde urethrography.

Treatment

- Fluid therapy.
- Treatment for hyperkalaemia if present (see 'Metabolic emergencies').
- Urinary catheterization – commonly requires sedation and should be carried out once the animal has been stabilized with fluid therapy.
- Urinary catheter should be left in place for 24–72 hours after initial decompression of the bladder. Urine production should be monitored during this time ideally by connecting the urinary catheter to a closed collection system.
- Analgesia/anti-inflammatories.

- If bladder stones are present surgery may be required to remove them. Longer-term medical treatment may be used to dissolve or prevent recurrence of calculi.

Uroabdomen

This condition occurs when urine leaks into the abdominal cavity, often secondary to a tear in the bladder wall (ruptured bladder). As in urethral obstruction, urine is not voided from the patient and high levels of potassium, urea and creatinine can build up in the blood, leading to severe clinical signs.

Causes

- Trauma.
- Following cystocentesis (this is most often a concern when a cystocentesis is performed while the urethra is blocked).
- Bladder neoplasia (cancer).

Clinical signs

- Distended and/or painful abdomen.
- Depression.
- Anorexia.
- Vomiting.
- Bradycardia.
- Lack of urination (as urine is leaking into abdomen). If the tear in the bladder wall is small, it is possible that the animal may still be able to void small amounts of urine via the urethra.

Diagnostic aids

- Blood tests (especially potassium, urea and creatinine levels).
- Abdominal ultrasonography.
- Analysis of fluid collected from the abdominal cavity by abdominocentesis.
- Radiography, including contrast studies.

Treatment

- Intravenous fluid therapy.
- Treatment for hyperkalaemia if present (see 'Metabolic emergencies').
- Surgical repair of the rupture.

Acute renal failure

This can happen if the kidneys suddenly fail. It is much less common than chronic renal failure in veterinary patients.

Causes

- Shock with significant reduction of blood supply to the kidneys (most commonly prolonged hypovolaemic shock).
- Infection (e.g. leptospirosis, bacterial pyelonephritis).
- Toxic damage (e.g. ethylene glycol).
- Metabolic (e.g. prolonged hypercalcaemia).
- Drug therapy (e.g. non-steroidal anti-inflammatory drugs, especially if given while the patient is in shock).
- Blood clots in the arteries supplying the kidneys (rare).
- Progression of chronic renal failure.

Clinical signs

- Depression.
- Anorexia.
- Vomiting.
- Uraemia (may be smelled on animal's breath).
- Abnormality in urine production, most commonly reduced (anuria/oliguria) but occasionally massively increased (polyuria).

Diagnostic aids

- Haematology and biochemistry.
- Urinalysis, including urine culture.
- Abdominal ultrasonography.
- Abdominal radiography.
- Serology (blood tests for infectious agents such as leptospirosis).

Treatment

- Intravenous fluid therapy.
- Treatment for underlying cause, if known (e.g. antibiotics for infection, specific treatment for hypercalcaemia).
- Drugs to encourage urine production (furosemide, mannitol).
- Peritoneal dialysis.
- Monitor urine production and blood tests.

Metabolic emergencies

Hypoglycaemia

This is a low level of blood glucose (sugar). It is the commonest reversible cause of collapse in neonatal/paediatric patients but can occur in older animals. It may also be seen in the smaller exotic species where metabolic rates are high.

Causes

- Young patient, especially toy breeds of dog.
- Insulin overdose in diabetic patients.
- Insulinoma (functional cancer of pancreas).
- Hypoadrenocorticism (Addison's disease).
- Liver failure.
- Sepsis or severe infection.
- Toxicity (xylitol – artifical sweetener used in human foodstuffs).

Clinical signs

- Weakness.
- Exercise intolerance.
- Collapse.
- Seizures.
- Coma.

Diagnostic aids

- Blood glucose level (glucometer).
- Haematology and biochemistry.

Treatment

- Intravenous (or intraosseous) glucose supplementation.
- Food offered as soon as able to eat.
- Rub glucose syrup on oral mucous membranes – unlikely to be effective if animal is severely hypoglycaemic, but may be attempted whilst intravenous access is obtained.

Hyperkalaemia

This is an increased blood potassium level. The normal level of potassium in blood is approximately 3.5–5.5 mmol/l. Levels >8.0 mmol/l may be fatal. Death occurs as the high potassium level leads to disturbances in electrical conduction within the heart initially causing bradycardia but ultimately asystole and death.

Causes

- Urethral obstruction.
- Acute renal failure.
- Uroabdomen.
- Hypoadrenocorticism (Addison's disease).
- Reperfusion injury.

Clinical signs

- Bradycardia (slow heart rate).
- Poor pulse quality.
- ECG changes.
- Other signs dependent on cause of hyperkalaemia.

Diagnostic aids

- Serum potassium level.
- ECG.
- Other tests dependent on underlying cause.

Treatment

Ultimately, successful treatment depends on identifying and treating the underlying cause of the hyperkalaemia. However, as it may be immediately life-threatening, the following therapies may be used to stabilize the animal, whatever the cause of the hyperkalaemia:

- Intravenous calcium gluconate
- Intravenous insulin and dextrose supplementation
- Intravenous fluid therapy.

Hypercalcaemia

This is an increased level of blood calcium.

Causes

- Neoplasia (cancer), especially lymphoma and anal sac carcinoma.
- Toxicity (e.g. human psoriasis cream, some rat poisons).
- Primary hyperparathyroidism (hormonal disease).
- Hypoadrenocorticism (Addison's disease).
- Granulomatous infections (e.g. lungworm, fungal disease).

Clinical signs

- Inappetence/anorexia.
- Polyuria/polydipsia.

- Depression.
- Vomiting.
- Tremors.
- Renal failure if prolonged.

Diagnostic aids

- Haematology and biochemistry.
- Urinalysis.
- Imaging studies (radiography, ultrasonography).

Treatment

As with hyperkalaemia, successful treatment requires identification and treatment of the underlying disease. However, while diagnostic tests are being carried out to allow this, the following medical treatments can be used to lower the calcium level and reduce the risk of renal damage:

- Intravenous fluid therapy with 0.9% saline
- Furosemide
- Bisphosphonates
- Calcitonin.

Hypoadrenocorticism (Addison's disease)

This is a disease where there is impaired secretion of hormones from the adrenal cortex. The animal becomes deficient in a number of hormones, most importantly aldosterone (a mineralocorticoid) and cortisol (a glucocorticoid). Aldosterone is a hormone that helps the body to maintain electrolyte balance (especially potassium), and cortisol is a hormone that helps the animal to maintain normal blood pressure and gastrointestinal tract function and to cope with stress. It is most commonly diagnosed in young to middle-aged female dogs and is very rare in cats.

Clinical signs

- Collapse.
- Weakness.
- Depression/lethargy.
- Polyuria/polydipsia.
- Intermittent gastrointestinal signs (vomiting, diarrhoea, inappetence).
- Bradycardia.
- Poor pulse quality.
- Pale mucous membranes with a prolonged capillary refill time.

Diagnostic aids

- Haematology and biochemistry.
- Urinalysis.
- ACTH stimulation test (this is the only way to make a certain diagnosis).
- ECG.

Treatment

- Intravenous fluid therapy.
- Treatment of hyperkalaemia if severe (see section above on hyperkalaemia).
- Hormone replacement therapy (both mineralocorticoid and glucocorticoid).

Diabetic ketoacidosis

This is a complication of diabetes mellitus where the body starts to produce ketones as an energy source. As these ketones are organic acids, if produced in large quantities they can cause the blood to become acidic, with severe systemic effects. Diabetic ketoacidosis may occur both in previously undiagnosed diabetics and in diabetic animals that have been on insulin treatment for some time.

Clinical signs

- Collapse.
- Inappetence/anorexia.
- Vomiting.
- Polyuria/polydipsia.
- Dehydration.
- Signs of shock (tachycardia, poor pulses).
- Tachypnoea (increased breathing rate).
- Ketones may be smelled on the breath (pear drop smell).

Diagnostic aids

- Haematology and biochemistry.
- Blood gas analysis (allows quantification of how acidic the blood is).
- Urinalysis and culture.
- Abdominal ultrasonography.

Treatment

- Intravenous fluid therapy.
- Insulin therapy – generally using a short-acting insulin by intravenous or intramuscular route for initial stabilization. A longer-term protocol of subcutaneous insulin for use at home can be introduced once the patient is stable.
- Antiemetics.
- Antibiotics.
- Careful monitoring of electrolytes with supplementation if necessary. Potassium, phosphorus and magnesium may all need supplementing.

Disseminated intravascular coagulation (DIC)

During DIC, the clotting system of the body becomes overactivated. This leads to consumption of the patient's clotting factors and the development of a generalized bleeding tendency. DIC always occurs secondary to a severe underlying problem such as septic shock, pancreatitis or heat stroke. It is a serious complication but can be reversible.

Clinical signs

- Petechiation/ecchymoses.
- Excesssive bleeding from catheter or venepuncture sites.
- Haemorrhage at mucosal surfaces.
- Presence of a severe underlying disease.

Diagnosis

- Platelet count (will be low with DIC).
- Clotting times (will be prolonged with DIC).
- Other clotting parameters such as D-dimers or fibrinogen degradation products.

Treatment

- Treatment of underlying disease.
- Fluid therapy to maintain tissue blood flow.
- Fresh frozen plasma transfusions.
- Medical treatment such as with heparin may be used dependent on the stage and severity of DIC.

Gastrointestinal and abdominal emergencies

Pharyngeal or oesophageal fish hook

Dogs or, less commonly, cats may ingest fish hooks either directly or by eating fish or bait attached to them. The fish hook commonly lodges in the pharynx or proximal oesophagus but occasionally more distally. If there is still a line attached to the hook, the owners should be instructed neither to pull it, as this may cause further damage, nor to cut the line, as it may help the veterinary surgeon locate the hook.

Clinical signs

- Drooling, possibly with blood-tinged saliva.
- Dysphagia (difficulty eating).
- Facial/pharyngeal discomfort (pawing at face).
- It is possible that the animal may display no clinical signs but simply be observed to have eaten the hook.

Diagnostic aids

- Radiography.

Treatment

- Removal of hook, usually under general anaesthesia.

The ease with which the hook can be removed depends both on its location (e.g. hooks lodged in the pharynx are easier to remove than oesophageal ones) and the number of barbs the hook has. Hooks with multiple barbs embedded in the wall of the oesophagus may require careful manipulation to remove. Most hooks can be removed under either direct or endoscopic visualization. Occasionally surgical removal is necessary.

Oesophageal foreign body

This occurs most commonly in terrier breeds, especially West Highland White Terriers. The foreign body is most commonly a bone.

Clinical signs

- Witnessed ingestion of a foreign object (often fed to the dog by the owners).
- Regurgitation.
- Retching/coughing.
- Hypersalivation.
- Inappetence.
- Depression.
- Pain or discomfort on eating.

Diagnostic aids

- Radiography.
- Endoscopy.

Treatment

- Removal of foreign object via mouth, aided by endoscopy.
- Removal of foreign object via mouth, aided by fluoroscopy.
- Pushing foreign object into stomach and either removal by laparotomy and gastrotomy or left to be destroyed by gastric acid.
- Rarely, surgical removal of the object via thoracotomy and oesophagotomy.

Complications

- Aspiration pneumonia.
- Oesophageal rupture.
- Oesophageal stricture (may occur up to several weeks later).

Megaoesophagus

This is a condition where the oesophageal muscle cannot contract normally and loses its tone, meaning that food is no longer pushed normally from the mouth to the stomach following swallowing. It can be congenital but is more commonly an acquired condition in older dogs and less commonly cats. Its main clinical sign is regurgitation, which is the *passive* process whereby food that remains in the oesophagus is brought back. Although a chronic condition, these patients commonly present as an emergency either as the disease worsens or if the patient develops pneumonia.

Clinical signs

- Regurgitation (may occur for up to several hours after eating).
- Weight loss.
- Commonly a good appetite is maintained.
- Coughing/dyspnoea due to secondary aspiration pneumonia.

Diagnostic aids

- Radiography.
- Haematology, biochemistry and other blood tests to try to identify an underlying cause.

Treatment

- Treatment of underlying cause if one is identified.
- Nutrition – often necessary to feed directly into the stomach via gastrotomy tube.
- Treatment of concurrent aspiration pneumonia with antibiotics.

Vomiting

This is the active expulsion of gastric contents (as opposed to passive regurgitation). There are many causes of vomiting but they can be subdivided according to whether the origin of the problem is within the gastrointestinal (GI) tract or outside it.

Causes of vomiting

Primary gastrointestinal causes:

- GI infection (viral, bacterial, parasitic)
- Dietary indiscretion
- Gastrointestinal foreign body
- Intussusception (telescoping of the bowel)
- Gastrointestinal neoplasia
- Pancreatitis.

Secondary causes:

- Renal disease
- Liver disease
- Infection (e.g. pyometra)
- Endocrine disease (e.g. hypoadrenocorticism)
- Neurological disease
- Drug therapy.

Vomiting is commonly (but not always) accompanied by diarrhoea. Vomiting and diarrhoea vary considerably in their severity: some patients with vomiting require emergency evaluation and treatment, whereas other patients have much milder signs, where emergency treatment is not necessary. When dealing with an owner whose pet is vomiting, the following questions should be asked and can be used to make an assessment of the severity of the problem and whether the animal should be seen on an emergency basis.

- How many times has the pet vomited in the last 12 hours?
- Is there any blood in the vomit? How much?
- Is the pet still keen to eat and drink? Are they able to keep down anything they eat?
- Is the pet significantly depressed? If the pet is significantly depressed it should be seen as an emergency regardless of the answers to the other questions.
- Does the pet have any other signs of abdominal pain (e.g. vocalization, abnormal position)?
- Has the pet been witnessed to eat any toxins or drugs or any objects of a size that might have become stuck in the GI tract?

Diagnostic aids

- Thorough history, including vaccination status and worming history.
- Physical examination.
- Haematology and biochemistry, including in-house blood smear evaluation to assess for neutropenia (low white blood cell count seen with severe GI infections, especially parvovirus).
- Urinalysis.
- Faecal analysis (both for parasites and culture).
- Abdominal radiography.
- Abdominal ultrasonography.
- Serological testing of both blood and faeces for infectious disease.

Treatment

- Intravenous fluid therapy.
- Treatment of underlying cause (may be medical or surgical).
- Nil by mouth until diagnosis made.
- Antiemetic therapy unless GI obstruction suspected.
- Good nursing care – warm comfortable environment.

Diarrhoea

Diarrhoea refers to the voiding of abnormal liquid faeces. Patients with diarrhoea may present as an emergency if the diarrhoea is severe (with significant fluid loss), if there is a large amount of blood in the faeces or if it is accompanied by marked vomiting and depression. Diarrhoea is commonly divided into:

- Small-bowel – large volumes of watery faeces passed with a relatively low frequency.
- Large-bowel – small volumes of semi-solid faeces passed frequently with straining. A small amount of fresh blood may be present.

When dealing with an owner whose pet has diarrhoea, the following questions should be asked and can be used to make an assessment of the severity of the problem and whether the animal should be seen on an emergency basis.

- How many times has the pet had diarrhoea in the last 24–48 hours?
- Is there any fresh blood in the diarrhoea? If so, how much?
- Is the diarrhoea black, very dark or tarry (suggestive of presence of digested blood)
- Is the diarrhoea associated with straining?
- Is there a large or small volume of diarrhoea produced each time the animal passes something?
- Is the diarrhoea watery or semi-solid?
- Is the pet still keen to eat and drink?
- Is the pet significantly depressed? If the pet is significantly depressed it should be seen as an emergency regardless of the answers to the other questions.
- Does the pet have any other signs of abdominal pain (e.g. vocalization, abnormal position)?
- Has the pet been witnessed eating any toxins or drugs or any objects of a size that might have become stuck in the GI tract?

Small-bowel diarrhoea is more commonly an emergency than large-bowel diarrhoea, especially if melaena (digested blood presenting as black, sticky or tarry faeces) is present.

Diagnostic aids

- Thorough history, including vaccination status and worming history.
- Physical examination.
- Haematology and biochemistry, including in-house blood smear evaluation to assess for neutropenia (low white blood cell count seen with severe GI infections, especially parvovirus).
- Urinalysis.
- Faecal analysis (both for parasites and culture).
- Abdominal radiography.
- Abdominal ultrasonography.
- Serological testing of both blood and faeces for infectious disease.

Treatment

- Intravenous fluid therapy.
- Treatment of underlying cause (may be medical or surgical treatment).

- Nil by mouth until diagnosis made.
- Good nursing care – ensure perineal area does not become sore or inflamed. This may require frequent bathing and clipping of hair in this region, or a tail bandage.

Gastrointestinal obstruction

Patients with GI obstruction most often present with vomiting and sometimes diarrhoea. They also commonly show signs of both hypovolaemic shock and dehydration. The obstruction may be complete or partial. Animals with complete obstructions have more severe and rapidly progressive signs than those with partial obstructions.

Obstructions may occur secondary to:

- Foreign body ingestion
- Intussusception
- GI neoplasia
- Incarceration.

Clinical signs

- Vomiting, sometimes with blood.
- Anorexia.
- Depression.
- Abdominal pain.
- Palpable abdominal mass (classically intussusceptions are sausage shaped).
- Hypovolaemic shock.
- Dehydration.
- Weight loss – especially with partial obstructions.
- Diarrhoea/melaena (digested blood in stool), especially with partial obstructions.

Diagnostic aids

- Abdominal radiography, possibly including a barium study.
- Abdominal ultrasonography.
- Haematology and biochemistry.
- Electrolyte and blood gas analysis.
- Urinalysis.
- Faecal analysis.

Treatment

- Intravenous fluid therapy for stabilization.
- Surgical removal of the obstruction – this may require resection of a portion of the bowel.
- Endoscopic removal may be attempted for gastric foreign bodies.

Postoperative monitoring and nursing care

This is crucial for a successful outcome. Patients should initially be maintained on intravenous fluids, with gradual re-introduction of water and then food over the 12–48 hours after surgery. Breakdown (dehiscence) of the incision in the bowel can occur for several days after surgery. Postoperative monitoring should include:

- Perfusion parameters (heart rate, pulse quality, mucous membrane colour and capillary refill time)
- Urine output

- Any vomiting or regurgitation
- Any faeces passed
- Bodyweight
- Hydration status
- Repeat electrolytes and acid–base status.

Gastric dilatation–volvulus

GDV is a condition of principally large-breed deep-chested dogs. The stomach becomes dilated with gas and then twists along its long axis. It typically causes a sudden onset of severe clinical signs.

Clinical signs

- Collapse.
- Severe hypovolaemic shock.
- Unproductive retching.
- Distended tympanic abdomen (though this can be hard to see in some of the most deep-chested dogs where the distended stomach is hidden under the ribcage).
- Tachycardia, possibly with arrhythmia.
- Pale mucous membranes with prolonged capillary refill time.
- Restlessness in early stages.
- Hypersalivation.
- Tachypnoea.

Diagnostic aids

- Abdominal radiography – right lateral view is most important.
- Haematology and biochemistry.
- Electrolyte and blood gas including lactate level.
- ECG (see Figure 21.15).

Treatment

- Intravenous fluid therapy for stabilization – shock doses of fluid via a large-bore catheter are often required.
- Gastric decompression via a stomach tube – this is not always possible and a stomach tube should never be forced in, as this may result in tearing of the oesophagus at the oesophageal gastric junction (cardia).
- Gastric decompression via percutaneous trocharization – a needle or catheter is inserted through the abdominal body wall in the area where tympany is detected, with the aim of entering the stomach and allowing gas to escape.
- Surgery – this is the definitive treatment and is typically performed as soon as the patient has been stabilized for anaesthesia with fluid therapy. At surgery, the stomach is derotated and then emptied (usually by passing a stomach tube following derotation). A gastropexy should then be performed. This involves anchoring the stomach in the correct position by suturing the stomach to the body wall.
- Good postoperative care is essential – the monitoring is as for the patient with GI obstruction.

Pancreatitis

This is a generalized inflammation of the pancreas. In most cases, it is unknown why it happens but it may be associated with obesity, a high-fat diet and certain diseases such as hyperadrenocorticism. One of the functions of the pancreas is to make the digestive enzymes. When the pancreas becomes inflamed, these enzymes are released into the circulation and can cause severe systemic signs, including shock and death.

Clinical signs

- Vomiting – may be severe.
- Anorexia.
- Collapse.
- Tachycardia.
- Severe abdominal pain – dogs may show the 'praying position'.
- Dehydration.
- Diarrhoea.

Diagnostic aids

- Haematology and biochemistry.
- Specific pancreatic blood tests, such as trypsinogen-like (TLI) and canine pancreatic lipase (cPLI) immunoreactivity.
- Abdominal ultrasonography.
- Abdominal fluid analysis (if present).
- Abdominal radiographs.

Treatment

- Intravenous fluid therapy.
- Antiemetics.
- Analgesia.
- Nil per mouth while vomiting is severe; small amounts of low-fat food can be introduced once vomiting has been controlled.
- Antibiotics.

Haemoabdomen

This occurs when an abdominal organ ruptures and the animal bleeds into its abdominal cavity. The spleen is the most common organ to rupture, often because there is a splenic tumour.

Clinical signs

- Collapse.
- Tachycardia.
- Poor pulse quality.
- Pale mucous membranes.
- Abdominal distension with a fluid thrill.

Diagnostic aids

- Haematology and biochemistry.
- Clotting profile.
- Abdominal ultrasonography.
- Abdominal fluid analysis.
- Thoracic radiographs to look for signs of metastasis (spread of cancer) to the chest.
- Abdominal radiographs.

Treatment

- Intravenous fluid therapy.
- Blood transfusion.
- Abdominal pressure wrap (see Figure 21.12).
- Surgery to identify and remove the bleeding organ.

Septic peritonitis

This is a condition where a septic (infected) fluid builds up in the abdominal cavity. The infection most commonly gains entry to the abdominal cavity from a ruptured GI tract, but other sources (e.g. ruptured urogenital or biliary tract) are possible.

Clinical signs

- Collapse.
- Tachycardia.
- Poor pulse quality.
- Red mucous membranes.
- Abdominal pain.
- Abdominal distension.
- Vomiting.
- Diarrhoea.
- Anorexia.

Diagnostic aids

- Haematology and biochemistry.
- Clotting profile.
- Abdominal radiography.
- Abdominal ultrasonography.
- Abdominal fluid analysis (cytology, biochemistry and culture).
- Urinalysis

Treatment

- Intravenous fluid therapy.
- Intravenous antibiotic therapy.
- Analgesia.
- Exploratory surgery to lavage (flush) the abdomen and identify and treat the source of infection.

Nursing care

Postoperative nursing care is vital to a successful outcome. Parameters to be monitored should include:

- Heart rate
- Pulse quality
- Mucous membrane colour
- Blood pressure
- Urine output
- Degree of pain
- Electolytes and acid–base.

These parameters can be used to guide postoperative fluid and analgesia requirements.

Hepatic failure

Animals with liver disease may present as an emergency, either because they have developed acute liver failure or have chronic liver disease with acute deterioration.

Causes

- Infection (e.g. leptospirosis).
- Toxin.
- Inflammation.
- Neoplasia.
- Acute deterioration of chronic disease.

Clinical signs

- Weakness.
- Inappetence.
- Vomiting, including haematemesis.
- Neurological signs (seizures, unusual behaviour, blindness).
- Jaundiced mucous membranes.
- Increased tendency to bleed.
- If underlying chronic disease, the animal may have weight loss, polyuria/polydipsia and/or abdominal distension.

Diagnostic aids

- Haematology and biochemistry.
- Clotting profile.
- Liver function tests (bile acid stimulation tests, ammonia level).
- Abdominal ultrasonography.
- Aspirate or biopsy of the liver.
- Urinalysis.

Treatment

- Intravenous fluid therapy.
- Antibiotics.
- Glucose supplementation.
- Lactulose to treat neurological signs (hepatic encephalopathy).
- Blood or plasma transfusion.
- Treatment of primary cause.

Ocular emergencies

Ocular emergencies are relatively common. Although they are rarely life-threatening, prompt action may need to be taken to prevent loss of sight in the eye. They are also often particularly distressing to owners, as they can look very dramatic, and it is recommended that the animal is admitted to the practice as soon as possible. As even minor ocular problems have the potential to deteriorate rapidly, with the possibility of loss of vision, all animals showing a sudden onset of signs related to the eye should be seen urgently.

With all ocular emergencies the following rules can be applied:

- Assess condition of the patient – abnormalities in the major body systems should always be addressed first, no matter how severe the injury to the eye
- Assess extent of ocular injury
- Prevent self-trauma (place Elizabethan collar)
- Give analgesia
- Keep the eye moist with a false-tear solution
- Keep the patient in a quiet dimly lit environment.

Traumatic proptosis

This represents the forward displacement of the entire globe, with entrapment of the eyelids behind the equator of the globe. It is most commonly seen following trauma and in breeds with shallow orbits, such as the Pekingese.

Clinical signs

- Anteriorly displaced globe.
- Swelling around the orbit.
- Signs of other head injuries (e.g. bleeding, bruising).

Treatment

The globe should be replaced into its correct position as quickly as possible if the animal is to regain vision in that eye; however, any concurrent injuries must be considered when deciding whether immediate replacement of the globe is the correct course of action.

- Sterile saline-soaked swab over the proptosed globe to keep eye moist – the saline may be slightly cooled to help to reduce periorbital swelling.
- Prevention of self-trauma.
- Analgesia.
- Sedation/anaesthesia with replacement of globe. Following replacement, the eyelids are commonly sutured closed for a period of time.

Ocular foreign body
Clinical signs

- Foreign body visible (Figure 21.20) or may be trapped under eyelids or third eyelid.
- Blepharospasm.
- Rubbing eye or face.
- Epiphora (excess tear production).
- Chemosis (conjunctival swelling).
- Photophobia.

Treatment

- Prevention of self-trauma (Elizabethan collar).
- Topical local anaesthesia.
- Flushing eye with large volume of sterile saline.
- Sedation or anaesthesia if foreign object lodged (especially under third eyelid).
- If foreign object does not appear to have penetrated the cornea, it should be gently grasped and removed.
- If foreign object has clearly penetrated the cornea, it should be left in place until it can be removed by a specialist veterinary ophthalmologist.
- Topical antibiotics.

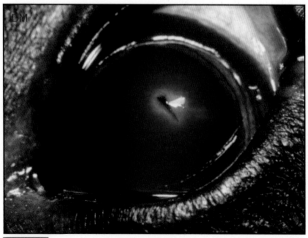

21.20 Corneal foreign body. (Courtesy of D Moore)

Corneal scratch/laceration

This is where the surface of the cornea is damaged. It occurs most commonly secondary to scratches from other animals or damage from vegetation.

Clinical signs

- Ocular pain.
- Blepharospasm.
- Photophobia.
- Epiphora.
- Squinting.
- Rubbing eye or face.
- Visible disruption of the corneal surface.
- Corneal oedema (blue discoloration of cornea) (Figure 21.21).
- If cornea is penetrated, there may be anterior uveitis (see below) or prolapse of the iris into or through the corneal wound.

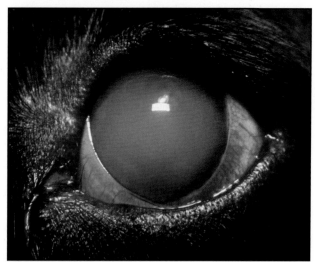

21.21 Blue discoloration of cornea indicative of corneal oedema. (Courtesy of D Moore)

Diagnostic aids

- Fluorescein stain of the eye – areas where the corneal epithelium is damaged will take up the stain.

Treatment

- Prevention of self-trauma.
- Topical local anaesthesia for analgesia and to allow a full examination.
- Topical medical treatment (antibiotics, treatment for uveitis if present).
- Deep scratches, especially if the cornea is penetrated, may require surgery.

Corneal ulcer

Causes

- Corneal trauma.
- Anatomical (e.g. exophthalmos, abnormal eyelashes).
- Breed-related (e.g. Boxer).
- Infectious.
- Lack of tear production.
- Chemical injury.

Clinical signs

- Ocular pain.
- Blepharospasm.
- Photophobia.
- Epiphora.
- Squinting.
- Rubbing eye or face.
- Purulent ocular discharge.
- Corneal oedema (blue discoloration of cornea) (see Figure 21.21).
- Secondary uveitis.

Diagnostic aids

- Full ophthalmological examination.
- Fluorescein staining – ulcerated areas will take up the fluorescein stain, unless the ulcer is very deep, with exposure of Descemet's membrane.

Treatment

- Prevention of self-trauma.
- Topical medical treatment (*not* corticosteroid).
- Treatment of underlying cause.
- Severe rapidly progressive ulcers (known as melting ulcers) may require surgical therapy.

Uveitis

This refers to inflammation of the uveal tract, which includes the iris, ciliary body and choroid layer. It may occur as a localized ocular problem or may be seen with a wide range of systemic infectious or inflammatory diseases.

Causes

- Ocular trauma.
- Infection.
- Inflammation.
- Neoplasia.
- Secondary to problems with the lens.

Clinical signs

- Ocular pain.
- Blepharospasm.
- Photophobia.
- Rubbing eye or face.
- Squinting.
- Miotic (constricted) pupil.
- Aqueous flare (cloudiness to anterior chamber).
- Secondary corneal oedema (blue discoloration of cornea) (see Figure 21.21).

Diagnostic aids

- Full ophthalmological examination.
- Careful full physical examination for signs of systemic disease.
- Haematology and biochemistry.
- Urinalysis.

Treatment

- Treatment of underlying cause.
- Analgesia (topical and/or systemic).

- Prevention of self-trauma.
- Topical anti-inflammatory.
- Topical mydriatic.

Glaucoma

This represents an increased intraocular pressure (i.e. pressure within the eyeball). It can be very painful and if not treated quickly can lead to permanent blindness in that eye. It is an inherited condition in some breeds (e.g. Cocker Spaniel, Springer Spaniel) due to anatomical abnormalities that pre-dispose to poor outflow of the aqueous humour. This is known as primary glaucoma. Secondary glaucoma may occur in any breed, secondary to a number of other ocular problems (e.g. lens luxation).

Clinical signs

- Often unilateral, sudden onset, severe ocular pain.
- Reduced or absent vision.
- Episcleral vascular congestion.
- Corneal oedema (blue discoloration to cornea) (see Figure 21.21).
- Dilated unresponsive pupil.
- Elevated intraocular pressure.

Diagnostic aids

- Full ophthalmological examination.
- Measurement of intraocular pressure using:
  - Indentation tonometry (Schiøtz tonomoter)
  - Applanation tonometry (Tonopen).

Treatment

- Prevention of self-trauma.
- Analgesia (topical or systemic).
- Topical treatment to:
  - Reduce production of aqueous humour
  - Improve outflow of aqueous humour.
- Systemic treatment to reduce pressure within globe (e.g. mannitol).
- Surgical intervention by a specialist ophthalmologist may be necessary.
- If the eye remains non-visual but painful, enucleation can be considered.

Hyphaema

This refers to bleeding within the anterior chamber.

Causes

- Trauma.
- Coagulation disorder.
- Hypertension.
- Neoplasia.
- Inflammation.

Clinical signs

- Blood visible in anterior chamber (Figure 21.22).
- Disturbed vision.
- Secondary uveitis.

Diagnostic aids

- Full clinical examination.
- Full ophthalmological examination.

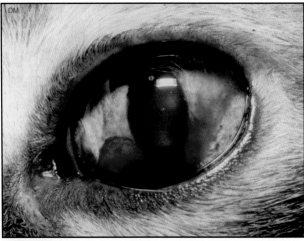

21.22 Hyphaema, with blood visible in the anterior chamber. (Courtesy of D Moore)

- Haematology and biochemistry.
- Clotting profile.
- Blood pressure measurement.

Treatment

- Treatment of underlying cause.
- Treatment of uveitis symptomatically if present.

Sudden-onset blindness

Animals that suddenly become blind may appear disoriented or confused or may become depressed and withdrawn. If the eyes appear outwardly normal, owners may not immediately realize their pet has become blind.

Causes

- Chorioretinitis (inflammation of the choroid and retina).
- Retinal detachment secondary to:
  - Hypertension (especially in cats)
  - Trauma.
- Retinal degeneration (e.g. SARDS in dogs).
- Optic neuritis (inflammation of the optic nerve).
- Intracranial disease (e.g. pituitary tumour).
- Glaucoma (although eye is usually painful).

Clinical signs

- Blindness.
- Bumping into things, especially in a new environment.
- Depression and unwillingness to move (especially cats).
- Inappetence/anorexia.
- Dilated non-responsive pupils.

Diagnostic aids

- Full ophthalmological examination.
- Full neurological examination.
- Blood pressure measurement (especially cats).
- Haematology and biochemistry.
- Urinalysis.

Treatment

- Treatment of underlying cause.

The animal may be very anxious, especially in a strange environment. To reduce its anxiety:

- Always use the animal's name whenever handling it
- Maintain a familiar smell if possible
- Reassure the animal verbally with a calm tone of voice as much as possible
- Move slowly and gently when handling the animal.

Nasal emergencies

Epistaxis

This refers to bleeding from the nostrils. It may be bilateral or unilateral. Although the volume of blood produced may seem to be large, it is rare for dogs or cats to become significantly anaemic or hypovolaemic following nasal bleeding. In small pets, however, even what appears to be a small blood loss may be more significant.

Causes

- Trauma.
- Nasal tumour.
- Infection, especially aspergillosis.
- Nasal foreign body.
- Coagulation disorder.
- Hypertension.

Clinical signs

- Nasal bleeding – always note if it is unilateral or bilateral.
- Stertorous breathing.
- Open-mouth breathing.
- Sneezing.
- Melaena (if blood is being swallowed).

Diagnostic aids

- Haematology and biochemistry.
- Clotting profile.
- Blood pressure.
- Nasal radiography.
- Nasal endoscopy plus biopsy.

Treatment

- Maintain a calm environment.
- Sedation.
- Cold compress externally.
- Topical application of adrenaline (either squirted into nostril or soaked on to a swab and placed in nostril).
- Absorbent dressing within nostril (e.g. tampon). It is vital to keep a record of the number of swabs/tampons used so it can be ensured that all are retrieved.
- Monitor for signs of hypovolaemia, which may occur if epistaxis is severe and/or prolonged. Treat with fluid therapy if it occurs.

Nasal foreign body

The commonest nasal foreign bodies are grass seeds, blades of grass and small pieces of wood.

Clinical signs

- Sneezing, may be paroxysmal.
- Nasal discharge, usually unilateral, occasionally blood tinged.
- Rubbing or pawing at nose.

Treatment

Removal of foreign body by:

- Endoscopy
- Flushing.

Nasal foreign bodies can be particularly hard to identify. They are rarely seen on radiographs. Endoscopy may be useful but the size of the endoscope often precludes a thorough and complete search of the entire nasal chamber, especially in small patients. If a foreign body cannot be seen and retrieved under direct visualization, nasal flushing should be performed.

Nasal flush procedure

1. Ensure that a cuffed endotracheal tube is in place, with cuff inflated.
2. Pack pharynx with swabs – count swabs and record. It is vital to double check that all swabs are removed before animal is recovered from anaesthesia.
3. Place animal in sternal recumbency with rostral end of nose tipped downward.
4. Fill 60 ml syringe with saline (20 ml for a cat).
5. Place nozzle of syringe up nostril that is most likely to be affected and squeeze both nostrils shut around.
6. Empty syringe with moderate force into nostril.
7. Hold empty bowl beneath nostril to catch any fluid.
8. Repeat multiple times and with both nostrils (recommend using at least 1 litre saline for a 20 kg dog).
9. Ensure that all swabs are retrieved from pharynx before patient is recovered from anaesthesia – the foreign material may sometimes be found on these swabs when they are removed.

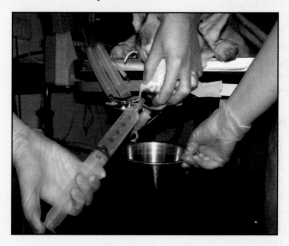

If foreign material is not found, it is possible that it had already been sneezed out before the animal reached the practice. However, it is also possible that it may remain *in situ*. This is unlikely to be dangerous for the animal, but a chronic nasal discharge may develop if any foreign material has been left behind. Owners should be warned of this possibility.

Aural emergencies

Although emergencies involving the ear are very rarely life-threatening, they can cause some distress to both the patient and the owner.

Aural foreign body

Clinical signs

- Head shaking.
- Rubbing or scratching ear.
- Pain on touching of head or aural region.
- Visualization of foreign body on auroscopic examination.

Treatment

- Removal of foreign body – invariably requires sedation.

Otitis externa and media

This is an infection of the external ear canal (otitis externa) or middle ear (otitis media).

Clinical signs

- Head shaking.
- Rubbing of head or scratching of ear.
- Self-trauma of aural region
- Vestibular signs (with otitis media – see Neurological emergencies).
- Aural discharge – may be waxy or foul smelling.
- Auroscopic examination confirms aural inflammation.

Treatment

- Emergency treatment rarely necessary unless neurological signs develop.
- Antibiotics (topical and systemic).
- Analgesia.
- Aural flush under anaesthesia.

Aural haematoma

This is a haematoma of the pinna. Although these swellings are never life-threatening, patients may present as an emergency as they can develop quite rapidly and be quite large.

Causes

- Head shaking.
- Self-trauma.

Clinical signs

- Soft non-painful swelling of the pinna.
- Scratching of the ear.
- History of head shaking or aural trauma.

Treatment

- Drainage of the haematoma.
- Bandaging of the ear following drainage has been recommended but is very difficult to achieve.
- Injection of corticosteroids following drainage

(sometimes used but is discouraged as it delays healing).
- Surgical techniques to maintain pressure across pinna whilst healing occurs.
- Reassurance to owners that it is not a life-threatening problem.

Environmental emergencies

Hyperthermia (heatstroke)

The normal body temperature of both the dog and cat is approximately 38.5°C. Dogs and cats are homeotherms and maintain this body temperature unless they suffer from hyperthermia or pyrexia. If a mammal is placed in a hot environment it will activate cooling mechanisms (e.g. panting, drinking cold water, moving to a cooler place, sweating in some species) that act to keep the body temperature close to this normal value. If these cooling mechanisms fail, then the animal's body temperature increases and can reach dangerously high levels (>41°C) and cause heatstroke.

Heatstroke *must* be distinguished from the other major cause of an elevated body temperature, which is pyrexia. In pyrexia, the animal's elevated body temperature is an appropriate response to an infection or inflammatory process and is actually a protective mechanism.

- In hyperthermia, cooling the animal is a vitally important part of treatment.
- In pyrexia, cooling the animal can place the patient under additional physiological stress.

Whenever an increased body temperature is found on examination, it must be decided whether it is elevated due to hyperthermia (in which case external cooling measures are appropriate) or pyrexia (in which case external cooling measures are inappropriate). Heatstroke is very rare in cats.

Causes

- Overexposure to a hot environment that the animal cannot remove itself from (e.g. locked in a car on a hot day, tied up outside in direct sunlight).
- Excessive exercise.
- Seizures (uncontrollable excessive muscle activity).
- Upper airway obstruction (inability to hyperventilate and thus loss of one of the dog's major cooling mechanisms).

Clinical signs

- Restlessness.
- Panting (or attempts to pant).
- Tachypnoea.
- Tachycardia.
- Poor pulse quality.
- Red mucous membranes.
- Markedly elevated body temperature (>41°C).
- Vomiting and diarrhoea.
- Ataxia.
- Collapse, coma, death.

Treatment

- Rapid-rate intravenous fluid therapy with fluids either at room temperature or slightly chilled.
- Active external cooling:
  - Wet animal's haircoat (running water will cool more efficiently than still water)
  - Clip animal's haircoat
  - Fan.
- Cold-water enema.
- Peritoneal lavage with cooled (not cold) fluids.

Aggressive cooling measures should be discontinued when the patient's body temperature reaches 40.5°C to avoid over-cooling and the development of hypothermia. Frequent and regular (every 10 minutes) monitoring of body temperature should then be performed in conjunction with less aggressive cooling measures until body temperature reaches 39.5°C.

A number of very serious complications can result from heatstroke, especially if the rise in body temperature has been prolonged. Once cooled, animals should be closely monitored for the development of:

- Disseminated intravascular coagulation
- Hypoglycaemia
- 'Shock gut' – with sloughing of the GI tract mucosa and development of haemorrhagic vomiting and diarrhoea
- Acute renal failure
- Cardiac dysrhythmias
- Pulmonary dysfunction.

If these develop, they should be treated symptomatically.

Hypothermia

This refers to a subnormal body temperature in mammals. Severe hypothermia is considered to be a body temperature below 28°C and is rare. Mild to moderate hypothermia is common. Smaller animals are more prone to becoming hypothermic, due to their high ratio of surface area to weight. Younger animals are also prone to hypothermia, as they are not yet able to generate body heat in the same way as adults.

Causes

- Severe disease/shock – especially common in cats.
- Sedation/anaesthesia.
- Prolonged exposure to low environmental temperatures.

Clinical signs

- Shivering.
- Depression.
- Slow breathing rate.
- Cardiac arrhythmias.
- Coma.
- Death.

Treatment

- Warmed intravenous fluids.
- Rewarming should only start once cardiovascular support (intravenous fluids) has been initiated.
- Passive rewarming – maintain warm ambient environment.
- Surface rewarming with circulating warm water or air blankets (Figure 21.23).

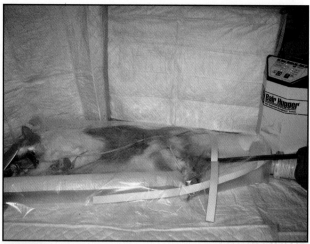

21.23   Warm-air blanket used for safely rewarming patients.

- If temperature less than 30°C, consider active core rewarming with warm peritoneal dialysis.
- Electric heating pads and heating lamps not recommended, due to potential for causing burns.
- Care should be taken not to warm the patient too rapidly, especially if they are also in shock. Rapid rewarming can worsen the signs of shock.

Burns

Burns result when intense heat (or, rarely, cold) damages the skin and subcutaneous tissues. Serum leaking from the damaged areas may lead to blister formation. Most burns seen in veterinary patients are iatrogenic (i.e. caused by veterinary intervention) – notably heat pads.

Burns can be classified by:

- Cause (Figure 21.24)
- Depth
  - Superficial – affecting only outermost layer of skin
  - Partial thickness – affecting slightly deeper layers of skin; blistering common
  - Full thickness – affecting all layers of skin
- Percentage of body surface affected.

Clinical signs

- Red, moist skin.
- Charred, leathery skin (seen with full-thickness burns).
- Pain (full-thickness burns are less painful, as nerve endings are destroyed).
- Heat.
- Signs of shock.

Type of burn	Potential causes
Dry	Hot objects, flames, friction, heat pads
Scald	Hot liquid, steam
Cold	Very cold objects, especially metals
Electrical	Chewing on electric cables
Radiation	Sun
Chemical	Caustic soda, paint stripper

21.24   Burns and potential causes.

Treatment

- Removing of the source of the problem, or moving the patient away from the source (taking care there is no risk to humans).
- Dousing the area in cold water for a minimum of 10 minutes (care should be taken not to overcool the patient and cause hypothermia).
- Very gently clipping the fur over a large area around the burn (burns can often be much larger than first thought).
- Covering the area, once cooled, with sterile non-adherent dressing or cling film.
- Analgesia.
- Elizabethan collar to prevent further self-trauma.
- Intravenous fluid therapy to treat concurrent shock.

WARNING

With electrical burns or electrocution, ensure that the electrical source is turned off before approaching patient. Do not put yourself at risk of being electrocuted – remember that both metal and water are good conductors of electricity.

Smoke inhalation

Animals are occasionally seen for evaluation and treatment of smoke inhalation after being trapped in fires.

Clinical signs

- Cough.
- Dyspnoea.
- Nasal discharge.
- Singed whiskers/evidence of burns.
- Brick-red mucous membranes if carbon monoxide has been inhaled.
- Neurological signs – may occur up to several days after smoke inhalation.

Diagnostic aids

- Arterial blood gas analysis.
- Co-oximetry.
- Thoracic radiographs.
- Pulse oximetry less useful.

Treatment

- Oxygen therapy.
- Supportive care.

Toxicological emergencies

A large number of substances may poison animals. Owners of animals with an acute onset of clinical signs often query whether their animal could have been poisoned. Although this may occur, malicious poisoning is rare.

Due to the large number of potential toxins and the wide variety of clinical signs exhibited, poisoning is a differential diagnosis for many emergency patients.

All substances have the potential to be toxic if given in the wrong amount or at the wrong time. Figure 21.25

Type of toxin	Examples
Veterinary prescription drugs	Insulin, NSAIDs, phenobarbital
Human prescription drugs	NSAIDs, human chemotherapy drugs, warfarin, human heart or asthma medication
Human recreational drugs	Cannabis, Ecstasy, cocaine
Human foodstuffs	Chocolate, onions, raisins
Household chemicals	Bleach, oven cleaner, antifreeze, paint
Garden chemicals	Herbicides, pesticides, molluscicides, rodenticides
Plants	Easter lily, foxglove

21.25 Categories of common toxicities, with examples.

summarizes the types of toxins that may be encountered. Toxins are most commonly ingested but may also be inhaled (e.g. carbon monoxide) or absorbed through the skin, e.g. permethrin toxicity in cats.

History taking for the suspected poisoned patient

Poisoning is more likely to be seen in certain groups of patients:

- Young dogs (due to their tendency to eat indiscriminately)
- Cats (many chemicals and drugs are not adequately detoxified by the feline liver)
- Animals that are free-ranging on farmland or wasteland where chemicals are stored or used.

Sensitive questioning is required as some owners may not wish to reveal what substances their pet has had access to or may not even know that a substance was toxic to their pet. If poisoning is suspected, the following questions should be asked.

Questions for suspected poisonings

- Is the pet on any medication? If so, when did it receive its last dose? How much did it receive?
- Has the pet been given any human medications? If so, what and how much?
- Has the pet had access to any human medications? If so, what?
- Has the pet eaten any human foodstuffs recently? If so, what?
- What chemical products are kept in the home? Garage? Garden? Is there any way the pet could have had access to them?
- Does the pet have access to any farmland, parkland or industrial land? Can it be checked whether any chemicals are stored or used regularly there?
- Has the pet had any access to illegal substances? (Reassure the owner that this information is given in confidence.)
- Has there been any building work or decorating at home with any unusual substances left around?
- Has the pet eaten anything unusual recently?
- Has there been anything on the pet's coat recently that it may have ingested while grooming?

If an owner has witnessed a pet eating a potential toxin, they should be asked to bring as much information as possible about the toxin to the practice. This could include any packaging and an idea of how much of the substance might have been ingested.

Veterinary Poisons Information Service

The VPIS is a 24-hour subscription-based helpline that supplies clinical information on possible animal toxicities. Practices must be registered to use the service and on calling will be asked for an identification number before information is supplied. The more detail it is possible to give the helpline, the more likely they are to be able to provide an accurate answer concerning possible complications and treatment for the toxicity.

Clinical signs

Toxicities can lead to a huge variety of different clinical presentations, but common clinical signs of poisoning include:

- Gastrointestinal signs
  - Profuse salivation
  - Vomiting
  - Diarrhoea
- Neurological signs
  - Behavioural change
  - Ataxia
  - Seizures
  - Collapse and coma
- Bleeding
- Unconsciousness and death.

The clinical signs and suggested treatments for some of the more common toxicities seen in the UK are summarized in Figure 21.26.

Diagnostic aids

- Haematology and biochemistry.
- Urinalysis (especially sediment examination).
- Clotting profile (for suspected rodenticide).
- Any vomit, faeces and urine produced should be kept and frozen in case it is required for future toxicological investigation.

Stabilization and treatment

The key aims in initial stabilization of any poisoned patient are to:

- Identify the poison and the amount ingested as accurately as possible

Toxin	Toxic dose (if known)	Principal clinical signs	Suggested treatment
Paracetamol	Cat 50–100 mg/kg Dog >200 mg/kg	Cyanosis (muddy mucous membranes), respiratory distress, facial swelling (cat), liver failure (especially dog)	Induction of emesis. N-acetylcysteine orally or i.v. Ascorbic acid orally Cimetidine i.v.
Ibuprofen	GI signs: Cat >50 mg/kg Dog >100 mg/kg Renal signs: >300 mg/kg	Gastric ulceration, vomiting, renal failure	Induction of emesis. Activated charcoal. Intravenous fluid therapy. Gastroprotectant drugs (e.g. H_2-blockers, omeprazole)
Anticoagulant rodenticides	Variable, depending on product	Haemorrhage – commonly starts 5–7 days following ingestion of toxin	Induction of emesis. Activated charcoal. Vitamin K (s.c. or orally). Whole blood or plasma transfusion
Metaldehyde (slug bait)	Median lethal dose (LD_{50}): Dog 210–600 mg/kg Cat 207 mg/kg	Severe seizures, depression, vomiting and diarrhoea, hyperthermia, metabolic acidosis	Gastric lavage. Activated charcoal. Control seizures. Cool
Organophosphates/ carbamate insecticides	Variable, depending on product	Salivation, lacrimation, urination, vomiting and diarrhoea, muscle tetany (twitching), depression	Activated charcoal. Prevent further grooming. Bathe (if topical exposure). Atropine. 2-PAM
Ethylene glycol (antifreeze)	Cat 1.5 ml/kg Dog 6.6 ml/kg	Vomiting, depression, ataxia, dehydration, oliguric renal failure	Induction of emesis. Intravenous fluid therapy. Administration of ethanol (alcohol). 4-methylpyrazole (specific antidote. for use in dogs)
Theobromine (chocolate)	Dog 250–500 mg/kg (NB 2.25 oz (64 g) cooking chocolate or 20 oz (560 g) of milk chocolate may be toxic in a 10 kg dog)	Restlessness, panting, vomiting, tachycardia, cardiac arrhythmias	Induction of emesis. Activated charcoal. Arrhythmia treatment
Paraquat (weedkiller)	LD_{50} 25–50 mg/kg	Vomiting, renal and hepatic signs, dyspnoea (pulmonary fibrosis)	No specific treatment. Supportive care
Easter lily	Unknown – toxic to cat	Acute renal failure	Supportive care
Permethrin (found in some over-the-counter flea treatments)	Toxic to cat – even small amounts topically can cause clinical signs	Twitching, muscular tremors, seizures	Heavy sedation/anaesthesia to control seizures required. Supportive care

21.26 Toxic dose, clinical signs and suggested treatments for some of the commoner toxicities seen in small animals in the UK.

- Prevent further absorption of the poison
- Treat any signs that develop symptomatically
- Administer any antidote or specific treatment (under the direction of a veterinary surgeon).

Preventing further absorption

Emetics

If an owner suspects that their animal has been poisoned, they should be asked to bring it to the practice immediately so that vomiting can be induced in a safe environment. Some owners may wish to try and induce vomiting at home but this is not recommended. Vomiting can be induced using a number of different emetics (Figure 21.27) under the direction of a veterinary surgeon.

Agent	Species	Dose	Route
Apomorphine	Dog	0.04–0.08 mg/kg	In conjunctival sac, s.c., i.m. or i.v.
Xylazine	Cat	1.1 mg/kg	i.m.
Washing soda crystals	Dog	1 crystal in small dog; 2 crystals in medium to large dog	Oral

21.27 Recommended compounds for induction of emesis.

Contraindications to emetics

Situations where vomiting should *not* be induced include:

- Where the toxin is a caustic or acidic substance or a volatile petroleum product that could cause further damage to tissues when it is vomited
- Where the patient is depressed or seizuring when there is a high risk of aspiration
- In species unable to vomit (e.g. rat).

When the administration of an emetic is contraindicated, gastric lavage may be employed. The animal is anaesthetized and the airway protected with a cuffed endotracheal tube.

Activated charcoal

Activated charcoal is administered in many patients following induction of emesis, as it adsorbs many toxins within the gastrointestinal tract and prevents further absorption of any remaining toxin. Some dogs will willingly eat activated charcoal mixed with food; in other patients the activated charcoal may have to be delivered by stomach tube. With some toxins, it is recommended that a dose of activated charcoal is repeated every 6 hours for 2–3 days.

Topical toxins

In patients where the toxin is on the skin (e.g. flea products, paint, creosote), the following steps should be followed:

- Inform the veterinary surgeon (drug treatments may be available for the toxicity seen with some flea products)
- Fit the patient with an Elizabethan collar to prevent any grooming and possible ingestion of the toxin
- Treat any systemic signs symptomatically
- Wear gloves

- Remove the contamination with a combination of grooming, clipping and bathing. Do not cool the patient too much while bathing it. Rinse the patient with copious amounts of warmed water. Specialist cleansers such as Swarfega are required for the removal of oily compounds such as creosote.

Symptomatic treatment

Most patients are treated symptomatically. The patient's cardiovascular, respiratory and neurological status and body temperature should be carefully monitored. Key treatments include:

- Intravenous fluid therapy to maintain intravascular volume and prevent dehydration
- Maintenance of normal body temperature
- Sedative or anti-seizure medication if neurological signs present.

Specific treatment

Specific treatments (antidotes) are available for only a small number of toxins. Some examples are given in Figure 21.26. It is only recommended that they are used if it is *known* that the toxin has been ingested. Antidotes may be expensive and may not be easily available in veterinary general practice.

Adder bites

The European Adder (*Viperis berus)* is the only native venomous snake present within the UK. Depending on geographical location, adder bites are not uncommon in dogs, especially in the warmer summer weather. Most bites occur on the limbs or muzzle. The incident is rarely witnessed by the owners as adders are very shy. The bites are rarely fatal.

Clinical signs

- Rapid swelling of bitten area.
- Fang marks may be present but are often difficult to identify.
- Depression.
- Rarely, distributive (anaphylactic) shock may occur.

Treatment

- Wound management – the adder bite should be treated as any other puncture wound.
- Fluid therapy if signs of shock are present.
- Medical treatment such as antihistamines.
- Cage rest.
- Antivenom if available.
- Techniques such as tourniquets, cutting the wound or attempting to suck the venom out are not recommended.

Insect stings (including bee and wasp)

Insect stings are a relatively common emergency. Although not life-threatening, they can be intensely irritating to the pet and distressing to the owner. They occur most commonly on the limbs or in the oral region. Rarely, if an animal is stung deep within the oropharynx, the associated swelling causes a degree of respiratory tract obstruction that may require emergency intervention.

Clinical signs

- Swelling and redness of bitten area.
- Pain.
- Pawing at mouth or chewing at limb.
- Development of distributive (anaphylactic) shock:
  - Tachycardia
  - Collapse
  - Dyspnoea
  - Vomiting
  - Seizures.

Treatment

- Local application of ice to reduce swelling.
- Antihistamines.
- Corticosteroids.
- Intravenous fluid therapy if signs of shock are present.

Toad poisoning

Toad poisoning that may be fatal occurs in the southern USA. In the UK, dogs will occasionally pick up and chew toads but, whilst this may result in local oral irritation and hypersalivation, it is not a life-threatening toxicity and is self-limiting. If the patient will allow, the mouth may be flushed with saline to speed resolution of signs.

Traumatic emergencies

Haemorrhage

Haemorrhage is defined as a loss of blood from the vessels. If haemorrhage is severe it leads to hypovolaemic shock and death. It is difficult to judge the severity of the haemorrhage simply from observing the amount of blood lost. The severity of the situation is best assessed by examining the animal's cardiovascular system parameters and assessing the patient for signs of shock. The principles of assessment and management of haemorrhage can be applied to all species.

Haemorrhage may be classified both by its location and by the type of vessel damaged:

- **External haemorrhage** occurs from wounds and is easily visible
- **Internal haemorrhage** may not be immediately obvious. Internal haemorrhage can occur in the thoracic or abdominal cavities, the gastrointestinal or urinary tract or in the muscle around a fracture site. Internal haemorrhage may be seen with:
  - Trauma
  - Clotting problems
  - Abnormalities of the internal organs, especially tumours.

Haemorrhage may occur from arteries, veins and/or capillaries:

- **Arterial bleeding** consists of bright red blood that spurts from the wound. It requires prompt recognition and urgent action to prevent significant blood loss. Haemorrhage from a major artery is seen uncommonly but can result in rapid blood loss and death

- **Venous and capillary bleeding** both consist of darker red blood that oozes rather than spurts from the wound. Differentiating between venous and capillary bleeding is often not possible and is rarely a clinically useful distinction.

In practice, most haemorrhage is a mixture of bleeding from different types of vessels. As the volume of blood lost can rarely be measured accurately, it is vital to assess the animal's perfusion parameters regularly. This gives an indication of the volume and rate of blood loss by the effect that it is having on the cardiovascular system (presence and severity of hypovolaemic shock). It also guides treatment (fluid therapy, see Chapter 22). Another useful assessment is the serial measurement of packed cell volume (PCV) and total solids/total protein.

Clinical signs

- Visible external blood loss.
- Bruising.
- Swelling of abdomen (if haemorrhage into peritoneal cavity).
- Dyspnoea (if haemorrhage into or around lungs).
- Melaena/haematemesis (if haemorrhage into GI tract).
- Signs of shock dependent on severity of haemorrhage.

Treatment

- Control of haemorrhage.
- Intravenous fluids.
- Blood transfusion.

Control of haemorrhage

Although external arterial haemorrhage is uncommon, prompt action is required when it is seen. The following methods may be used to control arterial haemorrhage:

- **Direct digital pressure** – ensure gloves are worn and apply pressure for at least 5 minutes
- **Artery forceps (haemostats)** – if the bleeding vessel can be seen it may be possible to clamp it directly with artery forceps
- **Pressure points** – firm pressure can be applied directly over an artery. With enough pressure, flow through the artery will temporarily stop and bleeding distal to this point will be reduced. Three potential pressure points are described although they are used rarely:
  - Brachial artery on medial aspect of proximal humerus
  - Femoral artery on medial aspect of femur
  - Coccygeal artery on ventral aspect of tail
- **Tourniquets** – with severe arterial haemorrhage in a limb it may be necessary to apply a tourniquet *temporarily* while the bleeding artery is located and ligated by the veterinary surgeon. Tourniquets can be applied anywhere on the limb proximal to the site of bleeding. Patients with tourniquets must be continually monitored and the tourniquet removed as soon as possible. If left in place there is a risk the limb may suffer significant compromise. A Penrose drain may be used as a tourniquet if a custom-made one is not available.

Venous and capillary bleeding is less likely to be imminently life threatening; however, if *continues* ▶

continued
severe, the following measures may be used to control the haemorrhage:

- **Pressure dressing** – apply direct pressure over the bleeding area using an absorbent pad and cohesive bandage
- **Abdominal pressure wrap** – if the patient is bleeding into the peritoneal cavity, an abdominal pressure wrap ('belly wrap') can be placed (see Figure 21.12). The increase in intra-abdominal pressure can aid haemostasis.

Wounds

Wounds are common emergencies. Most wounds are minor and do not put the animal at significant risk. However, some wounds can be life-threatening, especially if they are associated with significant blood loss or if they occur to the chest or abdomen and cause significant damage to underlying structures. The seriousness of a wound can be difficult to judge from its external appearance. An assessment of the animal's cardiovascular and respiratory systems gives a better indication of how life-threatening a wound is. Wounds can be described as shown in Figure 21.28 (see also Chapter 25).

Classification	Description	Notes
Incised	Clean cut caused by sharp object (e.g. glass, scalpel blade)	Bleeding may be profuse, especially if wound is large or deep
Lacerated	Wound causing tearing of tissue and uneven edges (e.g. barbed wire)	Bleeding likely to be less severe than with incised wound but more likely to be contaminated
Abrasion (graze)	Superficial wound where full skin thickness is not penetrated	Embedded dirt or foreign bodies may be present
Contusion (bruise)	Blunt blow that has ruptured capillaries below surface	May be associated with deeper injuries (e.g. fracture)
Puncture	Small external wound but often associated with significant deeper damage	Often caused by dog or cat bites
Gunshot	Nature of wound depends on type of gun	Entry wound may be small but associated with possible significant internal damage

21.28 Wound classifications.

Clinical signs

- Visible disruption of skin.
- Pain.
- Swelling.
- Haemorrhage.
- Shock.

Treatment

- *Always* treat shock or any other major body system condition first.

- Cover wound with sterile dressing to prevent further contamination whilst patient is being stabilized.
- Control haemorrhage.
- Analgesia.
- Once patient is stable:
  - Clip *wide* area around wound (especially bite wounds)
  - Remove any contaminating material
  - Flush wound copiously with sterile saline
  - Dress or suture wound (depending on nature of wound).
- Antibiosis.

If any large foreign bodies are present in the wound, or if there is a chance the wound penetrates the thoracic or abdominal cavity, the patient will require anaesthesia to explore the wound safely and so that all possible complications can be dealt with if they arise. Bite wounds also require surgical exploration with extensive flushing. Even if a bite wound looks small, the tooth may have caused minimal skin damage but surprisingly extensive damage to underlying tissues. There will also have been inoculation of bacteria from the attacking animal's mouth into the deeper tissues with a high risk of infection if extensive flushing is not performed. The animal should be stabilized before surgical exploration.

Fractures

A fracture occurs when there is a break in the continuity of the bone. It most often occurs after trauma, but pathological fractures may be seen. Pathological fractures are fractures that occur with minimal trauma, due to an underlying weakness in the bone. They are most often seen with bone tumours and metabolic bone disease.

For classification of fractures, fracture healing and fracture management see Chapter 25.

Clinical signs

- Lameness (usually non-weight-bearing).
- Swelling.
- Pain.
- Bruising over fracture site.
- Wound (if open fracture).
- Abnormal orientation to limb.
- Crepitus.

Diagnostic aids

Radiographs are necessary to classify the fracture and decide on a definitive treatment plan.

Treatment

Fractures most commonly occur following trauma but are rarely life-threatening. Concurrent injuries to the patient affecting the major body systems should *always* be addressed before specific treatment for the fracture is considered.

As the pain caused by the fracture is related to movement of the broken ends of the bone, the emergency management includes:

- Analgesia
- Immobilization of fracture site
  - Cage rest
  - Dressing – this should be applied as soon as possible to limit pain and further damage. The dressing *must* include the joint *both above and below* the fracture

site. If it is not possible to place this dressing with the animal conscious or lightly sedated, strict cage rest should be employed until the patient can be anaesthetized to allow safe placement of the dressing or fracture repair. Further information on dressings can be found in Chapter 25
- Preventing further patient interference with fracture site
- Ensuring patient comfort
  - If limited mobility, consider placement of urinary catheter.

Luxations

A luxation or dislocation occurs when the normal anatomy of a joint is disrupted so that the articular surfaces are no longer aligned normally. They generally occur secondary to trauma. Any joint can be affected but luxations of the hip, elbow, carpus and tarsus are most commonly seen.

For classification of luxations, treatment and complications, see Chapter 25.

Clinical signs

- Pain.
- Swelling of joint.
- Lameness.
- Abnormal angulation of the limb.

Treatment

- Provide analgesia.
- Limit patient movement.

- Do not attempt to reduce with patient conscious.
- Inform veterinary surgeon as soon as possible. Patients usually require general anaesthesia for reduction of the luxation, but reduction may be easier if the procedure is attempted soon after the injury.

Further reading

Battaglia AM (2001) *Small Animal Emergency and Critical Care.* WB Saunders, Philadelphia

Hackett T and Mazzaferro E (2006) *Veterinary Emergency and Critical Care Procedures.* Iowa State University Press, Ames, Iowa

King L and Boag A (eds) (2007) *BSAVA Manual of Canine and Feline Emergency and Critical Care, 2nd edition.* BSAVA Publications, Gloucester

Macintire DK, Drobatz KJ, Haskins SC and Saxon WD (2005) *Manual of Small Animal Emergency and Critical Care Medicine.* Lipincott, Williams & Wilkins, Philadelphia

Peterson ME and Talcott PA (2001) *Small Animal Toxicology.* WB Saunders, Philadelphia

Wingfield WE (2001) *Veterinary Emergency Medicine Secrets.* Hanlet & Belfus, Philadelphia

Useful websites

Veterinary Poisons Information Service:
www.vpis.co.uk

BSAVA/VPIS Poisons Triage Tool:
Available for BSAVA members at www.bsava.com

Self-assessment questions

1. List the three major body systems and explain why these should be evaluated before other systems in an emergency patient.
2. What is the commonest cause of shock in veterinary emergency patients?
3. A cat presents with dyspnoea and the veterinary surgeon tells you it has dull lung sounds. List four possible causes for this. What is the emergency treatment likely to be and what should you prepare?
4. A patient has just undergone cardiorespiratory arrest. There is not a veterinary surgeon present although you have called for help. Whilst waiting for the veterinary surgeon, what are the most important tasks you should perform?
5. What clinical signs are commonly seen with pyometra in the bitch?
6. A male cat presents with a history of straining to urinate and has a large firm bladder. His heart rate is only 80 bpm. Why is his heart rate so slow? Is this a worrying finding and if so why?
7. An owner calls your practice as they are worried that their dog is vomiting. What questions should you ask to help decide if the pet needs to be seen as an emergency?

Chapter 22

Small animal fluid therapy

Robyn Taylor, Paula Holmes and Shailen Jasani

Learning objectives

After studying this chapter, students should be able to:

- **Define terms used to describe the concentration and movement of fluid between body cavities**
- **Describe the distribution of water within the body and explain how the body gains, loses and regulates water**
- **Explain the differences between dehydration and hypovolaemia, and explain how both are assessed**
- **Describe the common types of parenteral fluids available and their uses**
- **Describe the steps involved in determining fluid plans and how these differ for dehydration and hypovolaemia**
- **Calculate fluid rates for the rehydration of small animals**
- **Discuss the advantages and disadvantages of different routes of fluid therapy**
- **Describe special considerations for, and complications of, fluid therapy; and explain how patients are monitored**
- **Describe techniques for the placement of intravenous catheters**
- **Correctly monitor patients receiving fluid therapy**
- **Describe the clinical signs associated with abnormalities in blood glucose, potassium and calcium concentrations, and explain their treatment**
- **Describe the different products available for blood transfusion and their uses**

Introduction

Fluid therapy is one of the most commonly used interventions in veterinary medicine. It is frequently a very useful and effective treatment, and can at times be life-saving. However, as with most drug therapies, fluid therapy also has the potential to cause harm if used incorrectly. In order to use fluid therapy most effectively and safely, it is necessary to have an understanding of the distribution and composition of body fluids, the types of therapeutic fluids available, the different routes and techniques for their administration, and how to monitor treatment.

Definitions and chemical symbols that will be useful when reading the rest of this chapter are listed in Figure 22.1.

- **Solvent**: a substance, usually a liquid, capable of dissolving another substance (the **solute**); water is the main solvent in the body
- **Solution**: a mixture in which a solute is dissolved and evenly distributed in a solvent
- **Diffusion**: the movement of particles from a region of higher concentration to one of lower concentration so that they become evenly distributed
- **Osmosis**: movement of water through a semi-permeable membrane from an area of low solute concentration to one of high solute concentration
- **Osmotic pressure**: the pressure that must be applied to a solution to prevent the inward flow of water across a semi-permeable membrane; this is related to the number (not size) of solute particles in the solution
- **Electrolyte**: a substance that breaks down into negative and positive ions when dissolved in water
- **Ion**: an atom or molecule that has lost or gained electrons so that it carries one or more negative or positive charges
- **Cation**: a positively charged ion (e.g. Na^+, K^+)
- **Anion**: a negatively charged ion (e.g. Cl^-, HCO_3^-)
- **Crystalloid solution**: an aqueous solution of electrolytes, mineral salts or other water-soluble molecules that can pass through a semi-permeable membrane into all body fluid compartments
- **Colloid solution**: a solution in which small particles are permanently suspended and which cannot pass through a semi-permeable membrane
- **Tonicity**: a measure of the osmotic pressure of two solutions separated by a semi-permeable membrane; the two solutions may, for example, be fluid administered intravenously and the body's extravascular fluid separated by the capillary membrane
- **Hypertonic solution**: a solution (administered fluid) that contains a greater concentration of impermeable solutes than the solution (extravascular fluid) on the other side of the semi-permeable membrane

22.1 Definitions and chemical symbols. *continues* ▶

- **Hypotonic solution**: a solution (administered fluid) that contains a lower concentration of impermeable solutes than the solution (extravascular fluid) on the other side of the semi-permeable membrane
- **Isotonic solution**: two solutions (administered fluid and extravascular fluid) that contain an equal concentration of solutes

Ca²⁺ = calcium ion
Cl⁻ = chloride ion
H⁺ = hydrogen ion (proton)
HCO₃⁻ = bicarbonate ion
K⁺ = potassium ion
Mg²⁺ = magnesium ion
Na⁺ = sodium ion
NaCl = sodium chloride

22.1   *continued* Definitions and chemical symbols.

Extracellular fluid (mmol/l)	Substance	Intracellular fluid (mmol/l)
145	Na⁺	12
110	Cl⁻	4
24	HCO₃⁻	12
4	K⁺	140
1	Mg²⁺	17
1.2	Ca²⁺	2
15 in plasma	Protein	50

22.3   Approximate composition of different body fluid compartments.

Distribution and composition of body fluid

The distribution of body water is shown in Figure 22.2 and the approximate compositions in Figure 22.3. Blood volume is equal to approximately 10% and plasma to 5–8% of a patient's bodyweight. Interstitial fluid is an ultrafiltrate of plasma. This means that it contains all the constituents of plasma except protein, which is too large to pass through semi-permeable membranes. Transcellular fluid represents specialized fluids formed by active secretory mechanisms, e.g. cerebrospinal fluid (CSF), synovial fluid. The positive and negative charges must be equal in each fluid compartment in order that no electrical gradients exist, as equilibrium must be maintained within all body fluids (see also Chapter 3).

Movement of fluid between compartments

Both the cell membranes that separate the intracellular and the interstitial compartments and the capillary membranes that separate the interstitial and intravascular compartments are permeable to water. Water movement into and out of cells is determined by tonicity and osmotic pressure.

Water movement across the capillary membrane is determined by the relative **osmotic** and **hydrostatic** pressures of the intravascular and interstitial fluids. The capillary membrane is readily permeable to ions but relatively impermeable to proteins, which are larger. Protein molecules, in particular albumin, are therefore the major contributors to the osmotic pressure of body fluids; this is called the colloid osmotic (oncotic) pressure (COP). Capillary COP is typically higher than interstitial COP and protein molecules are therefore very significant in the maintenance of adequate intravascular volume.

Hydrostatic pressure drives fluid out of compartments and therefore opposes osmotic pressure. Capillary hydrostatic pressure is greatest at the arteriolar end and lowest at the venule end. Overall this means that filtration usually occurs at the arteriolar end, supplying fresh fluid to the interstitial compartment, and reabsorption occurs at the venule end.

Body water balance

Body water content represents a balance between water intake and loss. A normal, healthy animal with free access to water is able to match intake and output and thereby maintain stable body water content.

The majority of **water intake** occurs via drinking and eating; metabolism of food also contributes a small amount. Causes of abnormal water intake include changes in diet, water deprivation (e.g. due to general anaesthesia) or psychogenic polydipsia.

Fluid loss

Normal water loss in dogs and cats occurs by the following methods:

- Urination: 24–48 ml/kg/day
- Defecation: 10–20 ml/kg/day
- Respiration: 20 ml/kg/day
- Sweating: negligible amounts.

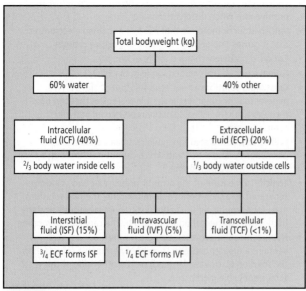

22.2   Distribution of body water into different compartments.

Fluid loss is categorized into **insensible** and **sensible** losses. Insensible losses are normal and inevitable, and they cannot be easily quantified; they are losses that occur through respiration (including panting) as well as in saliva and via the skin. Sensible losses are those that can be controlled (to an extent) by the animal and are losses that occur via urination and defecation.

Causes of abnormal fluid loss include:

- Altered urine production (e.g. kidney disease)
- Altered faecal losses (e.g. diarrhoea)
- Vomiting
- Excessive panting
- Body cavity effusions (transudates, modified transudates, exudates)
- Burns, open wounds
- Evaporative losses during surgery
- Blood loss
- Lactation.

The physiological responses to changes in the volume of the extracellular (interstitial and intravascular) compartment are summarized in Figure 22.4.

Indications for fluid therapy

The two most common indications for fluid therapy are the **replacement of fluid deficits in dehydration** and the **correction of perfusion deficits in hypovolaemia**. Other indications include the replacement of blood and blood components, the management of electrolyte imbalances and glucose imbalances and correction of acid–base balance.

Dehydration

Dehydration is a decrease in the patient's total body water content, with fluid being lost from *all body compartments*. Dehydration is classified into primary and mixed water depletion.

Primary water depletion occurs due to loss of pure water or lack of water intake. Causes include:

- Lack of water availability (e.g. forgetful owners, being trapped in garage)
- Prolonged inability to drink (e.g. jaw fracture, unconsciousness)
- Excessive panting
- Fever
- Diabetes insipidus.

Mixed water depletion is considerably more common and represents loss of both water and electrolytes. Causes include:

- Vomiting and diarrhoea: depending on cause and duration, sodium, chloride, bicarbonate, hydrogen ions and potassium may be lost
- Third-space fluid losses (e.g. into body cavities, gastrointestinal tract)
- Draining wounds.

Assessing fluid deficits in dehydration

Fluid deficits in dehydration are estimated using a combination of history, physical examination, and laboratory parameters.

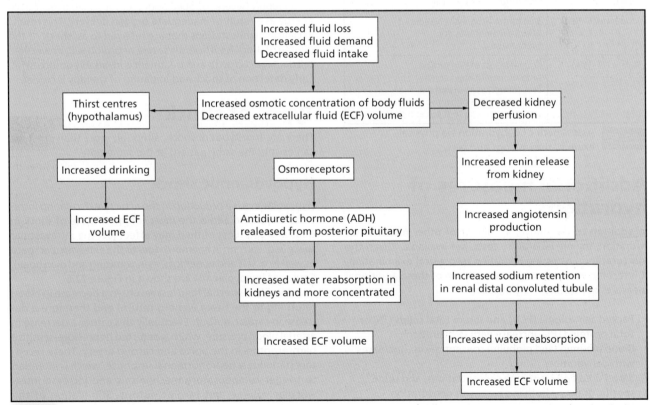

22.4 Mechanisms involved in the restoration of extracellular (intravascular and interstitial) fluid volume.

History

An indication of potential fluid deficits can be obtained by taking a thorough history. In the context of dehydration, the most important historical information includes:

- Food and water consumption
- Gastrointestinal losses, i.e. vomiting and diarrhoea: number of episodes and approximate quantities
- Urinary losses: frequency and volume of urination.

Physical examination

The physical examination parameters that are used to assess hydration are related to the fluid content of the interstitial compartment. They are: moistness of mucous membranes; skin turgor (elasticity); and presence and degree of globe retraction (sunken eyes). The perfusion parameters described later in this chapter become relevant if dehydration is severe enough to cause hypovolaemia.

There are a number of different versions of Figure 22.5 that are used to approximate dehydration on the basis of physical examination but these guidelines only provide a crude estimation of fluid loss in the dehydrated patient. This is useful for creating a fluid plan but a number of potential inaccuracies must be borne in mind. For example, skin turgor can be affected by the degree of subcutaneous fat present (with obese animals having increased turgor), and mucous membrane moistness can be affected by salivation (e.g. due to nausea).

Severity of dehydration (estimated % of bodyweight)	Progression of physical examination findings
<5%	Normal Assume dehydration based on history
Mild (5–6%)	Skin turgor mildly reduced
Moderate (6–10%)	Skin turgor progressively reduced Mucous membranes dry Eyes sunken
Severe (10–15%)	Complete loss of skin turgor Mucous membranes very dry Eyes severely sunken and dull Progressive signs of hypovolaemia, ultimately leading to shock and death

22.5 Assessment of dehydration via physical examination in dogs and cats.

Additional measures of hydration

In addition to the above, a number of other measures of hydration, mainly laboratory tests, are available. Given the inaccuracies in assessing hydration by physical examination, it is recommended to make as much use of these additional measures as possible. They include:

- Packed cell volume (PCV) and serum total solids (TS) or total protein (TP) – increase with dehydration
- Blood albumin (and globulin) concentration – increases with dehydration
- Blood urea and creatinine concentrations, and urine specific gravity – both increase with dehydration
- Short-term changes in bodyweight – reflect changes in fluid balance rather than nutritional status.

Packed cell volume and total solids/protein

Measuring PCV and TS or TP are invaluable, cheap and easy tests (see Chapter 19). Manual PCV is measured by centrifuging whole blood in capillary tubes and then using a PCV reader (haematocrit or microhaematocrit reader). Serum TS is measured using a refractometer and TP using a biochemistry analyser. In most cases TS and TP are the same, although TS measured using a refractometer may be higher, for example after colloid administration. Dehydration causes an increase in both PCV and TS or TP.

- Normal PCV in adult dogs is approximately 37–55% and in adult cats 24–45%.
- Normal TS or TP in adult dogs is approximately 50–70 g/l and in adult cats approximately 60–80 g/l.

It is important always to interpret PCV and TS or TP together, as each parameter can be affected by other changes in the body. For example, in anaemic patients PCV will be low but high TS or TP will allow dehydration to be identified. Sighthounds have a naturally raised PCV and so care must be taken when dealing with these patients not to over-estimate fluid loss.

Hypovolaemia and shock

Cells rely on sufficient delivery of oxygen and nutrients, and adequate removal of byproducts of metabolism, in order to function normally. This is dependent on an adequate blood supply (adequate perfusion). If there is a severe reduction in blood supply (severe hypoperfusion) cells are unable to produce energy as a result of inadequate oxygen delivery. This results in clinical manifestations that are referred to as '**shock**'. If the degree of shock is sufficiently severe or prolonged, irreversible cell damage can occur and treatment is invariably unsuccessful. Early detection of shock and initiation of therapy is crucial.

Types of shock

There are four types of shock, although more than one type can exist in the same patient at the same time.

Hypovolaemic shock

Hypovolaemia is a *reduction in the effective circulating intravascular volume* and is the most common cause of shock in dogs and cats. Loss of fluid may affect just the intravascular space (e.g. early on in haemorrhage) or the extravascular space as well (e.g. salt and water loss, as in vomiting and diarrhoea). Causes of hypovolaemia are shown in Figure 22.6.

Internal or external fluid loss results in a decrease in blood returning to the heart (venous return) and therefore a decrease in cardiac output. Eventually this causes a decrease in arterial blood pressure, which is detected by pressure-sensitive baroreceptors in the aorta and carotid artery. These receptors stimulate a neurohormonal response, which is intended to trigger compensatory mechanisms and increase intravascular volume and cardiac output. Stimulation of the sympathetic nervous system and release of catecholamines (adrenaline, noradrenaline) from the adrenal medulla cause

- Haemorrhage:
  - Trauma
  - Clotting disorder
  - Ruptured tumour
- Vomiting and diarrhoea
- Severe dehydration
- Third-space fluid loss:
  - Peritoneal
  - Pleural
  - Interstitial
  - Gastrointestinal
- Neoplasia
- Burn injury
- Severe polyuria

22.6 Causes of hypovolaemia in dogs and cats.

vasoconstriction and an increase in venous return to the heart, an increase in heart rate (positive chronotropy) and an increase in cardiac contractility (positive inotropy).

Other compensatory responses include: release of cortisol from the adrenal cortex that, in combination with circulating catecholamines, releases energy substrates; and sodium and water retention by the kidneys following release of anti-diuretic hormone (ADH) and aldosterone – this aims to help restore circulating blood volume to normal.

If hypovolaemia is left untreated the compensatory mechanisms may fail in time; the patient then moves from the *compensatory phase* through to *early* and then *late decompensatory phases,* resulting in shock.

Distributive shock

Distributive shock (also called maldistributive) is characterized by generalized excessive dilatation of blood vessels, which means that the blood volume is inadequate to maintain normal tissue perfusion. Causes include:

- Systemic inflammatory response syndrome (SIRS)
  - Sepsis
  - Severe pancreatitis
  - Major tissue trauma
  - Neoplasia
  - Burn injury
- Anaphylaxis/anaphylactoid reaction.

Cardiogenic shock

Cardiogenic shock results from an inability of the heart to pump blood adequately. Causes of cardiogenic shock include cardiomyopathy, heart valve disease and severe arrhythmias.

Obstructive shock

Obstructive shock is the result of obstruction of blood flow from the heart or of venous return to the heart. The most specific example of this in small animals is pericardial tamponade. Other causes include gastric dilatation–volvulus (GDV), constrictive pericarditis and pulmonary thrombo-embolism (PTE).

Hypovolaemia

Physical examination remains the most widely available means of assessing perfusion. The amount of information that can be derived from physical examination both at initial assessment and for subsequent monitoring should not be underestimated.

The physical examination parameters used to assess perfusion are:

- Heart rate (HR)
- Arterial (usually femoral and dorsal pedal) pulse quality
- Mucous membrane (MM) colour
- Capillary refill time (CRT)
- (Mentation)
- (Temperature of extremities).

Dogs

Most healthy adult dogs have a **heart rate** of 70–140 beats per minute (bpm) when examined in a veterinary practice. Resting heart rate is dependent on factors such as the individual animal's level of fitness and excitement/stress. The measured heart rate must be interpreted with consideration to the individual patient in question; for example a heart rate of >110 bpm is likely to be an abnormal finding in a calm healthy Greyhound and the same is true for a heart rate of <70 bpm in a Chihuahua.

The **dorsal pedal artery** is located just distal to the hock on the craniomedial aspect of the pelvic limb. It is useful to be familiar with palpating the dorsal pedal pulse both in terms of assessing perfusion and in other situations, e.g. obese animals, animals with pelvic or proximal pelvic limb fractures, some fractious animals.

Physical perfusion parameters are useful indicators of intravascular volume status in animals with uncomplicated hypovolaemia. They tend to change in a predictable way both as hypovolaemia progresses and as it is treated with fluid therapy. The expected findings in uncomplicated hypovolaemia in dogs are shown in Figure 22.7.

Perfusion parameter	Stage of hypovolaemia		
	Mild hypovolaemia *Compensatory*	*Moderate hypovolaemia* *Early decompensatory*	*Severe hypovolaemia* *Late decompensatory*
Heart rate	120–150 bpm	150–170 bpm	170–220 bpm
Femoral pulse	Bounding, snappy	Weak	Very weak or thready
Dorsal pedal pulse	Readily palpable	Just palpable	Not palpable
Mucous membrane colour	Normal, pinker	Pale pink	Very pale/white
Capillary refill time	≤1 second	1–2 seconds	>2 seconds or not detectable
Mentation	Usually normal	Depressed	Severely depressed
Extremities	Usually normal	Cool (or normal)	Cold

22.7 Perfusion parameters in different stages of uncomplicated hypovolaemia in dogs.

Cats

Healthy cats usually have a heart rate of 100–200 bpm in a veterinary setting, again varying with individual physiology and excitement/stress. However, cats are more susceptible to the stress of this environment and much higher heart rates (even up to 240 bpm) can be seen in cats that are completely healthy. The oral mucous membranes can appear pale in normal cats and another site (usually the conjunctival membranes) should be used to clarify the finding. Peripheral pulse assessment is not as reliable and repeatable in cats.

The common saying that 'cats are not small dogs' is very relevant when assessing hypovolaemia and the most common presentation for a hypovolaemic cat is as follows:

- 'Inappropriate' bradycardia
- Weak or absent pulses
- Pale mucous membranes
- Prolonged (>2.5 seconds) or undetectable capillary refill time
- Depression
- Hypothermia.

Types of parenteral fluid

Crystalloids

Crystalloids are electrolyte solutions that can pass freely out of the bloodstream through the capillary membrane. They are classified as *isotonic, hypertonic* or *hypotonic* based on how their tonicity compares to that of extracellular fluid (ECF) (Figure 22.8).

Crystalloid solutions are divided into replacement and maintenance solutions.

Replacement

The tonicity and electrolyte composition of **replacement** solutions are similar to those of extracellular fluid. They are an appropriate first choice in the vast majority of cases and are used in two main ways:

- At high rates to treat hypovolaemia, either alone or in combination with other fluid types (colloid, hypertonic saline)
- At low rates to replenish fluid deficits in dehydrated patients.

The two most commonly used replacement isotonic crystalloid solutions are buffered lactated Ringer's solution (LRS, also known as Hartmann's solution/compound sodium lactate) and 0.9% sodium chloride (NaCl) (normal or physiological saline). Following administration into the bloodstream, these fluids equilibrate relatively quickly with the fluid in the interstitial space (75–85% of the administered volume is likely to have left the bloodstream 30–60 minutes after infusion).

The compositions of buffered lactated Ringer's solution and 0.9% saline are not exactly the same; in particular LRS contains a small amount of both potassium and calcium. There are instances in which using one solution is more desirable than the other, but in reality in most cases it makes no clinically significant difference which is used. The small amount of calcium present in lactated Ringer's solution means that it should not be mixed with blood products.

Maintenance

Maintenance crystalloid solutions (e.g. 0.45% NaCl + 2.5% dextrose (glucose) + appropriate potassium supplementation; Normosol-M + 5% dextrose) have an electrolyte composition that is more similar to that of insensible electrolyte losses in healthy animals. There is therefore an argument for using these solutions in animals requiring maintenance fluid therapy only, i.e. once hypovolaemia and/or dehydration have been treated using a replacement solution.

However, the potassium content of maintenance fluids is relatively high and they are therefore limited to slow infusion rates. Furthermore, the majority of hospitalized patients are not 'healthy' and have ongoing electrolyte losses and reduced enteral intake. Maintenance crystalloid solutions are therefore very infrequently indicated for sole use, and replacement crystalloids supplemented with potassium are typically used throughout hospitalization.

Crystalloid solution	Na⁺ (mmol/l)	K⁺ (mmol/l)	Cl⁻ (mmol/l)	Ca²⁺ (mmol/l)	Tonicity relative to ECF
Replacement					
Hartmann's solution	131	5	111	2	Isotonic
Lactated Ringer's solution	130	4	109	1.5	Isotonic
0.9% NaCl ('normal' saline)	154	0	154	0	Isotonic
Maintenance					
0.45% NaCl + 2.5% dextrose (glucose) (requires additional potassium)	77	0	77	0	Hypotonic
Normosol-M + 5% dextrose (glucose)	40	13	40	0	Mildly hypertonic
Others					
0.45% NaCl ('half strength' saline)	77	0	77	0	Hypotonic
0.9% NaCl + 5% glucose	154	0	154	0	Hypertonic
7.2% NaCl (hypertonic saline)	1232	0	1232	0	Hypertonic

22.8 Composition and tonicity of some crystalloid therapeutic fluids.

Hypertonic saline

Hypertonic saline (e.g. 7.2–7.5% NaCl) causes plasma volume expansion, mainly by drawing water out of cells into the extracellular space down an osmotic gradient. Most of this fluid remains in the interstitial space but a proportion diffuses into the bloodstream, causing rapid and considerable intravascular volume expansion.

Hypertonic saline is used relatively infrequently but can prove invaluable in certain patients. It is used to treat hypovolaemia, especially in large/giant-breed dogs, where it may not be possible to administer isotonic crystalloids quickly enough. Hypertonic saline is also sometimes used to treat raised intracranial pressures, such as after head trauma. Recommended intravenous doses are 4–7 ml/kg for dogs and 2–4 ml/kg for cats, given over 5 minutes. Hypertonic saline must be followed by the use of a replacement isotonic crystalloid or colloid to rehydrate cells that have 'donated' fluid.

Hypotonic saline

There are two available hypotonic saline solutions: 0.45% 'half strength' NaCl; and 0.18% NaCl with 4% glucose. Sodium chloride 0.45% is used most commonly for the gradual correction of abnormalities in blood sodium concentration. Sodium chloride 0.18% is markedly hypotonic compared to extracellular fluid. It may occasionally be indicated in the treatment of severe acute hypernatraemia but this is a rare presentation in dogs and cats, and there is no indication for the routine use of this fluid.

Colloids

Colloid solutions consist of molecules of large molecular weight that do not readily leave the bloodstream and therefore increase the colloid osmotic (oncotic) pressure of the plasma. Colloid molecules generally remain in the bloodstream for up to several hours. This draws fluid into, and holds fluid in, the vasculature and causes plasma volume to expand. The volume and duration of plasma expansion depends in part on the specific colloid used – especially molecular size (molecular weight) – as well as the dose given and the species in question.

Proprietary synthetic colloid solutions are often made up in a 0.9% NaCl solution. Non-synthetic (natural) colloid solutions that are currently used therapeutically include plasma and human serum albumin (HSA) solutions.

Synthetic colloids

Synthetic colloids are used most commonly in the treatment of hypovolaemia, either when crystalloids are proving ineffective or in animals with hypoproteinaemia. Hypoproteinaemia results in reduced plasma COP, making crystalloids less useful. Colloids are also occasionally used more long term (e.g. for 24–48 hours) in animals with hypoproteinaemia or systemic vasculitis (e.g. in sepsis).

The three types of synthetic colloid solution in veterinary use currently are:

- Gelatines
- Dextrans
- Etherified starches.

At the time of writing, Gelofusine Veterinary (Dechra) and Haemaccel Infusion Solution (Veterinary) (Intervet/Schering-Plough) are the only synthetic colloids authorized for veterinary use. Both are gelatines and they have very similar properties. The molecules in these solutions are smaller than in other synthetic colloids and in general they cause the shortest duration of plasma volume expansion and are excreted most quickly from the body. Despite being unauthorized, other synthetic colloids may be preferred in certain circumstances due to greater perceived efficacy. Dextrans are solutions of glucose polymers and are commercially available in the UK, although more commonly used in the USA. They contain larger molecules than the gelatines and are therefore generally associated with a slightly longer duration of action and slower excretion from the body. Etherified starch (hydroxyethyl starch, HES) solutions are modified polymers of amylopectin (a plant starch), with the modification designed to increase their persistence in the circulation. Commercially available HES solutions include a variety of products with a wide range of molecular weights. Solutions are classified as of:

- High molecular weight, e.g. hetastarch
- Medium molecular weight, e.g. pentastarch
- Low molecular weight, e.g. tetrastarch.

In general, HES solutions cause longer plasma volume expansion and are excreted more slowly than other synthetic colloids; they are therefore considered more clinically useful. High-molecular-weight solutions have the longest duration of effect but are also associated with the greatest side effects.

The most significant side effect associated with synthetic colloids is their potential to cause multifactorial dose-dependent clotting abnormalities. Colloids also have a greater potential to cause intravascular overload. Allergic reactions have been reported, rarely. Gelatines are the colloid reportedly most likely to induce an allergic reaction, but they are generally considered to have little effect on clotting *in vivo*. Dextrans are considered more likely to cause clotting abnormalities than gelatines, and associated allergic reactions have also been reported. High-molecular-weight HES solutions are most likely to cause multifactorial dose-dependent coagulopathy; at the time of writing, tetrastarch is considered the safest HES solution in this respect. Allergic reactions occur very infrequently with HES solutions but they have been reported.

Synthetic colloid administration will affect serum total solids and urine specific gravity when measured using a refractometer.

Natural colloids

Haemoglobin–based oxygen–carrying solutions

Haemoglobin-based oxygen-carrying solutions (HBOCs) are not blood replacement solutions. They increase plasma haemoglobin concentration and therefore oxygen-carrying capacity but do not contain other blood constituents. The only HBOC authorized for veterinary clinical use is the haemoglobin glutamer Oxyglobin (Biopure USA). Production of this has currently ceased, and at the time of writing only limited stocks are available. Other HBOCs are under development and may become available in the future. Oxyglobin is a natural colloid based on polymerized modified bovine haemoglobin and is administered using standard intravenous fluid administration sets. It is currently only authorized for use in dogs but has been used extensively 'off-licence' in cats with great success.

The main indication is in the support of non-hypovolaemic anaemic patients while a diagnosis is achieved and treatment is implemented. Oxyglobin does not contain cellular antigens, so blood-typing and cross-matching do not need to be performed. It is supplied in a deoxygenated foil bag and has a long shelf-life of 3 years. Typical doses used in anaemic patients are 5–10 ml/kg at a rate of 0.5–1 ml/kg/h in cats and 30ml/kg i.v. at a rate of 0.5–3 ml/kg/h in dogs.

Oxyglobin also has a potent **colloidal effect** and it can therefore provide effective intravascular volume expansion. However, given that it is considerably more expensive than other proprietary colloids, its use in the treatment of hypovolaemia is typically not appropriate; the exception may be the treatment of hypovolaemia secondary to blood loss. The intravascular volume expansion that occurs is important to remember in non-hypovolaemic anaemic patients as there is a significant risk of fluid overload, especially in cats.

Some points to remember with respect to the clinical use of Oxyglobin include:

- Usually causes transient orange-yellow discoloration of mucous membranes, skin, urine and sclera
- Packed cell volume usually falls following administration secondary to intravascular volume expansion. It is therefore necessary to use free plasma haemoglobin concentration to monitor changes in oxygen-carrying capacity
- PCV (%) ≈ haemoglobin concentration (g/dl) x 3
- Will interfere with colorimetric serum biochemistry analysis, although the parameters affected will depend on both the analyser and the methodology
  - Peripheral blood smear evaluation is not affected
- Half-life can be dose-dependent but it has been estimated that at least 90% of the given volume will be eliminated from the body after 5–7 days.

Human serum albumin

Human serum albumin (HSA) solutions have been available commercially in different concentrations (e.g. 5%, 25%) for some time and there is some experience with the use of these products in veterinary medicine.

Albumin is a natural colloid and has a number of important functions, including:

- Responsible for the majority (75–85%) of plasma COP
- Contributes to maintaining the integrity of the capillary membrane
- Carries drugs and other molecules.

The therapeutic use of albumin has mainly focused on sick animals with marked hypoproteinaemia, sepsis or burns. At this time there remains much debate about the therapeutic use of albumin. It is also important to realize that albumin should rarely be used in stable animals with hypoproteinaemia (e.g. due to protein-losing enteropathy or nephropathy) in an attempt to increase plasma albumin concentration. The recommended approach in the management of such cases is to address the underlying cause of the hypoproteinaemia. The use of HSA in dogs has been associated with hypersensitivity reactions that may occasionally prove fatal.

At the time of writing, few general practices stock HSA solutions; however, it can usually be obtained from referral centres or pharmacies at human hospitals. An alternative approach to try and increase plasma albumin concentration is to transfuse species-specific plasma. However, this practice is generally discouraged because the albumin concentration of plasma is much lower than that of HSA solutions, which means that the volume of plasma required is comparatively much larger; this brings risks of volume overload and is expensive. In addition there are risks of transfusion reactions.

Blood and blood components
Fresh whole blood

Fresh whole blood (FWB) refers to blood as it is collected directly from the donor and usually includes the added anticoagulant without any other modification or separation. As long as it is transfused within 6 hours of collection FWB contains red blood cells, white blood cells, platelets, clotting factors and plasma proteins. Platelets and some clotting factors are rapidly inactivated during storage and it is therefore important to adhere to the 6-hour timeframe. Transfusion within 6 hours will also minimize the risk of bacterial growth in the whole blood. Whole blood can be stored in a refrigerator (1–6°C) and it is then classified as *stored whole blood*, which contains red blood cells and some plasma proteins only.

Packed red blood cells

Packed red blood cells (pRBCs) (Figure 22.9) are the erythrocytes that remain after plasma has been removed from whole blood; a unit of pRBCs contains no platelets, clotting factors or other plasma proteins. Plasma removal is most commonly done by centrifugation but can also be achieved by allowing the unit of whole blood to sit and settle, which will lead to separation. A unit of pRBCs with additive has a shelf-life of up to 42 days when stored refrigerated at 1–6°C; the exact shelf-life depends on the additive used. If no additive has been used, the cells are viable for 21 days. Once the transfusion begins, it should be completed within 6 hours to minimize the risk of bacterial growth whilst at room temperature.

Packed red blood cells are indicated for the treatment of anaemia and provide oxygen-carrying capacity.

Fresh frozen plasma

Fresh frozen plasma (FFP; Figure 22.9) refers to plasma that is extracted from fresh whole blood and frozen within 8 hours of collection from the donor. It is ideally stored at

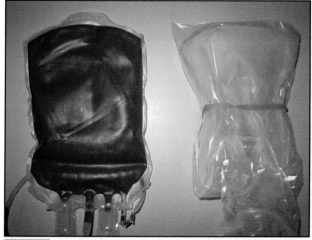

22.9 A unit of canine packed red blood cells (left) and a unit of canine fresh frozen plasma.

temperatures colder than −30°C, which allows clotting factors to be retained for 12 months; storage at less cold temperatures is likely to result in clotting factors being maintained for shorter periods. After 12 months FFP is reclassified as *stored frozen plasma* and can be kept for a further 4 years. Stored frozen plasma is not a source of factor V, factor VIII or von Willebrand factor (vWF); however, it does contain vitamin K-dependent factors (II, VII, IX, X) and can therefore be used, for example, to treat anticoagulant rodenticide intoxication. FFP should be transfused within 6 hours of thawing to minimize the risk of bacterial growth whilst at room temperature.

Fresh frozen plasma is used most commonly in the treatment of clotting factor deficiency, which may be acquired or congenital/hereditary. Plasma is a natural colloid; it contains proteins and will therefore cause some intravascular volume expansion in the recipient. Although it is generally not indicated for chronic support of protein-losing conditions (e.g. protein-losing nephropathy), plasma may be used during initial stabilization. It may also have a role in treating acute albumin loss, e.g. severe burn victims.

Clinical application: the fluid plan

So far in this chapter, the major indications for fluid therapy and the types of parenteral fluids available have been described. This section will explain how the two are combined in the clinical application of fluid therapy. A number of questions should be answered when determining the **fluid plan**:

- Is fluid therapy indicated? If so, what is/are the indication(s)?
- Which fluid(s) is/are appropriate?
- How should the fluid therapy be administered?
- How much should be given and for how long?
- Are there specific considerations for the patient in question?

It is also important that adequate monitoring is performed, both to ensure that fluid administration is successful and safe, and to assess the patient's response.

Dehydration

The aim in treatment of dehydration is to replace deficits in all fluid compartments that are affected. Dehydration is generally associated with minimal intravascular fluid loss and replacement is therefore aimed at the interstitial and intracellular compartments. Replacement isotonic crystalloids are used.

Administration of fluid therapy

In hospitalized patients, rehydration is usually performed via the intravenous route. In some cases other routes might be useful.

Volume and duration of fluid therapy

The equation that is traditionally used to calculate the fluid requirement of a dehydrated patient over a chosen period of time is:

Fluid requirement = Replacement volume + Maintenance requirement + Ongoing losses

where replacement volume = fluid deficit (ml) = percentage dehydration x bodyweight (kg) x 10.

Although there are inherent inaccuracies, estimating the patient's percentage dehydration on the basis of physical examination (see Figure 22.5) is useful as it allows the above calculation to be made.

Maintenance requirement

Maintenance fluid requirements are related to metabolic rate, which is a function of body surface area and varies with species and breed, and especially with age and size. Formulae are available for calculating maintenance fluid requirements in dogs and cats. Depending on which formula is used, different figures may be obtained. Probably the most common recommendations are as follows, where bodyweight (BW) is measured in kg:

- In animals weighing between 2 and 50 kg, use (BW x 30) + 70 ml/day
- In animals weighing <2 kg or >50 kg, use $BW^{0.75}$ x 70 ml/ day

However, the fact that there are different formulae shows that there is no definitive consensus on which is the 'most correct'. The authors therefore generally tend to use an empirical approach, with regular reassessment of the patient based on the commonly cited figures for maintenance crystalloid requirements of 2 ml/kg/h or 50 ml/kg/day.

It is important to remember that maintenance requirements for puppies, kittens and toy canine breeds are higher than for adult animals and larger breeds. In addition, maintenance requirements for overweight animals should be calculated using a reduced bodyweight. The authors generally use a range for fully grown dogs of 1.5 ml/kg/h (larger dogs) up to 4 ml/kg/h (very small dogs), and a range for fully grown cats of 2–3 ml/kg/h.

Ongoing losses

A number of sources describe different ways of estimating ongoing fluid losses (e.g. in vomitus, diarrhoea) in addition to those assumed in maintenance requirements. However there are both inherent inaccuracies and significant practical difficulties in the described methods.

The authors therefore prefer to estimate the contribution from these ongoing losses in terms of multiples of the patient's maintenance requirements. For example:

- A patient with no additional ongoing fluid losses has no additional contribution to the initial fluid plan
- A patient with occasional vomiting daily may have half a maintenance requirement added to the initial fluid plan
- A patient with multiple episodes of vomiting daily may have an extra maintenance requirement added to the initial fluid plan
- A patient with multiple episodes of vomiting and profuse diarrhoea daily may have two extra maintenance requirements added to the initial fluid plan.

The above are very much guidelines only, and ongoing losses are re-estimated on a daily basis. Although this approach is somewhat subjective, as long as ongoing losses and hydration parameters are reassessed daily and fluid rates are adjusted accordingly, the authors feel that this approach is both valid and clinically practical.

The initial fluid plan calculated for a dehydrated patient is an approximation and both the rate and the type of fluid used need to be reassessed. A range of different factors are taken into account, including:

- Changes in physical examination parameters and especially in other measures of hydration – PCV, TS, bodyweight, urea, creatinine
- Whether the animal is eating or drinking (if allowed)
- A subjective assessment of the degree of ongoing losses.

Due attention must also be paid to the provision of supplementary potassium in particular in appropriate cases. An example of calculating the fluid rate in a dehydrated patient is shown in Figure 22.10.

Hypovolaemia

The aim in treatment of hypovolaemia is to restore the effective circulating intravascular volume and thereby restore adequate tissue perfusion. Replacement isotonic crystalloids are the first choice in most cases but colloids, hypertonic saline and blood and blood components (see below) are sometimes used.

Fluid administration

Fluids are administered intravenously via one or more peripheral catheters of the shortest length but largest diameter available. Central lines take longer to place but may be necessary if a peripheral vein cannot be catheterized. Intraosseous fluid administration is indicated if vascular access cannot be established.

A 1-year-old male entire Labrador Retriever (25 kg) was presented with a 2-day history of vomiting and diarrhoea. On the basis of physical examination the dog was estimated to be 8% dehydrated.

The initial fluid rate for this dog is calculated as follows:

Fluid requirement = Replacement volume + Maintenance requirement + Ongoing losses

Replacement volume
Fluid deficit (ml)
= % dehydration x bodyweight (kg) x 10
= 8 x 25 x 10
= 2000 ml

A decision was made to replace this deficit over 24 hours.

Maintenance requirement
Given this dog's age, an estimated maintenance requirement of 2 ml/kg/h is used:
= 50 ml/h
= 1200 ml/24 h

Ongoing losses
Given this dog's presenting history, an additional maintenance requirement is added initially to allow for ongoing losses:
= 1200 ml/24 h

The dog's fluid requirement for the replacement period of 24 hours is therefore:
= (2000 ml + 1200 ml + 1200 ml) over 24 h
= 4400 ml over 24 h
= 183.3 ml/h
= ~7 ml/kg/h

If an infusion pump is not available, the following calculation is made:
A standard fluid administration set delivers 20 drops per ml
= 183 ml/h x 20 drops/ml
= 3660 drops/h
= 61 drops/min
= approximately 1 drop/second

At the end of the replacement period, the fluid rate should be reduced to meet maintenance and ongoing loss requirements. The rate should then be adjusted as necessary in accordance with regular assessment of both physical and laboratory parameters.

22.10   An example of calculating the fluid rate for rehydration.

Volume and duration of fluid therapy

Hypovolaemia is corrected over a short period of time, usually a few minutes to an hour. Traditionally, initial rates of fluid therapy for the treatment of hypovolaemia were quoted per hour. However, it is more appropriate to think in terms of *bolus administration and constant reassessment*. Fluid boluses are usually given over 15–20 minutes but in certain cases it may be appropriate to be more conservative (e.g. over 30–60 minutes). Guidelines for the use of replacement isotonic crystalloids are shown in Figure 22.11.

Fluid bolus	Species	
	Dogs	**Cats**
Initial bolus (ml/kg)	10–40	5–20
Total bolus (ml/kg):		
Mild hypovolaemia	20–40	10–20
Moderate hypovolaemia	40–60	20–40
Severe hypovolaemia	60–90	40–60

22.11 Guidelines for the use of replacement isotonic crystalloids in the treatment of hypovolaemia in dogs and cats.

In moderate to severe hypovolaemia, the following rates of colloid administration are applicable; these rates apply to all colloids currently used clinically:

- Dogs: 5–10 ml/kg boluses up to a total of 20 ml/kg
- Cats: 2–5 ml/kg boluses up to a total of 10 ml/kg.

Oxyglobin is given as 5 ml/kg boluses in dogs and 2–4 ml/kg boluses in cats. The manufacturer recommends a maximum total dose of 30 ml/kg in dogs. As mentioned previously, the product is not authorized for use in cats and there are therefore no manufacturer's recommendations; however, a smaller total dose is appropriate.

Routes of fluid administration

There are a number of routes by which fluid therapy can be administered and the most appropriate route depends on the patient's species, disease status and the length of time for which treatment is likely to be required.

Oral fluid therapy

If the patient's gastrointestinal tract is functioning, the patient is both willing and able to drink and there are no contraindications (e.g. protracted vomiting), the oral route should be considered, as it is the cheapest and least invasive. It is only appropriate, however, as initial therapy in patients that are *mildly dehydrated*. Oral fluids are also appropriate for ongoing maintenance in animals in which dehydration has been corrected using another route; recovery may also then be continued at home, which is less stressful. Some patients refuse to eat while hospitalized, and discharging these patients with oral rehydration preparations can facilitate full recovery.

Oral fluid therapy provides a wide margin of safety as the intestine acts like a barrier for selective electrolyte and water absorption. Sterile preparations are not required. Oral rehydration preparations are commercially available and may vary to some extent with respect to their glucose and electrolyte composition; the use of solutions specifically designed for small animals is strongly encouraged. A homemade substitute can be made by mixing one teaspoon of salt with a tablespoon of sugar in one litre of water; however, this solution is only suitable for short-term use as it lacks some of the other substances found in commercial rehydration solutions that are necessary for maintenance.

Subcutaneous fluid therapy

Subcutaneous fluid therapy is only really suitable for *mildly dehydrated* patients. Its sole use is inappropriate in patients with hypovolaemia as absorption is too slow due to poor peripheral perfusion. Only isotonic crystalloid solutions should be used and the total volume is typically divided between several sites. Depending on the species in question, a dose of 10–20 ml/kg is usually used and this route of administration is therefore most suitable for smaller dogs and cats and for exotic species. Suitable patient compliance is required. Fluids should be warmed to body temperature, as cold fluids will cause pain and vasoconstriction of the skin vessels, slowing down the rate of absorption.

Complications of skin sloughing, infection and pain are all potentially associated with repeated use of the subcutaneous route.

Other indications for subcutaneous fluid therapy may include patients whose owners are unable (or unwilling) to pay for intravenous fluid therapy and where owners are reluctant to leave their pets at the clinic. Subcutaneous fluid therapy is also used intermittently to provide fluid support in chronic illnesses such as chronic renal failure.

Intraperitoneal fluid therapy

Hypotonic or isotonic solutions can be used for intraperitoneal fluid therapy, as absorption is quicker and more efficient than using the subcutaneous route. Aseptic technique is required, however, to minimize the risk of infection, and care must be taken not to puncture any of the abdominal organs. Decreased ventilation can occur after administration due to the fluid within the abdominal cavity creating pressure on the diaphragm; however, this should only be transient and is usually insignificant unless excessive fluid volumes are used. Fluids should be warmed prior to administration.

The indications for intraperitoneal and subcutaneous fluid therapy are similar. Given the increased risks, intraperitoneal administration is rarely indicated in adult dogs and cats, though it can prove invaluable in very young animals and in exotic species.

Intraosseous fluid therapy

Intraosseous fluid therapy is typically resorted to when it is not possible to establish vascular access; examples include animals in severe hypovolaemic shock with collapsed veins, and neonatal animals. Intraosseous fluid therapy can be life-saving in such cases; it is usually stopped once venous access can be established in animals in shock. Suitable sites for intraosseous catheterization include:

- Proximal humerus
- Tibial crest
- Wing of the ilium
- Trochanteric fossa of the femur.

Special intraosseous needles (Figure 22.12) or infusion systems are available, but it is also possible to use spinal or hypodermic needles. Potential complications associated with intraosseous catheterization include osteomyelitis and fractures.

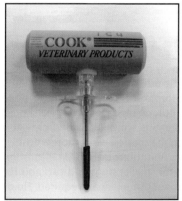

22.12

An example of an intraosseous needle.

Any fluid type and the majority of drugs can be given via the intraosseous route. Fluid is administered into the medullary cavity of the bone and absorption is as rapid as with intravenous administration. Aseptic technique is recommended for catheter placement. Maintaining an intraosseous catheter can be difficult and the catheter should be flushed with heparinized saline 3–6 times a day to prevent clot formation. The limb in which the catheter has been placed should be bandaged to immobilize it and prevent catheter displacement.

Intravenous fluid therapy

The intravenous route is the most widely used means of administering fluid therapy and is indicated in the treatment of both hypovolaemia and dehydration. A wide variety of veins can be catheterized depending on the animal in question and a wide range of catheters used.

Advantages of intravenous fluid therapy include:

- Rapid large volume fluid administration if required
- Administration of almost all fluid types, including blood products
- Patient more tolerant to long-term fluid therapy
- Constant rate of infusions can be administered.

Disadvantages of intravenous fluid therapy include:

- Learned technique is required
- Potential catheter-related complications, e.g. catheter site infection, thrombosis, phlebitis
- Patient may interfere with catheter
- Hyperosmolar fluids (e.g. total parenteral nutrition) should not be administered via the peripheral route and should be reserved for a central intravenous catheter.

Peripheral intravenous access

The most common peripheral vein used for catheterization in dogs and cats is the cephalic vein in the thoracic limb. The lateral saphenous vein in the pelvic limb is the next most commonly used site but should be avoided if possible, for example in animals with diarrhoea due to an increased risk of contamination. A variety of other veins (e.g. the carpal vein) may prove useful for short-term fluid administration in animals in which it is proving impossible to catheterize one of the more commonly used veins (e.g. in severe hypovolaemia).

Over-the-needle intravenous catheters are used most commonly and a variety exists (Figure 22.13).

Through-the-needle intravenous catheters are also available, although in the authors' experience they are used much less commonly than over-the-needle catheters.

Trade name	Company	Composition
Abbocath T	Abbott www.abbott.com	Teflon
Delta VenT	Delta Med www.deltamedit.com	Teflon
Surflo	Terumo www.terumomedical. com	Teflon
Angiocath	Becton Dickinson www.bd.com	FEP polymer
Jelco	Medex www.smiths-medical. com	FEP polymer
Optiva	Medex www.smiths-medical. com	Polyurethane
Neo Delta VenT	Delta Med www.deltamedit.com	Polyurethane

22.13 Examples of currently available over-the-needle peripheral intravenous catheters. Reproduced from the *BSAVA Manual of Canine and Feline Emergency and Critical Care*, 2nd edition.

Over-the-needle catheters

The following materials are required for over-the-needle catheter placement:

- Clippers
- Surgical scrub materials
  - e.g. three sterile gauze swabs soaked in chlorhexidine solution plus swabs soaked in spirit, or alcohol-based commercial pre-injection swabs
- Intravenous catheter:
  - Catheter size depends on the patient in question but also on the vein being used and the purpose for placement:
    - o A short large-bore catheter would be used for fluid resuscitation of hypovolaemia *versus* a smaller catheter for chemotherapy
    - o A 14 or 16 gauge catheter would be appropriate for a Great Dane requiring fluid resuscitation for gastric dilatation–volvulus (GDV), whereas a 20 gauge catheter would suffice for chemotherapy
    - o A 22 gauge catheter is used most commonly in adult cats, but a 20 gauge catheter may be more appropriate in a hypovolaemic cat

- T-connector, injection cap, or similar:
  - T-connectors or Y-connectors are of great use for connection to fluid giving sets for fluid administration
- A 5 ml syringe of heparinized saline 5 IU/ml
- Two or three strips of suitable tape:
  - The number depends on whether a T-connector (3) or a cap (2) is being used
  - The strips should be long enough to encircle the limb at least once
- Light dressing material
- Usually two individuals (it is possible in some animals for a single person to place a peripheral catheter using a tourniquet or similar device to raise the vein).

Through-the-needle catheters

These are divided into two types on the basis of how they are placed. In the first type the needle remains attached to the catheter following placement and is secured within a plastic guard outside the vein. In the second 'peel away' type, the catheter is inserted through a plastic sheath that can then be peeled away and discarded. Butterfly or winged needles have also been used for peripheral intravenous access. Although inexpensive, they are more irritant and carry a greater risk of puncturing vessel walls and are therefore not recommended for routine use.

Restraint

Depending on the patient and their clinical condition, variable degrees of manual restraint are required for peripheral intravenous catheterization. As always, excessive manual restraint is to be avoided in any potentially unstable or critically ill animal.

Sedation may occasionally be needed for intravenous catheter placement, such as in very boisterous or aggressive animals. It is far preferable to administer judicious but effective sedation in cases where it is needed than to persevere with repeated unsuccessful attempts at catheterization that may result in puncturing ('blowing') of veins and in patient and staff stress.

Intravenous catheter placement technique

1. An assistant restrains the patient.
2. Clip hair from the venepuncture site:
   - Remove hair from a generous area to minimize the risk of contamination
   - In animals with long hair/feathers, the area clipped/plucked should completely encircle the limb to prevent fur/feathers being caught up in the tapes used to secure the catheter.
3. Wash hands thoroughly to minimize contamination.
4. If using a connector, it should be flushed with sterile saline or heparinized saline prior to connection to the patient to remove the air.
5. Surgically prepare the venepuncture site:
   - Do not clean outside the clipped area, as this will drag contaminants into the venepuncture site
   - Any digital palpation of the vessel should be carried out before the skin preparation
   - Aseptic preparation may need to be very limited in an emergency situation; however, catheters placed without proper aseptic technique should be removed as soon as the patient has been stabilized and another catheter has been placed in a different vein. ▶

6. The assistant raises the vein by occluding it proximal to the site of venepuncture.
7. With the bevel of the catheter facing upwards, insert the catheter through the skin and into the vessel at an angle of 15 degrees. Ensure the barrel of the catheter is not touched.
   - Unless necessary, the catheter should not be placed too proximally as this increases the likelihood of catheter occlusion when the limb is flexed. Starting distally also allows further attempts more proximally if required.
   - It is generally helpful to place the thumb of the free hand adjacent to (but without compressing) the vein to minimize its movement during catheter insertion.

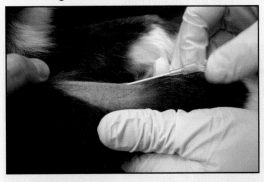

8. Blood will appear in the hub of the catheter when the vein has been entered successfully. Lower the angle of the catheter slightly and advance the catheter and stylet a little further (1–3 mm) as a single unit; this should ensure that the end of the catheter is fully inserted in the lumen of the vein.

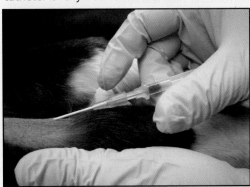

9. As long as the catheter continues to fill with blood, it can then be fully advanced over the stylet up to the hub. The stylet should be kept steady and this should be felt as a smooth movement with no resistance.

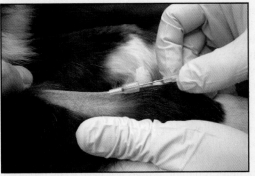

continues ▶

continued

10. Remove the stylet leaving the catheter in the vein, and attach the T- or Y-connector.
    – Before the stylet is removed, the person raising the vein should stop and move his/her thumb to apply pressure over the vein just proximal to the tip of the catheter. This will minimize the amount of blood that leaks.
11. If necessary, the leg and catheter are cleaned of spilt blood and the catheter and connector are then taped in position.
    – The first piece of tape should be placed under the catheter hub, passed around the circumference of the limb, and then wrapped over the catheter hub.
    – It is essential to make sure that the tape is not placed too tightly.

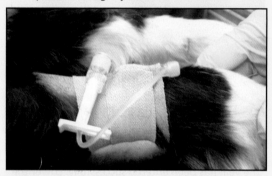

12. Flush the catheter via the connector/cap and ensure patency by feeling for fluid flowing proximal to the catheter; look for any swelling indicating perivascular fluid leakage.
13. Bandage the catheter with the dressing – again this must not be too tight and padding under and around T and Y connectors needs to be carried out carefully to avoid them digging into the skin.

Catheter care

If the catheter is not being used for fluid therapy or a constant rate infusion, it must be flushed regularly (typically every 4 hours) with heparinized saline to maintain patency. Pain during flushing or drug administration may suggest catheter failure and should prompt full evaluation and probable removal.

Intravenous catheters are observed casually many times each day during drug administration and patient interaction. At least once daily, the dressing should be removed, the site and taping examined, and the catheter assessed for patency and leakage. If the dressing becomes soiled between daily checks, it must be replaced to minimize contamination of the catheter site.

It is also important to monitor the limb distal to the catheter for swelling that may occur due to the tape or dressing being too tight. Swelling proximal to the catheter is usually due to 'blowing' of the vein and subcutaneous fluid/drug infiltration.

In the past it has been suggested that all peripheral intravenous catheters must be removed after 72 hours and another catheter placed in a different site. However, current recommendations support the view of removing catheters based on daily assessment for complications rather than after a fixed period of time – i.e. if the catheter site looks fine and the catheter is patent, it does not have to be replaced after 72 hours but can be left *in situ* for up to several more days.

Complications

Apart from failure of placement and premature occlusion or dislodgement, inflammation, thrombosis and infection are the most serious complications associated with peripheral intravenous catheterization.

Phlebitis (inflammation of the vessel wall) may be detectable as erythema (reddening) of the skin at the catheter site, pain, heat or swelling. **Thrombosis** (the formation of a blood clot in a blood vessel) may occur secondary to phlebitis (i.e. thrombophlebitis). If there is any suspicion of thrombophlebitis, a catheter should be placed in a different site and the offending one then removed. In the absence of infection, most cases of thrombophlebitis are self-limiting following catheter removal and resolve within a few days.

Thrombophlebitis in the presence of **infection** may be more severe, especially if a hospital-acquired (nosocomial) multidrug resistant infection is present (see Chapters 5 and 20). Signs of inflammation may be more obvious, possibly with cellulitis, and the patient may be pyrexic. It is important to evaluate all indwelling devices as a potential cause in any animal that develops pyrexia of unknown origin during hospitalization. Catheters should be replaced if there is any doubt.

If there is any suspicion of catheter-related infection, a catheter should be placed in a different site and the offending one then removed. The catheter should be removed aseptically and the tip submitted for culture and sensitivity. A decision to perform blood cultures and to institute empirical broad-spectrum antibiosis will be made on an individual patient basis. Some animals also require systemic analgesia and topical cooling treatment.

Central intravenous access

Long-stay central venous catheters are most commonly placed in the jugular vein (Figure 22.14), although central venous access via the medial saphenous vein for example is also used. A variety of different catheters are commercially available (Figure 22.15).

Indications or advantages associated with long-stay central venous catheters include:

- Long-term fluid administration – catheters can be left *in situ* for up to 21 days or in keeping with the manufacturer's recommendation

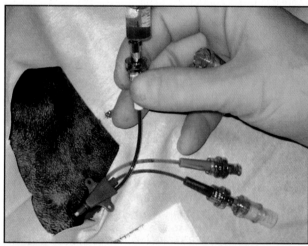

22.14   A triple-lumen jugular catheter being tested for patency before being sutured in place.

Trade name	Company	Composition
Centracath	Vygon www.vygon.com	Polyurethane
Hydrocath	Becton Dickinson www.bd.com	Polyurethane
Long-term catheter	MILA international www.milaint.com	Polyurethane
PICC	Arrow www.arrowint.com	Polyurethane
Long-term catheter with peel-away introducer	MILA international www.milaint.com	Polyurethane
Seldinger technique central catheter	Global/Surgivet www.surgivet.com	Polyurethane

22.15 Examples of commercially available long-stay/central venous catheters. Reproduced from the *BSAVA Manual of Canine and Feline Emergency and Critical Care, 2nd edition.*

- Multiple lumens allowing independent administration of more than one type of fluid
- Infusion of markedly hypertonic solutions such as total parenteral nutrition (TPN)
- Repeated blood sampling without the need for multiple episodes of venepuncture minimizes stress and trauma.

Description of the placement and maintenance of long-stay central venous catheters is beyond the scope of this chapter and readers are advised to consult the *BSAVA Manual of Canine and Feline Emergency and Critical Care*.

Complications and contraindications

Complications associated with long-stay central catheters include those described for peripheral catheters. The greater length and size of central catheters potentially increases the risks. This is especially true with respect to thrombosis and it is generally recommended to avoid central catheters in animals at increased risk of forming blood clots (hypercoagulable). There is also an increased risk of haemorrhage associated with central venous catheters and their use is ideally avoided in animals at increased risk of bleeding, for example due to thrombocytopenia or some other coagulopathy. The degree of blood loss following catheter dislodgement as a result of patient interference is in general also likely to be greater with central venous catheters.

Fluid administration equipment

Giving sets

Intravenous and intraosseous fluid therapy almost always require a fluid administration or giving set, of which there are three main types:

- **Standard (adult) giving set**: delivers 20 drops per ml of fluid
- **Burette/paediatric giving set**: delivers 60 drops per ml of fluid
  - Allows more accurate fluid administration to smaller patients
  - The burette chamber is pre-filled with the amount of fluid required to prevent accidental overadministration
- **Blood administration set**: delivers 15 drops per ml of blood
  - These are fitted with filters to prevent blood clots in the transfusion product reaching the patient.

Both standard and paediatric giving sets are available with a dial flow regulator fitted on to the tubing. The dials can usually be set to deliver fluid rates of 5–250 ml/h, with a relative degree of accuracy. Extension sets are also available to give patients more freedom and mobility whilst receiving fluid therapy. Both wide-bore and narrow extension sets are available (Figure 22.16).

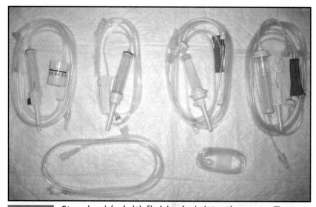

22.16 Standard (adult) fluid administration sets. Top row, left to right: wide bore with dial flow regulator; wide bore; two narrow bore. Bottom row: wide (left) and narrow (right) bore extension sets.

Infusion devices

Volumetric pumps (Figure 22.17) and syringe drivers (Figure 22.18) are a reliable and extremely useful way to deliver fluid therapy accurately. As well as controlling the rate of infusion, these devices are also usually fitted with alarms to signify occlusion or the presence of air in the giving set.

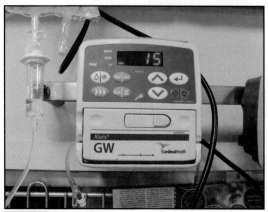

22.17 An example of an infusion pump.

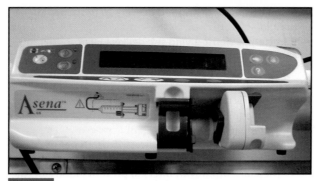

22.18 An example of a syringe driver.

Infusion pumps are very helpful when performing fluid resuscitation for hypovolaemia in smaller dogs and in cats. They allow an accurate infusion rate to be set, and most are designed with a 'volume to be infused' setting, which facilitates administration of fluid boluses. These devices are also extremely useful for increasing the reliability, accuracy and safety of more long-term fluid therapy in all animals.

The maximum infusion rate of most infusion pumps (generally 999 ml/h) is often too slow for fluid resuscitation in medium- to larger-sized dogs and their use may not be appropriate initially. Furthermore, for some bigger dogs the use of a pressure infuser (Figure 22.19) around the fluid bag can be invaluable in delivering the fluid within a suitable period of time; this can be mimicked by someone squeezing the bag if a pressure infuser is not available.

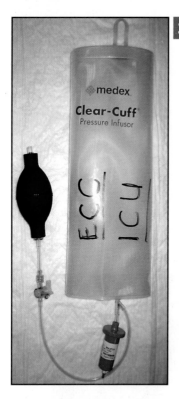

22.19 An example of a pressure infuser.

The maximum infusion rate of syringe drivers is lower but they offer a greater degree of control as the rate can be set with greater precision. They are most useful for administering fluid therapy to smaller animals such as neonates and small mammals, as well as for precise administration of other drug infusions.

Complications and monitoring

The most important complication of fluid therapy is **volume overload**, i.e. excessive fluid administration beyond that which the patient can excrete. In general, colloids are associated with a greater risk of volume overload. Volume overload results in tissue oedema as well as possible serous nasal discharge. Tissue oedema may be identified externally as chemosis (oedema and swelling of the conjunctiva) and oedema of the face or distal limbs. The most critical development, however, is pulmonary oedema, which may result in impaired oxygenation and has the potential to be fatal. Pulmonary oedema is detected by lung auscultation or thoracic radiography. Volume overload is treated by discontinuing or at least reducing the rate of fluid therapy and diuretic administration.

Air embolism

Care should be taken to minimize the risk of air entering the intravenous delivery system. This may occur prior to use of the administration set or if the bag is left empty after all the solution has been infused or during disconnection of the set.

Monitoring

Given the risk of volume overload with indiscriminate fluid administration, it is important to monitor animals receiving fluid therapy. The type and intensity of monitoring should be decided based on how susceptible each individual patient is thought to be to fluid overload.

Physical examination

Physical examination forms an important part of the monitoring. The following are assessed regularly:

- Perfusion and hydration parameters (plus PCV, TS)
- Bodyweight
- Respiratory rate, effort and lung auscultation
- Evidence of peripheral oedema (e.g. chemosis, distal limb oedema)
- Nasal discharge.

Urine output

Urine output is probably the most accessible way of quantifying fluid status, and placement of an indwelling urinary catheter attached to a closed collection system (Figure 22.20) is reasonably easy to achieve in most cases. The potential for discomfort and hospital-acquired infection should be borne in mind but urine output monitoring definitely has a role to play in a proportion of cases (e.g. very sick animals, postoperative cases).

Normal urine output in adult dogs and cats is 1–2 ml/kg/h. There is a degree of variation in urine specific gravity but normal ranges are approximately 1.015–1.045 in adult dogs and 1.035–1.060 in adult cats. Reduced urine production (oliguria) and increased urine specific gravity (hyposthenuria) are suggestive of fluid deficit and the need for more rapid infusion.

Although not ideal, if an indwelling urinary catheter cannot be used, it is possible to estimate urine output using pre-weighed incontinence pads. The patient is allowed to

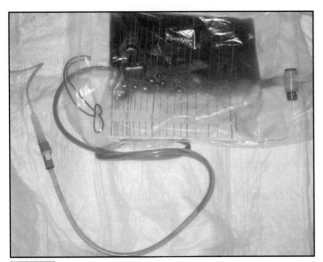

22.20 A closed urinary collection system.

urinate only on incontinence pads that are then weighed; each 1 g increase in weight is approximately equal to 1 ml of urine produced.

Arterial blood pressure

Measurement of arterial blood pressure can provide useful information, although it is important to realize that blood pressure usually does not fall significantly until later stages of hypovolaemia.

Central venous pressure

Central venous pressure measurement requires an indwelling central venous catheter and is greatly facilitated by having a transducer and multi-parameter monitor; however, it can be achieved using an improvised manometer (see Chapter 23). The pressure within the right atrium is measured and this is used as a guide to the pressure in the central venous system; it is therefore used to infer the patient's intravascular volume status. Central venous pressure monitoring is most robust using trends rather than single values, and is especially helpful in cardiac patients. There are significant practical issues with central venous pressure monitoring and it is not performed routinely outside of referral centres.

Special considerations

Heart disease

Patients with heart disease requiring fluid therapy need to be treated extremely carefully. Administration of fluids will increase the circulating volume and the diseased heart may not be able to cope with the added load, resulting in congestive heart failure. Hypovolaemia must still be treated but more conservatively than in an animal without heart disease, and fluid therapy should be discontinued as soon as possible.

In patients that require rehydration and maintenance fluid therapy, strategies such as using a low rate (0.5–1 ml/kg/h) infusion of 0.45% 'half strength' sodium chloride or subcutaneous fluid administration should be considered. These patients should be monitored very closely for signs of fluid overload.

Lung pathology

Lung pathology is a potential reason to be more conservative with fluid therapy. The lungs have extensive capacity to cope with fluid but diseased lungs may be more prone to oedema. This is a consideration for example in patients with pulmonary contusions following thoracic trauma.

Raised intracranial pressure

Causes of raised intracranial pressure include head trauma, intracranial masses and severe seizures. Overzealous intravenous fluid therapy can lead to brain oedema and thereby increase intracranial pressure further in such cases. This is most often a concern in patients with both hypovolaemia and head trauma. The hypovolaemia should be corrected as normal but then fluid therapy discontinued as soon as possible.

Chronic anaemia

Depending on the severity, animals with chronic anaemia may already be in a state of volume overload and are therefore at greater risk from aggressive fluid therapy. In addition, fluids will cause haemodilution; although the same number of red blood cells is still circulating in the body, a lower PCV is likely.

Renal insufficiency

Fluid therapy is an extremely important consideration in patients with renal insufficiency. This is especially the case in animals with acute renal failure that frequently have either oliguria (reduced urine production) or polyuria (excess urine production). Patients with oliguric renal failure are vulnerable to fluid overload (as well as hyperkalaemia), while those with polyuria are susceptible to dehydration and hypokalaemia. Monitoring of 'ins and outs' is very important in these cases, and intravenous fluid administration allows regular adjustment of 'ins' in response to 'outs'. Animals with chronic renal insufficiency may be anaemic and in some cases this can be moderate to severe. As described above, these patients may therefore be in a state of volume overload. Although this is unlikely to be a significant consideration when subcutaneous or low rates of intravenous fluid therapy are administered, it may be of importance during aggressive volume resuscitation.

Paediatric patients

Cardiovascular, renal and respiratory physiology is different in very young animals and may have implications in terms of fluid therapy. For example, puppies have less ability to concentrate their urine, resulting in the excess excretion of glucose and protein and the reduced excretion of sodium. This should be considered when managing concentrations of electrolytes and may determine fluid choice.

Very young animals have higher total body water content than adults and therefore a greater daily maintenance requirement. For mildly sick patients, oral fluid therapy should be sufficient via a tube or bottle, but the gag reflex should be confirmed first to avoid the risk of aspiration pneumonia. Subcutaneous fluid administration can also be effective as puppies and kittens have plenty of space for fluid via this route. Monitoring and maintaining body temperature is very important in young animals and the absorption of subcutaneous fluid is reduced in hypothermic patients.

For most critical cases, intravenous or intraosseous access is essential. A larger breed of puppy should have suitable peripheral vessels for intravenous access but the jugular vein may need to be used in smaller puppies and kittens. An over-the-needle intravenous catheter can often be placed in the jugular vein and maintained for a reasonable period of time. These catheters are not suitable for long-term use and should be managed in the same way as a normal central venous catheter.

The monitoring of fluid therapy is carried out as far as possible in the same way as for adult animals but can prove difficult in the very young. Other references should be consulted with respect to the differences in laboratory values in very young animals and it is also important to remember that these animals should be gaining weight daily – this is important when interpreting increasing bodyweight as evidence of rehydration.

Other indications for fluid therapy

Replacement of blood and blood components: transfusion therapy

Transfusion therapy is a growing discipline in veterinary medicine. Although still relatively confined to referral centres, the advent of national blood banks in the UK has led to an increasing availability of whole blood and blood components for transfusion. Blood transfusion can be life-saving and although it does not usually treat a disease directly, it can provide invaluable support to the patient while investigations are performed and treatment is given time to work.

As with all forms of fluid therapy, blood transfusion offers both benefits and potential adverse effects, and a good understanding of the indications for transfusion, appropriate use of individual blood components, and potential adverse effects is essential to maximize benefit and minimize risk.

Products available for transfusion include the following:

- Whole blood – fresh, stored (FWB)
- Packed red blood cells (pRBCs)
- Plasma – fresh frozen plasma (FFP), stored frozen plasma
- Cryoprecipitate
- Platelet-rich plasma/platelet concentrates.

It is important to use only the blood product that is indicated to minimize the risk of a transfusion reaction (and reduce the volume to be administered). Furthermore, use of blood components allows more than one patient to benefit from the whole blood donated. The most commonly used blood products have been discussed above. Although platelet-rich plasma is not available in the UK at the time of writing, it is expected to become available in the foreseeable future. This product is expensive and is only viable for 5 days; it must be stored at 22°C and agitated continuously.

Although component therapy is preferred and increasingly available from pet blood banks, FWB transfusion remains an important part of transfusion therapy. It is still very widely used in feline blood transfusions; although separation of feline whole blood into components is possible, appropriate storage conditions are not yet widely available. Fresh whole blood transfusion may also be appropriate for small dogs in which using a standard unit of packed red blood cells or plasma can be wasteful (i.e. as only a small proportion is actually given to the patient and the rest is discarded). At the time of writing many practices in the United Kingdom are still not readily supplied by a pet blood bank. Fresh whole blood is relatively easy to arrange in such areas using a staff or client dog and requires the blood collection bag and little else.

Fresh whole blood provides expansion of blood volume (plasma fluid), tissue re-oxygenation (red blood cells) and clotting factors.

Indications for transfusion

The two main indications for transfusion are anaemia and clotting disorders.

Anaemia

Anaemic patients generally fall into one of two categories – hypovolaemic and not hypovolaemic (i.e. normovolaemic). Causes of anaemia that do not result in hypovolaemia include chronic diseases (e.g. chronic kidney disease) and haemolysis (e.g. immune-mediated haemolytic anaemia). These patients are usually transfused if there are clinical signs caused by the anaemia or if significant intervention (e.g. surgery) is required. Treatment is with pRBCs or FWB depending on the animal in question, and is administered at a slow infusion rate, usually over 6 hours. Animals that suffer significant blood loss will become both hypovolaemic and anaemic. These patients are likely to need larger volumes of pRBCs or FWB given more rapidly along with replacement crystalloid.

Clotting disorders

Clotting disorders (coagulopathies) may be acquired or inherited. Acquired clotting disorders include anticoagulant rodenticide intoxication, liver failure, some forms of neoplasia, and severe thrombocytopenia. Inherited clotting disorders include vWF deficiency and haemophilia A (factor VIII deficiency). Plasma, cryoprecipitate or platelet-rich products may be indicated depending on the specific clotting disorder.

Blood types

Canine blood types

Canine blood types are named according to the presence or absence of antigens on the surface of red blood cells. The **dog erythrocyte antigen (DEA)** system is the most common way of classifying canine blood types. Blood types recognized under this system include DEA 1.1, 1.2, 3, 4, 5, 6, 7, 8 (a number of others including DEA 1.3 have also been defined). Other canine blood types that do not fit into this system have been described, such as the *Dal* blood type, and it is likely that more will be discovered.

Clinically, blood typing is usually restricted to testing for the presence or absence of DEA 1.1 (i.e. DEA 1.1 positive or negative). This is the most antigenic DEA blood type and the one most likely to cause a transfusion reaction. If blood typing cannot be performed, DEA 1.1-negative blood should ideally be given if available; in practical terms, DEA 1.1-negative dogs are considered universal donors.

However, dogs are not believed to have clinically significant naturally occurring antibodies against foreign RBC antigens (alloantibodies) and the first transfusion between two untyped dogs is therefore unlikely to incite an acute transfusion reaction. Hence, DEA 1.1 positive blood can be used for the first transfusion if necessary. A second untyped blood transfusion can be given safely within 4 days but thereafter anti-RBC antibodies may have formed and cross-matching is recommended.

It is best practice always to type both the recipient *and* the donor prior to transfusion, even if type-specific blood is not available and transfusion must still go ahead; this is because typing the recipient after a non-type specific transfusion can be more difficult if antibodies have begun to form.

Feline blood types

Feline blood types are named according to the presence or absence of antigens on the surface of red blood cells as type A, type B or type AB. *The vast majority of cats are type A* but type B is more common amongst certain breeds such as the British and Exotic Short-hair, the Devon and Cornish Rex, the Abyssinian, the Persian, the Maine Coon and the Norwegian Forest. There is marked geographical variation in the distribution of feline blood types. Type AB cats are relatively rare. Other feline blood types that do not fit into this system have been described, such as the *Mik* blood type, and it is likely that more will be discovered.

Blood typing of both donor and recipient is essential in feline transfusions as there is no 'universal donor'. Most (>95 %) type B cats have moderate to high levels of strong naturally occurring anti-type A antibodies; it is therefore very important not to give type A blood to a type B cat as there is a considerable risk of a severe acute and potentially fatal transfusion reaction. A small (25–30%) proportion of type A cats have some weak naturally occurring anti-type B antibodies; it is therefore less of a risk to give type B blood to a type A cat but type-specific transfusions are still very strongly recommended.

In-house blood typing

All practices that are likely to perform regular blood transfusions should invest in in-house blood typing equipment. Most methods involve applying red cells from the patient to antibodies built into the test device and looking for a reaction (agglutination) between RBC antigens and the antibodies. Blood-typing cards (Figure 22.21) are currently used most widely, but other systems are increasingly available and may offer advantages, especially easier interpretation (Figure 22.22).

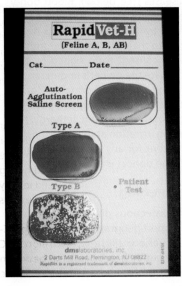

22.21 A blood-typing card showing a positive result for a type B cat.

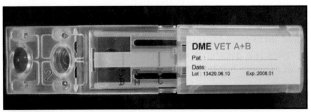

22.22 An alternative feline blood-typing system showing a positive result for a type B cat.

Cross-matching

Cross-matching is used to detect existing antibodies against red cell antigens; it detects **serological incompatibility**. Animals that have previously been transfused should always be cross-matched before receiving more blood products. Compatible cross-matches do not guarantee normal red blood cell survival in the recipient as a delayed transfusion reaction may occur. In-house testing is becoming increasingly available.

- **Major cross-matching** tests for antibodies in the *recipient's plasma* to *donor red cell antigens*. This type of incompatibility has the potential to be associated with the most severe transfusion reactions, as the recipient plasma volume and therefore antibody concentration is large (hence major).
- **Minor cross-matching** tests for antibodies in the *donor's plasma* to *recipient red cell antigens*. Transfusion reactions are likely to be less severe as the donor plasma volume and therefore antibody concentration is smaller (hence minor).

Controls

A donor and a recipient control test are usually also performed to check for any reaction between each individual's serum and *its own red blood cells.*

Preparation for transfusion and administration

It is increasingly possible to order required blood or blood components from pet blood banks. Nevertheless, it is essential to know how to administer these products correctly. A comprehensive discussion of the preparation and administration of blood and blood components is beyond the scope of this chapter. An overview is provided here and the reader is encouraged to consult the *BSAVA Manual of Canine and Feline Haematology and Transfusion Medicine* for further information.

Fresh whole blood

Fresh whole blood may be transfused immediately after collection if so required. If refrigerated for storage, the same recommendations apply prior to transfusion as for packed red blood cells. Refrigerated syringes of feline FWB must be warmed to room temperature prior to transfusion.

Packed red blood cells

Before using a unit of pRBCs, it is important to make sure that it is of the correct blood type, and to check both the unit's expiry date and its quality – if the bag is damaged or the product appears discoloured, it should be discarded. Packed red cells do not need to be warmed before transfusing a large dog, as the product will gradually warm to room temperature during transfusion; however, the unit should be warmed if rapid infusion is required or a small dog is being transfused as there is a greater risk of hypothermia. A warmed unit of pRBCs should not be returned to refrigerated storage.

Fresh frozen plasma

Fresh frozen plasma (FFP) needs to be thawed prior to transfusion. The most commonly recommended method is to place the unit in a plastic bag to prevent contamination of the injection ports, and then sit it in a warming bath set at 37°C; thawing usually takes approximately 30 minutes. If a warming bath is not available, various protocols using a microwave oven have been described. Thawed FFP that is then refrozen is reclassified as stored frozen plasma.

Administration

Dogs

All blood components must be transfused through a filter. Depending on the circumstances, it is possible to use either a blood administration set with an in-built 200 micron (μm) in-line filter or a standard fluid giving set to which a separate 18 μm filter is attached. Once blood products have been warmed or thawed they should be transfused within 6 hours to reduce the risk of bacterial growth. A dedicated intravenous catheter should be used for transfusions when possible and no medications should be added to any transfusion product.

Occasionally it is necessary to add fluid to a unit of pRBCs in order to decrease the viscosity. It is very important that fluids containing calcium, such as buffered lactated Ringer's solution, are avoided as the calcium will bind to the citrate in the anticoagulant and cause coagulation of the blood. Normal saline (0.9% NaCl) is calcium-free and can be used for dilution.

Prior to transfusion, it is best practice to check and record the patient's vital parameters (pulse rate and quality, mucous membrane colour and capillary refill time, respiratory rate and effort, and rectal temperature). These are then re-checked according to a defined transfusion protocol (e.g. after 15 minutes, after 30 minutes and then hourly) and aid in recognizing transfusion reactions. Pre-transfusion measurement of PCV and TS is also important, although they are usually known from the patient's preceding investigations.

The rate at which the transfusion is performed depends predominantly on the reason for the transfusion and the clinical status of the recipient. A typical starting rate for blood transfusion is 1 ml/kg/h and this is usually then increased gradually if there is no concern over a transfusion reaction.

Cats

Feline FWB transfusions are most commonly performed using the syringes into which the blood is initially collected from the donor. The authors usually attach two narrow-bore extension sets to the syringe with an 18 μm filter between the two sets. Each syringe should be transfused within 6 hours. Other considerations are the same as for canine transfusions.

Blood donor selection and management

There may be circumstances under which it is necessary to collect blood from donors within the practice environment. Even if blood bank products are used, it is important to have some understanding of the donor animals from which these products were obtained. Criteria for blood donor selection vary slightly between blood banks and hospitals; the following reflect the criteria used by the authors.

Canine blood donors

A dog must usually fulfil the following criteria in order to be considered suitable as a blood donor:

- 1–8 years old – some large breeds may stop being donors earlier
- >25 kg bodyweight – smaller dogs may be used for smaller units of FWB (usually direct collection of an accurately calculated volume into one or more syringes)
- Ready access to the jugular vein
- Packed cell volume ≥40 %
- Blood type (see above)
- Adequate vWF – donors are not routinely screened for vWF deficiency using vWF assays. Any dog with a history suggestive of possible vWF deficiency or of a breed with an increased incidence (e.g. Dobermann) should as a minimum have the buccal mucosal bleeding time (BMBT) determined prior to being approved as a donor
- Pregnant animals must not be used, although previous pregnancy no longer warrants exclusion.

Feline blood donors

A cat must usually fulfil the following criteria in order to be considered suitable as a blood donor:

- 1–8 years old
- ≥4.5 kg bodyweight
- PCV ≥35%.

Previous pregnancy is not a cause for exclusion in cats. Ideally indoor cats should be used; however, some centres will use cats that have outdoor access and test them for feline leukaemia virus (FeLV) and feline immunodeficiency virus (FIV) prior to each donation.

All donors

In general, all donors must receive regular preventive healthcare (vaccinations, worming, flea treatment) and be currently healthy, and should not be on medication (although the latter is discretionary). Blood donors should have annual haematology and biochemistry profiles and should be screened for infectious diseases (see below). Blood donors must have not received a previous transfusion and a good temperament is an essential trait. Ideally all blood donors should be blood-typed prior to their first use as a donor.

All donors should have a consent form signed by their owner which should clearly state the owner's understanding of consent for blood sampling and blood donation for the purpose of storage and transfusion, and any complications that may be expected (e.g. potential bruising, lethargy, haematoma formation and/or skin irritation at the venepuncture site). Clear indication of consent for any sedation and intravenous fluid therapy for feline donors is also required.

Infectious disease screening

To an extent, screening for infectious diseases depends on the risk of infection based upon geographical location and other factors. All animals are periodically re-tested. The number and prevalence of relevant infectious diseases is considerably less in dogs in the UK than it is abroad. It is therefore preferable not to use dogs that have travelled abroad as donors. Infectious diseases that may be screened for abroad include babesiosis, ehrlichiosis and leishmaniasis.

Feline blood donors are screened in the UK for FeLV, FIV, and *Mycoplasma haemofelis*. Negative antibody titres for feline infectious peritonitis (FIP) are preferred, but testing for *Toxoplasma gondii* is not routine.

Blood collection

A comprehensive discussion of blood collection is beyond the scope of this chapter. An overview is provided here and the reader is encouraged to consult the *BSAVA Manual of Canine and Feline Haematology and Transfusion Medicine.*

Prior to each blood donation, a full physical examination including temperature must be performed by a veterinary surgeon. The animal should be weighed and the PCV or blood haemoglobin concentration checked.

Dogs

The site most commonly used for blood collection is the jugular vein and strict aseptic technique must be maintained during the collection process to prevent contamination. The authors prefer the donor to be in lateral recumbency on a table but positioning should be decided on based on personal preference and especially patient compliance and comfort. Canine donors are usually not sedated for donation.

A human blood collection bag containing anticoagulant preservative (e.g. CPD (citrate, phosphate, dextrose) or CPDA (citrate, phosphate, dextrose, adenine)) is normally used. Proprietary bags are already attached to a needle when purchased; a 16 gauge diameter needle is standard. Blood can be collected successfully by gravity or via a suction system; the latter allows more rapid blood collection without the risk of haemolysis (Figure 22.23). If collecting blood via gravity, it is important that the collected blood is agitated regularly during the donation to ensure adequate mixing with the anticoagulant, thereby preventing clot formation.

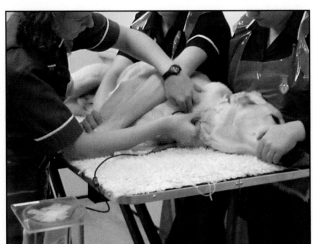

22.23 Blood being collected from a dog in lateral recumbency using a vacuum (suction) chamber.

Once the needle has been removed at the end of donation, direct pressure must be applied to the site to minimize bruising and haematoma formation. Fluid therapy is not necessary for the donor as long as no more than 15–20 ml/kg of blood is taken. The donor is then fed, and excessive exercise avoided for 24 hours.

Cats

The site most commonly used for blood collection is the jugular vein, and strict aseptic technique must be maintained during the collection process to prevent contamination. Sternal or lateral recumbency may be used as preferred by patient and phlebotomist. Unlike canine donors, it may be difficult to find a cat that does not require sedation for a blood collection. Ideally therefore the donor should not have eaten in the 8 hours prior to sedation. The authors prefer to administer intravenous sedation via a preplaced peripheral catheter and usually use a combination of ketamine and midazolam. This drug combination works quickly and it is therefore important to prepare all the equipment for blood collection prior to sedation.

At the time of writing there are no commercially available closed collection systems for feline blood donation. An open collection system is therefore used but blood collected in this way carries a greater risk of bacterial growth during storage. It is therefore preferable to collect blood for transfusion at the time it is required. This is usually carried out using a 19 or 21 gauge butterfly needle attached to a 20 ml syringe, to which the appropriate volume of anticoagulant has already been added. The maximum recommended volume of blood to be taken from a donor cat is 10–15 ml/kg and a total of two or three 20 ml syringes are therefore usually prepared in advance. Feline FWB transfusions are most commonly performed directly from these syringes without transferring the blood into a collection bag. Any syringes not being transfused immediately must be refrigerated, and all syringes must be transfused within 24 hours of collection or discarded.

Intravenous fluid therapy is usually administered to feline donors to replace the intravascular volume. The authors usually administer a replacement isotonic crystalloid solution at a rate of 10 ml/kg/h for 3 hours (i.e. total dose of 30 ml/kg). The donor cat can be fed when the effects of the sedation have subsided.

Transfusion reactions

Transfusion reactions are generally classified as acute or delayed, and immunological (due to antibodies) or non-immunological.

Acute reactions are those that occur during or shortly after transfusion. Acute immunological reactions are the most common form of transfusion reaction and include:

- Acute haemolytic transfusion reaction
- Allergic reaction
- Febrile non-haemolytic transfusion reaction.

There are a number of non-immunological acute reactions, although they are all generally uncommon. Examples include pre-transfusion haemolysis of donor cells, volume (circulatory) overload, citrate toxicity, hypothermia and bacterial contamination.

A full discussion of transfusion reactions is beyond the scope of this chapter. An overview has been included here and the reader is encouraged to consult the *BSAVA Manual of Canine and Feline Haematology and Transfusion Medicine.*

Acute haemolytic transfusion reaction

An acute haemolytic transfusion reaction is one that occurs when the recipient has sufficient pre-existing antibodies against antigens on the donor red blood cells; the antibodies bind to the antigens, causing the red blood cells to be destroyed. This type of transfusion reaction is of greatest concern in cats with type B blood that are transfused with type A; this can cause a severe and potentially fatal reaction. Clinical evidence of an acute haemolytic transfusion reaction in dogs and cats may include cardiovascular, respiratory and gastrointestinal signs, as well as evidence of red blood cell lysis (especially haemoglobinaemia and haemoglobinuria).

Acute allergic reaction

Acute allergic (hypersensitivity) transfusion reactions usually occur within seconds to 45 minutes of starting the transfusion. They are mostly mild and self-limiting, manifesting for example with erythema, pruritus and urticaria. Occasionally this type of reaction can be more severe, including full-blown anaphylaxis/anaphylactoid reactions, resulting in cardiovascular, respiratory or gastrointestinal signs that may be difficult to distinguish from an acute haemolytic transfusion reaction; a distinction can typically be made by looking for evidence of red blood cell lysis.

Febrile non-haemolytic transfusion reaction

This type of reaction describes an increase (of ≥1°C) in body temperature during or shortly after a transfusion that cannot be attributed to the primary disease or another process. A number of suggestions have been made as to the causes of febrile non-haemolytic transfusion reactions, but it is not usually possible to identify the cause in clinical cases. This type of reaction is typically mild and self-limiting.

Management of acute transfusion reactions

- The transfusion should be **stopped** as soon as there is a suspicion of a reaction and a major body system examination performed on the patient.
- If the reaction is severe, the intravenous catheter should be aspirated to remove any residual product before administering any intravenous treatment.
- A check should be made that the correct transfusion product is being used and it should be retained for possible analysis.
- Management of haemolytic transfusion reactions centres on providing appropriate symptomatic and supportive care, including intravenous fluid therapy and possible oxygen supplementation.
- Mild allergic reactions may benefit from the use of corticosteroids and/or antihistamines depending on their severity. In the case of allergic reactions or febrile non-haemolytic reactions in which the patient is stable and signs are resolving, the transfusion may be recommenced at a slower (e.g. 25–50%) rate with continued close monitoring.
- Severe allergic/anaphylactic reactions require aggressive intravenous fluid therapy and usually adrenaline administration; corticosteroids and antihistamines may be of some, albeit secondary, benefit in such cases.
- Administration of the same product should not be re-attempted in these severe cases.

Electrolyte imbalances
Potassium

Potassium is the major intracellular cation and up to 95% of total body potassium is located within cells. Potassium is essential for cell growth, nerve impulses, muscle contraction and cardiac function. External potassium balance consists of dietary input and absorption from the gastrointestinal tract, and output via urinary excretion. Internal potassium balance is maintained by the shift of potassium between extracellular and intracellular fluid. If the potassium concentration of the ECF rises acutely (e.g. due to impaired urinary excretion or accidental excessive intravenous potassium supplementation), potassium shifts into the intracellular space and the effectiveness with which this occurs determines the severity of hyperkalaemia in the short term.

Hypokalaemia

Hypokalaemia refers to a blood potassium concentration that is below the reference range for the particular analyser being used. Normal reference ranges vary to an extent between analysers and species, but hypokalaemia generally refers to a blood potassium concentration <3.5 mmol/l.

Causes

Hypokalaemia is most commonly diagnosed in animals that have a combination of:

- Decreased potassium intake due to inappetence
- Increased potassium loss due to vomiting and/or diarrhoea.

Increased urinary loss of potassium may also occur, for example, in chronic renal failure (especially cats) or secondary to medications such as non-potassium-sparing diuretics (loop or thiazide diuretics). An inherited condition in Burmese cats also results in episodic hypokalaemia.

Clinical signs

The clinical effects of hypokalaemia are largely determined by the severity. Blood potassium concentrations <3 mmol/l may be associated with muscle weakness and impaired contractility. Hindlimb weakness is often an initial sign of hypokalaemia in both dogs and cats, followed by weakness of the trunk muscles. In severe cases the respiratory muscles may be affected, resulting in the need for mechanical ventilatory support. Ventroflexion of the head is a common sign in cats and results from weakness of the neck muscles.

Severe hypokalaemia may also have major effects on the cardiovascular system. Cardiac arrhythmias can develop as hypokalaemia delays ventricular depolarization. Electrocardiogram changes associated with potassium concentrations <2.5 mmol/l include wide P waves, prolonged PR interval and prolonged QRS duration.

Treatment

Hypokalaemia is corrected most commonly with intravenous supplementation in the form of potassium chloride (KCl). A number of charts are available that provide guidelines with respect to potassium supplementation; one such table is shown in Figure 22.24. Note that 1 mEq of potassium is equivalent to 1 mmol of potassium. These guidelines are very much empirically derived and the amount of potassium

Serum potassium concentration (mmol/l)	Amount of potassium required (mmol)	
	Per 500 ml of crystalloid	*Per litre of crystalloid*
3.5–5.5	10	20
3.0–3.5	15	30
2.5–3.0	20	40
2.0–2.5	30	60
<2.0	40	80

22.24 Guidelines for intravenous potassium supplementation in dogs and cats.

delivered to an individual patient depends on the fluid rate as much as the potassium concentration. If a satisfactory response to empirical supplementation is not achieved, the actual rate of potassium administration should be calculated and used to guide subsequent therapy.

Intravenous potassium supplementation should not exceed 0.5 mEq (mmol)/kg/h (the use of enteral supplementation should not be overlooked if appropriate). In the exceptional circumstance where it is necessary to exceed this rate, continuous ECG monitoring should be used; great care must be taken to alert all staff to the use of such a high potassium, supplementation in order to avoid inadvertent bolus administration, which may be fatal. This rate of potassium supplementation must only be administered using an infusion pump or syringe driver, and the fluid bag and infusion device must be clearly labelled, e.g. *'high potassium concentration, do not bolus!'*.

Crystalloid solutions containing supplemental potassium should be mixed thoroughly to ensure even distribution of potassium within the fluid before administration to a patient. The intravenous catheter must be checked for patency as tissue necrosis can occur in the soft tissue if potassium leaks perivascularly. Regular blood sampling should be done to monitor blood potassium concentration during treatment.

In animals with mild hypokalaemia that are appetent or have an indwelling feeding tube, enteral potassium supplementation may be given. Potassium gluconate is commonly used.

Hyperkalaemia

Hyperkalaemia refers to a blood potassium concentration that is above the reference range for the particular analyser being used; this generally refers to a blood potassium concentration >5.5 mmol/l.

Causes

There are two major mechanisms of hyperkalaemia.

Decreased urinary excretion is the most common mechanism of hyperkalaemia and causes include:

- Urethral obstruction
- Uroperitoneum, e.g. due to bladder rupture
- Hypoadrenocorticism (Addison's disease)
- Anuric or oliguric renal failure
- Certain gastrointestinal disorders, e.g. trichuriasis (whipworm), salmonellosis
- Effusions

- Drug-related, e.g. ACE inhibitors, potassium-sparing diuretics.

Causes of **increased release of intracellular potassium** include:

- Insulin deficiency, e.g. diabetic ketoacidosis
- Acute mineral acidosis
- Significant cell death, e.g. heatstroke, severe trauma, reperfusion following thromboembolism, acute tumour lysis syndrome
- Pseudohyperkalaemia, e.g. haemolysis (especially in certain breeds such as the Japanese Akita), thrombocytosis.

Hyperkalaemia may also occur following excessive administration of potassium-containing intravenous fluids. Artefactual hyperkalaemia may be detected if the blood sample is contaminated with potassium–EDTA during transfer into sample pots.

Clinical signs

Although uncommon, hyperkalaemia is clinically significant; it may be associated with marked clinical signs and has the potential to be fatal. Muscle weakness can occur with hyperkalaemia as it does with hypokalaemia but it is usually only associated with blood potassium concentrations >8.0 mmol/l. The most severe and most recognizable signs of hyperkalaemia are those affecting the heart. An ECG displaying cardiac arrhythmias can be a good indicator of hyperkalaemia if serum potassium levels are not immediately available in an animal with suggestive history and physical examination findings.

ECG changes associated with hyperkalaemia include:

- Sinus bradycardia
- Prolongation of the PR interval
- Widening and bizarre appearance of the QRS complex, including sinoventricular rhythm
- Decreased amplitude, widening or complete absence (atrial standstill) of the P wave
- Tall/spiked T waves
- Asystole or ventricular fibrillation may be seen in association with cardiopulmonary arrest.

Treatment

Treatment of hyperkalaemia is determined predominantly by the severity of the associated clinical signs. Although it is important to know and monitor the actual blood potassium concentration, it is essential to *treat the patient rather than the potassium level itself*. Treatment of the underlying cause is also crucial.

In many cases **intravenous fluid therapy** alone is all that is required in conjunction with treatment of the underlying cause. Normal saline (0.9% NaCl) is usually used as it contains no potassium; however, the priority is very much to administer fluid therapy, and buffered lactated Ringer's solution is completely acceptable despite the very small amount of potassium it contains. Fluid therapy will dilute serum potassium and increase urine output, thereby reducing blood potassium concentration. In more severe cases it is necessary to administer additional drug therapy to help treat severe hyperkalaemia while the underlying cause is addressed; this is summarized in Figure 22.25.

Agent	Dose	Comments
10% calcium gluconate	0.5–1.0 ml/kg i.v. bolus over 30–60 seconds	Rapid onset of action and first line choice in a crisis Short duration of action (often 10–15 minutes) Monitor ECG during administration Does not lower serum potassium concentration but restores normal cell membrane excitability, stabilizing cardiac conduction Bolus can be repeated while other measures are used to reduce hyperkalaemia directly
Neutral (regular, soluble) insulin	0.25–0.5 IU/kg i.v.	Slower onset of action (can be > 15 minutes) Lowers serum potassium concentration by moving potassium into cells Intravenous glucose supplementation (0.25–0.5 g/kg i.v.) usually required for several hours (monitor and adjust accordingly)
Sodium bicarbonate	1–2 mmol/kg slow i.v. (repeat if necessary)	Lowers serum potassium concentration by moving potassium into cells Effect can persist for several hours Access to on-site acid–base analyser preferred

22.25   Additional drug therapy for clinically significant hyperkalaemia.

Potassium in diabetic ketoacidosis

Diabetic ketoacidosis (DKA) may occur as a result of diabetes mellitus: a relative or absolute insulin deficiency results in hyperglycaemia and in some cases excessive ketone body formation (see Chapter 20). Animals with DKA usually have complex potassium abnormalities and demonstrate the importance of distinguishing extracellular fluid potassium from total body potassium stores. At initial presentation serum potassium concentration may be normal or elevated in patients with DKA due to multiple factors, including:

- Dehydration
- Reduced renal potassium excretion
- Insulin deficiency (one of insulin's functions is to promote the uptake of potassium into cells)
- Acidaemia (leads to hydrogen ions moving into cells and potassium ions moving out of cells into the extracellular fluid).

However, this apparent normo- or hyperkalaemia may be masking a *depletion* of *total body* potassium stores which occurs in these patients for example due to inappetence, vomiting or osmotic diuresis. Once treatment for DKA is implemented, using fluid and insulin therapy, this total body potassium depletion may be detectable as hypokalaemia and potassium supplementation is then typically needed.

Calcium

Calcium is an important cation in both intra- and extracellular fluid, and it has many important roles in the body, including various cellular processes, neurotransmission, muscle contraction, blood clotting and as a cofactor for many enzymes. Calcium levels are tightly regulated, with bone acting as the major storage site. Calcium is released from bone into the bloodstream under controlled conditions, and it circulates in three forms: **ionized, protein-bound** and **complexed**. Ionized calcium is the biologically active form. The measurement of total calcium is widely available but may not reliably correlate with ionized calcium concentration. The use of albumin-based adjustment formulae to convert total serum calcium to ionized calcium is no longer considered reliable. Measurement of serum ionized calcium is recommended in all cases in which a clinically significant serum calcium abnormality is suspected.

Young dogs (typically <1 year old) may have serum calcium concentrations that are greater than quoted reference ranges for adult dogs. This is presumed to be due to normal bone growth and should not be overlooked when interpreting results from this patient population.

Hypocalcaemia

Causes

A large number of conditions are associated with hypocalcaemia. The more common ones include:

- Hypoalbuminaemia
- Renal failure (acute, chronic)
- Acute pancreatitis
- Puerperal tetany (eclampsia)
- Hypoparathyroidism
- Soft tissue trauma
- Rhabdomyolysis
- Ethylene glycol intoxication
- Transfusion of blood in citrated anticoagulant (the citrate binds to circulating calcium).

Clinical signs

Depending on the severity and rate of onset of hypocalcaemia, clinical signs may be vague and include inappetence, weakness, depression and vocalization. More severe signs of hypocalcaemia are neuromuscular and include nervous, restless or aggressive behaviour, facial rubbing, ataxia, stiffness, muscle twitching or tremors, tetany and seizures. Third eyelid prolapse may occur in cats and cardiovascular abnormalities may also be identified.

Treatment

Appropriate treatment for hypocalcaemia depends on the severity of the clinical signs and the underlying cause; the latter will affect the likely severity and also determines how long treatment will be required for.

Acute therapy involves administration of diluted 10% calcium gluconate solution as a slow intravenous bolus that can be repeated until clinical signs resolve. The patient must be monitored for bradycardia, and ECG monitoring is also recommended.

Sub-acute therapy involves administration of diluted 10% calcium gluconate as a constant rate infusion. Serum calcium concentration should be monitored daily initially during hospitalization or more frequently as dictated by clinical status.

Chronic treatment for hypocalcaemia usually involves short-term oral administration of elemental calcium and longer-term oral administration of vitamin D metabolites; a number of different proprietary vitamin D metabolite preparations are available to help maximize intestinal calcium absorption.

Hypercalcaemia

Causes

Hypercalcaemia may occur secondary to a number of disorders. A useful acronym for remembering the most common conditions associated with hypercalcaemia is HARDIONS:

- H: primary **H**yperparathyroidism
- A: hypoadrenocorticism (**A**ddison's disease): mild to moderate hypercalcaemia in a third of cases
- R: **R**enal failure: chronic or polyuric acute renal failure
- D: hypervitaminosis **D**
    - Vitamin D promotes intestinal absorption and renal reabsorption of calcium
    - Hypervitaminosis usually due to intoxication (e.g. rodenticides containing cholecalciferol, anti-psoriasis cream containing calcipotriol or calcipotriene)
- I: **I**diopathic: most common form in cats
- O: **O**steolysis
- N: **N**eoplasia
    - Humoral hypercalcaemia of malignancy is the most common cause in dogs
    - Commonly due to lymphoma or anal sac apocrine gland adenocarcinoma
- S: granulomatou**S** disease: e.g. panniculitis and angiostrongylosis.

Transient mild hypercalcaemia has also been associated with haemoconcentration, hyperproteinaemia and severe hypothermia.

Clinical signs

Hypercalcaemia can cause an osmotic diuresis, resulting in polyuria and polydipsia with possible dehydration. Signs of nausea, vomiting, abdominal pain and constipation can occur secondary to reduced intestinal motility due to hypercalcaemia. Other effects of hypercalcaemia are the result of interference with neuromuscular function and include agitation, lethargy, weakness and coma.

Deposition of calcium in tissues is a potentially very serious consequence of severe prolonged hypercalcaemia. Adverse pathophysiological effects most commonly occur in the kidneys, heart, central nervous system and gastrointestinal tract.

Treatment

Intravenous fluid therapy is the most effective means of addressing hypercalcaemia in conjunction with treatment of the underlying cause if possible. Normal saline (0.9% NaCl) is recommended as it is free of calcium (unlike buffered lactated Ringer's solution) and promotes urinary calcium excretion. Depending on the severity of the hypercalcaemia, additional drug therapy may be indicated, either at the outset or after assessing the patient's response to fluids. Furosemide is the usual first choice treatment; it is a loop diuretic and promotes calcium excretion. In a small proportion of cases further drug therapy is required, involving the use of glucocorticoids and bisphosphonates or calcitonin.

Glucose imbalances

Glucose is the end product of carbohydrate digestion. Any glucose not required for energy is stored in the form of glycogen in the liver and muscle cells, from which it is readily accessible. Once glycogen stores are full, surplus glucose is converted into fat. Blood glucose concentration is determined by a balance between insulin, which promotes glucose uptake from the blood, and its counter-regulatory hormones such as glucagon and adrenaline.

Hypoglycaemia

Causes

There are a number of causes of low circulating blood glucose levels; however, not all are usually associated with hypoglycaemia that is severe enough to require treatment. Causes of hypoglycaemia that frequently require treatment include:

- Excess circulating insulin levels: insulin-producing tumour (insulinoma) or accidental treatment overdose of diabetes mellitus
- Hypoglycaemia in neonates, juveniles or toy breed dogs and small pets with high metabolic rates
- Some liver tumours
- Pregnancy and lactation.

Other causes of hypoglycaemia include Addison's disease (hypoadrenocorticism) and sepsis, but the hypoglycaemia in these cases is usually less severe and does not typically require treatment.

Clinical signs

Depending on the severity of the hypoglycaemia, clinical signs range from mild (e.g. lethargy, weakness) to moderate (e.g. depression, ataxia, muscle tremors) to very severe (e.g. collapse, seizures, coma). Hypoglycaemia should be considered as a cause in any animal presenting for seizures or depressed mentation.

Treatment

The appropriate treatment for hypoglycaemia depends on the blood glucose concentration, the clinical signs and, in some cases, the cause. **Oral** therapy may be adequate in less severe cases; this consists of regular (e.g. every 1–2 hours) feeding of small amounts of food and in some cases sugar solutions, honey or similar.

More severe cases of hypoglycaemia require more aggressive intervention in the form of **parenteral** therapy; this is usually intravenous but intraosseous administration may be required in some cases.

Glucose is administered until clinical signs are controlled but a starting dose of 0.25–0.5 g/kg is usually recommended – this is equivalent to 0.5–1.0 ml/kg of a 50% glucose (dextrose) solution. Glucose should be diluted prior to administration as it can cause venous irritation and inflammation (phlebitis). The authors suggest diluting 50% glucose with an equal volume of any crystalloid solution.

Following bolus administration of glucose (which can be repeated), a glucose infusion is usually required to prevent recurrence of clinical signs. Some glucose solutions for infusion are available commercially (e.g. 0.9% NaCl + 5% glucose) but they can also be readily constituted. Glucose solutions for long-term infusion are usually of 2.5% or 5% concentration.

Treatment of hypoglycaemia should be guided by clinical signs and, if available, regular monitoring of blood glucose concentration. A glucometer is an inexpensive means of doing this, requires minimal blood to be taken and produces rapid results. However, it is important to try and ensure that the same device is used throughout, as different devices and models can generate different results. Electrolyte levels, in particular potassium, and acid–base balance should ideally also be monitored as these are affected by glucose levels.

Hyperglycaemia

Diabetes mellitus is the only cause of hyperglycaemia that requires specific treatment with exogenous insulin (see Chapter 20). Hyperglycaemia may be detected in other cases but treatment is not indicated; examples include other endocrine disorders (hyperadrenocorticism and acromegaly), secondary to stress (especially cats) and following seizures and head trauma.

The treatment of diabetic ketoacidosis (DKA) centres on intravenous fluid therapy, exogenous insulin administration and close monitoring of blood glucose concentrations, and close monitoring and supplementation as required of serum potassium and phosphate. Replacement isotonic crystalloid solutions are appropriate for use in DKA and both buffered lactated Ringer's solution and 0.9% NaCl may be used. There are theoretical pros and cons for each of these fluid types in patients with DKA but these considerations have not been shown to be of any clinical significance and either solution is appropriate. Most patients with DKA will benefit from an initial period of fluid therapy alone before insulin administration is commenced and it is noteworthy that fluid therapy often causes a decrease in hyperglycaemia for example due to dilution and improved renal perfusion increasing urinary glucose excretion.

Acid–base balance

The balance between acids and bases is instrumental in the maintenance of pH in the body; pH is calculated as the negative log (to the base 10) of the hydrogen ion concentration. The body is normally slightly alkaline at a pH of 7.35–7.45 (where a pH of 7 is neutral and a pH <7 is acidic). A number of terms are important when discussing acid–base homeostasis:

- **Acidaemia**: a blood pH <7.35
- **Alkalaemia**: a blood pH >7.45
- **Acidosis**: a process that pushes blood pH towards acidaemia (i.e. a process that results in an increase in blood H+ concentration)
- **Alkalosis**: a process that pushes blood pH towards alkalaemia (i.e. a process that results in a decrease in blood H+ concentration).

Acidosis or alkalosis will not necessarily result in a change in blood pH if the body is able to compensate adequately (see below). Acidosis and alkalosis may be either **metabolic** or **respiratory** depending on their origin. The following equation is also central to understanding the traditional approach to acid–base homeostasis:

$$H^+ + HCO_3^- \overset{\text{Carbonic anhydrase}}{\longleftrightarrow} \underset{\text{Carbonic acid}}{H_2CO_3} \longleftrightarrow CO_2 + H_2O$$

Compensation

Acid–base homeostasis is essential for normal cellular function as many enzymes and other proteins depend on pH being maintained within a strict range. On a daily basis the body produces large amounts of both carbon dioxide and hydrogen ions as byproducts of metabolism. Carbon dioxide is excreted via the lungs but acts as an acid (H+ donor) in solution, as shown in the equation above. Hydrogen ions are excreted via the kidneys. The body has three mechanisms for handling the daily acid load to prevent significant fluctuations of pH:

- Buffers: respond most rapidly
- Respiratory response: next mechanism to become effective; responds over minutes to hours
- Renal response: this is the slowest mechanism, occurring over several days.

Buffers

The body has several buffer systems to handle the daily acid load; the most important one is bicarbonate in a system that follows the equation above. Bicarbonate is constantly regenerated and added back to the bloodstream by the kidneys. Other buffers include haemoglobin and plasma proteins. Buffers can accept or donate H+ ions as required to minimize changes in pH. They trap the H+ ions until they can be delivered to either the lungs or the kidney for excretion.

Respiratory system

The respiratory system controls the level of carbon dioxide within the body. From the above equation it can be seen that removing more carbon dioxide by increasing ventilation has the net effect of reducing acidity, while decreasing ventilation retains carbon dioxide and therefore increases acidity. **Primary respiratory acid–base abnormalities** (respiratory acidosis or alkalosis) are the result of changes in carbon dioxide concentration (partial pressure) as a result of abnormal ventilation.

Renal system

The kidneys are able to generate both HCO_3^- ions and H+ ions: the HCO_3^- ions are absorbed into the extracellular fluid while the H+ ions are excreted in the urine. **Primary metabolic acid–base abnormalities** (metabolic acidosis or alkalosis) are the result of changes in levels of acids/bases other than carbon dioxide and result in changes in HCO_3^- concentration.

When a primary acid–base disturbance occurs, the consequences depend firstly on whether the buffers become overwhelmed. If they do, then a secondary respiratory or renal (metabolic) compensatory response occurs to try and minimize the effects of the primary disturbance on the body's pH. Causes of primary acid–base abnormalities and the anticipated compensatory responses are described in Figure 22.26. In most cases treatment of acid–base disturbances is aimed at resolving the underlying cause.

Metabolic abnormalities

Metabolic acidosis

Metabolic acidosis is the most common primary acid–base disturbance and in any individual patient a single or multiple mechanism(s) may be involved. For example, metabolic acidosis may occur in severe diarrhoea due to excessive loss of bicarbonate in intestinal secretions. However, some of these

Primary disturbance	pH	Primary change	Compensatory change	Common clinical causes
Metabolic acidosis	↓	↓ HCO_3^-	Respiratory response with increased ventilation leading to ↓ CO_2	Diarrhoea Diabetic ketoacidosis Lactic acidosis Uraemic acidosis
Metabolic alkalosis	↑	↑ HCO_3^-	Respiratory response with reduced ventilation leading to ↑ CO_2	Vomiting Diuretic therapy
Respiratory acidosis	↓	↑ CO_2	Metabolic (renal) response with increased acid secretion leading to ↑ HCO_3^-	Hypoventilation, e.g. upper airway obstruction, CNS disease, general anaesthesia, myasthenia gravis
Respiratory alkalosis	↑	↓ CO_2	Metabolic (renal) response with reduced acid secretion leading to ↓ HCO_3^-	Hyperventilation, e.g. lung disease, hyperthermia, pain, fear/stress, exercise

22.26   Causes of primary acid–base abnormalities and the anticipated compensatory responses.

patients also develop hypovolaemia with reduced tissue perfusion and consequent lactic acidosis.

In the vast majority of cases, treatment of metabolic acidosis is aimed at addressing the underlying cause rather than the acid–base disturbance itself. Typically this involves providing appropriate fluid therapy with a replacement isotonic crystalloid solution to correct hypovolaemia and/or dehydration; in some cases additional treatment is required for the underlying cause (e.g. insulin therapy in diabetic ketoacidosis).

There are theoretical pros and cons for the use of buffered lactated Ringer's solution *versus* 0.9% saline in patients with metabolic acidosis but these considerations have not been shown to be of any real clinical significance and either solution is appropriate. In exceptional cases where metabolic acidosis is severe (e.g. blood pH <7.15) and the underlying cause cannot be addressed sufficiently quickly, it may be necessary to administer intravenous sodium bicarbonate as an interim measure.

Metabolic alkalosis

Metabolic alkalosis is seen less commonly than metabolic acidosis and the two most common causes are vomiting and diuretic therapy. Excessive vomiting causes metabolic alkalosis as a result of the loss of hydrochloric acid in stomach contents, the net effect of which is to increase blood bicarbonate concentration. Potassium is also lost in stomach contents and this may result in hypokalaemia which worsens the alkalosis – potassium ions move out of the cells to compensate for the hypokalaemia and as a result hydrogen ions move into the intracellular fluid from the extracellular space to maintain electroneutrality.

Diuretics such as furosemide (a loop diuretic) and thiazides interfere with reabsorption of chloride and sodium in the renal tubules. Urinary losses of chloride exceed those of bicarbonate and there is also an increase in urinary excretion of hydrogen ions; the net effect is an increase in blood bicarbonate concentration, i.e. metabolic alkalosis.

These 'potassium-losing' diuretics also promote urinary potassium loss, potentially causing hypokalaemia that worsens the alkalosis. Treatment of metabolic alkalosis should address the underlying cause; this usually involves providing replacement isotonic crystalloid fluid therapy but also for example other medical or surgical interventions for vomiting or amending the patient's diuretic protocol.

Fluid therapy in exotic pets

Many of the concepts and principles described previously in the context of dogs and cats apply equally to exotic species. However, there are some important differences and additional points to bear in mind depending on the species in question.

Dosing of fluids based on accurate measurement of bodyweight is of even greater importance in smaller animals. Furthermore, because of the risks of excessive fluid administration, the use of an infusion device that can deliver small volumes of fluid – typically a syringe driver – is strongly encouraged.

As far as possible it is recommended to try and conform to the same approach advocated when considering fluid therapy in dogs and cats, namely:

- Is fluid therapy indicated? If so, what is/are the indication(s)?
- Which fluid(s) is/are appropriate?
- How should the fluid therapy be administered?
- How much should be given and for how long?
- Are there specific considerations for the patient in question?
- Monitoring.

This section will focus on the treatment of dehydration in exotic species. Although it is often more difficult to recognize clinically, these species may also suffer from hypovolaemia. Most hypovolaemic exotic patients are hypothermic and after fluid resuscitation has been commenced, warming is usually of paramount importance. Close monitoring is important to prevent hyperthermia. Due to the inherent difficulties in assessing perfusion in many exotic species, blood pressure monitoring (especially Doppler sphygmomanometry) can prove very useful in many cases.

The reader is reminded that providing adequate nutrition, in animals in which it is not contraindicated, is generally considered an even greater priority in exotic species than it is in dogs and cats. In addition, exotic species are frequently more prone to stress and this is an important consideration in many cases.

Fluid therapy in rabbits

Fluid therapy in rabbits is summarized in Figure 22.27 and some additional comments are made below.

Route of fluid administration	Types of fluid	Volume of fluid	Advantages	Disadvantages
Oral	Oral rehydration solution	10–15 ml/kg q 8 h	Relatively easy to do; potential to teach owners. Non-sterile solutions. Suitable for rehydration and maintenance	Absorption is slow and variable; therefore not suitable for treatment of hypovolaemia or very sick rabbits. Risk of tracheal intubation
Subcutaneous	Replacement crystalloid	Maximum volume depends on size; typically 30–100 ml Administer in two or more sites (e.g. under scruff of neck, lateral thorax)	Simple technique. Large overall volume. Suitable for rehydration. Useful for perioperative maintenance provision (e.g. neutering procedures)	Slow absorption, especially if poor perfusion; therefore not suitable for treatment of hypovolaemia or very sick rabbits
Intravenous	Replacement crystalloid, synthetic colloid, blood products	Maintenance: 60–100 ml/kg/day Hypovolaemia: suitable bolus over 10 minutes (e.g. 10 ml/kg crystalloid, 5 ml/kg colloid) Use of infusion device recommended	Rapid absorption of potentially large volumes. Relatively easy with practice. Suitable for rehydration and treatment of hypovolaemia	Painful – use topical analgesia. Potential for patient interference
Intraosseous	As for intravenous	As for intravenous	Rapid absorption of potentially large volumes. Relatively easy with practice. Reliable access to circulation in animals with collapsed or very small veins. Suitable for rehydration and treatment of hypovolaemia	Painful and requires good compliance; usually done under local or general anaesthesia. Strict asepsis required
Intraperitoneal	Replacement crystalloid	10 ml/kg	Simple technique. Large overall volume. Suitable for rehydration. Useful for perioperative maintenance provision	Absorption is slow and variable; therefore not suitable for treatment of hypovolaemia or very sick rabbits. Potential to damage intestines and other intra-abdominal structures. Not to be used if abdominal fluid or likely pathology is present

22.27 Summary of fluid therapy for rabbits

Indications

Fluid therapy may be indicated in rabbits for the following:

- Rehydration of dehydrated sick rabbits
- Maintenance of hospitalized sick rabbits
- Perioperative maintenance of healthy rabbits (e.g. routine dental treatment)
- Correction of hypovolaemia.

Assessment of hydration in rabbits is based on history, physical examination and clinical pathology findings (Figure 22.28) as described for dogs and cats. Useful areas of skin to check for loss of elasticity include the relatively hairless inguinal region, the inside of the pinnae and in males, the scrotal skin. Hypovolaemia is detected on physical examination in rabbits using the same parameters as described for dogs and cats. Significantly hypovolaemic rabbits are typically depressed, bradycardic with weak or absent peripheral pulses, and hypothermic (see Chapter 15 for normal values).

Fluid selection

Both replacement crystalloid and synthetic colloid solutions may be used in rabbits (Figure 22.27). Hypertonic saline has been used in rabbits and transfusion of blood products has also been described.

Fluid administration

Oral fluids

The reader is referred to Chapter 13 for further information on oral administration of fluids and nutrition in rabbits.

Species	PCV range (l/l)	Total protein (g/l)
Ferret	0.44–0.6	51–74
Rabbit	0.36–0.48	54–75
Guinea pig	0.37–0.48	46–62
Chinchilla	0.32–0.46	50–60
Rat	0.36–0.48	56–76
Mouse	0.39–0.49	35–72
Gerbil	0.43–0.49	43–85
Hamster [a]	0.36–0.55	45–75

22.28 Reference ranges for packed cell volume and serum total protein (solids) in rabbits, ferrets and rodents. [a] Average for Syrian and Russian hamsters.

Intravenous fluid therapy

The technique for intravenous catheter placement in rabbits is essentially the same as that for dogs and cats. Depending on the size of the rabbit in question, 22–27 gauge catheters are typically used.

The sites for intravenous access include:

- Marginal (lateral) ear vein (Figure 22.29)
- Lateral saphenous vein (Figure 22.30)
- Cephalic vein.

The use of topical anaesthesia (e.g. EMLA cream, Astra Zeneca) is very strongly encouraged in rabbits. The skin over the vein is clipped and the cream applied generously. The site

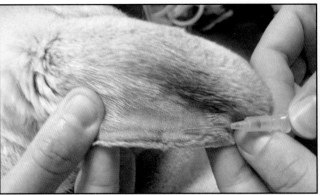
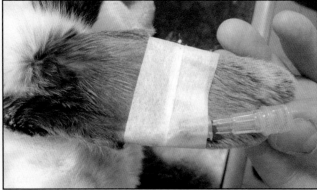

22.29   Venepuncture of the marginal ear vein in a rabbit. (Reproduced from the *BSAVA Manual of Rabbit Medicine and Surgery, 2nd edition*.)

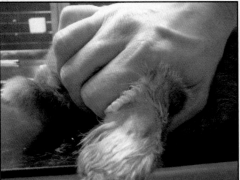
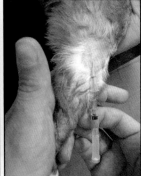
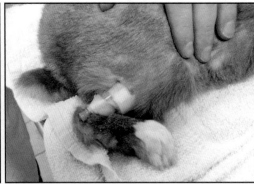

22.30   Venepuncture of the lateral saphenous vein in a rabbit. (Reproduced from the *BSAVA Manual of Rabbit Medicine and Surgery, 2nd edition*.)

is then covered with a non-adhesive dressing for 10–20 minutes before catheterization is attempted. As there is a delay for the topical anaesthetic to take effect, it is wise to apply the cream to at least two different sites from the outset, i.e. so that a second site is available immediately if catheterization of the first site fails.

If available, the use of an infusion device (in particular a syringe driver) is highly recommended.

Intraosseous

The intraosseous route is usually considered if intravenous access cannot be established. The two most common examples of this are very debilitated rabbits in which the veins are collapsed and very small rabbits in which the veins are too small. The vast majority of fluids and other types of drugs can be given via the intraosseous route. A 20–23 gauge hypodermic needle or spinal needle is usually used and sites for intraosseous catheterization include:

- Proximal femur
- Proximal tibia
- Proximal humerus.

Intraperitoneal

The procedure for intraperitoneal fluid administration is as follows:

1. Using aseptic technique, 10 ml/kg of warmed replacement crystalloid solution is drawn up into a syringe and connected to a 23 (or 25) gauge half-inch long needle.
2. The rabbit is positioned in dorsal recumbency with its head lower than its abdomen to allow the viscera to slide forward.
3. A generous area is clipped around the umbilicus and prepared aseptically using surgical scrub materials.
4. The needle is inserted just through the abdominal wall at a site lateral to the umbilicus in the lower right quadrant (Figure 23.31).
5. The syringe is drawn back to check that the needle has not punctured the intestines or another organ; if there is no concern, the fluid is slowly infused – there should be no resistance to injection.
6. The needle is withdrawn from the abdomen in one smooth movement.

Safe intraperitoneal fluid administration requires good patient compliance.

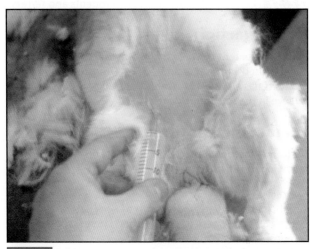

22.31   Intraperitoneal fluid administration in a rabbit.

Volume administered

A fluid plan for the rehydration of rabbits is calculated in the same way as for dogs and cats. It should be noted that the maintenance fluid requirement of rabbits is higher than for dogs and cats of a comparable age; a range of 60–100 ml/kg/day is generally used. Hypovolaemia is treated using fluid boluses as described for dogs and cats (see Figure 22.27).

Duration of fluid therapy

Rehydration is carried out for the period of time used in the fluid plan followed by maintenance therapy for as long as required. Fluid boluses are administered for hypovolaemia until perfusion is thought to have normalized.

Fluid therapy in rodents and ferrets

Indications

Indications for fluid therapy in rodents and ferrets are similar to those for rabbits. Assessment of hydration in these species is usually based on history and physical examination (Figure 22.32), although PCV and serum total protein/solids may be used in addition (see Figure 22.28). Assessment of perfusion is likely to prove challenging unless significantly abnormal, but hypovolaemic rodents are likely to be depressed, bradycardic and hypothermic (see Chapter 15 for normal values).

Severity of dehydration (estimated % of bodyweight)	Progression of physical examination findings
<5%	Not detectable Presumed based on history
Mild (5–6%)	Lethargic, dull Dry mucous membranes
Moderate (6–10%)	Depressed Dry mucous membranes Loss of skin elasticity (skin tenting)
Severe (10–15%)	Severely depressed – comatose Dry mucous membranes Complete loss of skin elasticity – sustained and obvious skin tenting Sunken eyes Progressive signs of hypovolaemia Eventually shock and death

22.32 Estimation of dehydration in rodents and ferrets.

Fluid selection

Both replacement crystalloid and synthetic colloid solutions may be used in rodents and ferrets. Transfusion of blood products has also been described, although this is harder to achieve in the smallest rodents.

Fluid administration

Fluids may be administered to rodents and ferrets via the following routes:

- Oral
- Subcutaneous (e.g. under scruff of neck, lateral thorax)
- Intravenous (especially cephalic and lateral saphenous veins) (Figures 22.33 and 22.34)
- Intraosseous (e.g. proximal femur, proximal tibia)
- Intraperitoneal.

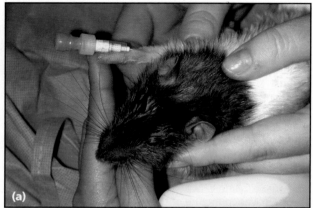

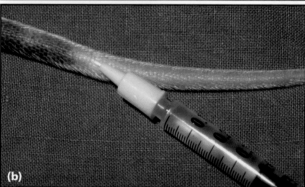

22.33 Intravenous catheterization in a rat. **(a)** Cephalic vein. **(b)** Lateral tail vein. (Reproduced from the *BSAVA Manual of Rodents and Ferrets*.)

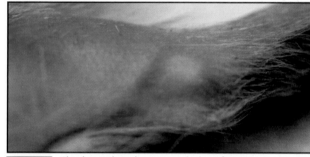

22.34 The lateral saphenous vein in a ferret. (Reproduced from the *BSAVA Manual of Rodents and Ferrets*.)

Many of the points made in Figure 22.27 about rabbits also apply to rodents and ferrets. Additional points to note include:

- Oral fluid dose in rodents and ferrets is 5–10 ml/kg as a maximum single dose; this is important to bear in mind when deciding how many treatments will be required per day to provide the daily maintenance requirement (see below)
- Suggested dose for subcutaneous or intraperitoneal administration is 15–30 ml/kg as a total single dose. Subcutaneous fluid administration under the scruff may be more painful for guinea pigs (highly innervated area in this species) and may be associated with fur slip in chinchillas
- Inhalant anaesthesia (or sedation) may be required to allow intravenous catheter placement but the risks associated with this must be borne in mind; topical anaesthesia is recommended in conscious animals

- In smaller rodents, peripheral vein catheterization is difficult due to the small vessel size, and jugular catheterization may be needed. This requires a surgical 'cut-down' procedure (see Chapter 25) under general anaesthesia and if the catheter is left *in situ*, the patient must be monitored very closely as fatal haemorrhage due to dislodgement or patient interference is a potential complication
- Rodents are likely to be very intolerant of bandages, dressings and indwelling devices
- A single 'off-the-needle' bolus (i.e. not placing a catheter but injecting via a needle and syringe) may be an option in smaller rodents, for example using a 25–27 gauge insulin needle or a butterfly needle
- All fluids should be warmed prior to administration and steps taken to keep the fluid warm during continuous administration
- The intraosseous route may be especially useful for catheterization in ferrets and can also be used in rodents.

Volume administered

Even more so than rabbits, rodents and ferrets generally have a higher maintenance fluid requirement than dogs and cats. This is due to a number of factors, most importantly:

- A greater body surface area to weight ratio and a higher metabolic rate
- Increased loss of fluid via respiration due to proportionally greater lung surface area
- Higher glomerular filtration rate in the kidneys.

Maintenance fluid requirement for rodents and ferrets is approximately 80–100 ml/kg/day. Fluid requirements for correction of dehydration are calculated in the same way as described for dogs and cats, and use of bodyweight to assess rehydration may be especially useful in rodents and ferrets, as repeated measurement of PCV and TS is usually not realistic. Hypovolaemia is treated with replacement crystalloid (e.g. 10–15 ml/kg) or synthetic colloid (e.g. 5 ml/kg) boluses.

Fluid therapy in reptiles

Reptiles can be assessed for dehydration in a similar way to the species previously described, although skin turgor is even less useful in reptiles. Assessments of thirst and urate (the chalky uric acid waste output of reptile kidneys) output can be made over 12–24 hours in hospitalized reptiles and will provide additional information.

The tonicity of reptile extracellular fluid, including plasma, is typically lower than that of mammals, and consequently solutions that are isotonic for mammals (e.g. 0.9% normal saline) are likely to be slightly hypertonic for reptiles. It is acceptable to use lactated Ringer's solution in particular (as it has a lower tonicity than 0.9% saline); alternatively a 2.5% glucose solution made up in 0.45% ('half strength') saline may be used. A rate of 10–40 ml/kg/day is usually used initially for rehydration depending on the species in question and the degree of dehydration suspected. Maintenance fluid requirement in reptiles is 5–15 ml/kg/day.

Perfusion can be difficult to assess; heart rate and blood pressure may be used but it is important to remember that normal values vary between species. Heart rate is also affected significantly by temperature and, unlike many other animals, reptiles should therefore be warmed before intravascular or intraosseous fluid administration. Standard replacement crystalloid solutions (e.g. 5–10 ml/kg bolus) are used for treatment of hypovolaemia and the use of synthetic colloid solutions (e.g. 3–5 ml/kg bolus) has also been described.

Fluid administration

Fluids may be administered to reptiles via the following routes:

- Oral (via intermittent stomach intubation or indwelling pharyngostomy tube)
- Soaking
- Intracoelomic
- Subcutaneous
- Intravenous
- Intraosseous.

Fluids should ideally be warmed to the reptile's optimal body temperature before administration.

Soaking

Soaking of reptiles in warm water (e.g. for 20 minutes twice daily) may allow a significant amount of water to be directly absorbed (especially via the cloaca) and also encourage drinking, appetite and defecation. This is likely to be minimally stressful to the patient and can contribute significantly to hydration; however, soaking is contraindicated in significantly depressed patients.

Intracoelomic fluid therapy

The abdominal cavity in reptiles is called the coelomic cavity. Reptiles do not have a diaphragm to separate the body cavities and therefore excessive fluid administration into the coelomic cavity may cause pressure on the lungs. The maximum recommended single fluid dose for intracoelomic administration is 20 ml/kg.

Subcutaneous fluid therapy

Suggested sites for subcutaneous fluid administration in reptiles include:

- Chelonians (turtles and tortoises): in the skin folds lateral to neck, just cranial to hindlimbs
- Lizards: lateral thorax
- Snakes: lateral aspect of dorsum in caudal third of body.

Intravenous fluid therapy

As always, intravenous fluid administration is the most direct route but intravascular access in reptiles usually requires a 'cut-down' procedure to be performed which is done under local anaesthesia, sedation and/or general anaesthesia. Sites for intravenous catheter placement include:

- Chelonians: jugular vein
- Lizards: cephalic vein, jugular vein, ventral coccygeal (tail) vein
- Snakes: jugular vein.

The dorsal tail vein in chelonians and the ventral tail vein or palatine vein in snakes may also be used for a single 'off-the-needle' fluid bolus.

Intraosseous fluid therapy

The intraosseous route is often preferred for fast access to the circulation in lizards and chelonians, especially smaller ones. As always, due consideration must be given to providing analgesia both during intraosseous catheter placement and while the catheter remains *in situ*. Sites for intraosseous catheter placement include:

- Chelonians: plastrocarapacial bridge/junction (Figure 22.35), proximal tibia
- Lizards: proximal femur, distal femur, proximal tibia, distal humerus
- Snakes: not possible.

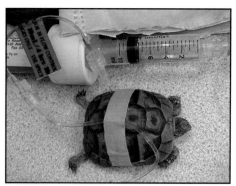

22.35 Intraosseous fluid administration into a septicaemic hatchling tortoise. (Courtesy of M Jessop)

Fluid therapy in birds

Birds have a high metabolic rate and fluid demand but they also naturally conserve water. Dehydration is assessed in a similar way to rodents and any sick bird is assumed to be at least 5% dehydrated. Reference ranges for PCV and TS are available for a number of species. Hypovolaemic shock may be identified by the presence of pale mucous membranes, a prolonged capillary or venous (basilic or ulnar vein) refill time and a fast heart rate. Routes of fluid administration in birds include:

- Oral
- Subcutaneous
- Intravenous
- Intraosseous.

Oral fluid administration is carried out via crop intubation. A maximum dose of 20 ml/kg is recommended but dosing may be repeated once the crop has emptied. The subcutaneous route can prove useful in birds and up to 20 ml/kg of fluid may be administered into the large precrural fold (Figure 22.36); other possible sites include the inguinal skin flap or lateral axillary areas. Veins that can be used in birds include:

- The right jugular vein in most species
- The basilic vein (wing or brachial vein) and the ulnar vein in larger birds
- The medial metatarsal vein in waterfowl.

Intraosseous administration is carried out via the proximal tibiotarsus or the distal or proximal ulna, and catheterization is usually performed under general anaesthesia or sedation. The femur and humerus should not be used as they connect to the air sacs and therefore the lungs. Fluids should not be given by intracoelomic injection because of the air sacs.

Maintenance fluid requirement for birds is 50 ml/kg/day, i.e. similar to dogs and cats, and the most commonly used fluids are warmed replacement crystalloid solutions or glucose saline if indicated. Synthetic colloids have also been used in birds. Intravenous or intraosseous fluid resuscitation for hypovolaemia should be performed using boluses of replacement crystalloid (e.g. 10–15 ml/kg) and synthetic colloid (e.g. 5 ml/kg); hypertonic saline has also been used in birds.

Further reading

Battaglia A (2007) *Small Animal Emergency and Critical Care for Veterinary Technicians, 2nd edn.* Saunders, Philadelphia

Boag AK and King LG (2007) *BSAVA Manual of Canine and Feline Emergency and Critical Care, 2nd edn.* BSAVA Publications, Gloucester

Brown D and Goodman G (2006) General nursing care and hospital management. In: *BSAVA Manual of Rabbit Medicine and Surgery, 2nd edn*, ed, Meredith A and Flecknell P, pp. 37–45 BSAVA Publications, Gloucester

Day MJ, Mackin A and Littlewood JD (2000) *BSAVA Manual of Canine and Feline Haematology and Transfusion Medicine.* BSAVA Publications, Gloucester

Hawkins MG and Graham JE (2007) Emergency and critical care of rodents. *Veterinary Clinics of North America: Exotic Animal Practice* **10**, 501–531

Hotston Moore P and Murrel J (2008) Advanced fluid therapy. In: *BSAVA Manual of Canine and Feline Advanced Veterinary Nursing, 2nd edn*, ed. A Hotston Moore and S Rudd, pp. 114–127. BSAVA Publications, Gloucester

Martinez-Jimenez D and Hernandez-Divers SJ (2007) Emergency care of reptiles. *Veterinary Clinics of North America: Exotic Animal Practice* **10**, 557–585

Self-assessment questions

1. List five causes of abnormal fluid loss.
2. How does the approach to treatment of dehydration differ from treatment of hypovolaemia?
3. Decide which fluid you would use to treat dehydration in an adult dog with anorexia. Calculate a fluid rate to rehydrate this patient intravenously over 24 hours; the dog weighs 15 kg, is estimated to be 7% dehydrated, and has no additional significant ongoing losses.
4. List five different routes of fluid therapy.
5. Name two conditions that often cause hypoglycaemia that is severe enough to require glucose supplementation.
6. List three causes of hyperkalaemia.
7. What is the normal pH of blood in the dog?
8. Which is the most common blood type in the overall cat population, type A, type B or type AB?
9. Which peripheral veins are usually used for intravenous catheter placement in rabbits?
10. What is the coelomic cavity in reptiles? Why do we need to be careful about how much fluid we administer into this cavity?

Chapter 23

Anaesthesia and analgesia

Jo Murrell and Vicky Ford-Fennah

Learning objectives

After studying this chapter, students should be able to:

- **Understand the principles of anaesthesia, including the physiological effects of anaesthetic drugs on body systems**
- **Understand the physiology and assessment of pain in animals**
- **Understand the principles of premedication, induction and maintenance of anaesthesia**
- **Understand the use of local anaesthetic techniques**
- **Describe the steps necessary to evaluate and prepare an animal for anaesthesia**
- **Understand the preparation and use of various types of anaesthetic equipment, including endotracheal tubes, equipment for administering inhalation anaesthetics, non-rebreathing and rebreathing circuits**
- **Understand the principles and risks of monitoring an anaesthetized animal, including the techniques and equipment required**
- **Support veterinary anaesthesia in dogs, cats, horses and exotic pets**
- **Prepare, operate and maintain anaesthetic equipment used in dogs, cats and exotic pets**
- **Assist with anaesthetic preparation, premedication and induction of anaesthesia in dogs, cats and exotic pets**
- **Monitor a small animal throughout anaesthesia and recovery**
- **Recognize and respond to anaesthetic emergencies**

Introduction

General anaesthesia is routinely carried out in small animal practice and most cats and dogs will receive at least one general anaesthetic during their lifetime, often for the purposes of neutering. Similarly, in equine practice general anaesthesia is an important clinical tool to ensure that safe surgical procedures may be performed. The use of local anaesthetic and sedative techniques also plays a large role in equine restraint.

Veterinary nurses play a critical role in the management of anaesthetized patients, commonly with responsibility for: the administration of premedication drugs; establishing intravenous access before induction of anaesthesia; maintenance and setting up of the anaesthetic machine and monitoring equipment; and monitoring the patient during the anaesthesia and recovery period. They are also critical in pain assessment during the perioperative period. It is therefore imperative that veterinary nurses have a good understanding of the principles of anaesthesia, including the pharmacology and the use of anaesthesia equipment for both maintenance and monitoring of anaesthesia.

Who may carry out anaesthesia in animals?

The RCVS has clearly defined what can and cannot be carried out by a qualified Registered or Listed Veterinary Nurse and by student veterinary nurses enrolled with the RCVS with regard to anaesthesia:

- Inducing anaesthesia by administration of a specific quantity of medicine directed by a veterinary surgeon may be carried out by a veterinary nurse or, under supervision by a veterinary surgeon, a student veterinary nurse
- Administering medicine incrementally or to effect to induce or maintain anaesthesia may only be carried out by a veterinary surgeon
- Maintaining anaesthesia is the responsibility of a veterinary surgeon, but a suitably trained person (such as a veterinary nurse) may assist by 'acting as the veterinary surgeon's hands', for example by moving dials
- Monitoring a patient during anaesthesia and the recovery period is the responsibility of the veterinary surgeon but may be carried out on his or her behalf by a suitably trained person (such as a veterinary nurse).

What is anaesthesia?

There are many different definitions of anaesthesia available in the literature.

Definition

For the purposes of this chapter, general anaesthesia is defined as a reversible **immobile** state that induces **amnesia** (loss of memory).

Both immobility and amnesia have useful clinical connections: the surgeon requires immobility, and the patients (certainly in the field of human anaesthesia) desire amnesia. The **triad of anaesthesia** has three components that contribute to the anaesthetized state:

- Muscle relaxation
- Unconsciousness
- Pain relief (analgesia/antinociception).

It is useful to think about the triad of anaesthesia when considering provision of a balanced anaesthesia protocol.

The principle of balanced anaesthesia

The underlying principle behind modern anaesthesia techniques is **balanced anaesthesia**. This can be defined as the use of multiple anaesthetic drugs in combination, in order to provide general anaesthesia. Instead of using a single anaesthetic agent for induction and maintenance of anaesthesia (e.g. the volatile anaesthetic agent isoflurane), for which high concentrations will be required to achieve the components of the anaesthesia triad, combinations of drugs are used. The side effects of most anaesthetic drugs are dose-dependent and the mechanisms by which these side effects occur varies for different classes of analgesic agent. Using combinations of drugs allows the dose of each individual agent to be reduced. Therefore, adoption of the principle of balanced anaesthesia usually allows for provision of better quality general anaesthesia associated with a reduction in cardiovascular and respiratory side effects.

Balanced anaesthesia may involve:

- Premedication with a sedative and analgesic drug
- Induction with an intravenous agent
- Maintenance with an inhalant agent
- Further analgesic drugs, if required (e.g. a constant rate infusion (CRI) of a short-acting opioid.

Effects of anaesthesia on major organ systems

Due to the profound effects of anaesthesia on most body organ systems, good preoperative assessment and the careful monitoring of animals during anaesthesia is vital in order to try and minimize physiological disturbances.

Brain

The mechanism by which most anaesthetic agents produce a state of anaesthesia is unknown, although it is suggested that agents act through a combination of effects on specific receptors in the central nervous system (CNS) and through an effect on the cell membrane of neuronal cells. Anaesthesia causes a reversible depression of CNS function, resulting in loss of consciousness.

Cardiovascular system

Depression of cardiovascular function is common during anaesthesia and may result from the central depressant effects of the drug (e.g. depression of the cardiovascular control centre in the brain) or through peripheral effects. This depression is usually manifest as a reduction in cardiac output and therefore blood flow to central and peripheral organs, with the potential to produce inadequate oxygenation of the tissues. Changes in the tone of blood vessels may also occur (peripheral vasodilation or vasoconstriction depending on the specific effects of the drugs that have been administered).

Respiratory system

Central depression of the respiratory centre in the brain is common during anaesthesia, leading to a reduced sensitivity to blood carbon dioxide (CO_2) concentration and reduced respiratory drive. This can result in:

- **Hypercapnia** (a higher concentration of CO_2 in the blood than normal)
- **Hypoxia** (when tissues receive an inadequate supply of oxygen, O_2).

Hypoxia occurs less frequently than hypercapnia because animals commonly receive >30% inspired O_2 during anaesthesia, which is higher than the O_2 concentration of room air. Reduced thoracic muscle tone can also reduce the effectiveness of ventilation, with the potential to cause hypercapnia.

Liver

The blood supply to the liver is via two routes: the hepatic artery and the portal vein. These two blood supplies work in tandem in order to maintain total liver blood flow within narrow limits. If portal blood supply decreases, the resistance in the hepatic artery is reduced in order to increase the blood supply via this route. All inhalant agents have the potential to reduce total liver blood flow through a reduction in cardiac output and through disturbing the reciprocal mechanism in the hepatic artery and portal vein. Halothane has a greater effect than other inhalant agents on liver blood flow.

Kidneys

The kidneys normally receive approximately 20% of total cardiac output, and adequate renal blood flow is essential to maintain normal renal function. General anaesthesia usually decreases renal blood flow, glomerular filtration rate, urine output and electrolyte excretion. These parameters usually return to normal a few hours after anaesthesia in healthy animals when the duration of anaesthesia is short.

Preparation for anaesthesia

Informed owner consent

Consent for carrying out an anaesthetic and the accompanying procedure must always be obtained (see Chapters 1 and 9). The purpose of the consent form is to record the client's agreement to treatment based on knowledge of what is involved and the likely consequences. The client may be the owner of the animal, someone acting with the authority of the owner or someone with other appropriate authority.

Before being asked to sign an anaesthesia consent form the person should be able to understand and retain the information provided and use it to come to a decision. Clients should be provided with the opportunity to read the form and ask questions before being asked to consent to the procedure or treatment. It is important to remember that children under the age of 16 should not be asked to sign a consent form.

Clinical history

It is important that, when possible, a full clinical history is obtained from the owner of every patient prior to anaesthesia. This will provide information on previous disease and anaesthetic history and will alert the anaesthetist to potential health problems at the time of presentation, which can be used to guide the clinical examination and the requirement for further evaluation before anaesthesia. Questions should be asked to obtain information on:

- The status of diagnosed chronic disease in the patient, including current medications such as non-steroidal anti-inflammatory drugs (NSAIDs), steroids, insulin, diuretics and cardiac medications
  - Generally, it is recommended that current medications are continued around the time of anaesthesia to avoid abrupt changes in drug regime; however, this must be determined on an individual animal and drug basis
  - It is important to question the owner carefully about concurrent NSAID administration (as this will influence administration of NSAIDs in the perioperative period) and steroids (as this will probably be a contraindication to the administration of NSAIDs in the perioperative period)
- Previous anaesthetic history
- Recent changes in bodyweight (may signal underlying undiagnosed disease)
- Recent changes in water consumption (increased drinking is a common sign of renal and endocrine disease)
- Recent changes in food consumption (may also be an indication of endocrine disease)
- Exercise intolerance (in dogs) – reduced willingness to exercise can be an indicator of underlying cardiovascular disease
- The temperament of the patient (useful to guide management of the patient while hospitalized)
- Vaccination status.

Clinical examination

A clinical examination (see Chapter 15) should be carried out before anaesthesia, with particular attention being paid to the systems affected by anaesthesia. It will also allow the temperament of the patient in response to handling to be assessed in a new environment, which may guide decisions about choice of premedication protocol and the requirement for sedation. Appropriate handling and safety measures should be observed at this time (see Chapters 2 and 10).

Pre-anaesthetic examination

The physical examination should concentrate on the body systems most affected by anaesthesia.

- Central nervous system:
  - Check that the animal has normal mentation (behaviour and level of consciousness), with no evidence of CNS depression
- Cardiovascular system:
  - Palpate the peripheral pulses, assessing pulse quality and regularity
  - Auscultate the heart and listen for murmurs; concurrent auscultation and palpation of the pulse will allow any pulse deficit to be detected
  - Check mucous membrane colour and capillary refill time
  - Carrying out an exercise test by walking the animal a short distance on the lead can be used to aid detection of marked cardiovascular abnormalities
  - Signs of dyspnoea, reluctance to move or collapse all signal that the animal will be at significant risk under anaesthesia and further investigation of the cardiovascular system is warranted
- Respiratory system:
  - Observe the respiratory rate and pattern when the animal is at rest, looking for signs of laboured breathing or abnormal respiratory rate
  - Auscultate the chest to detect abnormal lung sounds that may indicate respiratory disease

Additional pre-anaesthetic tests

Routine blood tests before anaesthesia should usually only be carried out on the basis of abnormalities detected on clinical examination or the clinical history. There is currently no evidence base to support routine pre-anaesthetic blood testing in healthy animals. In geriatric animals, where there is likely to be a higher incidence of concurrent disease, routine pre-anaesthetic blood testing may be more justifiable. Some equine hospitals will carry out a routine haematological examination prior to inducing general anaesthesia, justified on the grounds of the identified higher mortality rate in equine patients.

Anaemia may be detected by measuring haemoglobin concentration or packed cell volume (PCV) (see Chapter 19). A blood coagulation profile is warranted in animals with a suspected blood clotting disorder.

Biochemical testing can be used to assess liver disease (through measurement of liver enzymes and bile acid concentration); and serum urea and creatinine concentrations are used as a marker of renal function. Measurement of plasma total protein (TP) concentration will detect hypoproteinaemia.

Measurement of serum electrolyte concentration (sodium, potassium and chloride) is indicated in some animals with systemic disease.

If marked disturbances in fluid therapy or blood volume are expected during anaesthesia and surgery it is useful to take a baseline blood sample to measure PCV and TP. Changes in these parameters can then be used to guide fluid administration in response to disturbances in fluid balance during anaesthesia (see Chapter 22).

The cardiovascular and respiratory systems may require further evaluation using radiography, ultrasonography and electrocardiography.

Significance of clinical findings

Central nervous system disease

Systemic disease resulting in depression of the CNS can significantly reduce the amounts of anaesthetic agents required to induce and maintain anaesthesia: lower doses should be used and the agents given slowly and to effect, to reduce the likelihood of overdose. Seizures are common in animals with CNS disease and animals should be carefully monitored during the peri-anaesthetic period so that seizures can be managed promptly should they occur. Raised intracranial pressure resulting from space-occupying lesions in the cranium is associated with a number of specific anaesthetic considerations and knowledge of these is required before undertaking anaesthesia of this group of patients.

Cardiovascular disease

Cardiovascular disease is common in both cats and dogs and should not be considered a contraindication to anaesthesia. However, most cardiovascular diseases are likely to increase the risk of reduced cardiac output and hypotension during anaesthesia, increasing the likelihood of tissue hypoxia. Where possible, stabilization of the patient before anaesthesia is indicated, and the cardiovascular system should be monitored carefully so that derangements in cardiovascular function can be treated promptly.

Respiratory disease

Respiratory disease increases the risk of hypoxia and hypercapnia during anaesthesia. Supplementation with 100% O_2 is usually indicated immediately prior to induction of anaesthesia in patients with respiratory disease, in order to reduce the risk of hypoxia. Ventilation may require support with **intermittent positive pressure ventilation** (IPPV).

Hypovolaemia and dehydration

Reduced circulating blood volume predisposes the animal to reduced cardiac output and hypotension during anaesthesia. Correction of disturbances in fluid balance is indicated before induction of anaesthesia, using appropriate fluid therapy given intravenously (see Chapter 22).

Coagulation disorders

Abnormalities in blood coagulation promote blood loss during surgery. Correction of the coagulation disorder before surgery, by the administration of blood products or appropriate drug therapy, is indicated.

Liver and renal disease

Most anaesthetic drugs are metabolized in the liver, and therefore liver disease can prolong the duration of action of anaesthetic agents, leading to drug accumulation and a prolonged recovery time. Use of short-acting agents, given to effect, is recommended. Renal disease can be worsened by anaesthesia, particularly if adequate renal blood flow is not maintained, leading to renal ischaemia. Careful management of fluid therapy is required to prevent worsening of renal function.

Unstable blood glucose concentration

Common conditions leading to an unstable blood glucose concentration are diabetes mellitus and severe liver disease. Very young animals (<3 months of age) are also less able to regulate blood glucose concentration. Hypoglycaemia is a risk during anaesthesia, particularly as it cannot be detected by changes in mentation. Monitoring of blood glucose concentration during anaesthesia is recommended.

Electrolyte abnormalities

Disturbances in serum electrolyte concentrations are relatively common in animals suffering from systemic disease, particularly renal disease or some endocrine disorders (see Chapters 20 and 22). **Hyperkalaemia** (an elevated concentration of potassium in the blood) has particularly serious consequences during anaesthesia, as it results in heart conduction abnormalities and bradycardia. Normalization of blood potassium concentration is always indicated before induction of anaesthesia. This is particularly important for foals with a ruptured bladder and uroperitoneum. The temptation is to carry out emergency surgery immediately, but rebalancing electrolytes is always the priority.

Anaemia

Oxygen is mainly carried in the blood bound to haemoglobin; therefore severe anaemia will affect the oxygen-carrying capacity of the blood and may predispose the patient to hypoxia. Depending on the chronicity and severity of the anaemia, a blood transfusion may be indicated before anaesthesia.

Hypoproteinaemia

Most anaesthetic drugs are carried in the blood, bound to plasma proteins. It is only the unbound fraction of the drug that is active and able to cross the blood–brain barrier, in order to exert an anaesthetic effect. Drug doses should be reduced in hypoproteinaemic animals and drugs should be given slowly and to effect.

Pyrexia

Increased body temperature is a common finding in animals with acute illness, and detection during clinical examination should prompt further evaluation of the patient to establish the underlying cause. If pyrexia is severe (>40°C) it can result in increased heart rate and reduced myocardial contractility, decreasing cardiac output. If possible, body temperature should be normalized before the induction of anaesthesia.

American Society of Anesthesiologists (ASA) classification of anaesthetic risk

The information gathered from the patient history, clinical examination and auxiliary tests can be used to assign an ASA status to the patient. This system classifies the anaesthetic risk of the patient on a 5-point scale and can be used to guide selection of the anaesthesia protocol and the complexity of intraoperative monitoring.

ASA scale of anaesthetic risk

I: A normal healthy patient – e.g. a young dog presented for elective ovariohysterectomy

II: A patient with mild systemic disease – e.g. a dog with a low-grade heart murmur that is not showing any clinical signs of cardiac disease

III: A patient with severe systemic disease – e.g. a dog with a heart murmur that has resulted in reduced exercise tolerance

IV: A patient with severe systemic disease that is a constant threat to life – e.g. a dog with a cardiac arrhythmia that is causing severe circulatory compromise

V: A moribund patient that is not expected to survive without the operation – e.g. a dog with gastric dilatation and volvulus

E: Denotes that the procedure is an emergency

Specific risks associated with equine anaesthesia

A large study of perioperative equine mortality (Johnson *et al.*, 2002) identified that the risk of death related to anaesthesia was significantly higher in horses than in other species. The risk of death in healthy horses was approximately 1 in 100, and when data from abdominal surgeries (predominantly due to colic) and foals were included this rose to a death rate of approximately 1 in 55. This compares to recently reported death rates of 1 in 601 dogs, 1 in 419 cats and 1 in 72 rabbits. Three major causes (or groups of causes) of death were identified in horses: cardiovascular complications such as cardiac arrest during anaesthesia; post-anaesthetic myopathy or limb fracture in recovery (see later); and miscellaneous complications such as respiratory complications in recovery.

The risk was increased:

- In horses over 14 years old
- In cases of fracture surgery
- Where anaesthesia was of a long duration or carried out outside of normal working hours
- With certain anaesthetic drugs.

The increased anaesthetic risk in horses has led to the development of techniques to carry out procedures in heavily sedated, standing horses. Owners should also be made aware of the risks associated with anaesthesia when asked to give informed consent (see below) for an anaesthetic and surgical procedure.

Additional preparations

Fasting

Dogs, cats and ferrets

It is currently recommended that cats, ferrets and dogs are starved for a minimum of 3 hours prior to induction of anaesthesia or sedation; longer periods of starvation (>6 hours) may increase the incidence of gastro-oesophageal reflux and are not recommended. Puppies and kittens <12 weeks of age may be at risk of hypoglycaemia during pre-operative starvation and therefore should have food withdrawn for 3 hours only and should be observed for signs of hypoglycaemia during this period. Provision of glucose intravenously (via fluid therapy) should be considered in very young animals with limited glucose reserves. Some endocrine diseases can also predispose to hypoglycaemia during periods of starvation (e.g. insulinoma) and at-risk animals should be carefully monitored during starvation, and glucose support considered.

Horses

The issue of whether to starve horses prior to induction of anaesthesia is currently contentious. Traditionally, horses have been starved of hay at least overnight before anaesthesia the following day, with concentrate feed withdrawn on the morning of anaesthesia. This was to limit the volume within the gastrointestinal system and thereby reduce the potential for respiratory compromise, due to the pressure of the gastrointestinal tract on the diaphragm and lungs, and reduce the potential for compression of the great veins (such as the vena cava) by abdominal contents, decreasing venous return and cardiac output. However, this dogma has recently been challenged, particularly because horses that are not starved before anaesthesia, such as emergency cases, do not appear to have significantly impaired cardiopulmonary variables compared to starved horses.

The oral cavity of horses should be flushed out immediately prior to induction of anaesthesia to remove any food debris (see Chapter 10). Special large metal syringes are available to facilitate this process.

Rabbits

Rabbits do not need to be starved before anaesthesia as they are unable to regurgitate food. However, changes in diet during hospitalization should be avoided; it is therefore advisable to ask the owner to bring some of the animal's normal food to the surgery to ensure that a continued diet can be provided.

Rodents

Rats and mice do not vomit during induction of anaesthesia and so fasting is unnecessary.

Guinea pigs also do not vomit during induction but food is very occasionally retained in the pharynx during anaesthesia. Guinea pigs may be starved for approximately 2 hours before induction of anaesthesia; more prolonged fasting carries the disadvantage of an increased likelihood of gastrointestinal disturbances after anaesthesia. A pair of atraumatic forceps and a light source should also be readily available at the time of induction so that any food in the pharynx can be carefully removed.

Birds

The majority of birds, reptiles and amphibians do not need to be starved prior to anaesthesia. However, it is useful to check the size of the crop in birds before induction of anaesthesia, as regurgitation can occur. If the crop is very large and palpable, anaesthesia should be delayed until it has emptied.

Withdrawal of water

Water should not be withdrawn until the time of premedication, in order to prevent dehydration prior to induction of anaesthesia. For small mammals it is very important to withdraw the water bowl from the cage when the animal is premedicated, in order to prevent the possibility that they could become sedated with the head in the water bowl and drown. For horses, water should be removed immediately prior to induction of anaesthesia when the horse is moved from the stable to the induction box.

Weighing

All animals should be weighed before anaesthesia in order to calculate drug doses accurately. Weigh bands can be used to facilitate estimation of bodyweight in horses if a scale is not available.

Placement of intravenous catheters

Ideally, all animals should have some form of intravenous access established prior to anaesthesia, to allow administration of agents for induction, fluid therapy and additional drugs and in case of emergency. Placement of intravenous catheters is described in Chapter 22.

Small animals

In conscious cats and dogs the easiest vessels to catheterize are the cephalic (Figure 23.1a) and the saphenous (Figure 23.1b) veins. If these vessels are unavailable (e.g. due to previous catheter placement or the site of surgery) an intravenous catheter can be placed into the auricular vein that runs along the edge of the ear (Figure 23.1c). When using this site it is vital to palpate the area and ensure that there is no pulse to avoid placing the catheter in the artery. This site is most commonly used in rabbits but is also invaluable in Basset Hounds and Dachshunds (as the shape of their legs makes other sites less suitable).

The lateral tail vein is large in rats and an easy site for placement of an intravenous catheter (Figure 23.2), although placement usually first necessitates induction of anaesthesia so that the rat is immobile.

The brachial vein, which can be found on the medial aspect of the wing, is a useful route for catheterization in birds (Figure 23.3). It is also important to remember that the jugular vein is a potential site for intravenous access, although this can be more difficult in conscious animals.

When choosing a catheter it is important to consider the nature of the procedure to be carried out and the potential risks associated with the surgery, e.g. a 20 G catheter is suitable for a healthy 15 kg dog being castrated; however, if the same dog were having an exploratory laparotomy, an 18 G catheter would be more appropriate because of the higher risks associated with the procedure and the possible need to provide rapid intravenous fluid therapy.

Once the catheter is placed, it must be fixed securely in order to prevent displacement when the patient is moved.

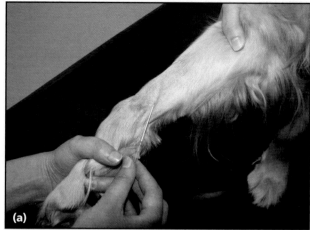
(a)

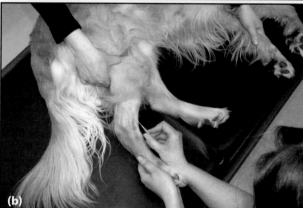
(b)

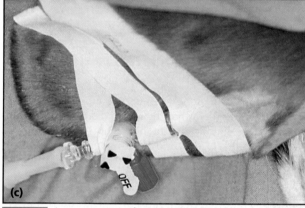
(c)

23.1 Intravenous catheterization sites in the dog. **(a)** Placement of a 20G catheter into the medial branch of the cephalic vein. **(b)** Placement of a 20G catheter into the saphenous vein. **(c)** Catheter in the auricular vein and connected to a 3-way tap.

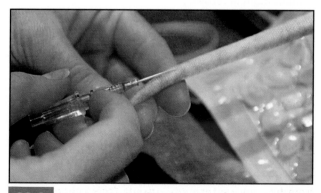

23.2 Catheterization of the lateral tail vein of a rat.

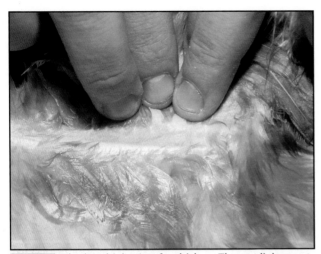

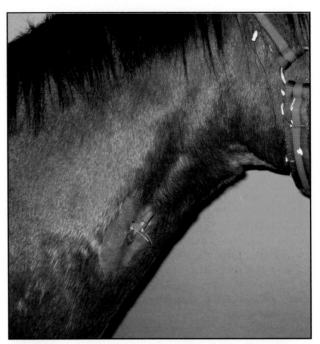

23.3 The brachial vein of a chicken. The medial aspect of the wing is shown, with the feathers dampened by surgical spirit to improve visibility of the vein. The vein is located just ventral to the fingertips.

Techniques vary depending on the species, site of placement and individual preference. If the patient is going to receive intravenous fluid therapy perioperatively (which is recommended), a T-port or similar system should be attached to allow fluids and drugs to be administered to the patient simultaneously (Figure 23.4).

23.5 Catheter placed in the jugular vein of a horse. A large area of hair has been clipped to facilitate aseptic placement. The catheter is secured in place by a suture to the skin and is capped with an injection port. (Courtesy of Carolyne Sheridan)

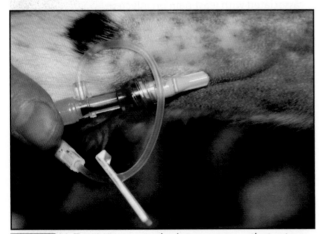

23.4 A T-port connects the intravenous catheter to a fluid administration set. This allows drugs to be injected through the rubber bung.

Horses

No horse should be anaesthetized without prior placement of an intravenous catheter in the jugular vein (Figure 23.5). The catheter must be placed in an aseptic manner and preferably before the horse is moved to the induction box.

It is unusual for an intravenous catheter to survive recovery from anaesthesia intact; therefore, if a longer-term catheter is required it is better to replace the catheter that was used during anaesthesia with a second long-stay catheter. Some clinicians adopt a policy of always placing the jugular catheter in the left jugular vein, so that the right jugular vein is preserved. This ensures that venous drainage from the head is never impaired by thrombophlebitis from bilateral catheter placement. The catheter can be placed 'upwards', with the tip pointing towards the head, or 'downwards', with the tip facing towards the heart. Placing the catheter upwards prevents air embolus should the cap of the catheter become dislodged, but major haemorrhage can result should the bung or cap become dislodged during recovery. Placing the catheter towards the heart means that air can be sucked into the venous circulation when the catheter is uncapped, which can, rarely, result in generation of air embolus and death.

Removal of shoes from horses

In order to prevent damage to the horse during induction and recovery from anaesthesia and to protect the floor covering of the induction box, shoes are generally removed before induction of anaesthesia. If this is not possible, due to the temperament of the horse or underlying disease (e.g. it might be difficult to remove shoes from a restless horse that is in pain), the shoes can be covered with durable tape or boots can be placed over the shoes during induction. The shoes can then be removed when the horse is anaesthetized and on the operating table. An alternative approach commonly employed is to use duct tape to cover the feet, thus avoiding sharp edges.

Rest and exercise

Immediate anaesthesia is not recommended for horses (or dogs) that have recently been subjected to hard exercise (e.g. racing), or horses that have been transported for long distances. Surgical repair of fractures that have been referred from gallops close to the hospital can, however, be carried out effectively relatively soon after the injury, which can reduce post-injury articular damage.

Where possible, dogs should be walked prior to anaesthesia, to allow them to pass urine and faeces. Cats should be provided with a litter tray.

Premedication and sedation

Premedication is an integral part of the total anaesthesia protocol. The choice of premedicant drugs will determine the characteristics of the ensuing anaesthesia. Therefore, when monitoring anaesthesia during the maintenance phase, vital parameters should be considered in light of the premedicant drugs administered.

Aims of premedication:

- To calm the patient prior to induction of anaesthesia
- To reduce stress during induction of anaesthesia for both the patient and staff
  - This is particularly important with horses where induction of anaesthesia in unpremedicated patients can be dangerous for both the horse and handlers
- To reduce the dose of anaesthetic drugs required for induction and maintenance of anaesthesia
- To contribute to a balanced anaesthesia technique
- To provide analgesia
- To counter adverse effects of other anaesthetic drugs
- To smooth recovery from anaesthesia through residual sedation and pain relief.

Sedation

Depending on the species and temperament of the patient, some procedures can be carried out under sedation rather than general anaesthesia. The drugs used for sedation are similar to those used for premedication, although higher doses are commonly used for sedation in order to achieve adequate chemical restraint. The principles of drug selection and monitoring are similar for sedation and premedication.

When deciding whether to sedate or anaesthetize an individual patient for a particular procedure, it is important to consider that sedation is not necessarily safer than

general anaesthesia. Generally, less cardiovascular and respiratory support can be given to a sedated than to an anaesthetized patient, particularly with respect to control of the airway. Therefore, in high-risk patients it is often better to elect for general anaesthesia rather than sedation, even though it might be possible to carry out the procedure under sedation alone.

In horses, sedation in combination with local anaesthesia and analgesia techniques is commonly used for significant surgical procedures. However, the increase in this practice is probably a result of the increased mortality risk associated with general anaesthesia in horses compared to other species.

Routes of premedication and sedative drug administration

Premedication and sedative drugs may be administered via several routes:

- **Intravenous**: Rapid onset of action but requires restraint of the patient and intravenous access to be established
- **Intramuscular**: Slower onset of action than the intravenous route but requires minimal restraint for injection. Large volumes injected intramuscularly can be painful. Site of injection does not appear to affect onset or depth of sedation
- **Subcutaneous**: Onset of sedation is slowest, but associated with least pain on injection.

Drugs used for premedication of small animals

Several classes of drug are commonly used for premedication in small animals, each with advantages and disadvantages (Figure 23.6). Most premedication protocols involve administration of a drug with sedative properties combined with an opioid analgesic drug. This usually increases the quality of sedation that is achieved, due to synergism between opioids and drugs with sedative properties. Synergism means that the

Class or drug	Advantages	Disadvantages
Phenothiazines, e.g. acepromazine	Synergism with opioids increases sedation (neuroleptanaesthesia). Provides reasonable sedation. Relatively wide margin of cardiovascular safety. Anti-arrhythmic action (mediated through an antagonistic action at alpha-1 receptors). Long duration of action (6 hours); can smooth recovery from anaesthesia. Can be given i.v., i.m. or s.c.	Relatively slow onset of action (30–45 min). Sedation not as profound as that provided by alpha-2 agonists; improved if environment is quiet and animal is left undisturbed. Long duration of action (may prolong recovery from anaesthesia). No antagonist available. Causes peripheral vasodilation through antagonism of alpha-1 receptors. **Do not use** in animals that are shocked or have significant cardiovascular disease. Peripheral vasodilation promotes heat loss and hypothermia
Alpha-2 agonists, e.g. medetomidine, dexmedetomidine	Profound sedation, synergism with opioids further increases sedation, allows a lower dose of the alpha-2 agonist to be used. Good muscle relaxation due to potency of hypnotic effect. Analgesia: contributes to a multimodal analgesia technique. Profound drug-sparing effect: contributes to a balanced anaesthesia technique. Peripheral vasoconstriction reduces heat loss and minimizes hypothermia. Antagonist available (atipamezole). Rapid, smooth recoveries from anaesthesia. Can be given i.v., i.m. or s.c.	Significant cardiovascular system effects: causes an intense initial vasoconstriction associated with a reduction in heart rate. Heart rate remains low due to central sympatholytic effects. Cardiac output is reduced. **Do not use** in animals with cardiovascular disease. Reduces liver blood flow: **do not use** in animals with significant liver disease. Can cause vomiting: **do not use** in animals where vomiting is undesirable, e.g. raised intraocular pressure or linear foreign body. Analgesia is of short duration (45–60 min) reversed by administration of atipamezole

23.6 Advantages and disadvantages of drugs used for premedication and sedation in small animals. *continues* ▶

Class or drug	Advantages	Disadvantages
Ketamine	Good sedation/anaesthesia when given in combination with another sedative drug: dependent on dose. Minimal effects on the cardiovascular system. Provides analgesia. Profound drug-sparing effect. Useful in cats where profound sedation is required, given in combination with a benzodiazepine. Can be given i.v. or i.m.	Causes excitation and muscle rigidity unless combined with another sedative drug, commonly a benzodiazepine. Poor quality of sedation in dogs, even when given in combination with another agent. Animals can be 'spacey' in recovery due to the hallucinogenic effects
Benzodiazepines, e.g. diazepam, midazolam	Sedation is enhanced by combination with an opioid. Good sedation in sick or young animals. Minimal effects on the cardiovascular system: useful in patients with cardiovascular disease. Midazolam can be given i.v., i.m. or s.c.	Sedation is minimal in healthy animals; combination with an opioid is required. Can cause excitement in healthy animals. Muscle relaxation may reduce ventilatory effort. Diazepam solubilized in propylene glycol causes pain on i.m. injection and thrombophlebitis i.v; use midazolam if possible
Opioids, e.g. buprenorphine, morphine (see also Opioid analgesics, later in chapter)	Enhance sedation when combined with acepromazine, alpha-2 agonists and benzodiazepines. Provide analgesia: choice of opioid depends on severity of pain expected from the procedure. Can be given i.v. (not pethidine), i.m. or s.c.	Morphine can cause vomiting when administered to animals that are not in pain. High doses of potent opioids may cause a reduction in heart rate; bradycardia can be managed by the administration of an anticholinergic if severe. Administration of a partial mu opioid agonist (e.g. buprenorphine or butorphanol) prior to induction of anaesthesia may reduce the effectiveness of full opioid agonists administered during anaesthesia
Anticholinergics; parasympatholytics, e.g. atropine, glycopyrrolate	Will counter bradycardia produced by potent opioids. Will counter bradycardia caused by stimulation of the parasympathetic nervous system during surgery, e.g. oculocardiac reflex, exploratory neck surgery. Can be given i.v., i.m. or s.c.	Rarely required as premedicant in modern anaesthesia protocols. Usually advisable to give in response to bradycardia rather than pre-emptively

23.6 *continued* Advantages and disadvantages of drugs used for premedication and sedation in small animals.

sedation is greater than can be achieved by simply summing the individual effects of the drugs. This protocol also ensures that analgesia is provided. Administration of NSAIDs prior to induction of anaesthesia can be helpful to provide improved intraoperative analgesia, but there are contraindications to this technique in some patients (see Analgesia, below).

It can be very useful to consider the ASA status of the patient (see above) when determining the premedication regimen (Figure 23.7). This takes the health status of the patient into consideration and allows some standardization of premedication protocols, which can be helpful within a busy practice situation. However, the individual requirements of each patient, such as the procedure to be carried out, must always be taken into consideration.

Premedication protocols in horses

The number of drugs that are authorized for administration to horses is significantly reduced compared to those for small animals because horses are classed as food-producing animals in Europe (see Chapter 8). However, a number of unauthorized drugs (for which minimum residue limits have not been established) can be given legally to horses that will not enter the food chain, as certified in the horse's passport.

In the UK, healthy horses are commonly premedicated with acepromazine, given intramuscularly 30–45 minutes before induction of anaesthesia and before the horse is moved from the stable to the induction box. Low doses of acepromazine

ASA status	Dogs	Cats
I: Normal, healthy patient	Acepromazine plus opioid Medetomidine/dexmedetomidine plus opioid	Acepromazine plus opioid Medetomidine/dexmedetomidine plus opioid
II: Patient with mild systemic disease	Acepromazine plus opioid Medetomidine/dexmedetomidine plus opioid (if no evidence of CVS disease)	Acepromazine plus opioid Medetomidine/dexmedetomidine plus opioid (if no evidence of CVS disease)
III: Patient with severe systemic disease	Acepromazine plus opioid Midazolam plus opioid	Acepromazine plus opioid Ketamine plus midazolam
IV: Patient with severe systemic disease that is a constant threat to life	Midazolam plus opioid	Ketamine plus midazolam Midazolam plus opioid
V: Moribund patient not expected to survive without the operation	Midazolam plus opioid, or either drug alone	Midazolam plus opioid, or either drug alone

23.7 Examples of premedication protocols for dogs and cats with differing ASA status.

capable of providing anxiolysis rather than overt sedation are usually administered. Widespread use of acepromazine reflects evidence that administration to healthy horses prior to induction of anaesthesia reduces equine mortality. Acepromazine should not be given to horses with cardiovascular disease or cardiovascular collapse (e.g. horses with colic) due to the vasodilatory properties of the drug. It can also cause priapism in male horses, which makes it less suitable for use in entire male breeding animals, for which damage to the penis could be disastrous.

Once the horse has been moved from the stable to the induction box (where general anaesthesia will be induced), further premedicant agents with more potent sedative properties, particularly alpha-2 agonists, are given intravenously. This is to ensure that the horse is adequately sedated before the administration of an induction agent.

Alpha-2 agonists in horses

Alpha-2 adrenergic agonists are widely used in equine anaesthesia because of their profound sedative and analgesic properties. They are the most widely used class of drugs for sedation of standing horses and are also commonly used for premedication immediately prior to induction of anaesthesia. The three alpha-2 agonists authorized for use in horses are romifidine, detomidine and xylazine. Romifidine and detomidine tend to be used interchangeably by equine practitioners depending on personal preference, although there are differences between them. The respective durations of action of the three drugs are:

- Romifidine: 45–60 minutes
- Detomidine: 20–30 minutes
- Xylazine: 15–20 minutes.

Xylazine is therefore often used for premedication prior to induction of anaesthesia in clinically unwell colic horses because the cardiovascular effects of the drug will be of the shortest duration. Analgesia provided by detomidine is considered to be greater than that provided by romifidine, although this is difficult to extrapolate through to clinical practice. The sedation and analgesia provided by alpha-2 agonists is significantly enhanced when this class of drug is combined with opioids (such as butorphanol).

Alpha-2 agonists are most commonly given intravenously, although intramuscular or buccal administration may be used in horses that are difficult to handle or needle-shy. A gel preparation of detomidine for oral/buccal administration has also recently become available. If injected intravenously, alpha-2 agonists should be given slowly in order to prevent adverse effects during injection, particularly when given during anaesthesia. Very rapid injection will result in a sudden peak in plasma concentration of the drug so that the cardiovascular side effects are likely to manifest themselves acutely and severely. For example, heart rate is likely to fall significantly (to a profound bradycardia) and cardiac output will markedly reduce. Apnoea may occur during anaesthesia, due to the sudden deepening in depth of anaesthesia following rapid intravenous injection.

Clinical signs associated with alpha-2 agonist sedation of a horse (see Figure 23.28a) include:

- Lowering of the head and drooping lower lip
- Wide-based stance
- Sweating (with high doses)

- Reduced respiratory rate
- Reduced heart rate (a second degree AV block is not uncommon).

Even though horses appear sedated, it is important to remember that they are still capable of kicking, particularly during examination of the hindlimbs. Care should be taken when working with sedated horses, and wearing a riding hat to protect the head is recommended. The combination of an alpha-2 agonist with an opioid will significantly reduce this risk but appropriate PPE should still be worn.

Monitoring premedicated patients

Drugs used for premedication can have profound effects on body systems, and careful monitoring of patients is therefore required. This should include:

- Monitoring the degree of sedation:
  - Marked sedation can result in airway obstruction in brachycephalic dogs and cats
  - Stretching out the head and neck can reduce respiratory obstruction in sedated patients
  - Acute respiratory obstruction is an indication to proceed directly to induction of anaesthesia and placement of an endotracheal tube
- Monitoring of body temperature:
  - Support body temperature to prevent onset of hypothermia, particularly in animals of low bodyweight and after acepromazine
- More invasive monitoring of high-risk patients after premedication, e.g. electrocardiography, pulse oximetry, oxygen supplementation.

In horses premedication with alpha-2 agonists is usually followed almost immediately by induction of anaesthesia. The horse is therefore under constant observation in the induction box following premedication and so considerations such as body temperature and more invasive monitoring do not apply.

Premedication tips

Premedication can be made safer and easier by remembering the following:

- Weigh all animals so that drug dosing is accurate. Dose recommendations for very potent drugs such as the alpha-2 agonists (dexmedetomidine) may be given based on body surface area rather than bodyweight (conversion charts are available). It is useful to have small scales available in the practice (such as digital kitchen scales) that are suitable for weighing rats and mice
- Give the premedication agents at the correct time relative to the expected onset of peak sedation and induction of anaesthesia
- Record the time of drug administration and the drugs given on the anaesthetic record on the front of the kennel/stable
- A quiet environment with minimal stimulation will promote good sedation following premedication.

Analgesia

Nurses play a huge role in both recognizing pain in animals and delivering analgesia protocols. It is therefore imperative that veterinary nurses have a good theoretical grounding in analgesic drug pharmacology as well as a sound practical knowledge of analgesia techniques.

Pathophysiology of pain

The neuroanatomy and pathophysiology of pain pathways are complex. Nevertheless, a basic understanding of these pathways is essential in order to understand the underlying principles of analgesic strategies and the mechanism of action of analgesic drugs. Informed decisions about different analgesic drug combinations and the timing of analgesic interventions can contribute to improved analgesia provision in veterinary practice. This section will focus on changes that occur in the pain pathway in response to noxious input, particularly the clinical relevance of these changes and how they might influence analgesia protocols.

What is pain?

The International Association for the Study of Pain defines pain in humans as 'a sensory or emotional experience associated with actual or potential tissue damage'. The absence of the ability to communicate does not negate the possibility that a person is experiencing pain or requires pain-relieving treatment. Recently this definition has been adopted for animals. It acknowledges that animals can also suffer as a result of pain. However, it is important to consider that pain is a *conscious* sensation or experience; therefore, when an animal is adequately anaesthetized and is unconscious, by definition it cannot experience pain.

What is a noxious stimulus?

A noxious stimulus is one that is damaging to tissues, for example a thermal, mechanical or chemical stimulus that is of sufficient magnitude to cause tissue damage. **Nociception** is activity in nociceptive pathways, caused by a noxious stimulus, which is transmitted to the CNS. Nociception usually results in pain perception in conscious animals; however, in an adequately anaesthetized animal nociception will not result in pain until recovery from anaesthesia.

Activation of the pain pathway

Large changes in pain sensitivity are recognized to occur after peripheral tissue injury. The resultant pain is not merely localized and short term at the site of the injury but surrounding tissues may also become painful following activation of the pain pathway. **Repeated activation of the nociceptive pathway results in a heightened sensitivity to pain.** Understanding these changes is important in order to manage clinical pain effectively.

Types of pain

It is now recognized that pain is not homogeneous (not a single entity); rather it comprises three categories – **physiological, inflammatory** and **neuropathic pain.**

Physiological pain

Physiological pain is an essential early warning device that alerts an animal to the presence of potentially damaging stimuli in the environment. An example of physiological pain is the response to a needle prick. The pain is 'appropriate' to the degree of stimulation, i.e. a stimulus–response relationship is maintained. If the force of the needle prick increases, the pain also increases in a linear manner. The pain stops when stimulation stops and the pain is localized; only the area that is stimulated causes pain. Physiological pain results from 'normal' activation of the pain pathways and is considered to serve a protective function.

Inflammatory pain

This type of **clinical pain** is initiated by tissue damage and inflammation and is the inevitable consequence of surgery or trauma to a patient. It differs from physiological pain in that it is associated with changes in the pain pathways that result in heightened pain sensitivity.

Neuropathic pain

This type of **clinical pain** is initiated by damage to the nervous system itself, such as damage to a peripheral nerve. An example of neuropathic pain in humans is 'phantom limb' pain, which commonly occurs following amputation of a leg or arm. Despite the large number of amputations carried out in a variety of veterinary species, the clinical significance of neuropathic pain in animals is not yet established and clinical management of chronic neuropathic pain can be extremely challenging.

How does clinical pain differ from physiological pain?

When clinical pain arises, there is hypersensitivity to pain at the site of tissue damage and in adjacent normal tissue. Pain may arise spontaneously. Stimuli that would not normally produce pain, such as touch, begin to do so (this is known as **allodynia**) and noxious stimuli evoke greater and more prolonged pain than in a healthy animal **(hyperalgesia).** Inflammatory pain hypersensitivity will usually return to normal if the disease process resulting in pain is controlled.

Why does pain sensitivity change?

Peripheral sensitization

Understanding **peripheral sensitization** is important because it is the mechanism by which noxious stimuli at the site of tissue injury produce a more intense and prolonged pain response once clinical pain is established. This is termed **primary hyperalgesia**.

Nociceptors are the free nerve endings of primary afferent nociceptive fibres, predominantly A and C fibres. These sensory fibres relay information from the periphery to the spinal cord (see Chapter 3); this is the first step in the relay of nociceptive information from the site of tissue damage in the periphery to the brain. The peripheral terminals of nociceptors (heat, mechanical, chemical and polymodal receptors that are activated in response to noxious stimuli) become more excitable following tissue damage, so that further noxious stimuli applied to the area are more likely to cause nociceptor activation and trigger activity in nociceptive pathways (which will usually ultimately result in pain). This modulation occurs following exposure of the nociceptor to sensitizing agents such as inflammatory mediators released during tissue damage. Administration of NSAIDs can be an effective strategy for reducing primary peripheral hyperalgesia because NSAIDs reduce the release of inflammatory mediators at the site of tissue damage, thereby decreasing nociceptor sensitization.

Central sensitization

Understanding **central sensitization** is important because it is a major mechanism by which increased pain sensitivity occurs following tissue damage and the onset of clinical pain. It results in **secondary hyperalgesia, allodynia** and **spontaneous pain**.

The spinal cord is the first site at which modulation of nociceptive information relayed from the periphery via A and C fibres occurs and, as such, is an important target site of many analgesic drugs. A and C fibres synapse with sensory neurons in the dorsal horn of the spinal cord and it is at this communication between primary afferent A and C fibres and spinal cord neurons that many of the changes associated with central sensitization occur. Modulation in central pain pathways is triggered by peripheral afferent sensory fibre input and results in enhanced responsiveness of pain transmission neurons.

The NMDA receptor

Neurotransmitters, including excitatory amino acids and peptides, ensure that an action potential arriving at the dorsal horn of the spinal cord via A and C fibres is transmitted to higher brain centres. The neurotransmitters released at the synapse between A and C fibres and the dorsal horn neuron are different in animals with physiological pain compared to those with clinical pain. The N-methyl-D-aspartate (NMDA) receptor plays a key role in clinical pain but is not normally activated during transmission of 'physiological pain'. Activation of the NMDA receptor is central to the development of central sensitization leading to enhanced pain sensitivity.

The conditions needed for activation of the NMDA receptor are complex, but essentially this receptor contributes to the transmission of noxious input from the periphery to the CNS following repeated input to the spinal cord by A and C fibres of noxious information caused by tissue injury and inflammation. Once the NMDA receptor is activated, there is a sudden augmentation of the amount of noxious input to the spinal cord that is relayed to the brain, where it is perceived as pain. This amplification of the response initiated by activation of the NMDA receptor seems to underlie central sensitization.

Pre-emptive analgesia

Pre-emptive analgesia can be defined as an analgesic treatment initiated before the start of surgery or tissue trauma. The underpinning theory behind this concept is that once peripheral and central sensitization have occurred, pain management becomes much more difficult because of the increased sensitivity to pain that results from the consequences of the activation of the nociceptive pathways. Administration of analgesic drugs 'pre-emptively' aims to prevent the development of sensitization and therefore make provision of effective analgesia easier to achieve after surgery.

An overwhelming amount of experimental data has demonstrated that various anti-nociceptive techniques applied before injury are more effective at reducing the post-injury central sensitization phenomenon than administration after injury. However, there is little evidence that this translates effectively to the clinical arena. Human clinical research studies over the last two decades have overwhelmingly demonstrated that pre-emptive administration of analgesics to surgical patients does not confer major benefits in terms of immediate postoperative pain relief or the need for supplementary analgesics. A number of caveats must, however, be considered: measuring postoperative pain in human patients is problematic; the requirement for analgesics after surgery is influenced by many psychological and physical factors, not only the degree of pain experienced by the individual; and pre-emptive analgesia in a clinical setting may not be adequate to prevent central and peripheral sensitization.

A few studies have investigated the effects of pre-emptive administration of analgesic drugs to dogs. Pre-emptive administration of opioids to bitches undergoing ovariohysterectomy has been shown to reduce secondary hyperalgesia, suggesting a positive benefit. However, caveats applied to the human studies are also applicable to studies in animals.

Despite the lack of clinical scientific evidence supporting pre-emptive analgesia, the general consensus amongst veterinary and medical professionals is that early administration of analgesics is good practice for the following reasons:

- No major deleterious effects from pre-emptive analgesic techniques have been identified
- Intraoperative analgesic administration will blunt the surgical stress response
- Intraoperative analgesics will reduce the requirement for other anaesthetic agents (balanced anaesthetic protocol)
- Pre-emptive analgesia may confer clinical benefits that cannot be detected by current study designs.

Multimodal analgesia

Multimodal or **balanced analgesia** is the principle of using different classes of analgesic drugs in combination. Because of the complexity of pain pathways, it is unrealistic to expect to achieve adequate analgesia by using single agents. Using drugs in combination causes pharmacological modulation of the pain pathway at different levels and sites, and is more effective at preventing pain sensation. There may also be synergistic benefits, as with premedication (see earlier). Drug combinations will usually allow the dose of individual agents to be reduced, which may reduce the incidence of side effects.

Recognition and quantification (scoring) of pain

Recognizing that an animal is in pain is probably one of the most challenging and important aspects of a veterinary nurse's role. Pain management in human medicine is challenging because the experience of pain is an emotion and is therefore difficult to measure and quantify and affected by many factors. Similarly, in veterinary patients it is vitally important to remember that pain is an emotional experience and varies greatly between individuals. **The mainstay of pain recognition is observation of the patient's behaviour. To assess this appropriately it is important to have a full appreciation of the full range of behaviours exhibited by different species and knowledge of what is normal behaviour for an individual patient.**

Pain-related behaviour

Variations in pain behaviour between different species are considered to be linked to whether they are a predator (e.g. cats, dogs) or prey (e.g. rabbit, horse) species in nature, and reflect the mechanism they employ for coping with dangerous situations. For example, dogs tend to fight whereas rabbits 'freeze'. Further, within each species different breeds also have different behavioural traits: Labradors tend to be stoical, while Whippets tend to be more sensitive and vocalize. It is essential to appreciate that all patients are individuals and have different perceptions as to how severe a pain is. Each patient should therefore be given analgesic drugs according to its own individual requirements for analgesia.

Dogs and cats

Typical behaviours that may be exhibited by dogs in pain:

- Sudden development of aggression – a previously friendly dog becomes aggressive or nervous, or a naturally aggressive or nervous dog becomes *more* aggressive or nervous
- Attention-seeking behaviour
- Guarding the site of injury or tissue damage
- Biting or scratching that may progress to extreme mutilation
  - A patient licking a wound could indicate that it is in pain (remember this postoperatively and consider additional analgesia rather than just applying an Elizabethan collar)
- Changes in sleep pattern and restlessness
- Posture: hunching; or the stereotypical 'praying' position typical of patients with abdominal pain (Figure 23.8)
- Anorexia or inappetence
- Vocalization, whimpering and whining, barking or growling
- Abnormal gait or movement – either non-weight-bearing or lameness on an affected leg or an abnormal gait when not wanting to stretch the abdomen or thorax
- Facial expression, including ear and eye position
- Weak or limp tail-wagging.

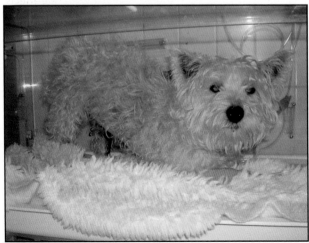

23.8 A dog in an incubator showing the 'praying' posture typically associated with cranial abdominal pain.

Although cats in pain exhibit many of the behaviours that are shown by dogs, signs of withdrawal and isolation are more common than attention-seeking behaviour.

Specific behaviours more likely to be exhibited by cats in pain:

- Posture, hunched in sternal recumbency rather than curled up and relaxed in lateral recumbency
- Immobility
- Anorexia
- Sudden development of aggression
- Cats in pain quite often bite themselves during their recovery from anaesthesia
- Lack of grooming
- Facial expression, ears rotated and flattened with 'frowning' expression
- Shying away from attention, sitting at the back of the kennel and hiding under bedding (although some cats will do this anyway as they find it reassuring)
- Spontaneous vocalization and hissing

Horses

Horses are a prey species and are very adept at hiding pain and discomfort. Visceral pain, such as that initiating from the gastrointestinal system caused by colic, may cause the following changes in behaviour:

- Pawing at the ground
- Turning to look at the flank
- Rolling in cases of severe abdominal pain
- Changes in ear position, e.g. the ears may point backwards
- Grinding of the teeth.

Musculoskeletal pain can be more obvious, particularly when it is associated with lameness due to pain originating from the limbs or feet. It may also be associated with subtle changes in behaviour, such as changes in ear position, teeth grinding, change in mentation or interest in the surrounding environment.

Rabbits and exotic pets

Rabbits are natural prey species and adept at hiding pain and discomfort. It is essential to remember that they find the veterinary environment particularly stressful and virtually all of the behaviours listed below could be caused by stress. Consequently, the hospitalization environment must be designed specifically to minimize stress, and the importance of this needs to be understood by the whole veterinary team.

Specific behaviours that may be exhibited by rabbits in pain:

- Anorexia (potentially leading to gut stasis)
- Reduced drinking
- Hunched up or awkward/abnormal position
- Reduced movement around the cage (almost frozen in position)
- Reduced interaction with environment
- Reluctance to being handled
- Limping or change in gait
- Licking or rubbing at a painful area
- Sudden development of aggression
- Squinting
- Teeth grinding.

Rabbits with foot pain often stretch their legs out behind them; however, this can also be a sign that the rabbit is content and relaxed. This is a good example of how challenging pain assessment in rabbits can be.

The effects of the veterinary environment on other pets such as small mammals, birds and reptiles are difficult to evaluate. It should be remembered that many of these animals use sensory systems that are different from those of cats and dogs and therefore they may be distressed by an environment that is appropriate for canine and feline patients. For example, rodents can hear very high frequency noises that humans are unable to detect and may find them distressing. Ideally, exotic species should be isolated from the main cat and dog ward areas and maintained in a quiet environment. Hospitalizing reptiles, rodents and birds in their home cage may reduce stress associated with transfer to a veterinary practice (see Chapter 12).

Other factors influencing the expression of pain behaviour

There are many factors that can alter both the expression of pain behaviour in a species and the experience of pain by individuals, making recognition of pain even more challenging, particularly in a hospital environment or following surgery. These include:

- **Age:** Younger patients may be more sensitive to painful stimuli. With the exception of neonates, this cannot be explained by differences in the pathophysiology of pain and nociceptive processing; it is more likely to relate to the perception or expression of pain by younger animals
- **Gender:** Females tend to be more sensitive to pain than males, except when pregnant. This is due to the effect of sex hormones on pain processing
- The **source** of the pain
- **Pain history:** Presence of CNS sensitization or a prior pain experience
- **Temperament:** A nervous patient may experience more pain and anxiety, increasing stress and fear
- Presence or absence of **additional stressors,** e.g. being away from their owner
- The patient's potential **inability to perform the pain behaviour** due to concurrent illness
- **Drugs:** Opioids and alpha-2 agonists often produce sedation, which can mask or prevent pain-related behaviour
- Presence of a **predator species** in the vicinity of a prey species (e.g. housing cats and rabbits next to dogs).

Physiological effects of pain

Pain may also result in physiological changes, primarily as a result of stimulation of the sympathetic nervous system. Physiological changes can be induced by many factors, however, including stress. It is therefore important not to rely on physiological changes alone as indicators of pain, but to combine these with behavioural assessment. Physiological signs can also be significantly affected by drug administration.

> ## Physiological changes induced by pain include:
> - Tachycardia
> - Increased blood pressure
> - Tachypnoea ▶

> - Changes in respiratory pattern, e.g. rapid shallow breathing caused by thoracic pain
> - Panting
> - Pyrexia
> - Salivation
> - Pupillary dilation
> - Shaking and shivering.

Recommended protocol for pain assessment

Assessing a patient for pain is a dynamic process, requiring interaction between the patient and the assessor. The best person to carry out pain assessment is the person who knows the patient best, having spent the most time with them during hospitalization. This person is often the veterinary nurse.

Pain assessment should involve identification of the behaviours described above and should follow a set protocol.

> ## Pain assessment protocol
> 1. Assessment/observation of behaviour and demeanour within the kennel/stable without any interference by the observer.
> 2. Observation of how the patient interacts with people when approached in the kennel/stable.
> 3. Assessment of patient movement outside of the kennel/stable (if appropriate).
> 4. Response to gentle palpation/manipulation of the site of injury and surrounding tissue.

Clinical use of pain scoring systems

Pain scoring systems are used for many reasons, the main one being to improve perioperative pain management. All patients are individuals and thus have different requirements for analgesia. A pain scoring system ensures a reflective approach, helping to improve standards, identify problem areas and optimize patient care. Patients that are in pain can pose a danger to personnel as they are more likely to be aggressive; improving their experiences within the veterinary environment should make them easier to manage on future occasions. A pain scoring system helps to assess the appropriate type, dose and frequency of required analgesic drug administration. It also standardizes care by reducing the interobserver variability of pain level. There are several different types of pain scoring systems.

Simple descriptive scale

In a simple descriptive scale (SDS), after pain assessment the observer rates the pain as follows:

- No pain
- Mild pain
- Moderate pain
- Severe pain.

Usually descriptors to aid classification are provided. Although this system is fairly crude, it is simple to use and can work well in a clinical environment.

Simple numerical rating scale

In a simple numerical rating scale (NRS) the observer assesses how much pain they think the patient is experiencing and then assigns a number appropriate to the degree of pain; usually this number is between 0 and 10. The system has been shown to be reasonably sensitive and appropriate for use by multiple observers; it is also simple to use.

Visual analogue scale

A visual analogue scale (VAS) is a simple method of recording pain (Figure 23.9). After pain assessment, the observer scores pain by marking a line that is 10 cm in length at a point corresponding to the degree of pain that the observer thinks the patient is experiencing. The line is anchored at two points:, 0 cm (no pain) and 10 cm (worst possible pain for that procedure).

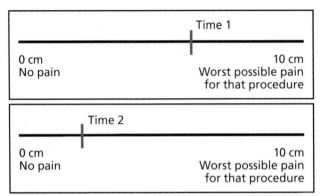

23.9 Example of a visual analogue scale for quantification of pain. A mark is made on the line by the observer according to their perception of the magnitude of pain experienced by the animal. At Time 2, following the administration of analgesia, this patient is perceived to be in less pain than at Time 1.

Advantages of this system are that the scoring system is continuous rather than having discrete categories (as in the NRS or SDS) and the result can be quantified numerically by measuring the distance of the mark along the line from the 0 mm anchor. The VAS is more sensitive than the NRS, but this is a disadvantage when used by more than one assessor. Therefore the VAS is often used for research studies carried out by a single observer but is not so helpful in a clinical environment.

Multidimensional or composite pain scales

Multidimensional or composite pain scales are more complex and try to take into account both the emotional effects of pain and its intensity. They comprise a number of separate assessments of different aspects of behaviour that can be associated with pain, e.g. posture, demeanour, attention to the wound. The **Glasgow Composite Pain Scale (GCPS)** is a composite pain scale that has been validated in dogs; no similar scales currently exist for cats.

The disadvantage of composite scales is that they are time-consuming and require a degree of knowledge. They can, however, provide more information about the pain experience of the animal, and the fact that the GCPS has undergone validation in a number of clinical research studies supports use of this scale. The short-form composite measure pain score can be downloaded from the University of Glasgow website.

Opioid analgesics

The opioid group of drugs is diverse, and the drugs within it differ with respect to their analgesic efficacy, duration of action and potential for side effects. Opioids are generally a very safe and versatile group of drugs to use. It is important to understand the differences in order to choose the most appropriate drug for a given situation. Opioids can be classified by which opioid receptor they bind to and according to whether they have **agonist**, **partial agonist** or **antagonist** effects (Figure 23.10). Opioids are Controlled Drugs (see Chapter 8).

Pharmacological effects of opioids

- **Analgesia:** Depending on the opioid chosen, different intensities of analgesia can be obtained. Opioids are a key element of perioperative pain control; mu (μ) agonists are the most effective analgesics. Generally the more potent the opioid (e.g. fentanyl), the greater the likelihood of clinically significant side effects.
- **Sedation:** The sedative effect of opioids is usually dose- and drug-dependent. Sedation from phenothiazines and alpha-2 agonists is enhanced when they are combined with opioids (see above).
- **Respiratory system:** Opioids such as methadone, morphine and buprenorphine do not cause clinically significant respiratory depression in animals at clinical dose rates. Fentanyl and remifentanil given intravenously during anaesthesia are likely to cause clinically significant respiratory depression, and animals may require support of ventilation.
- **Cardiovascular system:** Opioids have few negative effects on haemodynamics. They can cause a reduction in heart rate through stimulation of the vagal nerve, which can be managed by coadministration of an anticholinergic. The effect on heart rate is most apparent when the drugs are given intravenously or in high doses.
- **Gastrointestinal system:** Morphine directly stimulates the vomiting centre, and animals sedated or premedicated with morphine often vomit shortly after its administration. This effect is less apparent (or not evident at all) when morphine is used postoperatively for management of perioperative pain. Opioids stimulate the sphincters of the gastrointestinal tract, causing an overall action that is constipating; increased intestinal peristalsis tends to combat this effect.

Choice of opioid

The choice of opioid drug depends on a number of drug- and animal-related factors. The duration of action of different opioid drugs and their relative efficacy are shown in Figure 23.10.

Severity of pain

A full opioid agonist (morphine or methadone) should be given to animals that are likely to experience moderate or severe pain. These drugs have a relatively long duration of action and can be given repeatedly or by constant rate infusion (CRI; see below) if analgesia is of short duration or inadequate. Use of multimodal techniques may allow the dose of morphine or methadone to be reduced, or allow buprenorphine to be used instead. Fentanyl is an excellent

Drug	Opioid receptor effects	Analgesic efficacy	Duration of action	Routes of administration	Controlled Drug status
Morphine	mu receptor agonist	Potent analgesic agent	3–4 hours	i.v. (dilute with saline and give slowly; bolus or CRI), i.m., s.c., epidural (use a preservative-free solution)	Schedule 2
Methadone	mu receptor agonist	Equipotent to morphine	3–4 hours	i.v., i.m., s.c. Not routinely given by CRI or epidural	Schedule 2
Pethidine	mu receptor agonist	Potent but very short-acting	1–1.5 hours	i.m., s.c. Do not give i.v.	Schedule 2
Fentanyl	mu receptor agonist	More potent than morphine	10–20 minutes unless given by CRI	i.v. (CRI or bolus)	Schedule 2
Alfentanil	mu receptor agonist	Less potent than morphine, although clinical experience shows it is extremely effective in cats	Usually given by CRI	i.v. (CRI)	Schedule 2
Buprenorphine	mu receptor partial agonist	Significantly less potent than morphine	1–1.5 hours	i.v., i.m., s.c. (not recommended), oral, transmucosal	Schedule 3
Butorphanol	kappa receptor agonist	Potent analgesic agent	3–4 hours	i.v., i.m., s.c.	Not subject to Controlled Drug Regulations
Naloxone	mu receptor agonist	Antagonizes the analgesic effects of μ receptor agonists (e.g. morphine)	30–40 minutes	i.v.	Not subject to Controlled Drug Regulations

23.10   Characteristics of the commonly used opioid drugs.

analgesic drug but needs to be given continuously to provide effective analgesia postoperatively. Low doses given by CRI postoperatively can provide good analgesia without significant respiratory depression or bradycardia. When given intraoperatively, respiratory depression is more likely because of the concurrent anaesthesia.

Expected ongoing plan for pain management

Clinical evidence suggests that administration of a partial opioid agonist with a full opioid agonist (e.g. buprenorphine or butorphanol) with a full opioid agonist (e.g. morphine) does not produce additive analgesia. Therefore, if it is planned to use full opioid agonists intraoperatively or postoperatively, it is not ideal to premedicate with a partial opioid agonist.

Time of administration (premedication, intraoperative, postoperative)

Opioids given for premedication usually need to be longer acting. A choice is made between buprenorphine, butorphanol, morphine and methadone depending on the severity of pain and the overall analgesia plan. Sedation from buprenorphine is usually less than from the other drugs; therefore, if an animal is very excitable or aggressive, a higher dose of morphine or methadone should be given. Buprenorphine combined with alpha-2 agonists is a good combination for premedication. The analgesia and sedation provided by the alpha-2 agonist means that a full opioid agonist is often unnecessary.

When giving opioids intraoperatively to provide additional analgesia, good analgesia is required. It is therefore sensible to choose a full agonist (e.g. morphine, methadone, fentanyl, remifentanil). Fentanyl is ideally given by CRI; however, if only a short duration of additional analgesia is

required (e.g. during ovary removal in a spay procedure) then a single bolus dose is effective. Fentanyl CRI will also significantly reduce the amount of inhalant agent required to maintain anaesthesia, contributing to a balanced anaesthesia technique.

Ability to re-dose

If animals are not checked frequently overnight, then administration of a longer-acting opioid (e.g. buprenorphine) is desirable in order to achieve the longest duration of analgesia. This is also true for animals going home after surgery, when there is only a single chance to administer an injectable opioid.

Routes of administration

Fentanyl or morphine can be given by CRI, but animals should be monitored at regular intervals. Buprenorphine can be given sublingually in cats, which removes the need for repeated injections.

Opioid administration in horses

Traditionally there has been a reluctance to administer mu agonist opioids to horses due to concerns about possible motor stimulation. Opioids can cause 'box walking' in conscious horses, which manifests as deliberate and persistent walking around the stable or enclosure. It is more common when inappropriately high doses of opioids are given. Although it is more frequently reported following the administration of full mu agonists such as morphine, it is also reported after administration of butorphanol. Administration of potent opioids such as fentanyl to anaesthetized horses can also cause motor stimulation and limb movement, even in animals that are adequately anaesthetized; fentanyl is therefore usually avoided in both conscious and anaesthetized horses.

More recently, administration of morphine to horses in the perioperative period has become more common, in part due to the recognition that anaesthesia techniques in horses, in contrast to those used for small animals, are heavily dependent on the administration of high doses of volatile anaesthetic agents. There has also been a greater focus on the importance of effective perioperative pain management in this species. Morphine in horses is associated with a general concern about an increased risk of colic following administration due to the reduced gut motility induced by opioids. However, most clinical studies fail to show an increased risk of colic in the postoperative period following morphine administration during anaesthesia. Repeated morphine administration in the postoperative period may reduce faecal output, and feeding a laxative diet is therefore recommended. There is also limited clinical evidence to suggest that perioperative morphine is associated with improved recoveries from anaesthesia, presumably due to reduced pain during the recovery period, although larger studies are required to confirm this.

Butorphanol and buprenorphine are currently the only opioids authorized for administration to horses. Buprenorphine has a relatively long duration of action in horses (8–10 hours).

Non-steroidal anti-inflammatory drugs

NSAIDs are an important component of polymodal therapies aimed at providing perioperative analgesia in dogs and cats and are also used in the management of chronic pain, particularly osteoarthritis. Evidence suggests that the analgesic efficacy of most veterinary NSAIDs is comparable, so the most important factor in choice of NSAID is *safety*. Differences in the relative risk of side effects from different NSAIDs are apparent, particularly when used during the perioperative period.

NSAIDs inhibit the production of prostaglandins through inhibition of the **cyclooxygenase (COX) enzyme system**. Tissue damage causes the release of cell membrane lipids and prostaglandins are generated by the action of COX enzymes on products derived from those lipids. There are two isoforms of the enzyme: **COX-1 and COX-2**. Prostaglandins produced by the COX-1 pathway function largely (though not exclusively) in the gastrointestinal system, genital tract and brain. Many side effects of prostaglandins arise through inhibition of the production of such 'housekeeping' prostaglandins. Prostaglandins produced by the COX-2 pathway are largely (though not exclusively) generated following tissue damage and are termed **inducible prostaglandins**. It is these prostaglandins that are most important in mediating inflammation.

Side effects in dogs and cats

The most important adverse effects of NSAIDs are: impairment of renal function; and gastrointestinal irritation and ulceration. Although all NSAIDs can have antithrombotic effects by inhibiting the production of thromboxane A2, at therapeutic doses most NSAIDs (with the exception of aspirin) do not impair clotting mechanisms or impair bleeding time.

In the kidney locally produced prostaglandins are continually active in maintaining afferent arteriolar dilatation, and during periods of hypotension (such as may occur during anaesthesia) these prostaglandins assume an important role in the maintenance of normal renal haemodynamics. If the production of these prostaglandins is inhibited through the administration of an NSAID, renal hypoperfusion may occur with the potential to cause renal failure.

In the stomach and gastrointestinal system, prostaglandins promote the secretion of protective mucus, maintain mucosal blood flow and play a role in the modulation of gastric acid secretion. An NSAID-mediated decrease in prostaglandin production through inhibition of COX-1 can result in gastrointestinal ulceration (see Chapter 8).

Probably the most significant variation in NSAIDs lies in the safety of their administration during the perioperative period. The use of NSAIDs perioperatively has been shown to provide effective analgesia following a variety of orthopaedic and soft tissue procedures in both dogs and cats. Meloxicam, carprofen and robenacoxib (injectable form) are specifically authorized in the UK for perioperative administration to cats and dogs. Firocoxib is also authorized for preoperative administration in dogs but is not available as an injectable preparation. Administration of all other commercially available NSAIDs (e.g. ketoprofen, tepoxalin) should be delayed until the animal is fully recovered from anaesthesia and normotensive. Despite the increased safety of meloxicam, carprofen and robenacoxib, it is strongly advisable to avoid the perioperative administration of all NSAIDs in animals with impaired renal function. Gastrointestinal side effects are a particular problem during the chronic use of NSAIDs, for example in the management of osteoarthritis.

Clinical recommendations for perioperative NSAIDs

- Only administer NSAIDs that are authorized for preoperative administration in the perioperative period.
- Only administer an NSAID preoperatively to healthy animals undergoing routine procedures when hypotension during anaesthesia is not anticipated. Renal compromise is possible if an animal becomes hypotensive during anaesthesia when any NSAID has been given. If in doubt, delay NSAID administration until the animal is fully recovered from anaesthesia.
- Do not give NSAIDs to trauma or shock patients until they are normotensive and cardiovascularly stable.
- Do not give NSAIDs to animals with pre-existing renal disease.
- Do not give NSAIDs to animals with disorders of haemostasis.
- NSAIDs are liver metabolized, so liver dysfunction may alter the half-life of NSAIDs and lead to inadvertent drug overdose. Use carefully in animals with pre-existing liver disease and monitor the animal for altered liver function (blood biochemistry testing).
- Do not combine different NSAIDs or give NSAIDs and corticosteroids together.
- Check ongoing medications before perioperative drugs are administered.

NSAID administration in horses

NSAIDs are widely administered to horses for the management of pain. Horses appear to be more resistant than small animals to the renal effects of NSAIDs, which are therefore commonly given to anaesthetized horses despite the presence of concurrent hypotension or gastrointestinal disease (e.g. horses undergoing intestinal surgery).

Other drugs used for analgesia

Ketamine

Ketamine has been around for many years and is widely used in veterinary medicine for sedation and injectable anaesthesia. Use of ketamine in human patients had dwindled due to problems on recovery, such as hallucinations. However, interest in ketamine has recently resurged due to recognition of its profound analgesic properties, which are present at sub-anaesthetic doses. The use of low doses of ketamine to provide analgesia has been adopted into small animal and equine analgesic protocols. Ketamine is a Schedule 4 Controlled Drug with regulations affecting its storage and dispensing (see Chapter 8).

The principal analgesic action of ketamine is attributed to its NMDA receptor antagonist effects. Ketamine should be used as an adjunctive analgesic in combination with opioids, NSAIDs or other analgesics. It is not a drug that should be used alone to provide analgesia. It can be used safely in low doses to provide analgesia during surgery and during the postoperative period. At sub-anaesthetic doses, ketamine is not generally associated with CNS excitatory effects and concurrent sedation is minimal. CRI is advantageous to provide a stable background level of analgesia. Although a fluid infusion pump or syringe driver is not a prerequisite for this, it will allow more accurate and controlled administration. Ketamine by CRI is often used for 24–48 hours in dogs, cats and horses, despite limited data describing the pharmacokinetics of ketamine after prolonged infusions. Ketamine is metabolized to norketamine, which may contribute to the pharmacological effect.

Alpha-2 agonists in small animals

Alpha-2 adrenoreceptor agonists (alpha-2 agonists) are potent sedative, hypnotic and analgesic agents; these properties make them useful adjuncts for anaesthesia in small animal practice. They include the drugs medetomidine and dexmedetomidine. Medetomidine is a drug 'mixture', containing both levomedetomidine and dexmedetomidine in equal proportions. Levomedetomidine is considered to be pharmacologically inactive and so it is only the active form of this drug (dexmedetomidine) that has recently been authorized for veterinary use. It is likely that dexmedetomidine provides greater analgesia than medetomidine due to greater selectivity for the alpha-2 receptor; however, this has not been clearly demonstrated in the clinical arena.

Alpha-2 agonists have a potent antinociceptive action in experimental and clinical studies in animals and humans. The mechanism of alpha-2 agonist-mediated antinociception is not entirely understood; both supraspinal (brain) and spinal sites of action are involved. Extensive laboratory animal studies investigating the mechanism of alpha-2 agonist antinociception are confounded by the effects of sedation on behavioural evaluation of analgesia. Sedation complicates conclusions, particularly those involving supraspinally organized pain-related behaviours, upon which some experimental tests are based.

Medetomidine and dexmedetomidine are most commonly used for sedation or premedication but their additional analgesic effects should not be forgotten. Incorporation of an alpha-2 agonist into a premedication protocol will contribute to intraoperative analgesia, particularly if the alpha-2 agonist is re-dosed during anaesthesia. Dexmedetomidine has been recently evaluated as a postoperative analgesic in a clinical study in dogs; given by CRI it was found to be equally efficacious as morphine CRI. Sedation provided by the two drugs was also not different. Therefore, although dexmedetomidine by CRI is not a first-line drug for perioperative analgesia, it can be a useful adjunct where adequate analgesia is problematic. Due to the relatively short duration of analgesia from a single dose compared to the duration of sedation, CRI is required. It should be remembered that administration of atipamezole will reverse both sedative *and* analgesic effects.

Alpha-2 agonists for horses have been discussed earlier, in the section on Premedication.

Lidocaine

Systemically administered lidocaine has been shown to be effective in the treatment of acute postoperative pain and experimentally induced pin-prick pain and hyperalgesia in human studies. There are few robust clinical studies that have evaluated the use of systemic lidocaine for perioperative analgesia in animals.

The mechanism of analgesia following systemic lidocaine is not fully elucidated. Following peripheral nerve injury, sodium channel expression becomes modulated so that there is upregulation of sodium channel subtypes. This is associated with the presence of random and spontaneous ectopic discharges from injured nerves that occur in the absence of input from peripheral nociceptors. This abnormal activity causes abnormal input to the CNS and higher brain centres, which is interpreted as pain. Lidocaine is most effective at blocking sodium channels in a frequency-dependent manner. It is postulated that lidocaine may preferentially block the upregulated sodium channel subtypes, resulting in a reduction in perceived pain without any effect on normal conduction. Evidence suggests that the postoperative analgesic effect of an intraoperative lidocaine infusion cannot be simply attributed to residual plasma drug concentrations, suggesting the systemic lidocaine may have a pre-emptive analgesic effect.

Low-dose lidocaine by CRI is not associated with cardiovascular side effects, and heart rate and blood pressure have been shown to be well maintained in dogs; there are limited data describing the use of lidocaine by CRI in awake cats. More information on lidocaine is given under Local anaesthesia/analgesia, below.

Morphine/lidocaine/ketamine combination

A combination of morphine, lidocaine and ketamine (MLK) is relatively widely used for the provision of perioperative analgesia in cats and dogs, particularly in the USA. The drugs are usually mixed together in a single fluid bag and given simultaneously at a single rate that does not allow the rate of administration of the individual drugs in the mix to be adjusted. The underpinning rationale is that the combination is the ultimate multimodal analgesia protocol. There are, however, limited clinical data to support the use of this protocol.

Should a combination of drugs be required by intravenous infusion, it is optimal to give the drugs separately via separate infusion apparatus. This allows flexibility in dosing of the individual agents and also allows the animals to be weaned off the different drugs individually, rather than having to adopt an 'all or nothing' approach.

Gabapentin

Gabapentin, available as an oral preparation, has been proven to be effective for the treatment of neuropathic pain resulting from diabetic neuropathy and post-herpetic neuralgia in humans. Although its exact mode of action is not known, it appears to have a unique effect on voltage-dependent calcium ion channels at the post-synaptic dorsal horn. Other suggested mechanisms include enhanced inhibitory input of GABA-mediated pathways and antagonism of NMDA receptors.

Animal studies have shown that gabapentin does not alter acute nociception but suppresses experimentally induced hyperalgesia. There is strong experimental evidence that gabapentin prevents the development of neuronal sensitization and reverses established neuronal sensitization. This suggests that gabapentin may prove effective in acute pain disorders involving neuronal sensitization, such as post-operative pain.

There are no published clinical studies describing the use of gabapentin in cats or dogs for acute or chronic pain management. Anecdotal evidence suggests that it is widely used in specialist clinics in the management of osteoarthritis pain and cancer pain refractory to conventional analgesic strategies. In this setting it is used as an adjunctive agent with therapies such as NSAIDs, fentanyl patches and tramadol. The quoted dose range for gabapentin in cats and dogs is wide; it is advisable to start at the low end of the dose range and then increase the dose gradually until an effect is achieved. Gabapentin is metabolized by the liver and excreted via the kidneys, so that liver dysfunction may result in drug accumulation unless the dose is adjusted. Side effects include lethargy, sedation and ataxia, and sometimes nausea. The pharmacokinetics of gabapentin in cats and dogs have been described, but optimal dosing regimens to provide analgesia and the effects of prolonged gabapentin administration have not been investigated.

Tramadol

Although tramadol has been available as an analgesic drug for a number of years, it is only recently that the mechanism of action has been fully understood. Tramadol is a unique analgesic with opioid and non-opioid properties. Its action on mu opioid receptors is weak, and naloxone antagonizes only 30% of its analgesic activity. Alpha-2 antagonists significantly reverse tramadol analgesia, and therefore much of its analgesic action is thought likely to be via inhibition of reuptake of neurotransmitters such as noradrenaline. It is now accepted that in addition to a mu opioid agonist effect, tramadol enhances the function of the spinal descending inhibitory pathway by inhibition of reuptake of both 5HT (5-hydroxytryptamine, serotonin) and noradrenaline, together with presynaptic stimulation of 5HT release.

Similarly to gabapentin, tramadol is widely used as an adjunctive analgesic for chronic pain, yet there are limited published studies describing clinical use in cats or dogs. In contrast to gabapentin, tramadol is also used for perioperative pain management. It is available as a tablet and injectable formulation. It is not subject to the Misuse of Drugs Regulations and so can be dispensed for use in the home setting to improve analgesia, although the tablets are very bitter and cats especially find them distasteful. Metabolism is principally via hepatic biotransformation, with a small amount excreted unchanged by the kidneys. Side effects, though rare, may include gastrointestinal upset and sedation. Because of tramadol's monoamine reuptake inhibition, it should not be given to animals taking tricyclic antidepressants, serotonin reuptake inhibitors or monoamine oxidase inhibitors.

Pain management drugs used in exotic pets
Rabbits and rodents

The effects of drugs used in cats and dogs have been evaluated in rabbits, rats and mice, despite difficulties in assessing pain in these species and therefore the outcome of drug administration. It is recognized that opioids provide analgesia in these species, and buprenorphine is reported to be the most widely used opioid analgesic in laboratory small mammals. Buprenorphine has a wide margin of safety in these species, although the associated sedation may be disadvantageous in terms of prolonging recovery from anaesthesia in rabbits. It is therefore recommended to delay repeat doses of buprenorphine until rabbits are fully recovered from anaesthesia and awake. In rats, buprenorphine has been shown to cause pica (an appetite for non-nutritional objects), resulting in animals eating sawdust bedding with the potential to cause gastric obstruction. This can be overcome by using alternative bedding material. Buprenorphine is efficacious when given orally to rats in a 'jelly mixture' and dose rates are published for this technique in the laboratory animal literature.

NSAIDs are also very effective, although it is likely that doses to provide analgesia in rabbits and rodents are higher than in dogs and cats. Injectable carprofen has been shown to be effective given orally in a 'jelly mixture' to rats, avoiding the need for repeated injections. Oral meloxicam has been evaluated in rabbits but further work is required to establish the optimum dose.

Ketamine and alpha-2 agonists are commonly used as part of anaesthetic protocols for rabbits and rodents, although their specific actions as analgesic agents rather than anaesthetic agents have not been evaluated.

Birds

The most challenging part of the provision of effective analgesia is the ability to recognize pain in this diverse group of animals. However, adoption of a precautionary approach is recommended so that analgesia is always provided after carrying out procedures that are likely to be painful in other species, or when birds are presented with pre-existing tissue trauma or injury.

Opioids are frequently used in birds but unfortunately inconsistent experiences and species-specific differences in studies have led to controversial opinions about their use, effects and doses. It has been suggested that in birds the kappa opioid receptor is more important in providing analgesia, in contrast to mammals where the mu opioid receptor is predominantly associated with analgesia and the kappa opioid receptor plays a less significant role. The clinical significance of this is that butorphanol (predominantly a kappa agonist) might be more effective in birds than drugs that have a primary action at mu opioid receptors. Generally, butorphanol and buprenorphine are the most widely used opioids in birds; before using them for a particular clinical case it is important to research the literature regarding information for the particular bird species that requires analgesia.

NSAIDs have been widely used in birds but it is important to remember that doses for mammals may not be applicable to birds and side effects such as nephrotoxicity and gastric ulceration are common. This is unlikely to be a problem following administration of a single dose of a NSAID but should be considered for repeated administration.

Reptiles

Recognition of behaviours associated with pain is very difficult in reptiles, although a precautionary principle should again be adopted.

Routes of analgesic drug administration

In common with other drugs (see Chapter 8), the route of administration of analgesics is affected by authorization, pharmacological effects and onset of activity (see Figure 23.10).

- **Intravenous injection**: Best when analgesia is required quickly. Potent opioids such as fentanyl and alfentanil, when administered in the aqueous form, should only be given by slow intravenous injection. Pethidine cannot be given intravenously due to histamine release. Morphine must also be diluted and given slowly to prevent histamine release.
- **Intramuscular injection**: Care must be taken with the volume of drugs given and when choosing the injection site, as repeated injection at the same site will cause soreness. This is especially true for animals with low bodyweight and for exotic pets where a limited muscle mass increases the pain of repeated injection.
- **Subcutaneous injection**: Few pharmacokinetic data are available about the onset of action following subcutaneous injection of most drugs, although uptake is generally slower than with intramuscular or intravenous administration. The route is not recommended for buprenorphine, as current evidence suggests that uptake is slow, delaying the onset of action.
- **Transmucosal** (Figure 23.11): Shown to be effective in cats for the administration of buprenorphine (transmucosal administration is as effective as intravenous administration**).** The newer multidose formulation of buprenorphine appears to be unpalatable to cats when given transmucosally, and 1 ml vial preparations are preferred.

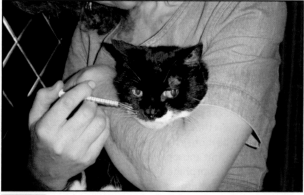

23.11   Oral transmucosal administration of buprenorphine. (Courtesy of Polly Taylor)

Transdermal administration

Both fentanyl and buprenorphine transdermal patches are available and can provide a valuable non-invasive source of long-term analgesia. Data surrounding the use of buprenorphine patches are limited and their effectiveness is currently unknown in dogs and cats. There is more research knowledge surrounding the use of fentanyl patches.

Most patches comprise a reservoir of the drug covered with a membrane that limits the rate of absorption, surrounded by an adhesive dressing with which to attach the patch to the patient's skin. Matrix patches, where the drug is embedded in the adhesive plaster, are also available. The patches are designed for human skin, and transdermal bioavailability of fentanyl is much lower in feline (34%) or canine skin (64%). The site of patch placement is also likely to be important, as the characteristics of the skin (such as thickness and vascularity) over different sites of the body are likely to affect the rate of drug absorption, although this has not been formally evaluated in a controlled clinical study.

Commonly used sites of patch placement are the lateral thorax, medial aspect of the thigh, and tail. The contact between the patch and the skin must be optimal to promote drug absorption. It is important that the patient is not able to gain access to the patch and ingest it. The site of application of the patch should be gently clipped, the skin cleaned using a detergent and allowed to air dry. Although patches have an adhesive strip this is not robust enough for veterinary patients, and a dressing should be applied over the patch (Figure 23.12) to promote adhesion; use of tissue glue can also be helpful.

Care should be taken when patches are used perioperatively as the patient's temperature and the temperature around the patch can affect the rate of drug absorption. If a patient is placed on to a warming device, e.g. a heat mat, the amount of drug released by the patch will increase. This can lead to severe respiratory depression in the case of fentanyl patches.

It takes approximately 24 hours in dogs and 12 hours in cats for the plasma concentration of fentanyl to reach therapeutic levels, so up until this time additional analgesia must be provided. There are many variables affecting the absorption of drugs via the transdermal route and using them as the sole method of analgesia is consequently unwise.

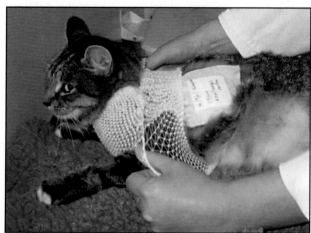

23.12   A fentanyl patch can be placed on clipped skin and covered with a flexible dressing to prevent the edges curling and excessive interference from the cat. It takes several hours to provide peak plasma fentanyl concentrations so it should be placed well in advance of surgery, and additional analgesia provided for the first few hours. (Courtesy of Polly Taylor)

Constant rate infusions

The use of CRIs has increased in popularity over the last few years, in both the peri- and postoperative periods. The main advantage compared to repeated injections is that peaks and troughs in plasma concentration, and therefore fluctuations in the level of analgesia provision, can be avoided. This reduces the risk of breakthrough pain and consequently minimizes stimulation of the pain pathways, potentially reducing further central and peripheral sensitization. Another advantage is that the patient does not need to have repeated injections, particularly intramuscular ones.

When using a CRI a 'loading' dose must first be administered to rapidly achieve plasma concentrations levels close to therapeutic levels. The infusion is started simultaneously to ensure that the therapeutic plasma concentration is maintained. The rate of infusion depends on the plasma concentration required as well as the rate at which the drug is redistributed and metabolized. The theory behind CRI is that as the drug is lost out of the circulation it is replaced, maintaining a constant plasma concentration.

CRI is mainly used for the intravenous administration of analgesics but is also useful for local anaesthetics, e.g. via epidural or wound catheters. When administering a drug by CRI, accuracy is vitally important. Although 'recipes' using only a standard giving set and a drip rate are available, they are not recommended, and use of either infusion pumps or syringe drivers is preferable (see Chapter 22). Selection of infusion apparatus with a high degree of accuracy for drug administration is important.

Considerations for preparing drugs for CRI

- The required rate of administration of potent analgesic drugs is often low, so diluting the drug with normal saline or lactated Ringer's (Hartmann's) solution will increase the accuracy of drug dosing. However, it is important to remember to *adjust the volume in the bag or syringe before adding the drug.* For example, for a 50 ml syringe, take up 45 ml of saline and then 5 ml of drug. If using a 500 ml bag of fluids and adding 5 ml of drug, remove 5 ml of the fluids from the bag *first* and then add the drug.
- Ensure that the drug solution is labelled with the patient details so that the infusion solution is uniquely linked with the patient for which it is intended.
- Ensure that the drug solution is clearly labelled with the date, drug name and concentration and intended infusion rate.
- Ensure that the extension set or giving set is long enough to prevent the lines from becoming disconnected and that they are long enough to allow the patient to move around in the kennel.
- Do not use needles to deliver the drug via an injection port but ensure that infusion lines are firmly connected using 3-way taps or via a T-port.
- Connect the infusion line delivering the drug as close as possible to the site of intravenous access in the patient. This reduces the time delay when the infusion is initially started.
- Ensure that connections and infusion lines are secured above ground level to prevent contamination of the infusion apparatus.

Nursing considerations for CRI

- As CRI relies on the patency of the intravenous catheter, good catheter management is vital (see Chapter 22).
- If CRI is being used in a non-anaesthetized patient it is important to remember that the drugs commonly given by CRI usually cause some degree of sedation and, consequently, recumbency. It is important to nurse these patients like any other recumbent animal (see Chapter 17).
- It is vital to ensure that no joints in the fluid line (e.g. where two extension sets join) or 3-way taps are on the floor, as this could be a source of contamination and could lead to a catheter infection.
- Remember to include the volume of fluids being used to administer the CRI in any fluid therapy calculation for the patient.

Local anaesthesia/ analgesia

Local analgesia/anaesthesia techniques are widely used in human medicine. Use of a local technique can often reduce the dose of other anaesthetic drugs required for maintenance of anaesthesia and can contribute to a multimodal analgesic technique. Use of specific nerve blocks to prevent the relay of nociceptive information from the site of injury to the spinal cord can also provide pre-emptive analgesia, and prevent or reduce the development of central sensitization. Specific nerve blocks are of particular value in equine patients, where they are used mainly to obviate distal limb pain and thereby reduce the dosage of anaesthetic agent required.

Local anaesthetic agents
Mechanism of action

Local anaesthetics reversibly block the conduction of action potentials in neurons by causing changes in the neuron membrane that prevent depolarization and thus block the propagation of an action potential; this is termed **membrane stabilization**.

An action potential can be described as a brief fluctuation in membrane potential caused by the rapid opening and closing of voltage-gated sodium ion channels. In resting mode nerve fibres are polarized, with higher concentrations of sodium ions outside than inside the nerve, with the reverse true for potassium ions. The sodium and potassium channels are closed. Depolarization is caused by the sodium channels opening, which allows an influx of sodium ions into the nerve fibre. Local anaesthetics prevent the sodium channels from opening so that depolarization and therefore action potential transmission is prevented. Sensory neurons are more sensitive to the effects of local anaesthetics than are motor neurons and are therefore blocked by lower concentrations of local anaesthetics. However, although it would be highly desirable to produce a blockade of sensory nerve fibres without any concurrent effects on motor nerves and therefore movement, achieving a sensory block without concurrent motor effects is rarely possible.

Characteristics of some local anaesthetic agents

Lidocaine:

- Extremely stable in solution
- Short duration of onset
- Duration of action 1–2 hours.

Bupivacaine:

- Very stable compound
- Slower rate of onset than lidocaine, duration of action 6–8 hours
- Four times more potent than lidocaine
- Shows good motor/sensory separation and does not require the addition of adrenaline to prolong its effects or reduce its systemic accumulation
- Greater potential for cardiotoxicity compared to lidocaine; do not give intravenously.

Systemic toxicity

These agents are lipid-soluble, have low molecular weight and readily cross the blood–brain barrier. At sub-toxic doses, local anaesthetics can act as anticonvulsants, sedatives and analgesics. At higher concentrations they can *cause* convulsions, and generalized CNS depression occurs. Due to a combination of slowing of conduction in the myocardium, myocardial depression and peripheral vasodilatation, hypotension, bradycardia and cardiac arrest can occur.

Systemic toxicity depends on:

- Site of injection: vascular sites lead to rapid absorption. Intercostal injections give much higher plasma concentrations than subcutaneous injections.
- Drug used
- Speed of injection: only important when given intravenously
- Addition of adrenaline: causes local vasoconstriction, resulting in slow absorption with reduction in peak concentration of up to 20–50%.

Cats and some exotic pets are considered to be more susceptible than dogs to local anaesthetic toxicity, but problems are uncommon if appropriate doses are given. Safe maximum doses of local anaesthetic agents are shown in Figure 23.13.

Local anaesthesia techniques

Topical anaesthesia

The application of local anaesthetics to mucous membranes (transmucosal) produces analgesia rapidly (within 5 minutes). Common areas for topical administration include the cornea (for ocular examinations), the nasal passages and the larynx (during intubation). The depth of analgesia produced in tissues is usually superficial (1–2 mm).

Absorption of local anaesthetic through the skin (stratum corneum) is poor. EMLA cream (APP Pharmaceuticals; contains lidocaine and prilocaine) and amethocaine are capable of producing anaesthesia if applied to the skin and covered with a non-permeable dressing for 30–60 minutes. In rabbits, topical application of EMLA cream can be very useful prior to placement of an intravenous catheter in the marginal ear (auricular) vein. Placing a latex glove over the ear and securing it at the ear base can improve drug absorption and therefore effectiveness.

Infiltration anaesthesia

The infiltration of local anaesthetics is commonly performed in veterinary practice; it is safe, reliable and does not require extensive experience. Sterile sharp needles should be used. If subsequent injections are made at the periphery of each wheal, then only one needle prick is felt.

- Local anaesthetic should be diluted with 0.9% sodium chloride and not sterile water.
- Adrenaline at a concentration of 1:200 000 may be used to delay the absorption of local anaesthetics and increase the duration of effect.
- Adrenaline should not be used where an end-arterial supply exists, as skin necrosis may result (ears, tails).

Regional anaesthesia

The principle underlying regional anaesthesia is that the nerve supply to a specific region or area is blocked where the nerves are easily accessible from the skin. The nerves must be readily palpable and follow a fixed course next to easily identifiable anatomical structures (usually bones) or be known to be found at fixed positions. Use of a nerve stimulator (Figure 23.14) to locate the peripheral nerve can significantly increase the accuracy of drug deposition and therefore effectiveness of the block. This can also allow a lower total volume of the local anaesthetic drug to be used, reducing motor side effects and the risk of toxicity due to absorption of local anaesthetic agents into the systemic circulation.

Patient type	Lidocaine	Lidocaine plus adrenaline	Bupivacaine
Cats and dogs	4 mg/kg	7 mg/kg	2 mg/kg
Horses	4 mg/kg	Because of licensing considerations, when a local anaesthetic with adrenaline is required in horses, Willcain (Dechra) – a preparation of procaine plus adrenaline – should be used (total dose 2–5 ml)	2 mg/kg
Rabbits and rodents	2 mg/kg	3 mg/kg	1 mg/kg
Birds	2 mg/kg	Do not use preparations containing adrenaline in birds	1 mg/kg

23.13 Maximum doses of local anaesthetics for infiltration. When performing intercostal or intrapleural injections, reduce dose by 25%. Reduce dose by 50% if injected into highly vascular area (e.g. brachial plexus) where systemic drug absorption is likely to be high.

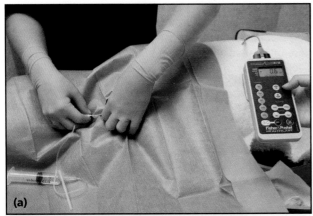

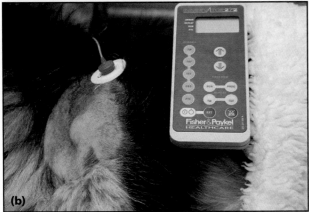

23.14 (a) Using a peripheral nerve stimulator to facilitate a brachial plexus block. The stimulating needle is being placed while an assistant holds the stimulator device. (b) The reference electrode is placed remote from the site of stimulation on a clipped area of skin.

Brachial plexus block

This block provides analgesia distal to the elbow and is therefore useful during distal forelimb surgical procedures.

Preparation of the patient

The patient is positioned in lateral recumbency. The site of injection is just proximal to the point of the shoulder (Figure 23.15); therefore a wide area should be clipped (approximately 6 cm x 6 cm) at this site, with the point of the shoulder at the centre. The skin should be prepared as if for surgery.

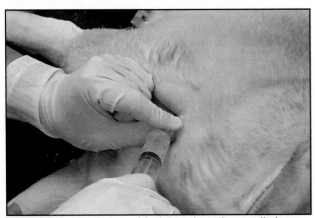

23.15 Brachial plexus block in a dog. The needle has been placed without using a peripheral nerve stimulator, and bupivacaine is being injected.

Clinical notes

The two most important complications following brachial plexus blocks are pneumothorax due to puncture of the cupulae (the apex of each pleural cavity lying at the thoracic inlet) and haemorrhage as a result of puncture of the axillary artery and vein. The needle should be aspirated prior to injection of the local anaesthetic block to prevent inadvertent intravenous injection of the local anaesthetic. This will also allow identification of needle placement in the cupulae. Some resistance should be felt during injection. Damage to the brachial plexus nerves themselves is also possible if the needle penetrates the nerve bundle. This is uncommon, particularly if a nerve stimulator is used to allow accurate location of the individual nerves that comprise the brachial plexus.

Epidural anaesthesia

Lumbosacral epidural anaesthesia may be used to provide analgesia for all procedures caudal to the thoracolumbar junction. It is especially useful for orthopaedic procedures in the hindquarters. Use of a combination of preservative-free morphine and bupivacaine is optimal. Morphine has a prolonged duration of action (18–24 h) and therefore provides significant postoperative analgesia. Veterinary nurses are not permitted to carry out epidural administration of drugs, as placement of catheters or needles for epidural anaesthesia involves entering a body space, which may only be carried out by a veterinary surgeon. It is important, however, that veterinary nurses have knowledge of the technique and the effects of drugs injected into the epidural space.

Preparation of the patient

Careful preparation of the patient to ensure that the epidural injection can be made aseptically is important. Epidural injection is usually carried out with the animal in sternal recumbency with the hindlimbs directed forward, although some people prefer to have the animal in lateral recumbency. The epidural space between L7 and S1 is identified in order to ensure that the site of clipping is correct. The dorsal spinous process of L7 is more pronounced than the preceding dorsal processes and immediately behind it a dip can be felt. A large window (approximately 6 cm x 6 cm) is clipped around the L7–S1 space and the skin prepared aseptically in a similar way to that for surgery. Drugs for administration into the epidural space should be drawn up and administered aseptically using sterile gloves, needles and syringes.

Technique

A spinal needle (22G) (Figure 23.16) or Tuohy needle (17G or 18G) (Figure 23.17), is placed perpendicular to the skin surface and slowly advanced through the skin by the veterinary surgeon.

Initially the stylet is left *in situ* in the needle, but as the point of the needle nears the anticipated site of the epidural space the stylet is removed. A popping sensation is felt as the needle penetrates the ligamentum flavum. Correct placement of the needle is checked in two ways:

- **Loss of resistance:** Correct placement of the needle is confirmed by a lack of resistance to the injection of either air or saline into the epidural space. Air may be associated with a patchy block as the air tends to localize around the nerve roots, resulting in an ineffective block.

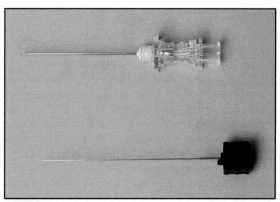

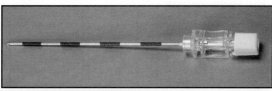

23.16 A 22 G short spinal needle suitable for use in a cat or small dog. The stylet has been removed from the needle.

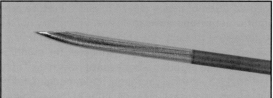

23.17 Tuohy needle, showing detail of curved distal end.

- **Hanging drop:** Once the epidural needle and stylet have been advanced through the superficial tissue, the stylet is removed and a drop of saline placed on the hub of the needle (Figure 23.18). The needle is then gradually advanced; entry of the tip of the needle into the epidural space is associated with the rapid movement of the drop of saline into the epidural space so that it can no longer be seen.

The presence of blood in the hub of the needle indicates that the needle has penetrated a blood vessel (usually the spinal ventral sinus), which typically occurs if the needle is not inserted in the midline. The needle should be withdrawn and

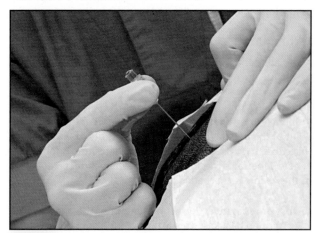

23.18 Epidural analgesia in a dog. The stylet has been removed from the spinal needle and a hanging drop technique is being used to locate the epidural space.

placement started again once the position of the animal has been checked and the location of L7–S1 confirmed.

If cerebrospinal fluid (CSF) is present in the needle, the dose of local anaesthetic should be reduced by 50% or the needle re-placed in a new space. Injection of local anaesthetic into the CSF is known as spinal anaesthesia, which has a more rapid onset than epidural anaesthesia.

Clinical notes

Epidural anaesthesia with local anaesthetic agents can induce vasodilatation of the mesenteric blood vessels due to blockade of sympathetic nervous system tone to the splanchnic vessels. Caution should be exercised in hypovolaemic patients, although fluid administration readily resolves the hypotension. Hypoventilation and paralysis may occur if the local anaesthetic spreads too far cranially (e.g. too large a volume has been injected). Artificial ventilation is instigated until the local anaesthetic block resolves and no adverse effects are seen. Epidural anaesthesia should not be carried out in patients with septicaemia or when the needle would have to traverse an area of infected skin. Coagulation disorders are also a contraindication to epidural anaesthesia due to the risk of continued bleeding around the spinal cord if a blood vessel is damaged during needle placement.

Morphine injected epidurally can be associated with urinary retention; therefore urination should be monitored in all animals for approximately 24 hours following epidural administration of morphine. If urinary retention occurs, placement of a urinary catheter to facilitate urination is likely to be indicated.

Local anaesthetics injected epidurally will cause motor effects and hindlimb paralysis for their duration of action (typically 6–8 h for bupivacaine). This should be considered when walking dogs that have received epidural local anaesthetics, and hindlimb support should be provided.

Hair regrowth at the site of epidural injection is more prolonged than for other body areas; it can therefore be prudent to warn owners that regrowth may take up to approximately 6 months after clipping.

Epidural catheters

Placement of an epidural catheter can be useful in patients that will benefit from a longer period of epidural analgesia, avoiding the need for repeat epidural injection. Kits are commercially available that contain all the equipment required for placement of an epidural catheter by the veterinary surgeon.

The first stage is the placement of a Tuohy needle in the epidural space. Tuohy needles have a rounded blunt-ended curved tip (Figure 23.17), so that there is no risk of damaging or cutting the catheter as it is threaded through the needle. The tip of the catheter is usually inserted up to the level of L3–L4, although more caudal placement may be required if the site of injury is distal to this. To prevent motor effects during catheter placement, usually morphine alone is injected into the epidural space for pain management. However, the catheters can become irritating after 12–24 hours, and injection of a low dose of lidocaine or bupivacaine *before* the injection of morphine can be helpful.

A bacterial filter is placed between the end of the catheter and the injection port to reduce the risk of infection being introduced into the epidural space. It is imperative that epidural catheters are managed aseptically and clearly labelled, so that other drugs are not inadvertently injected through the injection port.

Intercostal nerve block

Intercostal nerve blocks are useful for relieving pain following thoracic surgery and trauma. Following thoracotomy, the surgeon can easily place these blocks prior to closing the chest, using direct visualization of the intercostal nerve, artery and vein bundle. Bupivacaine is usually chosen because of its longer duration of action.

Intrapleural anaesthesia

Intrapleural application of local anaesthetics is a very effective technique for providing analgesia following thoracotomy or rib trauma. The local anaesthetic can be administered either through an over-the-needle catheter or through an indwelling chest drain (Figure 23.19). The site of injection is the cranial edge of a rib. The animal should be placed with the injured side downwards for the block to be maximally effective. Local anaesthetics are acidic and this route of administration is very painful in conscious animals. Diluting the dose of local anaesthetic with 0.9% saline (up to 40 ml total volume in a large dog) can reduce pain. Alternatively, sodium bicarbonate can be added to the local anaesthetic, though it is difficult to achieve physiological pH without generating precipitation. Bupivacaine produces analgesia of approximately 8 hours' duration.

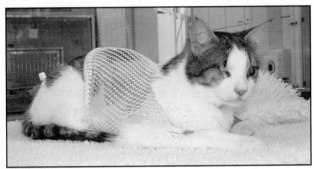

23.19 Cat with a chest drain placed after surgery. Intrapleural analgesia can be provided by injection of bupivacaine down the chest drain every 8 hours.

Maxillary and mandibular nerve blocks

These are extremely useful for analgesia for dental procedures or jaw surgery. The maxillary (Figure 23.20) and mandibular (Figure 23.21) nerves can be blocked as they exit from the infraorbital and mental foramina, respectively, or can be blocked more proximally, to provide a wider area of analgesia.

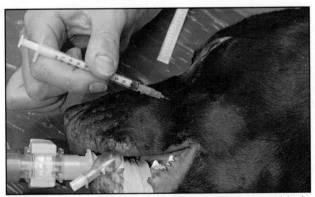

23.20 Site of injection for a distal maxillary nerve block, with the needle placed in the infraorbital foramen. Injection of local anaesthetic to block the infraorbital nerve will desensitize the ipsilateral soft tissues and upper incisor, premolar and canine teeth.

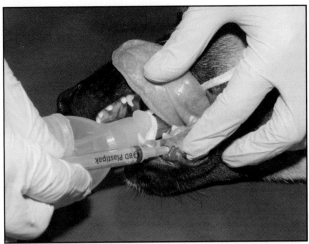

23.21 Distal mandibular nerve block. Local anaesthetic is being injected into the mental foramen. This will desensitize the ipsilateral lower incisors, premolar and canine teeth.

Intrasynovial analgesia

Injection of local anaesthetics and morphine is being increasingly employed to provide analgesia in small animals following joint surgery or arthroscopy. Generally it is recommended that these drugs are infused at the end of surgery so they are not flushed out of the joint prior to closure. The injection is usually made by the surgeon using sterile needles and syringes as aseptic technique is important. Intrasynovial analgesia has not undergone rigorous evaluation in the clinical arena, however, and information regarding clinical efficacy is lacking; it should therefore only be adopted as part of a multimodal analgesia protocol. The optimal doses of local anaesthetic and morphine have not been determined.

Wound catheters

Soaker or wound catheters are commonly used in human anaesthesia to provide postoperative analgesia following surgery. The catheters are placed by the surgeon at the end of the surgical procedure and sutured loosely in place (Figure 23.22). Postoperatively, local anaesthetic agents such as bupivacaine can be injected down the catheter to provide topical analgesia. The catheters come in different lengths and have holes along the distal third of the catheter to allow the

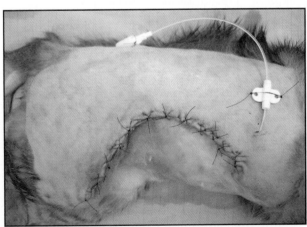

23.22 Wound catheter placed following reconstructive surgery in the flank of a cat. Bupivacaine administered through the wound catheter every 6–8 hours was used to provide analgesia.

injected local anaesthetic to spread into the area of surgical trauma. This technique usually allows the dose of systemic analgesics to be reduced, contributing to a multimodal protocol. A good example of a surgical procedure for which wound catheters can be very helpful is limb amputation. The catheter can be left in place for 24–36 hours after surgery and bupivacaine instilled every 8 hours to provide pain relief. It is important that the catheter is secured in place and covered to prevent removal by the patient.

Local anaesthetic blocks in horses

Concurrent use of local anaesthetic blocks and general anaesthesia for surgery in horses is gaining in popularity. Similar blocks to those in small animals can be performed. However, a major consideration as to whether a local anaesthetic block is appropriate for use in anaesthetized horses concerns the anticipated motor effects of that nerve block. This is particularly relevant when considering epidural administration or the use of distal limb nerve blocks to provide analgesia during surgery. Local anaesthetic nerve blocks are not recommended where they are likely to produce significant adverse effects on proprioception or motor function of the limbs during recovery from anaesthesia.

Induction of general anaesthesia

Induction of anaesthesia may be carried out using one of the following techniques:

- Injectable anaesthetic agent or combination of agents (usually short-acting) given **intravenously**
- Injectable anaesthetic agent or combination of agents given **intramuscularly**
- **Inhalant** agent given via mask or an induction chamber.

Placement of an intravenous catheter should be mandatory before induction of anaesthesia, whichever technique is used.

Choice of induction technique depends upon several factors:

- **Species**: In some species, such as the small mammals, intravenous access may not be easily achieved. In horses induction of anaesthesia is always carried out using injectable agents given rapidly intravenously, due to the dangers for both horse and handlers associated with a slow, uncontrolled induction of anaesthesia following intramuscular administration of induction agents
- **Temperament of the patient**: In some animals it may not be possible to administer an injectable agent. If gaseous anaesthesia is used for induction, temperament may influence the use of a mask or an induction chamber
- **Anaesthesia protocol**: The anaesthetist may choose to use a total injectable anaesthetic technique or maintenance with an inhalant agent (see below)
- **Age of the patient**: It may be preferable to avoid injectable agents in very young animals where liver metabolism of injected drugs will be slower, thereby prolonging recovery.

Drugs commonly used to induce anaesthesia
Injectable agents

Figure 23.23 gives the key pharmacological properties of commonly used injectable induction agents, together with the advantages and disadvantages associated with them. Further information is given on these agents in the section on 'Maintenance of anaesthesia'.

Use of inhalant agents to induce anaesthesia

Two methods are used to deliver an inhalational agent for induction of anaesthesia. The advantages and disadvantages of chamber *versus* mask induction techniques are described in Figure 23.24.

Drug	Formulations, preparation and storage	Routes of administration	Cardiovascular system effects	Respiratory system effects	Comments
Thiopental	Powder; dissolve in water for injection. Use 1.25% or 2.5% solution in small animals. Veterinary preparation no longer available	i.v. (causes severe thrombophlebitis if injected outside vein)	Myocardial depression, transient hypotension accompanied by compensatory tachycardia	Respiratory depression. May cause apnoea after injection	Repeat doses result in drug accumulation. Cannot be used for maintenance of anaesthesia
Propofol	Propofol solubilized in egg phosphatide and soya bean oil, with benzyl alcohol as a preservative, can be used for up to 28 days after the bottle is broached	i.v. (does not cause thrombophlebitis if injected outside vein)	Myocardial depression, vasodilation and bradycardia	Respiratory depression. May cause apnoea after injection	Relatively non-accumulative and can be used to maintain anaesthesia by incremental injection or CRI. The preparation containing preservative is not suitable for CRI
Alfaxalone	Solubilized in a cyclodextrin that does not cause histamine release; can be used in cats and dogs. No preservative so should be discarded or used immediately once bottle is opened	i.v., i.m.	Myocardial depression associated with compensatory increase in heart rate	Respiratory depression. May cause apnoea after injection	Recovery can be stormy if given to unpremedicated animals. Can be used to maintain anaesthesia by incremental injection or CRI.

23.23 Key pharmacology of injectable drugs used for induction of anaesthesia.

continues ▶

Drug	Formulations, preparation and storage	Routes of administration	Cardiovascular system effects	Respiratory system effects	Comments
Ketamine	Contains preservative; does not need to be stored in the fridge	i.v., i.m.	Stimulates sympathetic nervous system, increases heart rate. Minimal effects on cardiac output	Minimal effects; may cause apneustic breathing pattern	Can cause pain on i.m. injection. Only use in premedicated animals, commonly combined with a benzodiazepine. Low doses for induction; higher doses for period of anaesthesia as part of total injectable technique. Recovery can be 'spacey' or stormy, particularly in dogs. Analgesic

23.23 *continued* Key pharmacology of injectable drugs used for induction of anaesthesia.

Technique	Advantages	Disadvantages
Chamber induction	Does not require restraint of the patient	Depending on the size of the chamber it can take a relatively long period of time to build up a high concentration of inhalant agent inside the chamber; induction can be prolonged. Most animals find the technique aversive; injury may occur if the animal becomes excited and can move freely in the chamber. Movement can be limited by using a chamber size that is appropriate for the size of the animal. Significant environmental contamination occurs when the chamber is opened to remove the animal
Mask induction	Does not require any additional equipment, although suitably sized face masks must be available for delivery of the anaesthetic agent to the patient. Easy to deliver a high concentration of inhalant agent rapidly. The animal is restrained and cannot injure itself	Most animals find the technique aversive. Use of sevoflurane provides a faster induction than other agents. Difficult to restrain aggressive or unsedated patients. Use of 'cat bags' can be helpful to improve control of the patient. Leaking of inhalational agent around the face mask results in environmental contamination

23.24 Advantages and disadvantages of chamber and mask induction using inhalant agents.

Chamber induction technique

It is better to use a chamber that is as small as possible without compromising and squashing the animal. Use of a clear plastic chamber allows constant observation of the animal during induction, which is advantageous. An entry and an exit port are built into the chamber. The entry port (usually 15 mm in diameter) allows connection of an anaesthetic breathing circuit to the chamber for the delivery of inhalant agent and oxygen via an anaesthetic machine. The exit port (usually 22 mm in diameter) allows the connection of a scavenging system to the chamber to remove the inhalant agent.

1. First fill the chamber with oxygen.
2. Place the patient inside the closed chamber.
3. The inhalant agent is delivered via an anaesthetic machine (Figure 23.25). It is necessary to use a high percentage of volatile anaesthetic carried within high fresh gas flow in order to achieve anaesthesia in a timely fashion (for example 3–4% isoflurane or 7–8% sevoflurane).
4. Once the patient has lost the righting reflex (i.e. it does not try and correct its position when the chamber is tipped slightly), flush the chamber with oxygen to remove excess inhalant agent via the scavenging pipeline.
5. Open the chamber and remove the patient quickly before re-sealing the chamber.
6. Use a face mask to deliver further inhalant agent to maintain anaesthesia until a suitable plane has been obtained and the patient can be intubated. It is also possible to maintain anaesthesia via inhalant agent delivery by face mask, but this has health and safety implications for staff working in the area.

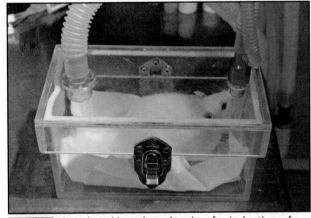

23.25 Rat placed in a clear chamber for induction of anaesthesia using an inhalant agent. The green tube is delivering halothane vaporized in oxygen into the chamber; the clear plastic tube is scavenging.

This technique is particularly useful for small mammals such as rats and mice but should not be adopted for rabbits. This is because rabbits hold their breath when exposed to inhalant agents when conscious and this can lead to hypoxia.

Mask induction technique

The animal is restrained and anaesthetic gases are delivered via a face mask and anaesthetic breathing circuit. There are two commonly used types of mask: clear ridged polycarbonate masks with a rubber diaphragm to provide a good fit of the mask over the nose and face of the animal (Figure 23.26); and flexible black rubber masks. Flexible rubber masks help

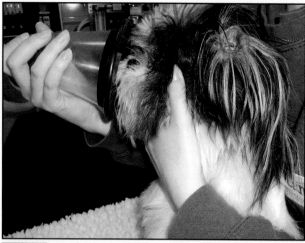

23.26 Mask induction of anaesthesia using an inhalant anaesthetic agent in a dog.

reduce the potential for trauma during induction of anaesthesia. This type of mask, however, tends to lack a rubber diaphragm where the mask fits over the face of the animal, making them inappropriate for use with inhalant agents due to the atmospheric pollution caused by not having a tight seal around the patient's nose and face. They are also not transparent, and so visual observation of the patient is impaired. The exception to this rule is use for induction of anaesthesia in ferrets, as they will usually position their face within the mask of their own accord due to it being dark; once within the mask they can easily be restrained to stay there.

Monitoring during induction

As the induction agent is being administered by the veterinary surgeon it is important to observe respiration and measure pulse rate by palpation (see later).

Induction of anaesthesia in horses

Induction of anaesthesia is a potentially dangerous period for both horse and handlers, although fractures are more likely to occur during the recovery period.

Drugs used for induction in horses

It is not appropriate to induce anaesthesia in horses using either inhalational techniques or injectable agents given intramuscularly; therefore only intravenous agents are used.

Ketamine

Ketamine is commonly used for induction of anaesthesia in horses because of its predictable effects and the smooth induction that it offers when given following sedation by an alpha-2 agonist. It causes CNS excitation in unsedated animals and therefore should never be given to inadequately sedated horses or a potentially dangerous situation – a horse that is ataxic, excited and uncoordinated – can arise. Ketamine may also be used for analgesia and maintenance of anaesthesia as part of total intravenous anaesthesia (TIVA) or partial intravenous anaesthesia (PIVA) techniques. Ketamine has relatively few cardiovascular effects and can support the cardiovascular system through stimulation of the sympathetic nervous system.

Thiopental

Historically, thiopental was used for induction of anaesthesia in horses, combined with premedication with either acepromazine or an alpha-2 agonist, or in combination with guiafenesin. Generally, induction of anaesthesia following thiopental is less smooth than following ketamine, or it requires more skill and a greater number of personnel to achieve a smooth, safe induction with thiopental. A veterinary preparation of thiopental is no longer available, although 500 mg vials of thiopental can be purchased through the human product market. This has led to thiopental only being routinely used as an emergency top-up drug to increase the depth of anaesthesia in horses that are moving. Onset of anaesthesia, or a deepening of anaesthesia, is more rapid with thiopental than with ketamine; therefore if a horse is actually moving, thiopental is preferred. As with small animals, thiopental can only be given intravenously. In horses a 10% solution is generally used. Due to the potential for drug accumulation, thiopental is not used to maintain or prolong anaesthesia by multiple doses.

Propofol

Propofol is not routinely used for induction of anaesthesia in adult horses because of cost and issues associated with speed of administration. The volume of propofol required to induce anaesthesia in an adult horse is such that it is difficult to give the dose rapidly as a bolus, leading to the potential for a slow and ataxic induction of anaesthesia. Propofol can be used to induce anaesthesia in foals, as their smaller body size means that a smooth and rapid induction can be achieved. Propofol has been used to maintain anaesthesia in horses when given by CRI but, because it is a poor reflex suppressant with minimal analgesic effects, depth of anaesthesia can be difficult to stabilize. It has also been given in combination with ketamine CRI for maintenance of anaesthesia but this technique has not been widely adopted.

Midazolam and diazepam

Benzodiazepines are commonly used during induction of anaesthesia in horses to provide improved muscle relaxation and therefore a smoother induction of anaesthesia with ketamine. Generally the benzodiazepine is given with ketamine, mixed in the same syringe.

Guiafenesin

Guiafenesin is a centrally acting muscle agent used in horses for induction of anaesthesia (in combination with thiopental or ketamine) or maintenance as part of TIVA. It also causes hypnosis and slight sedation. Guiafenesin causes intravascular haemolysis when given in concentrations >10%, limiting the concentration and therefore dose that can be administered quickly to horses. It is generally given by infusion via a drip bag and giving set until the horse starts to become ataxic, followed immediately by a bolus of ketamine or thiopental. Guiafenesin causes relatively few cardiovascular side effects and therefore can have advantages when used in horses with colic compared to the use of alpha-2 agonists. However, the longer time course of induction can be disadvantageous unless the horse is able to stand still during the induction progress.

Induction boxes

In a hospital situation, induction of anaesthesia should take place in a padded induction box (Figure 23.27). A number of different designs are available and there is no real consensus

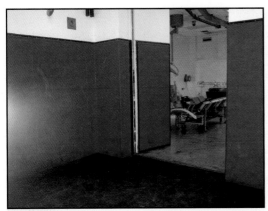

Equine induction box with one door open, showing the connection between the induction box and the equine theatre. The floor and walls of the box are covered with a compliant durable rubber-like material to reduce the risk of injury to the horse during induction of anaesthesia and also to facilitate cleaning. (Courtesy of Carolyne Sheridan)

on which is best in terms of reducing the potential for injury. Most induction boxes have an entrance from the outside and connecting doors to the operating theatre, allowing a one-way system, and padded floor and walls up to a height greater than the anticipated height that the horse could reach if it reared. The depth of the padding varies; some anaesthetists prefer a relatively hard padded floor to facilitate the horse obtaining its footing, whereas others prefer deeper padding. No objects should protrude from the walls or floor of the induction box in order to prevent injury. Some induction boxes have a pulley system to facilitate assisted recovery; these pullies are located high up on the walls to avoid the potential for damage to the horse.

Some induction boxes have half doors at the entrance into the theatre so that they can be shut in two phases (lower doors and then upper doors). This facilitates monitoring during the early phases of recovery. In addition to half doors, or instead of them, there is usually a small window that can be opened from the outside to look into the induction box during recovery for the purposes of monitoring. This can also be used to feed an O_2 pipeline into the box to supplement oxygen during recovery. Some induction boxes have a door that comes away from the wall of the induction box and can be closed against the horse, restraining it between one wall of the induction box and the padded door. This can facilitate a controlled induction of anaesthesia, particularly when using guiafenesin. The padded door can be re-placed to re-form the wall of the induction box during recovery from anaesthesia.

Procedure

Safety in equine anaesthesia (for both horse and handlers) can be assisted by having a strict protocol for the sequence of events that occur during the induction procedure. Ideally it is recommended that two people hold the horse during induction of anaesthesia with ketamine. For safety reasons, no people other than the anaesthetist and handlers should be present in the induction box during anaesthesia. Appropriate PPE should be worn if shown to be necessary by a risk assessment.

1. Lead the horse into the induction box and position it calmly. The optimal position within the box will be determined by box design and the choice of induction agents.

2. Use a padded headcollar to prevent damage to the facial nerves and face during induction. The nose and cheek areas of the head collar should be especially well padded (Figure 23.28).
3. Place an intravenous catheter, if not already in place. Flush the catheter with heparinized saline.
4. Attach two lead ropes to the head collar, one held by each person (Figure 23.28a).
5. Sedative and induction drugs are administered.
6. During induction, with help from the other handler, apply downward pressure on the horse's head to prevent it from lifting it up. This enables you to maintain the greatest control. Combine this with backward pressure on the brisket to prevent the horse coming forward.
7. Once the horse is recumbent, do not stand between its legs; ideally handlers should remain on the dorsal aspect of the horse (along its spine). Depending on the system being used to transfer the horse from the induction box to the operating room table, the horse's legs may need to be shackled or hobbled to allow attachment to a winch system.
8. The anaesthetist will check depth of anaesthesia to confirm that the horse is adequately anaesthetized for intubation and eventually movement to the operating room table. Maintaining control of the horse's head is important to ensure some restraint should movement occur during this phase.

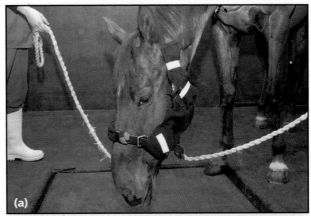
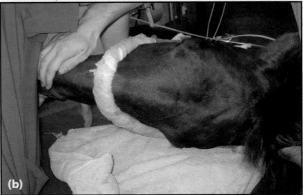

23.28 Induction of anaesthesia in horses. **(a)** A horse standing for induction after premedication with an alpha-2 agonist. The horse is wearing a padded headcollar. Two lead-ropes are attached to the headcollar, each held by a separate person to improve control. **(b)** The cheek pieces and strap running over the bridge of the nose of this headcollar have been padded with bandage material to reduce the risk of facial trauma. The towel placed under the horse's head is to prevent trauma to the eye. (Courtesy of Carolyne Sheridan)

Endotracheal intubation

Most patients should be intubated during anaesthesia, regardless of the technique being used to maintain anaesthesia, for the following reasons:

- To protect the airway during anaesthesia
- To maintain a patent airway
- To prevent soft tissue from obstructing the airway
- To prevent secretions (e.g. salivation and regurgitated material) from causing airway obstruction.

WARNING

Remember that an intubated airway can still become obstructed, as tubes can become kinked (especially red rubber-type tubes) or be blocked by plugs of secretions or lubricant. It is important to observe the patient's breathing pattern and tidal volume during anaesthesia to assess airway patency.

The intubation of very small patients with a narrow airway can result in trauma to the larynx and trachea; the costs and benefits of intubation must therefore be considered when attempting intubation of puppies, kittens and small mammals. As a general rule, intubation of patients with a bodyweight of <2 kg may be problematic and the placement of a very small endotracheal tube may increase respiratory resistance (due to the small tube diameter) compared to allowing the animal to breathe naturally through the mouth. Intubation of rats, mice and guinea pigs is a specialized technique and should not be undertaken without training and availability of appropriate equipment. Birds do not have an epiglottis, therefore visualization of the trachea is straightforward, and intubation is relatively easy compared to other species of a similar size.

Endotracheal tubes

There are a number of different types of endotracheal (ET) tube, each with differing advantages and disadvantages (Figure 23.29). They can be made of red rubber, PVC or silicone and be cuffed or uncuffed; examples of each are shown in Figure 23.30.

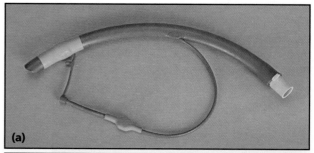

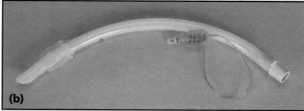

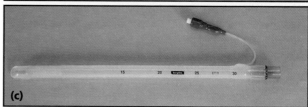

23.30 Endotracheal tubes. **(a)** Red rubber. The pilot balloon and cuff on the tube are maintained inflated using the cap on the pilot balloon. The cuff is a high-pressure, low-volume type. **(b)** PVC. This cuff is a low-pressure, high-volume type. The pilot balloon has a valve on it to maintain cuff inflation. **(c)** Silicone. This tube is much straighter than the other two types.

Cuffs may be of a high-volume, low-pressure or low-volume, high-pressure type:

- A **low-pressure, high-volume cuff** is safer in terms of the health of the tracheal mucosa, as the pressure of the inflated cuff is spread over a larger area; however, it does not provide such good protection of the airway as fluids can traverse folds in the cuff and enter the lungs
- A **high-pressure, low-volume cuff** provides more secure protection of the airway; however, there is a higher risk of tracheal necrosis due to the pressure of the cuff being exerted on a small band of tissue.

Tube type	Advantages	Disadvantages
Red rubber	Re-useable. Wide range of sizes available. Can be autoclaved. Easy to intubate, as pre-moulded	Fairly expensive (especially larger sizes). Perish with time. Not malleable. Kink easily (extreme care should be taken to ensure airway patency is maintained when the head is kinked, e.g. during cervical CSF taps). Irritant to the airway. Impossible to detect contamination without looking directly down the lumen. No self-sealing valve. Only available with low-volume, high-pressure cuff
PVC	Cheap. Although designed to be disposable, can be re-used. Malleable when warmed. Fairly kink-resistant. Non-irritant. Easy to place. High-pressure, low-volume and low-pressure, high volume cuffs available. Easy to see any contamination, e.g. plugs within the lumen. Cuffs are valved	Designed to be disposable. Cannot be repaired. Limited sizes available (no large sizes >11 mm internal diameter). Cannot be autoclaved. Connections can become loose once the PVC becomes warm
Silicone	Can be repaired (long life). Can be autoclaved. Malleable when warmed. Fairly kink-resistant. Non-irritant. Cuffs are valved. Wide range of sizes available. Possible to see contamination when examined carefully	Expensive to purchase. May require a stylet to facilitate intubation because the tubes do not have a moulded curve. Only available with low-volume, high-pressure cuff

23.29 Advantages and disadvantages of endotracheal tubes made from different materials.

Armoured or guarded ET tubes are usually made from PVC with a thick wall in which a wire coil is placed. They are designed to prevent kinking when the patient's neck is flexed, e.g. during a cisternal puncture to collect CSF. These tubes can become permanently occluded if over-flexed (unlikely to be possible with new designs) or if they are bitten by the patient.

A 'Murphy eye' may be present in some silicone and PVC tubes; this is an oval hole in the tube wall opposite to the bevel. The hole allows gases to enter and exit the tube if the end becomes occluded by sitting against the wall of the trachea or by secretions.

Choice of endotracheal tube

When selecting the size of ET tube for the patient it is important to consider both its diameter and length. The tube should be as big as comfortably fits down the trachea, to minimize the amount of air needed in the cuff (if a cuffed tube is being used) to provide a tracheal seal.

- Most adult cats can take a 4.5 or 5 mm uncuffed tube.
- In dogs, a rough guide for tube sizes are 8 mm for a 10 kg dog, 10 mm for a 20 kg dog and 12 mm for a 30 kg dog. However, it is important to consider tube size in terms of lean bodyweight and breed. Brachycephalic breeds often have a relatively narrow laryngeal diameter and trachea compared to their bodyweight.

Tubes that are too short displace easily, while overly long tubes carry a risk of one lung intubation due to the tube being placed down one bronchus. The tube end should be level with the front incisors and not sitting out proud of the mouth as this increases the equipment dead space (the volume of gas contained within equipment that is re-breathed without any changes in composition). To ensure tube length is optimal, the tube should be measured against the side of the patient, using the jaw and the thoracic inlet as marker points.

In cats, uncuffed tubes are generally preferred, except when it is known that a good tracheal seal will be needed (e.g. during IPPV) or if the patient is at a high risk of regurgitation (e.g. during dental procedures or cranial abdominal surgery). If a cuffed tube is used it is vital that the cuff is inflated carefully and not over-pressurized, because cats are at a high risk of tracheal necrosis. An alternative to using a cuffed tube in situations where the risk of regurgitation is high is placement of a throat pack (or rolled up swab attached to a piece of suture to allow easy retrieval) in order to prevent regurgitated material from entering the pharynx and the trachea. The throat pack must provide a good seal at the back of the mouth and must be removed at the end of anaesthesia.

Before using an ET tube:

- Visually inspect for any gross contamination and damage to the tube (e.g. bite marks)
- Check the lumen for contamination by holding the tube up to the light and looking down the lumen. Patency should never be checked by blowing down the tube, for reasons of health and safety
- Check the cuff. The cuff should be fully inflated and left for a few minutes to ensure that it stays inflated. If using a lubricant on the tube to aid intubation ▶

it is best applied at this time. Ideally, use a silicone spray designed specifically for this purpose. A water-based lubricant can be used; however, these can dry out and become sticky and may plug the tube if care is not taken during application. Fully deflate the cuff before intubation.

Cleaning ET tubes

- ET tubes should never be cleaned or come into contact with chlorhexidine-containing products as these cause tracheal irritation. ET tubes should be cleaned using a solution of washing-up liquid and water with a pipe cleaner brush to clean the lumen and a cloth to clean the exterior. They should then be thoroughly rinsed with copious amounts of water, including flushing down the lumen, and allowed to air dry. Once dried, they should be doused completely with surgical spirit, containing no additives, and allowed to air dry for a second time.
- ET tubes used for patients suffering from contagious diseases should either be disposed of or be sterilized (e.g. using an autoclave or ethylene oxide as per manufacturer's guidelines).

Endotracheal intubation
Intubation of dogs and cats

Following induction, once a suitable plane of anaesthesia to allow intubation has been achieved, cats and dogs should be positioned for intubation in the following way:

- Hold the upper jaw by the lateral aspect of the mucous membrane (gums) under the lips.
- Straighten and extend the neck to open the airway and facilitate intubation. Be aware that in some circumstances neck extension is contraindicated, e.g. cervical disc disease.
- Do not distort the soft tissues of the neck by pulling the scruff. Place the hand behind the base of the skull (feel for the bony prominence) and lift and extend the neck to place the head and neck in a straight line.

> **WARNING**
>
> To avoid the risk of being bitten, do not place your fingers in the patient's mouth.

Intubation is a procedure that veterinary nurses are permitted to perform and it is important that they are both proficient and confident in the technique. Intubation can be done either with (Figures 23.31 and 23.32) or without using a laryngoscope. Laryngoscopes facilitate laryngeal visualization and thus aid quick intubation and reduce the risk of laryngeal trauma. When using a laryngoscope, pull the tongue firmly out of the mouth between the canine teeth and place the blade of the laryngoscope at the base of the tongue (just in front of the larynx, **not on the epiglottis**); depress the blade downwards to improve laryngeal visualization. Two types of laryngoscope blade are commonly used in veterinary practice: Miller (straight blade) and Macintosh (curved) blade (Figure 23.33).

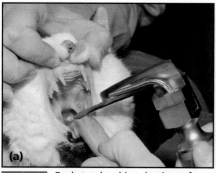
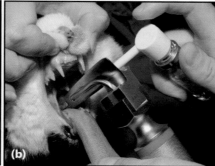
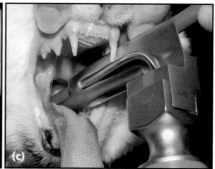

23.31 Endotracheal intubation of a cat. **(a)** Positioning the cat. **(b)** Using a largyngoscope to facilitate visualization of the larynx. Local anaesthetic spray is used to desensitize the larynx prior to intubation. **(c)** Placement of the endotracheal tube.

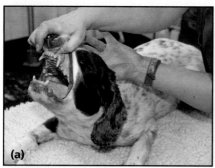
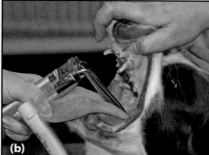
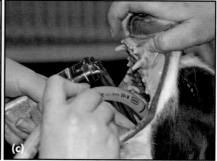

23.32 Endotracheal intubation of a dog. **(a)** Positioning the dog. **(b)** Using a laryngoscope to facilitate visualization of the larynx. **(c)** Placement of the endotracheal tube.

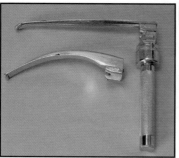

23.33 Laryngoscope with a Miller type blade (straight) attached. A Macintosh type blade (curved) is also shown.

Stylets can also aid intubation by stiffening the ET tube or acting as a guidewire. To stiffen the ET tube, the tube is threaded over the top of the stylet. A stylet can also guide placement of the tube by gently intubating the patient with the stylet and then threading the ET tube over it until the tube is introduced into the trachea. A polyurethane dog urinary catheter can be used as a stylet if plastic stylets are not available.

In cats, it is vital to spray the larynx with topical local anaesthetic (Figure 23.31b). This prevents laryngeal spasm during intubation. It is necessary to wait one minute after application of the local anaesthetic to allow mucosal absorption before attempting intubation. **Laryngeal spasm is an emergency as the patient is unable to open the larynx and breathe.**

Intubation of other species

Horses

The horse is an obligate nasal breather; therefore, although intubation is usually routine, it is important to stretch the neck out and disengage the epiglottis from the soft palate in order to facilitate intubation. A gag is placed to open the mouth prior to the start of intubation. A 26–30 mm diameter tube is usually appropriate for intubation of horses weighing 350–600 kg. It is important to check the integrity of the cuff before intubation.

The tube is placed blindly by advancing it midline between the teeth until the larynx is reached. Gentle rotation of the tube, combined with lifting the larynx from the outside of the neck, is usually sufficient to allow the tube to be passed successfully into the larynx. The cuff should then be inflated.

Left recurrent laryngeal nerve neuropathy is not uncommon in horses, particularly thoroughbreds. This reduces the ability of the horse to abduct the arytenoid cartilage during inspiration and can make intubation more difficult. It may be necessary to use a slightly smaller tube in affected animals. The same principles apply as with small animals in terms of making intubation atraumatic to prevent damage to the larynx that may present on extubation.

Rabbits

Intubation of rabbits may be achieved using either a 'blind' technique or using visualization with either an otoscope, a laryngoscope with a narrow blade or a rigid endoscope. In both cases it is imperative that the rabbit is already at an adequate depth of anaesthesia if intubation is to be successful. The internal diameter of ET tube appropriate for rabbits of 2.5–4 kg bodyweight is between 2.5 and 3.5 mm. Using an uncuffed ET tube will maximize the luminal diameter of the tube that can be placed, which is advantageous.

Blind technique:

1. Position the rabbit in sternal recumbency.
2. Use one hand to hold the rabbit's head so that the neck is straight and extended (this often requires the patient to be lifted up off its sternum, so the front legs are hanging).
3. Introduce the tube into the mouth using your other hand.
4. Whilst doing this, position your face (cheek and ear) close

to the patient's face and ET tube connector, looking towards the chest of the rabbit so you can see it breathing.
5. In time with inspiration, advance the tube gently but positively, listening for breath sounds.
6. If the tube enters the trachea the patient will often cough; consequently it is very important to keep a firm grip of the tube. You will also be able to hear and feel the passage of air in the tube. If the tube enters the oesophagus, no passage of air will be present.

Visualization technique:

1. Thread a dog urinary catheter down the centre of the ET tube to act as a stylet, so that the urinary catheter protrudes from the end of the ET tube.
2. Ask an assistant to position the rabbit in sternal recumbency and to extend the rabbit's head and neck.
3. Position the laryngosocope/otoscope/endoscope in the rabbit's mouth (a pair of atraumatic forceps can be very useful to pull the rabbit's tongue forward and out of the side of the mouth).
4. Once the larynx is visualized, pass the urinary catheter through the larynx and advance the ET tube down over the catheter.
5. If the tube enters the trachea the patient will usually cough.

The position of the tube can be checked by either feeling or looking for the passage of air:

- Pluck a small amount of hair from the rabbit and hold it firmly in front of the ET tube and watch for movement
- Attach the ET tube to the breathing system and watch for movement of the reservoir bag
- Give the rabbit a manual breath and watch for chest movement
- The preferred method is to attach a capnograph to the ET tube: if the tube is in the trachea CO_2 will be present when the patient exhales (or a breath is administered); if the tube is in the oesophagus no CO_2 will be present.

Birds

Intubation of birds can be relatively simple due to easy visualization of the trachea and glottis; however, use of a laryngoscope is still helpful to aid visualization and prevent trauma. Birds have complete tracheal rings, making the diameter of the trachea very inflexible and increasing the risk of tracheal necrosis if a tube of too large a diameter is placed. Use of cuffed tubes is not recommended in birds.

Management of ET tubes during anaesthesia

In most species, securing the ET tube in place is vital to ensure maintenance of the tube during anaesthesia. This can be achieved using gauze fixed to the tube and tied behind the patient's ears. Care should be taken to avoid nasal congestion if the tube is tied around the muzzle (in dogs) as this is not only uncomfortable for the patient but can result in respiratory distress during the recovery period. The ET tube is not commonly secured in place in horses.

Procedure immediately after intubation

1. Secure the ET tube in place.
2. Attach the ET tube to an appropriately sized ▶

breathing circuit and switch on the oxygen flow.
3. Attach the cuff inflation syringe to the pilot balloon.
4. Give the patient a breath via the bag on the breathing circuit and listen by the patient's mouth for any leaks around the tube. Inflate the cuff gradually until no leaks can be heard. The minimum amount of air needed to create a seal around the tube should be used during cuff inflation, to reduce the risk of tracheal necrosis.
5. Start administration of the inhalant agent (if applicable).

Periodically re-check for leaks around the tube, as the trachea can relax slightly and small movements in the tube can create spaces around it. It is important to remember that if gas can escape around the tube, regurgitant can also pass by the cuff, increasing the risk of regurgitation and aspiration.

If the patient has a history of regurgitation or has a condition that could increase the risk of regurgitation, e.g. myasthenia gravis or advanced pregnancy, the cuff should be inflated *immediately* after intubation, before the head and neck are lowered. This reduces the risk of aspiration.

If regurgitation does occur it is important first to drop the head of the patient down below the height of the thoracic outlet to facilitate drainage. The seal around the ET tube should be checked at the soonest opportunity and material sucked out of the patient's mouth and airway. This can be performed using a footpump-operated suction unit, a handheld suction device (widely available from medical equipment suppliers), or a surgical suction unit (care should be taken not to traumatize the soft tissues); alternatively, if these are not available, a 20 ml syringe attached to a 3-way tap and a 6 French dog urinary catheter may be used.

Heat moisture exchangers

HMEs (Figure 23.34) contain a porous material that absorbs the heat and moisture from exhaled air and then warms and moistens inspired gases as they pass through the chamber, thereby reducing tracheal drying and heat loss via the respiratory system. An HME is placed between the ET tube and the breathing system. Care should be taken when using HMEs in small patients as they increase dead space and resistance. They are designed for use in human medicine and different sizes are manufactured for different bodyweights. Animals of lower bodyweight have a relatively smaller tidal volume and choosing an HME with appropriate deadspace is important. HMEs are not used in horses. When using an HME the patient should be monitored for signs of increased respiratory effort that could indicate that the HME has become obstructed with secretions or become very wet, which can increase the resistance imposed by the device. HMEs are designed for single use only.

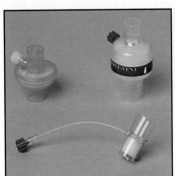

23.34 Heat moisture exchangers (HMEs) with different sized chambers and therefore deadspace. The capped ports are the sites of attachment for a gas sampling line for capnography.

Maintenance of anaesthesia

Anaesthesia can be maintained using a variety of different techniques and anaesthetic agents:

- Inhalant agents alone
- Total intravenous anaesthesia (**TIVA**) – injectable agents given intravenously in incremental doses or by CRI
- Partial intravenous anaesthesia (**PIVA**) – using a combination of intravenous injectable agents (e.g. propofol) and inhalant anaesthetics (e.g. isoflurane)
- Injectable agents given intramuscularly.

The advantages and disadvantages of total injectable versus total inhalant anaesthesia are shown in Figure 23.35. Total inhalational techniques are not appropriate in horses due to the dangers associated with induction of anaesthesia using inhalant agents in horses, nor for rabbits as breath-holding and subsequent hypoxia may be induced.

The advantages and disadvantages of TIVA *versus* PIVA are shown in Figure 23.36.

Inhalant agents

The inhalant agents, with the exception of nitrous oxide (N_2O), are all liquids at room temperature and are vaporized for use and mixed with carrier gas(es). Oxygen is the predominant carrier gas, but may be combined with nitrous oxide or medical air.

The vapour and carrier gas mixture are delivered to the patient via a breathing system into the respiratory tract and lungs. Absorption of the agent across the alveolar membrane allows the agent to be transported via the blood to the brain, where anaesthesia is induced or maintained.

Available inhalant agents differ in terms of their:

- Potency
- Volatility
- Solubility in tissues
- Inflammability
- Chemical stability
- Effect on organ function
- Metabolism
- Analgesic properties.

The pharmacology of the common inhalant agents is summarized in Figure 23.37.

Technique	Advantages	Disadvantages
Total injectable anaesthesia	No expensive equipment required Drugs may be given i.v. or i.m. (depending on agent) Induction usually rapid and stress-free Easy to induce and maintain: requires little technical expertise Although recommended, ET intubation and oxygen not mandatory No scavenging required	Difficult to regulate depth of anaesthesia if agents given i.m. I.V. access may be required Plasma concentration of drugs cannot be measured in real time Drugs must be metabolized before recovery can occur Duration of recovery depends on duration of anaesthesia if agents not rapidly metabolized
Total inhalational anaesthesia	Patient usually intubated and inhalant agent vaporized in oxygen: ensures airway is protected and oxygen supplementation provided Depth of anaesthesia easy to control by altering vaporizer dials Delivered concentration of agent can be easily measured by sampling airway gases Recovery not dependent on drug metabolism (inhalants largely excreted by exhalation) Long duration of anaesthesia does not necessarily mean a prolonged recovery time Useful for rats, mice and guinea pigs, when rapid recovery desired.	Requires anaesthetic machine and oxygen supply; equipment can be expensive Understanding of how anaesthetic machine works is required to use equipment safely Induction is relatively slow (compared to i.v. injection); can be stressful for patient and staff restraining them Waste anaesthetic gases must be removed from the immediate environment of the patient and staff Scavenging of waste gases is difficult during recovery period, leading to environmental contamination Inhalant agents are greenhouse gases and contribute to degradation of the ozone layer, as well as having potential health and safety risks for staff

23.35 Advantages and disadvantages of total injectable *versus* total inhalant anaesthesia techniques.

Technique	Advantages	Disadvantages
Total intravenous anaesthesia	Does not require anaesthetic machine and oxygen supply (although oxygen recommended) Useful when maintenance with inhalant agents problematic, e.g. during bronchoscopy Drugs with specific actions can be given to provide triad anaesthesia, e.g. propofol plus analgesic	Long duration of drug administration can result in drug accumulation and prolonged recovery time Plasma concentration of agent difficult to predict and likely to increase over time, even when given by CRI Unless given by CRI, peaks and troughs in depth of anaesthesia occur with redosing CRI requires controlled administration through syringe driver
Partial intravenous anaesthesia	Administration of selected injected agents usually provides analgesia and reduces concentration of inhalant required to maintain anaesthesia Balanced anaesthesia technique, often with improved cardiovascular stability	Injectable agents usually potent and require controlled administration through syringe driver More complex protocol necessitates experience Injectable agents can accumulate and prolong recovery time

23.36 Advantages and disadvantages of total *versus* partial intravenous anaesthesia.

Agent	MAC [a]	Blood/gas coefficient [b]	Pharmacological characteristics
Halothane	0.75%	2.3	Clear colourless liquid with sweet smell. Protect from light. Causes dose-dependent respiratory and myocardial depression and sensitizes myocardium to effects of catecholamines. Avoid in animals with arrhythmias or high circulating levels of catecholamines (e.g. very stressed animals, unstable hyperthyroid cats). Metabolized to some extent (30%) by the liver: increases recovery time after prolonged administration. Reduces liver blood flow: avoid in animals with liver disease
Isoflurane	1.15%	1.4	Pungent smell and irritant to airways: animals may resent induction. Dose-dependent respiratory and cardiovascular system depression. Reduces systemic vascular resistance, leading to vasodilation and compensatory increase in heart rate. Little liver metabolism; most excreted via respiratory system at end of anaesthesia. Minimal effect on liver blood flow
Sevoflurane	2.05%	0.6	Odourless, non-irritant. Lower solubility in blood than isoflurane or halothane. Agent of choice for induction. Dose-dependent reduction in myocardial contractility and mean arterial blood pressure. Very little liver metabolism; rapidly excreted via lungs. Unstable in presence of moist soda lime, producing small amounts of compound A, which is nephrotoxic in rats but not considered to be clinically significant in dogs and cats
Desflurane	5–10%	0.42	High saturated vapour pressure; vaporizes very rapidly at room temperature. Delivery requires special vaporizer that heats liquid desflurane to a constant temperature, enabling agent to be available at constant vapour pressure and negating effects that fluctuating ambient temperatures would otherwise have on concentration imparted into fresh gas flow of anaesthetic machine. Pungent smell; despite low blood solubility, rarely used for induction. Dose-dependent myocardial and respiratory system depression. Heart rate may increase due to stimulation of sympathetic nervous system. Very little liver metabolism; rapidly excreted via lungs

23.37 Key pharmacology of the common inhalant agents. [a] Values in humans given as examples; similar to MAC across veterinary species; [b] Solubility in blood: a higher coefficient indicates greater solubility.

Minimum alveolar concentration

Definition of MAC

The minimum alveolar concentration of the inhalant agent at equilibrium at 1 atmosphere pressure that is required to suppress movement in response to a supramaximal noxious stimulus in 50% of patients.

MAC is used as a measure of anaesthetic potency; inhalant agents that are more potent have a lower MAC value, i.e. a lower concentration of the agent is required to suppress movement. The mechanism of immobility caused by inhalant agents is considered to be at the level of the spinal cord, therefore potency as measured by MAC is a spinal cord rather than a brain phenomenon.

Solubility in blood

The solubility of an inhalant agent in blood (blood/gas partition coefficient) determines the speed of induction and recovery. The greater the solubility, the slower the onset of effect and the more slowly the patient goes to sleep. At the end of anaesthesia, agents that are highly soluble will have accumulated a large reservoir in the blood, fat and other tissues, and therefore blood levels of the agent fall slowly and recovery from anaesthesia is relatively slower. The newer anaesthetic agents (e.g. isoflurane, sevoflurane) are less soluble in blood than is halothane; therefore induction and recovery are more rapid, which is advantageous. Sevoflurane is the inhalant agent of choice for mask or chamber induction of anaesthesia because it is non-irritant and odourless and will produce the most rapid induction.

Health and safety considerations

Maximum workplace exposure limits for nitrous oxide, halothane and isoflurane have been established by nationalized agencies in many industrialized countries. It is a legislative requirement in the UK that practices carry out monitoring of anaesthetic pollutants in operating areas and maintain written records of this. It is also a legislative requirement that veterinary practices provide facilities for the scavenging of anaesthetic gases – passive, active (pump and air brake system) or charcoal absorbers (see Chapter 2).

The dangers to veterinary staff are difficult to quantify because most studies have failed to identify an association between waste anaesthetic gases and an increased incidence of adverse effects. Studies that have been carried out have focused on healthcare workers rather than members of the veterinary profession, so any findings of these studies can only be extrapolated to the veterinary workplace. A number of confounding variables usually affects these studies, including the effects of work stresses and long working hours.

The principal occupational health hazards associated with exposure of health workers to N_2O include the potential for effects on the bone marrow caused by depression of vitamin B12 function, diminished reproductive health and abusive self-administration. High concentrations of N_2O have also been shown to be teratogenic in experimental animals. Some studies have demonstrated that chronic exposure to inhalant anaesthetic agents is associated with physiological changes in healthcare staff, including an inhibition of neutrophil apoptosis, depressed central neurorespiratory activity and a higher incidence of DNA single strand breaks compared to controls. These findings should be balanced, however, against the findings of a systematic review of the subject which was unable to demonstrate an association between exposure and health risks. This study, however, still highlighted the importance of minimizing exposure to eliminate potential risks.

Nitrous oxide

N_2O is a vapour at room temperature and atmospheric pressure. It is not a potent enough anaesthetic agent to cause anaesthesia when administered alone, but is often used as a carrier gas. There are several reasons for including N_2O in the carrier gas mix:

- N$_2$O is a CNS depressant and is analgesic at concentrations >20%. Use of N$_2$O will reduce the concentration of inhalant agent required to maintain anaesthesia, contributing to a balanced anaesthesia technique
- N$_2$O has relatively minor effects on the cardiovascular and respiratory systems
- The second gas effect: N$_2$O is very insoluble in blood (blood/gas partition coefficient 0.47); its rapid absorption from the alveoli causes an abrupt increase in alveolar concentration of the administered inhalant agent, thereby also increasing the rate of uptake of that agent into the blood and increasing the speed of induction of anaesthesia or attainment of the desired brain concentration of the agent.

N$_2$O should not be administered at concentrations >70% in the inspired gas mixture (delivery of a minimum of 30% inspired O$_2$ concentration) in order to prevent hypoxia during anaesthesia.

When administration of N$_2$O is stopped, due to its very low solubility in blood, the volume of N$_2$O entering the alveolus from the blood is greater than the volume of nitrogen entering the pulmonary capillary. The N$_2$O effectively dilutes the alveolar air and if the animal is breathing room air at this point hypoxia can result due to dilution of the available O$_2$; this is termed **diffusion hypoxia**. To avoid this 100% O$_2$ should be administered for approximately 5–10 minutes after N$_2$O is discontinued.

Contraindications to nitrous oxide

- N$_2$O is 40 times more soluble than nitrogen in blood and therefore expands air-filled cavities because it passes from the blood into the cavity faster than nitrogen can diffuse out. This can double the size of a pneumothorax in 10 minutes when delivered at a concentration of 70%. N$_2$O should therefore not be used in patients with a gas-filled cavity, such as in cases of:
  - Pneumothorax
  - Bowel obstruction
  - Gas-filled eye, e.g. following intraocular surgery.
- Administration of N$_2$O should be avoided in animals with significant cardiovascular or respiratory disease and at high risk of hypoxia.
- N$_2$O is not usually used during maintenance of anaesthesia in horses due to the risk of hypoxia during anaesthesia and its propensity to accumulate in the gastrointestinal tract.

Injectable agents for use in small animals

Propofol

Propofol is used in TIVA in small animals, given as a constant rate infusion (CRI, see above) or by incremental injection. Low-dose CRI results in sedation (see above). Propofol is relatively non-accumulative in dogs and therefore can be used to maintain anaesthesia without a long duration of recovery. Cats metabolize propofol poorly and therefore prolonged administration may lead to a long recovery time. Propofol is not analgesic and is a poor reflex suppressant. A

better quality of anaesthesia, as well as provision of analgesia, can be ensured by combining it with an analgesic agent such as ketamine or a potent opioid.

Alfaxalone

Alfaxalone is used in TIVA, given by CRI or incremental injection. Low-dose CRI of alfaxalone results in sedation (see above). Alfaxalone has only recently become available in the UK (although it has been available for a longer period of time in Australasia) and therefore the clinical knowledge base associated with its use for maintenance of anaesthesia is relatively limited here. The drug is authorized for use in dogs and cats. It is rapidly metabolized by the liver; therefore repeated administration does not cause a prolonged recovery from anaesthesia.

Lidocaine

Lidocaine may be used in PIVA, given by CRI using a syringe driver. Systemic lidocaine provides analgesia and contributes to hypnosis; therefore administration is designed to provide analgesia and reduce the concentration of inhalational agent required to maintain anaesthesia, particularly in cardiovascularly unstable patients. Lidocaine may be continued postoperatively to provide analgesia.

> **WARNING**
>
> Lidocaine is not recommended for PIVA in cats, due to negative effects on the cardiovascular system when administered in combination with inhalant agents.

Potent opioids

Potent opioids are used in PIVA, given by CRI or incremental injection. The drugs used are usually short-acting mu agonists, such as fentanyl and alfentanil. Remifentanil is a new ultra-short-acting mu opioid that is metabolized extremely rapidly, regardless of the duration of administration. Opioids are commonly used to provide analgesia during inhalant anaesthesia, allowing the dose of inhalant agent to be reduced and contributing to a balanced anaesthesia technique. Administration by CRI will reduce drug accumulation and the potential for a prolonged recovery. Accumulation is less likely with alfentanil or remifentanil than with fentanyl. Potent mu opioids cause respiratory depression; therefore support of ventilation (IPPV, see later) may be required. Considerations for storage and record keeping of opioids are discussed in Chapter 8.

Ketamine

Low doses of ketamine given by CRI are used in PIVA, and higher doses can be used to maintain anaesthesia as part of TIVA. Ketamine is analgesic at subanaesthetic doses; therefore inclusion in the anaesthesia protocol will contribute to provision of perioperative analgesia. Low-dose ketamine infusion may be continued postoperatively to provide analgesia. Ketamine, given at low doses, does not cause excitation in cats or dogs. Considerations for storage and record keeping are discussed in Chapter 8.

Injectable agents used in horses

In recent years there has been a move away from maintenance of anaesthesia in horses using solely inhalant agents towards using PIVA. This development has been slow because of the traditional reluctance to use potent opioids in horses as part of anaesthesia techniques due to motor stimulation caused in anaesthetized horses, resulting in movement. Current techniques commonly involve the combination of an inhalant agent with a CRI of ketamine, lidocaine or an alpha-2 agonist such as medetomidine. All three drugs have the potential to accumulate and increase ataxia in recovery, thereby increasing the risk of limb fracture. Although used clinically in referral centres, PIVA techniques have not been widely evaluated in robust clinical studies, and data regarding optimal dose rates, duration of the infusion and effects on recovery are lacking. They should therefore be adopted with caution and the potential disadvantages considered before being used in individual cases.

TIVA is used in horses for procedures of short duration, particularly in centres where there are limited anaesthesia facilities (see Field anaesthesia, below). In its simplest form TIVA is achieved by maintaining anaesthesia with intravenous boluses of ketamine and an alpha-2 agonist. Usually half the induction dose of ketamine and alpha-2 agonist are used at top-ups, which need to be given at about 15-minute intervals depending on anaesthetic depth. More prolonged anaesthesia using this technique will prolong recovery and may decrease the quality of recovery due to ataxia.

An alternative means to maintaining anaesthesia without the use of inhalant agents is via a 'triple drip'. This is a combination of guiafenesin, ketamine and an alpha-2 agonist mixed together and delivered via a giving set. Guiafenesin provides muscle relaxation and usually the ketamine and alpha-2 agonist are added to the fluid bag containing guiafenesin in a fixed ratio. However, it is likely that guiafenesin will become unavailable in the UK within the next 12 months, in which case guiafenesin is likely to be replaced with midazolam. This combination has been adopted in continental Europe and some studies describing its use have been published. Maintenance using a triple drip is not recommended for longer than 1 hour, due to the effects of drug accumulation contributing to ataxia in recovery. Oxygen supplementation, via a nasal or endotracheal tube, should be routine. Monitoring depth of anaesthesia during TIVA can be problematic, due to the preservation of cranial nerve reflexes. Thus, blinking, lacrimation and nystagmus, all of which can be signs of inadequate anaesthesia in horses anaesthetized with inhalant agents, are normal in TIVA.

Field anaesthesia

The term 'field anaesthesia' generally encompasses situations where horses are anaesthetized in a 'non-theatre' environment. For example, a horse may be anaesthetized for short procedures such as castration in a field, stable or riding school. In these situations an anaesthetic machine and oxygen are not available; anaesthesia is therefore maintained using TIVA, either with repeat intravenous boluses of ketamine plus an alpha-2 agonist or by administration of ketamine plus an alpha-2 agonist plus guiafenesin in a 'triple drip'.

Considerations for field anaesthesia of horses

- Ensure that the people holding the horse for induction and recovery from anaesthesia are experienced and confident, as safety of the horse and handlers is paramount. Appropriate PPE should be worn as determined by risk assessments. ▶

- Ensure that the environment is free from objects that could cause trauma, e.g. the ground should be free from stones or hard objects that could damage the horse if it lay on them.
- Ensure that the horse's eyes are protected during recumbency; this can be achieved using topical lubrication and lifting the head slightly off the ground using a towel or other form of padding.
- It is important to establish intravenous access by placing an intravenous catheter before induction of anaesthesia.
- Ensure that the headcollar is well fitting and padded so that it does not loosen and come off during induction or recovery and that buckles do not cause trauma to the head. Attaching two lead ropes to the headcollar and having two handlers hold the horse during this period can achieve better control of the horse during induction of anaesthesia.
- Although oxygen is unlikely to be available, it is useful to have an appropriately sized ET tube available so that the horse can be intubated should respiratory obstruction occur.
- Ensure that one person is dedicated to monitoring depth of anaesthesia. This helps ensure that an adequate depth is maintained and that repeat doses of anaesthetic agents are given in a timely manner.
- Control of the horse is required during the recovery period. This is achieved by asking one handler to hold a rope attached to the headcollar and asking a second handler to steady the hind end of the horse by holding the tail. Application of downwards traction on the tail can stop the horse stumbling or swaying and becoming recumbent again after an attempt to stand. The handler holding the lead-rope can stop the horse walking forward and falling after a successful attempt to stand.

Management of the patient during the maintenance phase
Positioning

Care should be taken when positioning the patient on the surgery table:

- Overstretching limbs and tying them in a fixed position can lead to pain on recovery, particularly in patients with osteoarthritis
- Leg ties should be positioned carefully. On the hindlimbs they should be placed just above the stopper pad and not around the Achilles tendon. For the forelimbs, care should be taken when tying a leg back over the patient's thorax for some surgeries carried out in lateral recumbency. This is to prevent restriction of thoracic movement, which may impair spontaneous respiration
- Putting excessive pressure on superficial peripheral nerves can lead to nerve damage and neuropathy on recovery. Superficial nerves should not be placed against the hard edges of the table and ties should not be too tight around limbs
- Myopathy can occur in animals that are recumbent for a long period of time on an unsupported hard surface. Tables and table edges should therefore be padded

- Positioning for perineal surgery, where the hindlimbs hang over the end of the table and the patient is positioned with head down and the perineal area elevated, should be carried out very carefully. Adequate padding of the medial thighs is required to prevent damage to the superficial nerves in this region (Figure 23.38)
- Animals positioned in dorsal recumbency often have impaired ventilation due to the pressure of abdominal contents on the diaphragm. This is particularly the case in obese animals. The requirement for IPPV (see later) should be assessed rapidly after placement in dorsal recumbency
- The potential for skin burns in animals placed on heat pads or other contact warming devices should also be recognized.

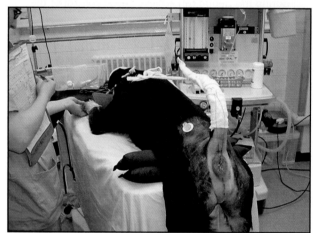

23.38 A dog positioned for perineal surgery showing how padding has been placed between the medial aspect of the thigh and the operating table. The perineal area of the dog is slightly elevated relative to the head and the tail elevated and fixed to allow visualization of the perineal area. A purse-string suture has been placed in the anus to prevent contamination of the surgical field with faeces.

Equine patients

Horses normally spend relatively little time in a recumbent position, and prolonged recumbency has serious implications. It can cause muscle and nerve damage, due to the effects of the pressure of the horse's own weight on large muscle masses and peripheral nerves. Post-anaesthetic myopathy is not uncommon in horses if they have been positioned poorly. Although this is a multifactorial syndrome, a major contributing factor is squashing of dependent muscles by the trunk or other large muscle masses. This leads to a build-up of pressure within the dependent muscle compartments, which compromises muscle blood flow, resulting in ischaemia ('**compartment syndrome**'). Post-anaesthetic myopathy can manifest with differing degrees of severity, ranging from muscle weakness to an inability to stand. It is extremely painful and in severe cases affected animals may require euthanasia. Correct positioning and padding can reduce the risk.

Most anaesthetic tables can be covered with thick padding approximately 10–12 cm thick, with a waterproof covering. Air beds can be used but may provide a less stable operating platform. It is important that the padding is not too hard; ideally the horse should sink into it slightly so that the padding is slightly compliant and wraps around to support the body.

Lateral recumbency

It is important that the entire body of the horse is placed on the padded surface (Figure 23.39). This prevents the development of pressure points, particularly over peripheral nerves. The head should be placed in a neutral position, not overly flexed or extended. The headcollar should be removed to prevent the development of pressure sores. The eyes should be protected, particularly the lower eye, to prevent corneal damage. Lubricating the cornea with a topical lubricant prevents drying of the corneal surface and should be repeated frequently during anaesthesia. The ear should be checked to make sure it is not trapped under the head, which might be a source of discomfort on recovery.

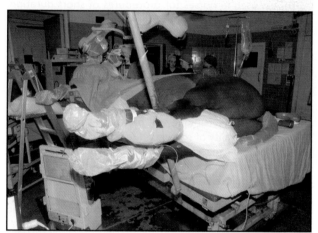

23.39 A horse positioned in lateral recumbency for surgery. A dedicated leg support is used to maintain the upper hindlimb parallel to the lower hindlimb. In addition, there is padding between the forelimbs and hindlimbs. This is to prevent the weight of the upper limb from causing nerve or muscle damage to the lower limb. The lower forelimb is pulled forward so that the weight of the upper forequarters of the horse is not pressing directly on the lower forelimb muscles.

The lower thoracic limb should be pulled forward to prevent damage to the triceps muscle from the pressure of the chest wall. The upper limbs (both fore- and hind-) should be supported in a position parallel to the table top, ideally using special leg supports. This is preferable to placing padding between the upper and lower limb to support the upper limb.

Dorsal recumbency

The horse should be placed squarely on its back (Figure 23.40). Careful attention should be paid to ensuring that the neck is straight, while not over-extended. The shoulder area should be well padded. The thoracic limbs may be allowed to rest on the sternal area, although some padding on the sternum may be required to prevent skin trauma. The pelvic limbs may be allowed to rest in a relaxed position. Sometimes the pelvic limbs may need to be held in extension using an overhead hoist (e.g. for arthroscopy procedures); however, a prolonged period of extension can increase the likelihood of femoral nerve damage and complications in recovery. The eyes and the ears should be checked to ensure they are protected while the horse is in dorsal recumbency; a topical eye lubricant should be used to prevent corneal drying.

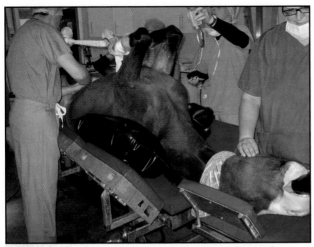

23.40 A horse positioned in dorsal recumbency for surgery. The fore- and hindlimbs are slightly flexed in a relaxed position. The horse is square on the table to ensure even distribution of weight over the lumbar muscles, the neck is straight to ensure even pressure on the neck muscles. (Courtesy of Carolyne Sheridan)

Muscle relaxation and neuromuscular blockade

Adequate muscle relaxation during surgery is vital. Reduced muscle tone decreases the requirement for traction on tissue during surgery, reducing pain and inflammation on recovery from anaesthesia. Prevention of movement may also be mandatory when sudden movement may be catastrophic, e.g. during intraocular (eye) surgery.

Muscle relaxation can be produced in four ways:

- **General anaesthesia**: High concentrations of anaesthetic agents are usually required to produce marked muscle relaxation and cannot guarantee prevention of sudden movement during anaesthesia
- Administration of a **local anaesthetic drug around a peripheral nerve**: Block conduction in motor neurons (see earlier)
- Administration of **local anaesthetic drug into the intrathecal or epidural space** (see earlier)
- Use of a **neuromuscular blocking agent (NMBA)**: This technique can be used to provide good muscle relaxation and prevent movement, while avoiding the need for a high concentration of inhalant agent which can have marked cardiovascular and respiratory system effects. It provides whole body muscle relaxation in contrast to techniques involving local anaesthetic agents.

Movement is the cardinal sign of inadequate anaesthesia; very careful attention should therefore be paid to monitoring depth of anaesthesia following administration of an NMBA in order to prevent inadequate anaesthesia and awareness in a patient that is unable to respond.

WARNING

- NMBAs must always be administered in combination with adequate general anaesthesia.
- Administration of an NMBA will stop respiration due to blockade of activity in respiratory muscles. The facility to support ventilation with IPPV must be available.

Indications for neuromuscular blockade

- **Intraocular surgery**: To prevent downward rotation of the eye and unpredictable body movement that might be catastrophic during surgery. The eye must be in a central position in order to allow surgical access.
- **Facilitate IPPV**: Respiration can be controlled without use of NMBAs, but in some animals their use is helpful to over-ride voluntary respiratory movements.
- **Laparotomy**: It can be helpful to reduce abdominal muscle wall tone and therefore reduce the traction required during exploration of the abdomen.
- **Cardiovascularly unstable patients**: NMBAs will contribute to a balanced anaesthesia technique and reduce the concentration of other drugs required to maintain anaesthesia, thereby reducing the negative cardiovascular consequence of anaesthesia. However, care must be taken to ensure that depth of anaesthesia is adequate.

Action of NMBAs

Muscle contraction is initiated by a nerve impulse or action potential in a motor nerve. The motor nerve connects with the muscle at the neuromuscular junction (NMJ) (Figure 23.41). Action potentials in the motor nerve arriving at the NMJ cause the release of acetylcholine (ACh) into the synaptic cleft. When activated by ACh, receptors on the post-synaptic membrane of the NMJ allow an ion channel to open which allows sodium ions to enter the muscle fibre. Sodium enters the muscle, resulting in depolarization of the post-synaptic membrane, generating a small action potential in the motor endplate and muscle fibre membrane, termed a motor endplate potential. This will result in muscle contraction. Neuromuscular blocking agents act at the NMJ to prevent action potential depolarization of the muscle fibre and muscle contraction.

Two classes of drug are used for neuromuscular blockade:

- **Depolarizing agents** (e.g. suxamethonium) bind reversibly to the ACh receptor to cause opening of the ion channel. This results in initial muscle contraction followed by muscle relaxation; further muscle contraction is prevented due to occupation of the receptor by the drug. Suxamethonium is rarely used clinically in veterinary practice.
- **Non-depolarizing agents** (e.g. atracurium, vecuronium) bind reversibly to the ACh receptor (but do not cause the ion channel to open and initiate muscle contraction) and prevent ACh from binding to the receptor. This prevents muscle contraction. Non-depolarizing agents are used clinically in veterinary practice.

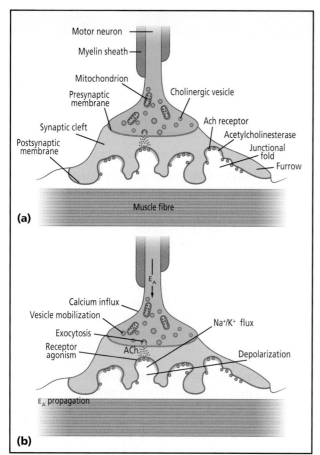

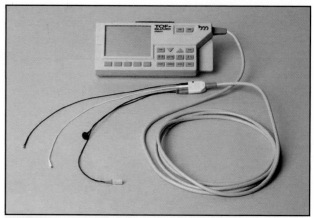

23.42 Peripheral nerve stimulator for monitoring neuromuscular blockade. The black and white leads with a 2 mm plug connector at their ends (on the far left of the picture) connect, respectively, to the negative and positive needle electrodes; these electrodes are placed subcutaneously over the peripheral nerve to be stimulated. At the end of another black lead is a small rectangular grey accelerometer that can be placed on the body part that will be moved as a result of stimulation of the muscle. A third black lead, between the white lead and the lead with the accelerometer, ends in a small round disc that is a temperature sensor. The accelerometer and temperature sensor are not essential.

23.41 Anatomy **(a)** and physiology **(b)** of the neuromuscular junction. E_A = action potential (Redrawn after *In Practice* (2007) **29**, 575)

Monitoring neuromuscular blockade

Monitoring is important because it allows the re-dosing interval to be determined and helps to ensure that return of respiratory activity is sufficient before ventilatory support is withdrawn. Neuromuscular blockade is monitored by electrically stimulating a superficial peripheral nerve and measuring the response in terms of resulting muscle contraction. This can be assessed by observation or palpation of a muscle twitch or by measuring movement resulting from the muscle contraction, e.g. by using an accelerometer placed on the body part that will move when the muscle contracts.

Peripheral nerve stimulators (Figure 23.42) can be purchased to monitor neuromuscular blockade. It is important that the electrodes used to stimulate the nerve are placed before the administration of the NMBA. This allows correct placement to be confirmed (by observation of the appropriate muscle contraction) before the onset of the blockade.

Superficial nerves commonly stimulated to assess neuromuscular blockade include:

- The **facial nerve** – to cause contraction of the dilator nasolabialis muscle and flare of the nostrils
- The **ulnar nerve** – to cause contraction of the muscles that flex the carpus; the site of placement of the electrodes for stimulation of the ulnar nerve are shown in Figure 23.43
- The **deep peroneal nerve** – to cause contraction of the digital extensors of the hindlimb.

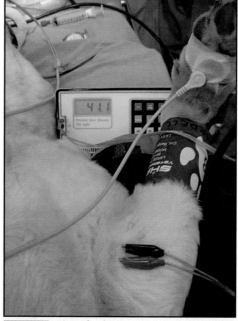

23.43 Site of subcutaneous placement of stimulating electrodes (needles) to stimulate the ulnar nerve to monitor neuromuscular blockade. The nerve runs medial to the olecranon and causes contraction of the carpal flexor muscles and flexion of the carpus. The electrodes are two 25 gauge 5/8 inch needles placed approximately 3 cm apart from each other. The black (negative) electrode is located distally to the red (positive) electrode. The electrodes are connected to a nerve stimulator. The display on the nerve stimulator shows the stimulating current in mA. A cuff for non-invasive measurement of blood pressure using the oscillometric technique is placed on the left forelimb. An ECG electrode and lead are also connected to the left forelimb footpad.

Reversal of neuromuscular blockade

Muscle contraction is normally terminated by the action of acetylcholinesterase. This enzyme breaks down ACh so that the ACh receptor is no longer occupied; the ion channels close and repolarization of the post-synaptic membrane occurs, resulting in muscle relaxation. Modern non-depolarizing agents are relatively short-acting (e.g. atracurium 45 min, vecuronium 20 min), and for many procedures duration is shorter than the anaesthesia period required. Duration of neuromuscular blockade is, however, unpredictable in some animals and reversal can be beneficial. Reversal also ensures that ventilatory function is returned to normal by the end of anaesthesia, so that the animal can safely recover from anaesthesia without respiratory compromise.

Reversal of non-depolarizing NMBAs can be achieved by administration of an anti-acetylcholinesterase such as neostigmine or edrophonium. These drugs block the activity of the enzyme so that the concentration of ACh in the synaptic cleft rises. ACh is then able to compete effectively with the NMBA for the ACh receptors, and muscle contraction can occur. In order to prevent unwanted systemic effects, an anticholinergic drug is administered concurrently (e.g. atropine or glycopyrrolate). This specifically prevents the bradycardia that would otherwise occur due to a prolonged activity of ACh on myocardial ACh receptors, causing increased parasympathetic nervous system effects.

Equipment for maintaining anaesthesia

The anaesthetic machine

A basic understanding of how an anaesthetic machine works is vital if the veterinary nurse is to assist in the safe administration of anaesthesia. Anaesthetic machines consist of several parts (Figure 23.44).

Gas supply

The gas supply can be from a cylinder, a pipeline or both.

Colour coding

The gas supply is colour coded for safety (Figure 23.45):

- Black cylinders with a white head and white pipelines for oxygen
- Blue cylinders and pipelines for nitrous oxide.

Another safety feature is the pin index system. This is the configuration of the pin holes on the cylinder and pins on the yoke (where the cylinder is attached to either the anaesthetic machine or the cylinder manifold on the pipeline supply). This prevents an oxygen cylinder being attached to an N₂O yoke or *vice versa*. Shrader probes (Figure 23.46a) and pipeline gas outlets also only fit the correct probe or outlet. On the yoke there is a Bodok seal (Figure

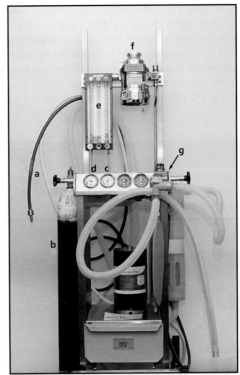

23.44 A simple anaesthetic machine. a = oxygen pipeline (white), nitrous oxide pipeline (blue); b = oxygen cylinder; c = pressure gauge for pipeline oxygen supply; d = pressure gauge for cylinder oxygen supply; e = oxygen and nitrous oxide flowmeters; f = isoflurane vaporizer; g = oxygen flush.

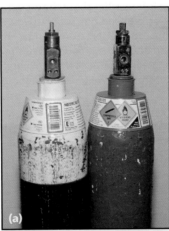
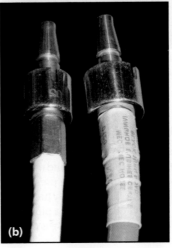

23.45 Colour coding. **(a)** In the UK, oxygen cylinders are black with a white neck, whereas nitrous oxide cylinders are blue. **(b)** Oxygen pipelines are white, whereas nitrous oxide pipelines are blue.

23.46b) that maintains a seal between the cylinder and the yoke. These often need changing. Before attaching a new cylinder it should be 'cracked' (turned on to allow a small amount of gas to escape, whilst holding the cylinder firmly and directing the gas exit point away from any personnel). This is to ensure that any contamination, e.g. dust, is not propelled into the anaesthetic machine or pipeline system.

> **WARNING**
>
> It is vital that no carbon-based oils and greases are used around the valves on cylinders and anaesthetic machines due to the risk of explosion.

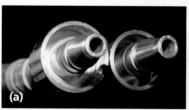

23.46 (a) Connection between oxygen and nitrous oxide pipelines to Schrader outlets; different gases have different sized connectors to prevent inadvertent misconnection of gas pipelines to the incorrect outlet. (b) A Bodok seal.

Pressure gauge

The pressure gauge provides information about the amount of gas left in the cylinder or pipeline gas supply (Figure 23.47). It should be remembered that pressure gauges do not give reliable information about the amount of gas remaining in N_2O cylinders or pipelines because N_2O is in liquid form; the cylinder must therefore be weighed to find out the content.

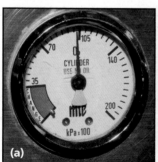

23.47 (a) Pressure gauge for a cylinder of oxygen.
(b) Pressure gauge for pipeline oxygen supply.

Pressure-reducing valve (regulators)

Regulators (pressure-reducing valves) (Figure 23.48) reduce the pressure of the gas coming from the cylinder and maintain a constant pressure to prevent any surges in the pressure of the gas being relayed to the patient. They are only present in anaesthetic machines that have cylinders. When a pipeline is used as the gas source, the pressure-reducing valve is present at the source of the gas.

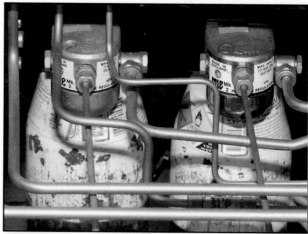

23.48 Pressure regulator attached to an oxygen cylinder on an anaesthetic machine.

Flowmeters

Flowmeters (rotameters) provide the final stage in the reduction of the pressure of the gas and allow manual adjustment of the volume of gas (O_2, medical air, N_2O) delivered to the patient (Figure 23.49). The flowmeter comprises a tube of tapered glass or plastic (narrower at the bottom and getting wider towards the top). Contained within the tube is a lightweight ball or bobbin that is moved within the tube by the gas passing around it (the movement of the gas is both laminar and turbulent, thus the flowmeter needs to be calibrated specifically for each gas). When setting the flow rate for a patient, the top of the bobbin or the middle of the ball should be used according to which is present on the anaesthetic machine in use.

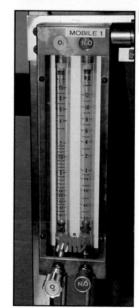

23.49 Oxygen and nitrous oxide flowmeters on an anaesthetic machine.

Back bar

The back bar supports the flowmeters and it is here that the vaporizers are mounted. Most anaesthetic machines in the UK use the 'Ohmeda selectatec' system. When using this system it is important that the vaporizer is 'locked' into place on to the back bar in order to ensure a seal and allow the vaporizer to work. Modern back bars that can mount more than one vaporizer have mechanisms to prevent more than one vaporizer being switched on at once, which would allow the potential for anaesthetic overdose.

Common gas outlet

The common gas outlet is the point at which the gases come out of the anaesthetic machine.

Additional features

Additional features that may be present on anaesthetic machines are:

- **Mini-Schrader sockets:** gas sockets that provide O_2 or air to power ventilators (Figure 23.50). They are usually found underneath the anaesthetic machine
- **Emergency oxygen flush** (Figure 23.51): provides O_2 directly from the cylinder or pipeline, bypassing the vaporizer. Care should be taken when using this function as the oxygen is delivered at high flow rates that could produce barotrauma
- **Oxygen failure alarm:** sounds if there is a drop in the pressure of the O_2 supply. This is a very important safety feature
- **Nitrous oxide cut-off:** if the oxygen fails and N_2O is also being used, administration of N_2O is terminated
- **Hypoxic guard:** the anaesthetic machine will not allow the delivery of N_2O without the concurrent delivery of O_2. It prevents accidental delivery of a hypoxic mixture by ensuring that there is always a minimum percentage of oxygen present in the delivered mixture
- **Pressure relief valve:** opens if the pressure at the common gas outlet is too high, i.e. if the common gas outlet is blocked. This is designed to prevent the pressure within the anaesthetic machine becoming too high and thus damaging the machine. It does provide a degree of protection to the patient; however, the pressure that needs to be reached before the valve is activated would cause substantial damage to the lungs of the patient.

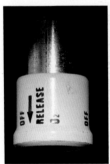

23.50 Mini-Schrader outlet used to attach a ventilator driven by oxygen to the machine oxygen supply.

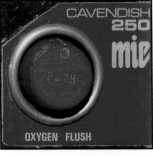

23.51 Oxygen flush on the front of an anaesthetic machine.

Vaporizers

The majority of vaporizers used in the UK are temperature-compensated (TEC) vaporizers. This means that they automatically compensate if the temperature changes, to ensure maintenance of a constant concentration of inhalant agent in the delivered gas mixture. Vaporizers work by splitting the gas into two channels: one channel passes through the vaporizing chamber and becomes saturated with anaesthetic vapour (with isoflurane this equates to a concentration of 32%); while the other channel bypasses the vaporizing chamber. The two channels are then combined before exiting the vaporizer. When the concentration of anaesthetic gas required is dialled up on the vaporizer, the amount of gas that is split off into the vaporizing channel is adjusted to achieve the required concentration. It is important not to tip vaporizers, to prevent contamination of the bypass chamber with inhalant agent that would make the output of the vaporizer unreliable and be potentially dangerous. It is important to follow the manufacturer's guidelines on servicing. Many vaporizers should not be used with fresh gas flow rates <0.75 l/min, as the output of the vaporizer may become inaccurate. Again, it is important to follow the manufacturer's guidelines.

Filling vaporizers

Due to the different physical properties of the agents it is important that each vaporizer is calibrated and designed to deliver a single gas. For example, using an isoflurane-specific vaporizer to deliver sevoflurane would result in concentrations different to those predicted. In order to prevent filling with the wrong agent, modern vaporizers have a keyed filling system. An agent-specific filler tube is used: one end slots into a fitting on the vaporizer and the other end slots on to a collar on the bottle of anaesthetic (Figure 23.52). Both the fitting on the vaporizer and the collar on the bottle are specific for one agent. This closed system, unlike older funnel fill systems, also minimizes environmental contamination. Nevertheless, vaporizers should still be filled at the end of the working day and with all ventilation systems for the room switched on, so that any waste gases are dissipated before the working area is used again.

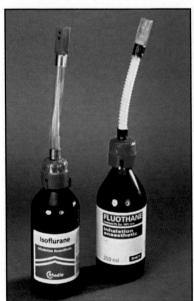

23.52 Bottles of isoflurane and halothane with the keyed anaesthetic vaporizer filling system attached.

Anaesthetic breathing systems

Anaesthetic breathing systems have several functions:

- Transfer of gases from the anaesthetic machine to the ET tube or face mask
- Removal of CO_2 breathed out by the patient, preventing rebreathing of CO_2
- Delivery of artificial breaths to the patient (IPPV, see later)
- Measurement of airway pressures, gas volumes and gas composition
- Scavenging of waste gases.

Some important definitions

- **Tidal volume (TV):** The volume of gas exhaled by the patient in one breath.
- **Minute volume (MV):** The volume of gas exhaled by the patient in 1 minute.
- **Rebreathing:** Inhalation of previously breathed gases that have taken part in gas exchange.
- **Reservoir bag** (rebreathing/breathing bag): An open-ended or closed bag that is attached to a breathing system.
- **Limbs of the anaesthetic breathing circuit** (breathing tubes): The tubing of the breathing system within which the gases are carried. These can be inspiratory or expiratory.
- **Unidirectional valves** (one-way valves): Ensure that the gases only flow in one direction.
- **APL (adjustable pressure limiting) valve** (pressure relief valve, pop-off valve, scavenging valve): Controls the amount of gas contained within the reservoir bag and how much gas escapes from the breathing system via the scavenging system. This valve commonly contains a plastic disc suspended on a spring that is depressed when a set pressure is exerted on it, causing the valve to open, thus allowing gases to escape. This acts as a safety feature, although the pressure that must be reached before the valve opens is quite high for some models, by which time barotrauma is likely to have occurred.
- **Fresh gas inlet:** The point where the gas enters the breathing system from the common gas outlet of the anaesthetic machine.
- **Anatomical deadspace:** The gas inhaled by the patient that does not undergo any gas exchange (i.e. the air within the upper airway and trachea).
- **Apparatus deadspace** (equipment deadspace): The volume of gas contained within the breathing system that is rebreathed by the patient and has not participated in gaseous exchange.
- **Open breathing systems:** These systems have no reservoir bag, unidirectional valves or carbon dioxide absorbent.
- **Semi-open systems:** These systems contain a reservoir bag and APL valve. They do not contain a CO_2 absorbent or unidirectional valve.
- **Closed systems:** Contain a reservoir bag, unidirectional valves, CO_2 absorbent and APL valve.
- **Semi-closed systems:** Same as a closed system except the circuit is used with the valve open or partially open.
- **Mapleson configuration:** A method of classifying ▶

non-rebreathing systems developed in 1954.

- **Coaxial system:** The inspiratory and expiratory limbs are contained one within the other. There is a possible advantage over parallel tubing in that the fresh gases are warmed; however damage/disconnection of the inner tube is not easily visible and this can make the circuit potentially hazardous to use.
- **Parallel system:** The inspiratory and expiratory limbs run side by side.
- **Compliance:** How well the lungs stretch to accommodate a change in volume in relation to the pressure applied.

Anaesthetic breathing systems are described as either **re-breathing** or **non-rebreathing** (Figure 23.53). The easiest way to distinguish between these is to identify whether there is any CO_2 absorbent present in the circuit. This absorbs the CO_2 that the patient breathes out, enabling this gas to be reused by the patient. In non-rebreathing systems the CO_2 is flushed out by the continued flow of fresh gas into the circuit. Non-rebreathing systems can be further classified as coaxial or parallel; there are advantages and disadvantages to each type (Figure 23.54).

Rebreathing	**23.53**
Circle To-and-fro Humphrey ADE–circle system	Breathing systems used in veterinary practice.
Non-rebreathing	
T-piece Bain (parallel or coaxial) Lack (parallel or coaxial) Magill Humphrey ADE	

System type	Advantages	Disadvantages
Rebreathing	Require low gas flow rates reducing cost associated with anaesthetic agent delivery and environmental contamination with waste gases. Reduced heat loss, as gases require less warming by the patient than in non-rebreathing circuits	Altering the concentration of volatile agent within the circuit takes time, depending on gas flow rate and volume of circuit. CO_2 absorbent and valves create resistance. Require an understanding of how the circuit works. Require maintenance associated with changing CO_2 absorbent. Can be expensive to purchase
Non-rebreathing	Concentration of inhalant agent can be adjusted rapidly. Minimal circuit resistance. Easy to use. Cheap to purchase	High gas flow rates increase costs associated with gases and inhalant agents and increase environmental contamination. Potential for rebreathing if patient breathes rapidly; gas flow rate must be increased. Significant heat loss through respiratory tract due to warming of inspired gases

23.54   Advantages and disadvantages of rebreathing and non-rebreathing systems.

Rebreathing systems

These systems allow the gases that have been exhaled by the patient to be re-used after the absorption of CO_2. They are economical when used in a 'closed' manner because the only gas that needs to be added is oxygen to compensate for that used by cells of the body during metabolism (**metabolic oxygen consumption**).

Circle system

The circle system (Figure 23.55) is the most commonly used rebreathing system. There are many different circle systems available, but they all work using the same principle. The main variation between models is the size of the soda lime canister and the tubing design. These factors determine the level of resistance to gas flow in the circuit and thus the size of patient the system can be used for. Most small circle systems are suitable for patients >10 kg. Circle systems contain **unidirectional valves** that ensure unidirectional gas flow. The gases that the patient breathes out pass through the canister containing the CO_2 absorbent before they are breathed again.

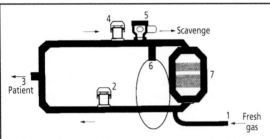

- *Fresh gas inflow* (1). This pipe connects the circuit with the common-gas outlet on the anaesthetic machine.
- *Unidirectional valves* (2 and 4). These are light transparent discs resting on knife-edge valve seats, enclosed within a transparent dome. Units should be easy to disassemble for drying and cleaning.
- *'Y' connector* (3). This connects inspiratory and expiratory limbs with endotracheal tube connectors or masks.
- *Adjustable pressure limiting (APL) valve* (5). This is opened to release surplus gas from 'low-flow' systems, during denitrogenation, and closed when lung inflation is imposed. APL valves should be shrouded for attachment to scavenging hoses.
- *Reservoir bag* (6). This allows IPPV; its volume should be 3–6 times the animal's tidal volume. Large bags increase circuit volume, make respiratory movement less obvious and are harder to squeeze. Inadequately sized bags collapse during large breaths and overdistend during expiration.
- *Absorbent canister* (7). Canisters for circle systems may have two compartments. When absorbent in one becomes exhausted, it is discarded; after refilling, the canister is replaced in the reverse direction. This allows optimal use of absorbent.
- *Hoses.* These are corrugated to prevent kinking.

23.55 Circle breathing system.

Practical considerations

When the patient is first anaesthetized and placed on to the circle system, high levels of nitrogen are exhaled due to the gas composition of room air breathed before induction. A higher gas flow, with the valve in an open or semi-open position, must be used for the first 15–20 minutes to allow **denitrogenation**, which prevents the development of a hypoxic mixture within the circle system. After 15–20 minutes the fresh gas flow can be reduced, either to the metabolic oxygen consumption rate (2–7 ml/kg), with the APL valve closed **(closed circle)**, or to a rate of 1 litre/min (for patients <10 kg), with the APL valve semi-open **(semi-closed system)**. The valve must be sufficiently open to prevent the bag from becoming overdistended.

Use of a truly 'closed' circle is not recommended for a number of reasons:

- Metabolic oxygen consumption is very variable, not only between individuals of different age, sex and breed but also due to changes in temperature and drug administration throughout the anaesthetic period. Maintaining the reservoir of gas at the correct oxygen concentration is therefore extremely difficult
- Most anaesthetic machines used in veterinary practice do not have flowmeters that allow accurate delivery of very low gas flow rates
- Most vaporizers used in veterinary practice are not calibrated to be accurate at very low flow rates
- Analysis of exhaled (end tidal) gases is needed to work out the concentration of inhalational agent that is being delivered to the patient, along with capnography (see below) to ensure that no rebreathing of CO_2 occurs
- Closed circle systems rely heavily on the CO_2 absorbent not being exhausted.

Advantages of circle systems

- Low fresh gas flow requirements, reducing medical gas costs.
- Decreased use of expensive volatile agents.
- Less environmental contamination.
- Reduced heat loss from the patient. The gases coming from the anaesthetic machine are cold but recirculation of gases though the soda lime (where an exothermic reaction takes place) warms the gases. The low flow rates also reduce the cold air being added to the system.
- Inspired gases are moistened as they pass through the soda lime because the reaction within the CO_2 absorbent produces water. Less new fresh gas and hence dry air is also added to the system.
- Ideal for IPPV.

Disadvantages of circle systems

- The canister needs to be filled with a CO_2 absorbent in accordance with the manufacturer's guidelines.
- Some canisters are fiddly to fill.
- Some canisters are difficult to clean.
- Canisters are often a source of gas leaks.
- Maintenance takes time and skill (it is vital to check the circle system before every use) and there is a cost associated with purchase of CO_2 absorbent.
- The CO_2 absorbent creates resistance.
- Relatively expensive to purchase.
- Water may collect in tubing and within the circle (must be allowed to dry out frequently).
- May be unsuitable for anaesthesia of hyperthermic patients or large-breed dogs as excessive heat may be generated, exacerbating or creating hyperthermia (although this effect can be reduced by using higher gas flow rates).

Maintenance of circle systems

Circle systems should be maintained following specific manufacturer's guidelines; however, there are a few basic principles that should always be adhered to.

Change the CO_2 absorbent frequently, following the absorbent manufacturer's guidelines. It is vital to be aware of the colour change that is present with that particular absorbent (see below).

- Change the CO_2 absorbent in a well ventilated room.
- Wear gloves (most CO_2 absorbents are caustic, especially when damp).
- Empty contents in accordance with local waste disposal regulations, taking care not to breath in any dust created.
- When the canister is empty, look for any small cracks or signs of damage.
- Check the circle system thoroughly after changing the absorbent:

1. Once the canister has been refilled, attach it to the anaesthetic machine and attach the Y-piece patient tubing.
2. Occlude the Y-piece at the patient end.
3. Close the APL valve.
4. Fill the circle with O_2 (using either the oxygen flush or flowmeter) until the reservoir bag becomes distended.
5. Listen and feel for any leaks, watching the reservoir bag for any signs of it deflating.
6. Open the APL valve to check that it is working and not sticking; this also prevents any accidents caused by inadvertently leaving the valve closed when the circuit is attached to the patient, such as possible barotrauma. Some gas will escape of its own accord and the rest should be removed by squeezing the reservoir bag. By keeping the Y-piece occluded during this process, all gases are removed from the breathing system via the scavenging, preventing environmental contamination from any inhalational agent residue within the system.
7. Date and initial the canister.

To-and-fro system

The to-and-fro breathing system (Figure 23.56) is no longer commonly used within small animal veterinary practice. The fresh gas enters the breathing system close to the patient. When the patient exhales, the gases pass through the Waters' canister, which contains the CO_2 absorbent, and into a reservoir bag. As the patient breathes in, the gases from the reservoir bag are drawn back though the Waters' canister, with any excess gas escaping though a pressure relief valve situated close to the patient.

To-and-fro systems have many disadvantages compared to circle systems:

- The bulky and heavy system is used close to the head of the patient:
  - This pulls on the ET tube, increasing the risk of accidental disconnection from the breathing system and accidental extubation, which can be damaging and dangerous due to the inflated cuff. There is also an increased risk of the ET tube becoming kinked
  - There is increased risk of caustic dust from the

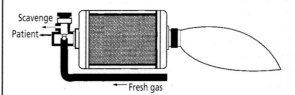

- *Fresh gas inflow.* This is situated adjacent to the endotracheal tube connector, allowing dialled concentrations of anaesthetic to be preferentially inspired and therefore giving greater control over anaesthesia.
- *Filter.* A metal gauze screen should be sited at the patient end of the canister to limit inhalation of alkaline dust.
- *Scavenging shroud.* Scavenging waste gas from a to-and-fro system relies on a suitable shroud on the adjustable pressure limiting valve.
- *Canister.* Transparent canisters allow absorbent colour and filling adequacy to be checked. Canisters in horizontal to-and-fro systems must be filled to capacity, otherwise the expired gas will 'channel', i.e. take the low resistance path over the absorbent, retaining CO_2.

23.56 To-and-fro breathing system.

absorbent entering the patient's lungs. This is especially problematic during IPPV
  - Location of the APL valve close to the head makes IPPV difficult, particularly during head and neck surgery
  - There is poor access for any surgery around the head and neck
- Due to the position of the canister in the circuit and the bidirectional flow of gases over the absorbent, the absorbent closest to the patient becomes exhausted first, increasing the equipment deadspace. This is especially problematical for smaller patients with a lower tidal volume
- There is a risk that gases can be channelled over the absorbent within the canister (particularly if the canister is not full), resulting in inefficient CO_2 absorption and the potential for rebreathing
- It is essential that the canister is filled correctly, as overfilling results in increased resistance and underfilling results in inefficient CO_2 absorption.

Carbon dioxide absorption

The CO_2 absorbent is integral to rebreathing systems. The individual designs vary between manufacturers, but the basic components are the same:

- Calcium hydroxide
- Sodium hydroxide
- Water
- pH indicator
- Silica
- Zeolite
- Calcium sulphate
- Calcium chloride.

The most important components are calcium hydroxide, sodium hydroxide and water.

The CO_2 absorbent may have granular or spherical particles which give a high surface area to volume ratio to maximize the surface exposed to the gas. The preparation must not be too dusty. Dust in the CO_2 absorbent has several effects:

- It increases resistance
- It damages the breathing system – the dust can settle within valves, making them inefficient, and can gather in seals, making leaks more likely
- It may reach the patient and cause caustic burns to the airway
- It may be an irritant to the operator refilling or emptying the canister.

The reaction with CO_2 takes place in two stages:

Stage 1

H_2O + CO_2 $\leftrightarrows$ H_2CO_3
Water   Carbon dioxide   Carbonic acid

Stage 2

$2H_2CO_3 + 2NaOH + Ca(OH)_2 \leftrightarrows CaCO_3 + Na_2CO_3 + 4H_2O + heat$

Carbonic acid + Sodium hydroxide + Calcium hydroxide $\leftrightarrows$ Calcium carbonate + Sodium carbonate + Water + Heat

Carbon dioxide absorption results in a pH change, signalled by a colour change in the pH indicator. It is important to refer to the manufacturer's guidelines in order to be aware of the colour change that occurs with a particular absorbent. The most commonly seen colour changes are from pink to white, and from white to purple. The colour change indicates that the absorbent has been exhausted and so must be changed.

Other indicators of exhaustion include:

- Increased end-tidal CO_2 (hypercapnia) as measured by a capnometer (clinical signs are increased heart and respiratory rates and blood pressure, brick red mucous membranes and bounding pulses)
- Increased inspired CO_2 (there should be no CO_2 present in the inspired gases)
- The canister of absorbent is cool to the touch (the reaction between the absorbent and CO_2 generates heat).

WARNING

A CO_2 absorbent that is left overnight after it has become exhausted will return to its original colour, and so the following day will appear as if it has not been exhausted. This occurs because the reaction between the CO_2 and absorbent is reversible. However, if this absorbent is then used it will change colour quickly, indicating its exhausted state. Exhausted absorbent should therefore be changed at the end of the day when the colour change is clear.

Absorbents can also release toxic byproducts. Dry sodium hydroxide can degrade isoflurane and halothane to produce carbon monoxide and can degrade sevoflurane to produce compound A, methanol and formaldehyde. Consequently it is very important that the absorbent does not dry out. This can be done by ensuring that the fresh gases and inhalational agent are switched off immediately after use to reduce drying by the fresh gases and exposure to the inhalational agent, and that the absorbent is regularly changed.

Non-rebreathing systems

Non-rebreathing systems are characterized by the absence of unidirectional valves and CO_2 absorbent. They require higher fresh gas flows than rebreathing systems because the expired CO_2 is removed from the circuit by new fresh gas flushing out the expired gases.

Features of non-rebreathing systems include:

- High fresh gas flow rates can exacerbate hypothermia – this is particularly problematic in patients of low bodyweight
- High fresh gas flow rates increase costs associated with both the anaesthetic gases (O_2 and N_2O or medical air) and inhalational agents
- High fresh gas flow rates lead to greater environmental contamination
- The patient receives the concentration of volatile agent that is dialled up on the vaporizer with no delay (i.e. next breath). Changes in depth of anaesthesia can be achieved quickly
- Optimal levels of N_2O can be used safely; total fresh gas flow can be divided in a ratio of 1:2 O_2:N_2O
- No changes in the fresh gas flow rate are required during the anaesthetic period (unless there are changes to the patient's minute volume due to changes in respiratory rate)
- A **circuit factor** (see Fig 23.57) is required to prevent rebreathing of alveolar gas.

Calculation of fresh gas flow rate

Due to the reliance on the fresh gas flow rate to prevent rebreathing, correct calculation of fresh gas flow rate is essential.

1. Calculate the patient's **tidal volume** (TV). This is the volume of gas exhaled in one breath and is considered to be between 10 and 15 ml/kg.
   - The size of the patient is the first thing to consider when determining which end of the 10–15 ml/kg range to use. Generally, use the high end of the range for small dogs and cats. For larger patients, e.g. Labradors, a tidal volume of 10 ml/kg is appropriate.
   - Consider the body condition of the patient. Only the lean weight, i.e. what the bodyweight would be at a body condition score of 3/5, should be used in the calculation.
   - Consider the shape of the patient's thorax. Deep-chested breeds such as Greyhounds will have a higher tidal volume than would be expected for their bodyweight (12–15 ml/kg).

   Tidal volume (ml) = 10–15 × bodyweight (kg)

2. Calculate the patient's **minute volume** (MV). This is the volume of gas expired by the patient in 1 minute and requires measurement of respiratory rate (breaths per minute). This should be done when the patient has been allowed to acclimatize to its environment. The best way of gathering this information is to observe the patient from a distance when it is in its kennel. If the patient is

panting, the respiratory rate should be estimated. Once the patient is anaesthetized the respiratory rate may be different to that used for the MV calculation. It is important to recalculate respiratory rate if it increases, as it will lead to increased MV.

Minute volume (ml/min) = **Tidal volume** (ml)
× **Respiratory rate** (/min)

3. Multiply the calculated minute volume by the **circuit factor** of the breathing system being used. The circuit factor varies between different breathing systems (Figure 23.57).

Fresh gas flow rate (ml/min) = **Minute volume** (ml/min)
× **Circuit factor**

Breathing system	Circuit factor
T-piece	2.5–3
Lack and Mini-Lack	1–1.5
Magill	1–1.5
Bain	2.5–3

23.57 Circuit factors for different breathing systems.

T-piece

Many different variations of the T-piece are used within veterinary practice. These differences are centred around the presence or absence of a reservoir bag and APL valve. The Ayre's T-piece (Mapleson E) (Figure 23.58a) has no reservoir bag or valve. An Ayre's T-piece with a Jackson–Rees modification (Mapleson F) (Figure 23.58b) has no valve but an open-ended reservoir bag. A paediatric T-piece (Mapleson D) contains an APL valve and a closed-ended reservoir bag.

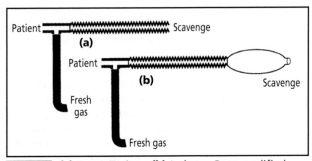

23.58 **(a)** Ayre's T-piece; **(b)** Jackson–Rees modified Ayre's T-piece.

Despite these variations, the principle of how a T-piece works is similar. Gases enter the breathing system close to the patient at the 'T' and fill all of the tubing from which the patient inhales. When the patient exhales, the gases move down the expiratory limb (the force of the fresh gas prevents the gases moving towards the anaesthetic machine) where they leave the system: directly into the scavenging system (Ayre's T-piece); through the open-ended reservoir bag and then the scavenging system (Jackson-Rees modification); or out of the APL valve (paediatric system). In the expiratory pause (the gap between breaths) the tubing fills with fresh gas in preparation for the next breath. A high flow rate is required to ensure all of the expired gases are flushed from

the system, preventing rebreathing; consequently a circuit factor of 2.5–3 times minute volume is required (the higher end of the range should be used for smaller patients).

The T-piece is a low-resistance circuit with a small amount of deadspace and is the breathing system of choice for small patients (<8 kg). It is not suitable for use in larger patients because the required high flow rates make it uneconomical and the narrow-bore tubing means that resistance will be created for larger patients during inspiration and expiration.

> **WARNING**
>
> Particular care must be taken when using the Ayre's T-piece with the Jackson–Rees modification due to the risk of the scavenging tubing dragging and causing the reservoir bag to twist and become occluded. This is extremely dangerous for the patient (possible pneumothorax, pneumomediastinum and decreased venous return).

T-pieces are suitable for IPPV. This is achieved either by closing the valve, applying positive pressure to the reservoir bag and then opening the valve, or by occluding the base of the reservoir bag as it enters the scavenging and then applying positive pressure. On the Ayres T-piece the end of the breathing tubing is occluded (e.g. with the thumb) creating positive pressure.

Bain

The principle of the Bain circuit (Figure 23.59) is similar to that of the T-piece. Two types of Bain circuit (Mapleson D) are available: coaxial and parallel. The coaxial Bain is more common, the inspiratory limb running inside the expiratory limb. The Bain has an APL valve and reservoir bag, but no unidirectional valves.

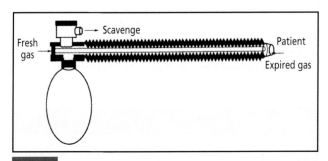

23.59 Modified Bain breathing system.

The tubing close to the patient is filled with fresh gas. As the patient inhales, gases are taken from both the inspiratory and expiratory limbs. When the patient exhales, gases flow down the expiratory limb (but not the inspiratory limb because of the resistance caused by the continued flow of fresh gas), into the reservoir bag and are expelled from the circuit via the APL valve and scavenging system. A larger reservoir bag than on the T-piece makes the Bain circuit suitable for larger patients, although the high flow rates required make it very uneconomical in patients >15 kg. This high flow rate is required to prevent rebreathing of CO_2 and is reflected by the circuit factor of 2.5–3 times minute volume.

The breathing system is suitable for IPPV, achieved by closing the valve, applying positive pressure to the reservoir bag and then immediately opening the valve. It is essential to open the valve immediately because the high fresh gas flow rates quickly create high pressures within the Bain circuit (often the valve will not need to be completely closed).

Lack

The Lack (Mapelson A) can also be either coaxial (Figure 23.60) or parallel (Figure 23.61); the parallel version is the more common. The circuit comprises an APL valve and reservoir bag. The reservoir bag is situated on the inspiratory limb of the system. As the patient inhales, gases are drawn from the inspiratory limb and reservoir bag. When the patient exhales, the first portion of expired gases (deadspace gases) enter the inspiratory limb before the rest (alveolar gases) pass down the expiratory limb and out of the APL valve into the scavenging system. The APL valve is situated next to the gas inlet on the anaesthetic breathing system. Rebreathing of the deadspace gases in the inspiratory limb at the start of the next breath means that the required fresh gas flow rate is lower than for the T-piece or Bain, and therefore the circuit factor is lower (1–1.5 times minute volume). The circuit is suitable for patients >10 kg.

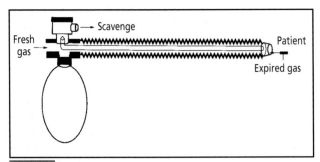

23.60   Coaxial Lack breathing system.

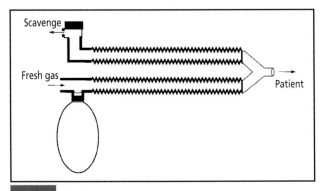

23.61   Parallel Lack breathing system.

Lack systems are not ideal for prolonged IPPV as this disrupts the pattern of gas flow within the circuit, resulting in rebreathing. However, if another breathing system that is more appropriate for IPPV is not available, rebreathing can be prevented by increasing the fresh gas flow rate.

Mini-Lack

This system has the same basic design as the conventional Lack, but is suitable for patients <10 kg because it uses narrow low-resistance tubing, with a narrower tubing connector and small reservoir bag. As with the traditional Lack, the design of the mini-Lack enables the use of lower flow rates compared with the T-piece, only requiring 1–1.5 times minute volume. However, this also makes it unsuitable for prolonged IPPV.

Magill

The Magill (Figure 23.62) also has a Mapleson A configuration. It consists of a reservoir bag that is situated by the fresh gas inlet on the breathing system, wide bore tubing, and an APL valve situated next to the patient's head, close to where the breathing system attaches to the ET tube.

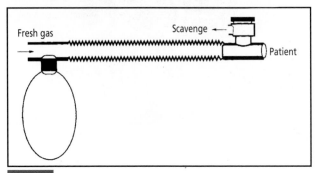

23.62   Magill breathing system.

When the fresh gases are switched on, the reservoir bag and tubing are filled. As the patient inhales, gases are drawn from the tubing and the reservoir bag. As the patient exhales, the first portion of the gas (deadspace gas) travels up the tubing before the pressure of new fresh gas entering the system forces the rest of the exhaled gases (alveolar gases) out of the APL valve and into the scavenging system (path of least resistance). This can occur due to the location of the valve next to the patient's head. The system is suitable for patients >10 kg. The circuit factor for the Magill is 1–1.5 times minute volume.

The location of the valve close to the patient's head has some additional disadvantages: it can increase the risk of accidental disconnection from the breathing system and cause accidental extubation; there is an increased risk of the ET tube becoming kinked; and the location of valve makes IPPV difficult and impractical for any surgery around the head and neck due to poor surgical access.

Humphrey ADE and Humphrey ADE–circle system

The Humphrey ADE breathing system (Figure 23.63) was designed to allow three breathing systems in one unit. The Mapelson A circuit is inefficient for controlled ventilation, as is the Mapleson D circuit for spontaneous ventilation. This single circuit can be changed from a Mapleson A system to a Mapleson D by moving a lever on the metallic block that connects the circuit to the fresh gas outlet on the anaesthetic machine. The reservoir bag is situated at the fresh gas inlet end of the circuit and gas is conducted to and from the patient down the inspiratory and expiratory limbs of the circuit.

* When the lever is in the 'up' position (Figure 23.63) the reservoir bag and respiratory valve are used, creating a Mapleson A type circuit that is ideally suited to spontaneous respiration. It is also suitable for manual ventilation with no change in the fresh gas flow rate, unlike a normal Lack or Magill. The Humphrey ADE–circle system is more efficient than a Magill, therefore average required fresh gas flow rates are 50 ml/kg/min.
* When the lever is in the 'down' position the bag and the valve are bypassed and the ventilator port is opened, creating a Mapelson D (Bain) system for use during IPPV. If no ventilator is attached and the port is left open the system will function like an Ayre's T-piece (Mapleson E).

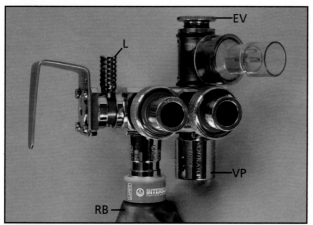

23.63 An ADE circuit. Depending on the position of the control lever (L) at the Humphrey block, gases pass through either the expiratory valve (EV) or the ventilator port (VP). RB = reservoir bag

The three modes centre around the use of the metal block section. The APL valve on this block is especially designed to provide minimal resistance, so the circuit is suitable for use in cats, but also has the benefit of providing 1 cmH$_2$O positive end-expiratory pressure (PEEP). The Humphrey ADE system uses 15 mm smooth-bore tubing, which encourages laminar flow and has a low resistance and a low volume, making it suitable for small patients when a small reservoir bag is used (e.g. 500 ml or 1 litre).

A later and very useful addition to the Humphrey ADE is that of a removable CO$_2$ absorber canister, which creates a fourth mode of breathing system: the circle mode (**Humphrey ADE–circle system**). The canister is easily attached to the main body of the ADE system using two lock nuts on the inspiratory and expiratory limbs. When the CO$_2$ canister is attached, during induction, when higher fresh gas flow rates are used, the fresh gases automatically pass over and not through the soda lime in the canister; the ADE therefore behaves more like a semi-closed system. Once the fresh gas is reduced, during the maintenance phase of the anaesthetic, the gases pass through the soda lime canister so that the breathing system functions as a circle system. Fresh gas flow rates as low as 1 litre/min can be used.

Before using this system it is important for the operator to understand fully how it works. Although a basic guide is described here, the authors recommend that the operator's manual is read thoroughly. A number of websites also describe the functioning of the Humphrey ADE/Humphrey ADE–circle systems.

Selection of appropriate circuit and calculation of fresh gas flow rate

Example 1: DSH cat, 4.5 kg, respiratory rate 32 breaths/min

Tidal volume = 4.5 × 15 = 67.5 ml
Minute volume = 67.5 × 32 = 2160 ml

T-piece circuit selected (low resistance, low deadspace, low TV).

Fresh gas flow rate = MV x circuit factor = 2160 × 2.5
= 5400 ml (5.4 litres) ▶

The veterinary surgeon requests that nitrous oxide is used.

O$_2$ flow rate = 5400 ÷ 3 = 1800 ml (c.2 litres)
N$_2$O flow rate = 1800 × 2 = 3600 ml (c.3.5 litres)

Once the cat is anaesthetized its respiratory rate reduces to 16 breaths/min, allowing recalculation of flow rate. This is not absolutely necessary and maintaining a high flow rate will do no harm, but will increase costs and increase environmental contamination.

Minute volume = 67.5 × 16 = 1080 ml
Fresh gas flow rate
= 1080 × 2.5 = 2700 ml (3 litres – 1 litre of O$_2$ plus 2 litres of N$_2$O)

Example 2: Labrador, 25 kg, respiratory rate 16 breaths/min

Tidal volume = 25 × 10 = 250 ml
Minute volume = 250 × 16 = 4000 ml

Lack selected due to lower requirement for fresh gas flow compared to a Bain and ease of circuit use compared to a Magill.

Fresh gas flow rate = MV x circuit factor = 4000 × 1
= 4000 ml (4 litres)

A circle system could also be used in a semi-closed configuration. This could be achieved by using a fresh gas flow rate of 3 litres/min for the first 20 minutes to ensure denitrogenation and then reducing the fresh gas flow rate to 1 litre/min.

Checking breathing systems

Breathing systems should be checked before every use. The basic principle is the same whatever the breathing system, with small variations towards the end of the check to test individual special features.

Checks to be performed on all breathing systems

1. Visually check for any contamination (e.g. blood) or obvious damage/holes in the tubing or reservoir bag. Dispose of damaged circuits or clean if necessary. Individual parts of systems can often be replaced without the need to replace the whole circuit.
2. Check that the components of the system are in the correct location, e.g. the valve and reservoir bag.
3. Attach the gas inlet on the breathing system to the common gas outlet of the anaesthetic machine.
4. Close the valve or, in the case of the Jackson–Rees modified Ayres T-piece, occlude the neck of the bag where it enters the scavenging system.
5. Occlude the patient attachment end, either with your hand or hold it against your leg (whichever method it is important to create an airtight seal).
6. Fill the system with O$_2$ (or medical air if available). This can be done either by using the oxygen flush or by the flowmeters. Stop gas flow once the reservoir bag is distended.
7. Listen and feel for any leaks.
8. Open the valve and squeeze the contents out of the reservoir bag to check that the valve opens fully. It is important whilst doing this to keep the patient attachment occluded.

Additional checks should be carried out for **coaxial systems**, to confirm that there is no damage to the inner limb.

- **Bain:** With the O_2 flowmeter set at 4 litres and the valve closed, use a pen (or disposable Bain breathing systems come with a plastic tool of the correct diameter) to occlude the inner limb. Observe the bobbin within the flowmeter – it will dip if there are no leaks in the system. It should only be transiently occluded as it causes back pressure within the anaesthetic machine, which could be damaging
- **Lack:** With the O_2 flowmeter set at 4 litres and the valve closed, use a pen (or disposable Lacks come with a plastic tool of the correct diameter) to occlude the inner limb. Observe the reservoir bag filling and becoming distended.

Anaesthetic machines and circuits for use with horses

In a theatre situation, where the duration of anaesthesia is likely to be prolonged compared to field techniques, the facility to provide oxygen support via an anaesthetic machine is vital. Dedicated large animal anaesthetic machines and circle breathing systems are used to deliver O_2 and anaesthetic gases to horses. The principles of using the circle system are similar to those for small animals but it must be remembered that, due to the larger body size and circuit volume, it can take longer to bring about changes in depth of anaesthesia in the horse unless higher flow rates are implemented. The use of a ventilator can facilitate this.

Scavenging systems

The scavenging of waste anaesthetic gases is controlled by the Control of Substances Hazardous to Health (COSHH) regulations (see Chapter 2). There are two types of scavenging system: active and passive.

Active scavenging

Active scavenging is the preferred technique for removing waste gases as it is the most reliable. It uses an extractor fan to create negative air pressure within the room. Ideally this should be used in combination with a pressure break such as a Barnsley receiver (Figure 23.64) to prevent excessive negative pressure from being exerted on the patient.

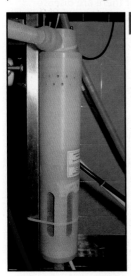

23.64 A Barnsley receiver.

Passive scavenging

Passive scavenging relies on gases moving either into a system containing activated charcoal or into a tube going outside the building; the latter is not really acceptable. Activated charcoal canisters should be weighed regularly to detect when the charcoal is exhausted, following the manufacturer's guidelines. The scavenging tubing should not be too long (ideally no longer than 1.5 m) and it is important that no resistance is created in the tube, e.g. through kinking. Activated charcoal does not absorb N_2O and so should not be used as the scavenging method for this gas.

Other ways of limiting environmental pollution

Along with ensuring that scavenging systems are adequate, other methods are used to decrease environmental contamination by waste anaesthetic gases. These include:

- Checking anaesthetic machines and breathing systems before every use
- Connecting the breathing system to the ET tube and inflating the cuff before switching on the volatile agent or N_2O
- Regularly checking for leaks around the ET tube cuff during anaesthesia
- Maintaining the animal on 100% O_2 for a couple of minutes once the volatile agent has been turned off, to flush anaesthetic gases out of the circuit via the scavenging system. The reservoir bag is disconnected and emptied several times
- Using a rebreathing system wherever possible, to minimize fresh gas flow rates
- Refilling vaporizers at the end of the day using key-fillers (see above). This should not be carried out by the same person every day, but on a rotational basis so as to minimize the individual exposure of staff
- Ensuring that recovery areas are well ventilated, as patients continue to breathe out inhalant agent during the recovery period
- Ensuring regular maintenance of anaesthetic machines
- Monitoring the concentration of inhalant agent in the environment regularly
- Only using inhalational techniques for induction of anaesthesia when absolutely necessary.

Environmental monitoring

Monitoring environmental contamination should be carried out routinely, e.g. every 6 months, using individual dosemeters worn by staff during a normal working day. These are widely available commercially.

Ventilation

The ability to provide patient ventilation manually, through the use of intermittent positive pressure ventilation (IPPV), is an important skill and one that all veterinary nurses should have. The basic technique is given below.

In order to perform IPPV optimally, capnography should ideally be used as it can help to tailor IPPV to the particular patient. For example, a steadily reducing $ETCO_2$ indicates over-ventilation (hyperventilation), due to provision of either a higher respiratory rate than necessary or a larger tidal volume, or both. Conversely, a steadily increasing $ETCO_2$ indicates under-ventilation (hypoventilation) through the provision of an inadequate respiratory rate or tidal volume.

A pulse oximeter is also an important piece of equipment, used to ensure that the IPPV is adequate to maintain the patient's oxygen levels.

IPPV technique

1. Close the valve (or occlude the neck of the reservoir bag as it enters the scavenging system if using an Ayre's T-piece with a Jackson–Rees modification).
2. Squeeze the reservoir bag while watching the patient's chest, to create a normal expansion.
3. Open the valve or stop occluding the reservoir bag.
4. Aim for a 1:2 ratio of inspiration to expiration to minimize the cardiovascular effects of IPPV.

WARNING

If a patient requires prolonged IPPV, this should be performed by a dedicated nurse rather than by the person monitoring the anaesthetic, as it is not possible to concentrate and perform both tasks adequately at the same time.

- The T-piece, Bain, circle and to–and-fro circuits are all suitable for prolonged IPPV with no change in fresh gas flow rate.
- The Lack and Magill can be used for short periods of IPPV but if prolonged IPPV is necessary the fresh gas flow rate should be increased to prevent rebreathing or, ideally, another breathing system should be used.

When to ventilate

The correct time to ventilate is ultimately the veterinary surgeon's decision but it is very important for nurses to be aware of the situations when a patient should receive manual IPPV or be placed on to a mechanical ventilator.

Indications for IPPV include:

- When the patient is unable to breathe adequately and spontaneously and to maintain normal CO_2 and O_2 concentrations in the blood, e.g. due to body position for surgery or obesity
- Thoracic surgery (including diaphragmatic rupture) that will impair normal respiratory function
- Pneumothorax
- Administration of an NMBA that will prevent spontaneous respiration
- During use of potent opioids that may cause apnoea
- Spinal cord damage or oedema that hinders respiratory drive or effort
- Diseases affecting respiratory muscle function, e.g. myasthenia gravis, phrenic nerve paralysis, botulism or tetanus
- Raised intracranial pressure (due to trauma or other disease processes). Prevention of hypercapnia is important to prevent a further rise in intracranial pressure
- Severe hypothermia.

Mechanical ventilators

Ventilators are becoming increasingly common in veterinary practice and there are a number of different models available. For the purposes of this chapter, only the basic principles will be explained. Any patient that requires manual IPPV will benefit from being placed on a mechanical ventilator designed for the size of patient. The advantages and disadvantages of using mechanical ventilators are listed in Figure 23.65.

Advantages
• Provide control over respiratory rate and volume
• Constant and regular rhythm help maintain a steady plane of anaesthesia
• No requirement for personnel to provide manual IPPV, allowing them to concentrate on monitoring the patient
• Special features may be used, i.e. PEEP

Disadvantages
• Reduced venous return (especially if there is a long inspiratory time and high airway pressures)
• High airway pressures may cause bradycardia
• Mechanical failure or faults may occur
• May cause harm to the patient if used incorrectly
• Expensive to purchase and require regular servicing to ensure safety

23.65 Advantages and disadvantages of using mechanical ventilators.

It is recommended that the ventilator parameters are pre-set prior to anaesthesia for cases that are likely to require IPPV in order to expedite a rapid transition to IPPV in an emergency. To test that the parameters are correct, a reservoir bag can be placed where the patient will be attached to the breathing system to act as an artificial lung.

Setting up a ventilator

Important principles to consider when setting up a mechanical ventilator include:

1. Estimate the tidal volume (TV) that the patient will require. For the purposes of setting up a ventilator the TV should always be set on the low end of what is expected for the patient (i.e. 10 ml/kg), as it is safer to increase TV to obtain optimal ventilation than to over-ventilate the patient initially. TV should be reduced if the patient is obese, because obesity decreases lung volume relative to bodyweight due to reduced compliance. This is also the case if there are disease processes present that may affect lung volume, e.g. a lung tumour. Some ventilators do not have a safety feature preventing over-ventilation (pressure cut off); therefore, setting the correct TV is vital.
2. Check that the ventilator and attachments on the ventilator are suitable for the size of the patient (e.g. correct size of bellows).
3. If there is a maximum pressure alarm/limit, set it appropriately. This should be a maximum of 15 cmH_2O for most patients.
4. Set the appropriate respiratory rate.
5. If possible set the inspiratory to expiratory ratio. This is the ratio of the time allowed for inspiration and expiration in one breath. Usually this is 1:2 or 1:3. Ensuring that the expiration phase of respiration is 2–3 times longer than the inspiration phase allows adequate time for venous return to the heart, reducing the impact of IPPV on the cardiovascular system.

Placing a patient on a ventilator

1. Ensure the scavenging system is connected correctly – this usually involves taking the scavenging tube off the breathing system and placing it on to an attachment on the ventilator.
2. Switch the ventilator on.
3. Check the pressure gauge to ensure that airway pressure is not excessively low or high. For most patients a pressure of 10–12 cmH$_2$O is appropriate.
4. Observe the patient's chest. Are there suitable chest movements? Change the tidal volume to gain the correct airway pressure and chest movement. Aim to create a breathing pattern that is as natural as possible.
5. Observe the capnogram if available.
6. If the patient is 'bucking' (breathing against) the ventilator, check depth of anaesthesia and increase the respiratory rate. Ventilation can be quite stimulating and the aim is to over-ride the patient's own respiratory drive. It is usually possible to achieve this by increasing the respiratory rate and ensuring an adequate depth of anaesthesia; however, it will sometimes be necessary for the veterinary surgeon to prescribe a drug to facilitate over-ride of spontaneous ventilation (e.g. a potent opioid such as fentanyl or a benzodiazepine such as midazolam).
7. Adjust the rate and volume of respiration in order to maintain optimal ETCO$_2$ (see Monitoring, below). The required rate will usually be around 14 breaths/min for cats and small dogs and 6–8 breaths/min for medium to large dogs. These are rough guidelines and it is important to remember that all patients are different.

Weaning a patient off a ventilator

1. Decrease the respiratory rate to increase ETCO$_2$.
2. If the ventilator has an assist mode or pressure trigger (the ventilator detects the patient taking a breath and completes a ventilator breath) switch to this mode first before switching the ventilator off.
3. Switch off the ventilator. If the patient does not start breathing spontaneously, provide occasional manual ventilation while closely observing the patient's O$_2$ saturation using a pulse oximeter.
4. Lighten the plane of anaesthesia.

Monitoring the anaesthetized patient

Monitoring during anaesthesia is one of the most common tasks performed by the veterinary nurse. If done well it can make a significant difference to case outcome; it may make the difference between an animal surviving anaesthesia or not. Anaesthesia has many negative effects on the body. Monitoring the patient effectively and providing appropriate support allows these negative effects to be minimized, reducing the risk of organ and tissue damage.

Anaesthetic records

Anaesthetic records, such as that shown in Figure 23.66, are legal documents and must give a true account of what occurred throughout the anaesthetic period. However, it is important to remember that monitoring the patient is the most important task to be undertaken and the anaesthetist should not become focused on filling in the record rather than monitoring the patient. Use of an anaesthetic record facilitates the detection of trends that are difficult to see unless parameters are recorded. The recommended format of an anaesthetic record card is graphical, to allow trends to be seen easily and problems to be identified promptly. The patient should be monitored continuously and each parameter recorded approximately every 5–10 minutes, depending on how stable the animal is under anaesthesia. There are many different anaesthetic record designs and choosing or designing a record card can be challenging.

Ideally, the following information should be included on an anaesthetic record:

- Date
- Patient name and case number
- Patient species, breed, age, sex, bodyweight
- History of previous anaesthesia
- Details of clinical examination and any problems or concerns
- American Society of Anesthesiologists (ASA) classification
- Drugs used for premedication, along with time, route of administration and effect
- Site of intravenous catheter placement
- Fluids given and the rate and total volume administered
- Estimation of blood loss
- Breathing system
- ET tube size
- Posture
- Monitors to be used
- Inhalational agent to be used.

Within the graphical section, the following should be included:

- Time of all drug administration and doses given (in mg not ml)
- Heart rate
- Respiration rate
- Other monitoring information, e.g. S_pO_2 (blood oxygen saturation), blood pressure, temperature, ETCO$_2$ (end tidal carbon dioxide)
- End tidal inhalational agent concentration or dialled vaporizer setting
- Fresh gas flow rate of the individual gases used.

There must be enough space available to record:

- Extra information, such as the time the patient is moved to theatre and the start of surgery
- Time of disconnection from the anaesthetic machine
- Time of extubation
- Immediate postoperative temperature, pulse and respiration
- Time that the patient lifts its head, moves into sternal recumbency and stands
- Quality of recovery
- General comments about the anaesthetic and the patient.

Anaesthetic Record-Langford Veterinary Services Ltd

Date: _____ Anaes.: _____ Case No: _____
Theatre: _____ Surg: _____ Species: _____
_____ WT: _____ Breed: _____
Diagnosis: _____ Age: _____
Procedure: _____ Sex: _____

PRE-OPERATIVE DETAILS:		E	GENERAL RISK
PREVIOUS ANAESTHETIC HISTORY:		G	
GENERAL PHYSIQUE:			
CLINICAL DATA T _____ P _____ R ____ Hb. _____ P.C.V. _____		F	
C.V.S.: ORDER:		P	
RESP. S:			
URINARY S.:		VP	

PREMEDICATION					E.C.G.
DRUGS: DOSE: ROUTE: TIME: EFFECT:					Catheter
1. ____ ____ ____ ____ ____					BP
2. ____ ____ ____ ____ ____					Other

TIME		DRUGS GIVEN	TOTAL DOSE	IV Fluids
1		1.		Blood –
2		2.		Colloids –
3		3.		Hartmann's –
4		4.		Naci/Dexi –
5		5.		TOTAL –
6		% AGENT		
O₂/N₂O L/min		Maintenance Flow	VT	Est Blood Loss

TUBE _____ MASK _____
SIZE
CIRCUIT _____
POSTURE _____ IPPV
NOTES:

(graph axis markings: 200, 180, 160, 140, 120, 100, 80, 60, 40, 20, 10, 8, 6, 4, 2)

Resp:- O
MAINTENANCE
CODE: Anaes:- Op.:- Ø B.P.:- > < Pulse:- •

| Disconnect |
| Head |
| Brisket |
| Stand |
| Quality |

TIME OF NOTES

POST OP. RECOVERY: T.   P.   R.

23.66 An example of an anaesthesia monitoring chart. (Courtesy of Langford Veterinary Services Ltd)

Anaesthetic records are not only important at the time of the anaesthetic but also afterwards. They can be vital for management of subsequent anaesthesia in the same patient and provide a source of information for both the veterinary surgeon and veterinary nurse to reflect upon in order to improve future case management (not only for that patient but others).

Key times to monitor anaesthesia

The anaesthetic procedure should be monitored throughout; however, there are some key times where monitoring is particularly important.

Premedication

Monitoring during premedication is discussed earlier in the chapter.

Induction

Induction of anaesthesia is a high-risk period. While anaesthesia is being induced the nurse should observe the patient's **breathing pattern** and **mucous membrane colour**. If intubation is prolonged the patient will benefit from provision of supplemental oxygen, delivered either by having a break in the attempt to intubate the patient and using a facemask, or by simple flow-by (holding the patient attachment of the breathing system close to the patient's nose).

Once the patient is intubated and the tube has been secured, the patient's **pulse** should be palpated immediately. Intubation can cause arrhythmias that can result in cardiac arrest (although this is extremely rare) and administration of drugs for induction of anaesthesia can cause marked changes in heart rate. It is also important to check that there are no problems before the introduction of an inhalational agent, i.e. excessive depth of anaesthesia following induction.

Maintenance

It is important to maintain the anaesthesia at an appropriate depth in order to avoid side effects associated with excessively high concentrations of anaesthetic. Although there are many different anaesthetic monitors available, the anaesthetist is the most important monitor and the most reliable. Selection of which parameters are monitored, and use of invasive monitoring techniques such as direct arterial blood pressure measurement, depends on the individual patient and procedure. Minimal monitoring in all patients should include pulse rate, respiratory rate and body temperature. Pulse oximetry is also starting to be considered part of a minimal monitoring protocol.

Monitoring the respiratory system

The rate, depth and characteristics of respiration should all be monitored. Further information on respiratory monitoring is given in the section on capnography.

A respiratory rate *higher* than expected is described as **tachypnoea** and may be indicative of:

- Inadequate depth of anaesthesia
- Noxious stimulation due to inadequate analgesia
- One lung intubation due to an excessively long ET tube
- Hypercapnia
- Use of an incorrect breathing system for that patient
- Low tidal volume.

A respiratory rate that is *lower* than expected is termed **bradypnoea** and may be indicative of:

- An excessive depth of anaesthesia
- Response to drug administration.

Apnoea – when the patient *stops* breathing – may be caused by:

- An excessive depth of anaesthesia
- Drugs (e.g. potent opioids)
- Inadequate depth of anaesthesia (breath holding)
- Impending cardiac arrest.

Whilst counting the breathing rate, the characteristics of the breaths should also be observed:

- If the patient has a slow respiratory rate but a large tidal volume (e.g. characteristic of a patient that has received an alpha-2 agonist and an opioid), this is likely to be adequate
- If the patient has a slow respiratory rate and a small tidal volume this is likely to result in hypercapnia and a reduction in O_2 saturation. This type of breathing is described as **hypoventilation**
- If the patient is breathing rapidly with a normal tidal volume, this is described as **hyperventilation** and will result in hypocapnia (a reduction in $ETCO_2$).

It is also important to take account of the amount of respiratory effort. If the patient is having difficulty in breathing this is described as **dyspnoea** and is often characterized by a large abdominal component to the respiratory effort. The size of the thoracic movement should also be compared to the volume of gas movement within the reservoir bag. **Dyspnoea represents an emergency and the veterinary surgeon should be informed immediately.**

Causes of dyspnoea during anaesthesia include:

- A problem with the breathing system, e.g. a sticking unidirectional valve on a circle circuit
- A problem with an ET tube, e.g. a very small tube for the size of patient, a plug of secretion, the bevel of the tube resting against the wall of the trachea, or a kink in the tube
- A concurrent problem, e.g. a pneumothorax.

If the patient appears to be breathing normally but there is no movement of the reservoir bag this could indicate:

- Oesophageal intubation. This can be confirmed with the use of a capnograph: if the oesophagus has been intubated no CO_2 will be detected
- Disconnection of the breathing system
- A fault in the breathing system.

Monitoring the cardiovascular system

Heart rate

Heart rate can be measured by auscultation using either a conventional stethoscope or oesophageal stethoscope and/or by palpation of the apex beat on the left-hand side of the patient's thorax.

A heart rate *higher* than expected is described as **tachycardia** and may indicate:

- Inadequate depth of anaesthesia
- Inadequate analgesia
- Result from drug administration, e.g. ketamine
- Presence of arrhythmias (abnormal heart rhythm on ECG)
- Hypercapnia
- Hypoxaemia
- Hypotension caused by shock and sepsis
- Concurrent disease, e.g. hyperthyroidism (these patients are normally tachycardic before anaesthesia).

A heart rate *lower* than expected is described as **bradycardia** and may indicate:

- Excessive depth of anaesthesia
- Result from drug administration, e.g. alpha-2 agonists and opioids
- Hypothermia
- Hypertension
- Vagal stimulation (stimulation of the vagal nerve caused by pressure or stimulation of the nerve during surgery). This is common during enucleation of the eye due to pressure on the eyeball, or during surgical dissection of the neck. If bradycardia occurs, the surgeon should be notified immediately so that they can stop what they are doing; this will normally lead to a rapid correction of the bradycardia. Administration of an anticholinergic (e.g. atropine) may be required to prevent recurrence of the bradycardia as surgery continues
- Hyperkalaemia (high levels of blood potassium)
- Severe acidosis (low blood pH)
- Severe hypoglycaemia (low blood glucose)
- Severe hypoxia.

Pulse

Pulse palpation (see also Chapter 15) provides information about the adequacy of cardiac output and the circulation. The most useful information is obtained from peripheral pulses, but if these are not palpable central pulses can be used. In this case, the underlying reason for a failure to palpate a peripheral pulse should be rapidly investigated.

Common sites of peripheral pulse palpation in anaesthetized dogs and cats include:

- **Metacarpal artery**: Palmar aspect of the forelimb, lateral to the dew claw

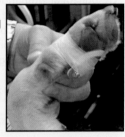

- **Dorsal pedal artery**: Medial aspect of the metatarsus

- **Lingual artery**: Midline on the ventral aspect of the tongue

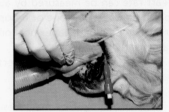

- **Labial artery**: Inside the upper lip, just behind the level of the canine tooth (the authors find this pulse particularly useful)

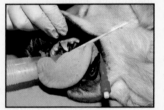

- **Coccygeal artery**: Ventral aspect of the base of the tail
- **Auricular artery**: Central ear pinna.

The femoral artery can be palpated but is a *central* pulse and provides less information than palpation of a *peripheral* pulse because peripheral pulse quality will be modified first as a result of hypotension or poor peripheral perfusion. It is often necessary to palpate the femoral artery, however, following administration of an alpha-2 agonist, due to peripheral vasoconstriction.

Common sites of peripheral pulse palpation in anaesthetized horses include:

- Transverse facial artery
- Facial artery
- Metatarsal artery
- Digital artery
- Coccygeal artery
- Auricular artery.

When palpating the pulse it is important to rest the fingers gently over the pulse point, palpate it and then apply pressure to see how easy it is to occlude. This process is important, as when the pulse is simply palpated, only the difference between systolic and diastolic blood pressure (pulse pressure) is felt. Seeing how easy it is to occlude the pulse provides information about vascular tone and mean arterial blood pressure. A hypotensive patient can have a pulse that is easily palpated but when pressure is applied it can be easily occluded.

It is also important to auscultate the heart and palpate pulses *at the same time*. If there is not a pulse for every heart sound this is referred to as a **pulse deficit**. The veterinary surgeon should be told immediately and an ECG obtained as the deficit is likely to indicate a cardiac arrhythmia (see later). The pulse should also be regular; an irregular pulse can indicate an arrhythmia. A commonly seen benign arrhythmia is **sinus arrhythmia**, characterized by an *increase* in heart rate on *inspiration* and *decrease* in heart rate on *expiration*. This is especially seen in fit dogs.

Mucous membrane colour and capillary refill time

Mucous membrane colour and capillary refill time (CRT) provide limited information about peripheral perfusion. Normal mucous membranes are described as salmon pink; when blanched (pressure applied), their normal colour returns within 2 seconds (see Chapter 15). Abnormal mucous membrane colours and their causes are shown in Figure 23.67. A prolonged CRT can indicate hypoperfusion, caused by hypovolaemia, hypotension, shock, hypothermia, cardiac failure/depression and vasodilation.

Colour	Possible causes
Pale pink	Vasoconstriction due to: surgical stimulation, e.g. surgeon pulling on a bitch's ovaries; lack of analgesia; haemorrhage or anaemia; drug administration, e.g. alpha-2 agonists; hypoperfusion
Red	Vasodilation, local congestion
Brick red	Severe vasodilation, sepsis, hypercapnia
Blue (cyanosis)	Hypoxia (NB An anaemic patient can be hypoxaemic without the presence of cyanosis due to the reduced oxygen-carrying capacity of the blood)

23.67 Mucous membrane colours during anaesthesia and their clinical interpretation.

Blood loss

Although the surgeon should also be monitoring the amount of blood lost by the patient, the anaesthetist is in the perfect position to monitor the volume of blood loss and provide the patient with necessary intravenous fluid support. Clinically significant blood loss will cause the following signs:

- Tachycardia
- Weak, rapid pulse (often described as thready)
- Hypotension (if using a blood pressure monitor)
- Prolonged CRT
- Pale mucous membranes.

Information on blood loss should be relayed to the veterinary surgeon and the appropriate action taken as prescribed by the veterinary surgeon. Generally blood loss <10% of circulating blood volume is well tolerated by healthy patients.

Estimating blood loss

1. Collect all used swabs.
2. Count them.
3. Weigh them.
4. Weigh the same number of dry new swabs (if only a couple of swabs have been used weigh 10 swabs and then divide the weight by 10 and multiply by the number used).
5. Subtract the weight of the dry new swabs from the weight of the used, bloody swabs.
6. Calculate the weight of blood contained in the swabs, assuming 1 g equates to 1 ml of fluid/blood.
7. Measure any blood in suction containers and estimate the blood on the floor, drapes and surgeon.
8. Establish the volume of any saline or other fluids used by the surgeon.
9. Add together the volume of blood loss calculated from the swabs, suction, etc., and subtract the volume of any other fluids used by the surgeon to establish the total volume of blood lost.
10. Estimate the patient's blood volume (88 ml × bodyweight (kg))
11. Divide the estimated blood volume by 100 and multiply by the estimated blood loss (ml).
12. This equates to % blood loss compared to the total blood volume of the patient.

Monitoring depth of anaesthesia

Cranial nerve and other reflexes provide information about CNS function and can be used to assess depth of anaesthesia. The *deeper* the plane of anaesthesia, the *greater* the depression of the central nervous system. Other information that should be included in the assessment of anaesthetic depth includes heart rate, respiratory rate and blood pressure.

Cranial reflexes commonly used to assess depth of anaesthesia

- **Palpebral reflex**: Assessed by brushing or lightly touching the medial canthus of the eye or the eyelashes. Brisk or spontaneous movement or blinking indicates a light plane of anaesthesia. As anaesthesia deepens, the palpebral reflex becomes more sluggish and is eventually abolished. A surgical plane of anaesthesia does not require the palpebral reflex to be abolished.
- **Eye position**: If possible, both eyes should be observed as they can be in different positions. A surgical plane of anaesthesia is usually indicated by the eye being in a ventromedial position with mainly the sclera visible. As depth of anaesthesia continues to increase the eye becomes central again. The use of ketamine can interfere with this pattern: the eye remains central regardless of anaesthetic depth.
- **Pupillary diameter:** With increasing depth of anaesthesia the pupil becomes more dilated.
- **Jaw tone:** Jaw tone becomes looser as depth of anaesthesia increases. This is difficult to assess in some breeds of dogs that have a very muscular jaw, e.g. English Bull Terrier. It is important to use a good

technique to allow sensitive analysis of this parameter and ensure the safety of the anaesthetist.
- **Pedal reflex:** This is assessed by application of a firm pinch between the patient's toes and observation of a withdrawal response. As depth of anaesthesia increases, the response will reduce until it is abolished.

Other cranial nerve reflexes can be used to indicate depth of anaesthesia; however, they tend to be seen at either inadequate or excessive depth of anaesthesia, thus limiting their routine use:

- **Corneal reflex:** Assessed using a damp cotton-wool bud to touch the cornea gently; the patient should blink in response. **This reflex should never be abolished as its absence is an indication of an anaesthetic overdose.**
- **Tongue curl:** When a patient is very lightly anaesthetized the tongue will curl when the jaw is opened.
- **Lacrimation:** This will reduce as the patient becomes more deeply anaesthetized.
- **Salivation:** Excessive salivation may occur with inadequate anaesthesia.

Monitoring depth of anaesthesia in horses

Depth of anaesthesia in horses is assessed using a combination of eye position, depression of reflexes, lack of movement, degree of anal tone, physiological parameters (heart rate, respiratory rate and blood pressure) and concentrations of inhalant agent measured in breathed gases.

Eye position

The eye may rotate ventrally and medially during the early stages of anaesthesia but returns to the centre of the globe as the level of anaesthesia deepens.

- **Nystagmus:** Lateral nystagmus is frequently observed during light anaesthesia but disappears as anaesthesia deepens.
- **Palpebral reflex:** Elicited by gently stroking the eyelashes along the upper and lower eyelids. The palpebral response is progressively depressed as anaesthesia deepens. It is generally present, but slow and sluggish, at surgical levels of anaesthesia.
- **Corneal reflex:** Closure of the eyelids in response to gentle pressure applied to the cornea. The corneal reflex should always be present during anaesthesia; absence indicates excessive anaesthetic induced depression of the CNS.
- **Lacrimation:** Common during light anaesthesia, reduced or absent at a surgical plane of anaesthesia.

Repeated stimulation of eye reflexes during a long anaesthesia may result in reflex depression. Usefulness of eye reflexes is also limited following the administration of ketamine or tiletamine. Characteristic effects of these cyclohexamine anaesthetics on the equine eye include:

- Blink response not abolished
- Lateral nystagmus
- Central eye position
- Lacrimation.

Anal tone

Touching the anus should cause contraction of the anal sphincter. Absence of anal tone indicates that anaesthesia is too deep. This is a crude method but may be useful when access to the patient's head is limited.

Physiological parameters

Heart and respiratory rate tend to remain remarkably stable in horses, despite sudden decreases in depth of anaesthesia, limiting their usefulness as a warning of impending inadequate anaesthesia or movement. Clinical experience suggests that sudden increases in arterial blood pressure commonly indicate a decrease in anaesthetic depth.

Monitoring depth of anaesthesia in exotic pets

Rabbits

Monitoring depth of anaesthesia in rabbits is very similar to the practice in cats and dogs, although the palpebral reflex is an unreliable guide. Absence of the corneal reflex is always a sign that depth of anaesthesia is excessive and should be lightened immediately. The hindlimb withdrawal reflex can be helpful; absence of a withdrawal reflex usually indicates a depth of anaesthesia suitable for surgery. Changes in respiratory and heart rate with depth of anaesthesia are similar to those in dogs and cats.

Rodents

Slowing of the respiratory rate can easily be assessed visually and will occur as anaesthesia deepens. Palpebral and corneal reflexes are difficult to assess in small rodents. As depth of anaesthesia increases following induction of anaesthesia there is loss of the righting reflex and of spontaneous movement. Presence or absence of a pedal withdrawal reflex to toe pinching is useful during the maintenance phase; at an anaesthetic depth suitable for surgery the pedal withdrawal reflex is abolished.

Birds

Monitoring depth of anaesthesia involves evaluation of muscle tone and various reflexes, including palpebral, corneal and pedal reflexes. At a depth of anaesthesia adequate for surgery, corneal and pedal reflexes will be present but very slow; the palpebral reflex will be absent. Changes in respiratory and heart rate with depth of anaesthesia are similar to those in dogs and cats.

Reptiles

Reptiles relax during anaesthesia from cranial to caudal; motor function returns in the opposite direction during recovery. The righting reflex is lost at light planes of surgical anaesthesia and is useful for monitoring during recovery. The palpebral reflex is generally lost at light planes of anaesthesia, but the corneal reflex persists; loss of the corneal reflex usually indicates excessive anaesthetic depth. At a surgical plane of anaesthesia the toe pinch or tail pinch withdrawal reflex should be abolished.

Monitoring body temperature

Anaesthesia inhibits the ability of the patient to thermoregulate. Hypothermia is a major concern with any anaesthetized patient, especially those with the following:

- A high surface area to bodyweight ratio (small patients)
- Very little body fat
- A thin coat
- A large area of fur clipped
- A large amount of internal tissues exposed, e.g. during laparotomy.

Hypothermia causes the following physiological changes:

- Reduction in metabolic rate leading to a decreased anaesthetic requirement and increased risk of anaesthetic overdose and a more prolonged recovery from anaesthesia
- Bradycardia with a potential reduction in cardiac output
- Increased risk of cardiac arrhythmias
- Increased blood loss during surgery due to impaired blood clotting mechanisms
- Shivering during recovery, increasing oxygen requirement
- Increased morbidity rate.

Normal body temperature ranges can be found in Chapter 15. To avoid hypothermia, body temperature should be monitored routinely throughout anaesthesia. This can be achieved using a conventional rectal thermometer. A more convenient method is to use a temperature probe that can be placed rectally, nasally or in the oesophagus (the most easy and convenient location). It also has the advantage of being continuous rather than intermittent, unlike manual measurement of rectal temperature using a conventional thermometer.

Preventing hypothermia

Heat loss from the patient can be minimized by:

- Reducing the preparation and surgery time
- Minimizing how wet the patient becomes during preparation of the surgical site
- Maintaining a high ambient temperature around the patient
- Use of heat and moisture exchangers
- Use of appropriate flow rates when using non-rebreathing systems
- Use of rebreathing systems when possible
- Providing the surgeon with warmed fluids to use during surgery, e.g. soaking swabs and lavage.

Methods for warming patients during anaesthesia

- **Electric heat mats:** These can be placed beneath the patient both perioperatively and postoperatively. They should not be left unattended with conscious patients due to the risk of the patient biting the mat and being electrocuted. The use of thermostatically controlled mats is recommended.
- **Hot hands:** These are examination gloves filled with hot water. Care should be taken when using these because of the risk of their bursting and getting the patient wet, accentuating any hypothermia, or causing scalding if the water is very hot. They also cool down very quickly and need to be replaced regularly; otherwise they will cool the patient.
- **Hot air blankets:** These are very safe to use. They

continues ▶

continued

work by blowing hot air into a disposable blanket that is placed around, under or on top of the patient. Eye lubrication is important to prevent the hot air from drying the cornea and causing a corneal ulcer.

- **Microwaveable warming aids:** It is particularly easy to overheat these, leading to thermal burns.

It is important to remember that an anaesthetized patient cannot move away from a heat source; measures must therefore be taken to ensure that the patient is not injured.

In adult horses, body temperature is not commonly monitored due to the reduced likelihood of hypothermia in large animals. A long duration of anaesthesia can predispose adult horses to hypothermia, however, and this should not be forgotten. Foals are at risk of hypothermia in a similar way to small animals.

Many exotic pet species are particularly prone to hypothermia due to their large body surface area to volume ratio. The principles of preventing hypothermia in small mammals and birds are similar to those for cats and dogs. Reptiles are exothermic and derive nearly all their body heat from the external environment. Most reptiles have a preferred body temperature (PBT) range that is associated with optimal metabolic function. During anaesthesia, reptiles should be maintained at a body temperature that is at the upper end of the PBT for that species.

Aids to patient monitoring

Monitors are becoming more common in modern veterinary practice, so it is vital for nurses to be able to use and interpret the information that they provide. It is not appropriate for every monitoring aid to be used on every patient; a cost/benefit analysis should be completed, particularly when using invasive monitoring techniques.

> **WARNING**
>
> The purpose of monitoring aids is to provide *additional* information about the physiological status of the patient. They should not replace the basic hands-on monitoring described above. **Monitors can, and do, go wrong.**

Cardiovascular system monitoring

Pulse oximetry

Pulse oximeters are probably the most commonly used monitors in veterinary anaesthesia. They provide a non-invasive method of measuring the percentage of oxygen bound to haemoglobin within arterial blood. It is important to monitor oxygenation saturation as this will detect tissue hypoxia, which is a common endpoint for many physiological disturbances (see later).

Pulse oximeters have a probe that emits red and infrared light at different wavelengths combined with a photodetector. Haemoglobin absorbs different wavelengths of the red and infrared light, depending on whether it is bound to oxygen. The amount of red and infrared light absorbed at each wavelength is measured by the photodetector and expressed by the pulse oximeter as a percentage of saturated haemoglobin (S_pO_2). This process only takes place for pulsatile blood flow, so only arterial blood is analysed. Pulse oximeters are

usually placed on the tongue (Figure 23.68) but can also be placed on other areas of non-pigmented skin, e.g. prepuce, vulva, between toes, ear pinnae; these are particularly useful if the tongue is not available as a placement site. Some probes cause trauma due to the strength of the spring that closes them. Damage can be avoided by moving the site of the probe frequently. A size of probe should be chosen that is appropriate to the size of the patient and to the area to which the probe will be attached.

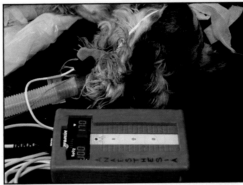

23.68 Pulse oximeter with the probe placed on the tongue.

All patients should have S_pO_2 >90%, as the amount of oxygen contained within arterial blood dramatically decreases when saturation falls below this value. The aim during anaesthesia should be to maintain S_pO_2 above 95%, to allow a safety margin. If N_2O is being used and S_pO_2 drops below 95% use of N_2O should be terminated and the reason for the reduction in O_2 saturation investigated.

Pulse oximeters often give anomalous results, however, so if S_pO_2 drops it is also important to look at the patient for signs of cyanosis to confirm the reading. Once checked, the probe should be repositioned. If persistently low readings are obtained the veterinary surgeon should be notified and IPPV performed until the cause is established. Anomalous results can be caused by:

- The probe squashing the tissue and preventing pulsatile blood flow
- Abnormal haemoglobin, i.e. carboxyhaemoglobin or methaemoglobin
- Intravenous dyes
- Patient movement (shivering)
- Vasoconstriction, e.g. when using alpha-2 agonists (this is a very common problem)
- Interference from ambient light
- Skin pigmentation
- Electrosurgical equipment, e.g. diathermy.

Pulse oximeters usually display a pulse rate; the accuracy of this should always be confirmed by pulse palpation. Some oximeters also provide photoplethysmography; the presence of a normal waveform helps to confirm that the reading is correct. The waveform should look like a direct blood pressure trace, as shown in Figure 23.69.

Pulse oximeters are reasonably reliable when used in horses, although the probe must be large enough to be placed on either side of the thick tongue and probes used for small animals are, therefore, usually inappropriate.

It is important to remember that some pulse oximeters are not effective at detecting the high heart rates that occur in rabbits, small rodents and birds, which also limits their

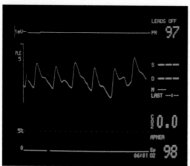

A normal plethysmograph trace from a pulse oximeter.

ability to measure haemoglobin saturation with oxygen. The specifications of pulse oximeters should be read carefully before they are purchased, to ensure that the model selected has the capability to provide accurate readings in a wide range of species.

Blood pressure measurement

Blood pressure measurement provides information about cardiovascular function and is an indirect measure of cardiac output and tissue blood flow.

Blood pressure = cardiac output x total peripheral resistance

It is important to avoid hypotension (mean blood pressure <60 mmHg) as it can have both short-term and long-term physiological effects (Figure 23.70).

Short-term effects
Accumulation of lactic acid, leading to metabolic acidosis Increased oxygen demand Increased glucose demand Increased cardiac work

Long-term effects
Ischaemic tissue damage, leading to organ damage (e.g. renal failure)

23.70 Short- and long-term effects of hypotension.

Blood pressure terminology

- **Systolic blood pressure** is the peak pressure within the arteries that occurs towards the end of the cardiac cycle, when the ventricles are contracting. It is determined by a combination of peripheral vascular resistance, stroke volume and intravascular volume. The normal range for cats, dogs and horses is 90–120 mmHg.
- **Diastolic blood pressure** is the minimum pressure within the arteries that occurs towards the beginning of the cardiac cycle. This is when the ventricles are filled with blood and is predominantly determined by the peripheral vascular resistance. The normal range for cats, dogs and horses is 55–90 mmHg.
- **Mean blood pressure** is the average arterial blood pressure during a cardiac cycle. This provides information about tissue perfusion. The normal range for cats, dogs and horses is 60–85 mmHg. It is important to maintain a mean blood pressure >60 mmHg to ensure adequate organ perfusion.

Two different techniques are used to measure arterial blood pressure: direct (**invasive**) (Figure 23.71) and indirect (**non-invasive**) (Figure 23.72). The relative advantages and disadvantages of direct and indirect blood pressure monitoring are listed in Figure 23.73. In cats and dogs, the decision to use a direct or indirect technique depends on the equipment available, the health status of the patient and the reason for anaesthesia. For indirect techniques, selection of cuff size is important. The cuff width should be approximately 40% of the circumference of the limb. A cuff that is too wide will artificially lower blood pressure; a cuff that is too narrow will artificially raise blood pressure.

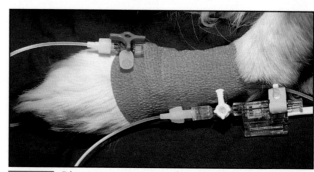

23.71 Direct measurement of arterial blood pressure. A catheter in the dorsal pedal artery of a dog is connected to an electronic transducer via non-compliant tubing.

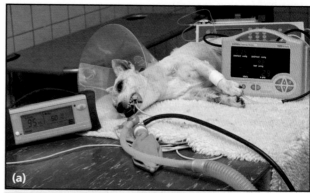

(a)

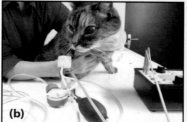

(b)

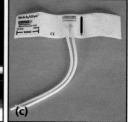

(c)

23.72 Indirect blood pressure measurement.
(a) Oscillometric measurement in an anaesthetized dog. The cuff is placed on the forelimb just proximal to the carpus and attached to the blood pressure machine via tubing. The dog is breathing anaesthetic gases via a Mapelson C circuit. A pulse oximeter probe is on its tongue and the monitor shows 95% haemoglobin saturation with oxygen. **(b)** Doppler technique in an awake cat. The Doppler probe is placed on the palmar aspect of the metacarpus and the cuff placed above the elbow. The sphygmomanometer measures the pressure in the cuff. **(c)** The width of the cuff for oscillometric and Doppler measurement should be 40% of the circumference of the limb at the site of cuff placement. This cuff is for use with an oscillometric machine. The bold black line across the width is placed over the artery.

Technique	Notes	Advantages	Disadvantages
Direct arterial blood pressure measurement (Figure 23.71)	Electronic transducer converts signal into waveform and blood pressure. Transducer must be placed at level of right atrium and zeroed relative to atmospheric air before use	Gold standard method; most accurate. Gives beat-to-beat assessment. Useful for assessing cardiovascular consequences of a cardiac arrhythmia	Technically demanding: requires placement of arterial catheter (most commonly in dorsal pedal artery). Failure to place catheter correctly can result in haematoma. Risk of sepsis or infection if not placed aseptically
Indirect arterial blood pressure measurement: Doppler technique (Figure 23.72b)	Cuff placed around distal limb or tail and manually inflated to occlude blood flow. Pressure in cuff released until blood flow can just be detected by Doppler probe over peripheral artery. This is systolic blood pressure, read from a pressure manometer that measures the pressure in the cuff	Non-invasive. More accurate than oscillometric technique in smaller patients. Can be useful for monitoring blood flow in other situations, e.g. during CPR	Less accurate than direct measurement. Does not give continuous reading. Must be measured manually. Most accurate measurement is systolic blood pressure; diastolic pressure not reliable
Indirect arterial blood pressure measurement: oscillometric technique (Figure 23.72a)	Uses same principle as Doppler technique but cuff is automatically inflated and deflated by the machine. Presence of pulsatile changes within cuff signals blood pressure	Non-invasive. Very simple to use. Automated and can be set to measure blood pressure every 3–5 min. Systolic, diastolic and mean blood pressure readings are measured or calculated	Less accurate than Doppler in small patients. Difficult to identify whether reading is accurate because process is automated

23.73 Advantages and disadvantages of direct and indirect blood pressure monitoring.

In horses, continuous measurement of arterial blood pressure using a direct technique (Figure 23.74) is considered mandatory in order to maintain a mean arterial pressure >60 mmHg.

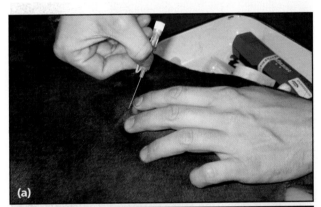

(a)

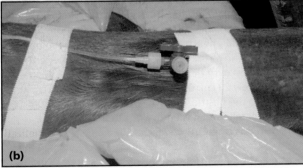

(b)

23.74 Direct blood pressure measurement in horses. **(a)** A 20G catheter being placed in the facial artery. The hair has been shaved over the artery and the site of placement cleaned gently with chlorhexidine and surgical spirit. The right hand of the anaesthetist is holding the catheter and the fingers of the left hand are palpating the artery to facilitate catheter placement. (Courtesy of Carolyne Sheridan) **(b)** Catheter placed in the metatarsal artery. The skin over the artery has been shaved and the catheter is secured tightly to the leg of the horse to prevent displacement.

Doppler ultrasonic probes can also be useful to provide an auditory monitor of heart rate and pulse quality in species where feeling pulse quality can be difficult, such as reptiles. The Doppler probe can be placed and secured over a peripheral artery or, for snakes, secured over the heart.

Electrocardiography

This is a non-invasive technique that provides information about the electrical activity of the heart (see also Chapter 20). It does not provide information about cardiac output (how well the heart is pumping) but does allow identification of arrhythmias and changes in heart electrical activity associated with other physiological abnormalities such as hypoxia, acid–base balance and electrolyte disturbances. The clinical significance of an arrhythmia can be assessed by concurrent pulse palpation or blood pressure measurement, in order to investigate the effect of the rhythm disturbance on cardiac output. A normal electrocardiogram (ECG) trace recorded during anaesthesia in a dog is shown in Figure 23.75.

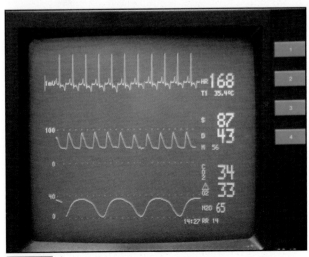

23.75 Monitor screen showing a normal ECG trace.

ECG monitoring during anaesthesia uses three electrodes, of which there are two types:

- Crocodile clips that are directly clipped to skin and then sprayed with surgical spirit
- Electrode pads that are stuck to the patient's paws.

Electrode connections in dogs and cats:
- Red: Right forelimb
- Yellow: Left forelimb
- Green: Left hindlimb.

Electrode connections in horses:
- Red: Right jugular groove
- Yellow: Apex of the left heart slightly above the left elbow
- Green: Ground electrode placed caudal to the heart (e.g. fold of skin on the flank).

Central venous pressure

Central venous pressure (CVP) measurement provides information about both the volume status of the patient and the ability of the right side of the heart to pump blood to the lungs. Monitoring of CVP is invasive, and placement of the jugular catheter requires skill. A long catheter is placed in the jugular vein so that its tip lies in the cranial vena cava (just past the level of the thoracic inlet). Several types of catheter are suitable, including Seldinger (Figure 23.76), peel-away and basic over-the-needle. If necessary, standard 20G or 18G catheters, as used for medium and large-breed dogs, can be used as jugular catheters in cats and small dogs. It is important that the site is prepared aseptically and the catheter placed using surgical gloves and a fenestrated drape.

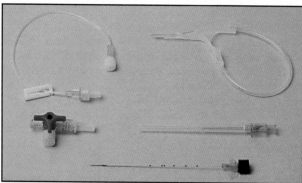

23.76 Central venous Seldinger catheter set, of suitable size for placement in a cat. The needle for jugular venous access has a green hub. The guidewire is at top right, coiled within the introducer device. The catheter, 3-way tap and extension set are also shown.

- The catheter should be measured up against the neck of the patient to ensure it is an appropriate length, with the tip extending just past the point of the thoracic inlet.
- A sandbag can be placed under the point of the shoulder or neck to aid visualization of the jugular vein and to help prevent development of an air embolus.
- Using a Seldinger technique, a needle is used to gain access to the jugular vein. Once the needle is successfully in the vein, a guidewire is placed through the needle to a suitable depth to allow the jugular catheter to be threaded over the guidewire to the correct depth. The tip of the jugular catheter should be placed at a depth to

ensure that it lies within the thoracic inlet. The proximal end of the guidewire is normally curved, with a J-tip, to prevent the sharp end of the wire from penetrating the wall of the jugular vein.

- Keeping the jugular catheter raised after placement until a bung has been inserted can reduce the risk of air embolus.
- The end of the catheter is attached either to a pressure transducer, which shows continuous readings, or to a water manometer or fluid column, which has to be read every few minutes. Measurement of CVP using a fluid column is relatively easy to perform using readily available equipment (Figure 23.77); this includes a bag of intravenous fluids (saline or Hartmann's solution), a giving set, a 3-way-tap, open-ended tubing and a ruler. Manometer kits containing these components can be purchased relatively cheaply.

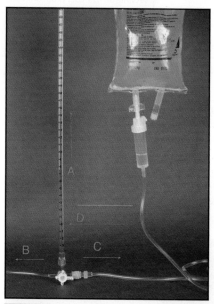

23.77 Measuring CVP using a fluid column. An open-ended section of drip line tubing is fixed in a straight vertical position (**A**). The red bobbin indicates the height of the water column above 0 cm (**D**, arrowed). A 3-way tap is connected to the bottom of the tubing and also to the jugular catheter (**B**) and bag of fluid (**C**). The open-ended drip line is then positioned so that D is level with the animal's heart; this can be achieved by taping the tube to the wall of the kennel. Before measurement, the tubing is filled with fluid from C to a height of approximately 20 cm, using the 3-way tap. The tap is then adjusted to the position shown. The height of the fluid column will fall until it is equivalent to the CVP of the animal. In this case CVP = +7.5 cmH$_2$0.

CVP can be measured in both awake and anaesthetized patients, although placement of a jugular catheter can be problematic in awake, unsedated animals. CVP measurement should be reserved for patients that will benefit:

- Patients that require aggressive fluid therapy – CVP can be used to guide fluid administration to maintain normovolaemia and ward off fluid overload
- Patients in which surgery is likely to cause marked blood loss and fluid replacement
- Patients with cardiovascular dysfunction that are at risk of fluid overload and pulmonary oedema.

The normal range for CVP in the cat and dog is 0–7 cmH$_2$O. If there is a sudden reduction in CVP this may indicate reduced cardiac output, reflecting decreased venous return to the right atrium. However, a low CVP is more usually indicative of reduced circulating blood volume due to hypovolaemia. A high CVP indicates either fluid overload or cardiac dysfunction.

Respiratory system monitoring

Capnography

Capnography involves the measurement of CO$_2$ concentration in inspired and expired gases and provides the anaesthetist with information about cardiovascular and respiratory function. To understand how this information is obtained it is important to understand the physiology of CO$_2$ transport in the body. Cells require oxygen and glucose for cell metabolism. These are delivered to cells by arterial blood and require adequate tissue perfusion. Cell metabolism uses the oxygen and glucose to create energy, forming CO$_2$ as a by-product. The CO$_2$ is transported from the peripheral tissues to the lungs by the venous circulation; this process requires adequate venous return. In the lungs, gaseous exchange takes place and the patient breathes out the CO$_2$; this process requires adequate ventilation.

End tidal CO$_2$ concentration (ETCO$_2$) is the peak concentration measured by the monitor during expiration. In a normal patient this should range between 35 and 45 mmHg (4.6–6 kPa or 5–6% depending on the units used by the monitor) (Figure 23.78a). Between breaths, CO$_2$ levels should be zero; however, this does not occur if the patient is rebreathing (see above).

If the patient has an ETCO$_2$ *greater* than the reference range it is described as being **hypercapnic.** This can indicate:

- Increased cardiac output and venous return
- Hypoventilation (Figure 23.78b)
- Increased metabolism (malignant hyperthermia or early sepsis)
- Rebreathing
- Laparoscopy due to absorption of CO$_2$ from the abdomen
- Exhausted CO$_2$ absorbent.

If the patient has an ETCO$_2$ *lower* than the reference range it is described as being **hypocapnic.** This can indicate:

- Decreased cardiac output and venous return
- Hyperventilation
- Severe hypothermia
- Rapidly reducing CO$_2$ indicates a failing circulation (impending cardiac arrest)
- Partial airway obstruction (Figure 23.78c).

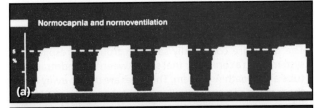

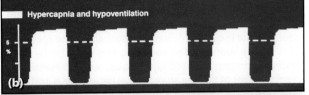

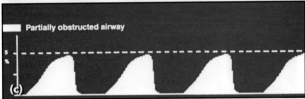

23.78 Capnograms; ETCO$_2$ is measured in %. **(a)** Normal. **(b)** Recorded from an animal with respiratory depression and hypoventilation: ETCO$_2$ is higher than normal. **(c)** Recorded from an animal with a partially obstructed airway. The rise in ETCO$_2$ is delayed due to airway obstruction.

Absence of CO$_2$ can indicate:

- Apnoea
- Disconnection from the breathing system, with the capnograph attachment being left attached to the breathing system
- Cardiac arrest.

Types of capnograph

Mainstream capnography

The measurement device is located in a small piece of tubing that connects between the endotracheal tube and the breathing system. This is ideal for measurement in small patients as the increase in deadspace is limited and gas sampling is not required. However, the probes are expensive and vulnerable to damage. They can also become contaminated during oral or head and neck surgery.

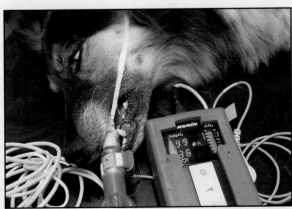

continues ▶

continued

Sidestream capnography

The gases are continually sampled from the respiratory system using a connector that sits between the endotracheal tube and breathing system. The gases are drawn away from the patient via a sample line, and taken to the analyser where measurement occurs. There is less risk of damage to the monitor because it is remote to the patient, but there is a time delay between gas sampling and read-out due to time required for gases to pass along the sampling line to the monitor. The sampling line can also become moist and contaminated with blood, which necessitates replacement of the line. In very small patients (e.g. rodents) the rate of gas sampling is not matched to the respiratory rate, and use in these patients is problematic.

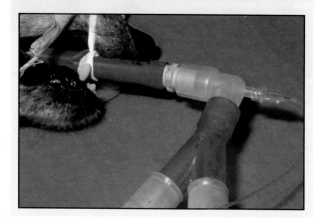

Capnographs also provide additional information about respiration, including:

- Respiration rate
- Apnoea
- Evaluation of respiratory depression
- Inspiratory or expiratory obstruction
- Breathing system leaks.

Airway gas analysers

Airway gas analysers are often found in combination with capnographs. They provide information about the concentrations of different gases in the inhaled and exhaled gas mixture, e.g. O_2 and N_2O concentrations, along with the inhalational agent that is being used. End tidal inhalant concentration, after a period of equilibration, is reflective of the concentration in the brain, and therefore can be useful in the assessment of depth of anaesthesia.

Other monitoring aids

Glucometers

Blood glucose can be monitored easily and cheaply using a hand-held glucometer (specific veterinary monitors are available). Perioperative use can be invaluable. Blood glucose should be routinely monitored in patients at risk of hypoglycaemia; this includes those <3 months old, with hepatic insufficiency or with diabetes mellitus (see later). These patients have a reduced ability to regulate their blood glucose when conscious, and anaesthesia exacerbates this further.

Urine output

Urine output is easily measured and provides important information about renal function. It can be measured either by manual expression of the bladder, so that urine produced can be collected and the volume measured, or by placement of a urinary catheter connected to a closed collection system (Figure 23.79), so that urine production can be assessed continually and non-invasively in the perioperative period. Urine output should be a minimum of 1–2 ml/kg/h.

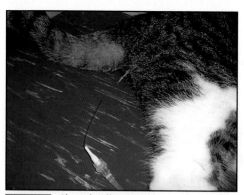

23.79 Closed collection system for monitoring urine output. The tube connects the urinary catheter to a syringe which is initially air-filled.

Electroencephalography

Electroencephalography is not routinely used in clinical practice. It measures the electrical activity of the brain and thus is an alternative method for evaluating depth of anaesthesia.

Blood gas analysis

A blood gas analyser is used to measure blood pH, partial pressure of oxygen (P_aO_2) and partial pressure of carbon dioxide (P_aCO_2) in arterial (most commonly) or venous (P_vO_2, P_vCO_2) blood samples. It can also calculate bicarbonate levels, base excess and saturation of haemoglobin with oxygen. These parameters provide accurate information about tissue oxygenation and respiratory gas exchange, and metabolic disturbances (e.g. metabolic acidosis). A sample of arterial blood is collected into a heparinized syringe, which can be quite challenging and painful for the patient unless an arterial catheter has been placed. During preparation of the site of arterial puncture using a needle stab, it is important to clip and prepare the site gently to avoid the artery going into spasm. Use of EMLA cream can reduce pain associated with sample collection in conscious animals.

Blood gas analysis in horses

Arterial blood gas analysis is very commonly used during anaesthesia in horses in order to monitor arterial O_2 and CO_2 (Figure 23.80). This is due to the high risk of hypoxia and the need to know accurately how blood O_2 tension is changing throughout the anaesthetic. Collection of arterial blood samples is usually simple due to the routine placement of an arterial catheter for direct arterial blood pressure monitoring. The frequency of blood gas analysis during an equine anaesthetic depends on factors such as:

- The health status of the horse
- The size of the horse and recumbency (may influence the likelihood of hypoxia)
- The oxygenation status of the horse measured during preceding samples.

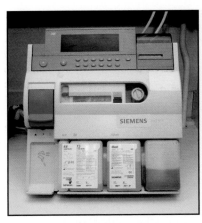

23.80 Blood gas analyser for measurement of blood oxygen and carbon dioxide. The red flap is lifted upwards in order to introduce the sample into the machine.

The anaesthetic recovery period

The recovery period is one of the most high-risk periods of anaesthesia. Reasons for this may include:

- Unless a nurse can be dedicated to the recovery area, observation is usually poor
- Monitoring during the recovery period is usually reduced
- Anaesthetic support such as oxygen supplementation is usually withdrawn, whilst the cardiovascular and respiratory depressant effects of the drugs remain
- Body temperature is poorly monitored and heat provision withdrawn.

Extubation

- **Dogs:** Extubation should take place once the patient has regained the ability to swallow. The ET tube cuff should be kept inflated until just before extubation, as the patient will be unable to protect its own airway until this point.
- **Cats**: Extubation should take place before the patient regains the ability to swallow due to the sensitivity of the larynx and the risk of laryngeal spasm. The correct time of extubation is often indicated by increased jaw tone, presence of a brisk palpebral reflex and an ear twitch when the hair is gently touched.
- **Horses:** There are differing opinions amongst anaesthetists about the optimal time to extubate horses. Most anaesthetists will wait to extubate the horse until swallowing has occurred and the depth of anaesthesia appears to be lightening, signalled by spontaneous blinking and eye lacrimation. The anaesthetist should position themselves carefully during this period to ensure that a quick exit from the box can be made should the horse suddenly attempt to stand, or leg movement occur. Oxygen (5–10 litres/min) is commonly supplemented during the recovery period via pipeline tubing from an oxygen source outside the box and delivered into the box via an observation window or specific port. The pipeline is fed up the ET tube before extubation and up one nostril after the ET tube has been removed. Once the horse is standing, the pipeline is voided from the nose, withdrawn from the box and the oxygen delivery stopped. The provision of a nasal tube

after tracheal extubation encourages a better airway until the horse is able to stand.
- **Rabbits and small rodents**: Extubation should take place once the patient starts to swallow or regain motor control.
- **Birds:** Extubation should occur when the patient is fully awake, breathing well and able to swallow.
- **Reptiles:** Similar to other species, extubation of reptiles should occur when pharyngeal reflexes have returned and the patient is breathing spontaneously.

Once extubated, the patient should be assessed to ensure that it can protect its airway adequately. This involves: assessing mucous membrane colour for signs of hypoxia; using a pulse oximeter on the tongue (if the patient will tolerate this) or earfold; monitoring respiratory rate and effort; and looking for signs of **paradoxical breathing** (asymmetrical chest movements or the chest expanding less rather than more on inspiration).

The recovery area

The recovery area for small animals should:

- Be warm (use of a paediatric incubator is ideal)
- Be well ventilated (to remove the anaesthetic gases being exhaled by the patient)
- Be quiet
- Be easily visible from main work area, so that help can be quickly obtained
- Have an available oxygen supply (either pipeline oxygen from the wall or a dedicated anaesthesia machine with an oxygen cylinder)
- Have accessible power points to allow warming devices and equipment to be plugged in
- Have padded bedding (ideally acrylic fleece bedding so that if the patient urinates it is drawn away from the patient).

The patient's body should also be covered by warm bedding to prevent any further heat loss and to correct any hypothermia. **Incubators** can be useful for small patients as they provide a warm environment, allow oxygen supplementation and are usually transparent, which enables easy observation of the patient.

Recovery in horses

Recovery from anaesthesia is a critical time, and careful management of the recovery period is essential in order to prevent complications. If the animal is being ventilated, some anaesthetists choose to ensure that spontaneous respiration has resumed before the horse is disconnected from the anaesthetic machine. However, this is controversial; there are some data to support the practice of disconnecting the animal immediately from the anaesthetic machine after cessation of IPPV and waiting for spontaneous respiration to resume in the recovery box. Demand valves can be used to deliver short-term positive pressure ventilation with oxygen via the endotracheal tube if spontaneous ventilation does not resume quickly in the recovery box.

Monitoring equipment should be removed in the order in which it was placed. Non-invasive monitoring equipment should be left in place the longest, as this equipment can be removed quickly, immediately before the horse is transferred. The horse should be disconnected from the anaesthetic machine and the administration of inhalant agents discontinued. It is important that the horse is anaesthetized adequately to allow safe transfer to the recovery box. It is common to give an alpha-2 agonist intramuscularly before the end of anaesthesia to provide additional sedation in the recovery period. This can prolong recumbency and contribute to a better quality of recovery. Horses that try to stand before they are fully awake are at greatest risk of self-injury. In this condition the horse has not regained coordination and motor function. Slower, more controlled recoveries should be encouraged.

The horse is transferred to the recovery box. The position in the recovery box will depend on the dimensions of the box and the surgery that has been carried out. If the horse has been placed in lateral recumbency during surgery it should be placed in the same lateral recumbency in the recovery box. This is to ensure that the inflated lung remains uppermost, reducing the risk of hypoxia during recovery from anaesthesia. If a horse has a bandaged limb it is usual to place that limb uppermost in recovery, in order to prevent the painful, bandaged, less flexible limb from jeopardizing attempts to stand. However, the consideration regarding lung function may outweigh this factor if the lower limb was operated on during surgery when the horse was in lateral recumbency.

The confidential enquiry into perioperative equine fatalities (CEPEF) showed that approximately one-third of perioperative deaths in 'healthy' horses were attributed to complications that occurred during recovery. Limb fractures caused by a 'stormy' recovery were particularly common, with pain suggested as a factor in horses attempting to stand prematurely. Due to safety reasons, once the horse is placed in the recovery box access to the animal is limited and monitoring of heart rate, respiratory rate, body temperature and perioperative pain is thus problematic. As the depth of anaesthesia becomes less and spontaneous movement occurs it is important that all personnel are outside the recovery box and that the doors of the box are bolted shut. This prevents the risk of the horse falling out through the doors should it make a sudden attempt to stand. In many practices the induction box also functions as the recovery box. Larger centres may have separate recovery boxes, in which case these may be slightly smaller than the induction box in order to restrict the movement of the horse during the recovery period. Limiting movement during recovery tends to reduce the horse's momentum, which can result in limb injury; however, it is important that the horse has adequate space to stand.

It is important that the horse is not squashed into the corner of a recovery box, without room to adopt sternal recumbency or stretch out its head. Most horses achieve the standing position by lurching forwards; therefore, room to allow this manoeuvre is important (Figure 23.81). The lower thoracic limb should be pulled forward so that it is not lying directly under the chest wall, as this could contribute to myopathy.

Following extubation, checks must be made to ensure that there is good airflow through both nostrils. Oedema of the dependent nasal passages is not uncommon during long procedures, necessitating placement of a nasal tube to ensure that the airway is patent during recovery. Nasal tubes should be made of a soft material and placed gently to prevent nasal bleeding, they should also be secured firmly to prevent inhalation of the tube. If the nasal airways are not patent, the ET tube may be secured in place during recovery to ensure that a patent airway is maintained.

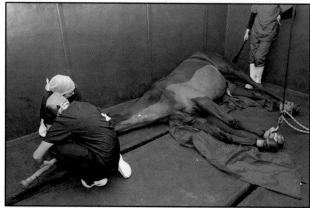

23.81 A horse in a recovery box at the end of anesthesia. The position of the horse allows space for it to roll into sternal recumbency, with room in front to allow forward movement as it attempts to stand. The lower forelimb has been pulled forward to minimize pressure on the lower limb muscles from the upper limb.

Assisted recovery

Assisting recovery in horses using head and tail ropes, either with or without a pulley system, is becoming increasingly common in equine anaesthesia. The principle underlying assisted recoveries is that the handlers exert tension on the ropes to prevent the horse from falling during an attempt to stand. It is not the aim to hoist the horse to its feet prematurely. Assistance can be useful for horses with limb abnormalities or that are fat and weak during the recovery period. The head rope is used to control the front end of the horse, but little tension should be applied on it during attempts to stand as that could unbalance the horse. Tension is maintained on the tail rope so that the horse cannot fall once in a standing position. It is important to remember that assisted recoveries carried out by inexperienced personnel can be dangerous to the horse as it can make recovery from anaesthesia more difficult.

Considerations for recovery in exotic pets

Rabbits and rodents

It should be remembered that cats and dogs are predators of rabbits and small rodents; allowing these species to recover in the same room as cats or dogs can therefore be extremely stressful for them. Recovery facilities should ideally be provided in an observed area away from noise. Achieving and maintaining normothermia is very important in rabbits and small rodents in order to prevent a prolongation of the recovery period. Monitoring body temperature as the animal awakens from anaesthesia is very difficult in rats and mice; a warm environment should therefore be maintained until normal activity resumes.

> **WARNING**
> - Never leave rabbits or small rodents unattended with electrical cables or water-filled warming devices, as they are very likely to chew through any unattended cables or rubbery materials.
> - Do not allow rabbits and rodents to recover on straw or wood shavings as these materials can easily damage the eyes when the animals are recumbent.

It is important to encourage eating and drinking as soon as possible after anaesthesia in order to reduce the risk of anorexia and gut stasis. Water and palatable food should be offered, and intake monitored, as soon as the animal is returned to the recovery environment.

Birds

Wing flapping and emergence delirium is common in birds, particularly after injectable anaesthesia techniques; preventing self-trauma during the recovery period is therefore vital. Wrapping the animal in a towel so that its wings are constrained is a useful way to control birds during the recovery period. As with other species, achieving and maintaining normothermia is important to hasten recovery. Food and water should be offered as soon as the bird is awake enough to be able to perch.

Reptiles

Prolonged recovery from anaesthesia is not uncommon in reptiles due to their low metabolic rate. In order to hasten recovery it is usually recommended to terminate delivery of inhalant agents 15–20 minutes before the end of anaesthesia. Reptiles should be maintained in a quiet environment during recovery, at a temperature in the upper end of their PBT range. Aquatic reptiles should not be allowed access to water until they have fully recovered from anaesthesia and are able to swim.

Monitoring during the recovery period

Patients should be closely observed for signs of postoperative complications, such as haemorrhage, with frequent assessment of vital parameters such as temperature, pulse rate and quality, respiratory rate, mucous membrane colour and CRT. Pain should also be assessed frequently. Water can be returned to the patient once it is able to move around the cage in a controlled manner.

The intravenous catheter should be removed once the animal is fully recovered from anaesthesia and there is no further requirement for intravenous fluid therapy. In some cases it is useful to maintain intravenous access for a longer period; for example:

- In high risk patients for which further intervention might be required (e.g. unexpected fluid support)
- In patients for which intravenous access is required for drug administration, e.g. to allow postoperative analgesia with intravenous opioids, therefore avoiding the need for painful intramuscular injections
- In patients at risk of seizures in recovery
- In patients at risk of airway complications in recovery.

Special considerations for recovery in small animal patients

CNS disease

Animals with CNS disease may have raised intracranial pressure (ICP), which can present problems during recovery from anaesthesia, particularly an increased risk of seizures. The following principles should be adopted:

- The patient must be closely observed throughout recovery so that seizures can be identified and managed promptly

- Ventilatory support must not be withdrawn until the patient's breathing is adequate and it is able to maintain normal ETCO$_2$. This can be monitored using capnography prior to extubation. The sampling line of the capnometer can be attached to a catheter and placed up a nostril to continue monitoring CO$_2$ concentration after extubation
- Care must be taken to avoid the patient coughing during extubation as this will raise ICP
- Administration of drugs that may elicit vomiting during the recovery period must be avoided, as vomiting will also raise ICP
- Measures to reduce ICP must be adopted. These include gentle elevation of the head (a triangular cushion can be useful to place under the head and neck). The neck should be stretched, to prevent obstruction of venous drainage from the head and to maintain normal ETCO$_2$
- Intravenous access must be maintained until approximately 12 hours after the animal is completely recovered from anaesthesia, to ensure that access can be rapidly achieved in the event of seizures
- Appropriate doses of anticonvulsant drugs, such as midazolam or diazepam, and of heparinized saline must be drawn up in a syringe next to the patient so that they can be given intravenously immediately following the onset of any seizure activity.

Animals that have undergone myelography as part of diagnostic testing for spinal disease are also at a high risk of seizure activity in recovery, due to the spinal and CNS effects of the contrast agents used. This is particularly the case when agents are injected into the cisterna magna rather than at L7–S1, due to the greater risk of cranial spread. The head should be raised during recovery to encourage distal movement of the contrast medium.

After intraocular surgery

Intraocular surgery can be painful; careful assessment of pain combined with the appropriate administration of analgesic agents is therefore imperative. Coughing and vomiting will raise intraocular pressure (IOP) and may compromise the surgery that has been carried out. Drugs that elicit vomiting must be avoided in the recovery period and care must be taken to avoid coughing during extubation. Placement of an Elizabethan collar can be useful to prevent trauma to the eye through scratching; however, Elizabethan collars should not be used as an alternative to adequate pain management.

After thoracotomy

This group of patients is at a high risk of hypoxia during recovery; therefore, monitoring of haemoglobin saturation with a pulse oximeter is extremely useful. Placement of the probe on a distal body part such as a teat, the vulva, the prepuce or a toe is usually well tolerated. Oxygen supplementation may be required, delivered using a strategy that is not stressful for the patient, e.g. facemask, nasal catheter or oxygen tent. Chest pain can decrease the efficiency of ventilation, so administration of adequate analgesia is vital.

After orthopaedic surgery

Following orthopaedic surgery, mobility may be impaired, particularly in animals with bandages or casts. Placing the patient on a padded mattress with soft bedding and turning it frequently (every 2 hours) will prevent discomfort in the recovery period and the development of pressure sores.

Catheterization of the bladder should be considered to prevent soiling of the bedding where patients cannot be walked outside due to paralysis or sedation. Bandages and casts must be checked frequently for signs of pressure sores or points of rubbing. Bandages or casts that are too tight or are rubbing should be replaced immediately. If necessary, patients should be supported when they are taken outside for a walk, to prevent scuffing of feet or limbs during walking.

Brachycephalic dogs and cats

Brachycephalic patients have a high risk of respiratory obstruction following extubation, due to excessive soft tissue at the back of their throats, which can obstruct the airway. The patient must be extubated as late as possible, although the likelihood of coughing following some types of surgical procedure where coughing is undesirable must be considered. The patient should be placed in the kennel with its neck stretched and the tongue pulled out of the mouth to minimize airway obstruction. Intravenous access must be maintained during the recovery period so that the animal can be rapidly re-anaesthetized and re-intubated if acute respiratory obstruction should occur. A tray containing all the equipment required for rapid re-intubation should be placed next to the patient; this should include heparinized saline, an induction agent such as propofol drawn up in an appropriate dose in a syringe, a laryngoscope, and a selection of suitably sized ET tubes.

Specific problems during recovery in horses

Post-anaesthetic myopathy

The incidence of post-anaesthetic myopathy in horses is approximately 7%. It manifests as muscle weakness, often leading to an inability to stand during recovery. Pain associated with the condition often leads to profuse sweating and the affected muscle group can feel hard to the touch.

Muscle damage is caused by inadequate oxygenation of the muscle tissue during anaesthesia, which also results in ischaemia. Large muscle masses such as the triceps, dorsal lumbar and gluteal muscles are most likely to be affected, depending on the position of the horse during anaesthesia and recumbency. The full pathophysiology of post-anaesthetic myopathy is unknown, but a major factor is the maintenance of adequate blood flow (and therefore oxygen) to the muscle tissue. The two most important factors that determine blood flow to the muscle tissue are **blood pressure**, which drives perfusion of the muscle tissue with blood, and the **intracompartmental pressure** inside the muscle tissue itself.

The intracompartmental pressure will oppose muscle perfusion, and can be minimized by careful positioning of the horse during anaesthesia to reduce excess weight being placed on the large muscle groups. This careful positioning, along with maintenance of a mean arterial blood pressure >60 mmHg (recommended to optimize blood flow to the muscles), significantly reduces the risk of post-anaesthetic myopathy.

Management of post-anaesthetic myopathy is supportive. Provision of analgesia to reduce pain is imperative. Strategies must also be implemented that help the horse to stand up and remain standing, in order to reduce the further effects of prolonged recumbency. This can involve supporting the horse in a sling in the immediate postoperative period.

Peripheral neuropathies

Peripheral nerves, especially those close to the skin, are at risk of damage during anaesthesia as a result of poor patient positioning, which can lead to excessive pressure on nerve fibres (see above). Peripheral neuropathy is indicated by reduced function of the muscle groups that are innervated by the affected nerve fibre. The facial, radial, femoral and peroneal nerves are most commonly affected. Most cases of peripheral neuropathy are mild in nature and resolve in the days following anaesthesia with appropriate supportive care. Pain is not usually a feature unless there is concurrent myopathy; this can be a useful diagnostic feature to differentiate between neuropathy and myopathy.

Limb fracture

Limb fracture can result from a 'stormy' or violent recovery or may be as a consequence of muscle weakness caused by post anaesthetic myopathy or neuropathy. If limb fracture is identified during the recovery period the horse should be re-anaesthetized as soon as it is safe to re-enter the recovery box. Management will depend on whether the fracture can be repaired and the prognosis for recovery following injury; however, limb fractures commonly necessitate euthanasia of the horse.

Nasal oedema

Horses positioned in dorsal recumbency for prolonged periods are at risk of head oedema due to the dependent position of the head relative to the body. Oedema can be minimized by lifting the head relative to the body, but is a common problem, particularly in horses with systemic disease caused by colic. Oedema can lead to partial or complete obstruction of the nasal passages, which can result in respiratory obstruction following extubation. The patency of the nasal passages should always be checked following extubation by placing a hand over the nostrils to detect whether airflow is present and whether it is bilateral. Partial obstruction can be relieved by careful placement of a nasal tube up one nostril. This must be done carefully in order to prevent nasal haemorrhage. Some anaesthetists will place a nasal tube before the onset of oedema (during anaesthesia) if they judge the risk of oedema to be high. It is important to secure the nasal tube in place to prevent inhalation during the recovery period. An alternative strategy is to recover the horse with the ET tube in place.

Spinal cord malacia

This is a relatively rare neuropathy that is usually associated with rapidly growing, well muscled horses placed in dorsal recumbency during anaesthesia. Typically, large-breed horses, such as shire or draught horses, are over-represented. Although the aetiology of the condition is unknown, it is thought to relate to hypoxic damage to the spinal cord during anaesthesia. Affected animals are unable to stand on their hindlimbs during recovery, and development of the condition usually results in euthanasia.

Postoperative colic

Mild postoperative colic is a relatively frequent occurrence following general anaesthesia in horses. Although the underlying cause is likely to be multifactorial, preoperative fasting, stress associated with anaesthesia and surgery and the potential movement of the gut during recumbency are all considered to have the potential to affect gastrointestinal function and therefore contribute to the development of postoperative colic. Management is largely based on symptomatic therapy, including the provision of analgesia and frequent reassessment.

Anaesthesia considerations for specific patient groups

Geriatric patients

It is difficult to define when an animal is geriatric. It depends on the species and breed, and there are no absolute values to define old age. It is more useful to classify animals as old depending on their clinical, rather than their chronological, age.

Geriatric animals do not have normal adult organ reserve function. Therefore, although they may appear to be clinically normal in a resting state prior to anaesthesia, they are less able to regulate organ function to maintain homeostasis in the face of stressors such as anaesthesia. Only drugs with minimal effects on the cardiovascular and respiratory systems should be given, and a balanced anaesthesia protocol should be used. Careful attention should be paid to monitoring during anaesthesia.

Geriatric patients have a high incidence of intercurrent disease. Careful history taking and clinical examination is important, and information must be obtained on current drug therapy. Osteoarthritis is common, and care is therefore required when moving animals during anaesthesia to prevent an exacerbation of pain on recovery from anaesthesia. Confusion and delirium during recovery is common in geriatric patients; good nursing care can reduce distress and disorientation in the recovery period.

Paediatric patients

Very young animals are not commonly anaesthetized in veterinary practice. Organ function typically matures when animals are around 3–4 months of age; animals younger than this can be considered paediatric.

Appropriately sized anaesthetic equipment must be available. The large body surface area to volume ratio predisposes young animals to hypothermia. Their body temperature must therefore be monitored and supported during anaesthesia.

Immature liver function results in prolonged metabolism of most anaesthetic agents. Short-acting agents should therefore be used, with a reliance on inhalational anaesthesia to avoid prolonged recovery. Immature renal function means that young animals are less able to regulate their fluid balance. Cardiac output is more dependent on heart rate than in adult animals; young animals therefore have a limited ability to respond to hypotension as they struggle to increase stroke volume. Paediatric patients also have a limited ability to regulate blood glucose concentration, predisposing them to hypoglycaemia during anaesthesia. Blood glucose concentration must therefore be monitored and supplemented intravenously if needed.

Brachycephalic patients

Major considerations relate to maintenance of the airway. The period prior to the induction of anaesthesia and intubation, and the recovery period following extubation (see above) pose the greatest risk. Animals must be closely monitored during these periods so that airway obstruction can be managed promptly.

- Intravenous access must be maintained with an intravenous catheter throughout the perioperative period so that rapid induction of anaesthesia and intubation is possible at all times.
- Animals should be extubated relatively late in the recovery period, when they are sufficiently awake to maintain a patent airway.
- The equipment for intubation must be kept available close to the animal both prior to intubation and following extubation, and should include a short-acting intravenous induction agent (e.g. alfaxalone or propofol), a laryngoscope, and a selection of suitably sized ET tubes. Topical local anaesthetic should be available for brachycephalic cats.
- Excess sedation after premedication can lead to airway obstruction due to the soft tissues surrounding the larynx and soft palate.
- Stress can exacerbate respiratory comprise. Mild sedation while in the hospital environment may therefore be required.
- Hyperthermia is common in brachycephalic dogs, particularly when they are stressed. Management of body temperature may therefore be required.

Obese patients

- Long needles are required for intramuscular injection of drugs, to avoid injection into fat depots and unreliable drug absorption.
- Obese animals should be weighed, but drug dose based on *estimated lean bodyweight* rather than actual weight. Fat is metabolically relatively inactive and dosing on 'obese weight' can lead to drug overdose.
- Obese patients are at risk of airway compromise due to fatty tissue around the larynx. Ventilation is often compromised, particularly when animals are in dorsal recumbency.

Patients with cardiovascular disease

Cardiovascular disease is relatively common in cats and dogs and is not a contraindication to anaesthesia. However, this patient group requires careful evaluation before anaesthesia in order to obtain information about the severity of the disease. This allows the anaesthetic protocol to be tailored to meet the demands of the individual patient.

- Animals with cardiovascular disease are generally less able to maintain normal cardiac output and blood pressure during anaesthesia. Monitoring of the cardiovascular system is vital to allow appropriate supportive measures to be implemented. Patients must be monitored from the time of premedication through to the postoperative period. Induction of anaesthesia is a particularly critical time; depending on the nature of the underlying disease, ECG monitoring during induction of anaesthesia may be advisable.
- Oxygen supplementation is important for all patients, but will be of particular benefit for patients with cardiovascular disease. Supplemental oxygen should be provided, to pre-oxygenate patients before induction of anaesthesia.
- Exacerbation of stress is particularly problematical as it increases the circulating levels of catecholamines that can promote cardiac arrhythmias (see later); careful handling and judicious use of sedative drugs is required.

Patients with renal disease

Chronic renal failure is common in geriatric cats. This is not a contraindication to anaesthesia but requires careful management of fluid therapy. Considerations for acute and chronic renal failure are different.

Acute renal failure

Acute renal failure is associated with high plasma concentrations of urea and creatinine, which can cause myocardial depression and altered acid–base balance. Plasma potassium concentration is often raised, which has the potential to cause cardiac arrhythmias, particularly during anaesthesia. Stabilization of the patient prior to anaesthesia with appropriate fluid therapy is paramount, particularly with regard to normalization of plasma potassium concentration.

Chronic renal failure

Animals with chronic renal failure maintain their glomerular filtration rate and stable urea and creatinine plasma concentrations by drinking more and urinating more; anaesthesia disrupts this mechanism. Plasma potassium concentration is likely to be low; supplementation of potassium (orally or through fluid therapy) is therefore advisable before anaesthesia. The patient must be checked for normal hydration before induction of anaesthesia; it can be useful to start intravenous fluid therapy before induction of anaesthesia. Fluids should be provided intravenously throughout the perioperative period until the patient is able to regulate its own fluid balance through drinking. Blood pressure must be monitored and mean arterial pressure maintained at >60 mmHg in order to reduce the risk of renal ischaemia and a worsening of renal function postoperatively.

Patients with liver disease

Most anaesthetic drugs are metabolized by the liver; hepatic disease will therefore slow drug metabolism, with the potential for drug accumulation and a prolonged recovery period. Short-acting agents should be used where possible, with reliance on an inhalational agent for maintenance of anaesthesia. Administration of halothane should be avoided. NSAIDs should be used judiciously; they have the potential to accumulate, leading to side effects in animals with reduced liver function, and may cause a further deterioration in liver function.

Patients undergoing caesarean operation

Anaesthetic considerations for a caesarean operation must include both the dam and the offspring. The following principles apply for all small mammals.

- Drugs that cross the blood–brain barrier to cause anaesthesia in the dam will also cross the placental barrier and affect the offspring. Premedication with an opioid drug is usually sufficient to provide sedation prior to induction of anaesthesia. Short-acting drugs, such as propofol or alfaxalone, should be used for induction of anaesthesia and inhalational agents for maintenance. Further administration of opioids should be restricted until the offspring have been removed from the uterus.
- Morphine is highly lipid-soluble and therefore less likely to be excreted in milk compared to other opioids such as pethidine, minimizing effects on the offspring after anaesthesia.
- Placing a pregnant dam on her back can compromise venous return to the heart and ventilation. The cardiovascular and respiratory systems must be monitored carefully; IPPV is likely to be necessary until the offspring are removed.
- Equipment needed for resuscitation of the offspring should be prepared. This should include: suction to clear the airway; towels to rub the offspring, to dry them and stimulate breathing; a warm environment in which to maintain the offspring until the dam is recovered from anaesthesia; and equipment for providing oxygen support (an oxygen tent is ideal).
- Veterinary nurses should be prepared to give the offspring a drop of naloxone under the tongue if they show signs of respiratory depression resulting from administration of opioids to the dam.
- If alpha-2 agonists have been administered to the dam as part of the anaesthetic protocol, the effects of the drug can be reversed in the offspring by administering a drop of atipamezole under the tongue.
- The dam must have sufficiently recovered from anaesthesia before she is placed with the offspring. She must then be monitored carefully so that she does not squash and injure the neonates if not sufficiently aware.

Patients with raised intracranial pressure

- If possible, raised ICP should be managed, using diuretic agents such as furosemide and mannitol, before induction of anaesthesia. Further exacerbation of raised ICP during anaesthesia can be prevented by ensuring that there is no obstruction to venous drainage from the head, e.g. placement of a jugular catheter should be avoided and the head and neck raised following induction.
- An elevation in $ETCO_2$ must be prevented as this will promote vasodilation of blood vessels and therefore raise ICP.
- Patients must be ventilated during anaesthesia, preferably using capnometry to ensure that $ETCO_2$ is maintained within the normal range.
- Generally, fluid replacement with 0.9% saline is preferred to other crystalloid solutions during anaesthesia because it is slightly more hypertonic than plasma and administration is therefore less likely to promote further increases in ICP.

Patients with diabetes mellitus

Management of blood glucose concentration is the most important consideration when anaesthetizing patients with diabetes mellitus. Low blood glucose will not be signalled by the onset of clinical signs (changes in mentation, loss of consciousness, seizure activity) in anaesthetized patients; detection and prevention of hypoglycaemia is therefore paramount. Hyperglycaemia is also associated with adverse effects and in human patients tight regulation of blood glucose within narrow limits is recommended; however, in veterinary practice, prevention of hyperglycaemia is currently perceived to be less important than prevention of hypoglycaemia.

For stable diabetic patients managed with insulin, the general recommendation is to advise the owner to give their pet half the normal insulin dose on the morning of anaesthesia. This is to prevent hypoglycaemia following insulin administration in patients that have been starved. This recommendation is not supported by clinical evidence, however.

- Premedication with alpha-2 adrenergic agents should be avoided as this class of drugs will result in an elevation of blood glucose. Surgery and anaesthesia alone will result in a destabilization of blood glucose concentration, and therefore administration of drugs with a specific effect on blood glucose regulation should be avoided.
- Following premedication, a blood sample should be taken for measurement of a baseline blood glucose concentration. If the patient is already hypoglycaemic (blood glucose <3 mmol/l) then intravenous glucose supplementation should be initiated.
- Blood glucose concentration should be monitored throughout anaesthesia and glucose supplementation initiated if required.
- Glucose is irritant when administered in high concentrations intravenously. Glucose solutions should therefore be diluted with saline or water for injection to 10–20% for administration via a peripheral vein. Glucose supplementation is more effective when a loading dose is given followed by a continuous rate infusion; administration of repeated bolus doses is inefficient and leads to peaks and troughs. The dose of the infusion can be adjusted according to the sequential results following monitoring of blood glucose concentration.
- On recovery from anaesthesia, blood glucose concentration usually returns to within normal limits, or hyperglycaemia develops. Blood glucose should be monitored periodically until the animal is fully awake and able to eat.

Anaesthetic emergencies

Commonly occurring anaesthetic emergencies usually involve disturbances in respiratory or cardiovascular system function.

Respiratory emergencies

Apnoea

Cessation of respiration is common during anaesthesia and can easily be recognized by an absence of chest movements, cessation of breathing bag movements and an absence of expired CO_2 (if respiratory function is being monitored using capnography). Apnoea will result in a fall in haemoglobin saturation with oxygen, although changes in O_2 saturation are likely to take a few minutes to occur in animals that have previously been breathing 100% O_2. The consequences of unmanaged apnoea are hypoxia and hypercapnia – potentially life-threatening.

Apnoea can be managed easily by instigating manual or automatic IPPV; however, at the same time as treating apnoea it is important to establish and manage the underlying cause. The most common reason for apnoea is an excessive depth of anaesthesia relative to surgical stimulation; therefore one of the first things to check is depth of anaesthesia. Other common causes of apnoea are given earlier in this chapter – see 'Monitoring of the respiratory system'.

Hypoventilation

Hypoventilation (inadequate ventilation) is very common during anaesthesia but can be difficult to assess by visual appraisal of chest movements alone. It is most easily diagnosed using capnography, where it will cause an elevation of $ETCO_2$. Hypoventilation does not usually result in hypoxia (unless very severe), but prolonged elevations in CO_2 can result in disturbances in acid–base balance, leading to respiratory acidosis. A severe acidosis may result in reduced myocardial function, leading to hypotension and reduced enzyme activity. Hypoventilation can be managed by supporting respiratory function by manual or automatic IPPV; however, it is also important to establish and manage the underlying cause. An excessive depth of anaesthesia is probably the most common reason for hypoventilation. Other common causes include body position (e.g. an overweight dog placed in dorsal recumbency) or administration of potent opioid drugs.

Cardiovascular emergencies
Bradycardia

Ultimately a severe reduction in heart rate will reduce cardiac output, due to the relation between heart rate, stroke volume and cardiac output. However, deciding the level at which bradycardia becomes clinically significant and requires management can be difficult. It is important to consider the preoperative heart rate, the species and breed, and the rate of reduction in heart rate; sudden changes may be more clinically significant than a gradual decline. Evaluation of blood pressure and the ECG can help in decision-making: hypotension or the presence of a 2nd or 3rd degree AV block indicates that the bradycardia should be managed and heart rate increased. A common cause of bradycardia is an excessive depth of anaesthesia; therefore it is important to check that anaesthesia depth is appropriate for the surgical procedure and to reduce anaesthetic depth by lowering the delivered concentration of inhalant agent if appropriate. Other common causes of bradycardia include the administration of potent opioids (which cause bradycardia by stimulation of the vagal nerve) or direct stimulation of the vagal nerve due to surgery. Anticholinergics can be administered to increase the low heart rate caused by vagal stimulation.

Tachycardia

Inappropriately high heart rates will ultimately reduce cardiac output due to inadequate time for cardiac filling between each beat, reducing stroke volume. Definition of tachycardia depends on the species, breed and preoperative heart rate, but in dogs heart rates >180 bpm will usually reduce cardiac output and have the potential to cause hypotension and hypoxia. Before managing a tachycardia it is important to establish the underlying cause. Inadequate depth of anaesthesia is an important cause of tachycardia; it is therefore important to evaluate depth of anaesthesia relative to level of surgical stimulation. The tachycardia may also be an appropriate compensatory response to hypotension and may be critical to preventing hypoxia and hypotension in the anaesthetized patient, in which case reducing heart rate may be inappropriate. This should be discussed with the veterinary surgeon in order to establish whether management of the tachycardia is appropriate for the particular patient. There is also a danger that tachycardia can promote cardiac arrhythmias due to myocardial hypoxia or the running of one ECG PQRS complex on to the next, in which case treatment to reduce heart rate is indicated. Pharmacological strategies to reduce heart rate include increasing depth of anaesthesia by the provision of analgesia or hypnosis, or administration of potent opioids specifically to cause vagal stimulation. Short-term specific antagonists of cardiac adrenergic 1 receptors such as esmolol can also be given intravenously in an emergency.

Cardiac arrhythmias

These are not uncommon during anaesthesia and can result from a multitude of reasons. Arrhythmias are usually classified as either atrial or ventricular in origin. Ventricular arrhythmias are usually more insidious and include ventricular tachycardia or ventricular extra systoles. Although abnormalities in the electrical activity of the heart may be detected by feeling for changes in the pulse rate or rhythm, the precise nature of the electrical disturbance can only be diagnosed by analysing an ECG trace.

Ventricular tachycardia

Ventricular tachycardia can be recognized by the presence of an increased heart rate or pulse rate and, on the ECG, QRS complexes at a higher than normal rate, without an associated P wave. In order to assess the clinical significance and determine whether treatment is required, the following must be evaluated:

- **Pulse rate** or **heart rate**: More severe tachycardias will have a greater effect on cardiac output due to the reduction in time for ventricular filling, thereby reducing stroke volume. Higher ventricular rates are also more likely to result in one QRS complex running into the next, which can promote ventricular fibrillation
- **QRS complexes**: Ventricular arrhythmias can be defined as unifocal (a single source of abnormal electrical activity) or multifocal (multiple sources of abnormal electrical activity driving the tachycardia). With unifocal abnormalities all QRS complexes look similar, whereas with multifocal abnormalities the QRS complexes look different. Multifocal abnormalities are generally considered to be more insidious due to the increased risk of ventricular fibrillation developing
- **Effect on cardiac output or pulse quality**: Some ventricular tachycardias are relatively benign, having minimal effects on cardiac output and blood pressure. It is important to assess whether there is a pulse deficit (i.e. whether there is a pulse beat for every QRS complex) and to assess pulse quality. The presence of a pulse deficit or poor pulse quality indicates that the cardiovascular consequences of the arrhythmia are marked, warranting prompt treatment. The effect of a ventricular tachycardia can be more readily assessed if blood pressure is measured using a direct technique. Direct arterial blood pressure monitoring allows blood pressure to be measured more accurately than an indirect technique or tactile assessment of pulse quality.

Treatment depends on the underlying cause, although this can be difficult to establish as ventricular tachycardia is commonly caused by myocardial hypoxia, which can develop for multiple reasons. Other common causes of ventricular tachycardia include splenic pathology (e.g. tumours of the

spleen necessitating removal of the spleen) and gastric dilatation–volvulus syndrome (GDV). Ventricular tachycardia can be managed pharmacologically by the intravenous administration of lidocaine, which decreases automaticity in ventricular muscle.

Ventricular extra systoles

These can be recognized on an ECG by the presence of intermittent QRS complexes without an associated P wave, indicating that the contraction of the myocardium resulting in a heart beat is initiated and generated by contraction of the *ventricle* only. A P wave may be seen on the ECG but it is usually dissociated from the QRS complex. The clinical significance of ventricular extra systoles depends on their effect on cardiac output and whether the QRS complex generates ventricular contraction adequate to cause a pulse. Other factors to consider are: frequency, presence of a pulse deficit and hypotension, and whether the extra systoles are multifocal or unifocal.

Common causes of ventricular extra systoles include myocardial hypoxia and severe bradycardia. Ventricular extra systoles represent escape beats where the intrinsic rate of electrical activity of the ventricles is faster than the intrinsic rate of electrical activity of the sinoatrial node. They can occasionally occur due to a severe bradycardia induced by the administration of an alpha-2 agonist. Management depends on the underlying cause. If the extra systoles result from a severe bradycardia, then management to increase heart rate is appropriate. Measures to improve myocardial oxygenation are required to correct myocardial hypoxia.

Atrial arrhythmias

The most common atrial arrhythmias are bradycardia and tachycardia, which are described earlier. Other common atrial arrhythmias are second- or third-degree AV blocks. This occurs when conduction of electrical activity through the atrioventricular (AV) node is slowed so that each P wave is not followed by a QRS complex. With a second-degree AV block there are some normal PQRS complexes and some P waves that are not conducted through the AV node. The pulse rate will feel irregular, as P waves alone will not result in ventricular activity and generation of a heart beat. A third-degree AV block occurs when no P waves are conducted through the AV node and there is complete dissociation between P waves and QRS complexes. Since no P waves are conducted through to the ventricle the intrinsic electrical activity of the ventricle takes over, generating QRS complexes that can be described as ventricular extra systoles or an escape rhythm. Usually each QRS complex is associated with a heart beat as they result in ventricular contraction. The pulse rate will feel irregular and pulse quality may be reduced.

Common causes of a second- or third-degree AV block include high vagal tone (which slows conduction through the AV node). This may be caused by drug administration (e.g. potent opioids or alpha-2 agonists) or by stimulation of the vagal nerve. Other causes of a severe bradycardia may also result in second- or third-degree AV block. Pharmacological management of an AV block involves administration of an anticholinergic such as atropine.

Hypotension

A low blood pressure is extremely common during anaesthesia due to the effects of anaesthetic drugs on the cardiovascular system to decrease cardiac output and cause vasodilation, combined with the potential for blood and other fluid losses. Although hypotension may be suspected from poor palpable pulse quality and the presence of an increased heart rate (as a compensatory response), it can only be identified definitively by measurement of blood pressure. Common causes of hypotension include excessive depth of anaesthesia, marked blood loss and inappropriate tachycardia or bradycardia.

Management of hypotension depends on the underlying cause. It is important first to check the depth of anaesthesia and adjust if appropriate. If the depth of anaesthesia seems correct for the surgical procedure, yet the patient requires a high concentration of inhalant agent to maintain anaesthesia, it is prudent to switch to a more balanced anaesthesia technique in order to reduce the concentration of inhalant required.

Hypotension in horses

Intraoperative hypotension is a common occurrence in horses. Although the underlying reason for this is not fully understood, myocardial depression caused by volatile agents is thought to be a significant contributing factor. Prompt management of hypotension is important because of the strong correlation between intraoperative hypotension and post-anaesthetic myopathy in adult horses. Neonatal foals have a lower mean arterial blood pressure than adults (50–60 mmHg) due to their lower vascular tone. The causes of hypotension in horses are similar to those in small animals and many of the management strategies are similar. However, in horses there is a greater reliance on positive inotropes (drugs that increase myocardial contractility) to increase blood pressure. Dobutamine is a synthetic catecholamine that is commonly used in equine anaesthesia to increase blood pressure. It has a primary agonist effect on beta-1 receptors in the myocardium, resulting in improved myocardial contractility. The drug is short-acting and potent, and is therefore infused intravenously to effect. Dobutamine is usually made up in solution with 0.9% NaCl, at a concentration of either 125 or 250 µg/ml. It is sensitive to light: pink discoloration of the solution indicates oxidation of the drug and a new solution should be made up for administration.

Hypoxia

Tissue or myocardial hypoxia is a common endpoint pathology resulting from a multitude of derangements. It is a life-threatening condition and has the potential to cause cardiac arrhythmias or permanent damage to vital organs, resulting in a reduction in organ function on recovery from anaesthesia. A pulse oximeter will detect tissue hypoxia, allowing prompt action.

When hypoxia is noted it is important to think about the multiple processes that could result in hypoxia in order to elucidate the underlying cause.

Actions to consider when hypoxia occurs

- Check that oxygen delivery via the anaesthetic breathing system is adequate. If <100% O_2 is being delivered then switch to 100% O_2 administration.
- Confirm that the oxygen being delivered to the patient by the breathing system is reaching the patient: Is the breathing system connected? Is the endotracheal tube blocked or kinked? ▶

- Check that the patient is ventilating adequately: Is the patient apnoeic?
- Is the oxygen that is delivered to the lungs being delivered to the central organs and peripheral tissues: Is the animal hypotensive? Is cardiac output adequate?

Hypoxaemia in horses

Hypoxaemia is defined as a subnormal P_aO_2; values <60 mmHg (measured by arterial blood gas analysis) are usually considered hypoxaemic. Hypoxaemia typically results in hypoxia.

Horses are particularly vulnerable to hypoxaemia during general anaesthesia due to the anatomy and physiology of their respiratory system. The major cause of arterial hypoxaemia in anaesthetized horses is the ventilation–perfusion ratio (V/Q) mismatch that occurs when there is an imbalance of pulmonary capillary blood flow and ventilation. In a normal standing horse ventilation and perfusion are coupled, meaning that blood flow to the different regions of the lung tissue and alveoli is matched to lung ventilation, or to alveoli that are inflated during inspiration. This matching ensures that blood leaving the lungs in the pulmonary artery is almost maximally saturated with oxygen.

During anaesthesia the functional residual capacity of the lungs is reduced and areas of the lung that are dependent (i.e. the lower regions of lung tissue when the horse is turned on its back) are poorly ventilated. In lateral recumbency the lower lung becomes relatively poorly ventilated, although the change in ventilation is less marked than when horses are placed in dorsal recumbency. In comparison, the lower regions of the lung tend to be preferentially perfused with blood, thus there is uncoupling of ventilation and perfusion. As a result, the blood leaving the lungs in the pulmonary artery is less well oxygenated than in a standing horse, leading to hypoxaemia. Although V/Q mismatch is a major cause of hypoxaemia in anaesthetized horses, there are also other contributing factors, of which atelectasis and hypoventilation are particularly important.

- **Atelectasis**: Defined as collapse of expanded lung tissue, atelectasis is common in anaesthetized horses. The two primary causes of atelectasis are compression of lung tissue by overlying abdominal contents, and absorption. Absorption atelectasis occurs when gases in an expanded alveolus are absorbed rapidly across the alveolar membrane into the blood stream, leading to alveolar collapse. Once alveolar collapse has occurred, re-expansion of the alveolus during the next inspiration is limited and the alveolus tends to stay collapsed. If this happens to a large number of alveoli it can lead to a significant area of atelectasis, which will impair gas exchange. Absorption atelectasis is most significant in horses breathing 100% inspired O_2 because oxygen is very rapidly absorbed across the alveolar membrane into the bloodstream. This has led to the practice of delivering gas mixtures to horses during anaesthesia that are composed of O_2 and 'medical air'. The nitrogen in medical air is slowly absorbed across the alveolar membrane and acts to 'splint' the alveolus open, preventing atelectasis. Atelectasis results in hypoxaemia because, similar to V/Q mismatch, it is associated with blood flow to lung tissue that is not ventilated with oxygen (areas of atelectasis), resulting in reduced O_2 concentrations in the pulmonary artery.

- **Hypoventilation**: Inadequate ventilation caused by respiratory depression induced by anaesthesia will increase the partial pressure of CO_2 in the lungs. In horses breathing <30% inspired O_2 concentration, an elevated partial pressure of CO_2 in the lungs can result in hypoxaemia because there is inadequate 'space' for O_2 in the lung tissue alongside the high CO_2 concentration. IPPV will rapidly correct hypoventilation, although it is important that the underlying cause (e.g. an excessive depth of anaesthesia) is also identified and corrected.

Improving arterial oxygen content in anaesthetized horses

- **Check that oxygen is being delivered** to the animal, the ET tube is positioned correctly in the trachea and there are no mechanical failures with the anaesthetic machine. Optimize the inspired O_2 concentration.
- **Instigate IPPV**: This will correct hypoventilation and may function to reverse atelectasis. In order to reduce the degree of atelectasis, however, IPPV is usually most effective when instigated immediately after induction of anaesthesia; initiation once hypoxaemia has been identified is commonly not effective at improving arterial O_2 concentrations. The negative effects of IPPV on the cardiovascular system must also be considered.
- **Administer aerosolized albuterol**: Albuterol is a beta-2 agonist that causes bronchodilation. Delivery of aerosolized albuterol into the trachea during inspiration has been shown to improve arterial O_2 content in some horses, although the underlying mechanism is not fully understood.
- **Improve cardiac output**: Optimizing arterial O_2 content is dependent on optimizing both lung function and the cardiovascular system. Cardiac output can be improved by ensuring an appropriate depth of anaesthesia, optimizing fluid therapy and cardiac function.

Cardiopulmonary arrest

Cardiopulmonary arrest is relatively uncommon in anaesthetized patients in general veterinary practice; therefore when it does occur it can be difficult to respond appropriately and rapidly due to lack of practice.

The **basic life support** techniques described in Chapter 21 are generally applicable to anaesthetized patients.

Basic life support sequence for an anaesthetized patient

1. Call for help.
2. Note the time.
3. Intubate patients that are not already intubated (most patients will already be intubated during anaesthesia). Check the patency and position of the ET tube in patients that are intubated.
4. Stop delivery of all anaesthetic agents and switch to ventilation with 100% O_2.
5. Give two rescue ventilations that are of sufficient magnitude to see a visible rise in chest position. ▶

6. Start chest compressions at a rate of 100–120 compressions per minute
   - Ensure the patient is on a hard surface to improve the efficiency of the compressions
   - Ensure that the height of the animal is low enough to allow you to carry out chest compressions effectively
   - When you are tired ask someone to take over from you.
7. Give 2 ventilations every 30 chest compressions; do not stop chest compressions during ventilation.
8. Assess the response to chest compression and ventilation:
   - Check for a palpable pulse. This can be difficult to assess frequently as it requires cessation of chest compressions
   - Use a Doppler probe placed on the eye to listen for blood flow in the retinal artery: this is a useful technique as the probe can be left in place to provide continuous monitoring
   - Check whether the animal is producing CO_2, assessed using capnography: production and exhalation of CO_2 during ventilation indicates that there is venous return to the heart
   - Check whether the animal is trying to breathe spontaneously. The return of spontaneous ventilation is a good sign!

The techniques used in cardiopulmonary resuscitation (CPR) are described in Chapter 21 and CPR technique should be practised using a critical care model (Figure 23.82). It can be helpful to create arrest scenarios and practise how to manage them. Careful monitoring of the patient during anaesthesia will facilitate the detection of problems early and hopefully allow measures to be put in place to prevent a cardiopulmonary arrest from occurring.

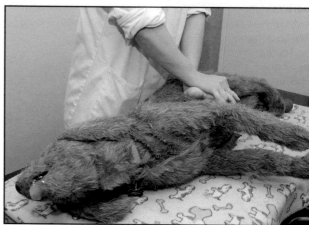

23.82 A critical care model that can be used for CPR training. This person is practising cardiac massage using the thoracic pump technique.

Advanced life support

This involves the administration of resuscitation drugs, the use of open chest massage and electrical defibrillation (if appropriate) as described in Chapter 21. Drugs used in advanced life support should be easily available (as a 'crash box') to all anaesthetists. ECG monitoring early in the resuscitation process will guide drug therapy and the requirement for defibrillation.

Death or euthanasia of anaesthetized patients and implications for carcass disposal

Anaesthetized animals may be euthanased by the veterinary surgeon as long as written consent for euthanasia has been obtained from the owner. It is normally expected that the veterinary surgeon will phone the owner to discuss euthanasia while the animal is still anaesthetized, especially if the recommendation for euthanasia is unexpected.

The most common means of achieving euthanasia under anaesthesia is with an overdose of pentobarbital. This can be administered intravenously to cats, dogs and rabbits. Intraperitoneal injection is appropriate for species where intravenous access is difficult to achieve, e.g. some rodents, birds and reptiles. Injection of pentobarbital into the heart is legal in unconscious animals as a means of euthanasia. It is important to ensure that adequate anaesthesia is maintained until death has been confirmed by the absence of spontaneous respiration and cardiac output (no palpable pulse) or by auscultation of the heart indicating no heart activity. It is prudent to increase the dose of volatile agent delivered to the patient during the process of euthanasia to safeguard against premature lightening of anaesthesia in the patient. If the patient is being monitored using ECG it is useful to note that the ECG may continue to appear normal despite the absence of any cardiac activity and the cessation of a peripheral pulse.

The owners of domestic pets (e.g. cats, dogs, rabbits, rodents, reptiles) are allowed to take their animal home, once euthanased, for burial. Other options for carcass disposal are cremation at registered premises with appropriate licensing.

Disposal of equine carcasses

Horses that have been euthanased during anaesthesia with an overdose of an injectable anaesthetic agent such as pentobarbital cannot be disposed of via a hunt kennels or zoo (where the equine carcass will be used for food). Therefore the options for carcass disposal are cremation or burial.

The European Union Regulations do not allow burial of pet horses as they consider the horse to be a food animal. However, at the time of writing, Defra does allow burial of pet horses at the discretion of the local authority; owners must check with the local Trading Standards Office. Each case is considered on an individual basis.

Acknowledgement

The authors would like to acknowledge the help and expertise of Tracey Dewey (Head of Photography, School of Veterinary Science, University of Bristol) for taking some of the photographs used in this chapter.

Further reading

Aspinall V (2008) *Clinical Procedures in Veterinary Nursing, 2nd edn.* Butterworth–Heinemanon, Oxford
Brodbelt D (2009) Perioperative mortality in small animal anaesthesia. *Veterinary Journal* **182**, 152–161
Challis K and Seymour C (2008) Advanced anaesthesia and analgesia. In: *BSAVA Manual of Canine and Feline Advanced Veterinary Nursing, 2nd edn,* ed. A Hotston Moore and S Rudd, pp. 128–144. BSAVA Publications, Gloucester
Doherty T and Valverde A (2006) *Manual of Equine Anaesthesia and Analgesia.* Blackwell, Oxford
Dugdale A (2010) *Veterinary Anaesthesia.* Blackwell, Oxford
Flecknell PA, Orr HE, Roughan JV and Stewart R (1999) Comparison of the effects of oral or subcutaneous carprofen or ketoprofen in rats undergoing laparotomy. *Veterinary Record* **144**, 65–67
Flecknell PA, Roughan JV and Stewart R (1999) Use of oral buprenorphine ('buprenorphine jello') for postoperative analgesia in rats – a clinical trial. *Laboratory animals* **33**, 169–174
Hall LW, Clarke KW and Trim CT (2001) *Veterinary Anaesthesia, 10th edn.* WB Saunders, London
Johnston GM, Taylor PM, Holmes MA and Wood JL (2002) The confidential enquiry into perioperative equine fatalities (CEPEF): mortality results of Phases 1 and 2. *Veterinary Anaesthesia and Analgesia*, **29**, 159–170
Meredith A and Johnson Delaney C (2010) *BSAVA Manual of Exotic Pets, 5th edn.* BSAVA Publications, Gloucester
Seymour C and Duke-Novakovski T (2007) *BSAVA Manual of Canine and Feline Anaesthesia and Analgesia, 2nd edn.* BSAVA Publications, Gloucester
Stanway G and Magee A (2007) Anaesthesia and analgesia. In: *BSAVA Manual of Practical Veterinary Nursing*, ed. E Mullineaux and M Jones, pp. 268–314. BSAVA Publications, Gloucester
Welch E (2009) *Anaesthesia for Veterinary Nurses.* Blackwell, Oxfordshire

Self-assessment questions

1. What are the aims of premedication?
2. What are the essential characteristics of red rubber and silicone tubes used for endotracheal intubation in cats and dogs?
3. Calculate the fresh gas flow rate required for maintenance of anaesthesia of an 18 kg dog with a respiratory rate of 13 breaths per minute, maintained on a Lack circuit.
4. Compare and contrast rebreathing and non-rebreathing anaesthetic circuits.
5. What are the advantages and disadvantages of total injectable and total inhalational anaesthetic techniques?
6. How can the respiratory and cardiovascular systems be monitored during anaesthesia?
7. What are the considerations when anaesthetizing a brachycephalic patient?
8. By which routes can resuscitation drugs be given during advanced life support?
9. What is multimodal analgesia?
10. What are the consequences of hypothermia during anaesthesia?
11. What are the significant factors to consider during the recovery period in the horse?

Chapter 24

Theatre practice

Dawn McHugh, Alison Young and Julie Johnson

Learning objectives

After studying this chapter, students should be able to:

- **Explain the principles of surgical asepsis**
- **Describe the role of the veterinary nurse in the establishment and maintenance of asepsis in the operating theatre**
- **Recognize a range of surgical instruments used in all types of veterinary surgery**
- **Describe the care and maintenance of surgical instruments/packs and equipment**
- **Describe the different methods of sterilization available and discuss their suitability and use for a range of surgical instruments and equipment used in veterinary surgery**
- **Describe the preparation of a patient for surgery and the intraoperative and immediate postoperative care of a patient**
- **Explain the roles of a veterinary nurse in the operating theatre as both a scrubbed and a circulating nurse**
- **Describe the ideal properties of suture materials and discuss the advantages and disadvantages of different types**
- **Recognize different suture patterns commonly used in veterinary surgery**

Introduction

The veterinary nurse is usually given the responsibility for running the operating theatre. This involves: maintenance of hygiene in the theatre; care and maintenance of instruments and equipment; preparation of theatre, the patient and the surgical team; and providing assistance as both a scrubbed and circulating nurse.

The most important factor in successful theatre practice is the establishment and maintenance of a good aseptic technique, i.e. all the steps taken to prevent contact with microorganisms.

Definitions

- **Sepsis** – the presence of pathogens or their toxic products in the blood or tissues of the patient; more commonly known as infection.
- **Asepsis** – free from infection, i.e. exclusion of microorganisms and spores.
- **Antisepsis** – prevention of sepsis by destruction or inhibition of microorganisms using an agent that may be safely applied to living tissue.
- **Sterilization** – the complete elimination of all microorganisms, including spores.
- **Disinfection** – the removal of microorganisms (but not necessarily spores).
- **Disinfectant** – an agent that destroys microorganisms – generally chemical agents applied to inanimate objects (see Chapter 12).

Factors influencing the development of infection

Infection of a clean surgical wound is always a matter of great concern. It is far better to prevent infection than to try and treat it. The use of antibiotics should not be relied upon to protect patients from the consequences of poor asepsis.

It has been established that most surgical wound infections occur at the time of surgery, not during the postoperative period. Poor aseptic technique will undoubtedly affect the success of any surgery and, in the long term, the success and reputation of the practice. Strict theatre discipline is essential if high standards are to be maintained. A specific protocol must exist, which should be respected and rigidly adhered to by everyone involved with surgery. The protocol should include:

- Correct theatre attire
- Scrubbing-up procedures
- Patient preparation procedures
- Draping techniques
- Sterilization information and procedures
- Organization of surgical lists, cleaning protocol and conduct during surgery.

Sources of contamination in the operating theatre include the operating room, equipment, personnel and the patient.

General rules for maintenance of asepsis in theatre

- Correct theatre attire should be worn at all times.
- There should be a minimum number of people present and movement should be kept to a minimum.
- There should be a new set of sterile instruments for each operation, even when dealing with a contaminated site.
- There should be a plan to perform 'clean' operations first, i.e. orthopaedic operations (especially when implants are used), and to carry out contaminated surgery last (e.g. aural and oral).
- Wherever possible there should be a room for 'dirty' procedures.
- An efficient sterilization programme should be adopted.
- The theatre should be maintained at an ambient temperature and the ventilation must be good. Hot, humid conditions will encourage the growth of pathogens, in particular *Pseudomonas* spp.
- Wherever possible, the patient should be clipped and bathed before it is taken to theatre.
- The surgical team must ensure that they do not touch any non-sterile surfaces during surgery. Any break in asepsis must be reported and rectified.
- No contaminated instruments or equipment should be returned to the sterile trolley.
- A record of all operations should be kept, so that if any sepsis problems arise the cause can be detected.
- A strict cleaning protocol must be maintained.
- Written standard operating procedures (SOPs) for maintaining asepsis in the theatre should be prepared.

Operating room and environment

Many microorganisms are airborne and any movement within the operating theatre will disperse them. Good ventilation is necessary as hot, humid conditions are a great threat to asepsis. Clean procedures should be performed first on the operating list because microorganisms from contaminated sites will remain in the air. The operating room itself must be easily cleaned and should contain minimal furniture.

Equipment and instruments

All equipment and instruments used in the operative site must be sterile. There must be a fresh set of instruments for each operation.

Personnel

The more people present in theatre, the greater is the likelihood of infection. All theatre personnel should wear theatre clothing: caps, masks, scrub suits and antistatic footwear (Figure 24.1). These are only worn in the designated theatre area. In addition, those who are in the surgical team should prepare their hands aseptically and wear sterile gowns and gloves.

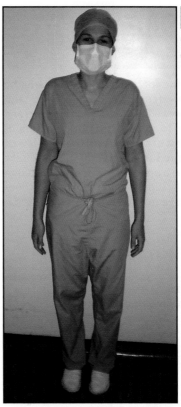

24.1

Correct attire for the operating theatre.

The patient

The patient is a source of contamination, especially as most animals are covered in hair. The source of microorganisms may be endogenous or exogenous:

- **Endogenous** – originate from within the body of the patient
- **Exogenous** – found on the outside of the animal, i.e. the skin and coat. This term is also used with reference to environmental sources of microorganisms (e.g. air, equipment).

It does not necessarily follow that introduction of microorganisms will result in an infected wound. Microorganisms can and will enter any wound that has been exposed to air, but whether infection follows depends on several variable factors.

Factors influencing wound infection

- **Virulence** (disease-producing ability) of the organism and resistance of the patient (see Chapter 5).
- **Duration of surgery** – bacterial contamination increases the longer the wound is open (infection rate doubles for every hour of operative time).
- **Surgical technique** – excessive trauma to tissues and damage to vascular supply may increase the likelihood of infection.
- **Impaired host resistance** – may increase the risk of infection if it is due to drugs, nutrition or underlying disease.
- **Contamination of the wound** – surgical wounds are classified with respect to their potential for contamination and infection (see Chapter 25).

The operating theatre suite

The design and layout of the operating theatre will rarely be within the control of the veterinary nurse. It is important, however, to have some knowledge of ideal requirements and desirable features in order to appreciate differing standards and to try to make the best of existing facilities. The layout of rooms within the theatre suite is important for the sake of asepsis. There should be a one-way traffic system, so that the surgical team and sterile supplies enter through one door and unscrubbed personnel enter and leave through a separate doorway.

The theatre suite components

- Operating theatre.
- Anaesthetic and preparation area.
- Area for washing and sterilizing equipment.
- Sterile storage area.
- Scrubbing-up area.
- Changing rooms.
- Recovery room.

The operating theatre

Many practices have just one operating theatre, which is used for all surgery. Larger hospitals may have theatres that are used specifically for particular types of surgery, such as orthopaedic work, general surgery and 'dirty' surgery (e.g. dental work).

The size of the theatre will depend on the purpose for which it is intended. If it is to be used for simple routine surgery, it can be quite compact; if it is to be used for orthopaedic surgery, a large amount of surgical equipment may be needed. If the theatre is too small, working conditions will be compromised and it may be difficult to maintain a high standard of asepsis. It has to be large enough to accommodate the patient, anaesthetic equipment, surgical instrument trolley, other equipment and personnel.

There are several other requirements that are essential, or at least desirable, as follows.

Basic design and materials

The operating theatre should be an end room, not a thoroughfare to other rooms.

It must be easy to clean. Walls and floors must be made of impervious non-staining materials; floors should be non-slip and hard wearing. Walls and ceiling should be painted with a light-coloured 'waterproof' paint. The corners and edges of all walls should be covered to facilitate cleaning.

Ceramic tiles are often used on walls in operating theatres. These are hard-wearing and easy to keep clean, but crevices between the tiles will be difficult to keep clean and may harbour dust and bacteria. The use of drains should be avoided within the operating theatre itself, but may be useful in a minor operation area.

Lighting and electricity

Good lighting is essential. Advantage should be taken of natural daylight. Ideally, lighting should be concealed within the ceiling, with additional side lights on the wall and an overhead theatre light.

There should be a good supply of electrical sockets (in waterproof casing), preferably recessed into the wall.

Heating and air-conditioning

Heating is an important consideration, since anaesthetized animals are unable to control their own body temperature. The ambient temperature should be between 15 and 20°C. Fan heaters cause air and dust movement and should be avoided. Modern wall-mounted radiators are widely available and a common choice for heating. They are, however, difficult to keep clean and will easily trap and harbour dust and dirt behind them. To avoid this, radiators should be included in the thorough weekly cleaning regime. Panel heating within the walls is ideal, but expensive.

A system of air-conditioning and ventilation is necessary. It is recommended that a positive ventilation system is used that can provide a minimum of 12 air changes per hour to ensure that a continuous fresh supply of air is provided to the theatre suite.

Doors and windows

The rooms should have double swing doors, which should normally be kept closed.

There should be no clear-glass window to the outside, as this will be distracting. Windows should not be opened, as this will be a threat to asepsis.

Operating table

The operating table should be adjustable to facilitate positioning of the patient and to suit the height of the surgeon. The base of the table may be static or maintained on wheels for easy moving. The table should be able to be raised and lowered and tilted as necessary. There is usually a hydraulically operated pump to adjust the height, and some electrically operated pumps are also available.

Operating tables for equine patients

It is important that special consideration is given to the operating table when carrying out equine surgical procedures as patients are likely to be large, heavy and difficult to move.

Choice will depend on:

- The number and type of surgeries performed
- The size of the operating theatre
- Financial considerations
- Personal preference.

There are a range of equine operating tables available:

- **Mobile** (Figure 24.2):
  - Most versatile and most popular in the UK
  - Needs to be easily movable by two or three people
  - Has battery- or mains-operated hydraulics
- **Fixed hydraulic:**
  - Not versatile
  - Positioning of horse, equipment or surgical access may be difficult
  - Usually there is an associated 'sump' in the floor, where the hydraulic ram and table are accommodated when not in use. This can become a haven for dirt, bacteria, etc.

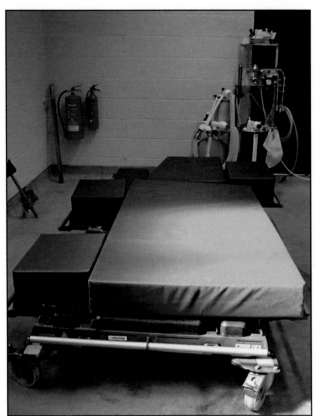

24.2 A mobile operating table suitable for equine patients.

- **Inflatable:**
  - Least expensive
  - Restrictive for positioning of horse, equipment and surgical access
  - Often too unstable for many procedures, especially orthopaedic surgery

Other equipment

There should be no shelving and minimal furniture as this will harbour dust. All equipment, including the operating table, must be easy to clean.

An X-ray viewer, preferably flush with the wall, is an important fixture in the operating theatre.

An air supply for power tools may be needed. This should ideally be piped into the theatre from cylinders housed outside it. Anaesthetic gases can be delivered in the same way. A scavenging system for anaesthetic waste gases will also be necessary (see Chapters 2 and 23). A wall clock is required to aid anaesthetic monitoring and timing of surgery.

A dry-wipe board is useful for recording details such as swab numbers, suture details and blood loss.

Anaesthetic preparation area

There should be a separate area where the induction of anaesthesia (see Chapter 23) and other preoperative procedures (e.g. clipping, catheterization of the bladder and preparation of the surgical site) can be carried out. It should lead directly into the operating theatre.

In the case of the equine patient, the anaesthetic preparation area should be large enough to accommodate horses of all sizes but not so large that a horse can move at speed when recovering from anaesthesia (Figure 24.3). The walls should be padded (usually PVC or rubber-coated), with

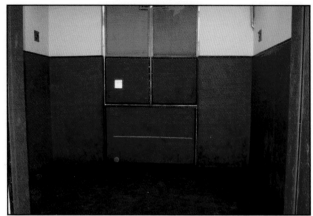

24.3 Induction box that can be used for safely inducing anaesthesia and for postoperative recovery of horses. (Courtesy of Carolyne Sheridan)

rounded corners and curved borders to the floor. The floor should be non-slip and slightly compressible (usually rubberized) to minimize potential injury during induction and recovery. Some clinics have a padded gate system to trap the horse during induction against the box wall. This swings on a set of robust hinges and can be opened as the horse gradually slumps to the floor.

Areas for washing and sterilizing equipment

There needs to be a separate room or area where dirty instruments are washed and another separate area where clean instrument kits and other equipment can be packed and sterilized. These areas should be situated close to the operating theatre but away from the sterile storage area. They should include sterilization facilities and possibly an ultrasonic instrument cleaner. A washing machine and tumble drier will be required to facilitate specific cleaning of theatre scrub suits, gowns and drapes. Ideally this should be in another closed room (possibly adjacent to the sterilization area), but situated furthest away from the operating theatres to confine the dust created when laundering such items.

Sterile storage area

Sterile supplies should be stored in closed cupboards away from the instrument washing area, but adjacent to theatre. Instrument trolleys can be laid out here prior to surgery. Entry should be directly into the theatre suite.

Scrubbing-up area

There should be a separate scrub room within the theatre suite, but outside the theatre itself. This should lead directly into the sterile preparation area and theatre. Swing doors, which can be foot operated, should separate the rooms.

Changing rooms

Changing rooms for personnel should be situated at the entrance to theatre. It is useful to have a red line delineating the sterile area and appropriate notices displayed to indicate these areas. Footwear for use in theatre should be placed at the entrance to theatre beyond the red line. This barrier should be adhered to at all times to ensure a high level of asepsis.

Recovery room

A room where the patient can recover following surgery may be situated near the operating theatre suite. It should be quiet and warm and should contain essential equipment to deal with any postoperative emergencies that might occur (see Chapter 23). Good observation of this area is also essential.

In equine patients the anaesthetic preparation area (see above) usually doubles as a recovery box. There should be some means of monitoring the patient during recovery safely from the outside of the box (e.g. CCTV or a porthole). Ropes and a pulley system can be used to allow assisted recovery in horses.

Hazards in the operating theatre

The avoidance of accidents to patients and staff in the operating theatre is of the utmost importance. The Health and Safety at Work etc. Act 1974 and the COSHH regulations (see Chapter 2) are designed to ensure safety in the workplace, including the operating theatre.

With the increasing use of new and sophisticated equipment, the risk of accidents has also increased. It is very important that all nursing staff are instructed in the use and maintenance of all new equipment. It is also important that all equipment is serviced regularly and tested for electrical safety to minimize risks.

- All staff should be aware of the dangers associated with inhaling anaesthetic gases. An anaesthetic gas-scavenging system must be fitted or absorptive filters used to minimize exposure to gases (see Chapter 23). In the operating theatre, nursing staff will be exposed to various chemicals. Appropriate protective clothing, masks and gloves should be worn.

Maintenance and cleaning of the operating theatre

A routine cleaning programme is essential for a high standard of asepsis to be maintained. Cleaning protocols should be adopted and strictly followed. These protocols should include details of all the daily, weekly and monthly tasks to be completed. Disinfectant agents are discussed in Chapter 12.

Cleaning equipment

Cleaning utensils should be designated specifically for use in the theatre suite only. They should be rinsed and allowed to dry after use. Buckets should always be emptied and rinsed out. All utensils should be stored in a separate cupboard or confined room away from the sterile area.

Cleaning equipment such as cloths and mop heads should be washed daily in a washing machine. Cloths should be discarded after a short time and replaced with new ones. Autoclavable mop heads are also available.

Routine cleaning of the operating theatre

- **At the beginning of each day:**
  - All the surfaces, furniture and equipment in the theatre suite should be damp-dusted, using a dilute solution of disinfectant (a dry duster would simply move dust around the room). Damp-dusting is performed to remove any traces of dust particles that may have settled overnight on the surfaces and equipment within the theatre.
- **Between cases:**
  - The operating table, stands, instrument trolleys, kick buckets, monitoring equipment and leads should be wiped clean using an appropriate disinfectant
  - The floors should be mopped clean if dirty. The operating table should be moved to allow cleaning if the floor has become contaminated with any fluid during a procedure
  - All waste material should be removed and disposed of appropriately.
- **At the end of the day:**
  - The floors in all rooms of the theatre suite should be vacuumed or swept to remove debris and loose hair
  - They should then be either wet-vacuumed or washed using disinfectant
  - All waste material should be removed and disposed of
  - Surfaces, equipment, operating tables, lights and scrub sinks should all be thoroughly washed down with disinfectant.
- **Once a week** there should be a more thorough deep cleaning session of the operating theatres:
  - All equipment should be removed from the room and the floors and walls should then be scrubbed
  - A disinfectant with detergent properties that will remove organic matter and that is active against a wide range of bacteria, including *Pseudomonas* spp., should be used
  - After removing any excess solution, the disinfectant should be allowed to dry on the surface rather than being rinsed off, for longer residual activity
  - All equipment should be meticulously wiped over.

Cleaning checks

A selection of swab samples for bacterial culture should be taken from a variety of sites in the operating theatre from time to time to ensure efficacy of the cleaning regime and to alert staff to any potential problems. There should be no growth of bacteria from sterilized equipment and most other sites (e.g. sinks, operating tables, trolleys, drains, positioning aids, surfaces, and lights).

The surgical patient

Surgical cases may be categorized as follows:

- **Elective** and **non-urgent** – the patient is usually healthy and often young (e.g. ovariohysterectomy, castration, corrective osteotomy)

- **Necessary** or **urgent** – not immediately life-threatening but requiring prompt attention (e.g. fracture repair, gastrointestinal surgery)
- **Emergency surgery** – life-threatening conditions (e.g. abdominal crisis), often traumatic (e.g. chest injury).

The time between admission and surgery will depend on various factors. In the simplest elective procedures, the patient is admitted on the morning of surgery and returns home later that day. Preoperative preparations in these cases are minimal. In others there may be a delay before surgery is performed. Reasons for this may include:

- **Investigative procedures**, e.g. diagnostic tests, radiographic and ultrasonographic studies
- **Fluid therapy or transfusion** – to improve the patient's physiological status before surgery
- **Presence of other injuries** that require treatment before surgery may be undertaken (e.g. thoracic trauma associated with a limb fracture)
- To allow **reduction of swelling/debridement** of wounds – bandaging of fracture site, application of wound dressings, etc.
- **Stabilization** of patient with concurrent metabolic disturbance (e.g. diabetes mellitus, renal disease, hyperadrenocorticism).

Admission of the patient

All relevant details must be recorded on the case records (see also Chapters 1, 9, 15).

- Check the reason for admission.
- Where relevant, identify the site (draw a diagram if necessary).
- Ensure that the owner understands what is to be done and how the patient will look when discharged (e.g. it will have a clipped area and may be wearing a bandage, cast, Elizabethan collar).
- Ensure that the patient is in good general health or that symptoms have not changed since last seen by a veterinary surgeon.
- Ensure that there is a contact telephone number and that an anaesthetic consent form is signed.
- Weigh the patient.
- Fit a plastic identification collar containing the patient's name/number, weight and reason for admission, to minimize the risk of mistakes occurring.

Preoperative preparation of the patient

Withholding food and water

Water should be available at all times up until the time of premedication, where the water bowl can be removed from the patient's kennel. Food is usually withheld for 6–12 hours prior to surgery. This is primarily to prevent regurgitation of food under general anaesthesia or during recovery. A full

stomach could also interfere with the surgical procedure in very young animals, very old animals and those with metabolic disorders, but prolonged withholding of food may be contraindicated. It is preferable for such cases to be placed as early as possible on the surgical list and then fed promptly afterwards to minimize metabolic disturbances and potential problems in the postoperative period.

For equine patients, water should also be provided until immediately prior to surgery. Feed is normally withheld for approximately 12 hours, although hay is sometimes withheld for longer. For some elective laparotomy procedures, e.g. ovariectomy, food may be withheld for 24 hours or more to facilitate surgical access.

Bathing and grooming

Ideally all patients should be bathed before surgery to decrease the risk of contamination, but this is not always feasible. It should be considered in elective orthopaedic procedures such as total hip replacement.

Horses should be groomed to minimize contamination and their tails plaited or covered. It is also advisable to plait manes if they are long.

Clipping the surgical site is necessary for most procedures (except intraoral). It may be carried out before or during anaesthesia (Figure 24.4), depending on patient cooperation, but should not be done more than 24 hours before the scheduled procedure, to avoid bacterial build-up on the patient's skin. Clipping is more commonly performed immediately prior to surgery under general anaesthesia.

Timing	Advantages	Disadvantages
Pre-anaesthesia	Shorter anaesthetic time. Improves asepsis: loose hairs generally shed before surgery. Can give initial skin preparation. Improves operating theatre efficiency	Patient may be uncooperative. Requires two or more people. Trauma to the skin may cause more irritation/site of infection. Clipping more than 12 hours before surgery may increase skin bacteria
During general anaesthesia	Often takes less time. Fewer people required to restrain animal. Desirable with fractious animals or painful/inaccessible sites	Decreases asepsis: small loose hairs are extremely difficult to remove, even with a vacuum cleaner Increases anaesthetic time

24.4 Advantages and disadvantages of clipping pre-anaesthesia and during general anaesthesia.

Considerations for preoperative clipping

- Clipping should be performed away from the operating theatre in a separate preparation area or room to minimize contamination by hair.
- Ensure that clipper blades are in good working order and are clean. Tears made in the skin will cause irritation, which may encourage postoperative licking and scratching and so will predispose the site to infection.
- Clip a large area around the surgical site. Ensure that the clipping is neat (this is what the owner will notice).

continues ▶

continued

- When clipping around a wound, a water-soluble sterile gel should be placed in the wound and on the coat at the edges of the wound to help prevent hair entering the wound. Individual sterile sachets of gel should be used for this, rather than tubes, to prevent contamination from, or of, the wound.
- Clean the clipper blades between patients using a bacteriocidal disinfectant. It may be necessary to sterilize the blades after clipping contaminated sites (e.g. abscesses).
- Do not allow clipper blades to become too hot during use, as this may cause inflammation or excoriation that will not be apparent until the postoperative period. Have a second pair of blades ready so that they can be swapped during procedures.
- Shaving the skin after clipping should be avoided as it can lead to severe excoriation, which encourages postoperative licking, scratching and soreness. Well maintained clippers should provide a close-enough clip to remove the hair adequately.

Administration of an enema

For some surgery (e.g. rectal/colonic) it is desirable to give an evacuant enema prior to surgery. A soap-and-water enema is simplest. The patient may need bathing afterwards to remove faecal contaminants from the skin. See Chapter 17 for more information on enemas.

Other possible preoperative procedures

Prior to anaesthesia:

- Placement of intravenous catheters
- Administration of a premedicant drug, 15 minutes to 1 hour before induction of anaesthesia (see Chapter 23)
- Covering of any wounds not associated with the surgery, to prevent contamination
- Application of a foot/hoof bandage to cover any unclipped areas where surgery involves a limb
- Administration of antibiotic drugs, if indicated; these are often given intravenously at the time of anaesthesia induction, to ensure effective concentrations at the time of surgery
- Flushing of the oral cavity with water to remove food particles and prevent these being introduced into the trachea during intubation. This is especially beneficial in horses.

Once anaesthetized:

- Placement of *additional* venous catheters (e.g. jugular) or of arterial catheters (for anaesthetic monitoring)
- Catheterization of the bladder may be required to:
  - Monitor urine output during and after surgery
  - Minimize risk of soiling during surgery
  - Facilitate access to abdominal organs
  - Prevent risk of bladder perforation or rupture during surgery
- Eye lubrication is necessary for all anaesthetized patients to prevent corneal drying during a procedure. A small amount of eye lubricant should be placed into each eye

prior to the surgery; depending on the length of the procedure, it may be necessary to reapply during surgery
- For perianal surgery, application of a purse-string suture around the anus to prevent contamination by faecal material. The nurse should ensure that this is removed at the end of surgery
- For surgery on distal limbs, application of an Esmarch's rubber bandage and tourniquet to give a bloodless operating field. The time of application must be recorded to ensure that the bandage is not left in place for >45 minutes and to avoid ischaemic injury to the limb
- For oral or nasal surgery, introduction of a throat pack (dampened conforming bandage) to prevent aspiration of blood, mucus, etc.
- For ophthalmic surgery, application of eye drops *immediately prior to* the surgery.

Preparation of horses' feet

Horses' feet are frequently grossly contaminated. It is therefore expedient to scrub and/or pare out the soles and to scrub the hoof walls of all four feet prior to surgery. Shoes are usually removed or padded for safety reasons. The feet may be covered to prevent contamination of the theatre area during surgery (Figure 24.5).

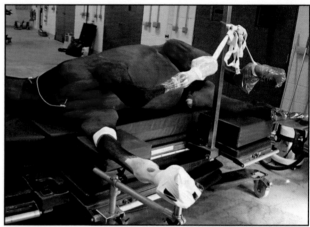

24.5   Preparing a horse for surgery may include covering its feet to prevent contamination of the theatre area.

Where surgery involves the hoof, it is usual to pack the sole and hoof wall. The foot may be prepared 12 hours in advance by a farrier, who will trim and rasp the hoof wall. The foot can also be soaked overnight in an iodine dressing (see Chapter 16), although this can leave deposits of iodine on the foot, which might interfere with radiographic imaging.

Aseptic preparation of the skin

The skin and coat are two of the greatest sources of wound contamination, as it is not possible to remove all bacteria from the skin. The aim is to reduce significantly the number present without damaging the skin itself. Skin bacteria include species of *Staphylococcus*, *Bacillus* and, occasionally, *Streptococcus*.

As antiseptic and detergent properties are required in skin-cleansing agents, surgical scrub solutions such as chlorhexidine and povidone–iodine are ideal. An antiseptic solution (which may be water- or alcohol-based) is then usually applied to give residual bacterial activity. Initial skin preparation should be done in the preparation room. This is not always possible with equine patients; often skin preparation must be completed once the horse has been positioned on the theatre table.

Surgical scrub solutions

The ideal properties of a surgical scrub solution are:

- Wide spectrum of antimicrobial activity
- Ability to decrease microbial count quickly
- Quick application
- Long residual lethal effect against microorganisms
- Remains active and effective in the presence of organic matter
- Safe to use without skin irritation or sensitization
- Economical
- Practical for veterinary use.

Examples of commonly used agents are given in Figure 24.6.

Agent	Properties
Povidone–iodine	Iodine combined with a detergent Broad-spectrum antimicrobial activity (bactericidal, viricidal and fungicidal) May cause severe skin reactions and irritation in some individuals Efficacy impaired by organic matter
Chlorhexidine	Effective against many bacteria (including *Escherichia coli* and *Pseudomonas* spp.) Viricidal, fungicidal and sporicidal properties Effective level of activity in presence of organic material Longer residual activity than povidone–iodine Relatively low toxicity to tissue
Triclosan	Newer agent, claimed to be antibacterial against both Gram-positive and Gram-negative bacteria

24.6 Commonly used surgical scrub solutions.

There are several different techniques that are commonly used.

Skin preparation technique

1. Put on surgical gloves, to prevent contamination of the patient's skin from your hands. It is not necessary, however, for the gloves to be sterile during the initial preparation.
2. Using lint-free swabs, a surgical scrub solution and a little warm water, clean the site, beginning at the proposed incision site and working outwards. Once the edges of the clipped area are reached, discard the swab and take a new one.
3. Continue this procedure until the area is clean, i.e. there is no discoloration or dirt visible on a white swab.
4. Avoid over-wetting the patient. For limb surgery that does not involve the foot, it should be wrapped in a non-sterile cohesive bandage to allow for draping once transferred into the operating theatre. Care should be taken to avoid soaking the coat, as this will increase the risk of 'strike-through' from the drapes, should material drapes be used, and may make the patient hypothermic, especially in the case of small pets. ▶

5. Move the patient into the theatre and position it for surgery. For limb surgery, a limb tie or tape is applied over the bandaged foot and attached to a transfusion stand. This allows preparation around all sides of the limb as the limb is suspended.
6. As the site is likely to have been contaminated to some extent in the transition to the theatre, clean the skin again in the manner previously described. Sterile gloves, saline and swabs are sometimes used, although this is not always necessary. Lint-free swabs should always be used, and never cotton wool, to prevent any residue being left on the skin.
7. The final stage of preparation involves application of an antiseptic skin solution that can ideally be sprayed over the surgical site and allowed to dry on to the skin, e.g. chlorhexidine isopropyl.

Preparation of eyes and mucous membranes

The solutions commonly used for preparation of the skin are likely to be irritant and cause damage to mucous membranes and, in particular, the eye. Dilute povidone–iodine antiseptic solution (0.1–0.2%) is commonly used to irrigate the eye and may also be used on oral and other mucous membranes. It is important to ensure the correct antiseptic solution is used; lathering scrub solutions must not be used as these will cause irritation. Chlorhexidine solutions have been shown to be more irritant to the surface of the cornea. Alcohol-based solutions should not be used on this sensitive tissue.

Some surgeons do not advocate clipping around the eye for intraocular surgery but instead use adhesive drapes to protect the eye from the hair and skin. Others prefer to clip a minimal amount of hair around the eye. A water-soluble gel can be applied to the hair and into the eye prior to clipping. Using clippers with a narrow fine blade will help to prevent hair being introduced into the eye. The skin around the eye is extremely thin and sensitive, and so it is important that the clippers are in good order and great care is taken when clipping. The eye should then be irrigated several times with saline to wash away any loose hair and remaining lubricant from the eye before irrigating with a dilute povidone–iodine antiseptic solution. Sterile cotton buds soaked in dilute povidone–iodine can be used very gently to clean inside the eyelids. The skin surrounding the eye should also be prepared with dilute povidone–iodine.

Positioning the patient for surgery

Patients should ideally be moved into the theatre on a stretcher or trolley ready to be safely positioned on the theatre table. For horses, overhead hoists are used to lift them safely from the induction/recovery box floor on to the operating table and later back to recover (Figure 24.7). Hoists are ideally electrical, with manual backup if necessary. This is particularly important if there is no emergency generator. The hoist is used to lift the patient following the placement of hobbles around the pasterns of the horse.

Most surgeons have individual preferences with regard to positioning of the patient for surgery, but there are some standard positions for specific operations. The veterinary nurse should be familiar with positioning for different surgical

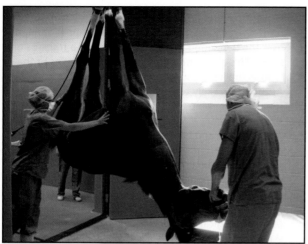

24.7 Using a hoist to move a horse from the induction box to the operating theatre. (Courtesy of Carolyne Sheridan)

techniques and individual variations. When there is any doubt, the nurse should check well in advance of surgery.

Some operating tables have adjustable sides and tilting facilities that assist in positioning the patient (Figure 24.8). If not, the use of additional restraining aids such as troughs, sandbags and tapes will be necessary. Care should be taken to avoid placing heavy sandbags over the limbs or tying tapes tightly, as this could occlude blood supply to the area. Because of the large size of the equine patient (an adult Thoroughbred horse weighs approximately 500 kg), careful positioning and adequate padding are essential, to minimize the risk of postoperative myopathy and neuropathy (see Chapter 23).

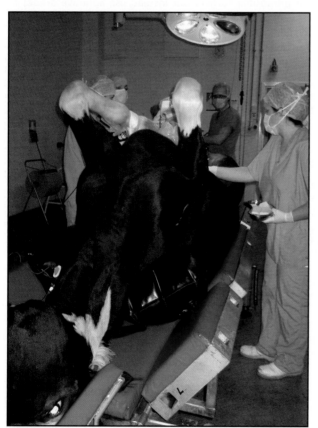

24.8 Adjustable sides and tilting facilities assist in positioning the patient on the operating table. (Courtesy of Carolyne Sheridan)

Preparation of the surgical team

Theatre attire

To maintain asepsis, all those involved in the surgery should change from their ordinary clothes into correct theatre attire before entering the operating theatre suite (see Figure 24.1).

- Theatre wear, which should be worn *only* within the theatre suite, usually consists of a simple two-piece **scrub suit**. A clean suit should be worn each day, and theatre clothing should be changed more frequently if it becomes contaminated.
- Theatre **footwear** should be antistatic and has traditionally consisted of white clogs or wellingtons. These have the advantage of being easy to clean. Canvas shoes are sometimes worn but have the disadvantage of being difficult to clean on a daily basis and should be covered by waterproof overshoes. All footwear should be wiped over with a disinfectant at the end of the day; plastic or rubber footwear can be more thoroughly cleaned in a washing machine and some theatre shoes may be autoclaved. Plastic overshoes are available that fit over normal shoes, but they are not recommended since they wear through in a very short time.
- All personnel should wear a **theatre cap** before entering the theatre suite. All hair should be neatly tucked away inside the hat. To accommodate longer hairstyles and beards, various styles of **headwear** are available. These are usually disposable and paper-based.
- The purpose of **masks** is to filter expired air from the nose and mouth and to prevent transmission of microorganisms from the surgical team to the patient. Masks are effective filters for relatively short periods only and therefore should be changed between operations.

Scrubbing up

Preoperative scrubbing up is a systematic washing and scrubbing of the hands and arms, which is performed by all members of the surgical team before each operation. As it is not possible to sterilize the skin, the aim of the scrubbing-up routine is to destroy as many microorganisms on the surface of the arms and hands as possible, prior to donning a sterile surgical gown and gloves.

Many different scrub routines have been described and no single technique is necessarily better than another. It is recommended that one of the tried and tested regimes is adopted and adhered to strictly.

The scrubbing procedure should take between 5 and 10 minutes: the clock should be checked at the start of the first stage and again at the start of the final stage, to ensure that the procedure has not been rushed and sufficient contact time with the surgical scrub solution has been allowed.

Before scrubbing up, fingernails should be cut short and any nail varnish removed.

Example of a scrub routine

1. Remove watch and jewellery.
2. Adjust the water supply (which should be elbow- or foot-operated) to a suitable temperature and flow.
3. Wash the hands thoroughly using an antimicrobial soap, adopting a good hand washing technique (see Chapter 5). At this stage, clean the nails using a nail pick.
4. Once the hands have been washed, wash the arms up to the elbows. Always keep the hands higher than the elbows so that water drains down towards the unscrubbed upper arms. The purpose of this stage of the procedure is to remove organic matter and grease from the skin.
5. Rinse the hands and then the lower arms, allowing water to wash away the soap from the hands towards the elbows.
6. Using a surgical scrub solution begin the surgical scrub. Use only sufficient water to produce a lather, as bactericidal properties of the scrub solution are dependent on contact time with the skin. Excessive amounts of water will rinse away the scrub solution before it has achieved its aim.
7. Lather the surgical scrub solution over the arms before scrubbing the hands. Take a sterile scrubbing brush and systematically scrub the hands. Scrub the palms of the hand, wrist and four surfaces of each finger and thumb (back, front and both sides) and the nails. Either rinse the brush and use it on the other hand or discard

it and take a second brush. It is not recommended that the backs of the hands and arms are scrubbed as this may lead to excoriation, which predisposes to infection.
8. When both hands have been scrubbed for the correct contact time, drop the brush into the sink. Begin to rinse the hands and arms as before, ensuring that the hands are constantly kept above the elbows to allow the water to drain away from the hands and off the elbows.
9. The final stage is to wash the hands and wrists in surgical scrub solution. This time the scrubbing process is not extended to the elbow, so that there is no danger that a previously unscrubbed area is touched.
10. Rinse the hands and arms as before.
11. Take a sterile hand towel, holding it at arm's length. Use a different quarter to dry each hand and each arm. Then discard the hand towel.

IMPORTANT NOTE
Once the scrubbing up routine has started, the hands must not touch the taps, sink or scrub dispenser. If these are inadvertently touched, the process must start again at Step 3.

Putting on a surgical gown

There are two different types of gown: back-tie and side-tie. The technique for putting on the gown is similar for both, with slight variations (Figure 24.9).

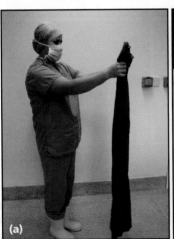
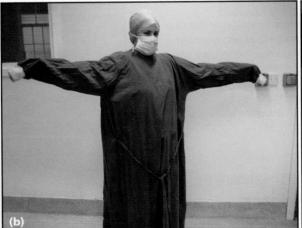
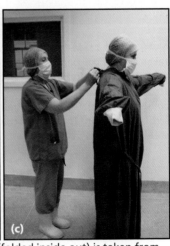
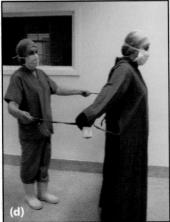

24.9 Putting on a sterile gown. **(a)** The sterile gown (folded inside out) is taken from its sterile pack, held at the shoulders and allowed to fall open. **(b)** One hand is slipped into each sleeve. No attempt should be made to try to pull the sleeves over the shoulder or to readjust the gown, as this will lead to contamination of the hands or outside of the gown. **(c)** An unscrubbed assistant should pull the back of the gown over the shoulders (touching only the inside surface of the gown) and secure the ties at the back. **(d)** With the hands retained within the sleeves, the waist ties should be picked up and held out to the sides. In the case of a **back-tying gown**, the unscrubbed assistant will then take the ends of the waist ties and secure them at the back. The back of the gown is now no longer sterile and must not come into contact with sterile equipment, drapes and gowns.

continues ▶

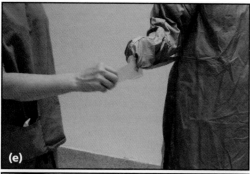

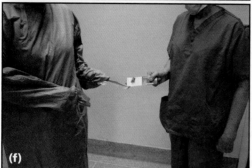

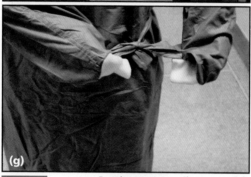

24.9 *continued* Putting on a sterile gown. **(e)** In the case of a **side-tying gown**, the unscrubbed assistant takes hold of the paper tape on the longer waist tape and takes the tie around the back to the opposite side. **(f)** The scrubbed person then pulls the tape, so that the paper tape comes away. **(g)** The gown is tied at the waist by the scrubbed person. This type of gown provides an all-round sterile field.

Putting on surgical gloves

Three methods are available: closed gloving, open gloving and the plunge method.

Closed gloving

The hands are kept inside the sleeves of the gown while gloving takes place. The outside of the gown never comes into contact with the hands. This technique has the advantage that it minimizes the chances of contaminating the gloves, since the outside of the gloves do not contact the skin. This method of gloving should be used for all surgical operations, to ensure a high level of asepsis is maintained throughout.

Open gloving

This method of gloving is used when only the hands need to be covered and is not routinely used for gloving and gowning. The technique has the disadvantage that the gloves are relatively easily contaminated by skin contact.

Closed gloving procedure

1. Hands remain within the sleeves of the gown. The glove packet is turned so that the fingers point towards the body. (The right glove will now be on the left and *vice versa*.)
2. The glove is picked up at the rim of the cuff of the glove.
3. The hand is turned over so that the glove lies on the palm surface with fingers of the glove still pointing towards the body.
4. The rim is picked up with the opposite hand.
5. It is then pulled over the fingers and over the dorsal surface of the wrist.
6. The glove is then pulled on as the fingers are pushed forwards.

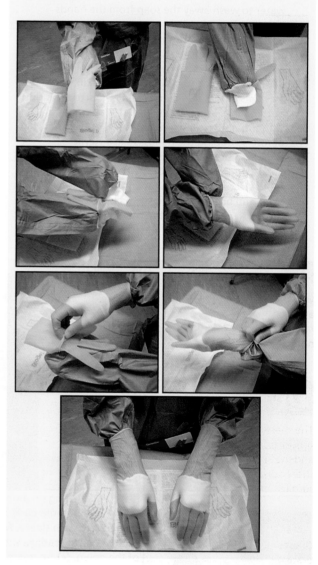

Open gloving is used for the following procedures:

- Jugular catheter placement
- Urinary catheter placement
- Administration of local blocks and epidurals
- Oesophagostomy and pharyngostomy feeding tube placement
- Draining any thoracic, abdominal or wound drains.

Open gloving procedure

1. The glove pack is opened by an assistant.
2. With the left hand, the right glove is picked up by the turned-down cuff, holding only the inner surface of the glove.
3. The glove is pulled on to the right hand. Do not unfold the cuff at this stage.
4. The gloved fingers of the right hand are placed under the cuff of the left glove and pulled on to the left hand, holding only the outer surface of this glove.
5. The rim of the left glove is hooked over the thumb whilst the cuff of the gown (if worn) is adjusted.
6. The cuff of the left glove is pulled over the cuff of the gown (if worn) using the fingers of the right hand.
7. The final steps are then repeated for the right hand.

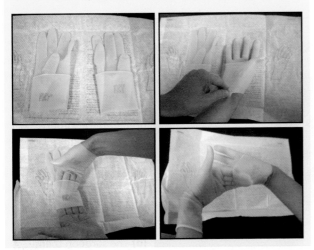

Plunge method

With this method the sterile glove is held open by a scrubbed assistant and the hand is inserted. There is a risk of contaminating both personnel involved; therefore this technique is not commonly employed in veterinary operating theatres.

Draping the patient

The reason for draping the patient is to maintain asepsis by preventing contamination of the surgical site from the hair and the immediate environment. Drapes must therefore cover the entire patient and operating table, leaving only the surgical site exposed.

Types of drape

Drapes may be disposable or re-usable. Ideally, disposable drapes should be used in preference to re-usable material drapes as they have many advantages. The relative advantages of each type are shown in Figure 24.10.

Disposable drapes

There are many different varieties available. Disposable drapes are usually paper-based and water-repellent and can be purchased pre-sterilized. Cheaper varieties tend to be non-conforming and may tear easily. Many commercial brands are of high quality, however, and reasonably affordable and their use is highly recommended for all surgical procedures.

Type of drape	Advantages	Disadvantages
Disposable	Labour-saving. Less laundry. Pre-sterilized. Usually very water-repellent. Always in perfect condition. Cost of drape charged to client	Initial outlay more expensive. Cheaper brands can be less conforming. Large stock needed
Re-usable drapes	Cheaper, although cost of laundering needs to be considered	Porous: all fluids leak through, leading to a break in asepsis. Time-consuming: washing and folding. Danger of threads detaching and gaining access to wounds. After repeated use quality becomes poor

24.10 Advantages and disadvantages of disposable and re-usable drapes.

Adhesive edges are useful for draping difficult areas. Good disposable drapes tend to be more conformable than cotton drapes and the high water resistance prevents bacterial strikethrough. They also help maintain body temperature during surgery.

Re-usable drapes

These are usually made from linen or cotton/polyester mixes. They may be custom-made to suit practice needs. Their main disadvantage is the higher risk of strikethrough when wet and thus increased risk of break in aseptic technique. This type of drape may appear to be more cost-effective than disposables but the expense of laundering and re-sterilizing after each use needs to be taken into consideration.

Draping the surgical site
Plain drapes

Four rectangular drapes are used to create a 'window' (**fenestration**) for the surgical site (Figure 24.11). The fenestration created can be of any size. The first drape should be placed between the surgeon and the near side of the table. A drape is then placed over the opposite side of the patient (i.e. away from the surgeon). Drapes are subsequently placed over both ends. They are then secured in place using towel clips.

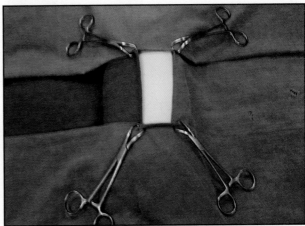

24.11 Draping the surgical site. Plain drapes are first placed longitudinally on both sides of the operating table. More drapes are then placed over each end and secured by towel clips.

Fenestrated drapes

Fenestrated drapes achieve the same effect as the plain drapes in leaving a surgery window, but the window is already formed in a single ready-made drape. Fenestrated drapes can be large enough to cover the entire animal and table top. A selection of different-sized fenestrations are needed to cater for different surgical sites.

Adhesive 'barrier' drapes

Sterile, clear, adhesive plastic sheets are sometimes placed over the surgical site. Standard drapes are applied in the usual way, and the adhesive drape is then placed over the skin and the entire draped fenestration. The skin incision is made through the adhesive material. These are particularly useful as they ensure a high level of aseptic technique is maintained,

as the patient's skin is completely covered by the drape and is therefore not touched by the surgical team. This type of drape is also completely water-resistant and helps to keep the patient dry during the surgical procedure. This is particularly useful when large volumes of fluid are required for lavage.

Draping limbs

There are various ways of draping a limb for surgery, one of which is shown in Figure 24.12.

Sub-draping

Additional towels are sometimes used to protect the incision site from contamination. They are applied to each side of the incision by towel clips. The towel is then folded back over the towel clips.

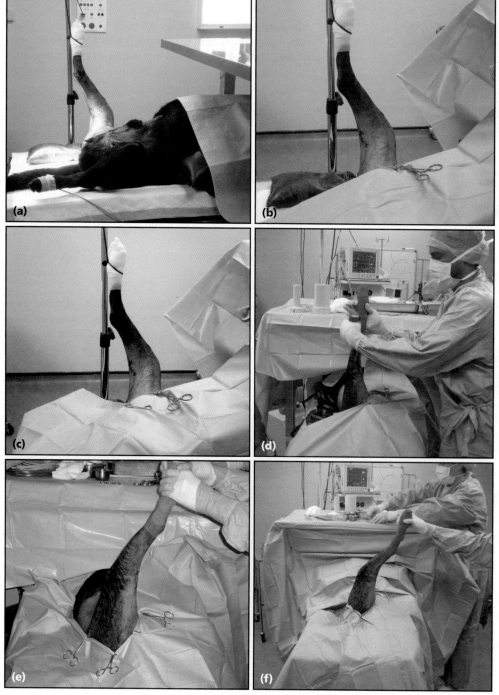

24.12 Draping a limb for surgery.
(a) The patient lies on the operating table with the limb suspended using a tie and transfusion stand. The patient is then prepared for surgery.
(b) The instrument trolley is covered and the first drape is placed between the surgeon and the operating table. **(c)** A second drape is placed over the end of the table.
(d) The surgeon then wraps the foot with sterile cohesive bandage. **(e)** The scrubbed assistant then continues to suspend the limb by holding the foot on the draped side of the table. A third drape is placed on the far side of the table. **(f)** The final drape is placed between the limb and the instrument trolley.

Surgical assistance

The theatre nurse has two main roles: as a scrubbed nurse and as a circulating nurse.

- A **scrubbed nurse** has scrubbed up for surgery and wears sterile theatre clothing so that they can work next to the operative field
- A **circulating nurse** has not scrubbed up with the surgical team.

Duties of a circulating nurse

- Helping to prepare theatre, instruments and equipment for surgery.
- Tying the surgical team into gowns.
- Helping to position the patient on the table.
- Preparation of the surgical site.
- Connecting the apparatus (diathermy, suction, airlines, etc.).
- Opening packs of sutures, instruments, etc.
- Counting swabs, sutures, etc. with the scrubbed nurse.
- Being in theatre at all times when surgery is in progress.
- Assisting the anaesthetist.
- Preparing postoperative dressings.
- Helping to move the patient to recovery.
- Helping to clear theatre at the end of surgery.

Scrubbed nurse

The role of the scrubbed nurse is an extremely important one and requires rigid adherence to a set of rules. It is very easy to make mistakes if corners are cut or changes made. It is important that the nurse possesses knowledge of the surgical procedure that is to be performed, so that the needs of the surgeon can be anticipated.

- It is essential to know exactly what instruments and equipment are on the trolley at the start and throughout surgery.
- All swabs, sutures, needles, etc., must be counted before surgery begins and again before the wound is closed, to prevent any items being accidentally left within a wound cavity.
- The nurse should watch the operation carefully in order to anticipate the surgeon's needs.
- Instruments should be passed to the surgeon so that they are ready to be used, i.e. not upside down.
- Instruments should be returned to the same place on the trolley each time so that the nurse knows exactly where they are. They should not be left around the surgical site, because they are likely to fall on the floor and because they will not be immediately to hand when needed.
- Instruments should be wiped over with a dry swab when they are returned to the trolley.
- Only one swab should be given to the surgeon at any time and the nurse must keep a constant check on the number of swabs used.
- Swabs should be applied firmly to a bleeding site, without wiping across the tissue, which may both damage the tissue and disturb a clot.

- All tissues should be handled gently to avoid trauma. Viscera in particular should be handled very carefully.
- One of the nurse's roles may be to irrigate the tissues with warmed saline to prevent desiccation, particularly during long operations.
- On completion of surgery, the nurse should ensure that all instruments, needles and swabs are returned to the trolley and that needles, blades and glassware are disposed of safely.

Preparing an instrument trolley

An instrument trolley is made from stainless steel and is used as either a dressing or surgical instrument trolley. It has removable and reversible shelves and a guard rail around it. The Mayo trolley is a type of instrument trolley with a tray that is removable for cleaning, is height adjustable and pivots. The framework of this trolley is normally mounted on four swivel brake castors.

Surgical instruments may be laid out on instrument trolleys, for use during surgery (Figure 24.13). A disposable water-resilient plastic drape should ideally be used to cover the trolley first; these can be purchased relatively cheaply and are available pre-sterilized. Should pre-packed plastic trolley drapes not be available, re-usable drapes can be used but, due to the higher risk of bacterial strikethrough, the top of the metal instrument trolley must first be covered with a waterproof sterile drape. Instrument sets may be packed in trays, complete with drapes, swabs, blades, etc.; in these cases the outer wrappings of the set can be unfolded to cover the surface of the trolley (see below).

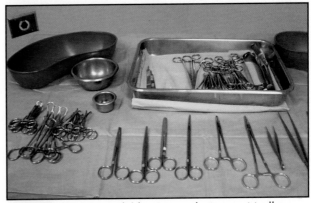

24.13 Instruments laid out on an instrument trolley, ready for use.

The trolley should be prepared immediately prior to use. The longer the instruments are exposed to air, the greater the chance of contamination from the environment or personnel. If there is a delay once the trolley has been laid out, a sterile drape should be placed over the top.

- Trolleys can be prepared by a scrubbed nurse at the beginning of a procedure, allowing the surgeon to scrub, gown and drape the patient in the meantime.
- Alternatively, a circulating nurse can lay out the instruments on the trolley using sterile Cheatle forceps. This is not the preferred method, however, as there is greater risk of the trolley becoming contaminated, as the circulating nurse is unsterile and would be leaning over the sterile draped surface to open instruments.

Care of the patient during surgery

It is important to remember that underneath the drapes is a live patient. Care must be taken by the surgical team to avoid leaning on the animal's chest, which may compromise breathing in a small patient. Careful positioning of towel clips is important to avoid delicate structures such as the eye, which cannot be seen once drapes have been placed.

Attention should be paid to the conservation of heat, especially in the small or very young. Warming devices should ideally be used in all anaesthetized patients; 'Bair Hugger' warming units work well by circulating warm air close to the patient via a blanket (Figure 24.14). Insulation (e.g. bubble-wrap) is useful, particularly around peripheral limbs and the tail, and warmed intravenous and irrigation fluids should be encouraged. Direct heat (e.g. hot-water bottles) should be avoided during both surgery and recovery periods, as the unconscious animal cannot move away if this is too hot. Serious burns can occur, which will not become apparent until the postoperative period.

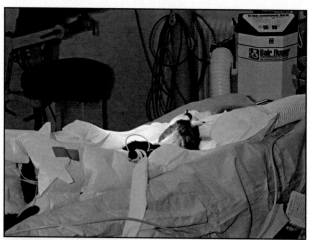

24.14 Warm air units, such as this Bair Hugger, may be used to keep the patient warm during surgery.

Careful positioning of the animal on the table is also important, to avoid postoperative complications. The patient's core temperature should be monitored throughout the surgical procedure. Other intraoperative care is described in Chapter 25.

Care of the postoperative patient

The patient should not be left unattended until it is conscious. The endotracheal tube is usually removed just before the cough reflex returns (see Chapter 23). The animal should be watched closely to ensure that an adequate airway is maintained once the tube has been removed, especially in brachycephalic breeds or following airway surgery. Cats should be observed closely for any signs of laryngospasm following endotracheal tube removal. A source of oxygen and a means of ventilation should be available during this time in case any problems arise. Colour of the mucous membranes and the presence or absence of respiratory noise and effort will be indicators of effective ventilation by the animal. The ability to maintain body temperature is lost under anaesthesia and so steps should be taken to prevent or reverse hypothermia.

Special considerations for the postoperative equine patient

Horses should not be left unobserved until they are safely back on their feet. The endotracheal tube is usually removed once the swallowing reflex has returned (see Chapter 23). A nasal tube is usually placed when the endotracheal tube is removed to ensure a patent airway. It is not unusual for a horse (especially when it has been positioned in dorsal recumbency) to develop pharyngeal or laryngeal oedema in the immediate postoperative period; placement of a nasotracheal tube enables passage of air. Oxygen is also often given in the early stage of recovery, ideally via a Hudson Demand valve. Horses that have undergone major nasal or sinus surgery, associated with major nasal haemorrhage, are usually fitted with an uncuffed recovery tube, with a heavy large end (made from plaster of Paris wrapped around the tube), that can be left in place until the horse is standing or at least in sternal recumbency. This will avoid inhalation of large blood clots, which can block the larynx and make the horse panic during recovery. Suction can also be used to maintain a blood-free airway.

A quiet recovery is desirable for all surgical cases and introduction of newer anaesthetic and sedation techniques has been of great benefit. The horse should be watched closely and there should be sufficient staff available to assist should unexpected problems arise. A headcollar with a long rope should be placed close to the recovery box to allow restraint of the horse should it be ataxic or excited when it rises. However, the risk of injury in the immediate recovery period remains much higher than that in small animals. This may be due to the horse's natural 'flight' instinct and, to some extent, temperament. Once the horse is safely back on its feet, it is usually ready to walk back to its box within 30–45 minutes. It is advisable to have at least two people to support the horse as it walks back.

A small feed or 'mash' is usually given soon after return to the box (once the horse has regained its composure, i.e. after the sedated effect period is over) and only small amounts of hay until normal droppings are passed. The horse should be monitored, as with small animals, for postoperative problems such as pain or haemorrhage, and for urine output. In the horse, particular attention should be paid to gut motility and the passage of faeces. It is not unusual for the horse to develop an impaction following anaesthesia and surgery, possibly associated with drugs administered and the withholding of food and water. If there is any doubt, regular 8-hourly administration of an electrolyte solution via nasogastric intubation may be carried out until faeces becomes normal in consistency. This can avoid a life-threatening caecal impaction.

Haemorrhage

During recovery, the patient should be observed for signs of external haemorrhage (which is usually obvious) or internal haemorrhage (signs of shock).

Recognition of pain

It is important to be able to recognize when an animal is in pain (see Chapter 23). The nurse should obtain instructions from the veterinary surgeon regarding postoperative analgesia.

Application of dressings or casts

Many orthopaedic and some soft tissue cases require post-operative bandages or casts (see Chapter 17). These should be applied before the animal regains consciousness. Care should be taken not to apply them too tightly (especially head and ear dressings). Bandages should be checked again once the patient is awake and in a normal upright position, as a change in position may make the bandage too tight or too loose.

Comfort

- Make sure that the animal has comfortable bedding, especially orthopaedic patients.
- Turn the animal regularly if it is disinclined or unable to turn over by itself.
- Give opportunities for the animal to urinate, or empty the bladder manually if necessary.
- Do not forget to offer food and drink if this is allowed, especially in young and old patients and those that are unable to move easily around the kennel.
- Make sure the area is quiet and warm but that the animal is well observed to monitor for signs of pain, shock, respiratory distress, etc.

Instrumentation

The cost of good-quality surgical instruments is extremely high but they will last for years if handled correctly, whereas cheaper instruments of poor quality will require early replacement.

- **Stainless steel** is the material of choice for most surgical instruments. It combines high resistance to corrosion with great strength and it has an attractive surface finish.
- **Tungsten carbide** inserts are often added to the tips of stainless steel instruments that are used for cutting or gripping, such as scissors and needle-holders. They are very hard and resistant to wear but tend to be expensive. Instruments with tungsten carbide inserts are often identified by their gold-coloured handles.
- **Chromium-plated carbon steel** surgical instruments are commonly used in veterinary practice because they are lower in price. However, they will rust, pit and blister when in contact with chemicals and saline and they tend to blunt quickly.
- **Titanium** is used in instruments for ophthalmic surgery. These instruments need to be handled delicately around the eye and are therefore much lighter in weight. Some ophthalmic surgery requires the use of an operating microscope; titanium instruments reduce the glare produced from the microscope light, allowing the surgeon to have increased visibility during the procedure.

Instrument sets

Instrument sets are made up to suit individual requirements and they vary from one veterinary practice to another. Some practices have sets for specific procedures (e.g. bitch spay set). Others have a standard instrument set that is used for all operations, to which other instruments will be added depending on the procedure. Often a smaller set will be available for minor procedures such as a cat spay. It is important that each of the standard instrument sets contains the same number and type of instruments so that the surgical team always knows what instruments they will have and so that it is easy to check that all are present at the end of the procedure. Instrument sets can be colour-coded by application of a piece of instrument identification adhesive tape. Figures 24.15 to 24.18 list suggested contents for various instrument sets required for soft tissue, orthopaedic and ophthalmic surgery, but these are only guidelines. Dental instruments are described in Chapter 27.

Instrument/equipment	Quantity
Scalpel blade handle no. 3	1
Dissecting forceps: • Rat-tooth fine (Adson) • Rat-tooth heavy • Dressing forceps (Debakey)	1 1 1
Mayo scissors – straight or curved	1
Metzenbaum scissors	1
Artery forceps	10
Mosquito forceps	5
Allis tissue forceps	4
Suture scissors	1
Needle holders	1
Langenbeck retractors	2
Gelpi retractors	2
Backhaus towel-holding forceps	10
Poole suction tip	1
Gallipot	1
Kidney bowl	2
Swabs (radiopaque) 10 cm x 10 cm	10
Additional instruments and equipment that may be required for general surgery	
Monopolar electrocautery handpiece	1
Scalpel blades no.10 and/or no.15	1 of each
Suction tubing	1

24.15 Standard instrument set.

Abdominal surgery
Self-retaining retractors; Doyen's bowel clamps; long dissecting forceps; long artery forceps (e.g. Roberts); towels to pack abdomen
Thoracic surgery
Rib cutters; Finochietto rib retractors; periosteal elevator; chest drain; suture wire; oscillating saw if sternotomy approach; lobectomy clamps; long-handled artery forceps (e.g. Roberts); rib raspatory

24.16 Additional instruments required for abdominal and thoracic surgery.

General
Osteotome; Gigli wire and handles; chisel; periosteal elevator; curette; hand drill; gouge; mallet; Hohmann retractor; putti rasp; hacksaw; Lister's bone cutting forceps; bone rongeurs
Power tools
Battery drill; air drill; mechanical bur; oscillating saw
Implants
Stainless steel wire; intramedullary pins; Kirschner wires; rush pins; staples; screws; plates
Bone pinning
Jacob's chuck and key; pin cutters; Steinmann pin
Wire fixation
Stainless steel wire; wire-holding forceps; wire-cutting forceps
Bone staples
Bone staples; staple introducer; staple remover
External fixator
Steinmann pins; Kirschner Ehmer rods; Kirschner Ehmer nuts; pin cutter; drill or Jacob's chuck
Bone plating or screw fixation
Venables/Sherman bone plates; Sherman screws; drill bit; air/hand drill; depth gauge; screw driver; plate bender
ASIF technique
(Association for the Study of Internal Fixation) Dynamic compression plates and screws; bone drills: standard and overdrill; bone tap and handle; drill guide – neutral and loaded; tap sleeve; drill insert; depth gauge; countersink; screwdriver; plate bender or irons

24.17   Additional instruments required for orthopaedic surgery.

- No. 3 scalpel handle
- Scalpel blade sizes 11, 15 or Beaver handle and blades
- Fine dissecting forceps
- Fine scissors
- Corneal scissors
- Capsule forceps
- Vectis
- Iris repositor
- Castroviejo needle-holders
- Eyelid speculum
- Irrigating cannula
- Distichiasis forceps

24.18   Additional instruments required for ophthalmic surgery.

General surgical instruments

There is a wide variety of different surgical instruments available. Veterinary nurses are not expected to be familiar with them all, but a broad knowledge of the names and appearances of the general instruments can be gained by reference to manuals and catalogues. Most of the surgical instruments and equipment used in equine surgery are the same as those used in small animal surgery.

Scalpel

The scalpel is the best instrument for dividing tissue with minimal trauma. Usually scalpel handles with interchangeable disposable blades are used (Figure 24.19). A size 3 handle is commonly used for small animal surgery with blade sizes 10, 11, 12 and 15. A size 4 handle is used for large animal surgery

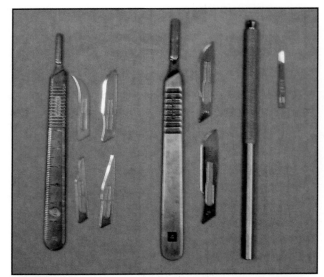

24.19   Scalpel handles and blades. From left to right: size 3 handle and sizes 10, 11, 12 and 15 blades; size 4 handle and sizes 21 and 20 blades; Beaver handle with one blade.

with blade sizes 20, 21 and 22. The primary advantage of disposable blades is consistent sharpness. A scalpel with a blade and handle as a disposable package is available, as is a small, rounded (Beaver) handle with smaller disposable blades, which has gained popularity with ophthalmic surgeons.

Dissecting forceps

These are commonly referred to as thumb forceps (Figure 24.20) and are designed to hold tissue. They have a spring action and the jaws are opposed by holding the metal blades

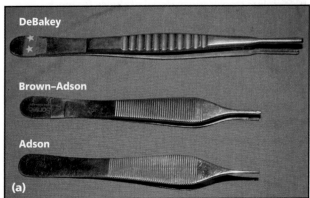

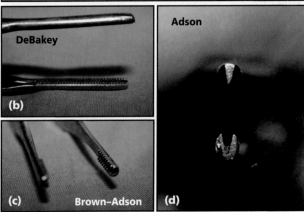

24.20   Dissecting forceps. **(a)** Thumb forceps. **(b–d)** Details of tips.

together. They may have plain or toothed ends. Generally, forceps with plain ends are used for handling delicate tissues such as viscera, whilst toothed forceps are used for denser tissues. Dissecting forceps should be held like a pencil.

Scissors

Operating scissors are available in various lengths and shapes (Figure 24.21). Mayo dissecting scissors are commonly used for routine surgery; the finer, long-handled Metzenbaum scissors tend to be used for more delicate work. Special suture scissors (e.g. Carless scissors) should be used for cutting sutures to prevent unnecessary blunting of dissecting scissors. For removal of sutures, Payne's scissors are used. These are small and curved with the cutting surface of one blade hollowed out to fit under the suture easily. Scissors should be held with the ring finger and thumb inserted in the ring of the scissor and the index finger placed on the shaft to guide the scissors.

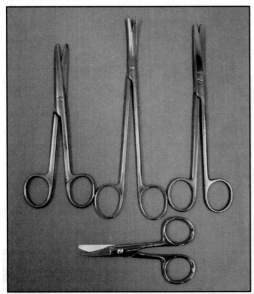

24.21 Surgical scissors. Clockwise from top left: Mayo; Metzenbaum; Carless suture-cutting; Payne's suture removal scissors.

Haemostatic or artery forceps

Artery forceps (Figure 24.22) are designed to clamp blood vessels and thus stop bleeding. They come in several different lengths and shapes. Most have transverse striations to facilitate holding tissue. There are many different patterns of artery forceps. Some of those commonly used include the Spencer Wells, Dunhill, Crile's, Cairn's and Kelly. Mosquito forceps are very small artery forceps for finer blood vessels, the most common type being the Halstead forceps. Like scissors, artery forceps should be held with the ring finger and thumb, using the index finger to steady the forceps.

Bowel clamps

These are designed to clamp bowel in an atraumatic manner. Several different types are available but the most common type used in veterinary surgery is the Doyen's bowel clamp (Figure 24.23).

Sponge-holding forceps

These are designed to hold sponges or swabs for skin preparation prior to surgery (Figure 24.23).

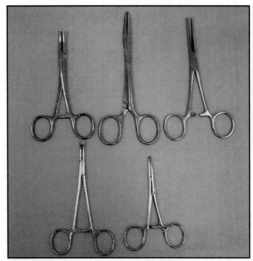

24.22 Artery forceps. Clockwise from top left: Dunhill; Spencer Wells; Kocher's; Criles; Halstead.

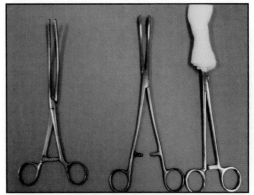

24.23 (Left) Doyen's bowel clamps. (Middle and right) Rampley's sponge-holding forceps.

Tissue forceps

Allis tissue forceps and Babcock's forceps are the most commonly used types of tissue forceps (Figure 24.24). They are designed to grasp tissue with minimal trauma but neither type should be used to grasp and hold viscera, for which more specialized forceps such as Duvall's should be used.

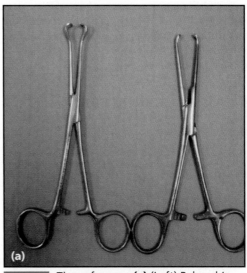

(a)

24.24 Tissue forceps. **(a)** (Left) Babcock's; (right) Allis.

continues ▶

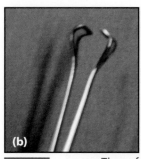
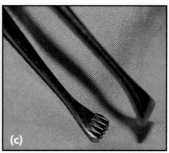

24.24 *continued* Tissue forceps. **(b)** Close-up of Babcock tip. **(c)** Close-up of Allis tip.

Towel clips

Towel clips (Figure 24.25) are used to attach drapes to the patient (see Figure 24.11) and to attach instruments to the operating site. Backhaus and Mayo forceps have a ringed handle and curved, pointed, tongue-like tips. Gray's cross-action forceps, commonly used in veterinary surgery, have a strong spring-clip attachment.

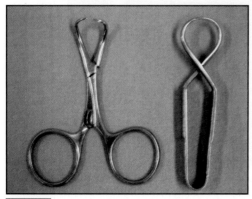

24.25   Towel clips. (Left) Backhaus; (right) Gray's.

Needle-holders

Needle-holders (Figure 24.26) are forceps that are specifically designed for holding suture needles during suturing and for knot tying.

- **Gillies** needle-holders are very commonly used in veterinary surgery. They have a scissor action as well, for cutting the suture ends. Their major disadvantage is that they have no ratchet, and so the needle has to be held in place by gripping the blades tightly.

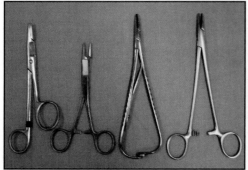

24.26   Needle-holders. From left to right: Gillies; Olsen-Hegar; McPhail's; Mayo-Hegar.

- **Olsen–Hegar** needle-holders also have a cutting edge but have the advantage of a ratchet to hold the needle securely in place. The disadvantage of the scissor edge is that the suture material may be inadvertently cut.
- **McPhail's** needle-holders traditionally have copper inserts in the tips, but those with tungsten carbide inserts are of superior quality. The handles have a spring ratchet so that by squeezing them together the jaws open and release the needle.
- **Mayo–Hegar** needle-holders resemble a pair of long-handled artery forceps. They have a ratchet but no scissor action. This is one of the most popular types of needle-holder.

Retractors

Retractors (Figure 24.27) are used to facilitate exposure of the operating field. They may be hand-held or self-retaining. Hand-held retractors include Langenbeck, Senn and Czerny, Army Navy and malleable. Muscle and joint retractors include Gelpi, West's and Travers. Examples of abdominal wall retractors are Gossett and Balfour; and Finochietto retractors are used for the chest.

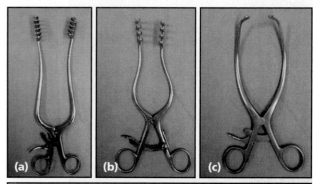
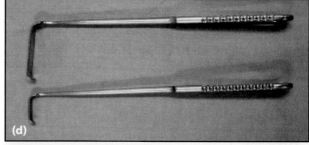
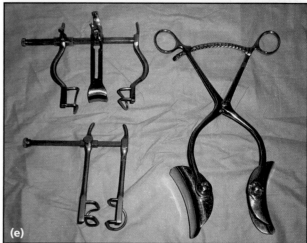

24.27   Retractors: **(a)** Travers; **(b)** Weitlaner; **(c)** Gelpi; **(d)** Langenbeck; **(e)** Abdominal retractors: (clockwise from top left) Balfours, Gosset, Possey. *continues* ▶

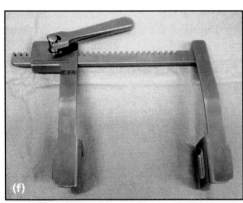

24.27
continued
Retractors:
(f) Thoracic
retractor:
Finochietto.

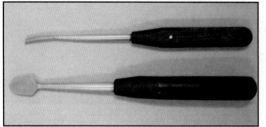

24.29 Small curved and large straight periosteal elevators.

Orthopaedic instruments

Osteotomes, chisels and gouges

These are used to cut or shape bone or cartilage. They are available in a wide variety of sizes. The cutting edge of the osteotome is tapered on both sides, whereas the chisel is tapered on one side only (Figure 24.28). The gouge has a U-shaped edge to remove larger pieces of cartilage or soft bone.

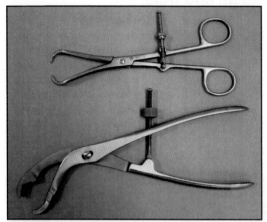

24.30 Bone-holding forceps. Top: Reduction forceps; bottom: Verbrugge.

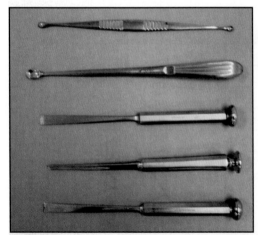

24.28 Some basic orthopaedic instruments. From top to bottom: Volkmann's scoop; curette; chisel; gouge; osteotome.

Curettes

Curettes have an oval-shaped cup (Figure 24.28). They scoop the surface of dense tissue to remove loose or degenerate tissue (e.g. cartilage flaps, necrotic bone). They are also useful for scooping cancellous bone material for a bone graft. The cup has a sharp cutting edge and is available in various sizes.

Periosteal elevators

Periosteal elevators (Figure 24.29) are used to lift periosteum and soft tissue from the surface of bone.

Bone-holding forceps

Bone-holding forceps (Figure 24.30) are designed to grip bone fragments during reduction and alignment in fracture repair.

Bone cutters and rongeurs

Bone rongeurs (Figure 24.31) are used to cut out small pieces of dense tissue such as bone or cartilage. Bone cutters (Figure 24.31) are designed to cut larger pieces of bone.

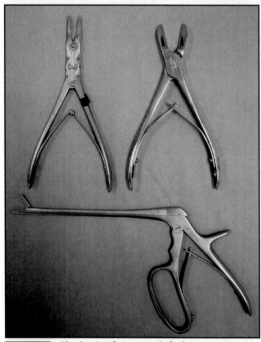

24.31 Clockwise from top left: bone rongeurs; Liston's bone-cutting forceps; arthroscopic rongeurs.

Bone rasps

Bone rasps may be used to remove sharp edges following arthroplasty procedures.

Retractors

Standard retractors are commonly used in orthopaedic surgery. In addition, hand-held Hohmann retractors (Figure 24.32) are often used for retracting muscle, tendons and ligaments.

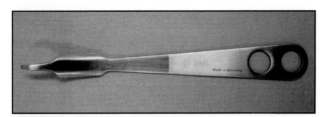

24.32 Hohmann retractor.

Drills, saws and burs

Hand, battery-operated and air drills (Figure 24.33) are commonly used in orthopaedic surgery. Hand drills are useful around delicate structures and when only minimal drilling is required, but for most major surgery a battery-operated or air drill should be a prerequisite. These allow more speed and precision than hand drills. Battery-operated drills tend to be slower and more cumbersome than most of the compact air drills available but they are suitable for most veterinary procedures and are less expensive. They should be recharged after each use.

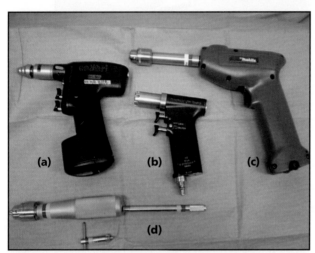

24.33 Orthopaedic drills. **(a)** Battery air drill – autoclavable. **(b)** Air powered drill. **(c)** Battery drill (chuck autoclavable). **(d)** Jacob's Chuck and Steinmann pin protector.

Oscillating saws and mechanical burs are either air or electrically driven. Great care should be taken when connecting attachments and during use. The power supply should not be applied until the couplings are assembled.

Wire forceps

Various wire-cutting and twisting forceps are available for applying cerclage wires and for stabilizing bones with wire.

Gigli wire and handles

These are used in osteotomy techniques to saw through bone with a cheese-wire effect.

Instrumentation for fracture repair

The instruments required for fracture repair depend on the technique that is to be used. Materials used to repair fractures

internally include Steinmann pins, orthopaedic wire, bone plates, screws and external fixator apparatus (Figures 24.34 and 24.35; see also Chapter 25).

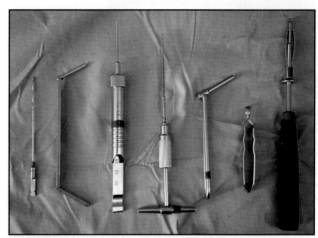

24.34 ASIF (Association for the Study of Internal Fixation) instruments for internal fixation. Instruments in order of use as per ASIF recommendations.

Screw dia. (mm)	Drill (mm) Gliding hole	Drill (mm) (Pilot hole)	Tap (mm)
5.5	5.5	4.0	5.5
4.5	4.5	3.2	4.5
3.5	3.5	2.5	3.5
2.7	2.7	2.0	2.7
2.0	2.0	1.5	2.0

24.35 Drill and bone tap combinations for ASIF screws commonly used in veterinary surgery.

Care and maintenance of surgical instruments

Surgical instruments should be handled carefully at all times. They should not be dropped into trays and sinks or on to trolleys. Special care should be taken of sharp edges and pointed instruments.

Care of new instruments

Most new instruments are supplied dry without lubrication. Before use, it is therefore recommended that they are washed and dried carefully and their moving parts lubricated with a proprietary instrument lubricant.

Cleaning after use

To comply with health and safety legislation, the veterinary nurse must wear protective clothing (i.e. a plastic apron and rubber gloves) when dealing with surgical instruments.

- Sharp items such as needles, glass vials and scalpel blades should be safely disposed of (see Chapter 2) before removing other disposable items such as suture packets and swabs from the instrument trolley.

- Any specialized or delicate equipment should be separated from the general instruments and cleaned separately.
- Large instruments, such as some orthopaedic instruments, should be washed separately from general instruments as they may cause damage to them or be damaged themselves.

Instruments should be cleaned as soon as possible on completion of surgery to prevent blood, tissue debris or saline drying on them, as this will lead to pitting of the surface and subsequent corrosion. Initial soaking or rinsing in cold water is highly effective for this. Hot water should not be used, as it causes coagulation of proteins (e.g. blood). Alternatively, instruments may be soaked in a chemical cleaning solution specifically manufactured for instrument cleaning.

Where indicated, instruments should be dismantled and ratchets or joints opened before immersion.

Instruments should then be cleaned under cool or warm running water, using a hand brush with fairly stiff bristles. Particular attention should be paid to joints, ratchets, serrations etc. Abrasive chemical agents should never be used as they may damage the surface of the instrument. Ordinary soap should also be avoided, as it causes an insoluble alkali film to form on the surface, thus trapping bacteria and protecting them from sterilization.

After this initial washing, instruments should be placed in an ultrasonic cleaner (see below). On completion of the ultrasonic cleaning cycle, the instruments are removed from the machine and are rinsed individually under running water – preferably distilled or deionized. After cleaning, each instrument should be inspected for distortion, misalignment, sharpness and incorrect assembly. Pivot movements, joints and ratchets should also be checked for correct function. The instruments are then dried prior to packing and re-sterilization, as water collecting in trapped areas may lead to corrosion.

Ultrasonic cleaners

Bench-top ultrasonic cleaners suitable for veterinary use are readily available and are relatively inexpensive. They are extremely effective at removing debris from areas inaccessible to brushes (e.g. box joints). They work by the production of sinusoidal energy waves with a vibration frequency in excess of 20,000 vibrations per second. This produces minute bubbles within the cleaning solution. These form on the surface of instruments. As the bubbles implode, energy is released and this breaks the bonds that hold debris on the surface.

Instruments are placed in the wire mesh basket of the ultrasonic cleaner and the unit is filled as per manufacturer's recommendation with a specific ultrasonic cleaning detergent. The basket is placed in the solution, the lid replaced and the unit switched on. Usually a period of approximately 15 minutes is sufficient, although on some machines altering the temperature can reduce this time.

Lubrication

Lubrication of instruments on a regular basis is recommended, particularly after using an ultrasonic cleaner. It is important to use lubricants that are recommended by the manufacturer. Mineral oils and grease must be avoided as they leave a film on the surface under which bacterial spores may be trapped, preventing adequate penetration during sterilization. Antimicrobial water-soluble lubricants (instrument milk) are available: instruments are dipped into the solution for a short period and then removed and allowed to dry. They do not need to be rinsed. Instruments that have been washed in a washer/disinfector that uses de-ionized water do not need lubrication.

Sharpening

- Scissors that become blunt should be returned to the manufacturer for sharpening or sent to a company that specifically offers an instrument sharpening service.
- Drill bits may be re-sharpened but replacement will give a more reliable instrument.
- Oscillating saw blades become worn and blunt and will require replacement.

Cleaning compressed air machines

Compressed air machines should never be immersed in water or put in ultrasonic cleaners. The machine should have detachable parts (drills, saw blades, etc.) that can be cleaned in a standard fashion as already described. The main handpiece should be detached from the air hose and cleaned according to the manufacturer's recommendations.

For metal air drills and oscillating saws it is usually possible to wash the outside of the body of the handset. Care must be taken to avoid water getting into the air hose attachment and internal mechanism of the handpiece. With more delicate air- or battery-powered tools, where this is not recommended, cleaning will usually involve wiping over the instrument thoroughly with a disinfectant cleaning solution, paying particular attention to triggers and couplings. Use of a small brush such as a nailbrush may be necessary to remove debris. The air hose should be wiped over with a damp cloth in a similar fashion and at the same time inspected to check that there is no damage to the outer sheath. The handpiece and hose attachments should be lubricated according to manufacturer's instructions. The machine should then be reassembled, attached to the air supply and run for approximately 30 seconds to allow oil to circulate and ensure patency of the equipment prior to packing and re-sterilization.

Surgical equipment

Suction apparatus

A suction unit in the operating theatre is important for several reasons. It may be used for: aspiration of the oropharynx and nasopharynx during or after surgery; thoracocentesis following surgery; or for suction of fluids and blood during the surgical procedure. Various suction machines are available and a size suitable for individual requirements should be chosen. It is sensible to choose a unit with two bottles (Figure 24.36) so that there is always a spare when one bottle becomes full. Fluid accumulated in a suction container should be disposed of in a sluice sink if possible to prevent the blocking and contamination of normal sinks.

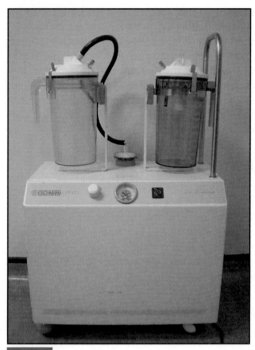

24.36 Suction apparatus with two bottles.

Diathermy

Diathermy is a useful method for coagulation of blood vessels or cutting of tissue during surgery by means of high-frequency alternating electrical current, which produces heat within the tissue at the point of application.

The advantages of diathermy are that it:

- Allows rapid control of haemorrhage and minimizes blood loss (particularly important in very small patients, where even small amounts of blood loss may be life threatening)
- Allows clear visualization of the surgical field
- Helps to minimize surgery time
- Reduces amount of foreign material in the form of ligatures that need to be left in the surgical site.

The nature of the waveform of the applied current used in diathermy can vary the effect from cutting to coagulation:

- Continuous waveforms are employed for cutting tissue
- Interrupted waveforms are used for coagulation.

Diathermy unit

There are several different types of diathermy machine available for surgical use. There are two common types of diathermy: monopolar and bipolar (Figure 24.37).

Monopolar diathermy usually involves a fingerswitch pencil used for cutting and coagulation. This type of diathermy requires the patient to be 'earthed' or 'grounded'. A ground or earth wire transfers the electrical current to a harmless place such as the ground. This 'earth' wire usually takes the form of a plate that is placed under the patient and is connected to the diathermy unit by a cable. If the patient is not sufficiently earthed, the electricity will pass along the line of least resistance, which may be the patient or the surgeon. This may lead to serious burning or electric shock to the patient or surgeon. The earth plate may be disposable or re-usable.

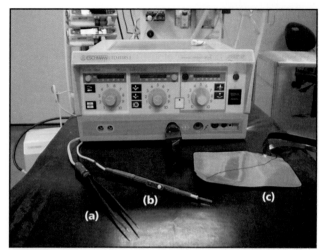

24.37 Diathermy machine. **(a)** Bipolar forceps. **(b)** Monopolar fingerswitch pencil. **(c)** Earth/ground plate.

There must be good contact between the plate and the patient but coupling gel is not usually necessary in animals.

With **bipolar diathermy** the current passes through the tips of the forceps across the tissue. This means a ground/earth plate is not required. The current is usually activated by depression of a foot pedal connected to the machine. Coagulation is achieved by applying the probe or forceps directly to the bleeding vessel or by touching the artery forceps clamping the vessel. Alcohol and other flammable materials should not be used with diathermy, because of the risk of fire.

Care of the diathermy unit

After use, the diathermy earth plate (if of the re-usable type) should be disinfected. The cable and lead should be washed, inspected for patency and re-sterilized. The unit should be serviced and maintained by a qualified engineer.

Endoscopes

There are two types of fibreoptic endoscopes in common use in veterinary practice (see also Chapter 18):

- **Flexible** – used for diagnostic examination of body tracts (e.g. upper respiratory tract, bronchi, urinary tract, oesophagus, stomach, rectum and colon)
- **Rigid** – used for diagnostic evaluation of trachea and bronchi, oesophagus, nasal cavities. Used for evaluation of joints (arthroscopy) and abdominal cavity (laparoscopy).

In small animal practice the flexible endoscope is more commonly used. Many instruments are obtained second hand from the medical field. Whilst this is an excellent source of good-quality inexpensive endoscopes, caution should be employed when purchasing such instruments as it may prove difficult to obtain spare parts for older models when repairs are necessary.

The fragile fibreoptic bundles contained within the endoscope are easily damaged by twisting and bending. The more fibres that are damaged, the less light will be transmitted. A second-hand instrument will almost certainly have some damaged fibres. A separate light source is needed to provide illumination. This may be purchased with the endoscope or separately. Relatively inexpensive portable light sources are readily available. These will usually incorporate an air pump for insufflation and a water bottle for flushing and washing the lens during use.

Video-endoscopes

Arthroscopy and laparoscopy are performed extensively in equine practice and are becoming more common in small animal practice. A video camera may be attached to the endoscope so that a remote and enlarged image is produced on a TV monitor. These video-endoscopes are expensive and require careful maintenance by a qualified engineer.

Care of endoscopes

Endoscopes should be cleaned as soon as possible after use, otherwise blood, mucus, etc. will become dried on and may block the air and fluid channels.

Flexible endoscopes

All modern flexible endoscopes are designed so that the whole instrument can be immersed to allow thorough cleaning. In most older endoscopes, although the tubing is immersible, the handset is not and the internal mechanism will be irreparably damaged if it is soaked. It is very important, therefore, to follow the manufacturer's recommendations with regard to cleaning.

Cleaning a flexible endoscope

1. With immersible endoscopes, a leak test should be performed after use to ensure that it is safe to soak the instrument when cleaning. A leak test kit and instructions will usually be provided by the manufacturer at the time of purchase. If there is evidence of fluid leakage within the endoscope, it should *not* be immersed but should be sent for repair immediately, otherwise the instrument may be permanently damaged. If the leak test is satisfactory, the endoscope may be safely immersed.
2. The outer surface of the endoscope should be wiped over with an instrument disinfectant. At this stage the instrument should be inspected for external damage.
3. The biopsy channel should be flushed with the disinfectant solution and a flexible wire brush introduced to clean the channel. It should then be flushed again.
4. The endoscope should be attached to its power source and the distal tip of the endoscope placed in disinfectant solution. Fluid is aspirated by depression of the suction button. This should then be flushed with distilled water.
5. The water and air buttons should be pressed to blow all water out of the system.
6. If the flush channel is blocked, the tip of the endoscope should be gently brushed with a soft toothbrush to try to dislodge debris from this tiny orifice.
7. It is recommended that the endoscope should be thoroughly dried. The instrument should ideally be hung up so that the tubing can hang straight down to allow drainage of any remaining fluid.
8. Once dry, the endoscope may be packed in its case or preferably hung in a cabinet so that the cable may remain straight.

Flexible endoscopes may be safely sterilized with ethylene oxide if desired. This is recommended, especially when the endoscopes are used frequently or where there is a risk of infection.

It is important to coil the fibreoptic cable in large loops when packing the sterilizer unit, to prevent risk of damaging the light fibres in the endoscope.

Rigid endoscopes

Rigid endoscopes are as easily damaged as flexible ones and they must be handled with care. Sterilization by ethylene oxide is recommended, but where several procedures are to be performed in one day it will only be possible to use cold chemical disinfection.

Cryosurgery

Cryosurgery is a technique used to destroy living tissue by the controlled application of extreme cold. The aim is to kill cells in a diseased target while producing minimal damage to normal surrounding tissue.

By the application of a refrigerant (usually liquid nitrogen) to the tissues, the temperature is reduced so that intracellular and extracellular water begins to freeze, with the formation of ice crystals. This eventually leads to cell denaturation and death. A rapid freeze followed by a slow thaw is recommended and usually 2–3 freeze–thaw cycles are necessary to achieve maximal effect. It is usually possible to approach a local hospital or research facility to obtain small amounts of the refrigerant as required.

Precautions

Liquid nitrogen is a harmful substance. To comply with COSHH regulations (see Chapter 2), a standard operating procedure (SOP) should be employed to prevent possible accidents when handling the substance. All persons involved in using liquid nitrogen should be trained and familiar with the SOP.

- Liquid nitrogen should be transported only in containers provided by the supplier of the liquid nitrogen or manufacturer of the cryosurgical equipment. These are insulated metal vessels of varying sizes.
- Protective eye goggles, an apron and insulated gloves must be worn when handling the refrigerant and equipment.
- The splashing of liquid nitrogen on to clothes, floors and equipment must be avoided, as it will disperse over a wide area.
- Skin contact with the refrigerant and probes must be avoided whilst in use.
- Care must be taken when filling the cryosurgical unit. A metal funnel should be used to pour liquid nitrogen from the reservoir vessel into the unit.

Cryosurgical units

In veterinary practice small thermos-sized units are normally used. These are easy to handle and manipulate. The liquid nitrogen may be applied via a probe that adheres to the tissue surface or from a more diffuse pulsating spray.

Care of equipment following use

Once the probe or spray attachment has thawed, it should be washed using an instrument disinfectant. Any remaining liquid nitrogen should be poured back into the reservoir vessel. Probes may be autoclaved if desired.

Preparation of the patient

- The hair around the site must be clipped to allow effective contact of the liquid nitrogen with the lesion.
- The site should have a basic skin preparation with a surgical scrub solution.
- The surrounding healthy tissue must be protected with insulation (e.g. polystyrene pieces). This is particularly important when using a spray around delicate structures such as the eye.

Postoperative care following cryosurgery

Initially there may be erythema and oedema, which should be monitored carefully in the immediate postoperative period. A slough will then follow, which may be moist. This should be cleaned once or twice a day. If there is any discharge, it is a good idea to apply petroleum jelly to the skin around the lesion to prevent excoriation.

Owners should be warned beforehand that following cryosurgery the affected area may be unsightly and there may be a copious foul-smelling discharge. They should also be told that the skin may become unpigmented, resulting in growth of white hair.

Suture materials

The ideal suture material should:

- Be suitable for use in any situation
- Be readily available and inexpensive
- Have a long shelf life and be easily sterilized if necessary
- Show high initial tensile strength, combined with a small diameter
- Have a good knot security (it should tie easily, with no tendency to slip or loosen, and the knot should hold securely without fraying)
- Produce minimal tissue reaction – it should be inert (i.e. not cause pain or swelling or delay healing), non-allergenic, non-carcinogenic and non-electrolytic
- Show good handling characteristics (it should be easy to handle when wet or dry and pass through tissue without friction or cutting)
- Not create an environment for bacterial growth, i.e. not show capillarity or wicking of fluids (ideally monofilament)
- Be absorbed after its function has been served.

No single suture material in the wide range available possesses all of these ideal characteristics. Selection tends to depend on the surgeon's training and preferences. Figure 24.38 explains the terms used to describe the characteristics of suture materials.

Suture material that is presented in a cassette reel should be avoided as sterility cannot be guaranteed. Suture material is the most commonly implanted foreign body into patients and should be thought of in such a way. The smallest size suture material suitable should be selected and as little as possible placed in the animal to try and minimize reaction.

Term	Meaning
Tensile strength	The breaking strength per unit area of tissue
Knot security	Related to the surface frictional characteristics of the material Every suture is weakest where it is tied. Often the strongest sutures have the poorest knot security
Tissue reaction	The response of the tissue to the suture material involved
Tissue drag	The degree of frictional force developed as the material is pulled through the tissue
Capillarity	The extent to which tissue fluid is attracted along the suture material. Materials with high capillarity act as a wick and encourage fluids to move along them. Such materials should not be used in the presence of sepsis
Memory	The tendency of the material to return to its original shape. A material with high memory tends to unkink during knot tying, i.e. knot security is poor with materials possessing high memory
Chatter	The lack of smoothness as a throw of a knot is tightened down
Stiffness and elongation	The less force required to stretch a suture, the more it will elongate before it ruptures
Sterilization characteristics	The ability of the material to undergo sterilization without deteriorating. Autoclaving is satisfactory for the nylon materials. Repeated autoclaving will, however, weaken them. The natural products and synthetic absorbable materials should not be steam-sterilized. Ethylene oxide sterilization is safe for all sutures provided the packs are sufficiently aerated

24.38 Characteristics of suture materials.

Classification of sutures

Suture materials are either absorbable or non-absorbable. They may be further classified as natural or synthetic, and as monofilament or multifilament (Figure 24.39; see also Chapter 25).

	Natural fibres	Synthetic
Absorbable	Multifilament: Catgut (plain/chromic)	**Monofilament:** Polydioxanone (e.g. PDS II) Polyglyconate (e.g. Maxon) Poliglecaprone 25 (e.g. Monocryl)
		Multifilament: Polyglactin 910 (e.g. Vicryl) Polyglycolic acid (e.g. Dexon)
Non-absorbable	Multifilament: Silk Linen (e.g. Supramid)	**Monofilament:** Polyamide (e.g. Ethilon) Polypropylene (e.g. Prolene) Polybutylester (e.g. Novafil) Polyethylene (e.g. Dermalene) Stainless steel (e.g. Flexon)
		Multifilament: Braided polyamide (e.g. Nuralon) Polyester (e.g. Mersiline) Coated polyester (e.g. Ethibond)

24.39 Examples of absorbable and non-absorbable suture materials.

Absorbable sutures

These materials are degraded within the tissues and lose their tensile strength by 60 days. Natural fibres (catgut) are removed by phagocytosis, which tends to produce some degree of tissue reaction. The synthetic absorbable materials are hydrolysed (broken down in the presence of water) and tend to produce minimal tissue reaction. In general, absorbable suture materials are used when closing internal tissue layers or organs that do not require long-term support.

Catgut

For many years, chromic and plain catgut have been used in both human and veterinary surgery. Catgut was made from the submucosa of sheep small intestine or the serosa of cattle intestines. 'Plain catgut' is untreated; 'chromic catgut' is tanned with chromic salts to slow its absorption, increase its strength and decrease the tissue reaction. Both still have disadvantages, including tissue reaction, poor tensile strength, poor knot security when wet and being prone to wicking. For these reasons synthetic suture materials are preferred. Following an EU ruling they have been withdrawn from manufacture and sale in the United Kingdom for use in human hospitals.

Polyglactin 910

This material is a copolymer of lactide and glycolide and is absorbed by hydrolysis. It is available in dyed and undyed preparations, the latter causing less tissue reaction. It is coated to improve its handling characteristics and it is braided.

- Polyglactin 910 has a higher initial tensile strength than catgut.
- It loses 50% of its strength in 14 days and is totally absorbed in 60–90 days.
- There is considerable tissue drag and careful placement of knots is necessary.
- It is commonly used for subcutaneous, intradermal and muscle layer closure as well as mucous membranes.

Polyglycolic acid

This is an inert, non-antigenic, non-pyrogenic polyester made from hydroxyacetic acid and it is braided. It is absorbed by hydrolysis; the hydrolysed breakdown products have been found to be bacteriostatic experimentally, so its use has been advocated in infected sites.

- Polyglycolic acid loses approximately 30% of its strength in 7 days and 80% in 14 days.
- Tissue drag is considerable even in the coated formulation and can cut through friable tissue.
- It has relatively poor knot security.

Polydioxanone

This is a monofilament absorbable suture that is absorbed by hydrolysis.

- Polydioxanone loses only 30% of its strength in 2 weeks and is minimally absorbed at 90 days.
- Tissue reaction is minimal.
- As it is monofilament, tissue drag is reduced.
- It is ideal in infected sites and where an absorbable material is required for a long period of time.
- Its main disadvantage is its springiness.

- It is commonly used for mucous membranes, subcutaneous, intradermal and muscle layer closure. It is used for closure of the linea alba after coeliotomy as it maintains its strength for a long period of time.

Polyglyconate

This synthetic monofilament absorbable suture is very similar to polydioxanone. It is slightly less springy and therefore easier to handle than polydioxanone.

Poliglecaprone 25

This new synthetic monofilament absorbable suture is similar to both polydioxanone and polyglyconate, but duration of tensile strength is shorter. It is broken down by hydrolysis.

- Poliglecaprone 25 is less springy than polydioxanone and polyglyconate.
- Tissue reaction is minimal.
- Tissue drag is minimal.
- Its main disadvantage is that although it has the highest tensile strength, by 14 days only 30% original strength is maintained.
- It is commonly used for subcutaneous and intradermal closure

Non-absorbable sutures

These maintain their strength for longer than 60 days. The material is neither hydrolysed nor phagocytosed: it becomes encapsulated within fibrous tissue. Non-absorbable sutures are used where prolonged mechanical support is required. The main indications for use are:

- In skin closure, where sutures are generally removed after 10 days
- Within slow-healing tissues.
- When the ligation required is permanent, e.g. patent ductus arteriosus ligation.

Silk

This is available as braided or twisted strands. It is obtained from threads spun by the silkworm larvae. It may be coated with silicone or wax to minimize the capillarity, which may promote infection.

Silk has good handling characteristics, excellent knot security and good tensile strength. It is relatively inexpensive. Its main uses include cardiovascular and thoracic surgery and it can be used on genital mucosa and adjacent to eyes as it is soft and causes less irritation to the surrounding tissue. It should not be used in infected sites, oral mucosa or hollow organs, where it may act as a focus for infection.

Linen

This is twisted from long strands of flax. It is easily sterilized, handles well and has excellent knot security. It does show capillary properties, however, and has been shown to contribute to sinus formation. It is now rarely used, if at all, as it has been largely superseded since the advent of the synthetic absorbable materials.

Polypropylene

This is an inert, non-absorbable monofilament material. It has high tensile strength but tends to stretch and is damaged if crushed by needle-holders. The suture material should only be grasped at the ends to prevent this. If it does require clamping then plastic tips ('shods') should be placed on the end of artery forceps to protect the suture material. The knot security is varied and a bulky knot may be formed. The strands flatten where they cross each other and this increases knot security. It is very springy but shows little tissue drag. It becomes encapsulated in a thin fibrous covering. It is the least thrombogenic suture material and is commonly used in vascular surgery.

Polyamide

This may be either monofilament or braided. The monofilament form causes little tissue reaction, has little tissue drag and is non-capillary. Its handling characteristics are not good and knot security can be poor. It loses approximately 15% of its tensile strength each year. It can be used on fascia and muscle, but the buried ends can be irritant in serous or synovial cavities. The braided form is usually sheathed in an attempt to decrease capillarity, but its use as a buried suture is not recommended. It shows more tissue drag than the monofilament variety, although it handles better.

Polyesters

Various braided polyesters are available. They are easy to handle and retain their tensile strength well. Some are coated with silicone, Teflon or polybutylate to reduce tissue drag. They tend to have poor knot-tying quality and some have shown signs of capillarity.

Stainless steel

This is available in monofilament or braided varieties. It is very strong, inert and non-capillary. It is relatively difficult to handle as the wire lacks elasticity and knots may be difficult to tie, but knot security is good. It is useful in slow-healing tissues such as bone, tendon and joint capsules, and in contaminated sites. It has become less popular in recent years as newer materials have become available; however, it is commonly used for the thoracic closure of median sternotomy wounds.

Alternatives to sutures

Staples

Metal clips or staples for use in skin and other tissues have gained popularity in the field of veterinary surgery over the last few years. Staples designed for skin closure are packed in a gun-like applicator for rapid insertion. These instruments are intended to be disposable, but they may be safely re-sterilized.

The main advantage of staples is speed of insertion. They are inert and well tolerated. Re-usable staple-removing forceps are available to remove metal skin staples.

Stapling instruments have also been designed for a number of soft tissue surgeries, including gastrointestinal anastomosis, splenectomy and lung lobectomy. Although designed for the human market, they are suitable for veterinary applications and are gaining popularity. They may permit resection of areas of bowel that are inaccessible to routine suturing, particularly in the equine abdomen. Their major disadvantage is cost, but their use can drastically reduce the overall surgery time/fee and so the cost difference is negligible. There may be indications for use in patients with high anaesthetic risks as they can significantly shorten surgery time.

Metal clips are also available for use as ligatures. They come in various sizes with re-usable applicators. They are simple and quick to use.

Tissue glue

Tissue glues are made from cyanomethacrylate monomers that polymerize on contact with moisture in the wound. IThey are especially useful in small animals, such as guinea pigs and rabbits, and can be used for wounds on pads, for holding catheters in position and in areas where there is limited room for suturing.

Adhesive tapes

Designed for use in humans, these have been of limited use in animals as they do not adhere well to moist skin.

Suture selection

The veterinary surgeon will normally select the suture material (see Chapter 25) but the veterinary nurse should be aware of which materials may be used in different tissues (Figure 24.40) and the sizes (Figure 24.41) that will be required.

Tissue	Suture materials
Skin	Monofilament nylon or polypropylene Metal staples Avoid materials with capillary action
Subcutis	Fine synthetic absorbable material with minimal tissue reaction, e.g. polydioxanone, polyglactin, polyglycolic acid
Muscle	Synthetic absorbable, non-absorbable, e.g. nylon
Fascia	Synthetic non-absorbable if prolonged suture strength required
Hollow viscus	Synthetic absorbable or polypropylene In bladder: monofilament synthetic
Tendon	Nylon, polypropylene, stainless steel
Blood vessels	Polypropylene: least thrombogenic is silk
Eyes	Synthetic absorbable, e.g. polyglactin, polydioxanone
Nerves	Nylon or polypropylene: minimal tissue reaction

24.40 Suture materials suitable for different tissues.

Metric	USP	Metric	USP
0.2	10/0	3	2/0
0.3	9/0	3.5	0
0.4	8/0	4	1
0.5	7/0	5	2
0.7	6/0	6	3 and 4
1	5/0	7	5
1.5	4/0	8	6
2	3/0		

24.41 Sizes of suture materials. In the metric system, each metric unit represents 0.1 mm.

Packaging of suture materials

Most suture materials are purchased in pre-sterilized individual packets. This guarantees a sterile suture (unless the packet is damaged) and a needle in perfect condition where one is attached. The only disadvantage is that of cost. Synthetic absorbable suture materials are only available packaged in this way.

Some suture materials are provided on a reel in surgical spirit, where the suture material is pulled off and a length cut as needed. This is a much less reliable way of storing suture materials and should be avoided for internal use.

Suture materials can also be purchased as lengths, which are then threaded on to re-sterilizable needles. This causes more tissue trauma, due to drag through the tissues where the suture material is doubled over through the eye of the needle. The needle is also more likely to become blunt.

Multi-use cassettes are still used in veterinary practice for packaging catgut (not UK), nylon and stainless steel sutures. The disadvantage of these is the likelihood of contamination of cassettes during use – they often become damaged. It is also easy to contaminate the material as it is cut from the reel and transferred to the instrument trolley. Their use is to be discouraged.

Suture needles

Suture needles are designed to pass through tissue easily. They must be sharp enough to penetrate tissues with minimal resistance, rigid enough to prevent excessive bending and yet flexible enough to bend before breaking. They should be made from corrosion-resistant stainless steel.

Swaged needles

Swaged or atraumatic needles are attached to the suture material, i.e. they do not require threading. The advantage of this is that a needle in perfect condition is available with each strand and tissue trauma is minimized by the passage of material and needle of a comparative size. All of the prepacked suture materials are available with a variety of different needle shapes and sizes.

Eyed needles

This type of needle requires threading. The primary indication for its use is economy of suitable material or use of special needles (e.g. for large-animal work). The disadvantages are increased tissue trauma due to the eye size, loss of sharpness of the needle tip, and bending and corrosion following repeated use. The needle shape refers to both the longitudinal shape of the shaft and the cross-sectional shape.

Longitudinal shape

Of the great variety of different sizes and shapes of needle that are available, some of those used in veterinary surgery are shown in Figure 24.42.

Cross-sectional shape

Round-bodied

These are designed to separate tissue fibres rather than cut them, and are used for soft tissue or in situations where easy splitting of tissue fibres is possible.

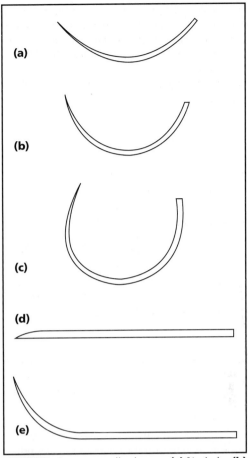

24.42 Suture needle shapes: **(a)** 3/8 circle; **(b)** 1/2 circle; **(c)** 5/8 circle; **(d)** straight; **(e)** 1/2 curved.

Modified point

The taper-cut needle has a cutting tip on the point of the needle and a round body. This provides increased penetration of the needle without increased tissue trauma.

The trocar-point needle has a strong cutting head and a robust round body. This is useful in dense tissue.

Cutting needles

These are required wherever dense or tough tissue needs to be sutured. The cross-sectional appearance of the needle is usually a triangular cutting edge, which extends at least half way along the shaft. The reverse cutting needle has the cutting edge on the outside of the needle curvature to improve strength and resistance to bending.

Micropoint needles

These are very fine needles with a sharp cutting edge. They are designed for ophthalmic surgery and microsurgery.

Selection of needles

The use of swaged needles is to be encouraged – their advantages far outweigh those of eyed needles. Other needles should be as close as possible in diameter to that of the suture. A large needle tract invites bacteria and foreign substances to enter the wound, thus delaying healing. The needle should be of the appropriate shape and size to enable the veterinary surgeon to close the wound accurately and precisely.

The smaller and deeper the wound, the greater the curve should be. Straight needles are designed to be handheld and tend to be used in the skin. Half-curved cutting needles have been commonly used in veterinary surgery but have little to recommend their use.

The tissue type will determine the necessary point of the needle. Generally speaking:

- Round-bodied needles are used for viscera, subcutaneous and friable tissue
- Taper-tip needles are used for easily penetrated tissue, i.e. for denser tissue
- Cutting needles are generally used in the skin.

Suture patterns

Veterinary nurses maintained on the Register held by the RCVS are legally allowed to perform minor acts of surgery, including the suturing of wounds. It is important that they should be familiar with basic suturing techniques. The veterinary surgeon should give practical instruction and reference should be made to surgical technique textbooks.

Suture patterns may be interrupted or continuous, and may be further classified as apposing, everting or inverting. However, a veterinary nurse would only usually perform apposing sutures, as this is the common pattern for wound closure. The other patterns are more commonly used during intestinal surgery.

- **Apposing** sutures bring the tissues in direct apposition.
- **Everting** sutures tend to turn the edges of the wound outwards.
- **Inverting** sutures turn the tissue inwards (e.g. towards the lumen of a viscus).

Surgical knots

A surgical knot has three main components:

- The **loop** is the part of the suture material within the apposed or ligated tissue
- The **knot** is composed of a number of throws, each throw linking the two strands of tissue around each other
- The **ears** are the cut ends of the suture that prevent the knot coming untied.

Knots can be tied by hand or by an instrument. Hand ties may be single or two-handed.

The basic surgical knot is the **reef knot** or **square knot**. A **surgeon's knot** has an initial double throw instead of a single throw. This reduces the risk of the first throw loosening before the second throw is placed but is usually only required for a wound under tension, which in itself is far from ideal.

Hand-tying helps to prevent slippage of the first throw, since tension can be kept on both ends of the suture throughout the procedure. However, it tends to be wasteful on suture material.

The knots of skin sutures should be pulled to one side of the incision and the suture loop should be loose. During the postoperative period the wound will swell and so sutures should be loose in anticipation of this. Sutures that are too tight compromise the vascular supply, promote infection and delay healing. They are also uncomfortable and encourage the patient to interfere with the wound.

Suture material should not be crushed in the jaws of needle-holders. When tying knots, only the end of the suture material should be grasped. Needle-holders should not be clamped on to the eye of swaged needles, as this will cause damage or breakage of the needle.

Interrupted sutures

The main advantage of the interrupted suture is its ability to maintain strength and tissue apposition if part of the suture line fails. Each suture is individually tied and cut distal to the knot. Its main disadvantage is the amount of suture material used and left within the tissue and the time required to suture.

Continuous sutures

These are neither knotted nor cut, except at each end of the suture line. The advantages of the continuous suture line are ease of application and minimal use of suture material. The main disadvantage is that slippage of either the beginning or end knot is likely to cause failure of the entire suture line, but as long as some basic rules are followed there should be little failure. At the start and end of a continuous suture line there should be a minimum of seven throws on the knot. Continuous suture patterns used in the skin are not ideal; when they are removed all of the suture material that has been on the outside of the patient, and therefore exposed to potential contamination, is pulled through the surgical wound increasing the risk of infection.

Common suture patterns

Common suture patterns used in the skin, in muscle and fascia, and in hollow organ closure are listed in Figure 24.43. Skin sutures (Figure 24.44) should be placed at least 5 mm from the skin edge and be placed squarely across the wound. The skin should be handled gently with fine rat-tooth forceps. The wound edges should be apposed or slightly everted with no gaping or overlapping.

In skin
• Simple interrupted
• Simple continuous
• Ford interlocking
• Interrupted vertical mattress
• Interrupted horizontal mattress
• Cruciate mattress
In muscle and fascia
• Simple interrupted
• Simple continuous
• Ford interlocking
• Cruciate mattress
• Horizontal mattress
• Vertical mattress
• Mayo mattress
In hollow organ closure
• Simple interrupted
• Parker–Kerr
• Purse-string
• Connell
• Cushing
• Lembert
• Gambee
• Halstead

24.43 Common suture patterns.

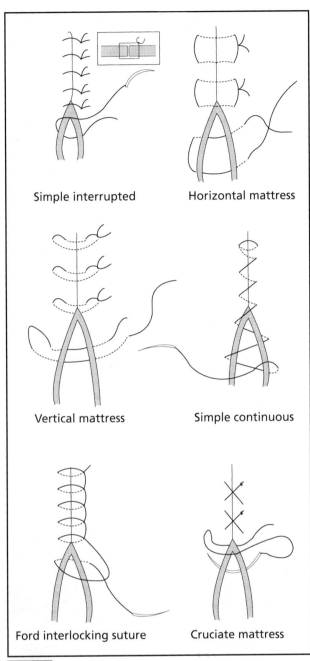

Simple interrupted   Horizontal mattress

Vertical mattress   Simple continuous

Ford interlocking suture   Cruciate mattress

24.44 Common suture patterns used in the skin.

Sterilization

Sterilization can be divided into heat sterilization and cold sterilization (Figure 24.45).

Heat sterilization

Steam under pressure (autoclave systems)

Steam under pressure is the most widely used and efficient method of sterilization. It is also the most economical, although the initial outlay may be large. Items that may be sterilized in the autoclave include:

- Autoclave (steam under pressure):
  - Vertical
  - Horizontal
  - Vacuum-assisted
- Dry heat:
  - Hot-air oven
  - High-vacuum oven
  - Convection oven

Cold sterilization

- Ethylene oxide
- Commercial solutions:
  - Chemical
  - Alcohol-based
- Gamma irradiation

24.45 Heat and cold sterilization.

- Instruments
- Drapes
- Gowns
- Swabs
- Most rubber articles
- Glassware
- Some plastic goods.

Heat-sensitive items that may be damaged in the autoclave include fibreoptic equipment, lenses and plastics (especially those designed to be disposable, such as catheters).

The three main types of autoclave are the vertical pressure cooker, the horizontal or vertical downward displacement autoclave and the vacuum-assisted autoclave.

Vertical pressure cooker

This very simple machine operates by boiling water in a closed container, like a household pressure cooker. It usually has an air vent at the top, which is closed once the air has been evacuated and pressure (15 psi) is allowed to build up. As the air vent is at the top, the main disadvantage of this type of autoclave is the danger that some air will be trapped underneath the steam. The temperature in this area will be lower and sterility cannot be guaranteed. It is also manually operated and there is room for human error in the sterilizing cycle.

Horizontal or vertical downward displacement autoclave

This type is larger and usually fully automatic. It uses an electrically operated boiler that is incorporated in the autoclave as a source of steam. Air is driven out more efficiently by downward displacement. There is an air outlet at the bottom and a steam outlet at the top.

Most of these machines are designed for loose instrument sterilization only, rather than packs, as they have insufficient penetrating ability and drying cycles: packs may seem to be dry but they remain damp, allowing entry of microorganisms during the storage period.

There is usually a choice of programmes on this type of autoclave, with temperatures of 112, 121, 126 or 134°C.

Vacuum-assisted autoclave (porous load)

This type of autoclave works on the same principle as the other two but uses a high-vacuum pump to evacuate air rapidly from the chamber at the beginning of the cycle. Steam penetration after evacuation is almost instantaneous and sterilization occurs very quickly. A second vacuum cycle rapidly withdraws moisture after sterilization and dries the load. It is suitable for all types of instruments, drapes and equipment and there is a choice of cycles using different temperatures and pressures.

Vacuum-assisted autoclaves are fully automatic, with fail-safe mechanisms (usually warning lights and alarms) that indicate whether the load is non-sterile or has been sterilized effectively. They are generally much larger and more sophisticated than other types and are invariably connected to a central boiler to supply steam. The cost of purchase and maintenance are higher, but the machine's efficiency and reliability in sterilization far outweigh those of the smaller types.

Principles of sterilization using steam under pressure

Although autoclaves vary in size and type, the basic principle of function remains the same. When water boils at 100°C some bacteria, spores and viruses are resistant to heat, and remain unchanged, even if exposed to such a temperature for a long time. By increasing the pressure, the temperature of the steam is raised and resistant microorganisms and spores will be killed by coagulation of cell proteins. It is the increased temperature, not the increased pressure, that leads to this destruction of microorganisms. The higher the temperature, the shorter the time needed to achieve sterilization (Figure 24.46).

Temperature (°C)	Pressure (psi)	Pressure (kg/cm²)	Time (minutes)
121	15	1.2	15
126	20	1.4	10
134	30	2	3½

24.46 Autoclave temperature, pressure and time combinations.

The autoclaving process

The central sterilizing chamber of the autoclave is surrounded by a steam jacket. The pressure in the jacket is raised (depending on the cycle). Steam then enters the chamber and, as it does so, air is displaced downwards, because steam is lighter. When all the air is evacuated, exhaust vents are closed and steam continues to enter until the desired pressure is reached. The more sophisticated types of autoclave have a vacuum prior to introduction of steam to displace air from materials to be sterilized. If any air remains in the chamber, the temperature will be lower than steam at that pressure and sterility cannot be guaranteed.

Once the air has been evacuated, steam that has entered the chamber begins to condense on the colder surfaces in the chamber, e.g. instruments. The steam produces heat, which penetrates to the innermost layer of the pack. The moisture increases the penetrability of the heat. After the given amount of time the steam is exhausted. As the temperature drops, the pressure returns to normal. In vacuum-assisted autoclaves the instruments are then heat dried, with filtered air replacing the exhausted steam. On modern machines the door cannot be opened until the end of this stage.

Effective sterilization also depends on correct loading of packs into the autoclave. There should be adequate space between them to allow steam to circulate freely. Care should be taken to avoid overloading and blocking of the inlet and exhaust valves. Before packing for sterilization, instruments must be free of grease and protein material to allow effective penetration of steam.

Maintenance of the autoclave

All types of autoclave should be serviced by a qualified engineer to ensure that they remain in good working order and remain electrically safe. Vacuum-assisted autoclaves with a separate boiler should be serviced every 3 months to comply with health and safety regulations. Thermocouple testing is recommended at least annually to ensure that effective sterilization is taking place.

Monitoring efficacy of sterilization in the autoclave

External sterility indicators should be used in all cases when sterilizing equipment; however, internal indicators must also be used when sterilizing bulky items so that penetration of heat/steam/chemical can be checked.

- **Chemical indicator strips** (e.g. TST Strips) show colour changes when the correct temperature, pressure and time have been reached. A strip is placed inside each pack. It is important that the appropriate strip is used for each different pressure/time/temperature cycle, otherwise a false result may be given.
- **Browne's tubes** work on the same principle, i.e. a colour change. Small glass tubes are partly filled with an orange-brown liquid that changes to green when certain temperatures have been maintained for a required period of time. Tubes are available that change at 121, 126 or 134°C. It is essential to ensure that the correct type of tube is selected for any particular temperature cycle. Browne's tubes are also available for hot-air ovens.
- **Bowie–Dick indicator tape** is commonly used to seal instrument and drape packs. It is a beige-coloured tape impregnated with chemical stripes that change to dark brown when a certain temperature is reached (121°C). As with ethylene oxide indicator tape, it is not reliable as an indicator of sterility as it does not ensure that the temperature was maintained for the required time.
- **Spore tests** are strips of paper impregnated with dried spores (usually *Bacillus stearothermophilus*). A strip is included in the load; on completion of the cycle it is placed in the culture medium provided and incubated at the appropriate temperature for up to 72 hours. If the sterilization process has been successful, the spores will have been killed and there will be no growth.

Spore systems are more accurate than chemical indicators but the delay in obtaining results is a major disadvantage. A combination of both systems is recommended: chemical indicators should be included in each pack and spore strips should be used at regular intervals.

Vacuum-assisted autoclaves will usually have visible temperature and pressure gauges on the front. Some systems have a paper recording chart that indicates the efficiency of sterilization.

Thermocouples (electrical leads with temperature-sensitive tips) are placed in various parts of the sterilizing chamber with the leads passed out through an aperture to a recording device outside. The temperature within the chamber can be constantly recorded throughout a cycle to check that required temperatures are achieved and held for the specified time.

Dry heat

Dry heat kills microorganisms by causing oxidative destruction of bacterial protoplasm. Microorganisms are much more resistant to dry heat than when heated in the presence of moisture and so higher temperatures are required (150–180°C). Dry heat below 140°C cannot destroy bacterial spores in <4–5 hours.

The range of equipment sterilized in this way is restricted: fabrics, rubber goods and plastic cannot withstand these high, dry temperatures and are easily damaged.

There are certain items for which dry heat sterilization is the method of choice. These include glass syringes, cutting instruments, ophthalmic instruments, drill bits, glassware, powders and oils.

Hot-air ovens

These are heated by electrical elements (Figure 24.47). They are usually small but are economical in terms of purchase and running costs. They have been largely superseded by the autoclave, which is more efficient and suitable for most types of material.

Item	Temperature (°C)	Time (min)
Glassware	180	60
Non-cutting instruments Powders, oils	160	120
Sharp-cutting instruments	150	180

24.47 Temperature and time ratios recommended for hot-air ovens.

A long cooling period is needed before the items may be used. The door should be fitted with a safety device to prevent it being opened before the oven is cool. It is important to ensure that the oven is not overloaded and that items are placed so that air can flow freely.

Spore strip tests and Browne's tubes are available that are designed specifically for testing sterility in hot-air ovens.

Moist heat (boiling)

Boiling is no longer considered as a method of sterilization. It cannot be guaranteed to kill all microorganisms and spores, because the maximum temperature of 100°C is insufficient to kill resistant spores.

Cold sterilization

Ethylene oxide

Ethylene oxide is a highly penetrative and effective method of sterilization. However, concerns have been expressed about its use in veterinary practice as it is toxic, irritant to tissue and a very inflammable gas. Its use is currently permitted and the danger to operators should be negligible as long as the manufacturer's recommendations are followed. COSHH Regulations may make its use impractical in some veterinary practices.

Ethylene oxide inactivates the DNA of the cells, thereby preventing cell reproduction. The technique is effective against vegetative bacteria, fungi, viruses and spores. Several factors influence the ability of ethylene oxide to destroy microorganisms, including temperature, pressure, concentration, humidity and time of exposure. As the temperature increases, the ability of ethylene oxide to penetrate increases and the duration of the cycle shortens. The only system available in the UK operates at room temperature for a period of 12 hours.

Use of the ethylene oxide sterilizer

The sterilizer consists of a plastic container fitted with a ventilation system to prevent gas entering the work area. It should be located in a clean, well ventilated area (e.g. fume cupboard) away from work areas. The temperature of the room must be at least 20°C during the cycle.

Individually packed items to be sterilized are placed in a polythene liner bag. The plastic bag is a gas diffusion membrane of known permeability, the function of which is to contain the gas given off by the ampoule and to release it at a controlled rate during the sterilization cycle. A gas ampoule containing the ethylene oxide liquid surrounded by a plastic shield is placed within the liner bag. Excess air is then pressed out before the mouth of the bag is closed. A flexible plastic purge tube protrudes into the sterilization unit. The end of this purge tube is placed in the mouth of the liner bag and, using a plastic locking bag tie, the neck of the liner bag is sealed around the purge tube. The top of the glass vial is snapped from outside the liner bag to release the sterilant gas. The door to the sterilizer unit is closed and locked, the ventilator switch is turned on and the items are left for 12 hours (the sterilization process is frequently performed overnight). At the end of the 12-hour period, the unit is unlocked, the liner bag is untied and a purge pump is switched on to aerate the chamber. The door may be opened after 2 hours and the load removed.

The latest model of the Anprolene ethylene oxide sterilizer has a 'cycle start' button, which is pressed when the glass vial is snapped. This then automatically begins a 2-hour purge at the end of sterilization. A green light indicates the end of that period and when the unit may be opened.

Preparation of materials for sterilization

Ethylene oxide is effective for the sterilization of many different types of equipment but its use is limited by the size of the container, the duration of the cycle and concerns about toxicity. Its use therefore tends to be restricted to items that are damaged by heat:

- Fibreoptic equipment
- Plastic catheters, trays, etc.
- Anaesthetic tubing, etc.
- Plastic syringes
- Optical instruments
- High-speed drills/burs
- Battery-operated drills.

Some commercially available products are sterilized by this method, e.g. syringes, synthetic absorbable suture materials and catheters, although most use gamma-irradiation. Equipment made of polyvinylchloride (PVC) should not be sterilized by this method as the material may react with the gas. Items that have previously been sterilized using gamma-irradiation should not then be re-sterilized.

Materials to be sterilized by ethylene oxide must be cleaned and dried. Water on instruments at the time of exposure may react with the gas and reduce its effectiveness.

Occlusive bungs, caps or stylets must be removed from instruments so that gas can penetrate freely. Syringes should be packaged disassembled.

Ethylene oxide penetrates materials more readily than steam and so a wider variety of packaging materials may be used when preparing items for sterilization and storage. However, nylon film designed for autoclaving should not be used, as it has been shown that there is poor penetration by ethylene oxide.

Testing efficiency of sterilization

- To indicate exposure to ethylene oxide, blue/green **indicator tape** (resembling Bowie–Dick tape in design) with yellow stripes that turn red following prolonged exposure to the gas may be used. It does not guarantee sterility as it gives no indication that exposure was for the correct length of time. In fact the colour change will occur after a fairly short period of time.
- **Indicator stickers** provided by the manufacturer have a yellow dot that turns blue following prolonged exposure to ethylene oxide. These are useful but not 100% reliable as sterility indicators, as the colour change will also occur following prolonged exposure to light. It is recommended that the box containing the roll of stickers is kept in a drawer or cupboard to prevent this change occurring before use.
- **Dosemeter strips** that undergo a colour change when exposed to ethylene oxide for the correct time may be placed in the centre of a pack or load to test the penetration efficiency.
- **Spore strips** placed into a load are added to a culture medium on completion of the cycle and are incubated for 72 hours. This is a useful test of the efficiency of the system but is obviously not suitable as an immediate indicator of sterility.

Hydrogen peroxide sterilizer

This system uses hydrogen peroxide gas plasma at low temperatures. It has a very short cycle time (between 28 and 60 minutes), allowing instruments and equipment to be sterilized and returned to use quickly. It does not require high temperatures and so is suitable for most items that previously used ethylene oxide. Another major advantage is that the only byproducts of the process are water vapour and oxygen. The system can be used for sterilizing endoscopes, arthroscopes and light cables, any plastic goods, batteries and power drills. It cannot be used to sterilize paper or wood products due to absorption.

Chemical disinfectant solutions

A number of chemical disinfectant solutions are produced commercially. Some are ready for use, others require dilution (usually with purified water) prior to use.

Until recently a solution containing glutaraldehyde was the most widely used product for chemical disinfection. Although it is still readily available, COSHH regulations may prevent its use in veterinary (and medical) practice.

The use of chemical solutions should really only be considered as a means of *disinfection*, although some manufacturers guarantee sterilization following prolonged immersion (usually 24 hours). It remains a useful method for surgical equipment that may not be sterilized by any other means. It has gained particular popularity for the disinfection of endoscopic equipment. There are several proprietary brands available.

Care should be taken to use the specific concentrations and immersion time stipulated by the manufacturer. Before immersion, a check should be made with the manufacturer that the equipment will not be damaged by wet disinfection. The chemical solution and the article to be disinfected should be placed in a tray or bowl, preferably with a lid to prevent evaporation and contamination by airborne microorganisms. Following immersion in chemical solutions, instruments should be rinsed in sterile water and dried before use. Chemical solutions should be discarded after use and a fresh solution made up each time.

Alcohol-based solutions

A variety of these have been used, such as ethyl alcohol and isopropyl alcohol. They work by denaturation and coagulation of proteins.

Irradiation

This type of sterilization uses a form of gamma irradiation and can only be carried out under controlled conditions. Many pre-packaged items are sterilized by this method, including suture materials and surgical gloves.

Packing supplies for sterilization

Various materials and containers are available for packing supplies for sterilization, each having advantages and disadvantages. Choice will depend on several factors:

- The packaging material must be resistant to damage when handled and not damage the equipment to be sterilized
- Steam or gas must be able to penetrate the wrapping for sterilization to occur and must be easily exhausted from the pack once sterilization is complete
- Microorganisms must not be able to penetrate from the outer surface of the wrap to the inner.

Other factors include:

- Size of autoclave/gas sterilizer
- Cost
- Personal preference
- Time taken to achieve sterility.

Materials and containers

Nylon film

Nylon film designed specifically for use in the autoclave is available in a variety of sizes. It has the advantages of being re-usable and transparent so that items can be easily seen. Its main disadvantage is that it becomes brittle after use, resulting in development of tiny unseen holes and therefore contamination of the pack. It is also difficult to remove sterile items from packs without contaminating them on the edges of the bag. The packs are often sealed using Bowie–Dick tape.

Seal-and-peel pouches

Disposable bags, consisting of a paper back and clear plasticized front with a fold-over seal, are available in a wide variety of sizes. They may be used with ethylene oxide or in the autoclave and there are also seal-and-peel bags made especially for hydrogen peroxide sterilization. The risk of contamination during opening is small. Double wrapping decreases the risk of damage to the instrument during storage or when opening the pack. They are most suitable for individual instruments, although large bags are available for small kits.

Paper

Paper-based sheets are used for packing instruments. The most suitable type consists of a crepe-like paper that is slightly elastic, conforming and water-repellent. It is therefore ideal as an outer dust layer for packs with a drape inner layer although it is acceptable to use these sheets for both inner and outer layers. It is intended to be disposable, but could be re-used if opened carefully and thoroughly checked for damage. It is available in different sized sheets that can be cut to the appropriate size.

Textile

Textile (drape) sheets, usually linen or a cotton/polyester combination, are used to wrap surgical equipment for sterilization. They are conforming, strong and re-usable but have the major disadvantage of being permeable to moisture. Usually a double layer of linen is covered by a waterproof paper-based wrap for surgical packs.

Drums

Metal drums with steam vents in the side, which are closed after sterilization, can be used for instruments, gowns and drapes. Their main disadvantage is that they are frequently multi-use and so there is a degree of environmental contamination each time the lid is opened. There is also a risk of contamination of items touching the edge or outside of the drum when they are removed. Initial outlay is relatively high but they will last for years.

Boxes and cartons

A variety of boxes and cartons are available for use in the autoclave. They are manufactured from non-toxic ethylene/propylene anti-static material to prevent dust attraction. They are designed for sterilization up to 137°C and for irradiation processes. They are useful for gown or drape packs and for specialized kits (e.g. orthopaedic kits). They are relatively inexpensive and may be re-used many times.

Care and sterilization of equipment

Gowns and drapes

After use, re-usable surgical gowns and drapes should be washed, dried and inspected for damage. Gowns should then be folded correctly so that the outside surface of the gown is on the inside (Figure 24.48). This is so that the surgical team can put on gowns in an aseptic fashion (see Figure 24.9). Plain drapes may be folded concertina style (Figure 24.49) or so that two corners are on the top surface (Figure 24.50). Fenestrated drapes are usually folded concertina style.

Both gowns and drapes may be sterilized by ethylene oxide but this method is often uneconomical in a large practice, owing to the small size of the sterilizer, duration of the cycle (12 hours) and the airing time (24 hours). Autoclaving is a quicker, more efficient method but it is essential that the machine has a porous load cycle to ensure complete penetration and drying of the load. A hot-air oven is unsuitable as it will lead to charring of the material.

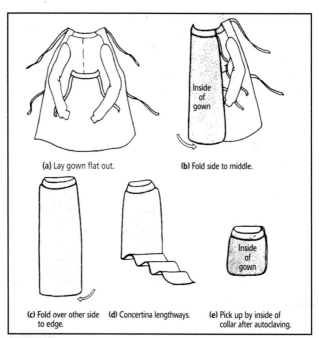

(a) Lay gown flat out. (b) Fold side to middle. (c) Fold over other side to edge. (d) Concertina lengthways. (e) Pick up by inside of collar after autoclaving.

24.48 Folding a gown.

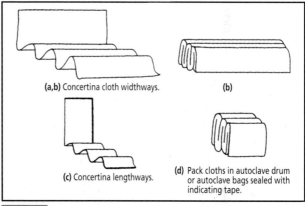

(a,b) Concertina cloth widthways. (b) (c) Concertina lengthways. (d) Pack cloths in autoclave drum or autoclave bags sealed with indicating tape.

24.49 Folding surgical drapes.

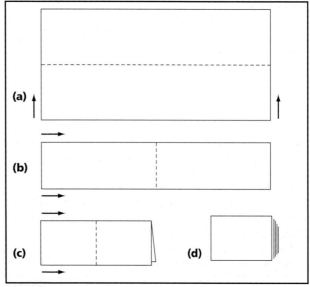

24.50 Folding a plain drape, corner to corner: **(a)** The drape is folded in half widthways, and then **(b–d)** folded in half lengthways three times, so that there are two corners at the top.

Gowns and drapes may be sterilized in drums, boxes, bags or packs. A handtowel is usually placed with the gown when packing for sterilization. Drapes are sometimes incorporated into the instrument pack.

Disposable sterile gowns and drapes are now widely used and are to be recommended (see above).

Swabs

Swabs may be purchased sterile or non-sterile. Each pack should have a consistent number that is known to all surgery staff (usually multiples of two or five). Swabs may be incorporated into the instrument pack, supplied in drums or packed individually.

Swabs should be sterilized in the same way as gowns and drapes.

Urinary catheters

Urinary catheters should not be re-used as it would be impossible to ensure they are free from any debris. They may be re-sterilized if opened in error but not used. They should be packed, without coiling if possible, in appropriate bags. Many brands of catheter may be sterilized by autoclaving but some will be damaged by heat. Ethylene oxide can be successfully used for all types of catheter. It is essential to ensure that they are aired for the recommended time before use.

Syringes

Plastic syringes are designed to be disposable. To ensure sterility after storage they must be packed individually. It is not economical to re-sterilize small syringes but some practices may choose to re-sterilize 30 and 50 ml syringes. If so, they should be disassembled, washed thoroughly and dried prior to sterilization.

Most plastic syringes can be autoclaved safely but some brands will be damaged. Ethylene oxide may be used effectively to sterilize syringes. The plungers should be removed from the barrel prior to this. Glass syringes may be sterilized using a hot-air oven, autoclave or ethylene oxide.

Liquids

It is usual to purchase liquids pre-sterilized, though more sophisticated autoclaves have a cycle for the sterilization of fluids. The risk of breakage of glass bottles is high and it is probably more economical to purchase fluids that have been commercially prepared.

Power tools

Air drills, saws and mechanical burs are usually autoclavable but individual manufacturer's instructions should always be followed. Autoclaving can, in some cases, lead to jamming of the motor. Ethylene oxide can be used for all air-driven tools. Battery drills frequently have a plastic casing that would melt in an autoclave but they can be sterilized by using ethylene oxide or hydrogen peroxide gas plasma.

Packing a surgical set

Instrument sets are often packed together with swabs, and sometimes drapes. They are usually wrapped so that, when unfolded, the layers of wrapping will cover the surface of the instrument trolley (see above).

A metal or plastic tray is first lined with a towel or linen drape sheet. The instruments should then be laid out in a specific order on the towel/sheet on the tray. This is generally the order in which they are likely to be used (see Figure 24.13). Swabs, drapes, etc. are then added. A water-resistant paper wrap is laid over the top of an instrument trolley, followed by two layers of linen sheet. The tray is placed on this and the pack is then wrapped, by folding the water-resistant paper wrap and two layers of linen sheet, as well as the towel lining the tray, up and around the instruments (Figure 24.51). The set is secured with Bowie–Dick tape. It should be labelled and dated prior to sterilization. Sharp or pointed instruments can be protected by application of autoclavable plastic tips.

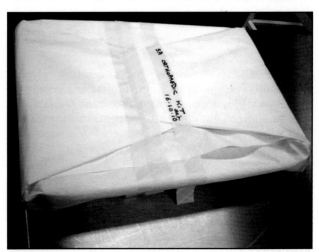

24.51 Instrument set wrapped in crêpe paper. The outer wrappings may be unfolded to cover the base of the trolley. The set has been labelled and dated.

Packing and sterilization of orthopaedic implants

Orthopaedic implants made of stainless steel or titanium are usually sterilized by autoclaving. They may be packed and stored in various ways, from individual packs for each plate, pin, screw or wire to complete sets. Choice will depend on individual preference, facilities and throughput of cases. The ends of Steinmann pins and Kirschner wires (K-wires) should be protected by plastic instrument tips or folded swabs secured with Bowie–Dick tape. All packs or items should be labelled clearly with name, size, length, diameter, etc. as relevant.

Storage after sterilization

There should be a separate area for storage of sterile packs. It should be dust free, dry and well ventilated. Ideally all packs should be kept in closed cupboards. They should be handled as little as possible to minimize risk of damage, and packed loosely on shelves so that bags are not damaged. The length of time for which packs may be safely stored after sterilization is the subject of much debate, with recommendations varying from a few weeks to 3 months. A sealed pack should remain sterile for a limitless period but it may become contaminated by excessive handling (resulting in damage to the pack) or moisture. NHS guidelines therefore recommend that unused autoclave packs should be repacked and re-sterilized after 1 year and items sterilized by ethylene oxide in seal-and-peel bags re-sterilized after 2 years. Packs that use any other type of packaging should be re-sterilized after 6 months.

Further reading

Auer JA and Stick JA (1999) *Equine Surgery*. WB Saunders, Philidelphia

Baines S, Lipscomb V and Hutchinson T (2012) *BSAVA Manual of Canine and Feline Surgical Principles: a Foundation Manual*. BSAVA Publications, Gloucester

College of Animal Welfare (1997) *Veterinary Surgical Instruments*. Butterworth-Heinemann, Oxford

Coumbe K (2001) *Equine Veterinary Nursing Manual*. Blackwell Science, London

Knecht CD, Allen AR, Williams DJ and Johnson JH (1987) *Fundamental Techniques in Veterinary Surgery, 3rd edn*. WB Saunders, Philadelphia

McCurnin DM (1990) *Clinical Textbook for Veterinary Technicians, 2nd edn*. WB Saunders, Philadelphia

McIlwraith CW, Nixon AJ, Wright IM and Boening J (2005) *Diagnostic and Surgical Arthroscopy in the Horse*. Elsevier, Philidephia

Scott K and Hotson-Moore A (2007) Surgical nursing. In: *BSAVA Manual of Practical Veterinary Nursing*, ed. E. Mullineaux and M. Jones, pp. 315–370. BSAVA Publications, Gloucester

Slatter D (2003) *Textbook of Small Animal Surgery, 3rd edn*. WB Saunders, Philadelphia

Tracey D (2000) *Small Animal Surgical Nursing*. Mosby, St Louis

Williams D and Niles J (2005) *BSAVA Manual of Canine and Feline Abdominal Surgery*. BSAVA Publications, Gloucester

Williams J and Moores A (2007) *BSAVA Manual of Canine and Feline Wound Management and Reconstruction, 2nd edn*. BSAVA Publications, Gloucester

Self-assessment questions

1. What factors can influence the development of wound infection?
2. How can postoperative myopathy related to the surgical period be avoided in the horse?
3. Identify ten procedures that may be carried out on a patient prior to surgery.
4. How does the role of the circulating nurse differ from that of the scrubbed nurse?
5. Identify three properties of the following suture materials:
   - Polyglycolic acid
   - Silk
   - Catgut.
6. What are the following surgical instruments used for:
   - Osteotome
   - Rongeurs
   - Gigli wire and handles?
7. What are the benefits of tissue glue?
8. How should surgical instruments be sterilized?
9. How long do instruments remain sterile following sterilization in an autoclave?
10. Describe how an arthroscope should be cleaned.

Chapter 25

Small animal surgical nursing

Davina Anderson and Jenny Smith

Learning objectives

After studying this chapter, students should be able to:

- **List the common surgical conditions encountered in the dog and cat**
- **Understand the common terms used to describe surgical conditions**
- **Describe the basic physiology and treatments of surgical diseases**
- **Describe the physical signs of normal and delayed healing of tissues and wounds**
- **Discuss the common complications and nursing requirements of surgical diseases**
- **Provide information to the owner on the postoperative nursing care required for surgical diseases**

Introduction

This chapter discusses the recognition of surgical diseases, surgical procedures, management and nursing of the post-operative patient, and the stages of normal and abnormal healing. The chapter relates predominantly to surgical conditions in dogs, cats and some exotic pets; however, the terminology used and many of the basic principles described may be extrapolated to other species. In order to understand this subject a basic knowledge of terminology is required; accurate communication between nursing staff and veterinary surgeons, and reliable record-keeping, can only be accomplished if correct terminology is used (Figure 25.1). Many terms used in the description of surgical diseases or procedures are created by the combination of two or more components. Knowledge of how these terms are created allows a new term to be understood without extensive learning by rote. The first part of the word usually describes the relevant anatomical area or structure whilst the suffix describes the nature of the procedure. For example, cystotomy, cystostomy and cystectomy all describe surgical procedures on the bladder.

Terminology	Meaning
General terms	
Prognosis	The prognosis is an indication of whether the animal is likely to survive the procedure – or at least how long the disease is likely to be controlled. For example a poor prognosis suggests that the animal will die fairly soon despite treatment, whereas an excellent prognosis suggests that the disease may be cured
Postoperative morbidity	This refers to the degree of complications that the animal may be expected to suffer after the surgery. High morbidity would suggest that an animal will need a lot of nursing care (e.g. paraplegics), whereas low morbidity suggests that the animal is expected to make a rapid and full recovery
Emergency surgery	Surgery that is performed immediately as a life-saving procedure despite increased anaesthetic and recovery risks in the ill patient
Elective surgery	Surgery that is planned and can be performed at a time convenient to the veterinary surgeon or owner
Stay sutures	These are long lengths of suture material temporarily placed in tissue so as to hold the tissue without causing bruising during surgery. Usually, the ends are held together with artery forceps, which are used as 'handles' to manipulate the tissue
Temporary openings	The suffix **-otomy** denotes a procedure for cutting open or dividing tissue during surgery. The tissue is then repaired to allow it to heal normally

Laparotomy or coeliotomy	A temporary opening into the abdomen. These are the standard terms of abdominal surgery. These terms can be further defined by identifying the site of the incision:
	    midline (linea alba)
	    paramedian (slightly to one side of the midline)
	    parapreputial (to one side of the prepuce)
	    paracostal (caudal and parallel to the last rib)

Rhinotomy	A temporary opening into the nasal cavity

25.1 Surgical terminology.

continues ▶

Terminology	Meaning
Temporary openings	
Tracheotomy	A temporary opening into the trachea
Thoracotomy	A temporary opening into the thorax
Gastrotomy	A temporary opening into the stomach
Enterotomy	A temporary opening into the intestine
Nephrotomy	A temporary opening into the kidney
Urethrotomy	A temporary opening into the urethra
Cystotomy	A temporary opening into the bladder
Hysterotomy	A temporary opening into the uterus (e.g. a caesarean)
Arthrotomy	A temporary opening into a joint space
Osteotomy	A temporary division of a bone
Myotomy	A temporary division of a muscle
Tenotomy	A temporary division of a tendon
Maintained openings	The suffix -**ostomy** denotes the creation of an opening or stoma ('mouth') which communicates with the outside through the skin. Usually a device is used to keep the stoma open, and then this is removed when the opening is allowed to close. Permanent stoma are sutured to the skin and allowed to heal open
Pharyngostomy	An opening in the pharynx, to allow feeding via a tube, or placement of an endotracheal tube bypassing the mouth
Tracheostomy	An opening in the trachea, to allow the animal to breathe when there is an obstruction in the larynx or pharynx, or when it is important not to have the endotracheal tube in the mouth during surgery. The opening may be maintained temporarily via a special tracheostomy tube, or it can be a permanent airway
Gastrostomy	An opening in the stomach to allow decompression or feeding bypassing the oesophagus, via a tube
Jejunostomy	An opening in the jejunum, to allow feeding bypassing the stomach and duodenum via a special feeding tube
Urethrostomy	A permanent opening in the urethra, to allow urination when there is an obstruction or stricture in the urethra distally
Cystostomy	An opening in the bladder, to divert urine from the urethra, via a drain
Removal of structures	The suffix -**ectomy** denotes the surgical removal of all or part of a structure. Where part of a structure is removed, the remaining part must be sutured back together. The point at which the tissue is rejoined is called the anastomosis
Tonsillectomy	Removal of the tonsils
Lung lobectomy	Removal of a lung lobe
Gastrectomy	Removal of part of the stomach
Pancreatectomy	Removal of part of the pancreas
Cholecystectomy	Removal of the gall bladder
Enterectomy	Removal of a length of intestine
Colectomy	Removal of part or all of the colon
Nephrectomy	Removal of a kidney
Cystectomy	Removal of part of the bladder wall
Mastectomy	Removal of some or all of the mammary glands
Orchidectomy	Removal of the testes
Ovariohysterectomy	Removel of the ovaries and uterus (spay)
Splenectomy	Removal of part or all of the spleen
Ostectomy	Removal of a section of bone

25.1 *continued* Surgical terminology.

Physiology of surgical nursing

Inflammation

Inflammation may be a normal physiological response to an injury or irritant, or part of a pathological process causing disease. An inflammatory response will be present as part of the healing process; it then persists for longer if disease develops. For example, the redness and swelling of the inflammation seen along the line of a surgical incision over the first 2–3 days after surgery are normal. If the animal licks the sutures or the surgical incision becomes infected, the inflammation will persist and then would be considered part of a pathological response to the continued injury.

The classical signs of inflammation are:

- Redness
- Swelling
- Heat
- Pain
- Loss of normal function of the tissue.

The redness, heat and swelling are due to an increase in the blood flow to the tissue. Swelling occurs as white blood cells and protein-rich fluid leave the blood vessels and accumulate in the tissue. Pain is due to stimulation of the nerve endings in the tissue as a response to the increased pressure due to the swelling, as well as inflammatory mediators and toxins released by the cells in the area. This fluid is known as inflammatory exudate and is an important part of the inflammatory process.

Inflammatory exudate serves a number of functions:

- Dilution of irritant substances in the tissues
- Delivery of immune cells to the tissues
- Delivery of immunoglobulins and other immune response substances
- Delivery of fibrinogen into the area to help with 'walling off' of the inflamed site
- Initiation of the response to injury and start of the healing process.

However, the inflammatory response can also lead to loss of function either due to destruction of the tissue (e.g. destruction of cartilage in erosive arthritis) or due to muscle spasm and pain.

Acute inflammation

Acute inflammation is the immediate and rapid response to injury (Figure 25.2). In ideal circumstances where the injury is self-limiting, the inflammation should settle down very quickly, i.e. within 2–3 days.

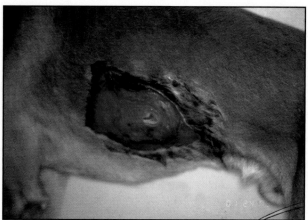

25.2   An acute avulsion of the skin on the flank of a Lurcher. The skin edges are painful and inflamed and there is serous ooze wetting the fur at the edges of the wound. This is a classic example of the very acute inflammatory phase of a wound.

There can be systemic signs of acute inflammation, including:

- Fever
- Increased pulse rate
- Increased circulating white blood cells, particularly polymorphonuclear leucocytes (PMNs).

In most circumstances, the acute inflammation resolves quickly once the injury is repaired or the initiating factor is eliminated. Where inflammation persists, it may become chronic and pathological (Figure 25.3). The acute inflammation seen in response to injury is a key stage in the development of normal healing.

Outcome	Notes
Resolution	No significant tissue injury
Healing	Tissues are slowly regenerated or repaired
Abscessation	An accumulation of pus that persists in a walled-off cavity
Degeneration	Damaged cells degenerate and are not repaired
Mineralization	Calcified deposits are laid down in soft tissues in response to chronic inflammation
Necrosis	Cell death occurs and the affected tissue is sloughed. Particularly seen in the skin or intestinal epithelium in response to severe inflammation
Gangrene	Cell death is associated with loss of the local blood supply and putrefaction of the tissues by anaerobic bacteria

25.3   Outcome of inflammation in tissues.

Chronic inflammation

Chronic inflammation refers to the fact that the inflammatory response has gone on for longer than expected, possibly weeks or months. These changes in the tissue may become irreversible and affect the normal function of the tissue permanently. The main difference in the tissue is that, instead of PMNs, a mononuclear cell population is seen together with proliferation of fibroblasts. There are three common situations where the inflammation persists and chronic inflammation results:

- Persistent low-grade infections (e.g. intracellular organisms or fungi)
- Prolonged exposure to foreign material (e.g. suture material)
- Autoimmune diseases (in these the inciting cause is the animal's own tissues and treatment aims to reduce the inflammatory response rather than remove the cause).

Inflammation of specific tissues

In different tissues the same basic processes occur, with production of fluid, swelling, oedema, increased blood supply and sometimes increased pain. For example, inflammation of the pancreas (pancreatitis) results in oedema and reddening of the pancreas with severe cranial abdominal pain. Peritonitis has been likened to an 'internal burn' as the peritoneum may become bright red, and produce large amounts of abdominal fluid.

Definitions: Inflammation of tissues

The suffix **-itis** indicates inflammation and/or infection of that tissue. This may be chronic (long term) or acute (sudden in onset)

- **Adenitis** – Inflammation of a gland.
- **Arthritis** – Inflammation of a joint.
- **Colitis** – Inflammation of the colon.
- **Conjunctivitis** – Inflammation of the conjunctiva of the eye.
- **Cystitis** – Inflammation of the bladder.
- **Dermatitis** – Inflammation of the skin. Specific terms may be used to describe the nature of the inflammation, e.g. pyoderma – an infected inflammation of the skin.
- **Enteritis** – Inflammation of the small intestines.
- **Gastritis** – Inflammation of the stomach.
- **Gingivitis** – Inflammation of the oral gingiva.
- **Hepatitis** – Inflammation of the liver.
- **Metritis** – Inflammation of the uterine lining. Pyometra denotes a concurrent infection of the inflamed uterus.
- **Nephritis** – Inflammation of the kidney, often called pyelonephritis to denote infection in the kidney.
- **Neuritis** – Inflammation of a nerve or nerve roots.
- **Orchitis** – Inflammation of the testes.
- **Otitis** – Inflammation of the ear. This may be the external ear canal (otitis externa) or the middle (otitis media) or inner ear (otitis interna).
- **Pancreatitis** – Inflammation of the pancreas.
- **Peritonitis** – Inflammation of the abdominal lining.
- **Pleuritis** – Inflammation of the thoracic lining.
- **Pneumonia** – Inflammation of the lungs.
- **Rhinitis** – Inflammation of the nasal cavity.
- **Tracheitis** – Inflammation of the trachea.
- **Urethritis** – Inflammation of the urethra.
- **Uveitis** – Inflammation of the iris of the eye.
- **Vaginitis** – Inflammation of the vagina.

Treatment of acute inflammation

The aims of treatment of inflammation are to remove the inciting cause and to prevent the development of chronic inflammation or long-term disease.

Removal of the inciting cause may be as simple as lavage (washing away) of debris or chemicals, or treatment of a bacterial infection with antibiotics. In the early stages, inflammation can sometimes be reduced by using cold compresses to reduce blood flow and thereby reduce swelling. Rapid treatment of burns (within 20 minutes) with cold water can reduce the extent of the injury by dissipating the heat and reducing the inflammatory response around the edge of the burn.

Sometimes it is necessary to limit the inflammatory response and drugs can be used. Drugs can reduce the inflammation and often have a secondary analgesic effect due to reduced stimulation of nerve endings and reduction of swelling. The commonly used drugs are corticosteroids and non-steroidal anti-inflammatory drugs (NSAIDs). These two groups of drugs have potential side effects; they should never be used together and are only used under the direction of a veterinary surgeon. If ongoing inflammation is caused by infection, topical antiseptics or systemic antibiotics may be used.

Fluid accumulation

Fluid can accumulate in tissues or in body spaces as part of a pathological process or as a response to injury and often is part of the inflammatory response. Analysis of the fluid is necessary in order to make a diagnosis of the disease process causing the fluid to accumulate.

Body fluid accumulations

- **Exudate** is the term used to describe inflammatory fluid that contains white blood cells and proteinaceous debris.
- **Blood** may accumulate in body cavities after organ haemorrhage or in tissue planes.
- **Serosanguineous exudate** is fluid that has the appearance of blood, but on analysis has a lower packed cell volume (PCV) than blood, and other inflammatory cells predominate.
- **Transudate** is fluid that has shifted across semi-permeable membranes and is largely acellular. It may accumulate due to loss of osmotic pressure (proteins in the circulating blood) or increased venous pressure.
- **Modified transudate**. When a transudate has been in the body cavity for a while, it causes irritation in its own right and some cells start to move into the transudate as part of the inflammatory response.
- **Physiological fluid** in an inappropriate space (e.g. urine, bile, chyle, saliva). The body produces some fluids that should always travel out through lined ducts. If there is a leak in the system, large volumes of these fluids may be identified in inappropriate spaces, such as free urine or bile in the abdomen.

Fluid-filled masses

Fluid-filled masses are often identified as part of investigation of disease, and they are differentiated according to the type of fluid within.

Seroma

Seromas are probably the commonest type of fluid-filled mass encountered in surgical nursing. A seroma is usually an accumulation of inflammatory exudate within the tissue underneath a surgical site. Some surgical procedures result in loss of normal tissue structure (**dead space**) and the spaces fill with fluid rapidly after the surgery. If measures are not taken to prevent this, the fluid may take a long time to resolve or may even need drainage.

Haematoma

This is the term used for a 'blood blister', where a blood vessel bursts due to trauma or surgery and the blood accumulates in the surrounding tissues (see Figure 25.27). It is important to differentiate between a haematoma due to direct trauma (or surgery) and a haematoma due to a clotting defect or vessel wall abnormality.

Abscess

An abscess is an accumulation of inflammatory exudate that contains dead and dying white cells (pus) in response to severe irritation or infection. It is usually walled off with a fibrous reaction (see below).

Physiological fluid leak

Sometimes normal body fluids can leak into tissue planes and become walled off by the inflammatory response to form a persistent fluid-filled mass. A good example of this is the salivary mucocele, where saliva leaks from the salivary duct and forms a fluctuant subcutaneous mass.

Abscesses and cellulitis

Abscesses and cellulitis are very common presentations of acute inflammatory disease in veterinary practice. When pyogenic organisms locate in a solid tissue, they cause cell death and a strong inflammatory response. This leads to the formation of pus. If this is not localized, it may distribute diffusely throughout the tissue and is known as **cellulitis.**

Abscesses are nearly always secondary to bacterial infection, and the pus is full of bacteria and dead bacteria inside white blood cells. An abscess can also be sterile when there are no bacteria involved but there is an accumulation of dead and dying cells and tissues within a fibrous capsule.

Within an abscess there are often several stages of inflammation going on at the same time, with pus in the centre, an acute inflammatory response around this with PMNs reacting to the toxins produced in the pus and, on the outside, a chronic inflammatory response with mononuclear cells and fibroblasts laying down a fibrous capsule. Sometimes the toxins produced by the abscess are not contained and they cause a **toxaemia**, which makes the animal systemically ill. The toxaemia can be life-threatening, causing pain, fever, vomiting, shock or even heart or kidney failure. Once the pus is discharged from the abscess, the systemic signs resolve and recovery is usually very rapid.

Abscesses that occur superficially (e.g. cat-bite abscess in the skin, Figure 25.4) often rupture spontaneously, releasing the pus through a hole in the overlying skin. Some abscesses occur internally (e.g. prostate, liver or peritoneal). If these abscesses rupture and release the pus throughout the abdomen, the consequences can be fatal.

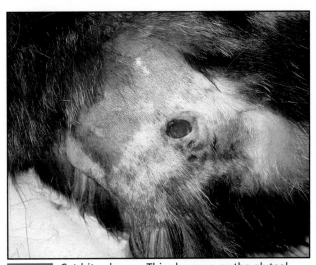

25.4 Cat-bite abscess. This abscess over the gluteal region has ruptured, releasing the pus. It has been clipped and cleaned and will now heal by second intention.

Treatment

Cellulitis is too diffuse to be treated except with systemic antibiotics, analgesics and anti-inflammatories. Abscesses can often be drained and this provides immediate relief from symptoms. Once the abscess is drained, the cavity collapses and the fibrous tissue granulates in and the hole heals over rapidly. If the diagnosis is not certain, a small needle and syringe can be used to aspirate some fluid from the abscess for analysis prior to treatment. Treatment is usually carried out under general anaesthetic, but at the very least, sedation and analgesics should be administered prior to treatment, as abscesses can be extremely painful.

- **Hot compresses** can be applied to very superficial abscesses. The principle is to soften the overlying skin and encourage rupture of the abscess through the surface. The use of poultices containing boric acid is not to be recommended, as they irritate the surrounding skin.
- **Surgical drainage** is a much quicker and more reliable way of treating abscesses. A hole is made in the skin at the most superficial point of the abscess, using a scalpel blade. The pus is allowed to drain and the cavity is lavaged with sterile fluids. The drainage hole should be encouraged to stay open for a few days, either by using a drain (see later) or by daily bathing with lavage of the cavity.
- **Resection** of abscesses. Deep abscesses or internal abscesses are not suitable for treatment by simple lancing. Deep abscesses may be dissected out around the fibrous capsule and removed in one piece. Internal abscesses may be either resected (e.g. a lung lobe abscess) or suctioned out under sterile conditions and the omentum used as a natural drain (e.g. prostatic abscesses).
- **Rabbits** can develop recurrent abscesses in the submandibular and cheek area. These are filled with a particularly thick type of pus that is very difficult to drain. It is important to open up the abscess adequately in order to allow treatments for some days afterwards. Compounds that debride the inside of the cavity, such as hydrogels or debriding solutions, are often used to

continue the cleaning process inside the cavity while it granulates. Sometimes the abscess is related to tooth root disease and this must also be treated in order to prevent recurrence. In some cases, there are multiple abscesses and it may be necessary to resect all of them.

Wound healing

Generally, acute inflammation of tissue is followed by healing. There are some basic processes that are common to all tissues:

- Removal of dead and foreign material
- Clearance of the inflammatory response
- Regeneration of lost tissue components if possible
- Replacement of lost tissue components by connective tissue.

The different outcomes of the healing process depend on the type of tissue and the degree of damage. There may be resolution, regeneration or organization.

Resolution

Where there is no tissue destruction and the inflammatory process is very mild (e.g. a superficial graze), the tissue can return to its original state prior to the injury.

Regeneration

The damaged tissue is completely replaced by proliferation of the remaining cells. This depends on the type of tissue, as regeneration can only occur if the lost cells can be replaced and if the connective tissue and vascular supply are still intact. In this context, cells are classified into three basic groups:

- **Labile cells** can divide and proliferate throughout life. They are highly capable of regeneration (e.g. epithelial cells, blood cells and lymphoid tissue)
- **Stable cells** do not normally divide, but can do so in response to certain stimuli, and may divide following injury to the tissue (e.g. cells in the liver, kidney, endocrine glands, bone and fibrous tissue)
- **Permanent cells** only divide during fetal growth and are incapable of regeneration (e.g neurons, cardiac muscle cells and, to some extent, skeletal muscle cells).

Organization

Where the cells cannot repair the damage by regeneration, the tissue heals by the formation of **scar tissue**, which is organized fibrous tissue with a large number of collagen fibres. Often this means that the tissue will lose its normal function, or be more susceptible to recurrent damage (e.g. scar tissue in skin) (see later).

Most tissues heal by a combination of these processes, with some parts capable of regeneration and others forming scar tissue. Skin is a good example of tissue that heals in the dermis by the formation of scar tissue (organization) and by regeneration in the epidermis.

Normal wound healing in skin

The normal process of healing follows a predictable pattern that can be used to determine the progress of any healing tissue. There is always overlap between the phases as they progress from one predominant cell type to another, and they are not distinct.

Inflammatory phase

After injury, there is an initial inflammatory phase triggered by activation of the platelets and fibrin in the blood clot, which in turn attracts neutrophils to the damaged tissue. The neutrophils will clear up bacteria, necrotic tissue and foreign material. They also release inflammatory mediators that attract macrophages into the tissue. Once the macrophages arrive, the final de-bridement process begins and the tissue starts to proliferate to repair the damage. The wound will look exudative, swollen and red during this phase (Figure 25.5).

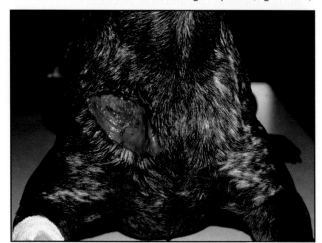

25.5 Gunshot wound across a dog's shoulder. The wound is peracute; there is tissue loss and inflammation and healing processes have not yet started.

Proliferative phase

The proliferative phase is triggered by the macrophages and involves fibroblasts that lay down the matrix of the tissue, endothelial cells that lay down new blood vessels, and epithelial cells that migrate over the top of the wound to reconstitute the epidermis (**epithelialization**). This phase is the most crucial part of wound healing, as it demonstrates that it is progressing normally. The classic appearance of this phase is the development of **granulation tissue** (Figure 25.6). Granulation tissue is bright red, very vascular and has a granular surface due to the capillary loops growing into the tissue. It is highly resistant to infection and is a sign that the wound is clear of bacterial infection. During the formation of granulation tissue, the wound starts to contract and this process alone can close a wound by up to 30% of its area. Gradually, the granulation tissue is replaced by collagen fibres and scar tissue is laid down.

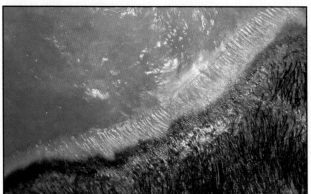

25.6 Close-up of a wound edge, showing healthy granulation tissue with an advancing epithelial edge.

Remodelling phase

Once the proliferation and repair of the tissue is complete, the scar will remodel and strengthen over a period of days to weeks as the hair regrows and the fibroblasts rearrange the matrix of the tissue according to the tensions during normal function.

In a clean surgical wound in skin, the inflammatory phase should last 24–48 hours; then a thin layer of granulation tissue develops between the edges of the surgical wound. By the time the sutures are removed at 7–10 days, the remodelling phase is well under way.

In larger skin wounds, the inflammatory phase may last longer due to infection or foreign material, and the granulation tissue may not start to develop until at least 3–5 days. Depending on how large the wound is, the proliferative phase (granulation, contraction and re-epithelialization) may take days to weeks to be completed.

Normal wound healing in other tissues

All tissues follow the same basic healing pattern as skin, with inflammatory, proliferative and remodelling phases.

Tendon and muscle injuries are often associated with trauma and other tissues may be simultaneously damaged, prolonging the healing process. The basic pattern is as for skin, but the remodelling phase is much more important as tendons and muscles have to retain function as well as strength. Muscle should heal quickly but may have to be immobilized to allow development of strength in the scar. Tendons take a very long time to develop strength; they have to be supported and only gradually reintroduced to weight bearing, otherwise they may stretch or rupture.

The gastrointestinal, urinary and reproductive tract tissues heal more rapidly than skin, with the fibrin clot helping to seal the wound initially, with the main support coming from the sutures for the first 3 days. The epithelium can regenerate and starts to close the wound almost immediately, with fibroblast proliferation giving the wound strength by 3–4 days after wounding. The urinary bladder heals the fastest and the colon the slowest. Normal healing in the gut depends on good nutrition and a good blood supply. Nutrition for the surgical wound comes from the lumen, and feeding the patient will also stimulate blood supply to the gut and accelerate healing. This simple concept emphasizes the importance of postoperative nursing and feeding of the patient.

Factors that affect normal wound healing

Normal wound healing in companion animals is reasonably efficient. Most wounds are delayed in healing either because the animal has another undiagnosed disease or because the management of the patient is poor (Figure 25.7). Sometimes treatments affect the rate of healing and these may have to be modified until the wound is healed.

Inflammation: a summary

- Inflammatory processes may be a normal part of the healing process but they can also be part of the pathology.
- Prolonged inflammation is usually a sign that the healing process is delayed.
- Responses to inflammation can aid in the diagnosis of the disease process.
- Some tissues can heal by regeneration, but others may have to heal by the formation of scar tissue.

Factors affecting healing	Clinical examples
Systemic diseases	Hypothyroidism, hyperadrenocorticism (Cushing's disease), protein-losing disease, renal or hepatic disease, diabetes mellitus, malnutrition, cachexia, cancer, severe cardiovascular disease
Wound management	Choice of wound dressing (primary layer), bandage technique, inadequate bandage protection, infrequent dressing changes, patient interference with the wound
Surgical factors	Prolonged anaesthetic time, wound infection, overly tight sutures, tension on the suture line, choice of suture material, poor surgical techniques, contamination of instrumentation or surgical site during surgery, inadequate closure or drainage of dead space. Foreign material left in the wound, including suture material may delay healing by increasing the inflammatory response
Therapy	Corticosteroids, antimetabolite chemotherapeutic drugs, radiotherapy

25.7 Causes of delayed wound healing.

Wounds

Classification of wounds

Wounds may be classified according to aetiology, depth of skin loss, contamination or infection, extent of soft tissue or bony involvement, duration since wounding, and site. For example: 'An abrasive, full-thickness, infected injury to the distal hindlimb with shear and fracture of the lateral metatarsal bone and loss of ligaments' (Figure 25.8). It is important to know how the wound was incurred in order to determine the extent of the injuries and the expected progression of the wound. Some types of injury affect the way in which the tissues heal and their susceptibility to infection.

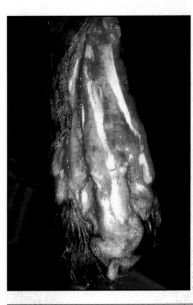

25.8 Traumatic wound on the distal limb as a result of a road traffic accident. The foot has been sheared, losing the skin and some soft tissue and damaging the collateral ligaments and metatarsal bones. (Courtesy of John Houlton)

Aetiology

There are 10 basic groups of wounds, classified by cause:

- Surgical (incisional)
- Surgical wound dehiscence
- Laceration
- Puncture
- Abrasion/shear
- Degloving/ischaemic/skin slough (avulsion)
- Burns – chemical, cold and heat, electrical
- Ballistic/gunshot
- Crush injury
- Chronic fistulae/sinuses.

These general groups are distinguished by the degree of tissue trauma, contamination and associated injuries. Identifying the cause of injury helps in determining appropriate wound management and also the expected healing time. Wounds that are heavily contaminated or have large amounts of tissue loss will have longer inflammatory phases and longer healing times. The category also helps to indicate the type and degree of contamination of the wound.

Degree of contamination

The only truly clean wound is a surgical wound; all other types of wound can be considered contaminated or infected. The optimal time for treatment of an open wound is within the first 6 hours. This is known as the 'golden period' and the wound is considered as contaminated, but not infected:

- 0–6 hours – little bacterial multiplication: contaminated
- 6–12 hours – bacteria beginning to divide: early infection
- Over 12 hours – bacterial invasion of tissues: (infection) established.

Surgical procedures are also classified according to infection and contamination (see later).

Viability and vascular supply to the tissue

Wounds may also be more susceptible to infection if there is associated tissue damage. Tissue that is devitalized (or necrotic) due to laceration or compression of blood vessels is more likely to become infected. Surgical wounds are more at risk of infection if a tourniquet has been applied, and cardiovascular disease may also delay healing due to poor blood supply to the limbs. Shock can result in vasoconstriction and if the circulation is not regained there may be reduced blood supply (and therefore increased risk of delayed healing or infection) to wounds in any area of the body.

Different types of tissue have a greater or lesser ability to resist infection. Well vascularized areas of skin have good bacterial defences; they should heal well and resist infection. Tissue may become devitalized due to poor surgical technique or desiccation during surgical debridement, which then increases the risk of infection or delayed healing.

Foreign material

All foreign material has to be removed before the wound is able to heal.

Healing of wounds (closure)

Primary closure (first intention healing)

Wounds that are closed surgically heal rapidly with a very short healing phase, because there is little foreign material or bacteria.

Delayed primary closure

Some wounds that are contaminated are better cleaned and managed as open wounds for 1–3 days in order to ensure that there is no residual infection. These wounds are then closed surgically once the earliest signs of granulation tissue formation are seen.

Secondary closure

A wound that is heavily contaminated, or where the surrounding skin is believed to be damaged, may be managed as an open wound for several days until it is possible to close the wound surgically. Such wounds will have well established granulation tissue and it may be necessary to excise some of this in order to close the wound.

Second intention healing

In some instances it is not possible, or it is unnecessary, to close a wound surgically and it is dressed and bandaged until it heals. In these cases, the wound heals by granulation (Figure 25.9), epithelialization and contraction. Large wounds may take weeks or months to close in this way and during this time the wound has to be regularly re-bandaged. It may be better for the patient and more cost-effective to attempt secondary closure using a reconstructive technique than continue with second intention healing.

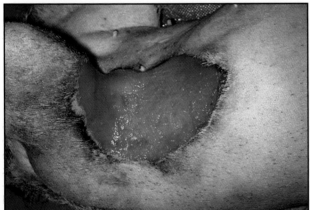

| 25.9 | Large burn wound in the flank fold of a dog. The wound is healing by second intention and has filled in with granulation tissue. The edges of the wound are beginning to epithelialize but there is little evidence yet of contraction. |

Management of primary closure wounds

This group of wounds covers all surgical incisions that are sutured, and will be the commonest wound management area that veterinary nurses have to provide advice on. Prevention of complications associated with surgical wounds relies on meticulous management in four main areas:

- Preoperative preparation of the patient
- Systemic or local wound factors that may affect wound healing (see above)
- Surgical technique and wound closure (see later)
- Postoperative management.

Preoperative management of the patient

The general principle behind preoperative management is that the patient should be as healthy as possible at the time of the surgery in order to reduce postoperative risks. Therefore elective procedures may be delayed if, on the day of admission, the animal has another incidental condition (e.g. diarrhoea). Patients that have concurrent injuries should be stabilized as much as possible prior to surgery, particularly if a long operation is necessary. Long periods of hospitalization before operations may also increase the risk of wound infection and breakdown. The specific reasons for this are not known, but may be due to increased stress during hospitalization and the colonization of the patient's skin with microorganisms other than its normal skin commensals.

Skin preparation and patient preparation are important in reducing the bacterial load and therefore also the risk of postsurgical inflammation and infection.

Prior to surgery, the number of microorganisms on the skin should be reduced as much as possible. Very dirty animals (e.g. farm dogs) may benefit from a general bath with non-medicated soap to remove dust and dirt that might contaminate the wound (as well as the operating theatre). With 'normal' levels of contamination, bathing makes no difference unless antiseptic solutions such as 4% w/v chlorhexidine are used. Generally, it is not necessary to bathe preoperatively; standard skin preparation at the time of surgery is adequate.

Clean wounds do not generally become infected postoperatively. The risks of infection can be determined by classifying the type of surgery and using an appropriate antibiotic protocol perioperatively if required (see later).

Hair removal

Ideally the hair is removed prior to anaesthesia after the premedication has been administered, thereby reducing the anaesthetic time; however, clipping often occurs after the patient has been anaesthetized. This also allows for loose hairs to fall off prior to skin preparation. The clipping should always be done outside theatre so that the contaminated hair can be removed from the vicinity of the surgery. Depilatories and shaving have been shown to increase wound infection rates and so clipping is the recommended technique for the removal of hair. Coarse hair is clipped with a No. 10 blade first and all clips are completed with a No. 40 blade. (Finer blades may be required for small mammals, see below.) The blade is held gently against the skin and run in the opposite direction to the lie of the hair. Lubricants and coolants are applied regularly to prevent overheating of the blade and it is important to ensure that the blade is sharp and has no missing teeth. Poor technique results in nicks in the skin, dermatitis and increased risk of postsurgical wound infection. A vacuum cleaner is often used to remove the loose hair from the patient and the table.

A generous area surrounding the proposed incision site should be clipped. This is essential to maintain sterility of the site and to allow the incision to be extended if required. For reconstructive procedures, the whole side of the animal may need to be clipped. For surgery on the limbs, the whole circumference and up to or beyond the adjacent joint should be clipped.

Small mammals have much thinner skin than dogs and cats, and extra care must be taken during hair removal (Figure 25.10). Although a No. 40 clipper blade is often used, variable high-speed clippers specifically designed for animals with fine hair are much better. These clippers make hair removal easier and cause less accidental cutting and burning of the skin. The amount of hair clipped in small mammals should be kept to a minimum to prevent hypothermia. Shaving should be avoided as there is evidence to suggest that this is associated with an increased infection rate (Alexander *et al.*, 1983; Willford, 1983).

Preparation of avian skin requires feathers to be plucked rather than clipped, in order to ensure regrowth of the feather.

For more information on hair removal see Chapter 24.

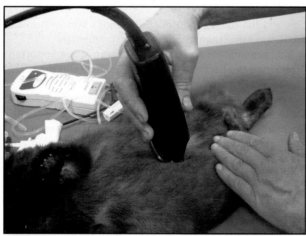

25.10 Rabbit fur should be clipped with very fine clippers to ensure that the underlying skin is not torn. The skin is gently held steady with the free hand.

Skin preparation

The patient's skin can never be made completely sterile. The aim of preoperative preparation is to reduce the bacterial count without damaging the skin's natural barriers to infection. Firstly, a surgical scrub solution is used that has antiseptic and detergent properties to degrease and kill bacteria on the skin surface. Secondly, a surgical antiseptic solution is applied to leave some residual activity to kill bacteria that may migrate out of the hair follicles or sebaceous glands during the surgery. For procedures that require particularly high standards of surgical asepsis for prolonged periods (e.g. specialist orthopaedic surgery), an adhesive impermeable transparent drape may be applied after the skin has been prepared. The surgeon then incises through the drape, which remains stuck to the edges of the skin incision, thereby protecting the surgical site from contamination during the operation.

For more information on skin preparation see Chapter 24.

Postoperative management of surgical wounds

When an animal is discharged, the owner should be given instructions for wound care, potential problems and when to seek advice. It is a good idea to explain the procedure that has been performed and to show the owner the wound before the animal goes home. Some practices will give specific instructions such as limited exercise, special diet, care of a bandage or physiotherapy. It is advisable that the owner is given written instructions on postoperative care so that there can be no misunderstanding at a later date if there is a complication associated with poor homecare.

Immediate perioperative care

At the end of the surgery, blood stains and clots should be gently wiped away using sterile fluid such as saline. Wetting of the surgical incision should be avoided if possible. Agents such as hydrogen peroxide solutions may be used to help to clean the haircoat, but should not be used on the perisurgical skin as it may cause dermatitis.

The main principles of managing a clean surgical wound are:

- Dressing the wound
- Observation of the wound and patient
- Prevention of self-mutilation
- Suture removal.

Dressing surgical wounds

Surgical wounds (Figure 25.11) are dressed, if required, for various reasons:

- To protect the wound from contamination or trauma
- To protect the wound from self-mutilation by the patient
- To absorb exudate from the wound
- To limit movement of the wound to reduce pain, or tension on the sutures
- To limit swelling of the surgical site.

Some surgical wounds do not require a dressing. Simple dressings consist of a non-adherent primary layer with a thin absorbent pad held in place by an adhesive tape. After 24 hours, this dressing can be removed as the wound will have formed a fibrin seal that is resistant to bacterial contamination. A commercial example of this kind of dressing is Primapore (Smith & Nephew) which has a strip of non-adherent dressing with an adhesive edge to hold it to the skin. Spray-on dressings can also be used to seal the wound in the first 24 hours with a waterproof and gas-permeable polymer layer.

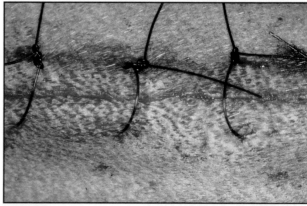

25.11 Close-up of a fresh surgical wound. The skin edges are gently apposed by the sutures and a thin line of blood clot is just visible. The edges of the wound are slightly swollen by the early inflammatory response. This swelling should be resolved by 2 days post surgery if the wound is healing well.

In some cases, additional padding is required and a thick cover of absorbent material such as cotton wool or gamgee may be used, which is held in place by tertiary dressings. Pressure bandages (e.g. Robert Jones) should always have substantial padding to prevent focal pressure points. All bandages should be replaced 24 hours after surgery to prevent the development of pressure injuries secondary to swelling under the dressing.

Wounds that are expected to exude heavily may need to be dressed more than once daily in order to ensure that the absorptive capacity of the dressing is not exceeded and the healthy tissues are kept dry and clean.

Monitoring of postsurgical wounds

Veterinary nurses are well placed to detect early signs of wound complications by careful observation of the surgical wound. If a dressing has been placed on the wound it may not be possible to observe the wound directly, but the skin surrounding the wound and the dressing itself can be observed.

The factors to pay particular attention to are:

- **Exudate** – Note the amount, colour and type (serous or purulent). If exudate continues to leak through a dressing, the dressing must be changed to observe the wound
- **Erythema** (reddening) – Note whether this is limited to the vicinity of the sutures or whether it extends further. Note whether the erythematous area has increased or decreased in size since the surgery
- **Oedema** – Note how severe the oedema is and whether it is increasing or reducing
- **Haematoma** – Note how severe the haematoma is and whether it is increasing or reducing
- **Pain** – Note the severity of the pain (a subjective score of 1–10 is sometimes helpful) and whether the pain is continuous, intermittent, only present when the wound is handled, or if there is no pain
- **Odour** – Note if there is a foul odour from the wound.

In addition to monitoring the wound, good post-surgical wound care also involves monitoring the patient for any signs of systemic illness that may be associated with wound complications. Both subjective and objective assessments should be performed:

- **Subjective assessment** – note whether the animal is bright, alert and responsive or whether there has been a change in demeanour since the surgery. Also note progressive changes in demeanour throughout the postoperative recovery phase
- **Objective assessment** – daily monitoring of temperature, pulse and respiration rates, food and water intake, defecation and urination and recording of clinical signs and treatments should constitute the minimum daily assessment of hospitalized patients in the postoperative phase. In some cases, a more detailed clinical examination including other factors such as water intake, neurological reflexes or blood parameters may be necessary.

Prevention of self-mutilation

Self-mutilation at the surgical incision often leads to wound dehiscence. Some tendency to lick the wound postoperatively is seen in almost all animals, but persistent licking or chewing at the wound may be an indicator of wound complications. Animals may also lick or chew at the wound because of concern at the foreign material on the skin (the sutures) or due to generalized skin disease causing pruritus.

Dressings will help to reduce self-mutilation, but a determined animal will soon destroy most bandages. Bitter sprays are available to protect either the bandage or the surgical site, but they are not as effective as preventing access to the wound altogether. The Elizabethan collar (see Chapter 17) is one of the most useful and commonly employed devices. These aids are available in opaque or clear plastic and are placed around the neck secured by a collar or harness. They must be large enough to prevent the nose from reaching over the edge of the collar and accessing the wound. Scratching with the hindfeet can be prevented using well padded bandages on the feet. Other devices available include neck braces or body braces that prevent the animal turning round to reach the wound. Basket muzzles are helpful in preventing animals from destroying bandages, but they must be carefully fitted to ensure that the animal can pant and drink water through the muzzle. Owners should be warned that other pets may interfere with the wound by grooming or playing.

Exotic species may require some ingenuity to prevent them interfering with sutures. The use of subcuticular sutures may be employed so that there are no skin sutures to irritate the fine skin. Elizabethan collars may be made out of light card or plastic, and splints can be made out of syringe cases or ice-lolly sticks. Care should be taken to ensure that the collar does not irritate the skin around the neck. Some species (e.g. rabbits) may 'freeze' on application of an Elizabethan collar and refuse to eat or drink. As it is important that herbivores eat as soon as possible after surgery, an 'anti-scratch' collar may be more appropriate in these situations.

It may be difficult to protect a laparotomy wound in rodents where the surgical site is in constant contact with the floor. These animals should be housed separately until the wound is healed and the bedding changed to a non-powdery form, such as shredded paper. The bedding must be completely changed daily to ensure minimal contamination of the wound with urine or faeces.

Removal of sutures

Sutures approximate the wound edges and this allows rapid first intention healing with minimal scarring. Sutures are removed as soon as the skin is healed and in most cases this will be in 7–10 days. Healing may be quicker in some young animals, whereas in older animals the sutures may be left in for a few extra days. Subcuticular sutures may be used to appose the skin edges using absorbable suture material. In these cases, the wound should still be checked 7–10 days later to ensure that the wound has healed normally.

If the wound has healed, the sutures should be easy to remove and this *should not be a painful procedure*. As the swelling resolves, the sutures become slightly loose and the tag can be lifted up with fingers or forceps, allowing a scissor blade to be slipped underneath, and the length entering the skin is cut, without needing to touch the skin surface. The suture then slides out of the skin. Skin staples require a special device for removal.

In snakes the sutures may remain in place until the next ecdysis (moult), as then the epidermis is more active and healing may be considered complete. In chelonians skin sutures are left in place for 4–6 weeks before removal.

Complications of surgical wounds

The main complication of surgical wounds is **dehiscence** (the breakdown of a wound along all or part of its length) (Figure 25.12). Factors that increase the risk of wound dehiscence are:

- Poor postoperative care of the wound
- Infection of the wound
- Seroma formation or haematoma
- Poor preoperative preparation of the patient
- Poor surgical technique
- Poor suture technique or inappropriate suture materials
- Decreased blood supply to the wound
- Poor general health of the patient.

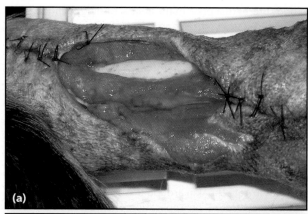
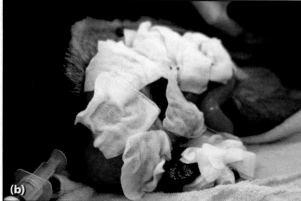

25.12 Surgical wound dehiscence. **(a)** A wound, sutured on the limb of a dog, that has been under too much tension. The central part of the wound has broken open and is now granulating slowly over the exposed bone. The edges of the sutured part are still inflamed. **(b)** A much more serious consequence of wound dehiscence in a bitch spay, where the midline repair has broken down and the abdominal contents (covered here by sterile swabs) have fallen out.

Infection is the most common cause of dehiscence and may be a result of either the poor postoperative care or the surgical preparation and technique. Other complications of wound healing include sinus formation, fistula and incisional hernia.

Sinus formation

This is a late infective complication. It is usually a small blind-ending tract lined with granulation tissue leading to an abscess cavity. Sinuses in surgical wounds are often focused around suture material or other foreign material inadvertently left in the wound at the time of surgery. Suture sinuses are often seen surrounding skin sutures if they are left in place for too long. They resolve on removal of the foreign material.

Fistula

This is an abnormal tract that forms between two epithelialized surfaces, or connects an epithelial surface to the skin. It can be a complication of wound healing, for example in anal or oronasal surgery. Occasionally it is seen as a congenital abnormality (e.g. rectovaginal fistula). Fistulae have to be surgically repaired.

Incisional hernia

This is a late complication of abdominal surgery where there is dehiscence of the incision in the muscle layers, while the skin repair remains intact. Abdominal contents may herniate out and lie in the space between the muscles or under the skin. It should be repaired as a matter of urgency in case the skin ruptures and the abdominal contents become contaminated.

Management of contaminated or infected wounds

Initial assessment

First aid measures are important in the initial assessment of the injury:

- Take brief details of the duration and site of the injury
- Assess bleeding and determine whether arterial or venous
- Arrest bleeding using a bandage or tourniquet if necessary
- Cover the wound with a sterile dressing to prevent further contamination in the hospital
- Assess the animal's general state of health; look for signs of shock
- Assess the animal for other life-threatening injuries
- Provide antibiotic cover and analgesia, as directed by a veterinary surgeon, and treat for shock if necessary
- Take a more detailed full history from the owner.

The history helps to determine the origin of the wound and the likely concurrent injuries. It will also determine whether the wound is classified as infected or contaminated.

Principles of management

The first stage is decontamination as far as possible, given the state of the wound and the condition of the patient. This also means prevention of further contamination in the hospital or by the animal. The second stage is debridement of necrotic or devitalized tissue and removal of any foreign debris. The final result should be control of infection and establishment of a healthy wound bed enabling closure of the skin deficit.

One of the important first steps is to clip and clean the surrounding undamaged skin (Figure 25.13). This not only helps to clean the wound, but also helps to assess the extent of the wound and viability of the skin. Ideally, the wound should be protected from further contamination, and it may

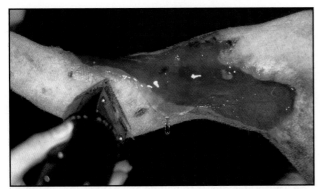

25.13 The skin surrounding a wound should be carefully clipped, using a covering such as K-Y jelly in the wound to protect it from contamination with hair clippings.

be closed using towel clips or a continuous suture. This is not always possible and so most wounds are packed with sterile swabs or filled with a water-soluble jelly (e.g. K-Y jelly, Johnson & Johnson) during clipping and cleaning. The jelly can then be washed away with any hair or dirt from the adjacent skin later on. The clipper blades must be properly disinfected and without chips that might cause dermatitis on nearby skin. Hair at the edges may be trimmed with scissors wetted with saline or dipped in mineral oil. Thorough and wide removal of hair is important in keeping the wound clean during the next phases of management.

Lavage of wounds

The aims of wound lavage are to wash debris out of the wound, to dilute the bacteria, and not to cause any further damage. It is therefore important to use large volumes of fluids and not to lavage too vigorously. This may be achieved by using a 20 ml syringe with an 18 gauge needle or catheter attached to a giving set and bag of fluid (Figure 25.14). Gross contamination or necrotic tissue may be washed away with gentle tap-water lavage using a hand shower. After this, the wound should be treated in a sterile manner to prevent further contamination.

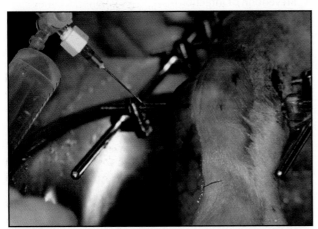

25.14 Once the surrounding skin has been clipped and cleaned, the wound itself can be irrigated or lavaged using sterile isotonic fluids (such as 0.9% saline). A 20 ml syringe is attached to a giving set and a three-way tap is used to fill the syringe with fluids from the fluid bag. The fluid is then sprayed on to the wound using an 18 gauge needle, as shown here. The procedure is repeated until the wound is completely clean.

Not all solutions are suitable for wound lavage; substances added to a lavage solution may damage the host cells and delay healing (Figure 25.15). Although it is tempting to use antiseptic solutions for infected wounds, they do not stay in the wound for long and may delay wound healing. In general it is better to use large volumes of sterile isotonic fluids to lavage wounds. If antiseptic solutions are used it is important to use the solution, rather than the surgical scrub, as the latter contains detergents that can irritate the wound.

Solution	Concentration	Indications
Sterile saline	0.9%	Any wound – no tissue damage; no antibacterial action other than dilution
Lactated Ringer's solution	As supplied	As above
Chlorhexidine	0.5%	Contaminated or infected wounds – *Staphylococcus aureus* often resistant. Toxic to fibroblasts. Residual activity good
Povidone–iodine	1%	Contaminated or infected wounds. Inactivated by debris, pus or blood. Broad spectrum, poor residual activity. Toxic to host cells
Hypochlorite	0.125%	Toxic to cells. Irritant for 4–5 days after use. *Not recommended*
Hydrogen peroxide	1–3%	No bactericidal activity. Very toxic to all cell types. *Not recommended*
Cetrimide/ chlorhexidine		Very toxic to cells. Irritant. *Not recommended*

25.15 Suitability of solutions for wound lavage.

Wound lavage procedure

1. Select at least a 1000 ml bag of warmed sterile isotonic fluid.
2. Attach a giving set with a three-way tap on the end.
3. Attach a 20 ml syringe and an 18 gauge needle or catheter to the three-way tap.
4. Lavage the wound over a bowl or tray to catch the fluid, using the 20 ml syringe to spray the wound surface.
5. Keep refilling the syringe from the fluid bag until all the fluids have been used to clean the wound or the wound fluid runs clear.
6. Carefully dry the healthy skin adjacent to the wound and cover the wound with sterile dressings.

Debridement of wounds

Debridement is the next crucial step in wound management. It involves removal of all infected, necrotic or contaminated tissue from the wound.

Antiseptics or antibiotics should not be a substitute for good surgical debridement. Debridement is the single most important step in the management of a wound and is often performed inadequately.

Surgical debridement

This is the best way to remove grossly contaminated tissue. The wound should be draped and prepared as for surgery and a scalpel used to cut away necrotic or dirty tissue. The instruments, gloves and drapes may be exchanged for sterile ones as the debridement progresses and the wound becomes cleaner. Surgical exploration of the wound also enables visualization of local anatomical structures and determination of the extent of the wound.

Debridement dressings

These are used in the initial stages until it is clear that there is no residual infection or necrotic material. Debridement dressings should not be left on the wound for more than 24 hours and in some instances may need to be changed twice daily. There are three main dressing types available for debridement (see later for details):

- Adherent dressings
- Hydrogels
- Hydrocolloids.

Other techniques

Commercial enzyme preparations can be applied to the wound to break down and allow removal of necrotic debris, but they are stopped once the granulation tissue is established.

Maggots have been used to debride wounds, allowing rapid establishment of healthy granulation tissue. Sterile maggots are produced commercially and are available at the correct larval stage for clinical use. They must be removed from the wound before they start to invade healthy tissue.

MRSA

Meticillin-resistant *Staphylococcus aureus* (MRSA) has been called the hospital 'superbug' by the Press. It is one of many bacterial strains often found in hospital environments that are resistant to a range of commonly used antibiotics (see also Chapter 5).

In veterinary care, the incidence of this infection has increased over the last few years and there have been a number of reports of MRSA causing clinical problems, particularly in orthopaedic cases.

MRSA is often found in the upper respiratory tract of healthy people and is a unique strain of *S. aureus* with a particular sensitivity pattern that makes it difficult to treat. Currently, most veterinary cases probably arise from MRSA acquired from the owner or veterinary staff. One study showed that hospital staff were two or three times more likely to carry MRSA and this suggests that pets belonging to people who work in hospitals may be more at risk of carrying MRSA.

When MRSA is identified during a routine culture test, it does not necessarily mean that the infection is untreatable. In many cases there is documented sensitivity to potentiated sulphonamides and human carriers can be treated with intranasal mupirocin. However, there is considerable evidence for MRSA protection in biofilm on orthopaedic implants or permanent suture materials, and resolution of the infection usually relies on removal of these implants. Even then, there is still a risk of septicaemia and death in cases that have not been dealt with early enough.

Currently the sample is tested *in vitro* against a number of antibiotics, one of which is oxacillin, and resistance to this suggests a phenotype consistent with MRSA. Some of the isolates will show sensitivity *in vitro* to other beta-lactam antibiotics, but it is important to be aware that this will not be the case *in vivo*.

Simple hygiene will make a large difference to transmission of MRSA to patients. This includes regular hand washing, alcohol rubs and wearing gloves as often as possible. However, evidence suggests that MRSA and other nosocomial organisms can be protected from disinfectants in live amoebae, thus avoiding the standard techniques for decontamination. Disposable gloves to handle any patient thought to be at risk, or for changing dressings and cleaning wounds, should be considered standard policy.

Some larger veterinary hospitals have considered screening staff for MRSA carrier status, but with employment rights this policy would have to be introduced with informed consent and members of staff could not be required to cooperate. Regular monitoring of culture results in practice, accurate theatre records and staff records will enable a rapid response in anticipating or monitoring outbreaks of MRSA infection.

Management of secondary closure wounds

Principles of wound dressings

Wound dressings are usually applied to the wound in three layers: the primary, secondary and tertiary layers. The general construction of the dressing depends on the location of the wound and the function of the dressing. Knowledge of the normal process of wound healing enables the veterinary nurse to choose the appropriate dressing at different stages of healing.

Wound dressing functions include:

- Absorption of exudate
- Analgesia
- Protection of the wound
- Prevention of infection
- Promotion of wound healing
- Maintaining a high humidity at the wound dressing interface.

Both the owner and the nursing staff should closely monitor all dressings for signs of complications. Poorly managed dressings will cause delayed wound healing and may cause further damage. Dressings that have been applied too tightly to the limb can cause damage ranging from areas of skin loss to loss of the whole limb or even death.

Reasons to remove the dressing

- Persistent chewing at the dressing.
- Foul smell from the dressing.
- Soiling or wetting of the dressing with water or urine.
- 'Strike-through' of exudate from the wound to the outside of the dressing.
- Slippage of the dressing from its original placement.

Written instructions should always be given to owners if an animal is discharged with a dressing in place.

Primary layer

The primary layer is the material that is placed in contact with the wound itself. The principle behind the primary layer is that it should *at least* not harm the wound and *at best* improve the rate of healing of the wound. Current thinking on wound management is that optimal healing occurs in a 'moist' environment. Dressings are therefore designed to provide a controlled environment that is not too 'wet' or too 'dry'.

There are numerous products available and it is important to realize that there is no perfect wound dressing. By understanding the way in which the different classes of dressings work, the veterinary nurse should be better equipped to use these dressings appropriately.

The functions of the primary layer will include some or all of the following at different stages:

- Debridement of necrotic tissue (this may require rehydration, lysis of fibrin attachments and physical removal from the wound)
- Absorption of fluid away from wound (if fluid is allowed to remain on the wound surface, it can macerate the tissues or provide a reservoir for infection)
- Stimulation of granulation tissue (some dressings actively promote and speed up the formation of granulation tissue)
- Promotion of epithelialization (epithelialization can only occur across healthy granulation tissue and is faster in a moist warm environment)
- Allowing contraction or controlled contraction of the wound.

Categories of primary layer dressings

Wound dressings can be described according to their basic characteristics. Some dressings may fall into more than one of the following categories, or dressings may be designed so that they have more than one general function:

- Adherent or non-adherent
- Absorbent or non-absorbent
- Passive, interactive or bioactive (passive: having no action on the wound; interactive: responding to the wound environment in some way; bioactive: having a biological effect on the wound)
- Occlusive, semi-occlusive or non-occlusive (this refers to the degree of the dressing's permeability to gas or vapour).

Adherent and non-adherent dressings

Saline-soaked gauze swabs are often used as passive adherent dressings in the early stages of wound management for debridement of necrotic tissue. These are cheap to apply and very effective; however, they may be painful to remove and can damage healthy tissue. They are often referred to as wet-to-dry dressings.

Passive non-adherent dressings are typically used over surgical wounds, skin grafts or granulation tissue. Perforated polyurethane membrane and paraffin gauze are common examples. These do not interact with the wound in any way, but prevent the secondary layers from sticking to the wound.

Absorbent dressings

Sometimes the secondary layer of the dressing is used to absorb exudate, but some primary layer dressings are specifically designed to absorb fluid and prevent it accumulating at the wound surface, causing maceration of the tissues.

Foam dressings (e.g. Allevyn, Smith and Nephew) usually have a semi-permeable membrane backing that allows absorption of fluid and some controlled evaporation, so that the wound environment remains moist without being too wet. These passive dressings can be useful for exudative granulating wounds, as they allow epithelialization in a moist environment.

Wounds that are producing copious amounts of fluid can be dressed with ordinary disposable baby nappies. These can be weighed to calculate how much fluid the animal is losing and to document improvement as the fluid exudate decreases.

Complex dressings

Alginate dressings are bioactive and interactive. They are sheets of a protein derived from seaweed and release sodium or calcium when in contact with body fluids. This results in the stimulation of haemostasis and inflammation. They are used to stimulate the formation of granulation tissue and for haemostasis in low-level bleeding. Once they are wet, they form a gel that keeps the surface of the wound moist. The disadvantage is that sometimes they cause the formation of excessive granulation tissue.

Hydrogel dressings are interactive, consisting of insoluble hydrophilic polymers. They are provided either as a sheet with a semi-permeable backing or as a gel. The hydrogel can rehydrate necrotic tissue, absorb exudate and reduce oedema. Where it is in gel form, a second primary layer must be put over the gel to prevent it from drying out and often the foam dressings are used for this purpose. It is useful where parts of the wound are granulating well and other parts require further debridement, as the gel will not harm healthy granulation tissue. The disadvantages are that the debridement process is very slow, and the combination of dressings may be expensive.

Hydrocolloids (dressings containing gel-forming agents such as sodium carboxymethylcellulose (NaCMC) and gelatine) are bioactive and interactive suspensions of polymers in an adhesive matrix. They are usually provided as a sheet with an occlusive backing that prevents dehydration of the wound. They can both rehydrate and debride necrotic wounds and will stimulate the formation of granulation tissue. Because they are adhesive, they may prevent contraction of the granulating wound by sticking to the edges and sometimes cause exuberant granulation tissue. They should not be used for infected wounds and they need to be changed regularly so may be expensive.

Topical wound treatments

- **Aloe vera** ointment actively stimulates the development of granulation tissue but only if very pure products are used.
- **Silver sulfadiazine** ointment (Flamazine, Smith & Nephew) is a topical broad-spectrum antibiotic with prolonged activity and is the agent of choice for prevention of sepsis from burns.
- **Zinc bacitracin** ointments may enhance epithelialization.
- **Malic, benzoic and salicylic acid solution** (Dermisol, Smithkline Beecham) has a very low pH and is a debriding agent; it is toxic to granulation tissue and should not be left in the wound.
- **Nanocrystalline silver** is used for infected wounds and is particularly useful in management of infections that are resistant to commonly used antibiotics. It also decreases the use of antibiotics and reduces the risk of multi-drug resistance.

Secondary bandage layer

The secondary layer of a dressing is used either to hold the primary layer in place, to provide padding to the wound underneath, to absorb exudate or to distribute the pressure of the bandage evenly. The secondary layer is most commonly an **orthopaedic wool**, which is available as rolls of viscose or polyester fleece in different widths. The bandage is applied evenly in a spiral with overlapping layers of 50% of the width of the material. If the bandage is required to distribute pressure (e.g. Robert Jones bandage, see Chapter 17), more substantial materials such as rolls of cotton wool are used. For heavy levels of exudate, cotton wadding such as gamgee may be incorporated into the secondary layer. The secondary layer is then stabilized using a conforming stretch bandage. This layer is again applied evenly with 50% overlap of width, only slightly compressing the wool layer underneath. It is important not to overstretch the bandage during application, particularly over narrow points in the limb, as pressure points may arise.

Tertiary bandage layer

The tertiary layer is primarily to protect the main functional layers of the bandage from soiling or mutilation by the animal. This outer layer is usually an elastic cohesive or adhesive bandage, applied in a spiral with 50% overlap of width. It is important that this layer is applied with even pressure, as the layers cannot slide over one another to relieve pressure points when the animal moves around in the bandage. At the top of the bandage, this layer must not extend over the top of the secondary layer padding as it will cause chafing of the skin. Finally, adhesive bandages should not be used to stick the bandage to the bare skin or haircoat as an attempt to help keep the bandage in place. The bottom of the bandage may be covered with an elastic adhesive bandage to increase wear. In order to keep the bottom of the bandage dry empty intravenous fluid bags or commercially available canvas boots may be used to protect a foot temporarily, but they should not be left on permanently.

Reconstructive surgery

General principles

Major reconstructive procedures are used when there is inadequate skin or other tissue available to close a deficit created by the surgery or trauma. Usually the surgical procedure is planned in advance so that the patient can be prepared and positioned appropriately. The general principles behind reconstructive surgery include the following:

- The patient should be haemodynamically stable prior to surgery
- The patient should be prepared for a long period of anaesthesia
- A very wide area of skin should be clipped and surgically prepared to allow for moving skin around into the wound
- The skin must be handled gently to prevent bruising that might damage its blood supply.

Reconstructive procedures require good wound management in advance of the surgical procedure. Often the success of the surgery relies on the elimination of infection and foreign or necrotic material prior to surgery.

When an incision is made in the skin, or a skin deficit occurs after trauma, the elastic recoil of the skin makes the edges gape apart. When the skin edges are advanced to close the large wound, there may be too much tension on the edges, causing delayed healing or dehiscence. The skin of the dog and cat generally is extremely mobile and can be manipulated to close skin deficits, but by taking into consideration the tension lines prior to surgery, sometimes the problems associated with the recoil of the skin edges can be avoided.

Suturing skin

Sutures are used to bring the tissues together so that they heal more quickly. Sutures in the skin should appose the tissues and not cause eversion or inversion of the skin edges. Generally:

- **Absorbable** sutures are used in deep tissues where they are not accessible for removal
- **Non-absorbable** sutures, which cause less tissue reaction, are used in the skin and then removed about 7–10 days after the surgery.

Sutures should not be placed too tightly, particularly in the skin, which swells slightly in the first 2–3 days after surgery. Tight sutures may either tear out as the skin swells, or cause itchiness, which encourages the animal to interfere with them. Finally, sutures that are placed too tightly may also constrict the vessels at the wound edge and delay wound healing.

Strategies to combat tension may be employed in most simple wounds either as a single procedure or in combination:

- **Subcuticular** sutures are used to hold the dermis together so that the skin sutures do not have to be too tight
- **Walking** sutures can advance skin towards the centre of the wound taking the tension off the main incision line
- **Vertical mattress** sutures can also be used as tension-relieving sutures to take the pressure off the incision line for a few days and then they are removed before the incision sutures.

Suture materials

There are many different types of suture material, all developed to perform different tasks in different surgical situations. They are divided into two main groups: natural and synthetic. Within these categories suture materials may be either **braided** or **monofilament** and either absorbable or non-absorbable (see Chapter 24).

Sizes

Suture materials are manufactured in different sizes (see Chapter 24). The **metric** gauge is the actual suture diameter in millimetres multiplied by 10. However, suture sizes are often referred to by the United States Pharmacopeia (USP) sizing, which has a different figure for the same suture material; for example, 2 metric is the same gauge as 3/0 USP.

Packaging

Suture material can be purchased in individual sterile packets, with a needle attached to the end of the material by a method known as **swaging**. This is ideal as it is known to be reliably sterile, the needle sharp and the material undamaged.

Selection criteria

When choosing a suture material, the following points need to be considered:

- **Security** of the knot – Monofilament materials have high memory (i.e. they are very springy) and therefore the knots are less secure than braided materials
- **Strength** of the suture material – Often braided materials are stronger than monofilament materials of an equivalent size
- **Longevity** of the suture material in the tissues – This may depend on the mechanism by which the suture material is broken down in specific tissues. Some materials (e.g. polydioxanone) are designed to be long lasting
- **Drag effect** when the material is drawn through tissues – Generally the braided materials drag through the tissues more than monofilament and are more likely to cause damage.

Tissues treat all suture materials as foreign material and mount an inflammatory response. Therefore it is a good surgical principle to use the minimum of suture material possible to achieve closure of the wound, and to use the smallest gauge of suture material that will be strong enough.

Natural materials cause much more inflammation and are less reliable than the synthetic materials.

Primary closure of large skin deficits

Large skin defects may not be amenable to simple closure and special reconstructive surgical techniques have to be used. These often involve moving flaps of skin around, and it is important that the blood vessels supplying the flap are carefully protected from damage during the surgery. Very fine rat-toothed forceps, stay sutures or specialist skin hooks may be used to handle the skin. The vessels should also be prevented from going into spasm during the surgery; hypotension, hypothermia, shock, dehydration and pain will all decrease blood flow to the skin and risk damage to the skin flap. These cases need very careful peri- and postoperative nursing:

- Clip and prepare very wide areas of skin surrounding the surgical site
- Protect the drapes from 'strike-through' that might compromise aseptic technique
- Monitor the patient for hypothermia and dehydration during surgery
- Count the swabs and estimate blood loss
- Provide soft bedding, good postoperative analgesia and close observation.

Some oncological surgeries will entail removal of part of the abdominal or thoracic wall. In these cases a synthetic mesh made of absorbable or non-absorbable material may be used to close the defect. These meshes are expensive and can result in the development of sinus tracts if aseptic technique is inadequate.

Skin flaps

Incisions are made, running away from the skin defect, to create a flap of skin that is then undermined so that it can be advanced to cover the defect. These flaps rely on the network of blood vessels in the dermis to supply the skin edges at the end of the flap. They have to have a wide base to ensure that enough vessels run into the flap to keep it alive and can only be moved into adjacent areas as far as the tension will allow.

Axial pattern skin flaps

These are specialist skin flaps that are defined and named by the specific artery and vein supplying that area of skin. The skin is elevated according to anatomical landmarks and the artery and vein are identified underneath. The flap of skin can then be moved as far as the vessels will allow. This kind of flap is very reliable as it has a well defined blood supply and can be used over wounds that have poor blood supply.

Free skin grafts

Skin grafts are pieces of skin removed from a donor site and then sutured in place on to a wound (Figure 25.16). They are usually used for wounds on the limbs that are difficult to repair using skin flaps. The skin graft is very susceptible to failure, as it has to rely on the wound bed for nutrition from the first day and has no independent blood supply. If the blood supply fails to grow into the skin graft within 3–4 days the graft will fail.

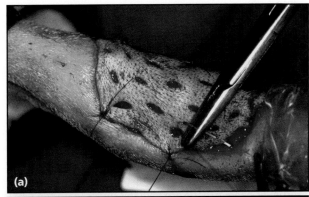

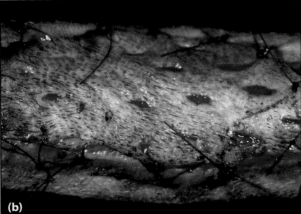

25.16 A free skin graft. **(a)** Graft in the process of being applied to the wound; sutures are being placed to secure it. The graft has been punctured with stab incisions so that fluid cannot accumulate under it during healing. **(b)** The same graft 7 days later; the hair is just beginning to grow, the stab incisions have almost healed over and the graft has healed on to the wound bed.

Skin grafts may be harvested as split-thickness grafts, which include only the epidermis and superficial dermis, or as full-thickness skin grafts (FTSGs), which include the whole of the epidermis and dermis. In animals, full-thickness pieces of skin are usually used, as this also transfers the hair follicles and so the final result is more cosmetic and hard wearing.

If it is difficult to harvest a large piece of skin from the flank, punch grafts or stamp or strip grafts may be taken and embedded into the wound, allowing the surface to re-epithelialize by growing out from the islands of little skin grafts.

- **Punch grafts** are usually taken with a skin biopsy punch and pushed into little holes in the granulation tissue.
- **Stamp or strip grafts** are small squares or strips of skin laid on to the granulation tissue with gaps between the grafts. These tend to have very sparse hair regrowth between the grafts and are quite fragile.

Usually FTSGs are **meshed** by making little stab incisions in the skin (see Figure 25.16) to allow it to conform better to the surface of the wound and also to allow drainage of fluid out from underneath the graft.

Management of free skin grafts

- A well padded bandage (Robert Jones) must be kept on for the first 5–7 days to immobilize the limb.
- Bandage changes must be carried out carefully in order that the graft does not move.
- Aseptic wound management is required to prevent infection.
- A non-adherent primary dressing layer is essential.

Postoperatively grafts are dressed with a non-adherent dressing such as paraffin gauze or silicone mesh and heavily bandaged (e.g. with a Robert Jones bandage) to prevent movement of the graft site. The dressing is changed as infrequently as possible, in order to minimize disruption of the fragile process of graft healing over the first 7 days.

Free skin grafts may fail due to inadequate preparation of the wound bed (e.g. chronic avascular granulation tissue), infection of the graft, failure to immobilize the graft or adherence of the primary dressing to the graft. They may also fail if serum or haemorrhage accumulates underneath the graft and lifts it off the wound surface so that the blood vessels cannot grow into the graft quickly enough.

Complications associated with reconstructive surgery

Many reconstructive procedures are long surgeries with large areas of tissue exposed for some time. Patients may dehydrate and also become hypothermic resulting in longer recovery times and poor skin circulation. If the surgical technique is poor these skin flaps have a high risk of failure. If the circulation fails in the skin flap it rapidly becomes ischaemic and over the first 3–4 days is cold to the touch, finally becoming hard and blackened as the skin dies.

Drains

Drains are used where there is a need to perform repeated lavage of a space, where there is a need for repeated aspiration of fluid (or air) from a space, or where the surgeon wants to prevent the accumulation of fluid in a space (e.g. seroma).

Passive *versus* active drains

Passive drains rely on gravity and capillary action, whereas active drains have a suction apparatus on one end – either intermittent or continuous.

Passive drains

The commonest passive drain is the **Penrose drain**, which is a soft latex tube (Figure 25.17) usually placed in the dead space created at surgery to allow drainage of fluid after surgery. One end of the drain is anchored in the wound with an absorbable suture and the other is anchored at the skin. The end of the drain should always exit through a separate skin incision site to the surgical incision so that it does not interfere with wound healing. As it relies on gravity, the drain should exit at the lowest possible point. To increase drainage, a larger drain or several drains may be placed (drainage volume depends on the surface area for the capillary action).

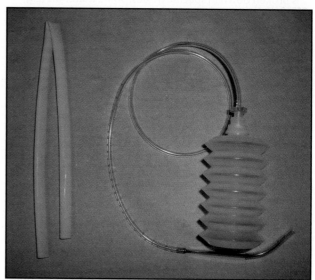

25.17   Drains can be used postoperatively to drain dead space and prevent seroma formation after reconstruction. **Penrose drains (left)** are soft latex tubes that allow fluid to drain out of the space along the surface of the drain (passive drainage). A dressing should be applied to protect the drain from contamination and to collect the fluid. An **active drain (right)** is a rigid tube in the wound with a device that exerts constant gentle negative pressure (suction). Active drains often have a sharp curved needle-like device on the end of the tube in order to place the drain through the skin. This 'needle' is then cut off and disposed of.

Active drains

Active drains usually have rigid walls and may have a radiopaque marker down the side so that their position can be checked. The most common is the **thoracic drain**, where a drain is placed through the skin, under a skin tunnel and then between the ribs into the thorax. The end of the drain is closed securely with clamps and bungs. The drain may be used to aspirate air or fluid out of the chest or to introduce treatment into the chest cavity (e.g. in pyothorax). The drain can be attached to a syringe for intermittent suction or to a suction device that continuously drains the chest. These drains have to be very carefully bandaged in as the animal could die if it chewed the end of the tube and the chest communicated directly with the outside.

Active drains are also used underneath surgical wounds, attached to suction devices that are little vacuum tubes. The continuous gentle suction applied to the dead space is a very effective way of preventing the formation of a seroma.

Closed *versus* open drains

The thoracic drain is always a closed drain and the system is sealed from the outside.

- Active drains are closed, as they collect the fluid in a reservoir bottle or tube.
- Passive drains will always be open, as they allow the fluids to drip out on to the patient or the floor.

When a passive drain is used, there is a potential risk of bacterial contamination of the wound as bacteria may migrate up the sides and lumen of the tube. In addition, there is increased nursing involved in keeping the skin clean and dry underneath the wound and preventing the haircoat from becoming matted with exudate. The skin may be protected by using either a thin layer of barrier cream under the end of the drain or a commercial synthetic spray that makes a breathable but waterproof barrier on the skin to help to prevent maceration, e.g. Cavilon (3M). Where possible the drain should be bandaged in place with a sterile dressing to absorb the fluid from the end of the drain. This has to be changed regularly to ensure that the skin does not become macerated.

Active drains still have some risk of bacterial contamination as there will be some migration of bacteria up the sides of the tube, but the risk is smaller, particularly as they can often be bandaged into place using antiseptic ointments and sterile dressings.

Care and management of drains

All drains should be handled in an aseptic manner and the animal treated with broad-spectrum antibiotics until the drains are removed. The animal must be prevented from interfering with the drain and the drain must be protected from the animal's urine or faeces. For removal, the skin suture is cut and the drain is then pulled out quickly with light pressure over the hole to help it to seal. Thoracic drains should have a purse-string suture pre-placed in the skin ready to close the skin on removal. With most other drains, the hole is allowed to granulate over after removal.

Wounds: a summary

- Wounds heal in a predictable manner, which can be manipulated by the veterinary surgeon or veterinary nurse to accelerate or delay the recovery of the animal.
- Classification of wounds is important in order to make a rational plan of approach to management of a case.
- Wounds allowed to heal by second intention should be assessed closely at each bandage change in order to determine what stage of healing the tissues have reached and to apply the appropriate dressing.
- Reconstructive surgery is the technique of choice where possible.

Fracture management

A fracture is a complete or incomplete break of bone continuity, with or without displacement of the resulting fragments.

Initial assessment and management

It is essential that the patient is adequately restrained before being examined or given first aid. However placid an animal is under normal circumstances it will often attempt to bite when in pain. A muzzle is often required.

Fractures may be accompanied by other injuries and some of these can be life-threatening. The fracture is of less priority and its repair (depending on its nature) can be left for several days until the patient is in a stable condition. It is important to prioritize these injuries and deal with the most life-threatening first (see Chapter 21). A full and careful examination can be carried out by the veterinary surgeon, analgesics administered and the limb temporarily supported with splints and bandages (see Chapter 17). When a fracture is suspected, two orthogonal radiographic views must be taken in order to make a specific diagnosis.

Fracture healing
Indirect fracture healing

This process was previously called secondary healing. Local events immediately after fracture are the same as in other tissues: haemorrhage, formation of a clot, and acute inflammation. The clot is gradually replaced by granulation tissue and blood vessels grow into the organizing clot from periosteal blood vessels and blood vessels in the medullary canal of the bone. Fibrous tissue is produced by fibroblasts in the organizing clot around the fracture and forms a cuff around the bone ends. This fibrous tissue is important: it stabilizes the fracture and allows cartilage to develop. This large cuff of stabilizing tissue is known as **callus** and is composed of fibrous tissue, cartilage and immature bone; this envelops the ends of the bone.

The cartilage is slowly replaced by bone in endochondral fashion. Cells called **chondroclasts** resorb cartilage and new bone is formed when **osteoblasts** line the surfaces and secrete a mineralized matrix. As this process progresses, the callus gradually contains more cartilage and bone and less fibrous tissue. The fracture becomes more stable until eventually the callus rigidly unites the bone ends and this is the point of **clinical union**. Callus is not always helpful; sometimes the callus formed may be disorganized and excessive and can interfere with the normal movements of muscle and tendons.

There is a long remodelling phase where the callus is replaced by mature bone. **Osteoclasts** are responsible for bone resorption in the remodelling phase; they remove the mineral part of the callus and degrade the collagenous and non-collagenous proteins. Simultaneously, mature bone is laid down by osteoblasts, thus recreating the original bony structure.

Haversian remodelling is a process of bone resorption and formation within the cortex and is the final step in restoration of the normal compact bone structure. The surface of the cortices becomes smooth and the bone's strength restored in response to normal weight bearing.

Direct fracture healing

Direct fracture healing (previously called primary healing) occurs when the bone edges are so close together that callus formation does not occur and the bone forms without the interim stage of fibrous tissue and cartilage. In cases where callus formation is detrimental to the return of function (e.g. joint surfaces), direct fracture healing is preferable and this usually requires surgical intervention as soon as possible after the trauma. The fragments must be held in rigid anatomical alignment (i.e. with plates, screws or wires, or a combination), and this allows Haversian systems to cross a minute fracture gap and repair the cortical bone directly with little or no callus formation.

Rate of fracture healing

Provided there are no complications, clinical union is usually achieved in 12–16 weeks in adult dogs and cats. Remodelling may continue for many months, or even years, after clinical union has occurred. The rate of fracture healing is assessed by clinical examination to detect the increase in rigidity and the firm swelling associated with union by callus formation. Radiographs are taken to assess the degree of callus formation and the extent of mineralization within the callus. Many factors influence the rate at which fractures heal and it is important to be aware of these when contemplating fracture repair.

- Fractures in immature animals heal more quickly than in adult animals.
- Fractures in geriatric animals heal more slowly.
- Fractures in debilitated animals heal more slowly. Debilitation may be due to poor nutrition or systemic illness such as hormonal disorder or kidney failure.
- Osteomyelitis interferes with healing and is one of the most common causes of poor fracture healing after surgical repair. Healing can progress normally once the infection is controlled.
- Fractures of cancellous bone heal more quickly than fractures in cortical bone.
- Fractures in bones that have a good blood supply heal more quickly than those in areas with a poor blood supply. For example, the pelvis and scapula are covered by large muscle masses which have a good blood supply and these bones heal well. The distal one-third of the radius and ulna has little muscle cover and a poor blood supply and fractures at this site heal poorly, especially in very small breeds of dog.
- Oblique fractures heal more quickly than transverse fractures, because there is a larger area of contact to promote tissue regrowth.
- Poor reduction or fixation of a fracture will result in a slow rate of healing.
- Movement of the fracture site delays or prevents healing.

Complications of fracture healing

- **Non-union** – complete failure of the fractured ends of the bone to unite.
- **Delayed union** – fracture healing progresses slowly. Clinical union is not achieved within the expected time.
- **Malunion** – fracture heals in an abnormal position. Untreated fractures and those not treated effectively often heal in an abnormal position. ▶

- **Shortened limb** – limb shortening occurs if there is healing with inadequate reduction of over-riding fracture fragments. Limb function may be severely compromised.
- **Osteomyelitis** – inflammation of the bone. Bacterial osteomyelitis is commonly caused by inadequate asepsis during surgery or in open fractures. It is more likely to occur if there is also damage to the local blood supply. This is recognized by heat, pain and swelling of the affected part, systemic illness, inappetence and fever.
- **Fracture disease** – a syndrome of muscle wastage and inability to flex joints in a limb after fracture repair. One or more joints in the affected limb may be held rigid due to scar formation within the joints or within muscles surrounding the fracture site. Fracture disease is more common after fixation by external coaptation or when there is inadequate reduction.
- **Sequestrum** – a necrotic piece of bone not incorporated successfully in the fracture repair.
- **Implant failure** – this can occur through poor choice of implants or technique, stress applied through the implant caused by overactive behaviour of the patient, or failure of the implant itself. This will result in a sudden deterioration, with instability and pain returning at the fracture site.

Classification of fractures

Modern classification of fractures provides information for both treatment and prognosis: the bone involved, type of displacement, direction of the fracture line and the number and type of fragments.

Open *versus* closed fractures

- A closed fracture describes a fracture with no break in the skin.
- An open fracture has a wound that has penetrated the skin and the fracture ends are open to the outside environment. This type carries a greater risk of infection and is often contaminated (e.g. a road traffic accident where the limb has been dragged along the road).

Anatomical description

- **Articular** – involving the joint.
- **Diaphyseal** – a fracture in the midshaft or diaphysis of the bone.
- **Metaphyseal** – a fracture of the area between the midshaft and the end of a long bone (epiphysis).
- **Physeal** – a fracture through the growth plate of an immature animal.
- **Epiphyseal** – a fracture of the epiphysis.
- **Condylar** – a fracture of the epiphysis when condyles are involved, e.g. the distal humerus or femur. Other common sites of fractures include the pelvis, the mandibles and the ribs.

Type of displacement

- **Greenstick** – an incomplete (i.e. only one cortex) fracture of a bone of an immature animal.

- **Fissure** – a fine crack, which may displace during surgery or when stressed.
- **Depressed** – especially fractures of the skull, where fragments may be pushed into the underlying cavity.
- **Compression** – often refers to fracture of a vertebral body where a compressive force has resulted in the shortening of a vertebra by a crushing effect.
- **Impacted** – cortical fragments forced into cancellous bone.
- **Avulsion** – a fracture in which a bony prominence has been torn away from the rest of the bone, usually by the pull of a muscle (e.g. fracture of the olecranon or avulsion of the tibial crest).

Direction of fracture line

- **Transverse** – fracture line is at 90 degrees to the axis of the bone (Figure 25.18a).
- **Oblique** – fracture line is at an angle of at least 30 degrees.
- **Spiral** – fracture line curves around the bone.
- **Longitudinal, Y or T** – refers to the appearance of the fracture lines on the bone.

Number or types of fracture

- **Simple** – one fracture line, creating two fragments (Figure 25.18a).
- **Comminuted** – more than one fracture line, creating more than two fragments (Figure 25.18a).
- **Wedge** – a multifragmented fracture with some contact between the main fragments after reduction.
- **Segmental** – one or more large complete fragments of the shaft of a long bone.
- **Irregular** – a diaphyseal fracture with no specific pattern.
- **Multiple** – more than one fracture in the same or different bones.

Other classifications

Some fractures are further classified to provide more detail about the appearance. Epiphyseal or growth plate fractures are classified by the Salter–Harris system, ranging from Type I to Type VI. Accessory carpal bone and central tarsal bone fractures are important fractures in racing Greyhounds and are each classified Type I to Type V.

Diagnosis of fractures

Clinical signs

Owners may have witnessed an incident and can give the veterinary surgeon vital information. A good clinical history may then give a good indication of the nature of the injuries.

The first signs, as with any injury, can be attributed to acute inflammation. The major clinical signs seen with fractures are:

- Pain localized to the affected bone
- Local swelling and heat
- Bruising at the fracture site leading to discoloration of the overlying soft tissues
- Marked loss of function (i.e. very lame or non-weight-bearing)
- Visible or palpable deformity of the affected bone
- Abnormal mobility at the fracture site
- Crepitus when the injured part is moved.

Radiography

General anaesthesia is usually necessary to obtain good quality radiographs. At least two views are essential to enable the veterinary surgeon to make a diagnosis and a plan for repair. Radiographs of the normal contralateral limb are useful in planning reconstruction of a severe fracture, e.g. comminuted or multiple fractures. Although it may be obvious that a limb is fractured, a good-quality radiograph will confirm details such as hairline fractures, small fissures and chips, or alterations in bone density, which could affect the treatment plan.

Principles of fracture repair

The primary aim of fracture fixation (Figure 25.18b) is to restore the functional anatomy of the fractured bone. This is achieved by:

- Restoring the continuity of the bone
- Restoring the length of the bone
- Restoring the functional shape of the bone
- Maintaining essential soft tissue function.

Essential soft tissues include the blood vessels supplying the bone, muscles acting on the bone and the nerves supplying the muscles. Any techniques for fracture repair must be sympathetic to these tissues because without them there is no chance of restoring function to the injured limb. Many techniques exist for successfully restoring bone continuity, length and shape. The same basic principles apply to all the techniques:

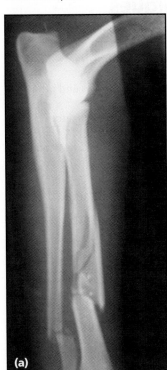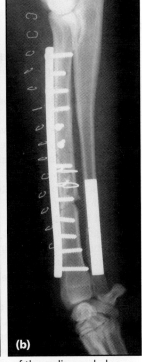

25.18 **(a)** A mid-shaft fracture of the radius and ulna. The ulna has a simple transverse diaphyseal fracture and the radius has a comminuted diaphyseal fracture; **(b)** The radius has been repaired with a 3.5 mm dynamic compression plate (DCP) and 3.5 mm cortical screws. Two lag screws have been placed (screws 5 and 6 from the top) and two cerclage wires have been placed around some of the fragments. The ulna has been repaired with a 2.7 mm DCP. The skin has been closed with skin staples.

- **Reduction** – the fracture fragments should be brought together in the correct anatomical alignment. This may be carried out 'closed' by traction and manipulation of the limb, or 'open' by performing surgery when the fracture is visualized and the individual fragments are manipulated back into position
- **Fixation** – the fragments should be immobilized in the correct alignment until clinical union occurs. The fragments may also be compressed together to narrow the fracture gap
- **Blood supply** – the blood supply to the bone fragments must be preserved. Fractures will heal only if there is an adequate blood supply.

Stabilization of fractures

After reduction of a fracture the bones must be held in position until healing occurs. Indications for immobilization at the fracture site are:

- To relieve pain
- To prevent displacement of the fragment (loss of reduction)
- To prevent movement that might cause delayed union or non-union.

In some cases, such as greenstick fractures and some pelvic fractures, immobilization may be unnecessary and simple restriction of activity will suffice.

Fixation techniques

Fracture fixation techniques are broadly classified into three groups:

- External coaptation, using casts or splints
- Internal fixation, using pins, plates, screws and other devices
- External–internal fixation using 'external fixators'.

There are a number of ways to repair fractures and there are a number of factors to be taken into account before deciding on the technique for repair:

- Classification of the fracture
- Age of the patient
- Size of the patient
- Temperament of patient
- Presence of any underlying disease
- Cost to owner
- Expectations of owner (e.g. working animal versus pet).

For example, a young dog's fractures will heal more quickly than an older dog's, and a fracture in a small breed, such as a Chihuahua, presents different problems than the same fracture in a Great Dane.

External coaptation

The aim of external coaptation is to limit motion at a fracture site by immobilizing the joints above and below the fracture. If the joints above and below the fracture cannot be immobilized, external coaptation is not suitable.

Methods of external coaptation fall into three main groups: casts, splints and extension splints.

External coaptation techniques

Advantages

- Technically simpler than some internal fixation techniques.
- Economical.
- Non-invasive.

Disadvantages

- They have limited applications. For example, casts are most useful for fractures below the stifle in the hindlimb and below the elbow in the forelimb.
- They do not provide sufficient stability for many fractures, particularly comminuted or severely oblique fractures
- They are at risk of causing decubital ulcers.
- Slower healing of fracture and greater callus formation.
- They restrict activity of joints and muscles in the limb and are therefore prone to causing fracture disease.

Types of fracture suitable for casting

Relatively stable fractures are ideal: greenstick fractures or simple oblique or spiral fractures that are stable after manual reduction. Where one bone is fractured close to an intact bone that provides a splint-like mechanism, a cast can be used (e.g. a fractured radius with an intact ulna). Casts are also used for postoperative support of arthrodeses, internal fixations or tendon repair.

Casting material should:

- Be conformable and easy to apply
- Reach maximum strength quickly.

The ideal finished cast should be:

- Hard wearing
- Radiolucent (to enable monitoring of fracture healing without removal of the cast)
- Strong and lightweight and not bulky
- Easy to remove
- Water resistant and 'breathable'
- Economical.

There are various types of casting materials available:

- **Polypropylene impregnated with resin** (e.g. Dynacast, Smith & Nephew) is easy to apply, radiolucent, strong, lightweight and hard wearing
- **Fibreglass impregnated with resin** (e.g. Vetcast Plus, 3M) is easy to apply, strong and lightweight. It is porous and allows the skin to breathe, which helps to reduce itching and odour. Softcast (3M) is made from knitted fibreglass material and is semi-rigid and flexible
- **Thermoplastic polymer mesh** (e.g. Vet-Lite, RUNLITE SA) is easy to apply, radiolucent (though the mesh creates a distracting pattern on the radiograph), strong and hard wearing. It is unaffected by contact with water, urine or faecal material. It can be reformed or reshaped with hot water
- **Plaster of Paris** is cheap and conformable but messy to apply. It makes a heavy, bulky and weak cast, is slow to reach maximum strength and loses strength when in contact with water. It is radio-opaque and has to be removed to monitor fracture healing.

Application of a cast

The casting material must be applied in close proximity to the bone to be able to give good support to the fracture. There is a fine line between using too much padding and too little. Too much will allow the fractured ends to move within the cast or cause the cast to slip. Too little casting material can lead to decubital ulcers. The cast must contain at least one joint above the fracture and one below, and prevent weight bearing across the fracture.

Applying a cast

The manufacturer's instructions should be followed closely. All the materials needed should be collected before applying the cast.

Equipment:

- Gloves
- Stockinette
- Synthetic cast padding, such as Soffban (Smith & Nephew)
- Sufficient rolls of casting material of appropriate size
- A bowl of water at the temperature recommended by the manufacturer.

Technique

1. Open or surgical wounds are covered with non-adherent dressing.
2. Stockinette is rolled up the limb, taking care to prevent any creases.
3. Cast padding is carefully and evenly wound on to the limb with 50% overlap at each turn, paying special attention to any bony prominence. Do not overpad these parts; instead use ring 'donuts'. Donuts can be made by cutting holes in small pads made out of cast padding; these are usually placed on the accessory carpal bone and olecranon of the forelimb or the calcaneus of the hindlimb. This prevents pressure ulceration on these structures
4. One roll of casting material is prepared by immersing it in the bowl of water and squeezing several times to allow the water to penetrate into the roll.
5. Excess water is squeezed out and the roll of casting material is applied to the limb in the same manner as the padding but with even tension. The casting material starts to set within minutes (depending on the type used), therefore it is important to work quickly.
6. Each roll is wetted individually just before application. Depending on the type of casting material used and the size of the patient, usually 2–3 layers are applied with 4–6 layers for larger dogs.
7. The pads and nails of the middle two toes are left exposed at the bottom of the cast.
8. A 1–2 cm length of padding is left exposed at the top and bottom of the cast.
9. Once the cast has hardened the stockinette and padding at each end are turned down over the edge of the cast and secured with tape.
10. A cast may be made stronger by applying splints made out of several lengths of casting material laid longitudinally down the compression side of the cast.

Splints

Gutter splints can be used as a fixation technique in some fractures, particularly those occurring below the carpus or hock in cats and small dogs. Splints can also be made from casting material (except plaster of Paris). A cast is applied as before, and then an oscillating saw is used to cut the length of the cast on the medial and lateral sides. The limb is dressed and bandaged appropriately and the two halves of the cast are reapplied to the limb and secured with an adhesive bandage.

Postoperative care of casts and splints

Owners should be given *written* instructions of how to look after the cast and what to look out for if complications arise.

- When the patient is taken outside, the bottom of the cast should be covered with a plastic bag (old drip bags are useful for this) and secured with tape – never elastic bands, as these may easily be forgotten and cause problems later on.
- Casts may have to be reapplied if the animal chews extensively or damages the cast. Growing animals will need a new cast every week to allow normal growth of the limb.
- Give medication as prescribed.
- Check cast daily and any of the following signs should be reported to the veterinary surgeon immediately:
  - Swelling of the limb or toes
  - Chafing at the edges of the cast
  - Staining of the cast with a discharge
  - A foul smell coming from the cast
  - Slipping of the cast from its original position
  - Chewing or other signs of discomfort
  - Collapse or bending of the cast (especially plaster of Paris)
  - General illness – depression, lethargy, lack of appetite.

Complications of casts

- Limb swelling – if the cast is too tight it restricts the lymphatic and venous drainage, which results in oedema of the lower limb. This is usually seen within 1 hour of applying the cast and needs urgent attention.
- Decubital ulcers – usually seen if the cast is poorly padded or is slightly loose and sliding on the skin.
- Cast loosening – if the cast was put on when the limb was swollen the cast may loosen once the swelling subsides.
- Prolonged immobilization of the limb may cause any of the following complications:
  - Joint stiffness and fibrosis
  - Cartilage degeneration
  - Muscle atrophy
  - Osteoporosis of disuse.
- Joint laxity – rapidly growing young large-breed dogs are particularly at risk.
- Delayed union, malunion and non-union may be seen with poor case selection, poor cast selection, poor casting technique or frequent reapplication of the cast and movement of the fracture site.
- Refracture on removal of the cast – provided that the limb has good callus formation (clinical union) on the radiograph at the time of cast removal this should not occur.

Removal of the cast

Generally limbs remain in a cast for 4–6 weeks. Radiographs are taken to establish the degree of healing and callus formation. The patient should be sedated or anaesthetized. An oscillating saw is the most suitable tool for removing casts. Two cuts are made in the cast with the line of cut carefully chosen to avoid bony prominences. The saw should never come into contact with the skin. The saw moves in an arc of 5–6 degrees and only cuts the solid casting material; the padding underneath catches on the blade and is not cut. The oscillating blade can become hot whilst cutting the cast and the saw should be rotated to use a cooler part of the blade. The padding underneath can be removed with scissors. Plaster shears can also be used: they are inserted at the distal end of the cast and the cut is advanced proximally in small regular steps.

Internal fixation

Internal fixation uses pins, plates, screws and wire to repair fractures.

Internal fixation

Advantages

- Suitable for fractures in any bone.
- Versatile and can handle the full range of fracture types.
- Allows accurate reduction and rigid fixation.
- Allows the limb to return to full function early, encouraging fracture healing and minimizing the risk of fracture disease.

Disadvantages

- Technique is relatively expensive and time-consuming.
- Some internal fixation techniques are technically demanding.
- There is capital expenditure on the equipment.
- The risks of surgery (wound healing problems, infection) are inherently greater in an open reduction and fixation than in closed reduction and fixation.
- Open fractures with extensive soft tissue injury may not be suitable.

Implants and techniques used in internal fixation

Intramedullary pins

These are called Steinmann pins; they are stainless steel rods with a sharp trocar point at each end, and it is possible to have one end threaded. They come in different widths ranging from 1.6 to 8 mm in diameter and are placed into the medulla of the bone that is fractured. They are inserted with a Jacobs Chuck or power drill.

- *Advantages:* cheap to purchase, quick to use, require minimal surgical exposure, easier to implant and remove than bone plates.
- *Disadvantages:* less stable fixation, slower return to function, secondary bone union (i.e. slower healing), greater aftercare required, not suitable for unstable fractures.

Postoperative management of intramedullary pins

- Two radiographic views are required to assess repair.
- Provide clients with written instructions outlining convalescent period and dates for follow-up examinations.
- Give medication (analgesics and possibly antibiotics) as directed.
- Exercise restrictions: lead-exercise only to allow patient to urinate and defecate. Cats should be restricted to a cage or a section of a room.
- Avoid stairs and prevent animal jumping on or off furniture.
- Sutures are usually removed after 10 days.
- At the first check, evaluate for limb function and assess joints adjacent to the fracture for range of motion. The point where the pin emerges from bone is examined for swelling or evidence of pin migration. There should be regular checks to monitor bone healing and possible pin migration.
- The pin is usually removed under anaesthetic once clinical union is achieved.

Interlocking nails

These are solid rods of 4, 4.7, 6 or 8 mm diameter, with holes through which interlocking nail bolts are inserted. The nails are placed in the medulla and the bolts fix the rod within the bone (Figure 25.19). Diaphyseal fractures are suitable for this method of repair and it gives a more reliable fixation than an intramedullary pin because the rotation and compression forces are resisted. It requires expensive equipment and technical expertise to insert. Equipment and implants are available in the UK but they are mostly used in specialist referral centres.

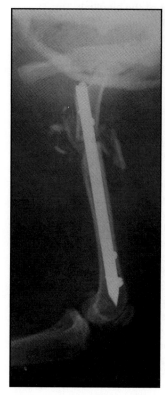

25.19 An interlocking nail has been used to repair this fracture of the femur. Two bolts have been placed in the distal fragment and another two bolts can just be seen in the proximal fragment.

Arthrodesis and Kirschner wires

These are smaller pins with diameters of 0.9 to 2 mm. Arthrodesis wires have trocar points at each end. Kirschner wires (K-wires) have a flattened bayonet point at one end and a trocar point at the other. These pins can be used as intramedullary pins in very small bones, as an aid in stabilizing a fragment while primary fixation is taking place or to create a tension-band wire (see below). They are also used in various types of fractures in small dogs and cats but not for midshaft fractures of long bones.

Cerclage wire

This is malleable monofilament stainless steel wire. It is often used to supplement the use of intramedullary pins, external skeletal fixators and bone plates (see Figure 25.18b). It compresses large fragments by encircling the bone and the fragment and then is twisted with wire twisters, pliers or special tighteners. It is also used to create a tension-band wire (see below).

Tension-band wire

This is used to fix an avulsed fracture. It uses two different directional forces to create compression of the fracture. Two K-wires are placed into the fragment and main bone. A cerclage wire is placed in a figure-of-eight pattern around the end of the pins and anchored through a predrilled hole to a solid part of the bone on the opposite side to the ligament or muscle that pulled off the fragment (Figure 25.20).

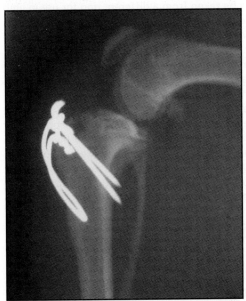

25.20 Two K-wires and a tension-band wire have been used to repair an avulsion fracture of the tibial tuberosity.

Venables and Sherman plates

A Venables plate is a rectangular bone plate with round holes. The number of holes varies from four to eight. A Sherman plate is similar to the Venables plate but narrows between the holes, making it lighter but not as strong. The plates are secured to the bone, bridging the fracture with Sherman self-tapping screws. Self-tapping screws differ from tapped screws by their slotted heads and two notches at the tip of the screw. They are available in two widths (7/64 and 9/64) and various different lengths. These plates are rarely used nowadays.

ASIF/AO systems

ASIF stands for the Association for the Study of Internal Fixation and is used in North America to name the patent and copyright of the system of orthopaedic equipment used for internal fixation. The European designation for the same equipment is AO, which stands for Arbeitsgemeinschaft für Osteosynthesefragen.

There is a wide variety of different plates and equipment for repairing every conceivable type of fracture. The most commonly used plate in veterinary practice is the **dynamic compression plate** (DCP; see Figure 25.18b). It is a strong plate with oval holes. These are available in different widths named by the size of screw they take and the length or number of holes. A 2.0 mm plate takes 2.0 mm screws; a 2.7 mm plate takes 2.7 mm screws; 3.5 mm and 4.5 mm plates come in narrow or broad widths and take 3.5 and 4.5 mm screws, respectively.

The DCP can serve various functions depending on how it is applied to the fractured bone. It can be used as a compression plate, as a neutralization plate, or as a buttress plate. A compression plate is used in simple transverse diaphyseal fractures to compress the ends of the bone together. A neutralization plate is used in oblique, spiral and comminuted fractures where compression is not possible and the fracture has been reconstructed with wires or screws but the repair needs additional support. A buttress plate is used to help to stabilize the fracture site and to bridge a fracture that is not reconstructable. The defect at the fracture site is usually filled with a cancellous bone graft.

Fracture management systems continue to evolve and specialist orthopaedic surgeons will use a wide variety of implant systems. Current thinking is that the fracture repair is better with minimally invasive techniques where the fragments and fracture site are handled as little as possible. These techniques use systems of plates and rods that stabilize the fracture without having to dissect down to the fracture site. Newer plates such as those with interlocking nail and locking head screws are developments that resolve issues that arise in specific situations.

Pre-tapped screws (AO type)

These screws are identified by the hexagonal head, which requires a special type of screwdriver to be able to place them. They are available in different widths and lengths and some larger screws are cortical or cancellous. Figure 25.21 is a guide to the sizes and drill bits to use.

Size of screw (mm)	Drill bit for core (mm)	Drill bit for gliding hole (mm)	Tap (mm)
1.5[a]	1.1	1.5	1.5
2.0[a]	1.5	2.0	2.0
2.4[a]	1.8	2.4	Self-tapping
2.7[a]	2.0	2.7	2.7
3.5[a]	2.5	3.5	3.5
4.0[b]	2.0	4.0	4.0
4.5[a]	3.2	4.5	4.5
6.5[b]	3.2	6.5	6.5

25.21 Sizes of AO-type screws and corresponding drill bits. [a] cortical; [b] cancellous.

After the plate has been contoured (bent to fit the shape of the bone), it is held in position with bone-holding forceps. A drill bit is selected to drill a hole the size of the core of the screw to include both near and far cortices; for example, if a 3.5 mm cortical screw is to be used, a 2.5 mm drill bit will be selected. The hole is then measured with the depth gauge and the correct length of screw is selected. The hole is then 'tapped' to create a thread for the screw. A tap is a special device designed to cut the thread in the bone. It is especially important to use the correct tap for the screw being inserted. The tap designed for the 4.0 mm cancellous screw cannot be used for the 3.5 mm cortical screw even though both screws are of similar widths, because the thread has a different pitch. The screw is finally driven into the hole using the hexagonal-head screwdriver.

Lag screw technique

A lag screw is not a specific type of screw but rather a technique. It is used to stabilize and compress fragments in a fracture (see Figure 25.18b). The fracture is reduced and held in place using bone-holding forceps. A hole the same width as the screw (the gliding hole) is drilled in the fragment, and the far cortex is then drilled with a drill bit the same size as the core of the screw. The far cortex is tapped, but the near cortex (in the fragment) is not. When the screw is driven into the hole it does not grip the fragment but just grips the far cortex; this has the effect of compressing the fragment into place.

Postoperative care after internal fixation

- Two radiographic views are required to assess the repair immediately postoperatively.
- Analgesia and nursing are aimed at a smooth and peaceful recovery from the anaesthesia.
- Early recovery of appetite and adequate nutrition is important.
- Long anaesthetic times and blood loss during reconstruction of the fracture may necessitate continuation of intravenous fluids into the recovery period.
- Assisted walking may be necessary to allow the animal an opportunity to urinate and defecate while limiting the use of the fractured limb.
- Daily monitoring of temperature, pulse and respiratory rates, food and water intake, urination and defecation and the recording of clinical signs and treatment is required during hospitalization.
- Give medication and analgesia as directed in the days following the surgery.
- Sutures are usually removed after 10 days.
- Clients should be provided with written instructions outlining the convalescent period and dates for follow-up examinations and re-radiography. These should be on a regular basis as directed by the veterinary surgeon. The owners should be instructed on how to recognize possible complications and how to seek veterinary advice if these occur.
- Exercise restrictions: cage rest is outdated with modern methods of rigid immobilization. It is considered to be beneficial to fracture healing and wellbeing of the patient to give short controlled ▶

bouts of lead-exercise: 10–15 minutes (on a lead) a couple of times a day for the first 3–4 weeks is usually sufficient. Hydrotherapy and physiotherapy are also of great benefit once any wounds have healed. This must be controlled in the early stages of healing to prevent overenthusiastic movements.

Complications associated with internal fixation

The most common complications are osteomyelitis and infection associated with the implants and implant failure. Both are often due to poor technique or poor choice of implants. In some cases, the postoperative care in the home environment is not sufficiently rigorous to protect the implants from failure.

Bone grafts

Bone grafts can be harvested from either cortical or cancellous bone. They are used to supplement fracture repair and accelerate healing across a wide fracture gap during reconstruction. The term **autograft** refers to bone taken from a site and used elsewhere in the same dog. An **allograft** refers to bone taken from one patient and transferred into another patient of the same species.

Cortical bone grafts consist of a whole segment of solid bone or chips of cortical bone either in a fracture or taken from a non-essential site. These bone grafts are very robust and can even be taken from a different dog for use in limb salvage although this is a specialised technique. It takes a long time for the cortical graft to become fully incorporated in the repair.

Cancellous bone is harvested from inside the medulla of long bones and the commonest sites used are the proximal humerus or the ilium. A drill is used to make a hole in the cortical bone and the cancellous bone is scraped out from the inside of the bone using a curette. Cancellous bone is very sensitive as it contains live cells. It should be handled in a sterile manner and stored in a blood-soaked swab on the trolley until used. Cancellous bone grafts are an essential part of the repair of complex fractures as they contribute cells and growth factors necessary for bone healing.

External skeletal fixation (ESF)

External skeletal fixation stabilizes fractures using pins that are inserted through a small stab incision in the skin and then into the bone. They usually travel through both cortices and are then fixed on the outside of the limb with bars and clamps (Figure 25.22) or acrylic resin. Different types of frame can be made according to the requirements of the fracture. A simple frame would consist of one bar and three or four pins exiting from the bone. A more complex frame could consist of multiple pins and three or more bars in three different planes.

Pins come in various sizes from 1.1 mm to 4 mm. Pins may be smooth with a trocar end or have threaded ends. End-threaded pins have either a **negative** thread, where the thread is cut out of the pin and the overall diameter of the pin remains the same, or a **positive** thread, where a thread is wound on to the pin and the overall diameter of the pin is slightly larger. Pins are also available with a positive thread in the middle of the pin rather than at the end. The advantage of a threaded

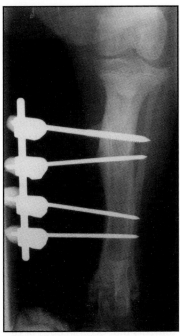

25.22 This radiograph shows an external fixator applied to a fractured tibia using one positively and one negatively threaded pin placed proximally to the fracture, and two negatively threaded pins placed distally. All pins are attached by clamps to a single bar.

pin is that it is less likely to loosen or be pulled out than a smooth pin. Pins are placed in both cortices of the bone but do not necessarily exit both sides. The centrally threaded pins are designed to exit both sides of the limb. Various sized clamps (single and double) and bars are available to fit the pins.

ESF: pros and cons

Advantages

- Minimal instrumentation required.
- Clamps and bars reusable.
- Minimal disruption of soft tissues.
- Minimal foreign body at fracture site.
- Open wound management easy.
- Easy to combine with other implants.
- Rigidity and alignment easily adjustable.
- Assessment of fracture healing easy.
- Easy to remove.

Disadvantages

- Soft tissue problems possible.
- Application technique requires practice.
- Premature pin loosening common.
- Difficult to apply to proximal limb.
- Can be difficult to obtain good radiographs of the limb.

Types of fracture suitable for external fixation

- Long bone fractures.
- Comminuted fractures.
- Open and infected fractures.
- Delayed unions and non-union.
- Mandibular fractures.

APEF system

The acrylic pin external fixator (APEF) system uses corrugated tubing which is filled with polymethylmethacrylate, a type of bone cement. All the pins are placed in the bone and the corrugated tubing is fixed to the ends of the pins. The cement is mixed and poured into the tubing. The tubing is then held in alignment until the cement has hardened. The hardening process is a chemical reaction between the liquid and powder components and intense heat is generated. It is important to protect the soft tissues (and fingers) from this heat. Heat can also be conducted down the pins and cause necrosis of the bone. Sterile swabs soaked in cool sterile saline can be placed on the tissues to help to protect them; saline can also be dribbled from a syringe on to the pins. The cement takes up to 10 minutes to set. Mandibular fractures are particularly suitable for this system; the acrylic can be formed around the pins and the shape of the jaw into a 'bumper bar'.

Postoperative care of external fixators

- Open wounds should be treated and dressed appropriately.
- The limb should have a compressive bandage applied for 2–3 days (changed daily) to minimize swelling. This bandage should go between the limb and the bars/acrylic and in between the pins and should include the toes.
- The ends of the pins protruding from the clamps or tubing should be covered with self-adhesive tape to prevent damage to furniture and owners.
- Air should be allowed to circulate between the skin and pins.
- Cats should be confined to cage rest.
- Exercise should be limited to lead-exercise only, taking care to avoid fences or other objects that are likely to catch the frame.
- Owners should be told to expect a small amount of scab formation at the site of the pin. This is normal and does not need to be cleaned on a daily basis. However, excess exudate does need to be cleaned and should be seen by the veterinary surgeon.
- Generally external fixators are well tolerated by the patient but an Elizabethan collar can be used to prevent the patient interfering with the frame.
- Written instructions should be given to the owner regarding medication, postoperative checks and radiographs.

Complications of external fixation

- Swelling of the soft tissues impinging on the clamps or acrylic bars.
- Excessive exudate from the pin site caused by movement of the skin and soft tissues.
- Loosening of pins (in some cases individual pins can be removed without losing the stability of the frame).

Luxations and subluxations

A **luxation** (also called a dislocation) is a displacement of articular surfaces from the normal position within a joint. The joint surfaces no longer touch each other. A **subluxation** is a partial dislocation of the joint surfaces.

Luxations and subluxations may be classified into two types: congenital and acquired.

- **Congenital** luxations or subluxations are anatomical abnormalities present at birth, which may or may not be inherited. The most common congenital luxation is that of the patella. In most cases a surgical procedure can replace the patella in its normal position. Some congenital luxations are so severe that they cannot be corrected. Some small dogs and cats may be able to cope with the permanently luxated joint, but in larger breeds severe congenital luxation may cause great disability.
- **Acquired** luxations and subluxations result from some form of trauma such as a road traffic accident. The ligaments keeping the joint in its normal position are damaged and the joint is forced out of alignment. Acquired luxations most commonly occur in the hip and elbow joints. Also affected but less commonly are phalangeal joints, the hock and shoulder joints.

First aid treatment for dislocations should follow that for fractures as presenting signs and trauma are often similar.

Clinical signs and diagnosis

The signs shown by the patient can mimic those of a fracture and it can be difficult to differentiate between them. Pain, deformity, loss of motion, non-weight bearing and crepitus are common signs to both. Sometimes typical stance positions are characteristic of an animal with a dislocation. Radiography is essential to confirm the diagnosis and also the presence or absence of other conditions, e.g. small fractures.

Treatment

Treatment of luxations requires the return of the joint to its normal anatomical position and repair of the damaged ligaments. Like fracture reduction, reduction of luxations may be achieved in several ways:

- **Closed reduction** is reduction of the joint by manipulation of the limb. This is the method that should be attempted first. Closed reduction should be attempted as soon as possible after injury as the longer the delay the less chance there is of successful reduction of the joint. Most joints are impossible to reduce under sedation, causing unnecessary pain and suffering to the patient, and reduction should be carried out under general anaesthetic. The joint should be re-radiographed afterwards to check that the reduction has been successful.
- **Open reduction** involves a surgical approach to the joint: the luxated bones are visualized and manipulated back into the joint. Some form of stabilization technique is usually required.

Postoperative care

Postoperative care is similar after both open and closed reductions, except that open luxations require the added precautions taken following surgery. The main postoperative aim is to avoid forces that could cause a recurrence of the luxation.

Once the joint is reduced, it must be immobilized. After a hip dislocation the hindlimb is supported in an Ehmer sling (see Chapter 17). After a shoulder dislocation the forelimb can be supported in a Velpeau sling (see Chapter 17). The slings are kept on for 5–7 days. Exercise should be restricted for 3–4 weeks and then slowly increased.

Complications

- Re-luxation is the most common complication especially if activity is not sufficiently restricted or if there is other pathology in the joint such as a fracture.
- Joint infection is a risk especially if an open reduction has been performed.
- There may be injury to surrounding soft tissues associated either with the original trauma or with the reduction of the joint. These injuries may not be obvious at first. They include damage to nerves in the region of the joint.

Oncological surgery

Oncology is the study of cancer and its related diseases. A **neoplasm**, or tumour, is an abnormal uncontrolled growth of cells that develop faster than the surrounding normal tissues. Most tumours arise as the animal ages and typically they are found in dogs or cats over 8–10 years of age. However, there are some very aggressive tumours that occur in dogs or cats as young as a few months old. Some breeds are specifically susceptible to certain tumours and may develop more than one tumour at the same time (e.g. Boxers, mast cell tumours; Flat-coated Retrievers, sarcomas). Many owners will be very concerned about the possibility that their animal has cancer, and they must be reassured that many tumours are benign and, if removed completely, will not grow again.

Neoplasia

Neoplasia is extremely common in small animal practice and all unexplained lumps on an animal should be investigated with the possibility of neoplasia in mind.

Tumours cause problems in a number of ways:

- The physical mass of the tumour presses on other structures and causes pain or loss of function (e.g. pressing on the pharynx and preventing swallowing)
- A rapidly growing tumour may use up energy resources and cause the animal to feel unwell and depressed
- Cytokines released by the tumour can cause distant physiological effects (see 'Paraneoplastic syndromes', below)
- The tumour may spread to other vital organs (e.g. heart, kidney, liver, lungs) and invade the tissues, causing loss of function and resulting in clinical signs.

Tumours may arise from any body tissue and the name of the neoplasm is derived from its tissue of origin. Very aggressive tumours may lose all their identifying characteristics because they are growing so fast, in these cases it may not be possible for the pathologist to identify the tissue of origin. It is important to know the tissue of origin as this enables the veterinary surgeon to predict how the tumour will behave and also to decide what treatment is most appropriate.

The terminology used in oncology is very specific and often describes both the type of tumour and how it behaves. Neoplasms may be benign or malignant and this description indicates whether or not the tumour is likely to spread to other organs or tissues in the animal and result in its death.

Benign tumours

Benign tumours usually grow quite slowly and are discrete and encapsulated. They are often freely mobile relative to neighbouring tissues.

- **Lipoma** – a benign tumour of adipose (fat) cells, very common in the subcutaneous tissues of older overweight animals.
- **Papilloma** – a benign wart-like tumour of epithelial cells, most often seen on the skin of cats and dogs (e.g. at the lip margins, eyelid and ear) but they also occur in the bladder and rectum.
- **Melanoma** – a benign pigmented skin tumour of melanocytes; some melanomas, however, are highly malignant, particularly if they arise in the mucous membranes of the mouth.
- **Fibroma** – a benign tumour of fibrous tissue present as firm superficial tumours of the skin, they may be difficult to differentiate from other more malignant skin tumours.
- **Adenoma** – a benign tumour of glandular tissue, it is quite common in older dogs (e.g. anal adenoma).

Malignant tumours

Malignant tumours may grow quickly or slowly. They may not have a definite capsule and may be closely attached to neighbouring tissue. Some malignant tumours will spread (**metastasize**) very readily to other organs such as the lungs, liver, spleen and bones. Metastasis may occur via various routes:

- In the circulation after invasion of blood vessels
- In the lymphatic system to the draining lymph node and beyond
- By direct contact of tumour cells with neighbouring organs by direct invasion (**extension**) or by exfoliation of tumour cells into a cavity such as the abdomen (**transplantation**).

Malignant tumours are also classified according to the tissue from which they arise:

- **Carcinoma** is a malignant tumour arising from epithelial cells:
  - **Squamous cell carcinoma** arises from squamous epithelium such as the oral cavity
  - **Transitional cell carcinoma** arises from the transitional epithelium characteristic of the bladder epithelium
- **Adenocarcinoma** is a malignant tumour of glandular tissue in epithelia
- **Sarcoma** is a malignant tumour arising from mesenchymal tissues (mainly connective tissues):
  - **Lymphosarcoma** is a tumour of the lymphoid tissues, common in dogs and may be seen in association with feline leukaemia virus in cats
  - **Fibrosarcoma** arises from fibroblasts and may be found in any connective tissue
  - **Osteosarcoma** is a malignant tumour of osteoblasts and is usually in the limb bones. In the dog, these tumours are commonly found in the distal radius or ulna, proximal humerus, distal femur or proximal tibia.

When the tumour is examined histopathologically, it can be further graded to determine its degree of malignancy by assessing its rate of proliferation and degree of differentiation of the cells.

Preparation for oncological surgery

Many forms of neoplasia are amenable to surgery. In order to plan treatment and advise the owner, a specific diagnosis of the type of tumour is necessary. This entails taking a sample from the tumour and submitting it for histopathology. Benign tumours may be completely cured by excisional surgery and a number of treatments are available for malignant tumours that will extend the lifespan of the animal while maintaining its quality of life.

Many animals are older and will require some investigation to establish whether there is evidence of other disease before the surgery is carried out. The animal should also be radiographed or scanned to check whether the neoplasia has spread to other sites. All animals should have a right and left lateral chest X-ray taken to check for metastases. Finally, many patients may be cachexic, malnourished or suffering from paraneoplastic disease that makes them increased surgical risks. Attention to nutrition and planned postsurgical care and nursing are important for successful oncological surgery.

Paraneoplastic disease

Tumours can cause other signs of illness apart from the physical effects of the mass itself. Some tumours secrete biologically active hormones that may cause generalized non-specific ill health or they may cause well defined disease syndromes. Sometimes the paraneoplastic syndrome is more acutely life-threatening than the tumour itself. For example:

- Anal adenocarcinoma and lymphosarcoma can cause hypercalcaemia, giving rise to polydypsia, polyuria and renal failure
- Insulinomas secrete active insulin which causes episodes of acute hypoglycaemia
- Mast-cell tumours can secrete histamine causing generalized or local acute inflammatory responses
- Thyroid adenomas secrete excess thyroxine, causing tachycardia, weight loss and hyperactivity.

Tumours can also cause pyrexia, cachexia and generalized poor nutrition due to other substances released into the circulation.

Biopsy
Fine-needle aspiration

This is the commonest and most useful method of obtaining tissue for diagnosis of tumours. It is also used to assess draining lymph nodes for evidence of metastasis. A fine-gauge hypodermic needle is inserted into the tumour to aspirate a few cells for cytological analysis (see Chapter 19). Sometimes ultrasound guidance is used to direct needles into intra-abdominal or intrathoracic tumours.

Bone marrow biopsy

Aspiration is also used to sample bone marrow using a special bone marrow biopsy needle. Usually the sample is taken from the wing of the ilium, under sedation with local anaesthesia or under general anaesthesia. The overlying skin is prepared as for surgery and a small skin incision is made over the bone. The bone marrow biopsy needle is driven through the cortex of the bone with the stylet in place. Once in the medullary cavity the stylet is removed and a syringe is used to aspirate bone marrow. The samples are dripped on to slides tilted at 60 degrees to the vertical so that they run down the slide forming a smear. These are air-dried and submitted for cytology.

Needle core biopsy

A small cylinder of tissue is obtained using a specialized instrument such as a Tru-Cut needle. There is a central notched obturator with an outer sleeve or cannula with an attached handle. General anaesthesia, or local anaesthesia of the overlying skin, is necessary. A stab incision is made in the skin to allow the loaded instrument to be introduced through the soft tissues, and ultrasound guidance may be used to direct the instrument into the centre of the tumour. Once the obturator is in the tumour the sleeve is pushed sharply over the notch in the obturator cutting out a tiny cylinder of tissue. The closed instrument is withdrawn and a hypodermic needle is used gently to dislodge the sample from the opened obturator.

Other biopsy methods

- **Punch biopsy** samples are taken from superficial lesions in the skin, using small circular cutters. The biopsy site may be closed using a single interrupted suture.
- **Trephine biopsy** samples are taken from bony tumours using a trephine or a Jamshidi needle. A core of bone/tumour a few millimetres in diameter is obtained and pushed out of the trephine or needle using a stylet.
- **Incisional biopsy** is used for tumours that are big enough to remove a piece of tissue from without affecting the ultimate surgical treatment. Usually a wedge of tissue is taken from a part of the tumour that appears to be actively growing and then the wedge is repaired with sutures. This is the most reliable way to obtain a diagnosis.
- **Excisional biopsy** is usually used for small tumours that are easy to remove with a margin of normal tissue particularly if they are suspected to be benign. It involves the complete removal of the tumour at the first surgery.

Principles of oncological surgery

The mainstay of any cancer therapy is to maintain the animal's quality of life. Side effects of treatment must be balanced by the clinical improvement – or cure. Most tumours are treated with surgical excision and usually the aim is to remove the entire tumour. Sometimes it is the mass of the tumour that is causing the animal discomfort and in these cases **debulking** surgery may be used to remove as much of the tumour as possible in order to improve the animal's quality of life until the mass regrows.

Well encapsulated benign tumours may be cured by simple excision of the tumour. However, many tumours require a **surgical margin** around the tumour in order to ensure that the tumour is entirely removed (Figure 25.23). Fibrosarcomas are a good example of tumours that are very invasive and require very wide margins of excision in order to attempt to effect a cure. This may in turn require complex reconstructive surgery to repair the defect made where the tumour was removed. Intraoperative techniques may be used to reduce the risk of spreading the tumour into normal tissues; for example, the surgeon may change gloves, instruments or drapes prior to closure.

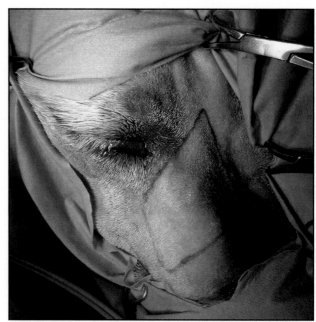

25.23 Skin tumours need to be removed with a margin of unaffected tissue, to ensure that the whole tumour is removed. Here a small mast cell tumour is to be removed with a margin of 2–3 cm. The surgeon has drawn the lines of incision on the skin with a sterile marker.

In some areas, a 'clean' surgical margin may not be possible and further types of therapy for the cancer may be indicated after the surgery. Some tumours are so malignant that postoperative chemotherapy or radiotherapy may be suggested even if the tumour appears to have been completely removed.

Palliative surgery may be used to remove a tumour to improve the animal's quality of life even though it does not alter the prognosis.

Submission of tissue for histopathology

All tissue removed from an animal should be submitted for histopathology or stored in formalin in case of recurrence.

Ideally all tissue removed from the animal should be submitted to the pathologist with a detailed history in order to maximize the information available with which to analyse the tumour. Large tumours may be difficult to submit by post, and representative samples may have to be taken from the mass; the main bulk of the tumour should be kept until the pathologist's report is complete in case more tissue is requested. Very bony samples have to be decalcified prior to cutting and this may result in a delay of up to 3 weeks before the report is received by the veterinary practice.

Where the tumour is malignant or locally invasive, the pathologist should be requested to assess the margins of the tumour in order to determine whether excision has been complete. Sometimes the surgeon may orientate the tumour by placing a marker suture at the cranial/caudal ends, or the edges of the mass can be painted with different colours of Indian ink, which are allowed to dry before fixation.

It is important that a clinical history is submitted with the sample in order for the pathologist to be able to provide accurate interpretation of the microscopic findings. In some cases, the pathologist may recommend immunostaining to further characterise the tumour for therapeutic purposes.

Fixation

Tissue should be fixed in 10% neutral buffered formalin in a volume ratio of 1 part specimen to 10 parts of formalin solution. Tissue >1 cm thick may need to be incised to allow more rapid access of the formalin to the deeper parts of the tissue so that adequate fixation occurs. Once the tissue has been fixed for 2–3 days, it can be posted with a 1:1 ratio of tissue to formalin. Formalin is carcinogenic and health and safety regulations must be observed during handling of the solution and preparing packages for posting (see Chapter 19). Some laboratories are now using FineFix, which is much less dangerous to handle and still fixes tissues adequately.

Other treatments

- **Cryosurgery** is where tumour tissue is destroyed by freeze–thaw cycles that cause the cells to rupture due to ice crystal formation. This is not very selective and normal cells are also killed.
- **Chemotherapy** is the use of cytotoxic drugs to kill tumour cells selectively; drugs are selected for specific tumour types.
- **Radiotherapy** is used in specialist centres to kill dividing tumour cells.
- **Hyperthermia** is a specialist technique that uses local application of heat via needles introduced into the tumour to try to kill the dividing tumour cells.
- **Photodynamic therapy** is a specialist technique using photosensitizing chemicals and light to kill tumour cells.

Often treatments may be combined with surgery. Adjunctive therapy in the form of analgesics, antibiotics, anti-inflammatories, specialist nutritional requirements and nursing care may be an important part of managing these patients.

Postoperative management and advice

Ongoing nursing and monitoring of cancer patients is often necessary (see *BSAVA Manual of Canine and Feline Rehabilitation, Supportive and Palliative Care*). Radiographs may be repeated at 4–6-month intervals to check for the development of metastases.

Oncological surgery carries with it the stigma of the dreaded word 'cancer' and many owners will continue to be concerned about the outcome long after the surgical wound has healed. Some animals have a very good quality of life for a considerable period of time even if the treatment has not been curative; owners may need reassurance that the animal is not suffering. Some tumours carry a poor prognosis, despite surgery, and owners may need extra time and advice on how to observe their animal for recurrence and quality of life. It can be very distressing for owners to think that the animal will die from the condition and be waiting for it to happen, all staff should be aware of the condition. Discussion about what to look for and how they might want to manage the euthanasia may be best carried out before the animal is terminally ill giving the owners time to come to terms with the inevitable. Many animals have 'good days' and 'bad days' towards the end and it is hard for the owner to understand that 'good days' do not necessarily mean that their pet is having a miraculous recovery.

Surgery and diseases of body systems

This section covers the main surgical diseases in the different body systems, and outlines the surgery and nursing implications of disease or potential surgical complications.

Nearly all surgical procedures are carried out under general anaesthesia and much of the postoperative nursing involves monitoring of the recovery from anaesthesia, and assessment and provision of analgesia (see Chapter 23). However, some surgical procedures also require postoperative monitoring for specific complications such as haemorrhage, infection, suture dehiscence or respiratory difficulties.

Surgical intervention in different areas of the body can be classified in terms of their potential for infection (Figure 25.24). Areas that can be prepared for aseptic surgery pose a different risk from those that are clearly infected and impossible to make aseptic.

These classifications of surgical procedures enable the surgical team to assess the risk of postoperative infection and treat appropriately. For example, category I does not require postoperative antibiotics and category IV may be treated with antibiotics before, during and after surgery. The most effective way to use antibiotics during surgery is to give an intravenous preparation before the first incision. Antibiotics given after the surgery has been completed will make no difference to the incidence of infection.

Category	Classification	Definition	Examples of surgical procedures
I	Clean surgery	A surgical wound made under aseptic conditions that does not enter any contaminated viscus, and where there is no break in sterile technique	Neutering. Uncomplicated hernias
II	Clean–contaminated surgery	A surgical wound made under aseptic conditions that enters the oropharynx, respiratory, alimentary or urogenital tracts, but where there is no other source of contamination	Lung lobectomy. Gastrotomy. Tracheotomy
III	Contaminated surgery	There is a major spill of contaminated material at surgery, or a break in sterile technique, or entry into a viscus with a high bacterial load (e.g. colon or rectum)	Abdominal surgery where gut contents spilled accidentally. Oral surgery. Wounds <4 hours old. Lower bowel surgery
IV	Infected surgery	The surgical site is known to be already infected	Aural surgery. Abscesses. Old wounds. Removal of necrotic tissue

25.24 Surgical classifications.

Reducing risk of infection

During surgery, the risks of infection can also be reduced by other means:

- Thorough lavage of contaminated tissue using sterile fluids
- Surgeon changing gloves or re-scrubbing after handling infected or contaminated tissue, prior to closing the unaffected tissue
- Changing instruments for fresh sterile ones
- Discarding suture material if used in contaminated areas and supplying fresh material for closure of clean areas
- Covering drapes with fresh sterile drapes prior to closure.

These techniques are commonly used after surgery on the gastrointestinal tract but the surgeon may also change gloves and instruments if concerned that they have been contaminated with tumour tissue, in order to reduce the risk of inadvertently spreading the tumour.

The eye

Ophthalmic surgery is one of the most meticulous areas of small animal surgery, where preparation, technique and postoperative care can have an enormous impact on outcome. General anaesthesia is required for all but the most minor procedures. Specialized instruments, theatre equipment and facilities for magnification (an operating microscope) may be necessary for some ophthalmic surgery.

General principles and preparation for eye surgery

The conjunctival sac is filled with a gel or lubricant and the haircoat is clipped very carefully from a small area surrounding the eye. The first stage is to clean any gross contamination or exudate off the eye and eyelids, using gauze swabs soaked in sterile saline. Skin preparation is completed using diluted povidone–iodine solution in preference to chlorhexidine solutions (note that surgical scrub solutions are not used in eye preparation). The corneal and conjunctival surfaces should then be irrigated with sterile balanced salt solutions or saline and a drop of broad-spectrum antibiotic solution may be instilled on to the surface prior to surgery. Alcohol solutions should not be used near the eye surface. During surgery, ocular lubricants may be used to keep the eye lubricated while the eyelids are held open.

Postoperatively, the eye is usually protected using an Elizabethan collar, and sometimes it is necessary to bandage the front paws. Bandages are difficult to keep secure over the eye and they limit postoperative monitoring and treatments.

Inflammation of the eye in the postoperative phase is often detrimental, particularly where specialist surgery has been performed on structures within the eye. In this regard ocular surgery is unusual, as corticosteroids may be used in the postoperative phase to reduce inflammation despite the delay in wound healing. Postoperative treatments may include topical ointments or drops for administration of antibiotics, steroids or cycloplegics (to reduce pupil spasm). In general, ointments can be applied less frequently than drops and may be easier for the owner to administer.

Analgesia is important and will make administration of treatments easier. Owners may need special advice and instruction on how to administer treatments safely.

Surgical conditions of the cornea and conjunctiva

Conjunctivitis

This is inflammation of the conjunctival membrane and is characterized by reddening of the conjunctiva. Usually the animal also shows increased tear production and overflow (**epiphora**). If the eye is very sore, the animal may hold the eyelids closed and be very reluctant to allow examination of the eye (**blepharospasm**). Conjunctivitis is not a surgical disease in its own right, but is often a sign of other conditions in the eye. In cats and rabbits it can be caused by a primary infection.

Keratitis and ulceration

Keratitis is inflammation of the cornea, which may be accompanied by ulceration. The inflamed cornea has a cloudy appearance due to the oedema. Using the dye fluorescein in the eye allows ulceration to be visualized, and this is important both for diagnosis and in monitoring healing of the ulcer. *Where ointments containing corticosteroids are to be used to treat keratitis, it is extremely important to ensure that no ulceration is present as the corticosteroid would prevent the ulcer from healing.*

Ulcers may be secondary to penetration of the conjunctiva by a foreign body or due to keratitis or exposure of the surface of the eye and drying out of the conjunctiva. Severe ulcers may cause erosion of the cornea and ultimately result in rupture of the eye.

Ulcers are treated using techniques to protect the surface of the eye while the ulcer heals by second intention. Small ulcers may be treated with removal of the initiating cause and antibiotic ointment. Large ulcers may require surgical treatment. Traditionally, the third eyelid used to be sutured across the front of the eye to cover the ulcer. However, newer techniques such as conjunctival flaps and corneal contact lenses provide better visualization of the ulcer to monitor healing and make it easier to apply treatments.

Keratitis can also be caused by the instillation of irritant chemicals on to the surface of the eye. This may be accidental, malicious or iatrogenic, and requires emergency treatment to prevent permanent scarring to the cornea. The eye should be irrigated with copious amounts of water or sterile saline to wash out as much of the chemical as possible. The eye should then be closely monitored for ulceration and treated appropriately.

Foreign bodies

Presentation with acute severe conjunctivitis may indicate the presence of a foreign body such as a grass seed trapped behind the eyelids. Careful examination of the inner surfaces of both eyelids and the third eyelid is necessary to identify and remove the foreign material. In calm animals, it may be possible to do this after application of local anaesthetic drops, but many animals will require sedation or general anaesthesia, as it can be very painful. After removal, the eye should be checked for ulceration.

Surgical conditions of the eyelids

Entropion

This is inversion of the eyelid margin such that the eyelashes rub on the cornea (Figure 25.25). There is often secondary conjunctivitis and keratitis. Entropion is treated by surgery to return the eyelid margin to its normal position.

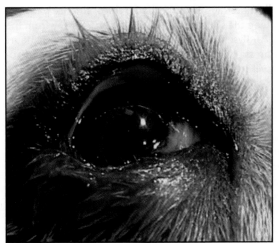

25.25 Entropion (shown here on the lower eyelid) is seen when the eyelid turns inwards and the eyelashes contact the conjunctival surface of the cornea causing constant irritation. (Courtesy of David Williams)

Ectropion

This is eversion of the eyelid margin. In most cases ectropion does not require surgical intervention, but in some dogs it prevents normal lubrication of the eye and gives rise to a chronic exposure keratitis. Certain breeds of dog may have both ectropion and entropion at different points along the eyelid margin.

Distichiasis

This is the most common of a group of disorders characterized by abnormal growth of hairs at the eyelid margin so that the hairs rub the surface of the cornea. In many cases the hairs do not cause a clinical problem but in some cases they cause a chronic keratitis requiring treatment. There are several surgical treatments described to remove the offending hairs and the follicle permanently.

Tumours

Tumours on the margin of the eyelid are very common in older dogs. They cause irritation by rubbing on the surface of the cornea and some are malignant. They are treated by excising a wedge of the eyelid margin containing the tumour.

Surgical conditions of the globe

Eyeball prolapse

Complete prolapse of the eyeball out of its socket (**proptosis** of the globe) can occur, particularly in brachycephalic dogs. First aid treatment is important if there is to be any chance of saving the eye. The eye must be kept moist using K-Y jelly (Johnson & Johnson) or Lacri-Lube (Allergan), supported by sterile saline-soaked swabs. Definitive surgery to replace the eye in the socket must be carried out as soon as possible.

Lens luxation

The lens is usually held in place by ligaments behind the pupil. If these fail, it can luxate either into the anterior chamber of the eye or caudally. This is usually a spontaneous event, often in terrier breeds, but can also be seen as a result of trauma. It requires emergency treatment to remove the lens, as the condition will lead to the development of glaucoma and blindness.

Glaucoma

This is an acute elevation in the pressure within the eye which can result in permanent blindness within 24 hours if not treated. There are several causes of glaucoma, but the commonest are anterior uveitis and lens luxation. The eye is extremely painful, the sclera engorged and the pupil is usually dilated. Emergency medical treatment includes analgesia and intravenous hypertonic fluids (mannitol) to try to draw fluid out of the eye. Surgical treatments are available in specialist centres.

Cataracts

A cataract is the opacification of the fibres or capsule of the lens of the eye, ultimately resulting in blindness. It should be distinguished from ageing changes in the lens that result in an apparent blue colour of the lens, but through which the animal can still see. Cataracts may be a primary disease or can be secondary to other conditions such as diabetes mellitus. They may be left untreated or can be surgically removed by specialist ophthalmic surgeons. Removal of the lens enables the animal to recognize objects and people as the lens is not as important in focusing as it is in humans. This restores quality of life to the older animal.

Ocular trauma

The eye may be penetrated by foreign bodies or lacerated by claws or teeth during fights with other animals. All these conditions may potentially result in loss of the eye and should be examined and treated as an emergency. Often animals benefit from referral to a specialist ophthalmic surgeon as they are more likely to have the skill to save the eye.

Retina

Most retinal diseases are not amenable to surgery in veterinary medicine, but the retina is an important site of disease in the eye. Of particular importance is a group of inherited diseases of the retina known as **progressive retinal atrophy** which are known to occur in certain breeds (see Chapter 4).

Skin

Skin biopsy

Skin biopsy is indicated for diagnosis of skin disease. Minimal preparation of the skin surface should be performed in order not to disrupt the surface cells that may aid the pathologist in making a diagnosis. The sample is taken using either a skin biopsy punch or just with a scalpel blade. Several samples should be taken from representative sites and the incisions closed with simple interrupted sutures. In severely diseased skin, there may be delayed wound healing.

Skin tumours

Skin masses should ideally be identified histologically prior to removal. The best way to identify the tumour is using fine-needle aspiration biopsy (see above). Surgery should be performed in the normal aseptic way and the skin closed with sutures. It is important to be aware that some small skin tumours may require tissue margins in three dimensions and therefore some fat and muscle may need to be removed along with the overlying skin.

Surgical management of local pyoderma

Some chronic local skin infections are related to long-term skin disease such as atopy (allergic skin disease) and are then exacerbated by the animal's anatomical skin folds. If the skin folds are not due to obesity, then it may be appropriate to resect the skin folds in order to prevent the recurrence of painful pyoderma. The common examples are vulval folds, screwtail folds and lip folds. Certain breeds, such as the brachycephalics and spaniels, are more likely to suffer from these conditions. Patients with allergic skin disease are most likely to interfere with their sutures as they are always itchy.

Urine/faecal scalding and decubital ulcers

Recumbent or incontinent patients are prone to soiling with urine or faeces and it is a failure of nursing management which then results in the development of decubital ulcers (pressure sores) or 'scald' (dermatitis). The skin and haircoat must be kept clean and dry at all times. In some cases this may involve several baths per day or clipping away haircoat to enable exposure of the skin so that it can be checked easily. Traditional treatments are to protect the skin with a thin layer of Vaseline or similar oil-based cream, so that the urine does not irritate the skin surface. However, this does not allow the skin to breathe and although the creams will prevent the skin from becoming worse, they will not help to treat any dermatitis. Commercial spray-on products are available (e.g. Cavilon) that provide a semi-permeable membrane under which the skin can heal while it is protected from the urine/faeces. The skin can also be covered with self-adhesive semi-permeable membranes.

Decubital ulcers (Figure 25.26) are much easier to avoid than to cure and this is an area where intensive nursing can really make the difference between survival and euthanasia. Padded bedding will help to prevent the development of pressure points in recumbent, obese or bony patients, and

25.26 Decubital ulcers are commonly a sign of poor patient care, but occasionally they are seen in dogs with medical conditions that predispose them to decubital ulcers. They are usually on pressure points where the bone is near the surface, such as the elbows or iliac crests. They often appear very round and have a variable depth of tissue loss. Sometimes they are so deep that the underlying bone becomes infected.

the use of material such as Vetbed or incontinence pads will help to keep the skin dry by wicking moisture away from the surface. Paralysed patients should be turned every 2–4 hours and all pressure points protected (see Chapter 17). Physiotherapy will encourage the blood supply to the skin and reduce the risk of necrosis (see Chapter 20)

Anal sacs

The anal sacs are situated on either side of the anus and contain anal glands, which produce a creamy coloured pungent exudate. The sacs are normally emptied on top of the faeces each time the animal defecates and should not swell up or cause irritation. If anal sacs become impacted they fill with fluid, which may then become secondarily infected, or they can eventually rupture and spill irritant infected contents into the tissues around the anus. This is often the case with animals that have chronic **anal furunculosis,** which is a deep-seated infection with sinus tracts in the skin around the anus and under the tail. It is very painful and usually associated with colitis, dietary intolerance and autoimmune disease.

The classic clinical sign of anal gland irritation is persistent chewing at the rump or tail and rubbing the perineum on the ground, particularly after defecation. Anal gland disease may be secondary to a number of non-surgical diseases such as obesity or diarrhoea. In some cases it is necessary to remove chronically diseased anal sacs to prevent recurrence of infection. When the anal sacs are emptied they should be palpated carefully to screen for anal sac neoplasia.

Anal sac adenocarcinoma is a malignant neoplasm, often seen in middle to older aged dogs, especially Cocker Spaniels. The tumour can cause hypercalcaemia (paraneoplastic disease) as well as spread to the sublumbar lymph nodes. The primary tumour may be tiny and even then the lymph nodes are very large. The treatment consists of removal of the primary tumour and these lymph nodes, and postoperative chemotherapy and remission of up to 3 years has been reported in some cases.

Interdigital disease

Interdigital disease may be part of generalized skin disease, although some breeds are particularly predisposed to the development of interdigital cysts or interdigital foreign bodies such as grass seeds. Dogs with long hair between the toes are particularly at risk of grass seeds becoming embedded in the thin interdigital skin. This causes painful swellings or abscesses. Sometimes it is possible to identify the end of the grass seed in the swelling and it is removed with forceps. If the seed has migrated into the leg, the sinus tract must be surgically explored. During the summer and autumn months, owners should be advised to check between and under the toes daily and keep the hair trimmed very short.

Abscesses

Long-haired breeds are particularly prone to migration of foreign bodies such as grass seeds and may then present with a painful swelling under the skin. The abscess may burst spontaneously but sometimes the grass seed continues to migrate and spreads the infection deep into the abdomen or chest. In these cases, advanced imaging such as MRI or CT may be necessary to locate the foreign body prior to surgical removal.

Aural surgery

The most common conditions of the ear are usually related to generalized skin disease. Recurrent shaking of the head and scratching at the ears can result in an aural haematoma, and persistent dermatitis may result in otitis externa.

Aural haematoma

This is the most common injury of the pinna. It is secondary to self-induced trauma and there is nearly always underlying otitis externa. A blood vessel bursts, usually on the underside of the pinna, and forms a large haematoma (Figure 25.27). This is painful and, if not treated, will cause the pinna to scar in a deformed shrivelled shape. Generally a haematoma is treated surgically. The haematoma is drained and cleaned allowing the skin to flatten again against the cartilage. Recurrence is prevented by suturing the skin to the cartilage to close the dead space with the knots tied on the outer surface of the pinna. Buttons, quills or X-ray film have all been used to help to flatten the skin and prevent the sutures from pulling out.

Postoperatively it is important to treat any underlying skin or ear disease and to prevent the patient from scratching at the ear again. This is achieved either with an Elizabethan collar or with a figure-of-eight head bandage (see Chapter 17).

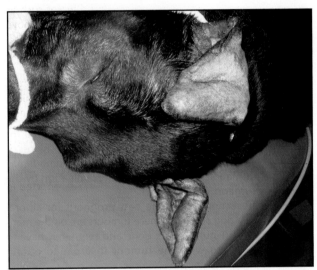

25.27 An aural haematoma forms when a blood vessel bursts and bleeds into the subcutaneous space between the skin and cartilage of the underside of the pinna. Often the pinna is heavy and painful, and drainage of the haematoma provides considerable relief. It is important to treat the underlying ear disease. This dog has been prepared for surgical drainage of bilateral aural haematomas, and the pinnae have been clipped.

Otitis externa

Otitis externa (Figure 25.28) is very common in both dogs and cats. There are many causes and these have to be investigated prior to treatment:

- Foreign bodies in the ear canal (e.g. grass seeds)
- Ear mites (*Otodectes*) (see Chapter 7)
- As an extension of generalized skin disease (e.g. atopy)
- Poor ear conformation, especially in the floppy-eared breeds or very hairy breeds
- Polyps or tumours
- Bacterial or yeast infection of the ears (this is usually secondary to one of the above).

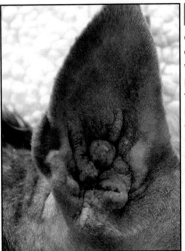

25.28 Chronic otitis externa. The external ear canal is completely obliterated with chronic greyish proliferative tissue. At this stage, it is not possible to salvage the ear by controlling the underlying skin disease and surgery would be recommended.

Animals usually present with head shaking, scratching at the ears, aural pain and there may be bleeding or discharge from the ear canals. It may be necessary to clean the ears with saline before they can be examined. They are often extremely painful and this procedure should be done with analgesia or under anaesthetic.

Tumours in the ear, or where cases of otitis externa have become very severe, are treated surgically:

- **Lateral wall resection**: the lateral wall of the vertical canal is removed so as to open up the ear to the air and allow better drainage and access for cleaning. This is only suitable for ears that have no disease on the medial wall of the vertical canal or in the horizontal canal
- **Vertical canal ablation**: the vertical canal is completely removed and the horizontal canal opening is sutured to the skin. This is only for ears where the disease is confined to the vertical canal
- **Total ear canal ablation (TECA)**: this procedure is most commonly used and is usually for severe long-term otitis externa. Often the infection has ruptured the tympanic membrane and there is also otitis media. The middle ear (**tympanic bulla**) is accessed at the time of surgery by enlarging the bony opening (**bulla osteotomy**) and the middle ear is scraped and lavaged clean. The whole of the vertical and horizontal ear canal are removed and the tissue and skin sutured closed over the top. This procedure is more challenging than the others but often is the only solution as it removes all the diseased tissue.

Ear surgery is regarded as infected and antibiotics are usually given both before, during and after the surgery. Ear infections are often longstanding, and opportunistic pathogens such as *Pseudomonas* or *Proteus* establish. They are difficult to treat as they are often resistant to most of the antibiotics commonly used. A foul-smelling greenish discharge may be an indication of these pathogens and a swab should be submitted for culture and sensitivity testing.

Postoperatively, the patients require analgesia and the ear must be protected from self-inflicted injury. An Elizabethan collar may be used, or a head bandage, or the pinnae may be bandaged together to stop them flapping against the wound. There is often a discharge of blood or exudate from the wound for several days and this must be gently cleaned away using sterile saline. The sutures may have to stay in slightly longer than usual, but small areas of dehiscence are allowed to heal by second intention.

Otitis media

In the dog this is usually an extension of otitis externa, but in the cat it may occur as a primary disease as an ascending infection via the eustachian tube. Access to the middle ear is either via a total ear canal ablation as described above if there is external disease or via a ventral approach (ventral bulla osteotomy). The animal is placed in dorsal recumbency and the dissection made directly over the tympanic bulla. A small drill is then used to make a hole in the bulla to allow drainage and lavage.

Otitis interna

Inflammation of the inner ear structures causes loss of balance, vomiting, head tilts, nystagmus and disorientation (vestibular syndrome). If this is secondary to severe middle ear disease, surgical management of the middle ear disease may be necessary to resolve the otitis interna.

Mammary tumours

Mammary neoplasia is the commonest tumour in the bitch, and the second most common tumour in all dogs. It is less common in the cat but it is seen in breeding queens (particularly Siamese) or cats that have been treated for oestrus suppression or skin disease using megestrol acetate.

In bitches the most commonly affected glands are the two caudal pairs, while in queens the cranial glands are most often affected. About 50% of mammary tumours in the bitch are benign but in cases with multiple masses they may all be different tumour types (Figure 25.29). In cats, over 80% of mammary masses are malignant and carcinomas tend to be particularly aggressive, most having metastasized by the time of presentation.

Fine-needle aspiration biopsy is rarely helpful except to differentiate mammary tumours from mastitis or hypertrophy. The type of tumour is rarely confirmed prior to surgery as it does not change the management of the disease.

Surgery is the treatment of choice for mammary tumours. In the bitch the type of surgery has little effect on the survival time, and radical surgery is generally unnecessary, as many tumours are benign. Surgery involves removing either just the affected gland (**mammectomy**) or that gland and an adjacent gland (**local mastectomy**) or all the glands on the affected side (**radical mastectomy** or **'mammary strip'**). In the cat, the tumours are usually aggressive and radical surgery is very important.

All mammary gland surgery is prone to dehiscence and ideally a drain should be used and postoperative antibiotic

![Mammary tumour photograph]

25.29 Mammary tumours in dogs may be benign or malignant and can grow to considerable size by the time the owner presents the animal for treatment. (Courtesy of Pierre Barreau)

therapy. To reduce the risk of wound complications surgery on both sides simultaneously is usually avoided.

Although in humans there are many other treatments used alongside surgery for mammary tumours, in dogs and cats there are currently no other treatments that are known to make a difference to survival after removal of malignant mammary tumours.

Digestive tract

Many diseases affecting the digestive tract have serious adverse effects on the fluid and electrolyte status of the patient. These deficits should be identified and stabilized prior to anaesthesia and surgery. Long periods of anorexia or vomiting and diarrhoea will cause the animal to be dehydrated and in a negative energy balance and therefore a poor candidate for surgery. Steps must be taken to replenish nutritional deficits and to maintain nutrition to minimize the effects of surgery on the patient. This may mean placement of feeding tubes prior to or during the surgical procedure to help with nursing the patient postoperatively. For example, an anorexic cat is likely to recover much more quickly if feeding tubes are placed at the time of surgery than if hand feeding or 'tempting' food is relied upon in the early postoperative stages.

Oral surgery

Oral tumours

These are generally seen in older dogs and cats. Tumours may arise on any structure of the oropharynx (tongue, gingiva, lips, palate, tonsils, etc.), and the prognosis depends very much upon both the site of the tumour and the type of tumour. As owners generally do not inspect their pet's mouth regularly these tumours may be large before they are presented for treatment. The first sign of a tumour may be halitosis, loss or displacement of teeth or facial swelling, and the tumour may only be identified at the time of dental examination by the veterinary surgeon.

Surgical resection carries the best prognosis for all oral tumours in the dog and cat. Where tumours are on the mandible or maxilla (Figure 25.30), bone and teeth may have to be removed along with the tumour in order to obtain

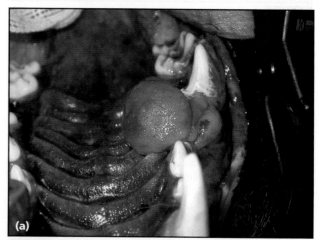
(a)

25.30 Maxillary tumours are usually seen in middle-aged to older dogs. **(a)** This dog has a tumour centred between premolar 3 and the carnassial tooth. The tumour must be removed with a margin of at least one uninvolved tooth on each side as well as the oral mucosa and underlying bone. *continues* ▶

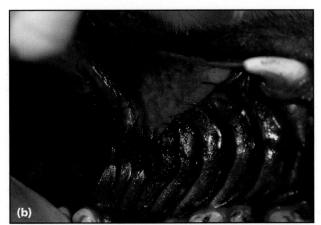

25.30 *continued* **(b)** The maxilla after the tumour has been removed along with all of the dental arcade up to the incisor. The defect has been repaired with a flap of mucosa from the lip.

adequate margins. The defect is then closed using flaps of mucosa from the lips and sutured with absorbable suture material. Postoperative nursing focuses on analgesia and ensuring that the patient can eat and drink easily. Food should be soft and formed not dry or abrasive (which might tear the sutures) or too sloppy (which might seep between the sutures). Tumours of the tonsils or palate often carry a worse prognosis particularly in cats.

Oronasal fistulae

These may be secondary to trauma, dental extraction or tumour resection. All fistulae should be repaired surgically to prevent food material impacting in the nasal cavity and causing a rhinitis. Preoperative preparation involves the use of saline and then dilute chlorhexidine or povidone–iodine solution to flush out debris accumulated in the cavity and nasal passages. Postoperatively, the defect should heal rapidly and may be kept clean with gentle oral lavage using chlorhexidine solutions.

Cleft palate

Puppies should always be checked for cleft palate at the time of birth, but it can also be traumatic in origin. Some clefts are repaired using simple advancement flaps; others require more advanced techniques, depending on the degree of involvement of the soft and hard palate. Protection of the suture line in the mouth is difficult and restriction of food intake or use of feeding tubes is counterproductive. The animal should be given soft formed food that will not get stuck in the suture line and is easy to swallow.

Foreign bodies and penetrating injuries

Foreign bodies such as sticks, bones, fish hooks, blades of grass or grass seeds may lodge in the soft tissues of the mouth and pharynx. All cause pain associated with the mouth, difficulty in swallowing and drooling.

The mouth can be opened in the conscious animal by using ropes behind the canine teeth of the upper and lower jaws, but the examination will be more effective under general anaesthesia. Penetrating injuries of the oesophagus and pharynx caused by sticks thrown for dogs by the owners can be potentially life-threatening and should be surgically explored as an emergency.

Oesophageal surgery

Oesophageal foreign bodies

Partial obstruction of the oesophagus with bones is common in terrier breeds and results in regurgitation of food and sometimes fluids. In cases where there is complete obstruction, dehydration is extremely rapid and hypovolaemia may be life-threatening. These cases are always emergencies. The foreign body is usually retrieved by extraction via the mouth through a rigid endoscope. Occasionally bones may have to be pushed down into the stomach. Digestible foreign bodies (such as bones) are not removed from the stomach but plastic toys or balls have to be removed via a gastrotomy. Postoperatively, the patient is treated with drugs to reduce gastric acidity in case of gastric reflux, which will exacerbate oesophagitis. The oesophagus is also assessed for tears and inflammation, using the endoscope. Small tears or bruising may be treated with nil by mouth and food and water via a gastrostomy tube for 3–5 days. Severe full-thickness tears may have to be explored via a thoracotomy to prevent development of sepsis, and the prognosis may be poor.

Oesophageal stricture

This condition may arise as a result of trauma secondary to an oesophageal foreign body but is also known to arise as a consequence of general anaesthesia. The animal presents 2–4 weeks after the initiating cause with a history of regurgitating all solid food. It is difficult to treat successfully. Therapy relies on stretching the stricture endoscopically and using steroid therapy to reduce the rate of recurrence of scar tissue. Animals may manage on a liquidized diet.

Gastric surgery

Foreign body

The cardinal sign of a gastric foreign body is persistent or intermittent vomiting. Diagnosis may be confirmed by radiography, contrast radiography or gastroscopy. Some foreign bodies may be retrieved endoscopically but many will require surgical removal. The stomach is accessed via a cranial midline laparotomy and pulled out of the abdomen as far as possible. The rest of the abdominal organs are packed off with sterile moist towels or swabs to protect them from contamination. The incision is usually made in an avascular area of the body of the stomach. The whole stomach should be inspected for other foreign bodies and mucosal damage prior to closure with a synthetic absorbable suture material.

Pyloric obstruction

This can be caused by a foreign body but more often it is because of pyloric thickening, due either to hypertrophy of the muscle or to neoplasia. These diseases are often known as **gastric outflow diseases** and congenital forms are more common in specific breeds such as brachycephalic dogs or Siamese cats. Once the diagnosis is confirmed, surgery is performed either to widen the pylorus (**pyloroplasty**) or to remove the pylorus altogether (**pyloric resection**).

Immediately postoperatively, small amounts of water are made available to the patient and then small quantities of a liquidized low-fat diet are offered 24 hours later. It is important to stimulate normal gastric motility without inducing vomiting, and some cases may have a gastrostomy tube placed at the time of surgery to help to decompress the stomach postoperatively for a few days.

Gastric dilatation–volvulus

This is a peracute rapidly fatal syndrome resulting from accumulation of food and gas in the stomach. The stomach dilates initially and this precipitates rotation of the stomach around its axis, resulting in occlusion of the oesophagus and the venous drainage. Severe hypovolaemic and toxic shock starts during the dilatation phase and escalates once rotation occurs. If not treated promptly, death results from the shock, gastric wall necrosis, ventricular dysrhythmias and disseminated intravascular coagulation (DIC). The specific aetiology is poorly understood, but usually the dogs are deep chested, often middle to older aged, and the condition may be associated with a nervous temperament. Preoperatively, nursing involves aggressive management of the shock and attempts to deflate the stomach either by passage of a stomach tube or by percutaneous needle gastrostomy (see Chapter 21).

Confirmation of rotation of the stomach is obtained with a right lateral abdominal radiograph (Figure 25.31) and indicates that surgical derotation is necessary.

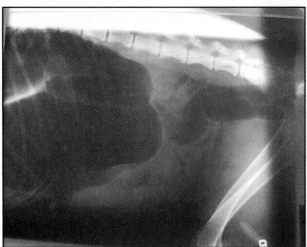

25.31 Right lateral abdominal radiograph of a dog with gastric dilatation–volvulus. The stomach can be seen hugely dilated with air and there is a characteristic fold of tissue crossing the dilated stomach, which indicates torsion.

GDV: treatment

1. Treat for shock with rapid administration of large volumes of intravenous fluids.
2. Intravenous antibiotics.
3. Decompression of the stomach via passage of a stomach tube.
4. Right lateral radiograph to confirm volvulus.
5. ECG – treat if necessary for ventricular dysrhythmias.
6. Surgery for decompression, derotation and assessment of stomach wall viability.

Usually a gastrostomy tube is placed at the time of surgery to allow decompression of the stomach if there is reduced gastric motility postoperatively, and the tube may be used for feeding if the animal is moribund. In order to prevent recurrence of the rotation, a gastropexy may be carried out where the pylorus is anchored to the body wall with sutures, but this does not prevent the recurrence of dilatation. Postoperative nursing continues treatment of fluid and electrolyte losses and in particular monitoring and treating ventricular arrhythmias.

Gastric neoplasia

Gastric neoplasms are often aggressive and may be very advanced before diagnosis. Clinical signs include haematemesis, weight loss and gastric pain. Some neoplasms can be resected if they are on the greater curvature of the stomach.

Tube gastrostomy

This is a useful tool for nutritional support (see Chapter 13) or decompression of the stomach. The tube is anchored in the stomach and exits through the body wall, where it is sutured to the skin and bandaged in place. The tube can be placed without surgery, using an endoscope to push the end of the tube through the skin (percutaneous endoscopic gastrostomy tube or PEG tube) or it is placed via a laparotomy. A mushroom-tipped catheter is usually used, although a Foley catheter may be substituted (Figure 25.32). It is important to protect the tube from mutilation by the animal, particularly if the tube was placed endoscopically, as it is less secure in the stomach wall than if sutured. Tubes are removed by pushing a probe into the end of the mushroom tip to straighten it out and allow the tube to be pulled through the abdominal wall. Tubes should not be removed too early (<3 days) before a seal has formed around the hole in the gastric wall. The resultant wound in the body wall may leak gastric contents for 1–2 days, but is kept clean with skin antiseptics and allowed to granulate closed.

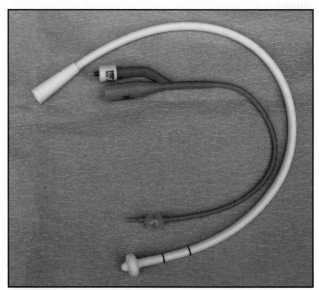

25.32 Depezzer (mushroom-tipped) and Foley catheters. These catheters can be used in situations where they need to be self-retaining (e.g. as a tube gastrostomy). To remove it, the Depezzer has to have the tip cut off, or straightened out. The Foley is removed by drawing the fluid out of the bulb.

Small intestine

Surgery on the small intestine (duodenum, jejunum and ileum) is common in small animal practice. The intestines are lifted out of the abdomen during surgery so that other organs are not contaminated if gut contents spill (Figure 25.33). They should be kept moist using sterile saline-soaked swabs or towels but this will mean that waterproof surgical drapes are necessary. Heat loss is rapid when the intestines are removed from the abdomen and it is necessary to provide a heating pad or warmed fluids.

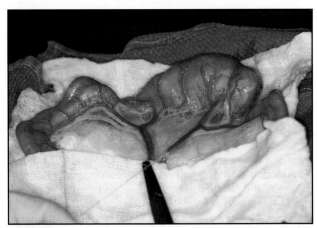

25.33 Intestinal surgery in a cat to remove a tumour in the small intestine (enterectomy). Note how the affected segment of intestine has been exteriorized from the abdomen and packed off with sterile swabs. The drapes underneath are also waterproof.

Biopsy

Intestinal biopsy is usually indicated when investigations of gastrointestinal signs such as persistent or recurrent vomiting or diarrhoea have been unrewarding. It is not possible to sample the jejunum or ileum via endoscopy and these have to be accessed via a laparotomy. Animals presented for intestinal biopsy may be poor candidates for surgery. Healing may be delayed due to hypoproteinaemia or cachexia. Small samples of intestine are taken from several sites all the way down the gastrointestinal tract and submitted in separate containers each labelled with the site of the sample. All the biopsy sites are sutured closed and wrapped with omentum.

Postoperatively, the animal is encouraged to eat and drink as soon as possible in order to encourage rapid healing of the biopsy sites.

Enterotomy: foreign body removal

Foreign bodies in the cat small intestine are often linear, e.g. string, wool, thread and needle. The material may be lodged behind the back of the tongue or trapped at the pylorus and travel all the way into the small intestine. Smooth muscle contraction of the gut wall then 'concertinas' the gut up the linear material and eventually either blocks the lumen or cuts through the wall of the intestine. Dogs more commonly ingest balls or plastic toys, which pass to a point along the jejunum and then become lodged.

Sometimes the foreign body can be palpated through the abdominal wall but often radiography is necessary to make the diagnosis. The animal is stabilized and the foreign body removed via a laparotomy.

Usually the foreign body can be removed via a scalpel incision in the gut wall and then the hole is closed with synthetic absorbable sutures. Sometimes the gut is very inflamed and appears necrotic, in which case an enterectomy may be necessary.

Enterectomy

Enterectomy is indicated where the gut is necrotic or there is a tumour in the wall. A section of the gut is removed and then the ends are sutured together to form an **anastomosis**. The affected section of gut is separated off, using Doyen bowel clamps or just an assistant's fingers to prevent leakage from the remaining bowel, and then cut with a scalpel to remove it. Once it is removed, the cut ends are held close together while the surgeon sutures the edges using synthetic absorbable suture material. Often the anastomosis is then wrapped in omentum to help to seal the surgical site. Postoperatively, healing is enhanced if the animal is encouraged to eat as soon as possible.

Intussusception

In this condition the small intestine invaginates into itself (like a telescope closing up). It is very rare in the cat but usually seen in young dogs often secondary to an episode of diarrhoea. The invaginated portion of intestine is called the **intussusceptum** and the outer part is the **intussuscipiens**. The blood supply to the intussusceptum is compromised and it often becomes necrotic. Symptoms are similar to those for intestinal obstruction and the diagnosis is usually made by radiography. Surgery to reduce the intussusception is necessary and if the intussusceptum is necrotic it is resected. Sometimes the disease recurs and the intestines may be sutured to each other (**enteropexy**) to prevent this.

Volvulus

Mesenteric volvulus is rarely reported in the dog or cat, though it is relatively common in horses. In all species it is rapidly fatal due to endotoxic and hypovolaemic shock secondary to death of most of the small intestine.

Large intestine

Surgery of the large intestine carries greater risk than surgery higher up the GI tract as there is an increased bacterial load and a slower rate of healing. Enemas near the time of surgery are detrimental to surgical asepsis as the slurry is more likely to spill and contaminate the abdomen. Preoperative oral antibiotics with anaerobic activity may help to reduce the bacterial load but perioperative antibiotics are essential and should be continued postoperatively. Hospital feeding should be careful not to induce a dietary enteritis, i.e. easily digested protein sources may be better than high-protein diets which may cause a nutritional diarrhoea. Often constipation or tenesmus is a sign of the disease and dietary fibre supplements and faecal modifiers such as ispaghula or sterculia are used to increase faecal mass and increase peristalsis. Paraffin pastes or liquids are less suitable as they only lubricate the faeces and do not alter the water content or soften impacted faeces.

Biopsy

Biopsy samples of the rectum and distal colon can be taken using rigid proctoscopy, but these are only of partial thickness. Full-thickness samples are taken via laparotomy, and carry an increased risk compared with small-intestinal biopsy. Strict aseptic technique, packing off the uncontaminated viscera and thorough lavage of the abdomen at the end of the procedure are important.

Colectomy

Removal of the colon is most often indicated for the treatment of chronic constipation in cats. Cats present with multiple episodes of complete obstipation requiring enemas and evacuation each time. Eventually the episodes become more frequent and the colon loses all function. It is important to check that the cat does not have an obstruction to defecation in the pelvic canal by rectal examination and radiography of the pelvis. Surgery involves careful identification and ligation of the vessels supplying the colon, and resection and re-anastomosis of the colon ends. In animals that are severely affected the ileocaecocolic valve may need to be removed as well. The animal is prepared for surgery with antibiotics but an enema is not performed as it is easier to prevent contamination of the abdomen during surgery if the faeces are dry and hard and can be removed within the colon.

These animals are often inappetent postoperatively and early nutritional support is important to healing in the colon. Dehiscence of the anastomosis is often fatal.

Rectal polyps/tumours

Rectal polyps (**papillomas**) cause faecal tenesmus, bleeding and discomfort and are often treated initially as colitis. Removal of the polyps is indicated because they are a pre-malignant change of the rectal mucosa. They can be removed by using a 'pull out' technique where the rectum is everted through the anus to allow removal of the polyp (Figure 25.34). The defect should be sutured using monofilament absorbable material and postoperative care is directed at reducing postoperative straining using analgesics, anti-inflammatories, local anaesthetic gel and dietary fibre. Where the tumour is identified as malignant or has invasive characteristics, a wider excision is carried out to remove the full thickness of the rectal wall.

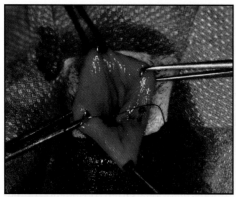

25.34 An intraoperative view of a rectal pull out procedure to remove a rectal polyp. The everted rectal mucosa is stabilized using Allis tissue forceps.

Rectal prolapse

This is eversion of the wall of the rectum through the anus. It is usually secondary to chronic straining and may be associated with a rectal tumour. Successful management requires treatment of the primary disease as well as reduction of the prolapse itself. The prolapse should be protected from self-mutilation and kept moist and lubricated, using lidocaine gel. Once the rectum is reduced it is maintained using a loose temporary purse-string suture around the anus. This may have to be loosened intermittently to allow defecation. Dietary faecal modifiers should be given to make the faeces soft and bulky.

Imperforate anus

This is a congenital condition where the anus fails to unite with the rectum, thus creating complete obstruction to the normal passage of faeces from the moment of birth. Sometimes it is possible to correct surgically.

Peritoneum

The peritoneum is the lining of the abdominal cavity and functions to help with healing of the intestinal tract and to protect it from infection if it becomes contaminated. Peritonitis occurs if there is contamination or irritation that results in an inflammatory response. Peritonitis can be due to surgical contamination, urine leakage from the bladder, intestinal content leakage due to perforation of any part of the GI tract, penetrating abdominal injury or leakage from the biliary or pancreatic systems. Initially, if there is no infection, peritonitis develops in response to the irritant nature of the fluid (e.g. urine or bile) and clinical signs may take a few days to develop. However, if the fluid is septic, or where there is leakage from the GI tract, the peritoneum becomes infected and this rapidly leads to severe illness, with septicaemia, shock and cardiovascular collapse within a few hours.

It is important for nurses to recognize peritonitis as part of postoperative monitoring of a patient, particularly after surgery on the GI tract. An animal may show some, or all, of the following clinical signs:

- Pyrexia
- Anorexia
- Depression
- Tachycardia
- Vomiting
- Ascites
- Abdominal pain.

The mainstay of treatment is to explore the abdomen surgically and find the source of contamination. In mild cases, or where there is no infection thorough lavage of the abdomen may be sufficient. Where there is infection the abdomen is best treated with open peritoneal drainage.

Abdominal lavage

Abdominal lavage involves pouring large volumes of warmed sterile isotonic fluids into the abdomen via a laparotomy and using suction to remove them until they come out clear. It is important to remove all the contaminated fluid to be effective and waterproof surgical drapes should be used.

Lavage technique

1. Give thorough abdominal lavage using sterile isotonic fluids (Hartmann's (lactated Ringer's) or saline) at body temperature.
2. Repeat lavage until the fluids come out clear.
3. All lavage fluid must be removed from the abdomen, as remaining fluid reduces the ability of the immune system to clear remaining bacteria.
4. Use omentum to cover any potential sites of leakage.
5. Change the surgeon's gloves and instruments. Re-drape with sterile drapes over the top of the contaminated drapes (preferably with waterproof drapes).
6. Topical antibiotics and antiseptics should not be used in the abdomen. Broad-spectrum bactericidal antibiotics are given intravenously pending the results of culture and sensitivity on a sample of abdominal fluid.

Open peritoneal drainage

Open peritoneal drainage is a technique whereby the abdomen is not fully closed after the lavage and is dressed with sterile dressings and a thick absorbent bandage (or disposable nappies). This dressing is changed using sterile technique 2–3 times per day while the infection drains from the abdomen. At each dressing change, the abdomen may be lavaged again through the open wound. Nursing of these patients is very complex and involves close monitoring of blood albumin and electrolyte levels, hydration and care of the bandage.

Respiratory tract

Respiratory distress is potentially life-threatening in any species and the veterinary nurse must be able to recognize respiratory difficulties quickly in order to respond with potentially life-saving first aid (see Chapter 21).

Respiratory difficulty arises from inadequate oxygen delivery to the tissues which causes hypoxia. There are a number of ways this can come about:

- Obstruction to the passage of air into the respiratory tract (e.g. laryngeal paralysis, tracheal collapse, foreign body)
- Inefficient oxygen exchange at the air–tissue interface (e.g. pulmonary oedema, pneumonia)
- Inadequate blood supply to the alveoli, despite normal delivery of gases (ventilation perfusion mismatch) (e.g. pulmonary thromboembolism, right-sided heart failure)
- Inadequate oxygen-carrying capacity (e.g. severe anaemia, carbon monoxide poisoning)
- Inadequate blood delivery to the tissues (e.g. hypovolaemia, circulatory collapse).

The clinical signs of respiratory distress will develop from an initial increase in respiratory rate and effort to visible cyanosis of the mucous membranes, loss of consciousness and death:

- Increased respiratory rate at rest
- Increased respiratory effort (there may be visible 'heaving' of the ribs)
- Exercise intolerance
- Open-mouth breathing (particularly cats)
- Cyanosis of the tongue and gingiva
- Collapse.

First aid treatment is essential even for only mildly affected patients. Animals that show any signs of respiratory difficulty may suddenly decompensate when they are stressed during examination and become profoundly hypoxic.

Respiratory distress

- Do not stress.
- Keep patient away from other animals.
- Monitor continuously.
- Provide oxygen supplementation.
- Sedate if necessary.
- Keep the patient cool (this prevents panting and improves ventilation).
- Be prepared for emergency tracheostomy, CPR or endotracheal intubation for ventilation.

Nasal disease

The dog and cat have different patterns of nasal disease, with the cat being predominantly affected by infectious agents causing acute or chronic rhinitis. Diagnosis of nasal disease can be very challenging and relies mainly on radiography, rhinoscopy, biopsy and in some cases MRI or CT scanning.

Rhinoscopy and biopsy

Rhinoscopy is used to visualize the nasal turbinates in order to take biopsies or look for a foreign body. Ideally a small rigid endoscope is used, but sometimes an auroscope is used or a small flexible endoscope to look behind the soft palate at the choanae.

Biopsy of the nose in most instances relies on radiographic diagnosis of a lesion and then taking a blind sample using biopsy forceps measured against the radiograph. In some cases, the sample may be taken using the rhinoscope to guide the biopsy forceps. Biopsy of inflamed turbinates causes profuse bleeding, and the pharynx must be packed. Usually pressure over the external nares is sufficient to arrest bleeding, but in severe cases adrenaline diluted to 1:100,000 may be sprayed up the nares to assist vasoconstriction of superficial vessels. Success in biopsy of nasal tumours often results in little haemorrhage.

Rhinotomy

Occasionally it is necessary to open the nasal cavity to take biopsies, remove foreign bodies or remove a benign tumour. This is done via an incision on the bridge of the nose and the nasal cavity is accessed through the nasal bones. Postoperative complications can include emphysema of the head and neck due to air leaking out through the rhinotomy incision.

Nasal aspergillosis

This is a fungal infection of the nasal cavity usually seen in younger dolichocephalic breeds of dog. It causes a purulent nasal discharge and often causes epistaxis, which can be very severe. Diagnosis is made sometimes on biopsy or rhinoscopy but it is more usually diagnosed by a blood test for anti-*Aspergillus* antibodies. Treatment usually involves treating the nasal cavity with an antifungal agent via tubes implanted through the frontal sinus. This may be done under anaesthetic, leaving the antifungal agent to soak in the nasal cavity for an hour, or the flushing may be carried out daily in the conscious animal for 5 days. The success rate of these techniques is about 70–80% but some dogs will need more than one treatment.

Nasal neoplasia

Nasal tumours tend to affect older dolichocephalic dogs and are most often carcinomas. In cats adenocarcinoma is the most common diagnosis but lymphoma is also seen. The Siamese may be more at risk. The diagnosis is made by radiography and biopsy of the abnormal region seen on the radiograph. Surgical treatment is not usually an option and nasal tumours are treated with a course of radiotherapy.

Stenotic nares (BAOS)

Brachycephalic airway obstruction syndrome (BAOS) affects brachycephalic breeds with deformed airways, resulting in difficulty with breathing. The commonest breeds affected are

Bulldog, Pekingese and Pug; occasionally Persian cats may be affected. The animal presents with noisy breathing which results from a combination of obstructions to the upper airway:

- Stenotic nares
- Overlong soft palate
- Tonsillar hypertrophy
- Pharyngeal hypertrophy.

Some dogs may also have a collapsed larynx and a narrow trachea.

Severely affected animals may have exercise intolerance and episodes of cyanosis and syncope. Animals may present as an emergency in hot weather when they may be suffering from heat stroke, dehydration, cyanosis and severe stress. Nursing requires oxygen supplementation, cooling, sedation and if necessary an emergency tracheostomy.

Surgical treatment depends on the most severely affected part of the airway: the stenotic nares can be widened and the tonsils and part of the soft palate resected to improve upper airway flow. Laryngeal collapse should not be confused with laryngeal paralysis (see below).

Laryngeal surgery

Surgery on the larynx is a complex procedure and can potentially result in severe difficulty during recovery due to mucosal swelling. The animal must be closely observed for signs of respiratory distress and facilities should be available for oxygen supplementation or emergency tracheostomy if necessary.

Laryngeal paralysis

This typically occurs in the older medium-sized breeds of dog. It is rarely seen in the cat. The disease results from paralysis of the recurrent laryngeal nerve, which means that the dog cannot abduct its arytenoid cartilages to open the airway on inspiration. The clinical signs range from increased noise on breathing when excited, panting on exercising, to cyanosis and collapse. These dogs often present in the summer when they are panting more to lose heat and the paralysed larynx becomes oedematous and swollen thereby further reducing airflow. They may collapse and be brought into the practice cyanotic and struggling to breathe. In hot weather they may also have heat stroke.

In an acute situation the animal may have to be anaesthetized so that the airway can be intubated and oxygen administered. Prior to recovery, the appropriate surgery is to 'tie back' the arytenoid cartilage so that it no longer obstructs the airway. If this is not possible, then it would be necessary to place a tracheostomy tube to bypass the larynx and allow the dog to breathe until surgery is possible.

Some breeds of dog are predisposed to laryngeal collapse, which is not amenable to laryngeal tieback and is treated with a permanent tracheostomy. The diagnosis is made on laryngoscopy. These dogs sometimes respond to weight loss and medical management.

Laryngeal tumours

These are rare, but also cause respiratory obstruction. Complete resection of the larynx is not very successful and there is little treatment possible, unless the tumour is sensitive to chemotherapy (e.g. lymphoma).

Trachea

The trachea is a rigid cartilaginous structure that prevents collapse of the airway when the animal creates negative pressure on inspiration.

Collapsing trachea

This is most often seen in toy or miniature breeds of dog, most notably the Yorkshire Terrier. The tracheal rings are not rigid, and when the dog is excited, or exercising, the trachea flattens and causes a harsh honking cough. Severely affected dogs may become cyanotic during coughing episodes, or even syncopal. Some dogs respond to medical management of weight loss, anti-inflammatories, antitussives and use of a harness rather than a collar. Dogs that are severely affected may require surgery to place rings around the outside of the trachea to provide a rigid support for the airway. An alternative is to place a stent along the inside of the trachea which holds it open and this has been very successful. The surgery is very complex and the postoperative period very risky, as the surgery can make the tracheal irritation worse.

Avulsion of the trachea

Typically this is seen in the cat after a road traffic accident. The trachea is torn apart usually quite distal within the thorax. The cat may initially appear normal, but becomes tachypnoeic over the first few days after the accident and may develop emphysema over the neck and shoulders. Surgical repair is urgent and involves a thoracotomy to re-anastomose the ends of the trachea. The surgery is technically difficult and the anaesthetic complicated by the fact that the cat requires IPPV during the surgery through a sterile endotracheal tube placed by the surgeon through the incision into the distal trachea. Postoperatively, a chest drain is placed to monitor for pneumothorax and the cat is closely monitored for signs of leakage from the anastomosis.

Ruptured trachea

Ruptured trachea can occur secondary to traumatic events such as road accidents or bite wounds; however, it is also reported subsequent to endotracheal intubation. In one study of iatrogenic tracheal rupture in cats, it was noted that it was more common after anaesthesia for routine dentistry. Inflation of the cuff and twisting of the head and neck during anaesthesia may be contributory factors. The cat presents either with subcutaneous emphysema 24 hours after the injury or with progressive dyspnoea 4–5 days later as the ends of the trachea narrow.

Tracheostomy

This may be temporary or permanent. It may be used for administration of anaesthetic gases during oral surgery or as a means of bypassing an obstructed upper airway. Most often it is used as a life-saving procedure in an emergency situation to bypass an obstructed upper airway.

Usually the airway is not completely blocked and administration of oxygen with a face mask provides some relief while the animal is prepared for tracheostomy. However, where the animal is unconscious or severely cyanotic, the veterinary nurse should be prepared to perform the tracheostomy using only local anaesthetic or no anaesthetic and no surgical preparation if the animal is likely to die with any delay. If airway obstruction is anticipated (e.g. after surgery on the upper airway), the ventral aspect of the neck may be prepared in readiness for an emergency tracheostomy. Tracheostomy tubes are illustrated in Figure 25.35.

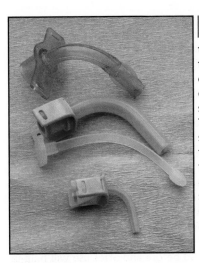

25.35 There are different types of tracheostomy tubes but all have a curved tube that enters through the skin into the trachea. The middle tube shown here also has a trochar that fits inside the tube. They are available in different sizes to accommodate different sizes of animal.

Emergency tracheostomy

1. Make sure that the oxygen delivery tube will fit the tracheostomy tube.
2. Clip and surgically prepare the ventral aspect of the neck.
3. Have a sterile surgical kit ready, together with the appropriate-sized tracheostomy tube and suture material to open up the tracheal incision.
4. Suction may be necessary for the lower airway.
5. Prepare for postoperative monitoring.

Management of a tracheostomy tube

- Constant monitoring for at least the first 12–24 hours.
- Regular suction of the tracheostomy tube every hour.
- Humidification of the trachea by instilling 2–10 ml sterile saline into the tube every hour.
- Changing the tracheostomy tube for a fresh sterile one every 2–6 hours, depending on the quantity of exudate.

Emergency airway

If an animal is very close to death and the materials are not immediately available, oxygen can be administered via a wide-gauge hypodermic needle or catheter pushed quickly through the ventral midline of the neck between the tracheal rings. This can then be used to administer oxygen via a narrow tube or urinary catheter.

Tracheal foreign body or neoplasia

Rarely an animal presents with obstruction of the trachea. If this is a foreign body it may be removed under anaesthesia using endoscopic forceps. Small tumours can be removed by resection of some of the tracheal rings and re-anastomosing the trachea.

Lungs

Principles of thoracotomy

The thorax can be approached either by entering the cavity between the ribs (lateral or **intercostal thoracotomy**) or by splitting the sternum and approaching the thorax from the ventral aspect (sternal thoracotomy or **sternotomy**). If more access is required, a rib can be resected.

Intercostal thoracotomy is the commonest approach and allows the surgeon access to the lungs, heart, oesophagus and pleural cavity on one side only. The advantage of sternotomy is that both sides of the chest can be explored at the same procedure. Sternotomy in large dogs requires the facilities to saw through the sternum. During the thoracotomy, the animal must be on IPPV continuously, and it should be monitored for heat loss and dehydration.

Following thoracotomy, great care is taken to close the incision with an airtight seal. A chest drain is used to remove the pleural air during closure and also postoperatively to monitor air or fluid leaks within the chest (Figure 25.36). A sterile drain is placed through a skin tunnel between the ribs and the other end is linked to a water seal which allows continual aspiration of air, or it may be occluded and drained intermittently (see 'Drains', above).

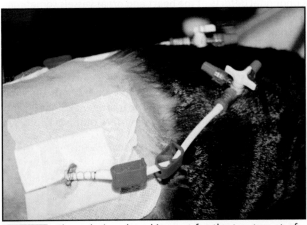

25.36 Chest drains placed in a cat for the treatment of pneumothorax. The drains are secured to the skin with a Chinese finger-trap suture. The drains should be further stabilized by a dressing and monitored continuously, as interference could be fatal. (Courtesy of C. Sturgeon)

Analgesia is very important after thoracotomy. It is also important to get large dogs up and moving around as soon as possible to reduce the risk of thromboembolism.

Lung lobectomy

Lung lobes are removed via an intercostal thoracotomy as this gives the best access to the arteries, veins and bronchus. The vessels and bronchus may be ligated and oversewn manually or a lung lobectomy stapling device can be used to perform the procedure in one step. After the lung lobe has been removed, the bronchus is checked for air leaks by filling the chest with warm sterile saline, inflating the lungs, and looking for bubbles.

Pyothorax

This is an infection of the pleura in the thoracic cavity. It is commonly seen in cats probably secondary to cat bites and in dogs probably due to migrating grass seeds. The animal presents with difficulty in breathing, due to large volumes of pus in the thoracic cavity. Mostly these cases are treated by placing thoracic drains in both sides of the chest and draining and lavaging the chest twice daily with sterile fluids and antibiotics. Persistent cases may require a thoracotomy to open up the chest cavity and debride infected tissue or look for the foreign body.

Cardiovascular system
Heart
Persistent ductus arteriosus (PDA)

This occurs when the ductus arteriosus fails to close at birth, and blood bypasses the lungs and left side of the heart, travelling from the pulmonary artery directly into the aorta. It creates a characteristic **heart murmur** that should be easily detected at the first vaccination check. If the condition is left untreated, the dog will eventually die from heart failure. The treatment is surgery via a left lateral thoracotomy to tie off the PDA. Alternatively, coils can be placed inside the PDA to occlude it.

Vascular ring anomaly

Congenital defects of the heart and great vessels sometimes occur and result in entrapment of the oesophagus between the ligamentum arteriosum (the remnants of the closed ductus arteriosum) and the other vessels. The commonest is a **persistent right aortic arch** (PRAA) when the aorta is found on the right side instead of the left and the ductus crosses the oesophagus and makes a constriction that prevents the normal passage of food on swallowing. The treatment is ligation and separation of the ductus from the surface of the oesophagus via a left-sided thoracotomy.

Arteries and veins
Vascular access: 'cut-down'

Intravenous treatments are usually given via an intravenous catheter placed in the cephalic vein. In patients that are collapsed, dehydrated or in severe shock it can be very difficult to identify the superficial veins in order to place the catheter. If it is not possible to place a jugular catheter, a 'cut-down' technique may be used instead to access a vein. The area over the vein is clipped and prepared surgically and a tourniquet is placed above the vein to increase visibility. An incision is made directly over the vein, and careful dissection down through the tissue planes is used to identify the vessel. The catheter is then placed routinely, flushed with heparin–saline and usually sutured in place. The skin is sutured over the surgical site and the wound is dressed.

Aortic thromboembolism

This is a serious emergency condition, usually seen in the cat, when a blood clot (**embolism**) breaks off and travels down the aorta to block the iliac arteries at the end of the aorta. This completely blocks the blood flow to one or both hindlimbs. The hindlimbs are cold, stiff and very painful and there is no palpable femoral pulse. Occasionally the condition is responsive to medical management; and surgical removal of the thromboembolism has been reported, but is only rarely successful. The condition is usually secondary to heart disease and the prognosis is poor.

Emergency vessel occlusion

Vessels may be lacerated or ruptured during the course of surgery or as a result of severe trauma. If the event occurs during surgery, small arteries (<2 mm) and veins (<4 mm) can be sealed using electrodiathermy, or may stop bleeding after a few minutes of direct pressure. Large vessels are ligated or double ligated, using absorbable synthetic suture material with good knot security. There are also commercial staples available to seal arteries and veins during surgery.

Traumatic haemorrhage may have to be stemmed prior to identifying the specific vessel. If the bleeding is clearly arterial (pumping), surgical exploration and ligation of the artery is a priority. However, the bleeding may be profuse and non-specific. Initially direct hand-held pressure on the wound using a sterile pack of absorbent material may be sufficient to slow the bleeding. If the bleeding continues to be profuse, other options are a tourniquet above the site of bleeding on a limb, application of a very heavily padded bandage or immediate surgical exploration under anaesthesia. It is very important to time the duration of a tourniquet to prevent ischaemic necrosis. It is also important to remove the bandage as soon as possible, otherwise high pressure underneath the bandage may result in the same effect. Weighing the material used to absorb the blood before and after use will help in estimating blood loss.

Major arteries may be repaired if necessary and blood flow can be temporarily stopped during the repair using bulldog clips or a Rommel tourniquet. Very fine-gauge polypropylene suture material is usually used to repair arteries or veins, as it causes very little tissue reaction.

Endocrine system
Thyroid gland
Thyroidectomy (dog)

In the dog, thyroidectomy is usually carried out as treatment for thyroid carcinoma. Small tumours may be easy to remove, but they can be very vascular and may be attached to vital structures in the neck.

Thyroidectomy (cat)

Hyperthyroidism is a common condition in the older cat. The majority of cases are due to a thyroid adenoma (a benign tumour) of one, or more usually both, thyroid lobes, which secretes excess thyroid hormone. It results typically in hyperactivity and restlessness, weight loss, polyphagia, polyuria/polydipsia, diarrhoea and tachycardia. Some cats may also have concurrent kidney disease and heart failure. The enlarged thyroid gland may be palpated in the neck, or the condition may be diagnosed from a blood sample. Initially, the cat is usually stabilized using an orally administered drug that controls the thyroid hormone levels, e.g. methimazole and carbimarcole, but ultimately surgery to remove the affected thyroid lobe or lobes is a curative treatment. The main risk associated with surgery is damage to the parathyroid glands, which are closely attached to the cranial end of the thyroid gland. This results in loss of control of calcium metabolism, and hypocalcaemia develops in the first 2–3 days after surgery. If the damage is severe, the cat may need calcium supplementation intravenously and then orally for 8–12 weeks until the parathyroid glands recover. Hyperthyroidism can also be treated in specialist centres with radiation therapy, using radioactive isotopes of iodine.

Adrenal glands

The adrenal glands in the dog and cat are sometimes removed as a treatment for hyperadrenocorticism (Cushing's disease) or phaeochromocytoma, where the adrenal gland is the primary source of the condition. Surgery involves deep dissection in the region of the dorsal abdominal vena cava and there can be severe haemorrhage. The patient may have delayed wound healing due to the medical condition and should be closely monitored for wound dehiscence. Sudden hormonal changes in the postoperative period can also destabilize a patient and they should be closely monitored for electrolyte abnormalities, hypotension and vomiting/diarrhoea. Adrenal tumours are common in ferrets and are often removed successfully.

Pancreas

The pancreas is a lobulated gland that is closely associated with the stomach and duodenum. The commonest disease is a sterile inflammation (pancreatitis), which causes severe abdominal pain and vomiting. This is not a surgical disease and surgical exploration will make the symptoms worse. Other conditions include pancreatic abscesses, damage due to abdominal trauma and pancreatic tumours.

Pancreatectomy

Abscesses and tumours may be removed by a partial pancreatectomy. If the lesion is in the body of the pancreas or involves the blood supply to the duodenum it is generally considered inoperable.

The most common tumour of the pancreas is an insulinoma. This is a tumour that secretes excess insulin and causes hypoglycaemia. After surgery the animal has to be carefully managed to ensure that acute pancreatitis does not occur. No food or water is given by mouth for the first 48 hours and hydration is maintained with intravenous fluids and electrolytes. Monitoring of the glucose levels is critical in postoperative management of insulinoma patients and they may need glucose or insulin therapy. When the animal is fed it should initially be given small quantities of a low-fat diet.

Pancreatic biopsy

In some patients with chronic low-grade pancreatitis, it is difficult to diagnose the disease without biopsy. Ideally, this is performed via laparoscopy to reduce the risk of a flare-up of the disease. Otherwise, a small piece of pancreas is removed via laparotomy and the patient is managed as for pancreatectomy.

Liver and gallbladder

Liver disease can potentially result in a number of medical conditions that would adversely affect the success of surgery. Many patients may have low levels of albumin and vitamin K and increased susceptibility to sedatives or anaesthetic agents. Animals with suspected liver disease should always have blood-clotting times tested prior to surgery and they may require a transfusion of plasma. The liver has remarkable powers of regeneration and can compensate for removal or damage to liver lobes.

Biopsy

The purpose of performing a liver biopsy is to achieve a specific diagnosis. Samples can be obtained either by laparoscopy or via a laparotomy incision. Usually just a small piece of the edge of a liver lobe is removed and normal clotting stops the bleeding spontaneously. Occasionally a Tru-Cut needle may be used with ultrasound guidance to obtain the sample.

Lobectomy

A whole liver lobe may need to be removed if it is diseased or damaged. The blood supply to the liver may be temporarily shut off using a small tourniquet during the surgery. Postoperatively, the animal must be monitored closely for haemorrhage into the abdominal cavity as this is the most common complication of the surgery.

Portosystemic shunts

A portosystemic shunt (PSS) is a congenital or acquired vascular anomaly that redirects blood flow in the portal vein so that it bypasses the liver. The clinical signs include poor growth, abnormal behaviour a few hours after feeding, seizures, urate calculi in the urinary tract and hypoglycaemia. The disease is usually diagnosed with blood tests and ultrasound scans of the liver. More detailed investigations such as a **portovenogram** (contrast material injected into a mesenteric vein) or contrast fluoroscopy may be necessary.

- Small breeds of dog are most commonly affected with **congenital shunts**; these are usually single large vessels draining into the abdominal vena cava (**extrahepatic shunts**).
- Large breeds of dog are usually affected with **intrahepatic shunts**.
- **Acquired shunts** are seen in older dogs or cats and are related to the development of veins that bypass the liver secondary to chronic liver disease that obstructs the normal flow of blood in the portal vein.

Only congenital PSS is treated surgically. The patient is usually stabilized with medical management first and then the shunt is tied off with silk via a laparotomy in one or more surgical procedures. Some referral centres use constrictor devices to occlude the shunt slowly, allowing the liver more time to adapt to the increased blood flow. Postoperative complications include abdominal pain, hypoglycaemia, diarrhoea, vomiting, hypotension, hypothermia, prolonged recovery time due to poor metabolism of anaesthetic drugs, seizures and shock.

Cholecystectomy

Cholangitis or **cholecystitis** (infection or inflammation of the biliary ducts and gallbladder) and **cholelithiasis** (stones in the gall bladder) may be treated by removal of the gall bladder. The surgery is carried out through a cranial midline laparotomy and the gall bladder is ligated and removed. The bile continues to drain into the duodenum through the bile duct, the only difference being that it does not collect in the gall bladder between meals. Postoperatively, the animal should be treated with antibiotics.

Spleen

The spleen is a large vascular organ in the abdomen on the left side next to the stomach. Although removal of the spleen in humans can result in the development of septicaemia, this has not been reported in dogs and cats and total splenectomy is not usually associated with any long-term problems.

Splenectomy

Indications for removal of the spleen include neoplasia, splenic torsion, trauma and haemorrhage. Haemangiosarcoma is the most common primary tumour of the spleen, and some tumours will be metastases from elsewhere. Up to half of splenic tumours may be benign or even just haematomas, and splenectomy can carry a good prognosis.

Sometimes patients present with acute haemorrhage from the spleen, and splenectomy is performed as an emergency procedure. More often, the bleeding is intermittent and the spleen is removed as an elective procedure to prevent a haemorrhagic crisis. If the haemorrhage has been severe, the animal may require a blood transfusion prior to surgery; if the haemorrhage is due to trauma and not neoplasia, an **autotransfusion** of blood can be carried out. At the time of the laparotomy the blood is suctioned via sterile apparatus out of the abdomen, mixed with the appropriate volume of anticoagulant, filtered and transfused into a peripheral vein. If there is any likelihood of neoplastic disease, autotransfusion should not be carried out.

Splenectomy may be performed using conventional surgical instruments and technique or using a stapler (Figure 25.37).

The most common postoperative complication is haemorrhage as a result of displacement of a ligature in the abdomen. The patient needs to be closely monitored for signs of intra-abdominal bleeding.

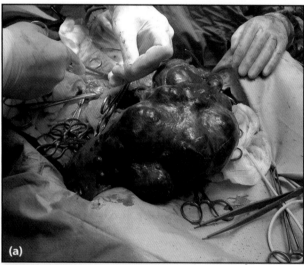

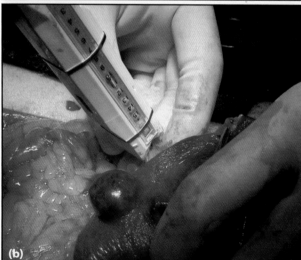

25.37 Splenectomy. **(a)** A splenectomy being carried out using conventional surgical technique, with hand-tied sutures and artery forceps for haemostasis. **(b)** A splenectomy being carried out using an LDS stapler. This is much faster but the stapler is expensive.

Urinary tract

All surgery of the urinary tract runs the potential risk of acute renal failure if kidney function is affected and urine production stops postoperatively. Urine production should be maintained at a minimum of 2 ml/kg/h using intravenous fluid therapy as required during the postoperative period. Urine needs to be collected and measured in order to monitor output. Diuretics or other treatments may be given if urine output is inadequate. Blood samples can also be analysed for urea, creatinine and electrolyte (potassium) levels, which also indicate renal function.

Kidney

The kidneys are **retroperitoneal**, which means that they lie outside the peritoneal cavity of the abdomen. They receive 25% of the total cardiac output and are one of the vital organs of the body. Surgical handling or trauma that might disrupt the blood supply or cause the artery to spasm could be potentially life-threatening.

Ureteronephrectomy

A kidney may be removed if there is severe trauma, neoplasia, **hydronephrosis** (enlargement of the kidney secondary to back pressure from the bladder), or severe **pyelonephritis** (infection). It is essential to be sure that the other kidney is functioning normally prior to this procedure otherwise the animal may go into postoperative renal failure. The kidney is removed together with its ureter, which is traced all the way down to the bladder and the arteries and veins are ligated. Postoperatively, intravenous fluids should be given until normal urine flow has been monitored and recorded.

Nephrotomy

Calculi can occasionally form in the kidney. These are very painful and may result in severe secondary infections of the kidney which may cause permanent damage. They are removed by a nephrotomy into the renal pelvis, when the calculus is removed and the incision repaired. Postoperative intravenous fluid therapy is important to ensure good urine production, along with close monitoring of blood urea and creatinine to check for evidence of urine leakage.

Renal biopsy

Biopsy of the kidney can be performed, but this is only done after extensive investigation of the renal disease as it carries considerable risks of haemorrhage and damage to renal function. Ideally, the sample is taken through a surgical incision, but sometimes it is carried out percutaneously using a Tru-Cut needle with ultrasound guidance. Postoperatively, pressure is used to stop bleeding and urine output is monitored and the urine analysed.

Ureter

The ureters travel in the retroperitoneal space from the kidney to the bladder. They can be imaged using intravenous excretory urography or ultrasound examination. They are not seen on plain radiographs.

Avulsion of the ureter

Rarely, the ureter may be torn secondary to abdominal trauma. This causes urine leakage into the retroperitoneal space, causing cellulitis with electrolyte abnormalities. In some cases the damage can be repaired surgically, but often ureteronephrectomy is necessary. It is important to stabilize the animal with respect to renal and electrolyte parameters prior to anaesthesia.

Ectopic ureters

This is a congenital condition where one or both ureters implant distal to the bladder, so that urine flows directly into the urethra. This results in a constant urinary incontinence, usually in a young dog. Golden Retrievers, Poodles and Labrador Retrievers are most commonly affected. The condition is diagnosed using excretory urography and ultrasonography. The ureters are often enlarged and abnormal due to ascending infections. In some cases, the ascending infection results in severe pyelonephritis and a ureteronephrectomy is carried out. Where the ureter and kidney are healthy it is possible to reimplant the ureter surgically into the bladder. Surgery on the ureter can result in spasm that causes the kidney to stop producing urine on that side for up to 48 hours. Ideally therefore, if both ureters require surgery, one side should be done at a time. As in renal surgery, urine production is carefully monitored postoperatively. In some cases, the incontinence may persist due to other bladder abnormalities.

Ureteric entrapment

The ureters run down to the bladder and in the female pass the uterine body and cervix. At this position they are at risk of entrapment in the ligature during routine ovariohysterectomy. This is life-threatening, particularly if both ureters are involved. If the ligature is removed within 7 days, little damage is done to the kidney and it should completely recover.

Urinary bladder

Surgery on the bladder is common in veterinary practice. The bladder lies in the caudal abdomen and can be accessed via a midline laparotomy. The bladder should be emptied prior to surgery, either using a catheter via the urethra or by cystocentesis using a small-gauge needle and syringe at surgery. The bladder wall is delicate and prone to oedema and bruising with rough handling, so it is usually held during surgery using stay sutures or fine forceps. Urine continues to collect in the bladder during surgery so it is important to protect the other abdominal organs from contamination with the urine during cystotomy.

Cystotomy and cystectomy

The most common indications for cystotomy are to remove calculi (stones) or tumours. Usually the incision in the bladder wall is made in the ventral aspect and more stay sutures may be placed lateral to the incision to assist opening the bladder for inspection. Sometimes the calculi are located far down the bladder neck and it may be necessary to place a urethral catheter and flush them into the bladder with sterile saline. For removal of neoplasms, the full thickness of the bladder wall is removed with a margin around the tumour and the bladder reconstructed. The incision is closed in two layers using a synthetic absorbable suture material. Postoperatively, the animal should be given the opportunity to empty the bladder as frequently as possible and monitored for normal urination and evidence of urine leakage (uraemia, hypothermia, abdominal pain) for 3–4 days.

Bladder rupture

This occurs either secondary to blunt abdominal trauma or due to prolonged urethral obstruction causing severe back pressure and accumulation of urine. Occasionally, bladder rupture occurs when attempts are made to express the bladder manually in paralysed patients. The condition may be diagnosed from the history, an absence of urine in the bladder or using diagnostic imaging. The immediate concern is the uroperitoneum and the metabolic consequences of the absorption of urine from the peritoneum. There may be uraemia, electrolyte imbalances, dehydration and shock, which may have to be treated prior to surgery. At surgery, the abdomen should be lavaged with sterile saline to remove urine and contaminants, and the bladder is repaired. Postoperatively, blood urea levels and urine production should be closely monitored.

Tube cystostomy (urinary diversion)

This is the placement of a drain through the abdominal wall in order to drain the bladder, bypassing the urethra. This may be used as a temporary measure prior to urethral surgery or after bladder or urethral surgery to divert urine flow. It can also be used for diversion of urine in patients with urethral obstruction due to tumours or paralysis of the bladder. A Foley catheter is drawn into the abdomen through a stab incision lateral to the midline (Figure 25.38). The tip is placed into the bladder, the balloon inflated with sterile saline and the catheter secured with sutures and omentum. The catheter is then secured to the outside of the body wall with sutures or zinc oxide butterfly tapes. In the hospital, this should be attached to a closed urine collection system to prevent the risk of ascending infections. In the longer term, the bladder is emptied at least four times daily by removing a bung from the end and attaching a syringe. When the drain is removed, the tip should be submitted for culture and then appropriate antibiotics used to treat any associated infection. Use of antibiotics while the drain is in place will not prevent infection and will only increase the likelihood of resistant strains developing.

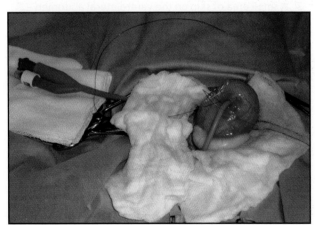

25.38 An intraoperative view of a bladder exteriorized for placement of a cystostomy tube using a Foley catheter.

Urethra

Surgery on the urethra is most often carried out following damage caused by calculi. Preoperatively, the systemic consequences of urethral obstruction may need to be addressed prior to anaesthesia, and often a urinary catheter is passed before surgery to make identification of the urethra easier.

Urethral obstruction

Blockage of the urethra in any species results in accumulation of urine in the bladder, which, if not relieved, causes back pressure on the kidneys and then bladder rupture. The urine spills into the abdomen and causes uraemia and death. The clinical signs may be severe abdominal pain with persistent straining to urinate.

Animals straining to urinate should be checked as an emergency to assess the bladder.

Cats are usually more severely affected than dogs, which may have only partial obstruction.

The urethra in the female is short and wide and unlikely to obstruct except secondary to neoplastic growth. In the male dog and cat the urethra is narrower, particularly at the tip in the male cat and at the level of the os penis in the male dog. This anatomical characteristic makes it prone to obstruction by urinary calculi. The type of stone that blocks the urethra depends on the disease and it should always be submitted for analysis in order to determine the most appropriate prophylactic treatment for the future.

Male cats also develop obstruction of the urethra secondary to feline lower urinary tract disease (FLUTD) and, in these cases, the obstruction is not always due to a calculus, but can be caused by a mucoid plug.

The priority is to stabilize the animal with intravenous fluids and decompress the bladder. If a urinary catheter cannot be passed, then it may be necessary to empty the bladder by cystocentesis. Once the pressure is reduced, it may then be possible to pass a catheter or to flush the urolith or plug back into the bladder with sterile saline (**retropulsion**). If it is not possible to remove the calculus in this way, urethrotomy is necessary.

Cystocentesis

1. Sedation is only necessary in fractious animals but analgesia should be provided.
2. The distended bladder is identified as a hard mass in the caudal abdomen.
3. A small area of skin on the ventrolateral abdomen directly over the bladder is clipped and surgically prepared.
4. A 20 G needle of the appropriate length for the size of animal is selected and attached to a 20 ml syringe via a three-way tap.
5. Sterile gloves are used or a short hand scrub is performed.
6. The bladder is gently held still with one hand and the needle is introduced into the bladder through the prepared area of skin.
7. The urine is drawn off and the three-way tap is used to expel the urine into a bowl. This is repeated until the bladder feels empty.
8. The volume of urine is recorded.

Urethrostomy

In some circumstances, either the cause of the urethral obstruction cannot be treated (e.g. calcium oxalate crystals) or the tip of the urethra is so damaged that it is prone to recurrent obstruction. In these cases, it may be necessary to create a new opening for urination through a wider part of the urethra. In the dog this is done at the level of the scrotum. In an intact male dog, castration and scrotal ablation are performed and then an incision into the urethra at that level is sutured to the skin edges (**scrotal urethrostomy**). In the male cat, the penis is amputated and the urethra is opened out and sutured to the skin edges (**perineal urethrostomy**). A urinary catheter should not be placed after surgery, and it is extremely important that the animal does not lick at the site at any stage during the healing process. Initially, there may be considerable bleeding associated with urination and it may be advisable to hospitalize the patient until this has reduced. Nursing involves keeping the site clean and free of urine or blood and preventing urine scald until the animal learns how to reposition during urination.

Urethral rupture

The urethra is exposed to damage in the male dog as it runs down the perineum and inguinal area and in all animals as it runs through the pelvic canal. The most common cause of rupture is trauma to the pelvic area and it is often seen secondary to pelvic fractures. The urine leaks out of the urethra and can cause severe inflammation of the pelvic tissues. Reabsorption of the urine then causes changes in the blood biochemistry such as uraemia and hyperkalaemia, which cause systemic illness. If the tear is small, the urethra may be treated with placement of a soft silicone indwelling urinary catheter, allowing it to heal by second intention. Larger tears or complete ruptures (avulsion) should be repaired surgically once the animal has been stabilized for the anaesthetic. Urine is then diverted through a cystostomy tube until the site is healed.

Urethral neoplasia

This is more common in the bitch than the dog and is occasionally seen in the cat. It usually presents with acute obstruction to urination although there may be a history of cystitis. Surgery can be performed to remove the urethra and reconstruct it using part of the vagina; however, the prognosis is very poor. It is important that a biopsy is done to confirm the diagnosis, as granulomatous urethritis can look very similar to neoplasia but can be treated successfully with steroids.

Urinary incontinence

Incontinence is most common in the bitch. It has to be investigated in order to determine the primary cause or causes:

- Ectopic ureter
- Pelvic bladder
- Short bladder neck
- Urinary tract infection
- Urinary sphincter mechanism incompetence (USMI).

The only condition that has to be treated surgically is ectopic ureter. The ureter is reimplanted into the bladder. The other conditions often present in a slightly older bitch or in the young bitch after spaying. They usually respond to medical management, but occasionally surgery is necessary to reposition the bladder neck and increase the pressure around the sphincter; this increases the holding capacity of the bladder and reduces incontinence. This surgery is usually carried out in specialist referral centres. Different techniques may be employed depending on the exact anatomical cause of the urinary incontinence, e.g. collagen injections into the urethral wall, urethropexy or colposuspension. Postoperative care involves carefully monitoring for urinary tract infections and ensuring that there is no retention of urine.

Incontinence in the male dog is usually secondary to prostatic disease. Castration may make the incontinence worse and it is very difficult to treat successfully, either with drugs or with surgery.

Reproductive system

Conditions are discussed in detail in Chapter 26.

Testes

The testes are the reproductive organ producing spermatozoa in male animals. They should normally descend after birth into the scrotum and remain externally located.

Elective castration (orchidectomy)

Castration may be carried out for therapeutic reasons (treatment of orchitis, perineal hernia, anal adenoma, testicular tumours or prostatitis), social reasons or as part of a neutering programme. Occasionally, castration is recommended to control behavioural abnormalities or difficulties such as roaming, excessive libido or aggression. Castration in the tomcat is usually carried out to prevent territorial spraying. Castration of the male dog at less than 6 months of age is associated with a decreased risk of prostatic neoplasia.

Castration in the cat is usually carried out via an incision in the scrotum; the testis is pulled out gently and then either it is ligated with suture material or the vas deferens and vascular bundle are tied in a knot to secure haemostasis. The vascular bundle is released into the scrotum and the procedure repeated on the other side. The cat is observed postoperatively for signs of haemorrhage, and then discharged with instructions for a litter tray to be used with shredded newspaper for 2–3 days. The wounds in the scrotum are not sutured, but allowed to heal by second intention.

Castration in the dog can be carried out either through a prescrotal midline incision or via scrotal ablation. **Prescrotal castration** involves pushing the testes forwards into the single incision and then the arteries and veins are ligated before removal of each testis. The skin incision is sutured closed, and the scrotum is left in place. **Scrotal ablation** involves removal of the scrotum and then the testes are removed with ligation as described above directly through the scrotal area. The skin is sutured closed. Prescrotal castration is quicker but leaves an unsightly scrotal sac behind and risks seroma or haematoma formation in the scrotum. Scrotal ablation takes longer, but has fewer complications associated with the healing of the surgical site.

Postoperatively, it is important that the owner is warned not to let the dog lick the sutures and that the dog is monitored for signs of ventral abdominal or scrotal swelling or bruising that might indicate ligature slippage.

Castration of rabbits may be carried out to reduce aggression and improve their behaviour as pets or in groups. Incisions may be made in a prescrotal or scrotal position and usually subcuticular sutures are used to close the incision. There is a theoretical risk of herniation through the inguinal canal and some surgeons will close the canal with one or two sutures before skin closure.

Retained testes (cryptorchidism)

Failure of one or both testes to descend is an inherited condition (see Chapter 26). It is more common in small-breed dogs, and is very rare in the cat. Both the retained testis and the descended testis are at risk of the development of neoplasia and they should be removed. Owners should be encouraged not to breed from affected animals.

The retained testis may be found at any point from the kidney down through the inguinal canal to just above the scrotal sac. The path is carefully explored surgically to locate the testicle, which is then removed in the standard way. The removed testis should be submitted for analysis to confirm that the correct tissue was removed.

Testicular neoplasia

These tumours are relatively common and are usually seen in older dogs. There are three main tumour types:

- Sertoli cell tumour (SCT)
- Seminoma (SEM)
- Interstitial cell tumour (ICT).

Sertoli cell tumours are more likely to metastasize than the other types to the lymph nodes, lung or liver. Sometimes SCT or SEM can cause a paraneoplastic syndrome associated with the production of hormones. Usually a feminization syndrome is seen that causes hair loss, **gynaecomastia** (enlarged mammary glands), prostatitis, atrophy of the unaffected testis and a pendulous prepuce, and the dog may become attractive to other male dogs. More severely affected dogs may also have bone marrow suppression, causing changes such as anaemia. Treatment with castration should carry a good prognosis.

Prostate

The prostate gland completely regresses after castration and should not develop disease later in life. Uncastrated dogs may develop prostatic disease secondary to the influence of the hormone testosterone. Symptoms may include infertility, impotence, incontinence, dysuria, haematuria, caudal abdominal pain and faecal tenesmus. The prostate can be examined by caudal palpation of the abdomen or rectal examination. Ultrasonography and radiography are also useful. Samples of the prostate gland can be taken by needle aspirates through the abdomen, alongside the rectum or via a urinary catheter. Ejaculation samples will also give some information about the fluid that the prostate is secreting.

Benign prostatic hyperplasia (BPH)

This occurs in the older male dog, when the prostate becomes acutely enlarged and very painful and secondary infection may occur. Castration may be indicated to prevent recurrence but in some cases may cause urinary incontinence. BPH may also be treated medically with drugs that inhibit the effect of testosterone, e.g. delamadinone acetate by injection or osaterone orally.

Prostatic cysts and abscesses

If BPH persists the prostate may develop cysts or abscesses, which can become enormous. Prostatic abscesses may be life-threatening, presenting with toxaemia and systemic disease similar to pyometra in the bitch. Cysts and abscesses should be operated on before they rupture and cause peritonitis. The approach is through a midline laparotomy; the abscess or cyst is drained and lavaged with sterile fluids until clean, and then packed with omentum before routine closure. Castration is recommended at the same time and a biopsy of the prostate is taken to screen for underlying neoplastic disease.

Prostatic neoplasia

Cancer can develop in the prostate gland of older dogs, whether castrated or entire. The gland is very painful and has similar signs to other prostatic diseases. Prostatic carcinoma rapidly spreads to the adjacent lymph nodes and sometimes the vertebral bodies. The prognosis is poor. Prostatectomy is unsuccessful at achieving a cure and results in complete urinary incontinence.

Penis

Amputation

Penile amputation is indicated where there is severe trauma to the penis or if there is neoplastic disease. The penis is extremely vascular and the procedure should be done under a tourniquet. Usually the whole of the os penis is removed and the urethra is reconstructed at the end of the inguinal part of the penis.

Mucosal eversion

Occasionally, hypersexed dogs may present with mucosal eversion of the tip of the urethra on the end of the penis. The mucosa is very vascular and bleeds because of the trauma. Castration may help, but usually the mucosa has also to be resected from the end of the penis. Again it helps to use a tourniquet during surgery and then absorbable fine-gauge suture material is used to resuture the mucosa at the end of the urethra. Postoperatively there may be some bleeding, and wadding may be used inside the prepuce to help to provide gentle pressure to stop this. The dog's behaviour has to be stopped and sometimes cold packing the swollen mucosa helps.

Ovaries and uterus

Elective ovariohysterectomy (spay)

In the UK, female companion animals are usually neutered (removal of the uterus and ovaries) to prevent unwanted litters and to prevent oestrous activity. Bitches are also neutered to decrease the risk of development of mammary tumours; the best effect of this is seen if the bitch is neutered before the first season. Bitches and queens are also neutered to prevent the development of pyometra (uterine infection) later in life. Female rabbits are neutered to prevent uterine neoplasia.

The ovaries are identified and the arteries tied off before cutting the ovarian ligament. A ligature is then placed around the uterine stump as close to the cervix as possible, to tie off the uterine arteries, before removal of the whole of the genital tract. The most important part of the procedure is to ensure that the ovaries are removed intact and no remnants are left behind that might secrete hormones. In some countries, only the ovaries are removed (**ovariectomy**); this is a shorter procedure and there is no documented increased risk of uterine disease. Laparoscopic techniques (see later) may be used to perform ovariectomies which result in much shorter recovery times and postoperative restriction. Bitches and many pedigree cats are usually operated from the midline and the majority of cats are operated on via a left flank approach with the patient lying in lateral recumbency. It has been suggested that spaying increases the likelihood of urinary incontinence in some breeds of dog but this is not proven and it is more likely that there is already an underlying bladder abnormality.

Postoperative analgesia and observation are important. The wound should be observed for signs of bleeding or bruising and the recovery monitored. Any postoperative spay patient that has a prolonged recovery from anaesthesia should be assessed for the possibility of intra-abdominal haemorrhage. Pale mucous membranes, generalized weakness, a rapid thready pulse, hypothermia, or bleeding from the laparotomy wound or vagina are all symptoms that should be investigated. Postoperative instructions relate to wound care and restricted activity to prevent dehiscence of the abdominal repair.

Pyometra

This is the accumulation of pus in the uterus (Figure 25.39), which may be infected or sterile. It occasionally occurs in the uterine remains in spayed females. It occurs most commonly in middle to older aged bitches. It is potentially life-threatening and often presents as an emergency. Disease occurs during metoestrus and the bitch may have a history of irregular oestrous patterns and of having been given oestrogens and progestogens. Clinical signs include depression, lethargy, anorexia, polydipsia and polyuria, vomiting and diarrhoea, and pyrexia. If the cervix is open (**open pyometra**), there is a vaginal discharge and the patient may be less ill than when the cervix is closed (**closed pyometra**) and all the pus is retained in the uterus.

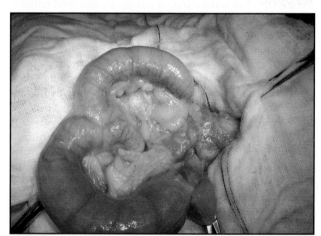

25.39 Intraoperative view of a pyometra. The uterus is grossly swollen and very vascular.

The animal may be in severe toxaemic shock and will often require intensive fluid therapy before being fit for anaesthesia. Ovariohysterectomy is required as a life-saving procedure as soon as the animal is stable enough for surgery. Intensive nursing is required in the postoperative phase. Fluid therapy should continue until renal function and urine output are normal.

Caesarean operation

This is removal of fetuses by hysterotomy. It may be necessary when a bitch or queen presents with dystocia (see Chapter 26).

Usually the caesarean operation is carried out under general anaesthetic, but epidural anaesthesia is the technique of choice where the facilities are available. Preparation for the caesarean operation focuses around the provision of enough personnel to resuscitate the puppies or kittens (see Chapter 21). Most veterinary surgeons use a midline approach to the abdomen, despite the possibility of subsequent interference with the sutures by the young. Preparation of the abdomen for aseptic surgery must be thorough, but the use of antiseptics that might cause dermatitis around the mammary glands should be avoided. The incision is closed routinely, though some surgeons may use a subcuticular closure in order that there are no skin sutures in the region where the offspring will be suckling.

Postoperative care involves close monitoring of the recovery from anaesthesia, and prevention of hypothermia. Regular postoperative checks are necessary to ensure that the dam is suckling and caring for the litter, despite the stress of hospitalization and surgery. Many cases will be discharged to their home environment as soon as possible after recovery and monitored with home visits. It is particularly important that the owner is given advice on postoperative nutrition of the dam and that frequent small meals are offered in the early stages postoperatively. Often these patients will develop transient diarrhoea due to hormonal influences. The litter and bedding must be kept as clean as possible to prevent postoperative sepsis.

In some circumstances an ovariohysterectomy will be performed at the same time as the caesarean operation. This is not ideal but is sometimes indicated where there is uterine rupture or risk of recurrent unwanted pregnancy (e.g. in 'stray' animals).

Neoplasia

Older animals may develop tumours of the ovaries or uterus. These can be very aggressive, but some are benign. Ovariohysterectomy is indicated.

Vagina

The vagina is usually only affected by disease in the entire bitch or queen. It rarely causes problems after neutering.

Hyperplasia

Vaginal hyperplasia is seen most often in brachycephalic breeds. The vaginal mucosa has an exaggerated hyperplastic response to the oestrogens secreted during oestrus, and excessive folds of vaginal mucosa protrude through the vulva. It often has the appearance of a tumour, but it regresses at the end of oestrus. The exposed mucosa must be kept clean and lubricated with K-Y jelly (Johnson & Johnson). Treatment to prevent recurrence is by ovariohysterectomy.

Prolapse

Vaginal prolapse is less common than hyperplasia, but occurs in the same breeds. Mild prolapses may not require treatment other than protection of the exposed mucosa. Spontaneous regression should occur during the dioestrous period. Vaginal prolapse may also occur in the post-partum period.

Neoplasia

Neoplasia of the vulva and vagina is seen occasionally. Most large fibrous tumours identified in the wall of the vagina are leiomyomas (benign), and are infiltrative hard nodules usually in the dorsal vaginal wall. The tumours are removed using an episiotomy to access the vaginal lumen from the perineum, and the bitch is also neutered. The urethra should be catheterized during surgery, so that the urethral orifice can be identified during the resection. Neoplasms of the vulva tend to be more aggressive carcinomas or mast cell tumours and require complex surgery for removal and reconstruction.

Hernias and ruptures

- A **hernia** is an abnormal protrusion of an organ or organs through a physiological opening in the lining of the cavity in which it is normally enclosed.
- A **rupture** is a pathological tear in the lining of the cavity through which enclosed organs may protrude.

Most hernias and ruptures affect the abdominal cavity, but a few occur elsewhere. An example outside the abdomen includes herniation of the occipital or temporal lobes of the brain under the bony tentorium cerebelli as a complication of space-occupying lesions of the cranium.

The openings through which a hernia may occur are either a normal opening that has enlarged to allow organs through (e.g. inguinal canal), or an opening that should have closed during normal development (e.g. umbilicus). Hernias and ruptures share some characteristics in terms of the risks associated with the protrusion of viscera; however, as hernias are physiological, they are usually lined by an outpouching of the cavity lining (e.g. the peritoneum). Ruptures are not lined and the cavity lining is ruptured along with the body wall.

Hernias and ruptures are further described by the following terms:

- **Reducible** – the contents of the hernia or rupture can be replaced in the original anatomical location by gentle pressure on the swelling to push the viscera back through the defect itself
- **Irreducible or incarcerated** – the contents of the hernia or rupture cannot be replaced, usually because of the formation of adhesions in chronic cases
- **Strangulated** – the contents of a hernia or rupture can become devitalized due to entrapment of the blood vessels passing through the defect. Strangulation is life-threatening and a serious emergency.

Umbilical hernia

This is a congenital condition where the umbilicus fails to close over and fat and abdominal contents protrude through under the skin. Small hernias are of no consequence as they usually do not increase in size as the animal grows. Large hernias should be repaired due to the risk of incarceration of small intestine or other abdominal organs.

Inguinal hernia

Herniation occurs through the inguinal canal, which is a physiological opening in the muscle of the caudal abdominal wall. It is more common in females than males, particularly in elderly overweight small-breed dogs. In the bitch a swelling may be seen in the groin extending towards the vulva. The hernia may contain fat in the broad ligament, uterus, intestines or bladder. If the bitch is pregnant, the gravid uterus can become strangulated. In male dogs, fat or intestine may herniate into the scrotal sac and can become strangulated because of the small opening.

The hernia should be scanned or radiographed to determine what structures it contains. The owner should be warned about the possibility of strangulation. All hernias should be surgically repaired and the inguinal canal narrowed to prevent recurrence. Ideally the animal should also be neutered.

Perineal hernia

Perineal hernia occurs almost exclusively in older male dogs. It is associated with degeneration of the muscles of the pelvic diaphragm (coccygeus and levator ani). Affected dogs have difficulty defecating and have an obvious swelling on one or both sides of the anus (Figure 25.40). The swelling is associated with impaction of faeces in the rectum as well as herniated abdominal contents. An important complication of perineal hernia is retroflexion and incarceration of the bladder and prostate. This can result in acute urethral obstruction and is an emergency.

There are a number of surgical techniques described for hernia repair that involve apposing the remains of the atrophied muscles using a monofilament long-lasting suture material (e.g. PDS (Ethicon) or polypropylene). Some techniques also involve transferring muscle flaps to help support the hernia repair and these techniques are usually more successful. All dogs are castrated to help to prevent recurrence.

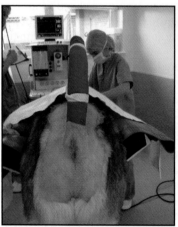

25.40 A bilateral perineal hernia. The perineal area is swollen with herniated contents of the caudal abdomen. Faeces are sometimes impacted in the caudal rectum, contributing to the perineal swelling. Rectal examination confirms the absence of the pelvic diaphragm.

Pre- and postoperative nursing

Preoperatively, the animal should be assessed for bladder position and the possibility that the bladder could be retroflexed into the hernia, obstructing the urethra. If there is doubt, the hernia may be radiographed or the urethra catheterized in order to empty the bladder. Sometimes the bladder has to be emptied by cystocentesis before it can be catheterized or reduced. The surgical site is considered contaminated and peri- and postoperative antibiotic cover is required. Before the surgical preparation, the rectal sacculation is manually emptied of faeces and a purse-string suture is placed to prevent faecal material contaminating the surgical site during surgery. Enemas are not used as they may result in loose slurry that could easily spill into the surgical site. Postoperatively, the purse-string is removed and faecal modifiers (ispaghula, sterculia) are given in the food to prevent straining against the hernia repair and also to improve rectal function. Bilateral hernia repairs sometimes develop rectal prolapse which requires a loose purse-string suture around the anus for a few days until the anus regains normal tone.

Diaphragmatic hernia

Diaphragmatic rupture is most commonly associated with trauma such as a road traffic accident, causing a sudden increase in abdominal pressure when the glottis is closed. The diaphragm tears either around the edge (**circumferential**) or across from the centre to the edge (**radial**). The loss of a functional diaphragm makes breathing difficult and this is coupled with herniation of abdominal contents such as intestine, liver, spleen or stomach into the pleural space. The trauma may also cause **pulmonary contusion** (bruising of the lungs) which adds to the animal's respiratory distress. Some cases are undiagnosed at the time of the original trauma and can present months later with dyspnoea when more abdominal contents herniate.

Congenital defects in the diaphragm are also seen, the most common of which is the pericardial–peritoneal diaphragmatic hernia. In this condition, the ventral portion of the diaphragm is absent and abdominal contents herniate into the mediastinum (not the pleural space). Often the animal also has a large umbilical hernia.

All diaphragmatic hernias are repaired surgically. Congenital defects are repaired as elective procedures, but ruptures may need to be repaired as an emergency if the stomach is in the chest and it begins to dilate. Ideally, the animal should be stabilized after the accident to improve the anaesthetic risk, but in some cases the dyspnoea is so severe that immediate surgery is necessary. The tear is sutured closed using long-lasting absorbable suture material. Chronic cases may be difficult to reduce due to adhesions to the pleura. Due to contraction of the abdominal muscles, the abdomen may be difficult to close once all the abdominal contents are returned. A chest drain may be necessary, particularly in chronic cases where there may be a pleural effusion.

Pre- and postoperative nursing

Preoperative nursing focuses on provision of supplementary oxygen, reducing stress on handling, analgesia and treatment of shock. The nurse should be prepared to provide IPPV during the anaesthesia (see Chapter 23) and to monitor for sudden changes in blood pressure when the abdominal viscera are moved back into the abdomen. A catheter may be used to aspirate air from the thorax as the rupture is closed or a chest drain may be used. Postoperatively, the animal should be watched carefully for signs of discomfort associated with increased abdominal pressure and evidence of continuing difficulty with breathing due to pulmonary contusions. Some cats may be inappetent after surgery, due to liver damage.

Prepubic tendon or abdominal wall rupture

This condition is usually seen as a consequence of abdominal wall trauma, most commonly a road accident, but also due to a blunt blow such as a kick. There may be other injuries associated with the trauma. Usually there is an extensive area of severe bruising over the rupture and the associated subcutaneous swelling.

The rupture is repaired surgically using long-lasting absorbable materials such as PDS (Ethicon). Macerated muscle tissue may not repair easily, and a synthetic mesh might be necessary to replace devitalized muscle. Where the prepubic attachment is ruptured, wire sutures may be used to reattach the ventral abdominal wall to the pubic bone.

Pre- and postoperative nursing

The animal should be stabilized and given analgesia prior to surgical repair. If the bladder is in the rupture, urine production should be closely monitored or the animal catheterized to ensure that the bladder neck is not entrapped. Analgesia is important as the abdominal wall is often bruised. Anti-inflammatories may help with resolution of bruising in addition to padded bedding and cage rest. Faecal modifiers should be given to assist with defecation so that the animal does not strain and put pressure on the abdominal repair. Animals that require a mesh implant should be closely monitored for signs of infection or sinus tracts associated with the implant. Postoperative exercise is restricted and the animal should be prevented from jumping up or stretching the abdomen.

Musculoskeletal system

Tendon and muscle repair

Tendon and muscle damage are usually secondary to trauma, unless a myotomy or tenotomy has been performed as part of a surgical approach to a joint.

Muscle damage is usually repaired as soon as possible after injury, using absorbable monofilament material. Trauma to muscle often results in macerated fragile tissue and it can be difficult to reappose successfully. Normal healthy muscle heals quickly after a myotomy as it has a good blood supply.

Tendons heal very slowly and have to be supported to ensure that they do not stretch and lose function. Orthopaedic implants may be used to protect the tendon until it has fully repaired and remodelled.

Limb amputation

Amputation is an unfortunate but not infrequent surgical procedure in all of the companion animals. It is a very difficult concept for many owners to come to terms with and they may need counselling and advice. Most animals cope with amputation much better than the owner expects (Figure 25.41) and some may even be walking and running within hours of anaesthetic recovery.

Amputation may be recommended for the following reasons:

- Curative removal of a benign tumour (e.g. haemangiopericytoma)
- Palliative removal of a malignant but very painful tumour (e.g. osteosarcoma)
- Injury to the distal limb that is beyond repair (e.g. shear injury)
- Nerve root avulsion resulting in permanent paralysis of the limb
- Economic reasons, if the complex fracture or soft tissue injury is too expensive for repair.

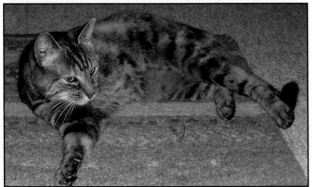

25.41 Animals frequently tolerate limb amputation remarkably well, as long as the remaining three limbs are free of any other orthopaedic or neurological disease. This cat has had her left forelimb amputated yet lives a full and normal life.

The most important aspect of assessment of a patient for amputation is establishing that the other three limbs are fit and free of arthritic or other disease. On admission it is important to check and state on the consent form which limb is to be amputated. Obese patients or very large breeds may not be suitable candidates for amputation as they will have difficulty shifting the centre of gravity over to the remaining legs and may be less agile.

Postoperative nursing

Surgery may be prolonged and there can be considerable blood loss from the cut muscle ends if diathermy is not available, so intravenous fluids are important to ensure a rapid recovery. Prevention of seroma formation at the site of the amputation can be achieved by bandaging or use of a drain. Postoperative nursing is important to help these patients to their feet as soon as possible in order that they can quickly adapt to a new gait. Walking must be assisted if the floor is slippery or rubber mats may be placed to give the animal confidence.

Arthrotomy

Some surgical conditions of the joints require surgery inside the joint itself (arthrotomy). The most common indications for joint surgery in the dog and cat are dislocations, ligamentous injuries (in particular, cruciate ligament rupture), **osteochondrosis** (abnormal development of cartilage in the joint), penetrating wounds of the joint and fractures involving the joint surface. The elbow, stifle and hip are the most commonly affected joints.

Strict asepsis is extremely important as postoperative infection in the joint is devastating. Equally important are haemostasis and meticulous repair of the surgical approach through the joint capsule. The joint is usually flushed with sterile saline at the end of the surgery, and the repair made using monofilament suture materials. Joint surgery can be very painful and good analgesia is important; some surgeons may use local anaesthetic into the joint. Seroma formation is a common postoperative complication and some veterinary surgeons will use a pressure bandage on the joint to prevent this and to immobilize the joint for a few days. However, it is difficult to immobilize the elbow and stifle and often bandages are ineffective. Exercise is usually limited to a strict regime and it is important that the owner is given clear written instructions.

In some specialist centres, joint surgery may be carried out using **arthroscopy.** This enables access to the joint without the disadvantages and postoperative complications of a surgical approach. The arthroscope must be sterile, and specialist instruments are used that are introduced into the joint via a separate opening. The joint is subject to a continuous high-pressure sterile fluid lavage during surgery. A sterile sleeve is used to cover the cable from the arthroscope to the viewing screen. This technique is often used in equine and farm animal joint surgery, as the joints are large. In dogs, only the stifle, elbow and shoulder are routinely investigated with arthroscopy and occasionally in larger breeds it is possible to scope the other joints. It is possible to remove fragments of cartilage or bone without opening the joint by using special instruments alongside the camera inside the joint.

Cruciate disease

The cruciate ligaments are two crossed ligaments within the stifle joint that stabilize the joint within its range of movement. There are also two C-shaped menisci that serve as 'shock absorbers' in the stifle. Disease of this complex joint is very common. It is often the cranial cruciate ligament that ruptures and the medial meniscus that is damaged. The instability results in the femur slipping on the tibia as the dog bears weight. The patient may be presented acutely lame, following trauma during exercise or with a low-grade, slowly progressing lameness of the affected hindlimb. Some breeds with upright conformation are prone to cruciate degeneration and may present with both hindlimbs affected. In dogs less than 15 kg bodyweight, the joint will eventually stabilize with rest and physiotherapy. In larger breeds, there is a better result if the joint is stabilized surgically. There are a number of surgical techniques that have been described and new methods continue to be developed. In all cases, the joint should be examined (sometimes using arthroscopy) to remove damaged meniscus prior to treatment for the instability. Veterinary nurses may encounter a number of surgical techniques, the most popular of which are listed below.

- Extracapsular techniques: These techniques use a lateral retinacular suture, where non-absorbable suture material is placed around the lateral fabella and through a hole drilled in the tibial crest, and then secured with metal crimps or a locking knot.
- Intracapsular technique: This is where a strip of patellar ligament and fascia is pulled through to the inside of the joint and secured with sutures.
- Tibial Plateau Levelling Osteotomy (TPLO): This procedure aims to make the stifle joint stable during weight bearing by changing the angle of the tibial plateau, allowing the dog to move without pain – although the ruptured ligament has not been 'repaired'. A curved cut is made with a saw and special radial blade in the proximal tibia. The tibia is then rotated through the appropriate number of degrees as measured from the radiograph taken prior to surgery. The bone is stabilized with a specially designed TPLO plate and screws to keep the tibial plateau in its new position.
- Cranial Closing Tibial Wedge Osteotomy (CCTWO): This procedure is similar to TPLO except that a wedge of bone is removed from the proximal tibia and a plate similar to a T plate is screwed into place over the cut.
- Tibial Tuberosity Advancement (TTA): This technique also aims to change the forces on weight bearing in the stifle. This is a simpler procedure than TPLO, but still requires special equipment, plates and screws.

Postoperative care after cruciate surgery depends on which technique has been used; however, there is usually a strict regime of rest followed by carefully controlled return to activity and fitness. The last three techniques (TPLO, CCTWO and TTA) require special training and should only be carried out by orthopaedic surgeons. The postoperative instructions must be carefully followed as the bone has been cut (fractured) and repositioned and there is a risk of severe complications if there is infection or overactivity postoperatively. All cruciate surgery is painful postoperatively and multimodal analgesia is an important part of nursing these patients.

Joint replacement

Dogs with chronically painful hips or elbows due to osteoarthritis may be candidates to have these joints replaced with artificial joints (prostheses). These are expensive procedures, but the success rate in experienced hands is as high as 90%

for hip replacement and 80% for elbow replacement. When there are complications, they are major and may result in loss of the joint function completely. These procedures are only carried out by specialist orthopaedic surgeons.

- Total Hip Replacement (THR): The diseased femoral head is removed and replaced with a metal femoral stem prosthesis, which is anchored into the femur (some systems use a special bone cement for this). The acetabulum is reamed out and a high-density polyethylene cup is anchored in position (again, with or without cement). A metal femoral head is then placed onto the femoral stem and this sits in the acetabular cup.
- Total Elbow Replacement (TER): This procedure is currently carried out at a few centres in the UK. The humeral joint surface is replaced with a metal component and the radius and ulna joint surfaces are replaced with high density polyethylene component. This technique is still being developed.
- Canine Knee Systems are currently in development and beginning to be performed in the UK, but there are few long-term data on their success.

Arthrodesis

Arthrodesis is the surgical fusion of a joint to prevent its movement, and is used when there is intractable joint pain, chronic instability of the joint or an irreparable joint fracture. The principle is that the joint surfaces are obliterated using curettes or power-driven burrs or saws, and then the joint is fused in a normal standing position, using plates or screws to compress the surfaces together. The joint is often supported with a cast postoperatively until the arthrodesis has fully healed and can support the animal's weight. Strict asepsis is essential to the success of the procedure. Sometimes the surgery is carried out using a tourniquet (e.g. carpal arthrodesis) to reduce blood loss and improve visibility during surgery.

Fractures

Fractures are usually the result of traumatic incidents. In small-breed dogs they can occur if the dog jumps down from a height (e.g. out of the owner's arms or off the sofa), or some dogs have a predisposition to certain spontaneous fractures (e.g. Springer Spaniels with elbow fractures). Some fractures are pathological and are associated with bone disease or neoplasia.

In most instances, fractures are repaired surgically, though this depends on the type of fracture (see earlier). It is important that two good quality orthogonal radiographs are obtained of the fracture prior to surgery, in order to plan the repair. Immediately postoperatively, two views are taken to assess the success of the repair and to determine the position of any implants. The healing is then followed up with regular radiographs in the weeks following surgery until evidence of union is seen.

Nursing the fracture patient

- Assessment and treatment of concurrent injuries.
- Provision of analgesia.
- Assisted walking to ensure that the animal does not slip when taken out.
- Provision of adequate dry bedding so that the animal remains dry and clean.

continues ▶

continued

- Monitoring for decubital ulcers.
- Monitoring the temperature, pulse and respiration rate as indicators of pain, infection or distress.
- Observation of the surgical wound for signs of postoperative infection.
- Detailed communication with the owner over the exercise regime and prevention of excessive use of the limb during the healing process.
- Regular radiography of the repaired fracture to monitor healing.

Physiotherapy by a qualified physiotherapist is sometimes used for fracture patients, but the programme must be assigned on an individual basis by a veterinary surgeon, as inappropriate manipulation may cause more harm.

Specialist orthopaedic surgery

Some orthopaedic surgery is only carried out in referral centres, such as TPLO, total hip replacement or very complex fractures. These procedures require detailed assessment of the animal and the surgery is performed under strict aseptic conditions. The equipment is expensive and the nursing staff must be experienced in the use and care of these instruments.

For example, when a total hip replacement is carried out, the animal is assessed for skin disease that may increase the risk of bacterial contamination at the time of surgery, obesity, and gastrointestinal disease that might cause diarrhoea during hospitalization, as well as its orthopaedic disease.

During surgery, the surgeons may wear two pairs of gloves. Adhesive waterproof disposable drapes are used and personnel in theatre are limited to reduce aerosol contamination. Often a culture swab is taken from the surgical wound just before closure to check for any contamination in the surgical wound during surgery.

Spinal surgery

Neurosurgical procedures require certain specialized equipment and skills and are usually carried out in referral centres. Diagnoses of spinal injuries or diseases are carried out using a combination of clinical examination and neurological tests and radiographs, contrast radiography (myelography) and advanced imaging techniques (e.g. MRI or CT). Samples of spinal fluid may be taken for analysis either from between the skull and first cervical vertebra (**cisternal puncture**) or from between the lumbar vertebrae (**lumbar puncture**).

Spinal cord injury arises from any pressure on the cord within the vertebral canal. The resulting inflammatory response can result in continued injury to the nerves even after the cause of the pressure has been relieved. Recovery from spinal injuries can be very slow and requires committed and caring nursing staff. Spinal patients are at risk from:

- Pneumonia
- Decubital ulcers
- Dermatitis due to urine or faecal skin soiling
- Limb oedema
- Muscle wasting
- Urinary tract infection.

Nursing spinal injuries

Recumbent animals are at high risk of a number of complications that can be alleviated or prevented by good nursing:

- Analgesia/pain management
- Wound management/assessment
- Ensuring that the bladder is emptied regularly
- Checking for decubital ulcers three times daily
- Turning the patient regularly – at last every 2 hours
- Monitoring conscious or unconscious defecation and urination
- Monitoring neurological reflexes and recording improvements
- Maintaining adequate nutrition
- Administering physiotherapy to all joints to prevent stiffness and cartilage degeneration
- Keeping the skin clean and dry
- Providing regular assisted walks and attention
- Moving the patient into a place where it can watch general activity.

Most dedicated owners can manage small to medium-sized recumbent patients at home once the animal is urinary continent, but will need detailed written guidelines on nursing care. Regular visits help to monitor the animal's progress and to provide support to the owners that they are doing everything correctly.

Spinal fractures

Spinal fractures are usually the result of trauma, and the radiograph may not accurately reflect the degree of spinal cord damage done at the time of impact if the spinal muscles have pulled the bones back into alignment. If a spinal fracture is suspected, the patient should not be sedated or anaesthetized for radiography, as the muscles may be holding the bones in place and preventing further spinal cord damage. Some fractures are managed with cage rest if the spinal cord injury is not severe. In other cases, the vertebrae have to be stabilized using pins, plates or external fixation.

Disc disease

The intervertebral discs can cause severe spinal cord injury if they dislodge and erupt into the spinal canal, contacting the ventral aspect of the spinal cord. This classically occurs in the small-breed dogs such as Dachshunds, Pekingese and Jack Russell Terriers, which have a defect in the cartilage component of the disc (Type 1). These disc protrusions can occur very suddenly and result in acute paralysis of the patient. Another disc disease syndrome is seen in ageing larger-breed dogs, which causes slow compression of the spinal cord and results in chronic nerve pain (Type 2).

Both types of disc disease are alleviated by surgery to open up the spinal canal (**laminectomy**) and to remove the fragments of disc pressing on the spinal cord. This is specialized surgery and careful assessment of the patient is necessary to determine which part of the spinal canal is affected. Postoperatively, the patient may be slightly worse before the neurological symptoms improve. They will require prolonged nursing care. Acute cases of paraplegia should be operated on as soon as possible to minimize the damage to the spinal cord.

Neoplasia

Tumours are occasionally diagnosed causing neurological symptoms secondary to slow compression of the spinal cord as they grow within the confined space of the spinal canal. Surgical removal of benign tumours of the meninges via a laminectomy can be successful, but tumours arising from the vertebrae themselves are usually inoperable.

Minimally invasive surgery (MIS)

Therapeutic techniques are constantly evolving and recent developments in veterinary surgery include the use of minimally invasive techniques.

Rigid endoscopes can be used to enter cavities such as the abdomen, thorax or joint space to visualize structures (see also Chapter 18) and to undertake diagnostic or therapeutic procedures. This enables procedures to be carried out using two or three small holes instead of large incisions. Laparoscopy relates to entering the abdomen and thoracoscopy is related to the thorax. Laparoscopy is routinely used to examine the abdomen in equine species and to take liver biopsy samples without the associated dangers of general anaesthesia and linea alba incision. In dogs and cats, minor procedures such as pancreatic, hepatic and lung biopsy, ovariectomy and gastropexy have been described, but in experienced hands it is also possible to carry out splenectomy, lung/liver lobectomy and pericardectomy.

These are difficult techniques to master and are generally carried out by surgeons who are in referral practice or institutions and are carrying out these techniques regularly. As with all surgery, there has to be a 'Plan B'. If the arthroscopy/laparoscopy/thoracoscopy does not go as planned, or it is not possible to complete the procedure using MIS, the surgeon has to have the skill and equipment to convert to a conventional surgical approach.

The surgical technique is based on the principle of triangulation. The telescope and instruments are introduced into the abdomen through trocars (cannulae) and form a triangle. At the base of the triangle, the surgeon and assistant manipulate the telescope (attached to the camera so the image is viewed on a screen) and an instrument, which meet at the tip of the triangle within the abdomen (Figure 25.42). Distension of the cavity with gas makes a space so that the surgeon can see the tips of the instruments and organs on the monitor.

Equipment

- Light source – The type of light source and the strength is important in the quality of the image obtained.
- Camera – This is attached to the end of the endoscope so that the surgeon can view the image on a screen.
- Trocars – These are used to make entry holes (portals) through which the instruments and endoscope can be introduced. Generally three portals are made; one for the camera and two for the instruments.
- Insufflator – This gently pumps carbon dioxide into the cavity (abdomen or thorax) which separates the organs so that the surgeon can see each one individually.
- Fluid pump – In arthroscopy, the joint space is separated for the camera by sterile saline (rather than carbon dioxide).
- Veress needle – This is a needle with a spring-loaded insert that slips out and covers the sharp tip after introduction into a cavity. This then enables the carbon dioxide to be introduced to make space in the cavity so that the other portals can be made safely (without the trocars damaging an organ).
- Endoscopes – These come in different sizes depending on the size of the patient and the cavity to be inspected. For example, the laparoscope used for an equine liver biopsy would be 10 mm, and for a Labrador ovariectomy would be 5 mm. Arthroscopes are usually between 2 and 4 mm in diameter. The endoscopes are also designed to have the view end-on or at an angle (10–40 degrees), which can make it easier to look around.

Surgical instruments

Special surgical instruments are used for MIS. These very fine, long-handled instruments fit down the trocars and are designed for specific purposes:

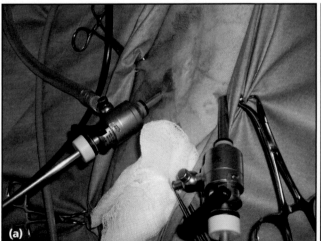
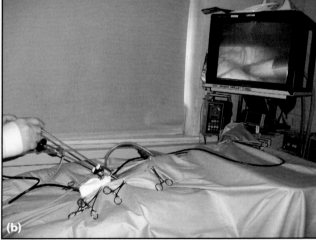

25.42 (a) Laparoscopy of an abdomen. Small incisions are made through which the laparoscope is inserted. Fine instruments are introduced through a trocar in another incision. (b) A light source and a camera are attached to the laparoscope and images appear on the monitor. Organs and abdominal contents can be inspected and the procedures being performed with the instruments through the other ports can be viewed in real time. (Courtesy of T. Charlesworth)

- Some can be attached to the diathermy unit so that they seal and cut at the same time
- Some are just for holding tissue
- Some are blunt ended and are used for moving tissue, as well as for other specialist applications.

Special diathermy units are used for MIS, as the power must be higher than in conventional surgery. A special unit called a Ligasure may be used to cut tissue by heat sealing. This unit can also be used to ligate vessels up to 7 mm in diameter.

MIS is a very advanced technique in human surgery but is in its infancy in veterinary surgery. There are specialist instruments for a variety of techniques; for example, special bags are used to hold removed organs, before they are pulled out through a small hole in the body wall.

Minimally invasive surgery involves expensive equipment and considerable experience. There is a risk of damage to organs or vessels when the sharp trocars are introduced. There are also reported risks associated with the insufflation of the cavity with CO_2, such as air embolism, hypercapnia, emphysema and peritoneal irritation.

Further reading

Alexander JW *et al.* (1983) The influence of hair removal methods on wounds. *Archives of Surgery* **118**, 347–352

Anderson DM (1999) Nursing patients undergoing skin reconstruction. *Veterinary Nursing* **14**, 52–61

Aspinall V (2003) *Clinical Procedures in Veterinary Nursing.* Butterworth-Heinemann, Oxford

Bojrab MJ (ed) (1993) *Disease Mechanisms in Small Animal Surgery,* 2nd edn. Lea & Febiger, Philadelphia

Bojrab MJ, Ellison GW and Slocum B (1998) *Current Techniques in Small Animal Surgery, 4th edn.* Williams & Wilkins, Baltimore

Coughlan A and Miller A (2006) *BSAVA Manual of Small Animal Fracture Repair and Management* (revised reprint). BSAVA Publications, Gloucester

Ellison GW (1993) Visceral healing and repair disorders. In: *Disease Mechanisms in Small Animal Surgery, 2nd edn,* ed. MJ Bojrab, pp. 2–6. Lea & Febiger, Philadelphia

Flecknell P (1988) Developments in the veterinary care of rabbits and rodents. *In Practice,* **20**, 286–295

Harari J (ed.) (1993) *Surgical Complications and Wound Healing in the Small Animal Practice.* WB Saunders, Philadelphia

Jeffery ND (1995) *Handbook of Small Animal Spinal Surgery.* WB Saunders, London

Lhermette P and Sobel D (2008) *BSAVA Manual of Canine and Feline Endoscopy and Endosurgery.* BSAVA Publications, Gloucester

Morgan DA (2000) *Guides for Health Care Staff, 9th edn.* Euromed Communications Ltd., Haslemere, Surrey

Piermattei DL and Flo GL (1997) *Handbook of Small Animal Orthopedics and Fracture Repair.* WB Saunders, Philadelphia

Pope ER (1993) Skin healing. In *Disease Mechanisms in Small Animal Surgery, 2nd edn,* ed. MJ Bojrab, pp. 151–155. Lea & Febiger, Philadelphia

Villiers E and Dunn J (1998) Collection and preparation of smears for cytological evaluation. *In Practice,* **20**, 270–377

Willford PS (1983) Hair removal – shave-preps, depilatories, and other preoperative considerations: are they really necessary? *Journal of the Operating Room Research Institute* **3**(3), 28–36

Williams J, McHugh D and White RAS (1992) Use of drains in small animal surgery. *In Practice* **14**, 73–81

Williams JM and Niles JD (2005) *BSAVA Manual of Canine and Feline Abdominal Surgery.* BSAVA Publications, Gloucester

Self-assessment questions

1. **What does the term pleuritis indicate?**
2. **What does the presence of bright red granulation tissue indicate?**
3. **How many days post surgery are skin sutures usually removed?**
4. **List three signs of wound complications.**
5. **Which type of drain requires suction?**
6. **What is the difference between a sequestrum and a sinus?**
7. **What is one of the most common causes of poor fracture healing after surgical repair?**
8. **For placement of a 2.7 mm screw what size drill bit should be selected to drill a pilot hole, a gliding hole for a lag screw and what size tap?**
9. **Is a fibrosarcoma a benign or malignant tumour?**
10. **List three complications specific to spinal surgery that a good nurse is able to prevent.**

Chapter 26

Reproduction, and obstetric and paediatric nursing

Wendy Adams, Gary England, Matthew Hanks and Simon Girling

Learning objectives

After studying this chapter, students should be able to:

- **Recognize typical behaviour and function of the reproductive system**
- **Understand the basic endocrine control of reproduction**
- **Be aware of the procedures involved in performing a clinical examination of the reproductive tract in males and females to enable detection of normal and abnormal function**
- **Appreciate which abnormalities are common, especially with respect to parturition**
- **Describe the unique physiology of neonatal animals so that care of the dam and neonate can be optimized at normal parturition, after assisted delivery and during the early neonatal period**

Breeding domestic pets

Breeding of domestic pets may occur as a planned event by the experienced breeder or by the novice but enthusiastic owner. Commonly, however, pet animals become pregnant as a result of an unintentional mating. Especially considering the thousands of unwanted pets that are destroyed by humane societies every year, it is the responsibility of the veterinary professional to educate owners of new pets so that they are fully aware of the reproductive physiology and the risks of pregnancy. In the majority of cases neutering of the pet is recommended.

Before breeding from a pet, the owner should give careful consideration to the quality of their animal, the availability of homes for the potential offspring and the potential costs involved, which may include a caesarean operation if the female has parturition difficulties.

Assessment of animals for breeding

Dogs and cats

Breeding should not be undertaken lightly. Potential breeders should take advice from many sources before breeding from any animal. The male and female should be carefully assessed before making the decision to breed. Both potential parents should be:

- Clinically sound (in good general health and wellbeing)
- Of suitable age for reproduction (the female should be skeletally mature, and both the male and the female should be of an age at which their temperamental and conformational qualities can be properly assessed)
- Free from hereditary diseases (all the necessary checks for the particular breed should have been undertaken)
- Of excellent temperament
- Free from infectious disease (in the UK, but not other countries, there are no bacterial venereal pathogens in dogs and therefore routine bacteriological swabbing of the prepuce or vagina is not necessary. In the cat, however, it is important to screen for feline leukaemia virus before embarking upon breeding).

Many animals that are used at stud do not meet these criteria; when this is the case it is the responsibility of the veterinary professional to ensure the owner is aware that their pet falls short of the required characteristics.

A dog breeder must obtain a breeder licence from their local authority if they breed five or more litters per year and/or they are carrying out a business of breeding dogs for sale/commercial gain. Under this licence, breeders must not whelp two litters from the same bitch within a 12-month period. Further details about breeder schemes, health schemes and licensing can be found at www.thekennelclub.org.uk. Breeders must also agree to adhere to a code of ethics set by the Kennel Club if they wish to register puppies.

The Governing Council of the Cat Fancy (GCCF) provides for the registration of cats and the production of certified certificates. In addition, it classifies breeds, licenses shows and publishes rules that control these functions. Whilst the GCCF publishes leaflets of general advice, it issues no specific guidelines regarding hereditary disease.

There are moral and legal responsibilities (under the Sale of Goods Act) for breeders of animals to ensure that the offspring are clinically healthy and have a sound temperament. There are many hereditary defects that should preclude animals from breeding (see Chapter 4). In the case of cryptorchidism, for example, the affected male and both its parents should be considered to be carriers and should not be used for breeding.

Control of hereditary disease in dogs

Three schemes, created in collaboration with the Kennel Club (KC) and the British Veterinary Association (BVA), aim to control the incidence of hereditary diseases in pedigree dogs. These are the BVA/KC Elbow Dysplasia Scheme, the BVA/KC Hip Dysplasia Scheme and the BVA/KC/ISDS (International Sheep Dog Society) Eye Scheme (see Chapter 4). There are also several health schemes that include DNA testing (see Chapter 4). Where they exist, it is strongly recommended that both the potential sire and dam are screened before breeding is undertaken. Other schemes have been adopted by certain breed societies to monitor the level of specific diseases.

Certain breed societies have established codes of conduct that aim to control the number of litters bred per bitch and the age of first mating. The Kennel Club may not register a litter of puppies born to a bitch if she:

- Was under a year old at the date of mating
- Had already reached 8 years of age at the time of whelping
- Has whelped more than six (from January 2012: more than four) litters
- Has previously had two caesarean operations (this will be implemented from 2012, although a reporting system for veterinary surgeons to the Kennel Club will be available in 2011)
- Was not resident in the UK at the time of whelping.

The Kennel Club may lift the second restriction if the bitch has previously successfully whelped at least one other litter of registered puppies and there is veterinary evidence that she is in good health and a suitable candidate to whelp another litter. A written application with supporting veterinary evidence must be submitted prior to the mating.

The Kennel Club may also refuse to register a litter of puppies if they are the result of a mating between father and daughter, mother and son or brother and sister. However, permission may be granted for such matings in exceptional circumstances if the mating was for scientifically proven welfare reasons.

Horses

Breeding soundness examination (BSE) of the mare

Although the full BSE is not required for every mare presented for breeding, clitoral swabbing is recommended for any mare presented for breeding in the UK. Examination of the internal reproductive tract and clitoral swabbing may only be carried out by a veterinary surgeon.

Indications for the BSE include:

- Mare >12 years of age
- Examination prior to undertaking expensive AI/embryo transfer (ET) programme
- In Thoroughbreds, most mares are examined at the beginning of the season and at various stages during ovulation and pregnancy

- Repeat breeder
- History of repeated early embryonic death
- History of problems in foaling
- History of endometritis/metritis
- Pre-purchase examination of a breeding mare.

The breeding soundness examination

1. History

- Age: fertility starts to decline at around 12 years of age.
- Number of foals, live or dead, dystocia, retained fetal membranes, etc.
- Breeding history with note of previous fertility or infertility, twins, endometritis.
- Sexual behaviour. Does the mare cycle normally and show oestrous behaviour?

2. General physical examination

The body condition and history of recent previous illness must be investigated. Laboratory tests may be indicated.

3. Examination of external genitalia

It is important to assess vulval/perineal conformation. This can be done by placing a finger horizontally on the posterior tip of the bony pelvic brim adjacent to the vulval lips. The dorsal vulval commissure is then assessed in relation to the bony pelvic brim and also the angle of the vulval commissure. The conformation will be: good, fair, or poor. Poor conformation will commonly lead to **pneumovagina**, which causes a foamy, frothy exudate in the vaginal cavity that can also lead to endometritis. If indicated (poor conformation/repeat breeder with fair conformation) then a **Caslick's vulvoplasty** may be required.

4. Clitoral swab for bacterial culture

It is important to test all breeding mares for contagious equine metritis (CEM) and other venereal pathogens. The clitoral sinuses and fossa can harbour the causative agents. The UK has a code of practice for CEM and other bacterial venereal diseases, which veterinary surgeons should follow when dealing with broodmares. **There is a statutory requirement to report any case of CEM to the appropriate authorities (Defra in England and Wales), as CEM is a notifiable disease.**

5. Examination of the internal reproductive tract

This is essential if AI is to be performed, to detect any pathology and confirm normality

- Manual palpation:
  - It is important that the mare is properly restrained
  - The nature of the cervix and uterine tone should be assessed (see Identification of oestrus, below)
  - Location and careful palpation of ovaries
- Transrectal ultrasonography:
  - Visualization of ovarian structures (size, corpora lutea, follicles, neoplasms, etc.)
  - Visualization of uterine horn diameter, free fluid, oedema/folds, cysts, etc.
  - The entire uterus should be evaluated. Unexpected pregnancies do occur! continues ▶

continued

6. Uterine swab for bacterial culture

It is important that the perineum of the mare is first washed and dried. A sterile double-guarded swab should then be passed directly into the uterine lumen. Sampling should be performed prior to any other invasive uterine procedure in order to minimize contamination. Samples for culture are best taken in early oestrus, when the cervix is relaxing, but they can be taken at any time. In general, pure heavy growths of organisms are more likely to be significant than light mixed growths, which are likely to be contaminants. The interpretation of culture results is best carried out in conjunction with the cytology and/or ultrasonography findings.

7. Uterine cytology

Samples may be collected in three ways:

- By uterine flush: 60 ml of sterile isotonic saline is flushed into the uterus and then aspirated. The aspirate is then centrifuged and placed on to a slide
- With a double-guarded swab, which is then 'rolled' on to a slide. It is also possible to use a swab sample for bacterial culture of the endometrium if the slide is sterile
- Using a gloved finger gently inserted through the cervix to collect a sample of endometrial cells, which is then smeared on to a slide.

The collected smears are stained using a rapid stain such as Diff-Quik and are examined for the presence of endometrial epithelial cells and neutrophils.

8. Vaginal examination

A vaginal speculum is used to visualize the vaginal mucosa and cervix. It is used to evaluate the presence or absence of pathology and to assess the stage of the oestrous cycle. Findings may include:

- Urine pooling
- Uterine or vaginal discharge
- Vaginal adhesions
- Persistent hymen
- Cervical trauma/adhesions.

Ancillary procedures

- **Endometrial biopsy:** Useful for diagnosis of endometrial pathology and for prognosis of future fertility, especially in aged mares or those with a history of pregnancy loss or chronic endometritis. Not carried out on every mare. A single sample taken from the base of one uterine horn is generally considered to be representative of the entire uterus. Collected tissue is fixed and examined for endometritis, periglandular fibrosis and cystic glandular distension. Classification, based on the severity of any changes, is associated with the expected ability of the mare to conceive and carry a foal to term:

  - Category I: 80–90%.
  - Category IIA: 50–79%.
  - Category IIB: 30–49%.
  - Category III: 10%.

- **Hysteroscopy (endoscopic examination of uterus):** Enables visualization of endometrial cysts and intra-luminal adhesions.
- **Endocrine assays:** Progesterone assays can be used to determine the presence or absence of luteal tissue. Testosterone, oestrone sulphate and inhibin assays are useful in the diagnosis of ovarian tumour, pregnancy (see below) and fetal viability.
- **Karyotyping:** Performed on animals suspected of having a chromosomal abnormality. Candidates are mares that have never cycled or that have 'infantile' reproductive tracts.

Breed societies and control of hereditary disease

There are many different breeds of horse and many are registered with their own breed society. Some breed societies have rules regarding the breeding of horses but others do not. For example, a Thoroughbred foal cannot be registered by Weatherby's, who hold the National Stud Book, unless it was conceived by a witnessed natural mating. Similarly, the Highland Pony breed society, while allowing artificial insemination (AI), may limit the number of mares a stallion inseminates using AI in any given breeding season.

The Thoroughbred Breeders Association insists that all registered Thoroughbred horses have a birth date of January 1st regardless of their actual date of birth. A foal born on December 31st will be considered to be 1 year old the very next day, i.e. on January 1st. To avoid this undesirable situation, in the UK a breeding season is imposed on Thoroughbreds that differs from the mare's physiological breeding season. The imposed breeding season starts on February 14th. Breeding after this date will ensure that all foals are born after January 1st the following year (gestation length approximately 342 days). This imposed birth date has another impact in that, as equids are seasonal breeders and breed only in spring and summer, only 30% of mares will be cycling by February 14th.

Some breed societies try to control unwanted traits in their breed of horse, e.g. stallions may be examined for unwanted traits such as 'parrot-mouth' (undershot jaw). Some breed societies have a 'grading' programme for osteochondrosis, which is considered to have a hereditary component, in an attempt to prevent affected animals from breeding. This requires the horse to be examined by a nominated veterinary surgeon and awarded a score. Only stallions that meet a certain grade may be registered with that breed society and have their offspring registered. Other breed societies have poor and unrealistic controls for hereditary disease, e.g. a veterinary surgeon or official is asked to state whether the stallion will ever develop arthritis. This is of course impossible.

No licence is required to breed horses.

Exotic pets

There are several organizations offering advice to those breeding and showing exotic pets, including the British Rabbit Council, British Cavy Council and British Bird Council. Such organizations promote breed standards and offer advice on breeding; however, there is little guidance relating to hereditary disease.

Male reproductive biology

The anatomy of the male reproductive tract is considered in Chapter 3.

Male dogs and tomcats

Male dogs and tomcats are sexually active throughout the year, although a minor seasonal effect may be noted in some countries. In the cat, the testes are descended into the scrotum at birth; in the dog, they descend into the scrotum by 10 days after birth. Puppies and kittens may show sexual activity from several weeks of age, but puberty does not occur until 6–12 months in the dog and 8–12 months in the cat. For both species, **spermatogenesis** (the production of spermatozoa) commences at approximately 5 months of age.

It is preferable not to use a male at stud until he is at least 12 months of age, as it is not possible to evaluate his qualities fully until this time; even then the occurrence of certain hereditary diseases may not be apparent. It is advisable that the first mating attempts should be with an experienced female.

The fertile lifespan of a male varies considerably and is probably related to the longevity of the breed. It is certain that average seminal quality of male stud dogs is reduced from 7 years of age onwards.

In many cases, behaviour that may be normal for a male animal is considered to be antisocial by humans. These 'problems' include territory marking, mounting inappropriate objects and aggression towards other males. They often necessitate treatment, which may include behavioural modification therapy in conjunction with drugs that inhibit male hormone production, such as progestogens. Castration may be required in certain cases.

Endocrinology

The production of hormones from the testes is under the control of the hypothalamic–pituitary–gonadal axis. The interstitial (Leydig) cells are the source of testosterone production from the testes. Luteinizing hormone (LH), a gonadotrophic hormone released from the pituitary gland, stimulates the production of testosterone. A second pituitary gonadotrophin called follicle stimulating hormone (FSH) appears to increase the process of spermatogenesis directly via the Sertoli cells. Testosterone has a negative feedback effect upon the release of FSH and LH, which is mediated by gonadotrophin-releasing hormone (GnRH) (Figure 26.1).

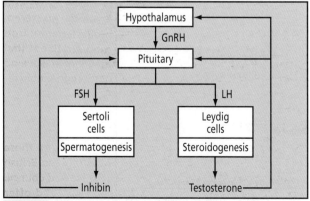

26.1 Schematic representation of the endocrine control of testicular function in the male.

Stallions

Despite horses being seasonal breeders, stallions are able to produce usable semen throughout the year. Some components of the semen will differ depending on time of year, but it remains basically the same.

Endocrinology

The endocrinology of reproduction in the stallion is very similar to that in other male animals. As equids are seasonal breeders, the reproductive hormones increase during the period from April to September. Because of this increase in hormones, the stallion's testes become larger. This increase in size improves semen quality and quantity, as daily sperm output is very closely correlated to testicular volume.

Female reproductive biology

The anatomy of the female reproductive tract is considered in Chapter 3.

The domestic bitch

The oestrous cycle

In the bitch, the onset of cyclical activity (puberty) is normally between 6 and 23 months of age, with most bitches having their first oestrus by the age of 12–14 months. Bitches that do not exhibit oestrous behaviour by the anticipated age are considered to have delayed puberty, but it should be remembered that many normal bitches will not cycle until they are 2 years old. The majority of bitches start to cycle about 6 months after they have reached adult height and weight, which may explain some of the variations exhibited between breeds.

Bitches generally have one or two oestrous cycles per year. Each oestrus ends with spontaneous ovulation, which is followed by the luteal phase. A variable period of acyclicity (called anoestrus) follows the luteal phase.

The bitch is **polytocous** (produces numerous offspring in each litter) and the oestrous periods are non-seasonal. The interval between each cycle can vary between 5 and 13 months but the average is 7 months.

The end of each oestrous cycle is signified by the presence of the '**season**', the onset of which is signalled by the presence of a bloody vulval discharge. During this time ovulation normally occurs, followed by the luteal phase or metoestrus (dioestrus). Each 'season' will normally last an average of 3 weeks in the domestic bitch, but they can be shorter or can extend to 4 weeks or more in some cases. The season length can be variable between bitches and can vary from season to season. The bitch is said to be '**out of season**' once the vulval discharge has stopped.

The stages of the oestrous cycle in the bitch are pro-oestrus, oestrus, metoestrus (dioestrus) and anoestrus (Figure 26.2). The terms '**in season**' or '**in heat**' are both used to indicate the stage of the cycle when the bitch is receptive to the male dog, i.e. oestrus.

Late anoestrus

During late anoestrus two hormones are released from the pituitary gland: **follicle stimulating hormone (FSH)** and

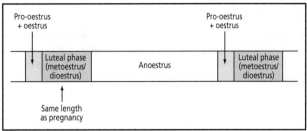

26.2 Sequence and length of various stages of the oestrous cycle of the bitch.

luteinizing hormone (LH). These initiate the growth of follicles within the ovaries and cause the follicles to produce the hormone oestrogen.

Pro-oestrus

During pro-oestrus the bitch will not allow mating but may show increased receptivity to the male. Pro-oestrus is characterized by increased plasma concentrations of **oestrogen**, causing swelling of the vulva and the development of a serosangineous (bloody) vulval discharge. Oestrogens also induce the release of specific pheromones, which are responsible for attracting male dogs. This period lasts for approximately 7 days. Oestrogens also cause thickening of the vaginal wall and an increase in the number of epithelial cell layers. During pro-oestrus the elevated concentrations of oestrogen have a negative feedback effect upon the release of the gonadotrophin hormones from the pituitary gland, and the concentrations of FSH and LH are reduced compared with late anoestrus.

Oestrus

During oestrus the bitch demonstrates characteristic behaviour towards the male dog, including deviation of the tail and presentation of the vulva and perineum. The bitch will stand to be mated (**standing oestrus**). The oestrous period lasts for approximately 7 days. The onset of oestrus is related to a decline in the concentration of plasma oestrogen and at the same time the production of the hormone **progesterone**. The bitch is unusual in that progesterone is produced in low concentrations by luteinization of the follicle, a process that occurs before ovulation. (In many species progesterone is only produced after ovulation.) It is this decline in the concentration of oestrogen and the slight increase in the concentration of progesterone that is responsible for stimulating a surge in both FSH and LH. This surge is the trigger for the release of eggs from the ovaries (**ovulation**), which occurs

spontaneously approximately 2 days later, towards the end of oestrus. The bitch is said to be a **spontaneous ovulator**. It can therefore be seen that the hormonal stimulus for ovulation occurs during standing oestrus and that the release of eggs also occurs during this period. Each egg is contained within a fluid-filled structure called a **follicle**. After ovulation, the follicle develops into a solid structure called a **corpus luteum**. One corpus luteum forms from each follicle that has ovulated and the corpus luteum produces progesterone. The end of standing oestrus is associated with relatively high concentrations of progesterone in the blood.

The average length of the oestrous cycle is 7 months, roughly divided into pro-oestrus (10 days), oestrus (10 days), luteal phase (pregnancy or non-pregnancy) (2 months) and anoestrus (4.5 months). For individual bitches, cyclicity may range from highly variable to almost regular.

Metoestrus (also called dioestrus)

In many species the phase of progesterone production (the **luteal phase**) is divided into two phases: the early luteal phase (termed **metoestrus**); and the mature luteal phase (termed **dioestrus**). In the bitch, however, the early luteal phase occurs during standing oestrus, making this terminology difficult to adopt (since metoestrus would then be occurring during oestrus). In the bitch, the terms metoestrus and dioestrus are therefore often used synonymously to reflect the luteal phase of the cycle after the end of standing oestrus. This phase is characterized by the presence of the corpora lutea upon the ovaries and the presence of the hormone progesterone in the blood.

The period of metoestrus lasts whilst the corpora lutea continue to produce progesterone and it is approximately 55 days in length. In the pregnant bitch, the period of metoestrus is synonymous with **pregnancy**. The bitch is unusual when compared with females of other species, in that the duration of metoestrus is similar whether she is pregnant or not (Figure 26.3). The birth of puppies occurs when progesterone secretion is terminated. In the non-pregnant bitch the corpora lutea persist for a similar period of time.

Towards the end of metoestrus another hormone, called prolactin, is released from the pituitary gland. This is responsible for the development of mammary tissue and the onset of lactation. Prolactin is produced in both the pregnant and the non-pregnant bitch, and is the reason why false or **pseudopregnancy** is a common event in the bitch (see later).

The hormonal changes of the oestrous cycle of the pregnant bitch are summarized in Figure 26.4.

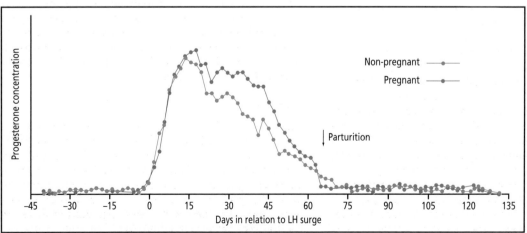

26.3 Changes in plasma progesterone concentration in the pregnant and non-pregnant bitch.

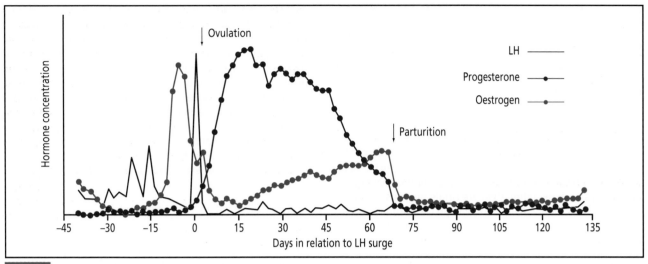

| | 26.4 | Changes in plasma hormones during the oestrous cycle of the pregnant bitch. |

Anoestrus

Metoestrus is followed by a period of quiescence, during which time there is effectively no hormonal activity. In the non-pregnant bitch there is no sudden decline in the concentration of progesterone but values gradually reduce and the transition to anoestrus is smooth. The situation is slightly different during pregnancy because progesterone concentrations rapidly decline, and it is this event that stimulates the onset of parturition. The length of anoestrus varies considerably between bitches, but on average it is 5 months.

The domestic queen

The oestrous cycle

Female cats generally exhibit their first oestrus at 6–9 months of age, but this is dependent upon photoperiod. Those that are born in the summer frequently commence cycling at the first spring; those that are born in the winter may not cycle until they are at least 12 months of age.

Queens have multiple oestrous cycles each year. They typically cycle from February to September and are seasonally polyoestrous. Ovulation is not spontaneous as for the bitch, but is induced by coitus. Queens are said to be **induced ovulators.** The interval between each oestrous cycle varies depending upon whether the queen has ovulated, or fails to ovulate either because she is not mated or because there is insufficient hormone release at mating. Unmated queens return to oestrus at intervals of 14–21 days. Queens that ovulate but do not become pregnant generally return to oestrus after approximately 45 days.

The stages of the oestrous cycle in the queen are anoestrus, pro-oestrus, oestrus and interoestrus (Figure 26.5). The terms 'in season' or 'in heat' are used to indicate the stage of the cycle when the queen is receptive to the male, i.e. oestrus. During winter there is essentially no hormone activity; the queen is in anoestrus. In springtime, cyclical activity commences and, in the unmated queen, periods of sexual activity (pro-oestrus and oestrus) are interrupted by periods of non-receptivity (interoestrus). If the queen is mated and ovulation is induced, she enters metoestrus or pregnancy.

Pregnancy follows a fertile mating; metoestrus (also called pseudopregnancy) follows a sterile mating. The duration of

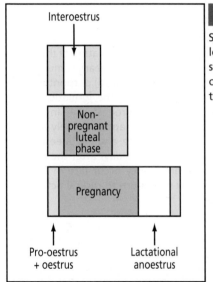

| | 26.5 |

Sequence and length of various stages of the oestrous cycle of the queen.

pseudopregnancy in the queen is shorter than that of pregnancy, unlike the situation in the bitch.

Pro-oestrus

Follicular development occurs during this phase due to the release of LH and FSH. This causes the secretion of oestrogen that is responsible for the development of the signs of pro-oestrus, including attraction of the male and the changes in the vaginal epithelium similar to those seen in the bitch. Pro-oestrus in the queen is often poorly recognized unless a male is present, but during this stage the queen will not accept mating. Pro-oestrus lasts for 2–3 days.

Oestrus

The exact hormonal changes that cause the onset of standing oestrus are uncertain, but may be associated with increasing concentrations of oestrogen. The clinical signs of oestrus (also termed **calling**) include persistent vocalization, and rolling and rubbing against inanimate objects. In the presence of the male, the queen may show persistent treading of the hind feet, lateral deviation of the tail and lordosis of the spine. Oestrus lasts between 2 and 10 days.

Interoestrus

In the absence of mating, or when mating does not result in ovulation, the signs of oestrus gradually decline and the queen enters a stage of non-receptivity. This period may last for between 3 and 14 days. After this time the queen returns to pro-oestrus and oestrus.

Pregnancy

Ovulation in the queen is caused by the release of LH, which is stimulated by mating. Each mating results in a surge of LH, but there appears to be a threshold value below which ovulation will not be induced. Multiple matings are therefore more likely to result in ovulation than are single matings.

Ovulation is followed by an increase in the plasma concentration of progesterone released from the newly formed corpora lutea. Peak progesterone concentrations are reached approximately 1 month after mating and are maintained for the duration of the pregnancy, which varies between 64 and 68 days. It is not uncommon for queens to have an absence of cyclical activity during lactation. This has been called **lactational anoestrus**.

Metoestrus (pseudopregnancy)

Non-fertile matings result in ovulation without conception. Ovulation may also occur following stimulation of the vagina (e.g. following collection of a vaginal smear), stimulation of the perineum (which may be self-induced) or spontaneously in some queens. Ovulation results in the formation of corpora lutea and the production of progesterone in a similar manner to early pregnancy. After approximately 40 days, progesterone concentrations decline, and the queen returns to cyclical activity approximately 45 days after the previous oestrus. Should pseudopregnancy occur late in the year (autumn), the queen may not return to cyclical activity but may enter anoestrus.

The mare
The oestrous cycle

Mares are seasonally polyoestrous, meaning that they have multiple cycles (every 21 days) during a 'breeding season', which in the northern hemisphere starts around March/April and finishes around September/October. Mares are 'long day' breeders, although about 15–20% of mares continue to ovulate throughout the winter months. In the UK, it is mainly 'native' ponies and horses that make up the small percentage of equids that cycle all year round. Photoperiod is the most important factor influencing this seasonality but the process is gradual rather than being an 'all or nothing' situation. Mares seem to respond best to a photoperiod of around 16 hours.

During the winter months the mare is said to be **anoestrous**. No follicles develop on her ovaries and she does not ovulate. She is therefore unable to conceive. As the days become longer her ovaries start to function again. Before the mare enters her breeding season she goes through a period called the **transitional period**. The transitional period describes the period of resurgence of **hypothalamic–pituitary–ovarian function** as the mare approaches her first ovulation of the year. It is characterized by:

- Multiple follicles on both ovaries, which grow and regress
- Irregular response to teasing, often with prolonged periods of 'behavioural oestrus'
- Failure to ovulate.

Increasing GnRH produces increases in LH and FSH. FSH reaches high levels early in the transitional period. FSH causes follicular development. However, a threshold of FSH and LH is required for ovulation to occur. Immature follicles on the ovaries produce oestrogen but regress without ovulating. The production of oestrogen causes the mare to show oestrous ('heat') behaviour. Once ovulation has occurred the mare will continue to ovulate regularly for the remainder of the breeding season.

The importance of the spring transition lies in the fact that, although the mare may be showing signs of 'heat', she is NOT ovulating. She cannot therefore be successfully bred.

Summary of the equine oestrous cycle

- **Oestrous cycle** – average length 21–22 days.
- **Oestrus** – average length 5–7 days. Ovulation occurs approximately 24 hours before the end of oestrus. The mare's cervix becomes pink, moist, flaccid and open. The uterus also becomes relaxed.
- **Dioestrus** – average length 14–15 days. The mare's cervix becomes dry, pale and firm. The uterus becomes firm.

Diseases of the male reproductive tract and assessment of fertility

Dogs and cats

There are a variety of conditions that may affect the reproductive organs of the tomcat or male dog.

Endocrinological abnormalities

Primary abnormalities in the secretion of pituitary hormones may result in poor development of gonadal tissue, a condition called **hypogonadism**. This is rare but has been reported in both species.

Diseases of the testes
Cryptorchidism

An absence of the testes (**anorchia**) is very rare; in most cases the testes are retained within the abdomen. These undescended testes belong to the condition known as **cryptorchidism** (literally, 'hidden testicle'). Often the condition is unilateral, with one testicle present within the scrotum and the other retained within the abdomen. These cases are often wrongly called monorchids; **monorchidism** actually refers to an animal with a single testicle. Some cryptorchid animals are bilaterally affected and no testes are seen within the scrotum. The treatment for all cryptorchids is removal of both testes, because of the high incidence of neoplasia within the abdominal testicle, and the fact that the condition is likely to be inherited.

Orchitis

This is inflammation of the testes; it is rare but may follow trauma (particularly in the tomcat) or ascending bacterial infection. In some countries (but not the UK) orchitis may be caused by the bacterium *Brucella canis*, which is a venereal pathogen transmitted at coitus.

Testicular tumours

Testicular tumours are the second most common tumour affecting the male dog but are rare in the tomcat. There are three common tumour types: those affecting the Leydig cells (Leydig cell tumour); those affecting the Sertoli cells (Sertoli cell tumour); and those affecting the germ cells (**seminoma**). Some of these tumours may be endocrinologically active and secrete female hormones (oestrogens), which produce signs of feminization.

Diseases of the accessory glands

The prostate gland in the male dog is the only accessory sex gland. The tomcat has both prostate and bulbourethral glands, but disease of either is rare. Prostate abnormalities in the dog are common and include benign enlargement (hyperplasia), bacterial prostatitis, prostatic cysts and prostatic tumours. The clinical signs of these diseases may be similar and include difficulty urinating and defecating and the presence of blood within urine or semen.

Diseases of the penis and prepuce

It is common for there to be a creamy discharge from the prepuce of the male dog and this should be considered normal unless it is excessive. It is not seen in the tomcat.

Phimosis

Phimosis is a condition where there is inability to extrude the penis, due to an abnormally small preputial orifice. This may occur either congenitally or as a result of trauma or inflammation, and may result in pain during erection. **Paraphimosis** is a failure to retract the penis into the prepuce and may also be due to a small preputial orifice. The penis becomes dry and necrotic and urethral obstruction may result. **Priapism** refers to the persistent enlargement of the penis in the absence of sexual excitement.

Lymphoid hyperplasia

This is a relatively common condition in the male dog, where the bulbus glandis is covered with multiple nodules 2–3 mm in diameter. These are usually smooth and do not cause any significant disease, but they may be traumatized at the time of mating or semen collection.

Assessment of fertility

Male fertility may be assessed by the evaluation of semen quality. Semen may be collected by stimulating the male dog to ejaculate by hand (artificial vaginas are no longer used for this purpose). Semen collection is more difficult in the tomcat and may require general anaesthesia and electroejaculation. A special artificial vagina may be used to collect from trained tomcats. Collection equipment should be warmed before use.

Once collected, semen should be placed into a water bath at body temperature to prevent damage to the sperm. The second fraction of the dog ejaculate (Figure 26.6) and the entire cat ejaculate should be used for evaluation.

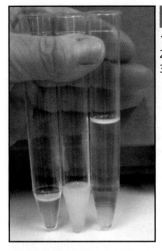

26.6 Dog ejaculate (from left to right): 1st fraction, prostatic fluid; 2nd fraction, semen-rich; 3rd fraction, prostatic fluid.

Examination of canine ejaculate

1. The volume should be measured and the colour recorded. Normal semen volume is up to 2.0 ml for the dog and 0.1–0.5 ml in the tomcat. Normal semen is white and milky.
2. After gently mixing the sample, a drop should be placed upon a warmed microscope slide and a subjective assessment made of the percentage of sperm with vigorous forward progression.
3. A small portion of the sample should be diluted with water to kill the sperm and therefore stop their movement. The spermatozoal concentration can then be measured using a haemocytometer counting chamber. The total sperm output should be calculated by multiplying this value by the volume of the sample.
4. A portion of the sample should be stained to allow the differentiation of live and dead sperm and the assessment of spermatozoal morphology. A combination of the stains nigrosin and eosin is suitable for this purpose. Normally, four parts of stain are mixed with one part semen, and a smear is then immediately made on a glass microscope slide. When examined under high magnification, nigrosin appears as a background stain. The eosin is a vital stain – it stains only sperm with a damaged membrane, i.e. dead sperm (Figure 26.7). When using nigrosin and eosin, sperm are either stained pink (these are termed dead) or are unstained (these are termed live).

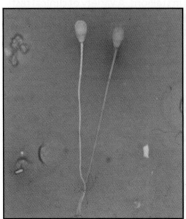

26.7 Photomicrograph of dog sperm: (left) live, and (right) dead sperm with clamped acrosome.

The semen characteristics of fertile dogs are given in Figure 26.8.

	Normal progressive motility (%)	Volume (ml)	Concentration (x 10⁶/ml)	Total sperm output (x 10⁶)
Mean	85.2	1.3	310.5	403.4
S.D.	6.2	0.4	82	120
Range	42–92	0.4–3.4	50–560	36–620

26.8 Characteristics of the second fraction of the ejaculate from 53 fertile dogs.

The stallion

Diseases of the scrotum

Any inflammation or swelling of the scrotum increases the temperature and adversely affects spermatogenesis. After the lesion resolves, it takes approximately 2 months for the animal to produce normal ejaculates.

Acute trauma

Intrascrotal haemorrhage can lead to permanent testicular damage due to the insulating properties of the resultant fibrous tissue. Surgical removal of the organized blood clot or hemicastration (removal of affected testicle) can be performed in an attempt to save the unaffected testis. Stallions that have had one testicle removed may still be able to have a productive breeding career. The remaining testicle will undergo hypertrophy to produce more spermatozoa, but this will never be as much as a stallion with two testicles.

Hydrocele

A hydrocele is an abnormal collection of fluid between visceral and parietal tunics and affects fertility by increasing testicular temperature. The condition is not usually painful. If unilateral and persistent, the affected testis and tunics are removed to save the contralateral testis from heat-induced degeneration.

Diseases of the testes

Cryptorchidism

Cryptorchidism presents in a similar way as for other species. The condition may be inherited but this has not been proven. The animal may be presented as castrated, which is of concern as stallion behaviour can be dangerous; this is the main reason cryptorchidism is treated in stallions. A variety of clinical tests, including hormonal assays, are performed to ascertain whether there is active testicular tissue in the horse.

Some abdominal testicles become neoplastic, and others do not descend because they are teratomatous.

Trauma

Testicular haematoma is rare, usually following a major injury such as a kick. Extensive scar tissue formation can lead to complete loss of testicular function. The condition is usually acute and very painful. Ultrasonography can reveal the extent of the damage. If haemorrhage is contained within tunica albuginea, adhesions may not occur. If testicular damage is severe, hemicastration may be required.

Torsion

A stallion's testicles are quite movable and some slight rotation of the testes is commonplace. Rotation >270 degrees is usually required to produce torsion and stop blood flow. The affected testicle can be saved only if the condition is identified and surgically corrected promptly. Otherwise hemicastration will be required if the other testicle is to remain functional.

Orchitis

Primary orchitis (inflammation of the testis) is rare. The affected testis is hot, swollen, tense and acutely painful. The stallion may also have a fever and scrotal oedema and may walk with a stiffened hindlimb gait. If left untreated, testicular degeneration and permanent infertility can develop.

Tumours

Stallions rarely suffer from testicular tumours but when they do occur the tumour types are very similar to those seen in other species.

Small testes

- **Congenital hypoplasia** is relatively common in stallions, affecting approximately 3%. It is possibly hereditary and so the affected stallions should not be selected for a breeding programme.
- **Testicular degeneration** is a major cause of subfertility/infertility and can be a sequel to many of the conditions described above. Testicular degeneration is an acquired condition, caused by chronic inflammation of 2–6 weeks' duration.

History is important for differentiating between these two conditions. Unlike testicular hypoplasia, mild cases of degeneration may be reversible, but it may take several months for semen to return to normal. Treatment with GnRH has been tried but remains controversial. As it takes approximately 60 days from the development of spermatogonia to sperm ejaculation, it is possible for acute testicular degeneration to be present and yet for the ejaculate to be fairly satisfactory. It may take 2–6 weeks for the infertility to become apparent.

Diseases of the epididymis

- **Large epididymis:** Epididymitis is very rare in the stallion and is usually associated with orchitis. Chronic epididymitis leads to obstruction of the epididymis and so produces an aspermic ejaculate. This blockage leads to pressure degeneration in the testes.
- **Sperm granuloma:** Spermatozoa in the seminiferous tubules are kept separate from blood vessels because they are not recognized as 'self'. When they do cross into the local blood vessels following trauma, specific anti-sperm antibodies are produced. This produces inflammation and a sperm granuloma is created.

Diseases of the accessory sex glands

Problems with the accessory sex glands are very rare in stallions. They can be a reservoir for viruses such as equine viral arteritis (EVA).

Diseases of the penis and prepuce

Deviation of the penis

This may be congenital, associated with a persistent frenulum (penis and prepuce normally separate at puberty) or acquired after traumatic injury, with scar tissue formation on the ventral aspect of the penis. Sometimes surgery can correct deviation. Without correction, natural mating can be problematic.

Phimosis

As in other species, **phimosis** is caused by a constriction of the preputial orifice, which may be congenital or acquired. It prevents the penis extruding. The passing of urine may also be a problem when voided directly into the prepuce. **Paraphimosis** often follows acute preputial trauma or the use of phenothiazine tranquillizers (acetylpromazine, ACP). The condition is also sometimes seen in stallions/geldings suffering from chronic grass sickness.

Haematoma of the penis

This often follows a kick from a mare at breeding and is a serious problem if it involves a rupture of the tunica albuginea. If only the superficial vessels of the penis are affected and the tunica albuginea is intact then the prognosis is good. Ultrasonography can help show the extent of the damage.

Infection (balanoposthitis)

(Balanitis = inflammation of the glans penis; posthitis = inflammation of the prepuce.) The preputial cavity contains a wide variety of microorganisms. Trauma can allow introduction of bacteria into deeper tissues, which can lead to local infection. This results in swelling, inflammation, pain and preputial discharge. Stallions can develop an iatrogenic balanoposthitis if they are over-washed with medicated soaps. The natural flora can be upset and an overgrowth of a single bacterium can ensue, sometimes causing pain and swelling. The treatment may involve the inoculation of 'normal' bacteria taken from another stallion that has tested negative for sexually transmitted disease. One primary cause of balanoposthitis is **equine coital exanthema (equine herpesvirus-3, EHV-3).** This virus causes blister lesions on the penis that cause pain and inflammation. The virus is sexually transmitted but has no effect on fertility. It does not cause abortion or affect semen quality. The condition is self-limiting and complete resolution occurs in 3–5 weeks.

Inapparent venereal pathogens are another important source of infection. There are three bacteria that can reside on the stallion's penis and, while they do not cause balanoposthitis, they can cause serious uterine disease in mares and so seriously affect fertility. The three bacteria are:

- *Taylorella equigenitalis* – This bacterium is not native to the UK, which means it is a statutory requirement to report it to Defra when isolated from a swab taken from a stallion's penis. It causes contagious equine metritis (CEM), a notifiable disease; the bacterium is also known as the contagious equine metritis organism (CEMO)
- *Pseudomonas aeruginosa.* See the mare section below for more information
- *Klebsiella pneumoniae* (capsule types 1, 2 and 5). See the mare section below for more information.

Penile neoplasia

This is quite common and can be difficult to treat. Removal of the penis is possible, but obviously adversely affects the breeding capability of the stallion. Three of the most common forms of penile neoplasia are described below.

- **Fibropapilloma:** Rare and usually regress spontaneously in 1–6 months. Because of this, treatment is rarely undertaken.
- **Squamous cell carcinoma:** Not uncommon in stallions. Penile sebaceous material is thought to predispose to the development of precancerous lesions. In non-breeding stallions the penis may be rarely seen, so this condition may go undiagnosed until quite severe and extensive. If localized to a small area in the glans, local removal with cryosurgery or by using a surgical laser can allow the horse to return to stallion duties. However, the condition is often not detected until later and a partial amputation is necessary.
- **Sarcoids:** These are the most common tumours found on equids; they are almost always benign, and frequently occur on preputial skin. They can also ulcerate and need to be differentiated from a squamous cell carcinoma. Sarcoids can be removed in a variety of ways but recurrence is likely.

Loss of libido

Loss of libido can be a serious problem. The causes are largely genetic, although environmental influences can also play an important role:

- Nutrition – if the horse is too thin or too fat
- Systemic disease
- Age
- Management:
  - Harsh handling
  - Poor restraint of the mare
  - Improper footing, causing the stallion to slip or become unbalanced on his hindlimbs
  - Pain when mounting the mare
  - Overuse
- Psychological factors – can result from a previous painful experience, overuse or excessive discipline
- Musculoskeletal – especially if it involves the hindquarters, e.g. lameness
- Hormonal:
  - Impotent stallions tend to have lower blood concentrations of LH and oestradiol, whereas concentrations of testosterone are normal
  - Administration of low levels of testosterone appears to increase the sexual interest of 'slow starter' stallions within 10 days. Novice stallions generally do not need further treatment after the first ejaculation, although the treatment may adversely affect semen quality.

Ejaculatory dysfunction

Ejaculatory dysfunction can be caused by psychological factors (see above) or by physical problems such as nerve damage or blocked ampullae.

Assessment of fertility

Fertility can only be truly proven by the production of offspring, but it is possible to examine a stallion to try and identify any conditions that may affect it. The stallion can be checked for sexually transmitted diseases (STDs) and for any unwanted heritable conditions.

The evaluation procedure is very similar to that in the dog, with only a few differences. All stallions must be screened for pathogens, namely CEMO (see above), *Klebsiella pneumoniae* (capsule types 1, 2 and 5) and *Pseudomonas aeruginosa*. A blood sample may also be taken for serological testing for equine viral arteritis. The libido is assessed using a mare in oestrus: the stallion should obtain and maintain an erection within 5 minutes of the mare being present.

A semen sample is taken using an artificial vagina. This is a latex tube kept warm by filling the outside of the tube with warm water. After collection the semen is filtered to remove the gel fraction of the ejaculate. The volume is then measured. A healthy stallion will produce between 40 and 100 ml of filtered semen. If <30ml is obtained, this does not count as a full ejaculate.

The semen's motility is quickly assessed in two ways:

- The percentage of spermatozoa that are moving (total motility)
- The percentage of spermatozoa that are moving progressively, i.e. in a straight line (progressive motility).

Normal stallion sperm should have a progressive motility of 60%. This figure is effectively the live:dead ratio. The sperm are then counted, either by using a slide called an 'improved Neubauer' or by using a densimeter, which uses light adsorption. A healthy stallion will generally have a concentration of around 175–200 million sperm per ml of semen.

The pH of the semen can be checked and should be 7.4. Any change may indicate infection or contamination with urine. Sperm morphology is evaluated using a killed sample of the semen. This is a very important component of the breeding soundness because sperm morphology is closely related to fertility. At least 100 sperm cells (ideally 200) should be assessed for normal morphology. The morphological defects assessed are similar to those for other species. Finally, a sperm longevity test is performed by leaving the sample at room temperature. There should be at least 10% progressive motility after 6 hours.

Diseases of the female reproductive tract

The domestic bitch

Endocrinological abnormalities

The common endocrinological abnormalities of the bitch include:

- **Delayed onset of puberty** – cyclical activity is not present at 24 months of age
- **Prolonged anoestrus** – failure to return to cyclical activity, resulting in a prolonged interoestrus interval
- **Silent oestrous cycles** – normal cyclical activity, including ovulation, but without the external signs of oestrus
- **Split oestrus** – signs of pro-oestrus but this does not terminate in ovulation and is followed 2–12 weeks later by a normal cycle
- **Ovulation failure** – when bitches have apparently normal oestrous periods with an absence of ovulation; these bitches often return to oestrus with shorter than normal intervals.

Pseudopregnancy

One specific endocrinological condition frequently seen in the bitch is pseudopregnancy (false pregnancy, phantom pregnancy or **pseudocyesis**). The signs of the condition may include anorexia, abdominal enlargement, nest making, nursing of inanimate objects, mammary development and lactation. False pregnancy should be considered normal in the bitch, because the changes in plasma hormones are similar in both pregnant and non-pregnant individuals. It has been wrongly thought that pseudopregnancy is produced by either an overproduction of progesterone or abnormal persistence of the corpus luteum. The actual mechanism is related to the decline in plasma progesterone concentration during late metoestrus, which is associated with an increase in plasma concentrations of prolactin.

In many cases, therapy is not required because the signs will gradually decline. Often, removal of the bedding material that the bitch is using to make a nest or removal of the toys she is nursing will be enough to help the bitch to overcome a false pregnancy. In certain cases it may be necessary to use hormonal therapy to reduce the plasma concentrations of prolactin.

Diseases of the ovary

There are few abnormalities of the ovary. An absence of ovarian development (**ovarian agenesis**) may occur; this usually affects one side only and may affect fertility. **Ovarian cysts** are rare and may be associated with signs of persistent oestrus, but most cysts originate from the ovarian bursa and are not endocrinologically active. **Ovarian tumours** are also rare.

Occasionally, bitches with both ovarian and testicular tissue are seen. These animals are termed '**intersex**' and may be recognized because of the appearance of their external genitalia. The vulva may be cranially positioned and an os clitoris may develop. The gonads may be found in a normal ovarian position or within the scrotum. These animals are usually sterile.

Diseases of the uterus

Developmental problems of the uterus include **aplasia** (abnormal development) or **agenesis** (failure of development); in these cases reproductive cyclicity will be normal but the bitch may fail to become pregnant. Intersex animals may have the presence of both uterine tissue and vasa deferentia.

Cystic endometrial hyperplasia and pyometra

The most common uterine disease of the bitch is cystic endometrial hyperplasia (**CEH**), which may develop into pyometra. Hyperplasia of the endometrium occurs in response to progesterone during normal metoestrus. In young animals the hyperplasia resolves at the end of the luteal phase. This is not the case in older bitches and small cystic regions develop within the glandular tissue. The uterus in this state is probably more prone to infection than the normal uterus, and should bacteria enter during oestrus (when the cervix is open) they may proliferate. The accumulation of pus within the uterus (**pyometra**) leads to the bitch becoming unwell.

Clinical signs may include the presence of a malodorous, creamy yellow to blood-stained vulval discharge (pus), lethargy, inappetence, pyrexia, vomiting, polydipsia and polyuria. In some cases the cervix is not open and a vulval discharge is absent; these cases are called **closed pyometra**.

In all cases of pyometra the treatment of choice is ovariohysterectomy following stabilization of the patient using appropriate fluid therapy. Medical treatment (with combinations of prolactin inhibitors and prostaglandins or with progesterone receptor antagonists) has been advocated and success rates can be up to 80% for resolving the acute problem, although in up to 50% of cases pyometra returns after the next oestrus. In most cases the best option is surgery.

Treatment of bitches with progestogens for the prevention or suppression of oestrus, or with oestrogens for the treatment of unwanted matings, may predispose to the development of pyometra.

Diseases of the vagina and vestibule

Congenital abnormalities of the caudal reproductive tract include segmental aplasia and hymenal or vestibular constrictions.

Vaginitis (inflammation of the vagina) is sometimes seen in prepubertal bitches and usually resolves after the first oestrus. Specific infectious causes of vaginitis include *Brucella canis* (not present in the UK) and canine herpesvirus. Many bacteria are found within the vagina as normal commensal organisms (including beta-haemolytic streptococci), which many dog breeders wrongly consider to be venereal pathogens. There is little value in routine bacteriological swabbing of the vagina before breeding, since usually only these commensal bacteria are isolated.

Diseases of the external genitalia

Congenital abnormalities such as vulval atresia and agenesis are rare. Clitoral hypertrophy may occur associated with intersexuality.

The domestic queen
Endocrinological abnormalities

Delayed puberty may be difficult to assess in the queen, since the onset of cyclical activity is related to the season of the year at birth (see above). Delayed puberty and prolonged anoestrus have been seen but they are rare.

The most common abnormality is ovulation failure, which often results from insufficient reflex release of LH at mating. The majority of queens will ovulate if 4–12 matings are allowed in a 4-hour period.

Pseudopregnancy also occurs in the queen. This condition is dissimilar to that seen in the bitch and usually follows a sterile mating (or occasionally spontaneous ovulation). After ovulation there is an increase in plasma progesterone (Figure 26.9), which does not occur in the absence of mating, and no return to oestrus for a further 35–40 days. The major clinical sign is an absence of oestrus; treatment is not required.

Diseases of the ovary

Congenital diseases of the ovary such as ovarian agenesis and ovarian hypoplasia are rare. Ovarian cysts and neoplasms may develop similar to those seen in the bitch but are also rare.

Premature ovarian failure may be seen in queens aged 8 years and above; these animals stop cycling for an unknown reason.

Diseases of the uterus

The range of uterine abnormalities seen in the cat is similar to that seen in the bitch. Pyometra may be less common, because in the absence of mating ovulation does not occur and the luteal phase is therefore absent. Spontaneous ovulations or the common use of progestogens may cause the development of CEH and pyometra.

Diseases of the vagina, vestibule and external genitalia

Congenital abnormalities of the vagina, vestibule and external genitalia are rare but include vaginal and vulval aplasia and defects associated with intersexuality. Vaginitis is uncommon.

The mare
Small ovaries and not cycling

Small ovaries and a lack of cycling may be caused by the following:

- **Mare still in 'winter anoestrus':** The mare has not ovulated during the current breeding season. It may simply be a matter of time until the mare enters the 'transitional period' and then finally ovulates, signifying entry into the ovulatory season for this mare. It is important to check there is a good level of nutrition and good health. Both of these can prevent a mare from cycling

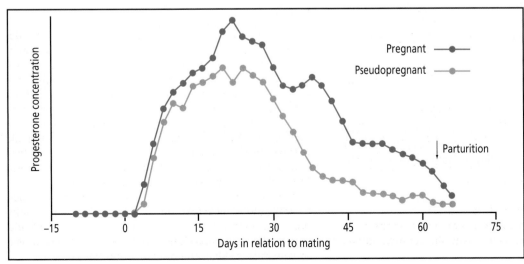

26.9

Progesterone profiles in the pregnant and pseudopregnant queen.

- **Pregnancy:** This is a surprisingly common reason for a mare not to ovulate during the ovulatory season, especially in poorly managed breeding herds. It is essential to rule out pregnancy before any invasive uterine investigations are carried out
- **Hypoplasia – Chromosomal abnormality (63 XO),** *Turner's syndrome:* Diagnosis involves repeated palpations of the reproductive tract, which shows a lack of ovarian activity. Ovaries are small, smooth and firm. Karyotype examination is needed for definitive diagnosis.

Enlarged ovary and not cycling

Cystic ovarian disease does not occur in equids, so an enlarged ovary may be caused by one of the following conditions.

Ovarian neoplasia

The most common tumour is granulosa thecal cell tumour (GTCT). Although uncommon in horses (2.5% of all equine neoplasms) it is relatively common compared to other species and accounts for 87% of equine ovarian tumours. GTCTs are usually, in some way, endocrinologically active. They are normally unilateral, multicystic and are rarely malignant.

Other ovarian tumours include dysgerminoma and cystadenoma.

A GTCT will generally destroy the affected ovary and will very often cause atrophy of the contralateral ovary. Because of this, the mare will cease to have normal ovarian activity and mares with a GTCT will show one of the following types of abnormal sexual behaviour:

- Anoestrus
- Stallion-like behaviour, including aggression, mounting and teasing.

A number of GTCTs are discovered as incidental findings.

Secretion of inhibin by the neoplastic granulosa cells is thought to be partly, if not wholly, responsible for the atrophy of the contralateral ovary. Inhibin has the effect of inhibiting FSH secretion. Diagnosis is usually made on clinical signs, manual palpation, ultrasound examination per rectum and blood hormonal assays. GTCTs have been recorded in mares of all ages (2–20 years), but the highest frequency appears to be between 5 and 9 years. They have even been recorded in pregnant mares. Surgery is the only option available for the treatment of GTCTs in the mare, and removal under laparoscopic control is proving more popular, as this can also be carried out in the standing horse. With the removal of the affected ovary, the mare will return to normal cyclical activity should in about 6–18 months. Fertility will be good.

Ovarian haematoma/haematocyst

These occur following haemorrhage into the follicular cavity or excessive haemorrhage following ovulation. They can persist for many months and can become very large. Some may luteinize, but they generally do not interfere with the normal oestrous cycle.

Anovulatory haemorrhagic follicles

These are most common during the autumn transition and are thought to occur due to an insensitivity or reduction in LH secretion.

Transitional ovary with multiple, non-dominant follicles

These ovaries can become quite large but are always <10 cm in diameter.

Ovarian abscess

These are very rare and usually only occur as a result of surgical follicular aspiration.

Normal sized ovaries and not cycling

The most common cause during the breeding season is prolonged dioestrus. This is a failure of luteal regression at day 14 of the oestrous cycle. It can be quite common, with up to 25% of cycles affected. Prolonged dioestrus can also result from 'dioestrus ovulation' on day 9–14 or early embryonic death at any time from day 20–60. Some mares simply do not show good oestrus behaviour. These mares require a good teaser stallion or more regular examinations to determine the stage of the oestrous cycle.

Diseases of the uterus and vagina

Endometritis

Inflammation of the endometrium (endometritis) is considered to be one of the most common causes of subfertility in the mare. Recent advances have improved our understanding of endometritis. There are four types of endometritis.

Persistent post-mating induced endometritis (PMIE)

The incidence of PMIE after natural mating and frozen semen insemination is 15% and 28%, respectively. If it occurs, subfertility can result if not treated. At the start of the breeding season, a thorough history may help to identify a mare that develops PMIE. Otherwise the diagnosis is made post-service.

Chronic uterine infection

Chronic uterine infection can be introduced by:

- Pneumovagina due to abnormal conformation or injury to vulva or perineal region.
- Parturition
- Copulation
- Veterinary gynaecological procedures.

Not all endometritis is caused by infection. For example, PMIE may simply be an accumulation of sterile fluid. However, if there is microbial involvement the most commonly isolated organisms are:

- Beta-haemolytic streptococci (e.g. *Streptococcus zooepidemicus*)
- *Escherichia coli*
- *Pseudomonas aeruginosa*
- *Klebsiella pneumoniae*
- Fungi, including yeasts.

In the UK, endometritis can rarely be caused by *Taylorella equigenitalis* (CEMO). This disease is notifiable by law.

Chronic degenerative endometritis

Chronic degenerative endometritis (also known as endometrosis) describes the accumulation of scar tissue (fibrosis) within the endometrium. The condition is diagnosed following an endometrial biopsy (see also above). The aetiology of this type of endometritis is not understood. It mainly affects older mares (>12 years of age) but has been seen in younger mares. There is no treatment.

Sexually transmitted diseases

The organisms that are responsible for this type of endometritis are *Taylorella equigenitalis* (CEMO), *Klebsiella pneumoniae* (capsule types 1, 2 and 5) and *Pseudomonas aeruginosa*. Their diagnosis in the mare is described above.

Urovagina

Poor conformation can lead to urine flowing back into the vagina. The urine can irritate and cause inflammation of the cervix and can also flow back into the uterus producing a urometra. Both conditions can seriously affect fertility. The condition can be resolved by carrying out a urethral extension procedure.

Vaginal varicose veins

These are surprisingly common in older mares. The mare will present with a small amount of blood at the vulva that may coincide with her oestrus. On examination, one or more dilated engorged mucosal veins may be seen. These veins can easily rupture, causing bleeding. They do not generally require treatment and often regress during the winter anoestrus. If they are a persistent problem the veins may be ligated. Other treatments such as topical application of formaldehyde can also produce good results.

'Pseudopregnancy'

A small percentage of mares will have what some practitioners describe as pseudopregnancy. It is accepted that true pseudopregnancy does not occur in the mare. Any mare that fails to show signs of oestrus after being in oestrus 18–20 days previously should receive an ultrasound examination to check for pregnancy, as this is the most common reason for mares not to show oestrus during the breeding season.

If no pregnancy is seen the most likely reason for the mare not to show oestrus is dioestrous ovulation. This may be definitively diagnosed using serial ultrasound examinations of the ovaries or serial progesterone assays. Dioestrous ovulations may be treated using PGF2-alpha.

Control of reproduction in males

Dogs and cats

The majority of male dogs do not cause problems if they remain entire, but there are situations where control of 'antisocial' behaviour may be necessary. The situation in the entire tomcat is rather different, because the problems of territory marking, roaming and aggression are greater (for owners) than in the dog.

Surgical contraception

The most common method of regulating sexual activity is castration, which is not reversible. More information on the surgical procedure for elective castration of the dog and tomcat can be found in Chapter 25.

- Castration of the domestic dog is generally carried out at 8–12 months of age, after the dog has reached puberty. Castration before puberty may result in failure of development of the secondary sexual characteristics. In some males a change in metabolic rate may result in increased bodyweight. Castration after puberty together with correct dietary control eliminates the majority of problems associated with canine castration.
- Castration of the tomcat is normally performed at approximately 5–6 months of age, just prior to puberty; although in some centres castration is undertaken as early as 8 weeks of age.

Vasectomy is rarely performed in the dog or tomcat. It involves removal of part of the vas deferens, thus preventing ejaculation of sperm. The procedure does not interfere with sexual behaviour. Since in many cases the latter is the primary aim, vasectomy has no advantages over castration.

Exogenous hormones

Chemical control of reproductive function can be achieved in both species on a short-term basis using hormones that suppress the normal release of testosterone. The most commonly used agents include the progestogens (drugs with progesterone-like activity), which may be administered daily orally (e.g. megestrol acetate) or as a depot injection (e.g. proligestone or delmadinone acetate). These drugs do not produce infertility, only a reduced libido. There is also interest in the GnRH-agonist drugs, which, when administered as depot preparations, cause an initial stimulation of the pituitary–gonadal axis and then a long duration (for as long as the product is active) of downregulation. Recently, an implant containing the GnRH-agonist deslorelin has become commercially available. This preparation (Suprelorin 4.7 mg Implant) is authorized for the induction of temporary infertility in male dogs. Approximately 6 weeks after placing the implant the dog becomes infertile and this situation is maintained for at least 6 months after the initial treatment.

Vaccination

As technology advances it is becoming more likely that vaccines will be developed against components of the reproductive system. Currently, whilst some experimental vaccines are available for use in females in other species (directed against the zona pellucida), there are none available for use in the male dog or cat.

The stallion

Surgical contraception

Stallions can be very dangerous animals and the vast majority are neutered at a young age. Castration is either performed under local analgesia in the standing patient or under a general anaesthetic. The blood vessels and spermatic cord are either ligated before sectioning or are crushed using a surgical instrument called an emasculator. This piece of equipment simultaneously crushes and cuts the blood vessels and cord. There is no need for sutures to be placed after emasculation.

The surgery can be performed from around 6 months of age. The vaginal tunic may be left open (i.e. no ligatures) after emasculation in animals up to 2 years of age, or when the procedure is carried out in the standing animal. This allows drainage of the wound, which reduces the chance of infection. However, a semi-closed technique is more commonly used under general anaesthesia, when the incisions are closed after meticulous haemostasis. This procedure reduces the risk of evisceration (intestinal prolapse through inguinal ring) and major haemorrhage. However, such a semi-closed castration does risk incisional swelling; hence the need for meticulous haemostasis.

Chemical contraception

This is not available for the stallion. While exogenous progesterone has been shown to reduce libido in stallions, it has not been shown to render them infertile.

Control of reproduction in females

Many methods have been employed to control the reproductive cycle of the bitch and queen. These include surgical methods and medical control of cyclical activity. More recently, advances have been made in the induction of oestrus and in the termination of pregnancy.

The domestic bitch

Surgical neutering

Ovariohysterectomy is the removal of both ovaries and the uterus to the level of the cervix. The term 'spaying' is commonly used to describe this procedure. In some countries it is more common to remove only the ovaries (ovariectomy). Either technique should be considered in any bitch not required for breeding. Both have several advantages, including a reduction in the incidence of mammary tumours, and elimination of the problems of false pregnancy and of pyometra, as well the obvious advantages of absence of oestrous behaviour and inability to produce offspring. See Chapter 25 for more information.

There are several claimed adverse effects, including an increased incidence of incontinence, changes in coat texture and a tendency to gain weight. Whilst little can be done regarding the former two conditions, the latter may easily be controlled by correct dietary management.

Age for neutering

There is considerable discussion concerning the correct time to perform the procedure on a bitch. Some veterinary surgeons operate before puberty when there is no doubt that the surgery is technically easier and recovery is more rapid than in older animals; some veterinary surgeons operate as early as 4 months of age. It has been suggested that when the surgery is performed before puberty (the first oestrus) there is an increased chance that the external genitalia will be underdeveloped (resulting in a recessed vulva for example) and there may also be effects on the closure time of the animal's growth plates (resulting in the animals having long limbs). However, it is important to note that prepubertal neutering does significantly protect the female against the development of mammary tumours later in life. Other veterinary surgeons wait until after the first oestrus to avoid some of these possible adverse effects, although waiting increases the risk of pregnancy and false pregnancy. There are some specific conditions for which it is not advisable to perform surgical neutering before puberty. These include bitches with prepubertal vaginitis, bitches with urinary incontinence and bitches of certain breeds where changes in coat colour are common after neutering (e.g. some red-haired breeds).

Medical inhibition of cycling activity

A variety of compounds may be used to inhibit cycling activity, including progesterone or progesterone-like compounds (**progestogens**), testosterone or other male hormones (**androgens**) and GnRH agonists and antagonists. Drugs may either be administered during anoestrus to prevent the occurrence of an oestrus (the term **prevention** is used), or be given during pro-oestrus or oestrus to abolish the signs of that particular oestrus (the term **suppression** is used).

The most commonly used compounds are the progestogens, which are formulated as depot injections or as oral tablets. Depot injections (e.g. proligestone) may be used during anoestrus to prevent the occurrence of the next anticipated oestrus. Oral tablets (e.g. megestrol acetate) may be used either during anoestrus for oestrus prevention, or during pro-oestrus to suppress the signs of that oestrus.

These drugs are not recommended for use before the first oestrus or in an animal that is required for breeding. The side effects of these drugs may include increased appetite, weight gain, lethargy, mammary enlargement, coat and temperament changes and the risk of inducing pyometra.

Termination of pregnancy

Unwanted matings are commonly seen in general practice. The term **misalliance** is often used to describe such cases. There are several treatment options should pregnancy termination be necessary. If the bitch is not required for breeding, an ovariohysterectomy may be performed early in metoestrus, approximately 2–4 weeks after the end of oestrus. Medical therapy using oestrogens on several occasions after mating or using progesterone receptor antagonists is usually successful in preventing conception. In later pregnancy it is possible to use various drugs (e.g. progesterone receptor antagonists or prolactin inhibitors and/or prostaglandins) that lower the concentration of progesterone in the blood or block its actions and therefore induce resorption or abortion.

Induction of oestrus

With the development of new drugs and new drug regimes it has become possible to induce an oestrous cycle in the bitch. The best success rates occur with prolactin inhibitors such as cabergoline. These methods may be useful in bitches that have longer than average interoestrus intervals, those that are slow to reach puberty and those that do not exhibit behavioural signs of oestrus.

The domestic queen

Surgical neutering

The indications and potential adverse effects of ovariohysterectomy and ovariectomy in the cat are similar to those in the bitch. The procedure is usually performed when the queen is 5–6 months of age, regardless of the onset of puberty; poor development of the external genitalia does not cause problems. In the UK the surgical procedure is frequently performed through a flank incision, but this approach is best avoided in oriental breeds where coat colour is temperature-dependent and clipping of the coat may result in the growth of dark-coloured hairs. See Chapter 25 for more information.

Medical inhibition of cycling activity

The drugs available for use in the queen are similar to those described for the domestic bitch. Long-term drug therapy is less commonly used, because queens that are not wanted for breeding are usually surgically neutered.

Termination of pregnancy

Treatment of an unwanted mating can be achieved by the administration of progestogens if the queen is still in oestrus, or progesterone receptor antagonists if she has ovulated. In many cases pregnancy termination is performed a month after mating, using similar drug regimes to those described for the bitch.

Induction of oestrus

Various drugs may be used for the induction of oestrus and ovulation. In most cases it is important to remember that the queen is a seasonal breeder, and that her cyclicity is governed by photoperiod.

The mare

Advancing the breeding season

The breeding of horses is a multi-million pound industry and getting mares in foal as quickly as possible is an active area of research. Advancing the breeding season by only 30 days will allow the breeder to produce an early foal that is well developed at sale time.

Artificial lighting

Daylength is an important stimulus for the oestrous cycle in the mare. Several methods have been described to offer the mare artificial lighting conditions; however, 24 hours of lighting is detrimental.

- A 16-hour light period starting in late November (before 1st December) is able to advance the first ovulation by around 60–80 days (16 hours light : 8 hours dark).
- Adding 2–3 hours of light at the end of the day (as dusk falls) is also effective; although the mare must be kept outside to receive as much natural light as possible.
- Another method reported is the 'flash' or 'pulse' system, which delivers 1 hour of light 9.5 hours after the onset of darkness. This system is not widely used commercially.

NB If the lighting system fails for more than 2–3 days the mare will go back to where she was before the light treatment.
Artificial lighting is considered the most effective method for advancing time to first ovulation.

Dopamine antagonists

Experimentally, drugs such as domperidone and sulpiride have the effect of reducing dopamine, which in turn allows the release of prolactin from the anterior pituitary. High levels of prolactin naturally occur during the summer months and are thought to play a reproductive role in mares.

Progestogens

Once the mare is in the transitional period, the administration of exogenous progestogen has been shown to shorten the time to first ovulation. The hormone can be given orally in the feed.

Inducing or delaying oestrus

It may be desirable to inseminate or cover a mare on a specific day, particularly if chilled semen is being flown over from another country or a stallion is competing and is only available for a very short period. Two basic approaches involve either *extending* or *shortening* the luteal phase of the cycle.

Exogenous progestogens

These drugs are commonly used to extend the luteal period. They produce two important effects on the cycling mare:

- Inhibit behavioural oestrus. Mares will begin to 'tease-out' after 2–3 days of treatment
- Diminish LH levels and block final maturation of follicles and therefore ovulation. This is not 100% effective in the mare.

After cessation of progestogen treatment, on average the mare will show signs of oestrus in 5 days (3–6 days) and will ovulate in 10 days (8–15 days).

Prostaglandin F2-alpha

PGF2-alpha is used to shorten the luteal period. It causes the lysis of the corpus luteum, resulting in a decline of serum progesterone. A corpus luteum will only regress in response to exogenous PGF2-alpha >5 days after ovulation. Oestrous response starts at about 3–4 days after injection, with ovulation occurring about 7–12 days after injection.

Induction of ovulation during oestrus

Controlling when a mare ovulates during oestrus can significantly improve conception rates and in some cases reduce the incidence of endometritis.

Human chorionic gonadatrophin

hCG has an LH-like effect, helping to mature and ovulate a dominant follicle. hCG is given when the mare has a follicle of 30–35 mm or more. Under these circumstances, 90% of mares ovulate within 48 hours of injection.

GnRH implant/injections

GnRH injected into the mare when she has a follicle >30 mm produces a very similar response to injection with hCG but the treatment is comparatively expensive.

Inhibition of cycling activity

There may be situations when it is desirable for a mare not to cycle normally, such as during competitions, and there are a few ways of achieving this:

- **Progestogen treatment:** As described above, progestogens stop mares showing oestrous behaviour and ovulating. Their use can be expensive and, because they are given orally in the mare's feed, there is a public health concern as the preparations will have an effect on humans if the product comes into contact with their skin
- **Ovariectomy:** Removal of the ovaries is a permanent solution to prevent a mare cycling. The procedure can be performed with the mare standing, using keyhole surgery techniques. The mare's uterus is not removed
- **Uterine marbles:** Recently it has become fashionable to insert a 35–45 mm glass marble into the uterus of mares. This seems to stop cycling in around 40–50% of mares although the mechanism is not fully understood. The author does not recommend this treatment as the long-term effects have not yet been studied and removal of the marble once in the mare's uterus can be difficult.

Assessing the optimum time for mating

The domestic bitch

Determination of the time of ovulation in the bitch is important because the bitch is monoestrous (has one oestrous cycle followed by an obligatory period of anoestrus). The clinical signs of oestrus are not always reliable indicators of the time of ovulation; in many bitches the behavioural signs do not correlate well with the changes in hormone concentration. There are two factors that increase the likelihood of conception despite these potential problems: the relatively long fertile period of the eggs; and the relatively long survival of spermatozoa within the female reproductive tract.

There are several methods by which the optimum time for mating can be detected, including clinical assessments, measurement of plasma hormone concentration and vaginal cytology.

Clinical assessments

The clinical signs of oestrus do not correlate well with the underlying hormonal events. The 'average bitch' ovulates 12 days after the onset of pro-oestrus and should be mated from day 14 onwards, when oocytes have matured. In some bitches ovulation may occur as early as day 5 or as late as day 32 after the onset of pro-oestrus, and these bitches would be unlikely to become pregnant if mated on the 12th and 14th day, which is common breeding practice.

Studies on laboratory dogs have shown that the LH surge often occurs around the same time as the onset of standing oestrus. Although there is some variation of this event, commencing mating 4 days after the onset of standing oestrus may be a suitable time in many bitches.

One clinical assessment that may be useful in the bitch is the timing of vulval softening (Figure 26.10). This often occurs during the LH surge when there is a switch from oestrogen dominance to progesterone dominance of the reproductive tract.

If only clinical assessments are available, the combination of the onset of standing oestrus and the timing of distinct

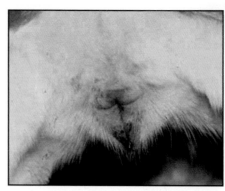

26.10
Bitch's softened vulva, just after the LH surge.

vulval softening may be useful in the prediction of the best mating time, since each event occurs on average 2 days before ovulation.

Measurement of plasma hormone concentration

The three relevant plasma hormones are LH, oestrogen and progesterone.

- Plasma concentrations of **luteinizing hormone** would detect impending ovulation, as the fertile period is between 4 and 8 days after the LH surge. Unfortunately, there is no simple method by which plasma LH concentrations can be readily measured.
- There is little value in the measurement of plasma **oestrogen** concentrations because the oestrogen plateau is not predictive of the timing of ovulation.
- Plasma **progesterone** concentrations are very useful, since this hormone is absent during pro-oestrus and begins to increase at the same time as the plasma surge of LH. Thus, detecting a rise in the concentration of plasma progesterone is predictive of ovulation.

Progesterone can be easily measured in the practice laboratory within 30 minutes of sample collection, using a commercial enzyme-linked immunosorbent assay (ELISA) test kit. This method simply involves comparison of a colour change in the sample with the colour change in low- and high-progesterone controls.

Vaginal cytology

The changes in the concentration of plasma hormone concentrations have a marked effect upon the vaginal mucosa. When the bitch is in anoestrus, there are approximately two or three layers of cells lining the vagina. During pro-oestrus, the vagina develops many cell layers in order to protect itself during mating. The cells within these layers differ from each other in their shape and size. When cells are collected from the vagina (the technique called a **vaginal smear**), only the cells on the surface of the vagina are removed. Different cell types are therefore collected at the various stages of the reproductive cycle. Staining of these cells and subsequent microscopic examination allows an assessment of the underlying hormone changes to be made. Cells can be collected either by aspirating vaginal fluid using a pipette, or using a cotton swab. Once collected, cells are placed on a glass microscope slide, spread into a thin film and stained so that they can be individually examined.

- During anoestrus (Figure 26.11a) the vaginal wall is only a few cells in thickness and these cells are small and spherical in shape. Because they are positioned close to the basement membrane they are called **parabasal** cells. The anoestrus vaginal smear is characterized by the presence of these cells. There are also normally a few white blood cells (**neutrophils**), which remove cell debris and bacteria.

- During pro-oestrus (Figure 26.11b) the vaginal mucosa increases in thickness under the influence of oestrogen. The mucosa may be up to five or six cells thick. The cells further away from the basement membrane are larger in diameter than those nearer to the membrane. These cells have a large area of cytoplasm surrounding the cell nucleus and are called small intermediate cells. When the surface cells are collected during pro-oestrus they are therefore predominantly these **small intermediate cells**, although there will also be a small number of the parabasal cells present. White blood cells are also present during pro-oestrus, but numbers are reduced compared with anoestrus. This is because the increased thickness of the vaginal mucosa prevents movement of the white blood cells into the lumen of the vagina. Red blood cells are also present in the vaginal smear during pro-oestrus. These cells originate from the uterus and pass into the vagina via the cervix.

- During oestrus (Figure 26.11c) the vaginal mucosa continues to thicken and the number of cell layers increases. There may be up to 12 cell layers during oestrus. Surface cells are large and irregular in shape and are called **large intermediate cells**. Cells of this size may accumulate the material keratin and are then termed keratinized. The nucleus of these large **keratinized** cells often disappears. The cells are then called **anuclear** because of the absence of the nucleus. White blood cells are not found in the vaginal smear during oestrus because the thick vaginal wall does not allow them to penetrate. Red blood cells are present in large numbers during oestrus.

- During metoestrus (Figure 26.11d) there is sloughing of much of the vaginal mucosal epithelium. This is caused by the increasing concentrations of the hormone progesterone. The number of cell layers is reduced and the surface cells are again the small intermediate epithelial cells or parabasal cells. Several of the epithelial cells may have vacuoles within the cytoplasm, giving the cell a 'foamy' appearance. **Foam cells** and epithelial cells with cytoplasmic inclusion bodies are characteristic of metoestrus. Because of the large amount of degenerate cellular material within the vaginal lumen, there is a rapid influx of white blood cells as soon as the mucosa is thin enough to allow their penetration. Large numbers of white blood cells are therefore found in the metoestrus vaginal smear. Few red blood cells are present during metoestrus.

The bitch should first be mated when the percentage of anuclear cells is maximal (usually 80% or above) (Figure 26.12). There are variations from the normal: some bitches may have two peaks of anuclear cells and some have a low percentage of anuclear cells during the fertile period.

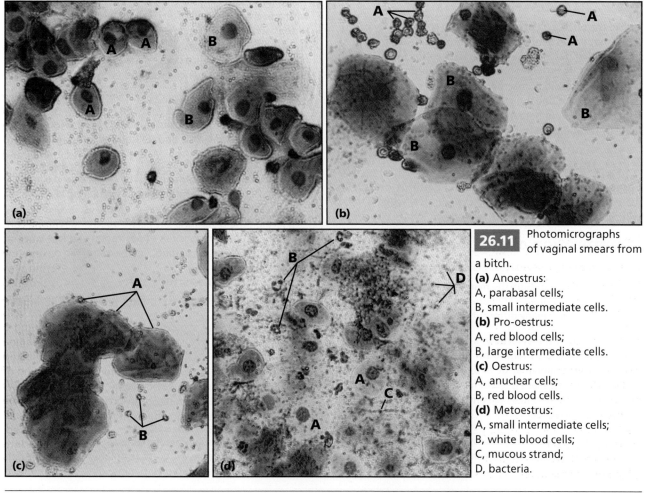

26.11 Photomicrographs of vaginal smears from a bitch. **(a)** Anoestrus: A, parabasal cells; B, small intermediate cells. **(b)** Pro-oestrus: A, red blood cells; B, large intermediate cells. **(c)** Oestrus: A, anuclear cells; B, red blood cells. **(d)** Metoestrus: A, small intermediate cells; B, white blood cells; C, mucous strand; D, bacteria.

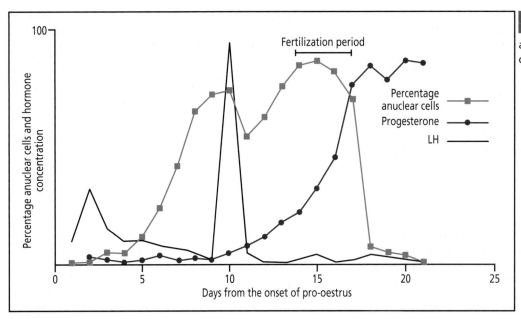

26.12 Changes in percentage of anuclear cells during oestrus in the bitch.

Other tests

A number of other tests have been evaluated in the past, including the measurement of electrical resistance, pH and glucose concentration in the vagina. None of these methods is reliable. Examination of the vaginal wall using an endoscope (**vaginoscopy**) may be valuable for identifying the optimal time for breeding, as the vaginal wall undergoes specific changes around the time of ovulation.

The domestic queen

Unlike the bitch, ovulation in the queen is induced by coitus. After mating, assuming that a sufficient release of LH has occurred, follicles increase in size and ovulation follows 24–36 hours later. Mating is best planned during the peak of oestrus, and vaginal cytology may be used to assess this time, but collection of the smear may itself induce ovulation. Multiple copulations should be permitted to ensure an adequate release of LH and therefore ovulation.

The mare

Because of the potentially variable length of oestrus in mares, it can be difficult to predict accurately when a mare will ovulate.

Identification of oestrus

Behaviour in response to teasing

This is elicited by exposing the mare to a teaser stallion. Most studs use a non-valuable stallion as a teaser, such as a pony stallion. There are many different teasing methods:

- The mare may be let loose in a field, with the teaser stallion in a smaller fenced off area in the centre
- The teaser stallion may be in a stable looking out over the door as the mare is led in front of him
- The mare is placed in a race and the teaser stallion introduced outside.

Daily or every-other-day access will determine when the mare is ready to mate. The mare may give the following signs if she is in oestrus:

- Quiet and calm
- Ears forward
- Nuzzling
- Posturing
- Moving to stallion
- Squatting and urinating
- Raising tail
- Clitoral winking (everting vulva and pushing forward the clitoris).

Maiden mares (mares that have never bred), and mares with a foal at foot, will often respond poorly to teasing due to fear and uncertainty. It is important to note that teasing is a poor predictor of ovulation but is very useful in differentiating oestrus from dioestrus. Inadequate teasing can affect reproductive performance on broodmare farms.

Rectal palpation

This method is commonly used to identify oestrus in the mare. Cervical and uterine tone and follicular size and firmness are determined.

- Uterine tone is prominent and the cervix closed (cigar-like) when there are high levels of circulating progesterone, i.e. the mare is in dioestrus.
- Uterine tone is soft and the cervix open and relaxed when there are high levels of oestrogen and low levels of progesterone circulating, i.e. the mare is in oestrus.

Transrectal ultrasonography

This technique (see Chapter 18) has revolutionized equine reproductive management and is used in conjunction with rectal palpation. Ultrasonography can provide the following information:

- Presence or absence of a corpus luteum
- Follicle size, shape and echogenicity
- Endometrial oedema in response to circulating oestrogen
- Pathology such as uterine fluid, endometrial cysts, etc.

Early oestrus is usually accompanied by a follicle of around 20–30 mm in diameter. Progressive enlargement of the follicle to >40 mm is associated with impending ovulation.

Vaginoscopy

A speculum can be passed into the vagina and a visual inspection of the cranial vagina and external os of the cervix can be made. See above for details on how the cervix changes according to the stage of the cycle.

Hormonal assays

A blood sample can be taken and tested for progesterone, which is the hormone produced by the corpus luteum following ovulation. Serum progesterone concentration should be >1 ng/ml in dioestrus and <1 ng/ml in oestrus.

Detection of ovulation

The mare has a relatively long oestrus (5–7 days) and ovulation normally occurs at approximately 24 hours before the end of the oestrus period. No single method exists to reliably predict the precise moment of ovulation. However, the following criteria are of use:

- **Size of ovulating follicle.** Follicles grow at 3–5 mm/day during oestrus and very few follicles ovulate within 24 hours when <33 mm in diameter. The size of the follicle at ovulation is NOT determined by the size of the mare. Small ponies will ovulate from the same size follicles as large shire breeds
- **Change in consistency** of the ovulating follicle from a tense tight sphere to a soft fluctuant structure
- **Change in shape** of the ovulating follicle on ultrasonography from round to a pear or conical shape indicates impending ovulation. However, this may not be seen in all follicles
- **Change in endometrial oedema** on ultrasonography, appearing like a 'halved orange'. Oedema is maximal at around 1–2 days prior to ovulation and starts to decline in prominence around 24 hours prior to ovulation.

It is important to collate all information to help make an estimation of when the mare will ovulate and thus when to mate/inseminate her. Fertility is highest when mares are bred within a window from 48 hours prior to ovulation and 6 hours post-ovulation (although it is possible to achieve conception 12 hours post-ovulation).

Normal mating behaviour

It is important that the events of natural mating are understood so that abnormalities can be recognized, while remembering that the mating environment is often artificial. On the day of mating, bitches and queens are frequently transported large distances, are introduced to the male briefly and then expected to mate immediately. This situation eliminates the normal courtship phase associated with pro-oestrous behaviour and may result in mating problems. In addition many females are presented to males at inappropriate times, either because this is convenient for the owner or because of inexact assessment of the stage of the oestrous cycle. On such occasions sexual behaviour of both males and females may not be optimal.

Dogs

The dog and bitch will normally exhibit play behaviour when they are first introduced to each other. Generally the bitch should be taken to the designated area first. The dog can then be introduced. He should be restrained on a lead to ensure that the bitch is happy for the dog to be there and is receptive to him. Once this has been established the dog can be allowed off his lead. The dog and bitch will normally play for a few minutes (Figure 26.13a). Very experienced studs may forego this playtime and mount the bitch straight away, so it is important to establish the willingness of the bitch to be mated in the first instance. The bitch will normally settle and stand with her tail deviated to one side in order to allow mating to take place. This tail deviation is known as 'flagging'.

The dog may ejaculate a small volume of clear fluid either before mounting the bitch or whilst he is trying to gain intromission into the bitch. This fluid is the **first fraction** of the ejaculate and does not contain sperm. It originates from the prostate gland and its function is to flush any urine or cellular debris from the urethra. The dog will continue to mount, thrust and dismount until his position allows the tip of the penis to enter the bitch's vagina. This is known as **intromission** (Figure 26.13b). The dog will now achieve a full erection. The dog appears to move much closer to the bitch and the thrusting movements increase rapidly. He will now ejaculate the **second fraction** of ejaculate, which is sperm-rich (see Figure 26.6).

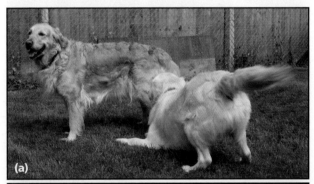

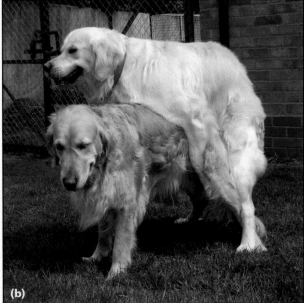

26.13   Normal mating behaviour in the dog: **(a)** playing prior to mating; **(b)** intromission.   *continues* ▶

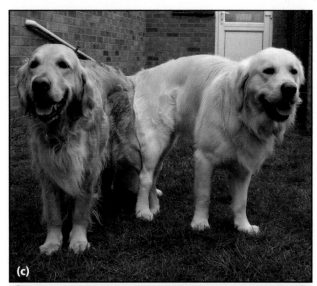

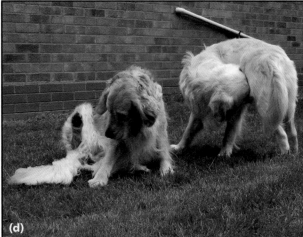

26.13   *continued* Normal mating behaviour in the dog: **(c)** the 'tie'; **(d)** separation after mating.

Once thrusting has subsided the dog will turn through 180 degrees and dismount the bitch whilst his penis remains within her vagina. The dog and bitch will now stand tail-to-tail and this is called the **tie** (Figure 26.13c). The tie is associated with the dog ejaculating the **third fraction** of ejaculate. This is again clear fluid and prostatic in origin and its purpose is to flush the sperm forwards through the cervix into the uterus. The tie will last on average for 20 minutes but varies considerably between dogs and can be as short as 5 minutes or over an hour in length.

Once the swelling of the bulbous gland subsides, the dog and bitch will separate and the mating is finished (Figure 26.13d). The bitch should be checked for any bleeding. There is normally a small amount of fluid that comes away when the tie ends; this is just the last portion of prostatic fluid and is normal. The fluid can sometimes be bloodstained, depending on the bitch's discharge. Bitches with a coloured discharge tend to have a heavier staining of this fluid. If this fluid is very heavily bloodstained, the bitch and the dog should be checked thoroughly.

If all is normal, the bitch is taken away from the area first. The dog will usually lick at himself to help the penis re-enter its sheath. At this time the dog should be checked to ensure that his penis has returned to its sheath correctly. Occasionally, during the mating process, small blood vessels in the dog's penis will burst, resulting in a small amount of bloody discharge. This should subside quickly.

Cats

The period of sexual introduction and play is variable in the cat, depending upon the experience and aggression of the male. The normal sequence of events occurs rapidly compared with the dog. The male usually approaches the female from the side or back and grasps her neck in his mouth. Whilst maintaining this grasp he mounts the female and positions himself to align the genital regions. The queen normally lowers her chest and elevates the pelvic region whilst deviating her tail. Pelvic thrusting and ejaculation occur rapidly. During intromission the queen often emits a cry and attempts to end mating by rolling, turning and striking at the male. The female then exhibits a marked postcoital reaction consisting of violent rolling and excessive licking. She will not allow further mating at this time.

Horses

A good stallion can naturally cover two mares per day, 6 days per week (approximately 150 mares in one season). Requirements for mating are:

- A good teaser stallion
- A teasing system suited to the management system
- An experienced observer and recorder.

Once the mare is considered to be cycling:

- Mares should be teased (see above) three times per week or preferably every other day during the breeding season
- Those that respond positively to teasing are traditionally covered on day 2 or 3 of oestrus and then every other day until the end of oestrus
- Mares should be covered prior to ovulation when the mare has a dominant follicle (>30 mm) present. If it is necessary to limit the number of matings, the ovaries should be palpated daily and mating should take place just prior to ovulation
- If ovulation has occurred then reasonable conception rates may still be achieved by breeding <12 hours after ovulation; however, the mare will probably not stand to be mated and may require AI. It has been shown that there is a greater incidence of early embryonic loss associated with post-ovulation inseminations due to the fertilization of an aged ovum.

It is important to restrain the mare adequately for mating (see Chapter 10). Use of a headcollar and/or Chifney (anti-rearing) bit is recommended. A twitch can be used on the mare to keep her still. Some studs place hobbles on the hindlimbs of the mare or tie up a foreleg. The mare's tail should be wrapped in a bandage or plastic bag.

The perineal region must be washed three times with mild soap or povidone–iodine scrub, rinsed and dried prior to mating. To minimize contamination and the chance of endometritis:

- Mating should take place as few times as possible
- Optimal hygiene should always be employed (stallion and mare).

Problems in mating

Dogs

The mating of dogs and bitches always seems a straightforward process, but there can often be problems. The most common difficulty is that the dog does not tie with the bitch. This is not considered a satisfactory outcome, although it is quite possible that such matings will still result in the bitch conceiving if the dog has ejaculated. The most common reason for a mating with no tie is that there is a height difference between the dog and the bitch. The dog must be able to enter the bitch as straight as possible and this could be difficult if he is too short or too tall. If the dog is too short, a step should be used to make him 'taller'; a step can be used by the bitch if the stud is too tall. Sometimes the dog will not tie because he has had an unpleasant past experience that has resulted in a loss of confidence, often causing a failure to achieve a full erection. In these instances, holding the dog and bitch together as soon as the dog's thrusting has stopped may be helpful. This is known as a **held tie**, but this in itself can be very difficult to achieve. The dog should not be allowed to mate the bitch too many times without achieving a tie. It is better to try a few times and then rest the dog until the next day.

Often the bitch's position can be a problem: she may not elevate her vulva correctly, she may not deviate her tail very well, or she may keep moving her tail from side to side. In these instances elevating the bitch's vulva to the correct position or holding her tail out of the way can help the dog. These problems are commonly associated with inexperienced bitches. **Maiden bitches** (bitches that have not been mated before) can be a little overwhelmed by the whole process and require much more support than an experienced bitch. Inexperienced bitches will often stand at first but then appear to change their minds. In these cases, the owner must be patient. Often the bitch just requires a little more time to get used to the stud and the idea of being mated. These matings can sometimes take several hours to achieve, but the bitch should not be rushed and must not be forced to stand. This can result in her not standing to be mated at all.

Some bitches can be difficult if the stud dog is playing too much and leaping on the bitch. The more inexperienced stud will exhibit this type of behaviour. The problem is rectified by gentle restraint of the bitch, ensuring that the human presence does not upset the stud. Whenever possible a new stud dog should be put with an experienced bitch, and a new bitch with an experienced stud.

Cats

In the cat, it is frequently very difficult to be present during a mating since this puts off all but the most experienced males; in the majority of cases, it is necessary to observe from a distance. It is always better to have an experienced partner when a queen or tomcat is mated for the first time.

Assisted reproduction

Dogs

Several techniques may be used to assist reproduction in the bitch. These include the induction of oestrus (see above) and artificial insemination.

Artificial insemination

Artificial insemination (AI) is the technique of placing semen collected from a male into the reproductive tract of the female. It may involve the use of freshly collected semen, semen that has been diluted and chilled, or semen that has been frozen and then thawed.

Advantages of AI in dogs

- Reduces the requirement to transport animals.
- Is an acceptable way of overcoming, to some extent, quarantine restrictions that may prevent the movement of animals from one country to another.
- Increases the genetic pool available to an individual breed within a country.
- Reduces the disease risk that is always present when unknown animals enter a kennel for mating. (In some countries the use of AI may reduce the spread of infectious diseases.)
- May be useful when natural mating is difficult:
  - Bitches that ovulate when they are not in standing oestrus
  - Bitches with hyperplasia of the vaginal floor
  - Male animals that, due to age, debility, back pain or premature ejaculation, are unable to achieve a natural mating.

The greatest area of interest is probably in the storage of genetic material by freezing semen for insemination at a future date. This may be necessary in male animals that are likely to become infertile due to castration or to medical treatments with certain hormones. The more common reason is the preservation of semen from superior animals for use in future generations.

Collected semen may be deposited easily into the vagina of the bitch using a long inseminating pipette that is gently introduced near to the cervix. When semen is placed in this position, spermatozoa must swim through the cervix, into the uterus and up the uterine horns. During a natural mating, contractions of the vagina and uterus help in transporting semen. These contractions generally do not occur during insemination, though some may be produced by stimulating the vagina. Vaginal insemination is therefore not ideal, but usually when fresh or chilled semen is used the spermatozoa will live long enough to fertilize the eggs. In the case of frozen semen, the spermatozoa do not live for long after thawing and so vaginal inseminations are not very satisfactory.

The chance of pregnancy can be improved if the semen is placed directly into the uterus rather than into the vagina. It is very difficult to place a catheter through the bitch's cervix into the uterus (a technique that is simple in many other animals) because the vagina is long and narrow and because the cervical opening is small and at an angle to the vagina. A special insemination pipette has been developed for this purpose. Some research workers have been able to catheterize the cervix using an endoscope. However, in certain countries the commonest way of performing uterine insemination is surgically via a laparotomy. In the UK the ethics of this procedure have been questioned.

Because of the short lifespan of the preserved sperm, it is most important that inseminations are accurately timed in relation to ovulation. The ideal time is 2–5 days after ovulation, and this is best assessed by using the measurement of plasma progesterone concentration and the study of vaginal cytology (see above).

In the UK, puppies that are the result of artificial insemination can only be registered if the Kennel Club has given prior permission. The permission of the Kennel Club is not required before semen is imported or exported. There are specific regulations set by Defra in the UK and by similar organizations in other countries, which aim to prevent the introduction of infectious diseases. Import regulations vary between countries but are particularly stringent for the UK. Import permit requirements usually include: health certification before, and a set time period after, semen collection; quarantine of semen until the second health examination, and various serological tests.

Cats

Whilst artificial insemination has been widely practised in the domestic cat as a research model for wild cats, the technique is not commonly used in the UK. Techniques used in the cat are further advanced than those in the dog and include the induction of ovulation, *in vitro* fertilization and embryo transfer.

Horses
Artificial insemination

AI can be used in all horse breeds except Thoroughbreds. Chilled or frozen semen can be used and, with recent advances, conception rates are virtually the same as for natural mating. Indeed, in certain mares breeding using chilled semen AI can produce better conception rates than natural breeding.

Advantages of AI in horses

- Possible to have an increased conception rate.
- Mares can be bred to stallions that would otherwise be geographically inaccessible.
- Mares and foals are not subject to transport stress.
- Mares can remain in training/work.
- Mare owners save on transport costs.
- Reduction in spread of some venereal diseases.

Disadvantages of AI in horses

- Veterinary costs are higher.
- Mare owners must tease mares, arrange semen shipment and communicate with the veterinary surgeon and the stud farm.
- Repeat inseminations lead to increased semen costs.
- Frozen semen conception rates can be poor (30–50% average conception rates per cycle).

The cost of some AI programmes may mean that a full breeding soundness examination (see earlier) is indicated to avoid insemination of a mare that does not have a uterus capable of facilitating conception and pregnancy. See earlier for information on predicting ovulation, and therefore the optimum time for insemination.

Procedure for inseminating a mare by AI

1. Wrap the tail.
2. Empty the rectum.
3. Wash the perineal region with mild soap, ▶

such as povidone–iodine, and dry.
4. A clean plastic rectal sleeve and sterile glove should be worn.
5. A non-spermicidal lubricant is used.
6. Semen is drawn into a latex/silicone-free syringe and the insemination pipette attached.
7. The hand and pipette are passed into the vagina and the cervix located.
8. The pipette is passed through the cervix and the semen deposited into the uterus.

Embryo transfer

In recent years, embryo transfer has become a relatively common procedure and is a natural extension of AI. The mare is inseminated in the usual way and the embryo is collected as it enters the uterus at around day 7. This embryo is then transferred to a recipient mare that carries and gives birth to the foal. Generally, a recipient is cyclically 48 hours behind the donor at time of transfer.

Other reproductive procedures
Oocyte collection

The mare's oviduct does not allow unfertilized ova to enter the uterus. The unfertilized ova are retained within the distal oviduct and broken down. Therefore oocyte recovery is performed surgically. Follicular puncture and aspiration is required. Transvaginal, ultrasound-guided follicular puncture is used. The collected oocytes are most commonly used for GIFT (see below).

Gamete intra-fallopian tube transfer (GIFT)

GIFT has been successful and is offered commercially by a few institutions. GIFT involves the surgical deposition of an oocyte and sperm into the oviduct of a recipient mare. It seems the oviduct plays a crucial role in providing the correct environment for conception.

Embryological development

Dogs and cats
Fertilization

The **egg** (ovum), which is released at ovulation from the follicle, is surrounded by a thick protective coat. The inner layer comprises glycoprotein and is called the **zona pellucida**, whilst the outer layer is made up of small follicular cells and is called the **corona radiata** (Figure 26.14).

The egg is fertilized during its passage through the uterine tube. Just before fertilization, sperm change their type of motility so that they are able to burrow through the cells surrounding the egg. During this process a reaction occurs in the head region of the sperm, resulting in the release of an enzyme that starts to digest the zona pellucida. These sperm are said to be **acrosome-reacted**. The sperm is then able to penetrate into the egg (the process called **fertilization**).

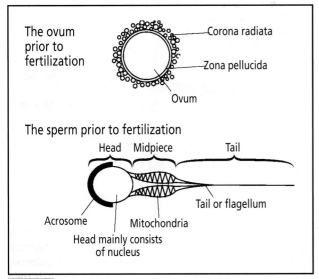

The ovum prior to fertilization
- Corona radiata
- Zona pellucida
- Ovum

The sperm prior to fertilization
- Head
- Midpiece
- Tail
- Acrosome
- Mitochondria
- Tail or flagellum
- Head mainly consists of nucleus

26.14 Structure of ovum and sperm. (Not to same scale)

The fertilized egg is often called a **zygote** or **conceptus.** It is sometimes also called an embryo, but this term needs to be differentiated from the embryo proper, which is the mass of cells that form the true body of the developing animal – see below.

The conceptus

After fertilization the conceptus continues to travel down the uterine tube towards the uterus and generally reaches the uterus by day 7 after ovulation. During its journey, the cells of the conceptus begin to divide (Figure 26.15). By doubling at each division the conceptus has two, then four and then eight cells, before forming a solid ball of cells called a **morula.**

The spherical morula develops a central fluid-filled cavity. The cells lining the cavity are called the **trophoblast.** Cells tend to accumulate at one end of the conceptus and are called the **inner cell mass.** This gathering of cells will eventually form the **embryo proper.** Three separate layers then develop and these will finally form specific recognizable areas of the body.

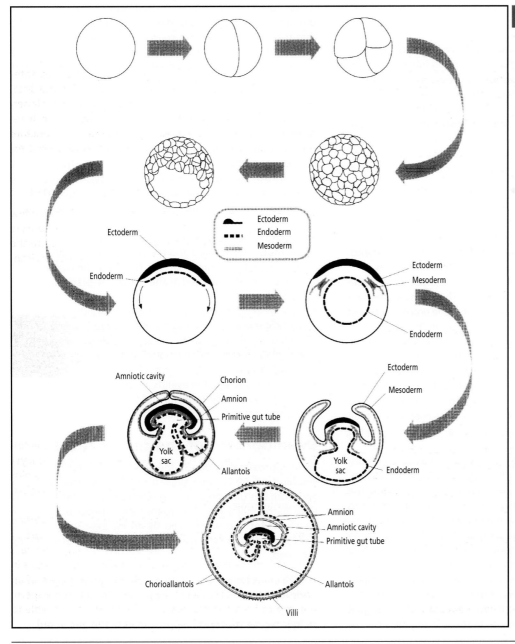

26.15 Early embryonic development.

- The outer layer of the inner cell mass is called the **ectoderm** – this will form the skin and the nervous system.
- The middle layer of the inner cell mass is called the **mesoderm** – this will form several organ systems and the musculoskeletal system.
- The inner layer of the inner cell mass is called the **endoderm** – this will form the lining of the gastrointestinal tract and of other visceral organs.

Two long blocks of mesoderm develop. Underneath these, the endodermal cells spread out and form a lining to the trophoblast which is called the **yolk sac**. In birds (and also in reptiles) this contains a true yolk, which provides nourishment, but in mammals it is a fluid-filled sac for nutrient transfer. The two blocks of mesoderm then align themselves, one next to the ectoderm and one next to the endoderm. A cavity forms between these two layers of the mesoderm. The inner cell mass curls around and encloses the mesoderm and endoderm layers, which will then form the internal organs of the embryo. The yolk sac and the trophoblast form the **placental membranes**.

Implantation

During the period of maturation of the conceptus it has been slowly moving down the uterine tube and has entered the uterus. Usually there are multiple conceptuses, which tend to move around within the uterus and become relatively evenly spaced apart. The conceptuses lie close to the wall of the uterus and the process of **implantation** starts at approximately day 14 in the bitch and day 11 in the queen. During implantation the conceptus partly destroys an area of the uterine wall (the **endometrium**) and becomes firmly attached.

The placental membranes

The placental membranes form around the embryo and are therefore called the extra-embryonic membranes. There are four basic components to the **extra-embryonic membranes**: the yolk sac, the chorion, the amnion and the allantois.

As the gut starts to develop (from the endoderm), a specific part of this forms the allantois. The **allantois** receives urine from the kidneys via a special tube (the **urachus**) present only in the embryo and fetus (it regresses in the adult).

Whilst the allantois is developing, the trophoblast continues to expand and it spreads around the embryo as a double sheet. The outer membrane is called the **chorion** and the inner layer is called the **amnion**. Throughout the period of this development the allantois continues to be filled with fetal urine and ultimately the allantois comes into contact and then fuses with the chorion. This combined structure is called the **chorioallantois**.

The **placenta** is the thickened area of the extra-embryonic membranes that attaches the fetus to the endometrium. The placenta is an interface between the fetus and the mother that allows transmission of oxygen and nutrients to the fetus whilst ensuring the elimination of waste products. To do this the fetus develops a blood supply to the placenta (actually within the chorioallantois), which has a large surface area of contact with the maternal tissue.

In the bitch the placenta is described as having a **zonary** nature, because it forms as a broad belt around the fetus (Figure 26.16). At the edge of the placenta is the **marginal haematoma**. This is a region where there is degeneration of

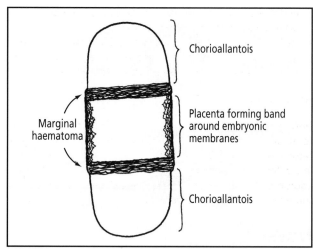

26.16 The extra-embryonic membranes in the zonary placenta of the bitch.

the maternal endothelium with a resultant bleeding into the spaces formed by the degeneration. Substances secreted by the chorion prevent the blood from clotting, and it is thought that this blood may form a source of iron for the fetus. The fluid in the marginal haematoma is green in bitches and brownish in queens. These are the colours that are noted at the time of placental separation in these species.

Development of the canine embryo

As the cells of the inner cell mass multiply and then start to curve underneath themselves, they form the head and trunk of the embryo. Within the embryo an inner cavity forms, which is called the **coelom** (the main body cavity). The coelom is divided into two separate zones by the diaphragm. The cranial zone is the thorax and the caudal zone is the abdomen.

- Generally by 3 weeks after ovulation the amnion and the allantois have formed and the embryo (in the dog) is approximately 5 mm in length. Normally the uterus itself is now slightly enlarged at the site of the placental attachment.
- By 4 weeks of age it is possible to identify the forming vertebrae and limb buds and the embryo is approaching 20 mm in length. Usually at this stage there is the first evidence of ossification (though this is not yet visible on a radiograph).
- By 5 weeks of age the eyelids, internal ears and canine teeth have started to form, and the embryo is approximately 35 mm in length.

Development of the canine fetus

From approximately day 35 the external features of the developing canine embryo allow it to be recognized as a dog and from this time onwards it is referred to as a **fetus**. By this time all the major internal organs have formed, and further development is characterized by an increase in size, especially elongation of the trunk and an increase in diameter of the head.

- By 6 weeks the digits and the external genitalia are well developed and the fetus is approximately 60 mm in length.
- By 7 weeks the fetus is approximately 100 mm in length

and there is significant ossification of the vertebral bodies and some of the long bones.

- At 8 weeks the fetus is approximately 150 mm in length and has hair and pads. Fetuses are normally delivered at approximately 9 weeks (65 ± 1 days after ovulation).

Placental membranes at birth

During birth the chorioallantois is recognized as the outer fetal sac (often called the '**water bag**'), which ruptures as the fetus moves into the birth canal. The amnion, which is the inner fetal sac, is designed also to rupture and provide additional lubrication, but it does not always rupture and in some cases the fetus may be delivered within the amnion.

Horses

Uterine changes and placental development

The embryo enters the uterus at around day 6 post-ovulation, having moved through the oviduct following the secretion of prostaglandin E2 (PGE2). This hormone elicits peristalsis in the oviduct, which 'wafts' the embryo down to the uterotuberal junction. At this stage, the embryo is either a late stage morula or an early stage blastocyst.

Maternal recognition of pregnancy prevents the production of PGF2-alpha. This is thought to involve:

- Movement of the embryo around the uterus, allowing the embryo to contact *every part* of the endometrium
- Secretion by the embryo of anti-luteolysins/luteotropic substances, which are taken up by the endometrium. The exact nature of these anti-luteolysins is not fully known.

Extensive placentation in the mare is driven by the production of epidermal growth factor (EGF), which occurs between days 35 and 40 in the epithelial lining in the apical portions of the endometrial glands. EGF is also likely to be responsible for stimulating the considerable growth and remodelling of the endometrium that must occur between days 40 and 150 to create the elongated and, eventually, very branched and complex endometrial crypts into which the equally complex and branched allantochorionic villi will interdigitate during development of the microcotyledons.

The equine placenta is classified as a **diffuse** placenta and is actually relatively poor in the transfer of nutrition, etc., to and from the fetus. Because the equine placenta is so poor, twins are very rare and often result in abortion.

At day 35 the trophoblast proliferates at an area mid-way around the embryonic vesicle. This area is called the chorionic girdle. These proliferations invade the endometrium and produce **endometrial cups**, which are unique to equids. Endometrial cups can range in size from small, isolated structures of only 0.5–1.0 cm in diameter, to long ribbons of tissue that may be as large as 20 cm in length and 1.5–3.0 cm in width. Increasing numbers of T lymphocytes, plasma cells, eosinophils and other mononuclear cells accumulate in the endometrium at the edge of the cup tissue and appear to 'wall off' the mass of fetal cells from the surrounding maternal tissue. The endometrial cups secrete hormones (such as eCG) that aid in the maintenance of pregnancy. Strangely though, these endometrial cups are not thought to be essential for pregnancy to continue to term.

Pregnancy in the domestic bitch

Pregnancy diagnosis

The clinical signs of pregnancy may include:

- Increased bodyweight and abdominal enlargement (these signs may not be obvious if the number of puppies is small)
- A reduced food intake and a vulval discharge – these are common approximately 1 month into the pregnancy
- Enlargement and reddening of the mammary glands – may be noted especially from 40 days after mating (but may also be present in bitches with pseudopregnancy)
- Production of milk – a variable finding (some bitches produce serous fluid from day 40 and milk from day 55 onwards, whilst in others this may not occur until just before parturition).

As well as observation of the clinical signs (noting that mammary gland development, increased weight and abdominal enlargement may be present in pseudopregnancy as well as in pregnancy), there are several methods for pregnancy diagnosis in the bitch.

Abdominal palpation

This is best performed approximately 1 month after mating, when the conceptual swellings are approximately 2 cm in diameter. The technique can be highly accurate but may be difficult in obese or nervous animals, and may be inaccurate if the bitch was mated early such that pregnancy is not as advanced as anticipated. After day 35 individual conceptuses cannot easily be palpated and diagnosis becomes more difficult.

Ultrasound examination

Diagnostic B-mode ultrasonography is now commonly used for pregnancy diagnosis (Figure 26.17). The technique is non-invasive and without risk to the puppies, dam or veterinary surgeon. The bitch can be examined in the standing position with minimal restraint. Using ultrasound it is possible to diagnose pregnancy as early as 16 days after ovulation, but in most cases this time is not known and so it is prudent to wait until 28 days after mating. At that time the fluid-filled conceptuses can be imaged easily and embryonic tissue identified. It is possible to assess the number of conceptuses, though this can be inaccurate, especially when the litter is large. Movement of the fetal heart can be seen and this confirms fetal

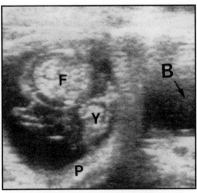

26.17

Ultrasound image of a pregnant bitch. F, fetus; Y, yolk sac; B, urinary bladder; P, placenta.

viability. It is possible to examine the bitch at any time after day 28 to diagnose pregnancy and to confirm fetal viability and growth. With later examinations it is less easy to estimate the number of puppies.

Radiography

From day 30 it is possible to detect uterine enlargement with good-quality radiographs. This is not actually diagnostic of pregnancy, since pyometra may have a similar appearance. Pregnancy diagnosis is not possible until after day 45, when mineralization of the fetal skeleton is detectable radiographically. At this stage it is unlikely that there will be radiation damage to the fetus, but sedation or anaesthesia of the dam may be required and is a potential risk. In late pregnancy the number of puppies can be reliably estimated by counting the number of fetal skulls.

Identification of fetal heart beats

In late pregnancy it is possible to auscultate the fetal heart beats using a stethoscope, or to record a fetal ECG. Both of these methods are diagnostic of pregnancy; fetal heart rate is more rapid than that of the dam.

Hormone tests

Plasma concentrations of progesterone are not useful for the detection of pregnancy in the bitch. Measurement of the hormone **relaxin** is diagnostic of pregnancy, and there is now a rapid ELISA test kit that can be run within the practice laboratory to measure this hormone. Alternatively, a blood sample can be sent away to a commercial laboratory.

Acute phase proteins

The rise in the concentration of acute phase proteins has been used as the basis of a commercial pregnancy test in the bitch. Concentrations of these proteins (including fibrinogen and C-reactive protein) increase from approximately 25 days onwards. The test is reliable, although these proteins are also released in inflammatory conditions such as pyometra.

Uterine changes during pregnancy

Under the influence of progesterone, the uterus becomes prepared to accept and nourish a pregnancy. This occurs in both pregnant and non-pregnant bitches, since both have elevated concentrations of progesterone. The specific change that occurs is an increased thickness of the uterine wall (the endometrium) associated with enlargement of specific glandular regions.

Overall, the uterus increases in diameter only slightly under the influence of progesterone and it is not until approximately 21 days that there is any enlargement related to the presence of a pregnancy. At this time there is slight swelling at the site of each pregnancy. By approximately 4 weeks the uterine swellings are significant in size and can be readily detected by palpation: the swellings are approximately 4 cm x 7 cm in size at 5 weeks and 5 cm x 8 cm at 6 weeks. Normally by 7 weeks the uterus has enlarged to such a degree that the individual swellings are no longer apparent and the adjacent fetuses are in contact with one another. From here onwards the uterus is very large and the fetuses can move freely within the allantoic fluid.

Duration of pregnancy

The length of pregnancy in the bitch is relatively consistent, at 64, 65 or 66 days from the pre-ovulatory LH surge. However, the *apparent* length of pregnancy, assessed from the time of mating, may vary between 56 and 72 days, since both early and late matings may be fertile.

- Early matings require sperm survival within the female reproductive tract until ovulation and egg maturation; such matings produce an apparently long pregnancy.
- Late matings occur when eggs are waiting to be fertilized for some time after ovulation; such matings produce an apparently shorter pregnancy.

Care of the bitch during pregnancy

Food intake does not increase during the first 30 days of pregnancy. After this time the absolute requirement for carbohydrate and protein increases. During the last half of pregnancy, food consumption may be doubled. Provided that diet is well balanced and contains suitable amounts of vitamins and minerals it is not necessary to provide extra supplementation, but it may be necessary to divide the food into two or three meals during the day. Supplementation with calcium and vitamin D should be avoided, since this does not prevent eclampsia and can be dangerous.

Regular exercise should be provided throughout pregnancy, limited by the amount the bitch is willing to undertake.

For the control of ascarid infections (see Chapter 7) it is necessary to administer medication during pregnancy to reduce or prevent perinatal transmission. Various drugs (benzimidazoles, milbemycin) and treatment regimes have been advocated for the treatment of pregnant bitches. Many veterinary practices would advise that ascarid control should be undertaken prior to mating and after parturition, normally carried out at the same time that the puppies are treated. If it does become necessary to treat the dam, then this can be done during pregnancy.

It is advisable to ensure that routine vaccination has been performed before mating. Vaccination during pregnancy is unlikely to be damaging to the fetus and therefore may be undertaken if necessary, but no live vaccine is licensed for this purpose.

Certain physiological changes occur during pregnancy and include the development of a normochromic, normocytic anaemia and a reduction of the packed cell volume; these changes are normal.

Pregnancy in the domestic queen

Pregnancy diagnosis

The clinical signs of pregnancy include increased bodyweight and abdominal enlargement (these signs are often apparent in all but young queens) and mammary development, which is obvious from approximately day 40. These changes are usually diagnostic for pregnancy, since pseudopregnancy is not common and is not usually associated with clinical signs.

Abdominal palpation

Conceptual swellings can be palpated from approximately 21 days after mating. These are discrete until 30 days after mating but become more difficult to palpate from this time onwards.

Identification of fetal heartbeats

In late pregnancy the fetal heartbeats may be auscultated using a stethoscope. At this time it is also usually possible to palpate the fetus in all but the most obese cats.

Radiography

From day 30 it is possible to detect uterine enlargement with good-quality radiographs. Mineralization of the fetal skeleton is detectable radiographically from 40 days after mating.

Ultrasound examination

Diagnostic B-mode ultrasonography may be used for pregnancy diagnosis in the cat. The pregnancy length can be assessed from mating time, unlike in the bitch. Conceptuses can be imaged from 12 days after mating and embryonic tissue can usually be seen from day 14. From this time onwards it is possible to identify pregnancy, confirm fetal viability and assess fetal growth. It is more difficult to assess the number of kittens in later pregnancy.

Hormone tests

Plasma concentrations of progesterone are elevated in both pregnancy and pseudopregnancy, therefore measurement of this hormone is not diagnostic. Plasma relaxin concentrations are elevated from day 25; this hormone is diagnostic of pregnancy and can be measured as described for the bitch.

Duration of pregnancy

The average length of pregnancy in the queen is 65 days, with a range of 64–68 days.

Care of the queen during pregnancy

During the second half of pregnancy there is an increase in food intake and in the requirement for both carbohydrate and protein. Provided that diet is well balanced and contains suitable amounts of vitamins and minerals, it is not necessary to provide extra supplementation.

Many queens continue to be active during pregnancy and the amount of exercise is best limited by the individual cat.

It is advisable to ensure that routine vaccination has been performed prior to mating.

Pregnancy in the mare

Pregnancy diagnosis

Ultrasound examination

Ultrasound examination per rectum (see Chapter 18) has become the most reliable technique and can be used from day 10 post-ovulation. In reality, ultrasound examination at day 14–16 is used to diagnose pregnancy most effectively and to manage mares that present with twin embryos. In the mare the embryonic vesicle stays spherical for much longer than in other species.

- **Days 10–16:** At day 10, small vesicles are spherical and can be found anywhere in the uterus. At day 16 the vesicles are still spherical and are usually found at the caudal portion of one of the uterine horns. During these early days of pregnancy the vesicle will have bright echogenic poles. These are not associated with the embryonic disc and are an imaging artefact. During these early days the vesicle grows very quickly.
- **Days 17–22:** The vesicle has a growth plateau between days 17 and 26. After day 17 the vesicle is often irregular in shape (Figure 26.18). This is thought to be due to increased tone and thickness of the uterine wall. Using ultrasonography, the embryo is first visualized within the vesicle at day 20–25, and is most commonly observed in the ventral position. The heartbeat is usually detected after day 22 and is used to determine embryonic health and wellbeing.
- **Days 22–55:** At day 24, the allantois can be seen. As the allantois expands, the yolk sac contracts and so, by day 40, the embryo is lifted dorsally in the vesicle. After day 40, the yolk sac degenerates and the umbilical cord is formed, which allows the embryo to drop down to the ventral portion of the vesicle once again by day 50.

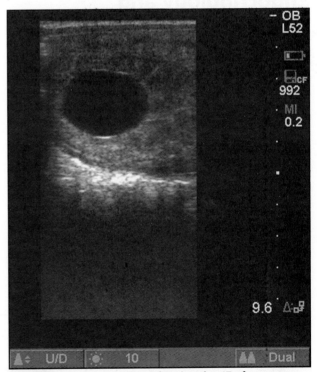

26.18 Ultrasound image showing day 17 of pregnancy in a mare. The embryo appears as a fluid-filled (black) vesicle. The bright areas at the top and bottom are enhancement artefacts.

Indirect pregnancy tests

The first maternal recognition of pregnancy is thought to occur at about 48 hours post-fertilization with the production of a protein called 'early pregnancy factor' (EPF). This protein has been detected in horses, humans, sheep and mice. It may prove useful in the future for detecting early pregnancy but is NOT used at this time.

- **Equine chorionic gonadatrophin (eCG):** This hormone, also known as PMSG, is produced by the endometrial cups (see below). eCG is used as the basis for a pregnancy test in mares from day 40. The test can have false positives, with pregnancy having been lost but the endometrial cups remaining. It is useful for wild equids and very small ponies.
- **Oestrone sulphate:** This assay can be used from day 60–70 onwards, although laboratories will recommend samples be taken at 100–120 days of gestation. The oestrone sulphate is produced by precursors from the fetal gonadal tissue and is then converted into oestrogen sulphate in the placenta. It is an indicator of fetal viability since it is only produced in the presence of a viable fetus.
- **Progesterone:** This may be used for pregnancy diagnosis but it is important to note that elevated progesterone levels are an indication of luteal tissue and NOT of pregnancy itself. However, if blood taken from a mare 18–22 days after the last ovulation still shows elevated progesterone levels, it suggests that an active corpus luteum is still present and therefore the mare may be pregnant, as she would otherwise be in oestrus at this time.

Endocrinology and maintenance of pregnancy

The hormonal changes that occur during pregnancy are shown in Figure 26.19. Endocrinological assays have been outdated by ultrasonography in determining pregnancy in the mare (see above). They are, however, a useful tool in some situations.

Progesterone

This hormone is essential for the maintenance of pregnancy in horses (and other species).

- **Primary corpus luteum** describes the corpus luteum that is present following the ovulation that led to the pregnancy. The primary corpus luteum persists because of the inhibition of PGF2-alpha secretion described above.
- After day 35–40 of pregnancy, ECG stimulates the production of additional follicles on both ovaries, which lead to **secondary corpora lutea**.

- Primary and secondary corpora lutea persist until after day 160 but are virtually gone by day 210. Both produce progesterone.
- The fetoplacental unit begins to secrete progesterone from day 60 and by day 100 is producing sufficient progesterone to maintain pregnancy. Pregnancy in the mare, therefore, is maintained by the placenta after day 100–120 of gestation.

Equine chorionic gonadatrophin (eCG) – also known as 'pregnant mare serum gonadatrophin' (PMSG)

- Cells from the embryo attach to the endometrium at about day 35, and form endometrial cups, which produce eCG.
- In the mare, eCG has mainly LH-like effects. It causes resurgence of the primary corpus luteum and luteinization of the secondary corpora lutea. It is also involved in the maternal immunotolerance of foreign antigens produced by the fetus.
- In other species, eCG also has FSH activity and it is widely used as a 'superovulatory' drug in sheep, cattle, goats, deer, dogs and cats. It is marketed as 'PMSG'.

Oestrogens

- Maternal serum oestrogen levels rise from about day 35 of pregnancy. This rise does NOT occur unless there is a functional corpus luteum. eCG from the endometrial cups apparently stimulates luteal steroidogenesis, resulting in increased oestrogen synthesis and secretion from corpus luteum tissue.
- After day 45, additional oestrogens are produced by the fetoplacental unit and released into the maternal circulation. Oestrogen levels peak at around 210–250 days and then slowly decline.
- Oestrogens are thought to play a role in the development of the vascular supply and endometrial hypertrophy during pregnancy.

Duration of pregnancy

The gestation of a mare is approximately 342 days, although mares can go >12 months and still produce a normal foal. If a foal leaves the uterus at 300 days or less it is considered to be an abortion. The minimum gestation that is required to have any hope of a viable foal is 330 days.

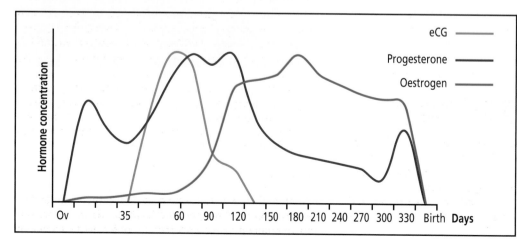

26.19 Hormone concentrations during pregnancy in the mare. Ov = ovulation. Adapted from McKinnon and Voss (1993).

Care of the mare during pregnancy

Trace element supplementation

A mare that receives a balanced diet does not strictly require any extra trace element supplementation; however, commercial feeds are available for the pregnant mare.

Vaccinations

A mare should have equine herpesvirus-1 (EHV-1) vaccinations at 5, 7 and 9 months of gestation. This is to avoid abortion caused by EHV-1. Mares should also receive a tetanus booster at around 4 weeks prior to parturition. This is to ensure good levels of tetanus antibody in the colostrum. Some studs also vaccinate mares for rotavirus if this has been a problem in the past. Rotavirus can cause diarrhoea in young foals and there are commercial rotavirus vaccines available; these should be given according to the manufacturer's recommendations.

Anthelmintics

Most anthelmintics are authorized for use in pregnant mares. While there is little evidence to suggest that a periparturient rise in faecal eggs occurs in the mare, regular worming is very important as foals can be infected and have a worm burden as young as 2 weeks. Clean pastures are therefore essential on a stud farm. When using anthelmintics in foals it is important to check the datasheets before use.

Abnormalities of pregnancy in the bitch and queen

Resorption and abortion

A great concern for owners is the risk of resorption or abortion during pregnancy. To understand the differences in these processes, it is necessary to define the stages of development. In general the term **embryo** is used when the characteristics of the conceptus are not discernable. From approximately 35 days after ovulation the characteristics of a puppy become obvious and the term **fetus** is used.

- **Resorption** refers to the resorption of the entire conceptus and occurs during the embryonic stage of development.
- **Abortion** refers to the expulsion of the fetus and the fetal membranes before term (i.e. before 58 days after ovulation).
- A **stillbirth** is the expulsion of the fetus and fetal membranes after day 58 (i.e. close to term).

The incidence of resorption or abortion of the entire litter is not known, but it is certain that up to 5% of bitches and queens suffer isolated resorption of one or two conceptuses, with continuation of the remaining pregnancy.

There are many potential causes of resorption and abortion, including infectious agents, trauma, fetal defects and maternal environment.

- In the dog, the infectious agents *Brucella canis* (not present in the UK), canine distemper virus, canine herpesvirus and *Toxoplasma gondii* have all been implicated as causes of abortion and resorption. It is possible to vaccinate the bitch against canine herpesvirus (see Chapter 5); the vaccine is given on two occasions during pregnancy and is very effective in reducing subsequent pregnancy loss, stillbirths and fading pups.
- In the cat, feline herpesvirus 1, feline panleucopenia virus, feline leukaemia virus, feline coronavirus (FIP) and *Toxoplasma gondii* infection may produce abortion, resorption or stillbirths.

In many cases embryonic death and pregnancy loss are best assessed using real-time diagnostic B-mode ultrasonography. Resorptions may not be recognized by the owner unless associated with a period of illness. Abortion of fetal tissue may be obvious, but may not be noticed should the dam eat the aborted material. In the face of an abortion, there is little that can be administered to the patient except supportive therapy.

Hypoglycaemia

Pregnancy hypoglycaemia has been reported in the bitch and is associated with reduced blood glucose concentrations during late pregnancy. The clinical signs include weakness that may progress to coma. The condition may be confused with hypocalcaemia, which occurs at a similar time (see later).

Parturition in the bitch and queen

Preparation for parturition in the bitch

In the last few weeks of pregnancy, attempts should be made to encourage the bitch to accept a nest in a suitable place for parturition and rearing. Ideally, this should be a warm, clean, draught- and damp-proof room that can be heated. The room is best isolated from the main thoroughfare of the household, where the bitch can rest quietly, but it is beneficial for socializing the litter if noises from washing machines, radios and people talking can be heard. The room should be of a sufficient size to allow the growing litter to play and, where possible, for puppies to have access to an outside area (should the weather permit).

The room should contain a whelping bed. The bed should be large enough to allow the dam to stretch and have sufficient room for a large litter. The sides should be high enough to prevent the puppies escaping until they are approximately 4 weeks old.

In some cases, particularly in a bitch with a long or thick hair coat, it might be useful to remove some of the coat from around the perineum and ventral abdomen prior to the whelping. This will help the puppies gain access to the nipples and allows cleaning of the dam after parturition.

Heating

Hypothermia is a major cause of neonatal mortality and so the environmental temperature is critical. Neonates are unable to regulate their own temperature for the first week of life and rely on the dam and other neonates to keep warm. A chilled neonate will not respond normally, move properly or be able to suck, and this may result in it being neglected by the dam. It is therefore recommended that the room must be able to be heated to 25–30°C for the first few days of the neonates' life. This temperature is often unbearable for the dam and so can be safely reduced to approximately 22°C after this time. It is most important that the litter is kept well away from any draughts that might chill them.

The room can easily be warmed using a thermostatically controlled heater. A heat lamp can be suspended over the bed, but care must be taken to ensure that the neonates do not overheat. It is recommended that perhaps only half the bed or box is heated, so that the dam can move out of the heat if she wishes. Well protected hot-water bottles or circulating water blankets provide good alternatives.

Useful equipment

A plentiful supply of newspaper is necessary for the area. Plenty of bedding that can easily be removed when soiled should be available. Shredded paper can be used but with care, since very small neonates may get caught up in it. If using a fabric bedding material, then at least three or four of these will be needed. A supply of blankets will suffice.

Scales, a clock and a notepad are useful, to enable a record to be kept of the times of birth and weights of neonates. A thermometer should be kept in order to record the dam's rectal temperature prior to parturition.

Sometimes dams can be clumsy at the time of parturition. If there is a large litter, it may be useful to put some of the neonates out of harm's way in a small box within the nesting bed. It is important to ensure that the neonates are kept warm whilst away from their mother. This can be achieved by wrapping a hot-water bottle in some towels and placing it in the bottom of the box.

A supply of milk substitute can be offered to the dam during parturition. No food should be offered at this time, in the event that the dam gets into difficulty and requires veterinary intervention.

There should be suitable equipment to facilitate the artificial rearing of the neonates should this be required. This should include small syringes, feeding bottles and teats and substitute milk for feeding the neonates, along with cotton wool for cleaning any spilt milk off them and to aid urination and defecation if the dam is unable to care for them at all.

Stages of parturition

In the last week of pregnancy it is prudent to record the dam's rectal temperature at least twice daily. This is to detect the prepartum hypothermia that precedes the onset of parturition by 24–36 hours. This decline in body temperature is mediated by a sudden reduction in the plasma concentration of progesterone. The rectal temperature usually changes from approximately 39°C to below 37°C.

There are five stages of parturition:

- Preparation
- First stage (onset of contractions)
- Second stage (propulsion of fetus)
- Third stage (passage of placenta)
- Puerperium (after parturition).

Preparation stage

The preparation stage is associated with the decline in plasma progesterone concentration and hence the decrease in rectal temperature. At this time the vaginal and perineal tissue will relax and the dam may show some signs of impending parturition.

She may start to prepare her nest by shredding and ripping up the bedding and may be more restless than usual. She may also show an increased mucous discharge from her vulva, which will probably be slightly more swollen. It is important to remember that some bitches may show no signs of preparation at all.

Some bitches may seek the company of others, while some will try to find solace in a quiet place on their own. Few bitches will be happy with an audience for whelping and so it is best if just one person can stay with the bitch for the birth. Many queens will seek seclusion to give birth to their kittens, preferring not to have people around them at this time.

First stage of parturition

The first stage of parturition commences with the onset of uterine contractions and can be 1–12 hours in duration, but this is very variable. By this time, milk is usually present within the mammary glands or should appear at this stage.

With the onset of contractions the bitch might become increasingly restless, pant and/or shiver and her nesting behaviour might become more frantic. Some bitches will refuse food at this time or may vomit their last meal. Most cats will seek seclusion at this time.

The uterine contractions will push the fetus against the cervix, which has begun to dilate. This may result in the rupture of the allantochorion and so allantoic fluid may then be produced from the vulva.

Second stage of parturition

The second stage is characterized by an increase in uterine contractions; the onset of abdominal contractions and propulsion of the fetus through the cervix into the vagina. These will begin when the first fetus enters the pelvic canal. The contractions are normally quite noticeable. The bitch will appear to squeeze from her ribs towards the perineal area and then relax.

The time of the first contractions should be recorded, in case there is any delay in the whelping. The time between the onset of straining and the birth of the first puppy is variable. It can be as short as 10 minutes or up to 30 minutes or longer, particularly in maiden bitches. If the bitch continues to have contractions as described earlier, for more than one hour without producing a puppy, or if her waters have broken and a puppy has not been produced, the veterinary surgeon should be contacted. It may be necessary for the veterinary surgeon to attend the bitch to assess whether she is experiencing dystocia and whether assistance is required for the delivery.

Most bitches will be in lateral recumbency during whelping, but some prefer to stand. Delivery of the head is often the most difficult part of the birth and may be associated with some pain, but once this is delivered the rest of the puppy is usually delivered rapidly.

A membrane, the amnion, surrounds the fetus and is often seen at the vulva during straining. It may appear and then disappear with the contractions, and it may rupture spontaneously or be broken by the dam. The puppy may also be born within it.

After delivery, the dam will normally commence vigorous licking, removing the membranes and clearing fluid from around the neonate's face. If the dam fails to remove the membranes immediately after the birth, it must be done for her swiftly. Occasionally young or inexperienced bitches may need help and encouragement with the immediate licking and cleaning. This can be achieved using a clean soft towel. The neonate should be given a vigorous rub with a towel to stimulate it, to help to clear the airways of any fluid and to dry it so as to avoid chilling. When rubbing a neonate it is recommended that the animal is held with its head lower than its bottom (to aid the drainage of fluid from its lungs).

The birth of the fetus is usually followed by the passage of the allantochorion or placenta (**afterbirth**). Normally a dam separates the neonate from the placenta by chewing through the cord and then eating the placenta when it is expelled. It is important to ensure that the dam does not chew the umbilicus excessively, as this can cause damage to the neonate. If the dam does not sever the umbilicus, the placenta can be separated by tearing or cutting the cord using scissors. Care must be taken if the cord is to be torn. The procedure can be achieved by holding the cord an inch or so away from the neonate's abdomen and tearing the cord with the other hand. The dam should be given every opportunity to clean and fuss over the neonate before it is removed for weighing and checking, etc. (see below).

Once all the procedures have been carried out, the neonate can be returned to the dam. The neonates are best left with their mother during the remainder of the delivery, as removing them might distress the dam, inhibiting further straining. If the dam is young, inexperienced or particularly clumsy, it can be a good idea to put a few of the neonates in a warm box, once the dam has attended to them. This will keep them safer whilst the dam continues giving birth.

Third stage of parturition

The third stage is the passage of the placenta. In the bitch and the queen the passage of the placenta occurs usually during the second stage of parturition, but occasionally one or more young are delivered without their placenta one each, which is expelled at a later stage or delivered with subsequent young. It is useful to count the number of placentas passed, as a larger number of young compared with the number of placentas may indicate that the dam has retained one or more placentas; this condition is rare however.

After a bitch has finished whelping, there is normally a dark vulval discharge. This contains a green pigment that originates from the placenta. This discharge should normally decline after about a week.

Puerperium

The puerperium is the period after parturition during which the reproductive tract returns to its normal non-pregnant state. During this time the uterus starts its involution and it is common to see a mucoid vulval discharge that may last for up to 6 weeks.

Parturition in the mare

The foaling environment

A foaling mare should not be placed in a strange environment or be handled by strangers immediately prior to parturition. Any sudden changes may delay foaling. Ideally, mares should be placed in the foaling environment 2–3 weeks prior to their expected foaling date. Mares can foal in a variety of locations, depending on the weather and facilities available. Whatever the choice of foaling location, the environment should be clean, have adequate space, and be reasonably quiet.

- Mares due to foal during the cooler months will require a large (14 ft x 14 ft (4.27 m x 4.27 m minimum), clean foaling stable. For mares foaling in a stable, the stable should be freshly bedded with clean, dry straw. An 20–25 cm thick bed of straw will decrease chances of infection, and is easier to clean. Safety of the mare and foal should be kept in mind when selecting a foaling stable. Stables should be constructed to allow isolation of the mare and the safety to the newborn foal.
- During warm weather, many breeders choose to allow their mares to foal in the paddock. Mares foaling in paddocks should either be isolated or have sufficient space to separate themselves from any other horses in the pasture. Additionally, the pasture should be examined for possible hazards to the foal. A shelter should be provided in case of wet or cold weather.
- Regardless of the location, the foaling area should be isolated and quiet. In a bid to minimize disturbances, many breeders install CCTV to watch their mares. This is especially useful considering that the majority of mares foal at night.

Signs of impending parturition

Due to the variable gestational length shown in horses, it can be difficult to predict exactly when the mare will give birth. Mares vary tremendously in the signs that they exhibit; some show many signs of impending parturition, whereas others show none at all. Signs that can help include the following:

- Mammary development begins 2–6 weeks prepartum. Major changes normally occur within 2 weeks of term. The mammary gland distends with colostrum 2–3 days prepartum and the teats accumulate a 'crusty' golden/yellow substance on their tips, called 'wax'
- Electrolyte measurements in mammary gland secretions will often show decreasing sodium and increasing potassium concentrations (Figure 26.20) 48 hours prior to parturition. At term, calcium concentration in the secretions will be >40 mmol/l

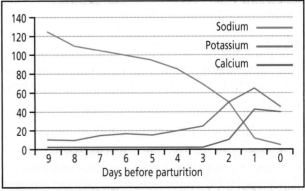

26.20   The changes in electrolyte concentrations that occur towards the end of pregnancy can be used to detect impending parturition in the mare.

- Relaxation of sacrosciatic ligaments (ligaments next to tail) and vulva, so the 'tail head' appears to rise
- Relaxation of the cervix (may occur 0–30 days prepartum).

The stages of parturition

First stage

This involves the mare getting up and down, which is *thought* to play an important role in getting the fetus into position. A radiographic study showed that the full-term equine fetus lies in a ventral position (i.e. upside down) with its poll/neck and forelimbs flexed. With the progression of first- stage labour, the foal rotates the front of its body 180 degrees and then extends its neck and forelimbs. Mare movement possibly aids this re-positioning. Mares have control over first-stage labour and are able to interrupt this stage if they feel disturbed.

Second stage

The best way to describe second stage labour is 'explosive'. The time from chorioallantoic rupture and the appearance of amnion should take as little as 10 minutes, with the foal delivered within 20–30 minutes. The same principles of presentation apply to the foal compared to other farm species; that is to say, 'normally' presented foals are delivered with their forelimbs just before their heads. One front limb should also be slightly ahead of the other, to narrow the width at the shoulders. This is called an anterior presentation. A posterior presentation, which accounts for around 1% of all foalings, is hindlimbs first.

Third stage

Expulsion of membranes takes place within 2–3 hours. **Retention of fetal membranes for more than 4–5 hours is considered a veterinary emergency.**

Dystocia in the bitch and queen

The term **dystocia** literally means difficult birth; it is used to indicate any problem that interferes with normal birth. Dystocia is rare in the queen but problems are not uncommon in the bitch, especially in brachycephalic breeds such as the Bulldog and Boston Terrier. The two main causes of dystocia are maternal factors and fetal factors.

Maternal dystocia

Maternal dystocia may be divided into two categories: poor straining efforts by the dam and obstruction of the birth canal.

Poor straining efforts of the dam

Poor straining may be the result of nervousness or pain that inhibits normal parturition, but it is more commonly the result of poor myometrial contractions, a condition that has been termed **uterine inertia**. Inertia may be primary, in which case parturition does not commence, or may be secondary to some other factor occurring during parturition.

Primary uterine inertia

This is rare in the queen but is seen not uncommonly in young bitches with only one or two puppies, or in older overweight bitches with large litters. The cause of the condition is unknown, but it may relate to poor condition of the uterine musculature in fat or debilitated animals, overstretching of the uterus when the litter size is large, poor stimulus for parturition when there are only a few fetuses or low plasma calcium concentrations.

The endocrinological events of parturition are usually normal, but subsequent uterine contractions are not fully initiated and parturition does not follow. A green vulval discharge, which indicates placental separation, may be seen some days after the expected date of parturition. In some cases the owner may have observed initial weak uterine contractions or have noted the decline in body temperature. At this stage the administration of the hormone oxytocin may stimulate uterine contractions. Some cases may respond to the intravenous administration of calcium borogluconate. Repeated doses of oxytocin may be necessary but oxytocin should only be given when it is certain that there is no obstruction to the birth canal. It is not possible in the bitch to assess the patency of the cervix by digital palpation (the vagina of an average 20 kg bitch is 20 cm long). In certain cases a caesarean operation may be necessary.

Primary uterine inertia may be anticipated in some bitches because of a previous history of this problem or because of their age, physical condition or the number of puppies. The best assessment of the bitch is to monitor the rectal temperature twice daily during the last 7–10 days of pregnancy.

Secondary uterine inertia

This is the cessation of uterine contractions after they have started. Most commonly it is the result of uterine exhaustion following obstructive dystocia, but it may occur spontaneously during the second stage of parturition, presumably because of factors similar to those seen with primary uterine inertia. If the cause of the dystocia can be relieved, the administration of oxytocin and calcium may be suitable. In some cases caesarean operation may be necessary.

Obstruction of the birth canal

Obstruction may be the result of abnormalities of the birth canal, such as:

- Deformity of the pelvic bones – these may be congenital malformations, developmental abnormalities or the result of previous trauma, commonly following a road accident
- Soft tissue abnormalities within the pelvis which press against the reproductive tract – they might include pelvic neoplasms, though these are rare in animals of breeding age
- Abnormality of the reproductive tract itself – for example, torsion of the uterus or congenital vaginal or uterine constrictions.

Fetal dystocia

Fetal oversize

Oversize of the fetus relative to the birth canal may be the result of:

- Breed conformation – dystocia may be considered almost normal for certain breeds with exaggerated physical characteristics such as a large head size
- Actual fetal oversize – when the litter size is small and large fetuses develop within the uterus
- Fetal abnormalities – including fetal 'monsters', resulting in relative oversize and dystocia.

In the majority of these cases a caesarean operation is necessary for delivery of the fetuses, whether normal or abnormal.

Abnormalities of fetal alignment

Variation from the normal presentation, position and posture of the fetus during delivery may result in dystocia. This may be corrected in certain cases by manipulation via the vagina; however, caesarean operation may be necessary.

- The **presentation** of a fetus is a description of the direction of its long axis in relation to the long axis of the dam (Figure 26.21). Puppies and kittens can only be delivered in longitudinal presentation (i.e. the long axis of the fetus is parallel to the long axis of the dam) but may have either anterior (fetal head delivered first) or posterior (fetus delivered backwards) presentation.
- The **position** of a fetus is a description of its dorsal axis with respect to the dorsum of the dam; this describes the degree of rotation of the fetus. Most species are normally born in dorsal position; i.e. the back of the fetus is uppermost in the same orientation as the dam.
- The **posture** of a fetus is a description of the orientation of the head and legs, which may be extended or flexed. For anterior presentation the head must be extended, and this occurs naturally during a posterior presentation.

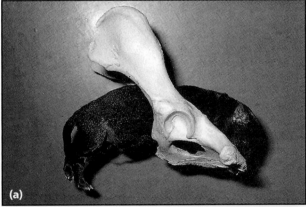

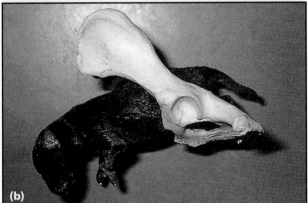

26.21 Presentation of a fetus: **(a)** normal anterior presentation; **(b)** normal posterior presentation. continues ▶

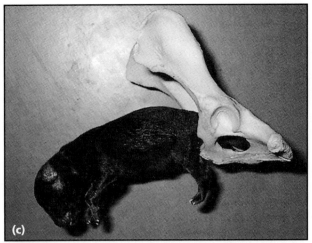

26.21 *continued* Presentation of a fetus: **(c)** breech presentation.

A **breech birth** refers to a fetus delivered in posterior longitudinal presentation, usually in dorsal position with the hindlimbs flexed. This means that the fetus is presented 'bottom first' with its hindlimbs directed towards the dam's head. A fetus delivered in posterior presentation with the legs extended is not a breech presentation.

Recognition of dystocia

The normal events of parturition, as outlined above, should be clearly understood so that recognition of dystocia can be achieved rapidly, allowing prompt intervention.

Collection of a relevant history is essential in the evaluation of a potential case of dystocia. This includes the estimation of the stage of pregnancy. Determination of the mating time is most helpful for establishing the stage of pregnancy in queens but is not very useful for bitches, where apparent pregnancy length can vary between 56 and 72 days from mating (see above). Regular monitoring of rectal temperature is therefore essential in the bitch. It should be established whether this has been done by the owner and, if so, what changes were observed.

Of particular importance is the time course of events from the onset of parturition, e.g. the onset of behavioural changes such as restlessness, nest making and panting. The time when straining first occurred and the character of the straining efforts may also be useful as an indicator of dystocia, as will the times that any young were produced.

It is not possible to give definite guidelines regarding potential cases of dystocia but examination of the patient is warranted in certain situations:

- A bitch that has exceeded 70 days from the last mating and has no signs of impending parturition
- A queen that has exceeded 65 days from the last mating and has no signs of impending parturition
- The dam is unsettled and strains forcefully but infrequently
- There are signs of straining which then cease
- There is a black/green vulval discharge with no signs of parturition
- There has been a decline in rectal temperature and parturition has not commenced within 48 hours
- There has been ineffectual straining for 1 hour or more, i.e. the bitch has been having regular contractions, but a puppy has not been produced

- Several young have been produced, the last more than 2 hours ago and the dam is restless
- Several young have been produced, the last more than 2 hours ago and a larger litter is expected (may not be known by the owner).

Investigation

In most cases it is necessary to ensure that the animal is pregnant and/or that viable fetuses remain within the uterus. This can be achieved by transabdominal palpation, auscultation of fetal heartbeats, real-time ultrasonography and radiography, as described earlier for pregnancy diagnosis.

Further investigation involves digital examination of the vagina to assess whether a fetus is present and to establish fetal alignment. This should only be performed after cleaning the vulval area thoroughly with an antiseptic solution and scrubbing the hands or wearing surgical gloves. A water-soluble lubricant should be applied to the fingers, and the vestibule and vagina should be carefully examined. The presence of bone or soft-tissue abnormalities of the pelvis should be noted. The presentation, position and posture of the fetus should be established before any further intervention is contemplated.

For normal presentations, delivery can be assisted using the thumb and forefinger placed in a cradle manner around the fetal head (anterior presentation) or pelvis (posterior presentation). Traction should only be applied during the straining effort of the bitch, but pressure on the roof of the vagina may be applied with the finger to stimulate straining. Sterile gauze or similar fabric may help to grip the puppy or kitten when assisting delivery. Undue force should never be applied to the feet, as these are easily damaged or deformed.

Caesarean operation

There are a number of reasons for performing a caesarean operation. In many cases this may be for the relief of dystocia, whilst occasionally it may be an elective procedure when there is concern over fetomaternal disproportion. Surgical factors are considered in Chapter 25.

Anaesthesia

It is important to remember that there are several marked physiological changes during pregnancy that may affect the requirements for anaesthesia. These physiological changes result in decreased minimum alveolar concentrations of anaesthetic gases, an increased oxygen requirement, and commonly hypoventilation and subsequent hypoxia and hypercarbia. In addition, in cases of dystocia, the animal may be debilitated and may have recently been fed.

The general aims are to:

- Ensure adequate oxygenation (intubation and oxygen administration)
- Maintain blood volume and prevent hypotension (intravenous fluid therapy)
- Minimize depression of the fetus and dam during and after surgery (reduce the dose of anaesthetic agents used).

There are many anaesthetic regimes suitable for this procedure, including the use of volatile agents for induction and maintenance of anaesthesia and the use of rapid-acting intravenous induction agents (such as propofol) followed by maintenance of anaesthesia using a volatile inhalational anaesthetic (see Chapter 23).

Complications

Complications of caesarean operation in bitches and queens include:

- Anaesthetic risks in the dam and the neonate
- Risks during surgery of uterine rupture and haemorrhage resulting in hypovolaemia
- Postoperative risks, including wound infection and wound breakdown
- Interference with the wound by neonates trying to suckle
- Problems in the dam of accepting the litter.

Some veterinary surgeons prefer to perform the operation via a flank incision to avoid the problem of wound interference when the neonates try to suckle.

The problem of rejection of the litter by a young dam after a caesarean operation may be overcome by placing the offspring with the dam as soon as possible after surgery. The mother's milk should be squeezed on to the newborn's heads if rejection is a problem. The dam should be carefully observed until she is able to coordinate sufficiently not to damage them and she must not be left unattended until successful suckling has been noted.

Dystocia in the mare

The incidence of dystocia is very low in horses when compared to other farmed species, but does vary from breed to breed. Thoroughbreds are thought to have an incidence of 4–5% compared to 8–12% for draught breeds and Shetlands. Long fetal limbs and necks are usually the cause of the problem. **Equine dystocia is a true emergency and is the difference between a live and a dead foal.** This is in contrast to bovine practice, where the practitioner would not be unduly concerned if a cow had been calving for 2–3 hours, as a live offspring is still likely. A combination of powerful abdominal contractions and early separation of the placenta ensure this is virtually never the case with equine dystocias.

The causes of dystocia are similar to those for other species, and the basic approach is also similar. Sedation is often required to facilitate a thorough examination and, due to the size of the mare, anaesthesia may be employed to allow the foal to be delivered. Hygiene is of utmost importance if metritis is to be avoided.

The commonest cause of dystocia in the Thoroughbred is 'contracted foal syndrome'. Such cases always require a caesarean operation to minimize injury to the mare's reproductive tract. The expulsive efforts of the mare and the length of fetal limbs make catastrophes quite common. Foals die very quickly and a caesarean operation will at least preserve the mare.

Manipulation of the fetus

Once the mare has been restrained, manipulation (repositioning of the foal) may be undertaken. This is very difficult in fetuses near the end of gestation. It is most frequently carried out under a general anaesthetic with the hind end of the mare hoisted high, allowing repulsion and repositioning of the foal's limbs. In **repulsion**, the fetus is pushed back into the uterus, where space is available, and the position or posture is corrected. It is always necessary to repel before attempting manipulations. In **rotation**, the fetus is turned on its long axis to bring it into a dorsal position. The hind end of the mare is then lowered prior to traction and, hopefully, delivery. In the mare there is a high risk of uterine rupture because of the long neck and limbs of the fetus. If the foal cannot be delivered within 15 minutes, another option should be considered.

Caesarean operation

This is a major procedure in the mare and must be performed in a hospital environment if a good prognosis is to be achieved. Indications include:

- Transverse presentation
- Uterine torsion
- Malposture of living fetus that cannot be corrected rapidly
- Maternal pelvic deformities.

The time from induction of anaesthesia to foal removal should be <20 minutes. The usual approach is through a mid-line laparotomy. Postoperative complications may include infection, laminitis and retained placenta.

Embryotomy

Embryotomy refers to the sectioning of a dead foal *in utero* to facilitate vaginal delivery. Specialized tools are used to minimize damage to the reproductive tract but almost invariably some trauma does occur to the mare. The cervix is the most likely structure to be affected, which can have a serious effect on the mare's future fertility. Embryotomy should therefore be an act of 'last resort', when a caesarean operation is not an option.

The postpartum period

The bitch and queen
Postparturient care of the dam

Once the dam has finished giving birth she should be cleaned, paying particular attention to her perineum. This will make her feel more comfortable. She should now be given the opportunity to exercise and urinate or defecate. Usually the dam will then settle with her litter during feeding. Soiled bedding should be changed for clean, fresh material.

The dam should then be offered some food. It must be remembered that, depending on the amount of afterbirths she has eaten, if any, she may be prone to gastrointestinal upset. It is therefore recommended that for the first day or so she should be offered something nutritious but 'light'. Chicken, fish, rice and pasta are all suitable. The dam should be offered her diet in five or six small meals. This can be a pre-prepared diet specifically suitable for lactation. The amount she receives should depend on the litter size. A dam with a large litter will need significantly more food than one with only a small litter. The dam should remain on five or six small meals per day for the first few weeks. The diet should

not be altered too quickly, as this may worsen any gastrointestinal upset.

During the first 2 weeks after the birth of the litter, the dam will spend much of her time with the litter and therefore it may be preferable to feed her close to the nest. A readily accessible supply of fresh water should be close by. Once weaning begins, the dam should be encouraged to leave the nest for increasingly longer periods.

The dam should be encouraged to exercise during lactation. Where possible, to minimize the risk of infection of the litter, this should be where she will not come into contact with other animals.

Once weaning has begun and is well underway, the demands on the dam start to reduce and therefore her relevant food intake should also gradually begin to fall. If the dam has lost a great deal of weight through her efforts to feed the litter, then her food intake should remain high so that she can replace some of the lost bodyweight. When she has regained some weight her food intake can be reduced.

Normally a veterinary surgeon should be called to examine the dam when parturition is finished, in order to check her health and that of her newborn litter. Thereafter the dam's general health should also be closely monitored throughout lactation. Common problems to look for are signs of eclampsia (see later), mastitis (see later), pyrexia, and a foul-smelling vulval discharge. If any of these are observed, veterinary attention should be sought. The litter should also be closely monitored for fading syndrome (see later).

Lactation

The development of the mammary gland after puberty is under hormonal control. During pregnancy, **progesterone** from the corpus luteum causes the glands to enlarge; this is sometimes also seen in false pregnancies. Hormones are responsible for the **initiation** of milk secretion (see below). They also play a vital role in the **maintenance** of milk secretion after it has been established. The terminology used to describe the various aspects of lactation is often confused:

- **Milk secretion** refers to the synthesis of milk by the epithelial cells and the passage of milk from the cytoplasm of the cells into the alveolar lumen
- **Milk removal** includes the passive withdrawal of milk from the cisterns and sinuses and the ejection of milk from the alveolar lumina
- **Lactation** refers to the combined processes of milk secretion and removal
- **Lactogenesis** is the initiation of milk secretion
- **Mammogenesis** describes the development of the mammary gland
- **Galactopoiesis** refers to the enhancement of established lactation.

In the bitch, there is a long luteal phase in both pregnancy and non-pregnancy. Progesterone primes the mammary glands; mammary gland secretion and the development of obvious clinical signs of pregnancy (and pseudopregnancy) is associated with a rise in plasma concentration of prolactin, which commences at 30–35 days after the LH surge. Prolactin is the principal luteotrophic factor in the bitch. Prolactin concentration continues to increase during late pregnancy to a plateau at approximately day 60. Prolactin concentration surges during the prepartum decline in progesterone, and reaches a peak at or shortly after parturition.

Initiation of milk secretion

The hormonal control of the initiation of lactation has not been fully investigated in the bitch and queen. It is likely to be either a rise in the blood concentrations of prolactin and glucocorticoids at the time of parturition, or a decrease in the concentrations of compounds that have an inhibitory effect on the milk secretion process, namely progesterone and transcortin.

Prior to parturition, lipid and protein granules form in the epithelial cells and accumulate in the lumen of the alveolus as colostrum. **Colostrum** is the first milk produced and is a source of antibodies for the neonate. In the bitch and queen, antibodies are present in the milk for several days after parturition. Antibodies are readily absorbed on the first day after birth, the rate of absorption varies for different antibodies and the intestinal tract ceases to absorb different antibodies at different times. As a general rule, puppies and kittens should have sucked (or be given colostrum) within 8 hours of birth, ideally within the first few hours.

Oxytocin secreted by the posterior pituitary gland in the few hours around parturition enables the release or 'letdown' of milk in response to sucking by the neonate. Continuation of sucking is necessary to maintain the production of milk.

Milk

Milk is the liquid produced after the colostrum. The composition of milk varies between species: milk produced by the bitch and queen is more concentrated and contains more protein and twice as much fat as cow's milk. The average composition of canine and feline milk is shown in Figure 26.22. The basic milk sugar is lactose. A variety of milk substitutes are commercially available and these are discussed later.

Constituent	Quantity
Water	70–90%
Fat	0–30%
Protein	1–15%
Carbohydrate	3–7%
Minerals	0.5–1% calcium phosphate, magnesium, sodium, potassium and chloride. Deficient in iron and copper. Traces of iodine, cobalt, tin and silica
Vitamins	A, B2, B5, E, K. Low in C and D

26.22 The average composition of canine and feline milk.

The mare

Uterine involution occurs by 6–10 days postpartum. Little endometrial tissue is lost following parturition; vaginal discharge should therefore be scant. Mares are able to be re-bred after only 10 days. Delayed involution is a problem that can be identified when the mare is examined prior to breeding.

Periparturient abnormalities in the bitch and queen

There are several conditions that may occur during late pregnancy or soon after parturition in both the domestic bitch and the queen. Some conditions are emergencies; prompt recognition of the clinical signs is essential to allow successful treatment.

Hypocalcaemia (eclampsia, puerperal tetany)

Low plasma concentrations of calcium are related to calcium loss in the milk and poor dietary calcium availability. The condition can be seen during late pregnancy or early lactation but is most common 10–30 days after whelping. It is rare in the queen. The clinical signs include restlessness, panting, increased salivation, tremors and a stiff gait that may progress to muscle fasciculations, pyrexia and tachycardia. If untreated, seizures and death result. The slow administration of calcium borogluconate by intravenous injection produces a rapid resolution of the clinical signs. During administration, cardiac rate and rhythm should be monitored. Calcium supplementation may then be given orally or by subcutaneous injection to prevent recurrence of the condition. The litter should be hand-fed and older litters weaned.

Placental retention

The retention of placental tissue is uncommon in both the bitch and the queen. Placentas are normally delivered following each puppy or kitten (see above) and may be quickly eaten by the dam. If a placenta is retained, the clinical signs are a persistent green vulval discharge. This should be differentiated from the normal haemorrhagic discharge that may persist for 1 week after parturition (a mucoid discharge may be present for up to 6 weeks). If a retained placenta is diagnosed by either ultrasound examination or palpation, the administration of oxytocin will usually allow its delivery.

Postpartum metritis

Infection and inflammation of the uterus may occur following prolonged parturition, abortion, fetal and/or placental retention or obstetrical manipulation. The clinical signs commonly include a persistent purulent vulval discharge, lethargy and pyrexia. Treatment with broad-spectrum antibiotics should be instituted immediately; fluid replacement therapy may be required. In some cases the condition may be acutely septic, resulting in dehydration and collapse, and requires aggressive treatment to prevent mortality.

Postpartum haemorrhage

Excessive blood loss after parturition may indicate uterine or vaginal tearing, or an underlying coagulation disorder. A vaginal tampon can be useful when the lesion is within the wall or the vagina, and oxytocin administration may be useful to promote uterine involution. The dam should be monitored for signs of shock and a blood transfusion may be necessary. In severe cases an exploratory laparotomy may be required.

Subinvolution of placental sites

The persistence of a blood-coloured vulval discharge for more than 6 weeks after parturition may indicate subinvolution of placental sites. This is where one or more areas of the uterus fails to involute completely and there is continued blood loss, often until revascularization at the subsequent oestrus. Most cases resolve spontaneously and require no treatment.

Uterine prolapse

Uterine prolapse is a very uncommon complication that occurs within a few hours of delivery of the last neonate. The condition requires urgent treatment, usually via a laparotomy. Trauma to the uterus means that ovariohysterectomy is frequently required.

Agalactia

Agalactia is the term often used to describe absence of milk after parturition. It is important to differentiate two conditions:

- Failure of milk production (true agalactia)
- Failure of milk letdown.

Whilst failure of milk letdown can be treated by the administration of oxytocin, this drug is not effective when there has been failure of milk production. Some success has been reported in treating bitches with failure of milk production using metoclopramide, but careful management of the litter will be required as they will require supplementary feeding with an alternative source of colostrum until lactation commences. Alternatively, the puppies may be fostered, if possible.

Mastitis

Inflammation of the mammary gland is not common in the bitch or queen, but it may have disastrous results should the dam reject the litter because of pain when suckling. It is usually the result of bacterial infection, either bloodborne or through the teat. The mammary glands are tender, warm and firm upon palpation and the milk may be contaminated with blood and inflammatory cells so that it becomes yellow, pink or brown. The dam may become lethargic and anorexic if the condition is not treated. Bathing and massaging the gland with warm water and gently removing the infected fluid may be helpful, but antibiotics are usually required. It should be remembered that these agents will be excreted in the milk and ingested by the neonates.

Postpartum complications in the mare

Postpartum pain

Most postpartum pain is associated with normal uterine contractions that probably make the mare feel 'crampy'. This seems to be most common in primiparous mares, and tends to be intermittent. There is usually a moderate increase in heart rate (although the whole process of foaling can increase the mare's heart rate), with some sweating. Administration of analgesics is indicated if the mare is getting distressed. The pain usually subsides within 1–2 hours, possibly because of the demands of the newborn foal. Severe persistent pain may be due to large colon torsion; however, this condition is usually seen 1–3 days postpartum.

Retained placenta/fetal membranes

The equine placenta is considered to be retained when it has not been passed by 3–5 hours after parturition. **It is an equine medical emergency and should be dealt with as such.** The equine placenta covers every part of the endometrium, including the non-pregnant horn, which is the most common site for retention. The retained placenta causes the rapid build-up of bacteria and their associated toxins. The proliferation of bacteria leads to the development of metritis and endotoxaemia. These conditions produce the metritis–laminitis syndrome that can lead to severely debilitating illness or death. Retention occurs in 2–10% of mares. Some mares seem to have a propensity to retain placentas after each labour. Retention of the placenta will affect fertility at the 'foal heat', i.e. the first oestrus postpartum. Oxytocin is the treatment of choice, but uterine lavage with 10 litres of sterile saline can also be performed to cause distension of the uterus and so cause release of endogenous oxytocin, which allows fetal membranes to be released and expelled.

Uterine artery rupture

Rupture of the uterine artery following parturition is thankfully not a common occurrence in brood mares. Nevertheless, most practitioners that are involved in stud medicine will have experience of this condition. The incidence seems to increase in older multiparous mares. Mares can collapse with little warning so, when dealing with this condition, personnel must be aware of the location of the exit and should avoid coming between the mare and a wall or corner. The precise aetiology is unknown, but low plasma copper concentration has been suggested as a predisposing factor. It is believed that the condition is a 'sporadic event' that cannot be predicted the first time it occurs. Most cases will bleed within 12 hours of foaling, although bleeding can occur days later.

The rupture can produce rapid fatal haemorrhage into the peritoneal cavity within an hour or two of parturition. The mare will show signs of colic, have a rapid heart rate and be sweating. Mares with very pale mucous membranes are often beyond help and so have a poor prognosis. It is, however, possible that the haemorrhage is contained in the broad ligament. Anecdotal reports of mares presenting at foal heat with large abdominal masses (haematoma) on rectal examination show the variation in clinical signs that this condition can produce.

The diagnosis is made on the basis of the clinical signs. Rectal examination in the *acutely* haemorrhaging mare would, in this author's (MH) opinion, not only be pointless but would also be dangerous to the examining veterinary surgeon. A mare that has unrelenting colic with no other significant signs would benefit from a rectal examination, and a broad ligament haematoma should be considered at this time. Ultrasonography per rectum will also be useful if a mass is palpated.

Mares that survive with haematomas in the broad ligament have been bred on the second heat postpartum with no ill effects. Some practitioners take a more conservative approach and only breed mares again when they are satisfied that sufficient repair has occurred as detected by ultrasonography before mating. The chance of the mare having another bleed in the future is debatable. In practice, it would be unlucky to see a mare twice with this condition.

Uterine artery haemorrhage can occasionally occur prepartum.

Uterine prolapse

This is an uncommon but potentially life-threatening condition that should be treated as an emergency. It has been reported in mares that have been anaesthetized to facilitate fetal delivery and presumably occurs due to the relaxation produced by the anaesthetic. The presentation the practitioner is more likely to see is prolapse due to natural foaling.

Uterine prolapse can occur following dystocia and retained fetal membranes, and starts with the inversion and prolapse of a uterine horn. It can also occur following late gestation abortion. The uterus is often damaged to some degree and must be carefully assessed for tears before replacing. Uterine artery rupture can even occur, which can lead to fatal haemorrhage. Any damage and/or infection caused by the prolapse will have a negative effect on the mare's future fertility.

Rectal prolapse

This is a very rare but serious life-threatening complication that can often lead to peritonitis. Due to irritation and prolonged abdominal effort, the caudal rectum may protrude from the anus. Damage to the rectal vasculature is common following rectal prolapse, leading to necrosis and peritonitis. A short length of prolapsed rectum has a better prognosis than a long length that involves avulsion of small colonic vessels.

Some texts suggest using epidural anaesthesia followed by replacement of the rectum. These same texts seem to state that the condition has a very poor prognosis despite therapy. Other texts describe surgical treatment with reasonable success rates.

Regardless of therapy, oral laxatives, antibiotics and anti-endotoxic medication is indicated.

Perineal lacerations and rectovaginal fistula

These may occur when there is damage to the birth canal and/or perineum during unassisted foaling or during prolonged obstetrical manipulation. Although damage often requires some sort of treatment, the injuries often look worse than they are and life-threatening injuries are rare. Due to the powerful expulsive forces that occur during equine parturition, fetal malposition can cause significant damage to the vagina, vestibular sphincter and labia. Foal hooves can get pressed against the dorsal vaginal wall, leading to laceration of the vagina and rectum. The damage is usually obvious on gross examination. Injuries are classified as:

- **First-degree lacerations** – involving the vaginal mucosa and skin at the dorsal commissure of the vulva
- **Second-degree lacerations** – involving the vaginal mucosa, submucosa and perineal musculature
- **Third-degree lacerations** – involving damage to the vagina and anus, so that the rectum communicates with either the vagina and/or vestibule. This damage produces a common opening for the vagina and anus (Figure 26.23).

A rectovaginal (rectovestibular) fistula is a 'hole' between the rectum and the vagina or vestibule. The vulva and anus may appear undamaged externally.

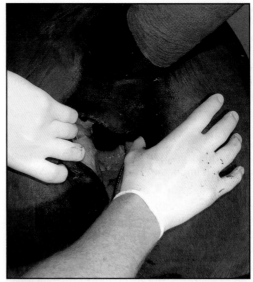

26.23 Third-degree postpartum perineal laceration in a mare.

Third-degree lacerations will be immediately obvious, whereas first- and second-degree lacerations will become apparent during the postpartum examination. A vaginal and rectal examination will aid in the diagnosis of a rectovaginal fistula. More subtle damage to the cranial vagina may require examination using a speculum. It is normal for mares to have some vulval and perineal swelling immediately postpartum. Treatment of these wounds varies according to the severity of damage sustained. The basic approach in the acute stage is similar to that for other traumatic wounds, in that it should involve assessment of the structures involved, decontamination, and antimicrobial and anti-inflammatory administration. The mare should also be given tetanus prophylaxis following recommended guidelines.

The short-term objective is to minimize pain and infection so as to allow the development of healthy granulation tissue. This is best achieved with daily or twice daily lavage with dilute povidine–iodine. The longer-term objective is to retain as much healthy tissue as possible between the rectum and vestibule, so as to facilitate surgical repair at a later date. Aggressive surgical debridement is not generally required or advised, and only obviously non-viable tissue should be removed. In the very early stages, this author (MH) may leave tissue until it is clear that the area is devitalized. It is recommended that the mare's diet is designed to keep the faeces as loose as possible. This minimizes impactions and pain during defecation. Surgical repair can take place in 4–8 weeks and is generally only necessary in third-degree lacerations and rectovaginal fistulas. Repair should take place once healing has finished and certainly before any mating takes place. The surgical repair for third-degree lacerations can consist of two stages, 4–6 weeks apart. The first stage involves the repair of the rectovaginal shelf and the second stage repairs the perineal body and vulva. The anus may not be functional but this does not seem to affect the mare. Surgical repair of rectovaginal fistulas can have the added benefit of retaining a functional anus, depending on the technique chosen for repair. The prognosis for future breeding is good to guarded, with around 70–80% of mares with third degree lacerations able to carry a foal through to term. A thorough breeding soundness examination is recommended prior to embarking on any future breeding with the mare. Recurrence is of course possible, and so care should be taken at subsequent foalings.

Cervical lacerations

A competent closed cervix during gestation is arguably one of the most important factors in a pregnancy continuing to term. Ascending uterine infections leading to a placentitis is a significant cause of infectious abortion in mares. A significantly damaged cervix can lead to the mare being retired from breeding duties. Cervical damage is most commonly associated with dystocia and prolonged fetal manipulation, but can also be caused by large foals (especially in maiden mares) and late gestation abortions. Mares that abort a late-gestation foal do not have the benefit of the tissue relaxation that occurs in a normal prepartum mare.

Excessive traction applied to the foal during early second-stage labour can also lead to cervical tearing. There is a balance between achieving good progress during parturition and pulling the foal out before the cervix has fully dilated. Embryotomy in the mare (see above) also has the very real risk of damaging the mare's cervix, thus potentially rendering her unsuitable for future breeding. Cervical fibrosis and adhesion to the cranial vagina or fornix can also occur. Pathology of this kind carries a poor prognosis for future breeding.

Manual palpation of the cervix during dioestrus is the best method of diagnosing cervical lacerations. Passing an index finger part way into the external os of the cervix and then feeling the outer surface of the cervix with a thumb should make tears apparent. Relating their location to the face of a clock allows positions to be recorded. Tears involving <25% of the cervical length carry a good prognosis and usually do not require surgical treatment. Lesions involving ≥50% of the cervical length require surgical repair.

Colonic rupture

The mare will show signs of colic, acute peritonitis with injected mucous membranes. In all but a few exceptional cases, rupture will require euthanasia of the mare.

Colonic torsion

This may be seen 1–3 days after foaling, but can occur as late as 4–6 weeks postpartum or after a caesarean operation. There is severe colic with cardiovascular clinical signs. An early diagnosis and surgical correction is required if the mare has any hope of survival.

Vaginal haematoma

A red blister-like structure is seen protruding through the vulva. This usually resolves without any specific treatment.

Breeding exotic pets

Many of the reproductive principles described for dogs and cats also apply to many exotic pets, in particular mammalian species. However, each species may differ considerably in other ways. Only basic details of reproduction of the individual exotic species can be covered in this chapter and the reader is referred to other texts such as the *BSAVA Manual of Exotic Pets*.

Small mammals

Descriptions of the basic reproductive parameters for a variety of common small mammals are given in Figure 26.24.

Ferrets

The male ferret (hob) is often twice the size of the female ferret (jill). It is also simple to differentiate the sexes by inspection of the external genitalia.

Testicular size of the hob varies during the year and can be very small during the non-breeding season. The use of GnRH implants to prevent breeding in hobs and reduce their odour is now favoured rather than surgical neutering, due to the association between neutering and the development of adrenal neoplasia.

Jills are sexually mature in the spring after their birth. The breeding season for ferrets in the UK stretches from February/March to September/October and the jill is in a near-permanent (persistent) state of oestrus, as she is an induced ovulator. Persistent oestrus may result in bone marrow suppression and potentially lethal pancytopenia. Mating with a vasectomized male ferret provides a short-term solution in females that may be required for breeding in the future, as does the use of proligestone. Surgical neutering is no longer recommended as a method of preventing oestrus in jills unless there is evidence of uterine disease, as such neutering has been associated with endocrinopathies. Proligestone injections or GnRH-agonist implants (lasting 18–24 months) are preferred.

Rabbits

Sexual maturity in rabbits varies between breeds but is typically reached at 4–5 months in females (does) and 5–8 months in males (bucks). Rabbits are seasonally polyoestrus and are induced ovulators. Both males and females may be territorially aggressive during the breeding season and this, as well as unwanted litters, is a major reason for neutering pet animals. Neutering is usually carried out from 5–6 months of age. Importantly, early neutering of female rabbits prevents uterine adenocarcinoma, the most common neoplasia in female rabbits, in addition to other uterine and mammary conditions.

Pregnancy can be detected by palpation or ultrasonography from approximately 14 days gestation. Average gestation is around 31 days. Parturition is called kindling.

Rodents

Sexing

Female rodents have separate external orifices for their urinary and reproductive systems. This can be used for sexing the animals, in conjunction with the spacing of the urinary papilla (the nodule-like lump on the ventrum through which the urinary tract exits in the female rodent) from the anus. In females, the urinary papilla is closer to the anus and, if care is taken, the entrance to the genital tract may be seen between the urinary papilla and the caudally situated anus (Figure 26.25). In males, the prepuce is spaced at a greater distance from the anus. There are also prominent testes in adult males, but these may be retracted into the caudal abdomen. The testes may be encouraged to descend by gently holding the male rodent vertically, with head uppermost and resting its rear on the palm of one hand.

Species	Sexual maturity	Oestrous cycle interval	Duration of oestrus	Ovulation	Gestation length	Pseudopregnancy	Litter size
Rat	8–10 weeks	4–5 days Non-seasonally polyoestrous	10–20 hours	Spontaneous	21–23 days	Approx. 14 days after non-fertile mating	8–18
Mouse	6–7 weeks	4–5 days Non-seasonally polyoestrous	10–20 hours	Spontaneous	19–21 days	Approx. 14 days after non-fertile mating	5–12
Syrian hamster	6–12 weeks	4 days	8–26 hours	Spontaneous	15–18 days	Approx. 8–10 days after non-fertile mating	5–10
Gerbil	8–10 weeks	4–7 days	12–18 hours	Spontaneous	23–26 days (42 days if delayed implantation)	Approx. 16 days after non-fertile mating	3–8
Guinea pig	1.5–3 months	15–17 days	6–11 hours	Spontaneous	59–72 days (average 63 days)		1–6 (average 3–4)
Chinchilla	6–9 months	30–50 days Seasonally polyoestrous	40 hours	Spontaneous	111 days		2
Rabbit	4–8 months	Seasonally polyoestrous	Variable during the breeding season	Induced	29–35 days (average 31 days)	Approx. 16 days after induced ovulation	4–10
Ferret	4–8 months First Spring after birth	Seasonally polyoestrous	7 months. Persistent according to day length	Induced	41–42 days	Approx. 42 days after induced ovulation	2–14

26.24   Reproductive parameters for small mammals.

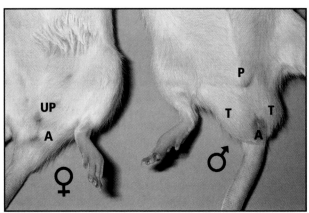

26.25   Differences in anogenital distance in rats: (left) female; (right) male. A = anus; P = prepuce; T = testes; UP = urinary papilla. (Reproduced from *BSAVA Manual of Exotic Pets, 4th edition*)

Guinea pigs

Guinea pig sows have a higher risk of complications during parturition because the piglets are large and fully formed at birth. If a sow is to be bred from, she should have her first litter prior to 8 months of age. Upon reaching adulthood her pelvic symphysis will stiffen and she may not be able to deliver her piglets, resulting in dystocia and requiring a caesarean operation.

Birds

Many bird species will breed predominantly at one time of the year. Some seasonal breeders are triggered to start breeding by an initial decrease in daylength, as is seen over the winter, followed by an increase, as occurs in the spring. This daylength variation stimulates the pineal gland, which is connected to the pituitary gland, to alter levels of melatonin and GnRH; this can stimulate the reproductive cycle. Other seasonal breeders are stimulated to cycle by other external stimuli, such as rainfall and food availability. Sexual maturity may be reached quickly in smaller species, such as finches, or may take several years, as with many of the larger parrots.

Some bird species are sexually **monomorphic**, i.e. the two sexes look physically identical (e.g. Amazon parrots, macaws). In other species there is a distinct difference: they are sexually **dimorphic**. For example, in budgerigars the male has a blue cere and the female a brown or pinkish one. In many birds of prey, the female is up to twice the size of the male.

Mating involves the male mounting the female and pressing his vent to hers. Following mating, the sperm may be stored in the oviduct for a short period. The whole process from shedding of the oocyte to laying of the egg takes approximately 2 days. The number of eggs laid in a 'clutch' varies between species.

Occasionally a female will not pass an egg efficiently, resulting in her becoming **egg-bound**. The fully formed egg may lodge in the vagina or in the shell gland. This may also happen as the result of trauma to the vent.

Incubation of the eggs may be performed by just the female or just the male or by both parents, depending on the species. Incubation periods vary between species, as do weaning ages (Figure 26.26). Artificial incubation may help increase hatching rates. Parent-reared birds take longer to wean on average than hand-reared ones and are usually less hand-tame.

Species	Incubation period (days)	Weaning (days): parent-reared	Weaning (days): hand-reared	Sexual maturity
African Grey parrot	26–28	100–120	75–90	4–6 years
Amazon parrot	26–29	90–120	75–90	4–6 years
Barn owl	30–31	70–75		1 year
Budgerigar	16–18	30–40	30	6–9 months
Canary	12–14	21		< 1 year
Cockatiel	18–20	47–52	42–49	6–12 months
Cockatoo: large spp. Cockatoo: medium spp.	23–30 (depending on spp.)	60–80 45–60	95–120 75–100	5–6 years 3–4 years
Harris hawk	32	35–45 (fledging) [a]		> 3 years
Lovebird	18–24	45–55	40–45	6–12 months
Macaw: large spp. Macaw: small spp.	26–28 23–26	120–150 90–120	95–120 75–90	5–7 years 4–6 years
Peregrine falcon	29–32	35–42 (fledging) [a]		> 3 years
Pheasant	22–24	Precocial [b]		
Pigeon	16–19	35		1 year
Zebra finch	12–16	25–28		9 months

26.26   Reproductive parameters for selected bird species. [a] Fledging refers to time when bird can first fly. [b] Self-feeding from hatchling.

Reptiles

Reptiles are classified as:

- **Oviparous**: Lay eggs externally
- **Ovoviviparous**: Produce live young instead of laying eggs, but the eggs are produced internally
- **Viviparous**: A form of placenta/thin-walled egg structure is produced in the reproductive system, which allows the fetus to develop and live young are produced.

Reptile eggs are generally soft-shelled and more leathery than birds' eggs, although egg production in lizards is similar to the process in birds. Incubation length depends upon the temperature at which the eggs are kept. Unlike birds' eggs,

reptile eggs should not be moved during incubation but kept with the same side up as when they were deposited. Figure 26.27 gives an idea of some common incubation lengths, or, where the species is viviparous, the gestation length.

Chelonians

Male chelonians often have longer tails, as the vent is found here, caudal to the edge of the carapace, and houses the single phallus (Figure 26.28). In some species the male and female vary significantly in size (e.g. Indian star tortoise, striped mud turtle, red-eared terrapin); in others there are other differing secondary sexual characteristics, such as longer claws in females (e.g. leopard and Indian star tortoises) and differing eye colours (box turtle). Males of many

Species	Method of reproduction	Incubation/gestation period (days)	Incubation/ temperature ranges (°C)
Boa constructor	Viviparous	100–200	28–32.5
Burmese python	Oviparous	55–65	28–32
Corn snake	Oviparous	55–70	28–30
Garter snake	Viviparous	90–100	24–29.5
Kingsnake	Oviparous	55–70	28–30
Bearded dragon	Oviparous	65–115	28–32
Green iguana	Oviparous	60–70	25–30
Jackson's chameleon	Ovoviviparous	90–180	27–29
Leopard gecko	Oviparous	150–170	28–32
Hermann's tortoise	Oviparous	85–100	30–33
Leopard tortoise	Oviparous	140–155	28–32
Red-eared terrapin	Oviparous	54–80	28–29
African spurred tortoise	Oviparous	120–170	28–32

26.27   Reproductive parameters for selected reptiles.

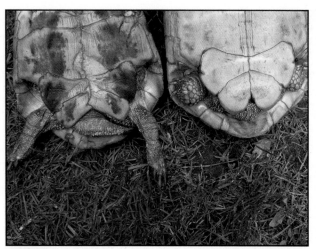

26.28   Sexual dimorphism in Hermann's tortoise: the male (left) has a longer tail and wider anal scutes than the female (right). (Courtesy of Alan Humphreys.)

Mediterranean species of tortoise and turtle possess a dished (concave) plastron, to make mounting the female easier, and often have a narrower angle to the caudal plastron in front of the cloaca than the egg-bearing females. Some female Mediterranean species have a hinge to the caudal part of the plastron to allow easier egg-laying.

In the colder northerly climes of the UK the incubation of chelonian eggs in an outside environment is not possible. It is necessary to remove the eggs from wherever they have been laid by the female and transfer them to a purpose-built incubator for hatching. Incubators may be purchased from many reptile outlets, or from commercial poultry or cagebird suppliers.

Egg binding may occur in chelonians, often caused by the development of an abnormally large egg but sometimes due to a damaged pelvis, which results in an inability to pass even normal-sized eggs. Another cause of egg binding is egg retention, which can be related to behavioural stress, often due to an unsuitable habitat.

Incubation temperature control is important in sex determination. For example, the eggs of the spur-thighed tortoise will produce males if kept at 29.5°C and females if kept at 31.5°C. This principle seems to apply to a large number of tortoise species, with males being predominantly produced at lower temperatures than females. If the temperature range is kept at 28–31°C, a mixture of sexes is likely to be achieved.

Lizards

In most species of lizard there are external physical differences that allow differentiation of the sexes. These include: prominent prefemoral pores in male iguanids; larger scales caudal to the vent in male anoles; wider tail bases in male green iguanas; greater ornamentation such as larger crests in plumed basilisks; horns in Jackson's chameleons; and larger crest spines in male water dragons. In other species, such as the beaded lizard, some monitors and the Gila monster, sexual identification must be performed by surgical probing.

Sexual maturity varies according to the species and also according to the husbandry provided, as poor nutrition and poor heat or ultraviolet light provision may lead to delays in maturation.

Lizard eggs may be incubated in vivaria. Incubation periods vary from 45–70 days for smaller lizards to 90–130 days for larger lizards (see Figure 26.27). A few species are parthenogenetic, i.e. females give birth to females with no need for male fertilization.

Obstructive (eggs too large) and non-obstructive (insufficient nesting site, digging substrate, poor physical condition or infection of the oviduct) dystocia are common problems in the egg-laying lizards.

Sex determination in most lizards is dependent on genetic factors, with the exception of some geckos, for which sex determination is temperature-dependent.

Snakes

Telling the sexes apart can be difficult in snakes and is best performed by surgical probing. A fine sterile blunt-ended probe is inserted through the vent and advanced just to one side of the midline in a caudal direction. If the snake is a male, the probe will pass into one of the inverted hemipenes and so will insert to a depth of 8–16 subcaudal scales. In females there are anal glands in this region and so the probe may be inserted to a depth of only 2–6 subcaudal scales. In some species, such as boas, males possess a paracloacal spur (the remnant of the pelvic limb) on either side of the body ventrally at the level of the cloaca. In very young snakes it may be possible to evert the hemipenes manually, with care, in a technique known as 'popping'.

Sex determination in snakes is entirely chromosomally dependent; the process is not influenced by temperature, as it is in chelonians and geckos.

The average incubation period in snakes is generally 45–70 days (see Figure 26.27); artificial incubation improves hatching rates. Temperatures for incubation vary from 24 to 32°C; it is important to have a thermometer and humidity gauge within the incubator. When eggs are retrieved from the nest site, particular care should be taken to maintain the same position of the egg in the incubator. The eggs should not be turned or touched during the incubation process, as this can cause significant fetal mortality.

Egg impaction, which is thought to be a result of exhaustion or calcium deficiency, may occur in egg-laying species.

Care and management of neonatal puppies and kittens

The neonatal period is characterized by complete dependence of the newborn on its dam, and is generally agreed to be the first 3 weeks after birth.

When a neonate is born it is essential to:

1. Establish a clear airway and stimulate respiration.
2. Cut the umbilicus.
3. Keep the neonate warm until active.
4. Encourage the neonate to feed.

It is essential that a clear airway is established as soon as a neonate is born (or delivered via a caesarean operation). This is usually done by the dam but should be done by the nurse if necessary (i.e. if the dam fails/is unable to establish a clear airway). This involves removal of the surrounding fetal membranes using a soft dry towel. This will usually stimulate respiration. The mouth and nose can be cleared of fetal fluid by suction. **The practice of swinging the neonate in an arc should be avoided because of the risk of cerebral haemorrhage.** If vigorous rubbing does not stimulate respiration, positive pressure ventilation using a snug-fitting mask may be started, ensuring that the head and neck are extended. If the heart is not beating, external cardiac massage combined with artificial respiration may be attempted.

The umbilicus should be clamped and cut approximately 3 cm from the puppy's or kitten's abdomen; excessive bleeding can be prevented by the application of a ligature.

Once regular respiratory efforts are maintained, the neonate may be placed into a prewarmed box or incubator until it is active, when it may be returned to the dam and encouraged to feed. Suckling normally occurs immediately after birth and at intervals of 2–3 hours for the first few days.

Once the dam is sufficiently happy for the neonate to be removed, it should be checked for abnormalities.

Examination of the neonatal puppy or kitten

- Record the birth weight. Normal neonates will increase their bodyweight by 5–10% per day; a failure to do so may indicate poor health.
- Check the neonate for congenital abnormalities, such as cleft palate or harelip.
- Check the umbilicus for herniation. The umbilicus should be clean and show no evidence of further bleeding. If the umbilicus is bleeding, it can be ligated to prevent further blood loss.
- Breathing should be regular and even. The normal respiratory rate for a neonate is 15–40 breaths per minute. There should not be excessive noise. If there is excessive noise, this may indicate that the neonate still has fluid in its lungs and the appropriate action should be taken.
- There should be no discharge from the eyes or ears.
- Record any other birth defects, as well as the neonate's colour and gender.
- The neonate's rectal temperature could also be taken and recorded at this time, but in reality this is unnecessary. The normal rectal temperature for the first week after birth should be 32–34°C.

Neonatal characteristics

Neonatal puppies and kittens are unable to stand at birth but should be quite mobile, using their limbs to crawl. Neonates need to be assessed for their general strength. The weakest must be carefully observed, since they do not feed adequately and may fail to thrive. Standing may be seen from 10 days after birth and most should be able to walk at 3 weeks of age.

Puppies and kittens are born with their eyes closed; separation of the upper and lower lids with opening of the eyes should occur by approximately 10–14 days after birth. The cornea at this stage may appear slightly cloudy, but this will disappear over the first 4 weeks. Many kittens are born with strabismus (a squint), which persists until they are 8 weeks old.

Care of the litter

During the first few weeks of life the dam will take care of the needs of the litter. However, the litter must be checked regularly for signs of problems, ensuring that all of them are receiving an adequate supply of milk from the dam and that no individual is missing out on feeding opportunities. There should be a plentiful supply of clean bedding available, so that the dam and her offspring are comfortable and not lying on soiled or wet bedding.

Normally the dam will lick the perineal region in order to stimulate the neonates to defecate or urinate and she continues to do this for the first 2–3 weeks after birth. After this time the neonates will urinate and defecate voluntarily and therefore the amount of soiling in the nest will increase and it will require more frequent changing.

The litter should be weighed on a regular basis, usually weekly, to ensure that all of them are gaining weight adequately. At 10–14 days, when the eyes of puppies and kittens should open, they will gradually be able to focus on objects. They will become stronger on their legs and begin to crawl around. At this time it is advisable to ensure that all the puppies are able to use their hindlegs properly; sometimes very large or fat puppies fail to get up on their hindlegs and will haul themselves around on their front legs and bellies. If this becomes apparent, the puppy should be checked to ensure that there is nothing physically wrong with the legs, and then be encouraged to use its hindlegs by placing a hand under its bottom and pushing it on to its hindlegs. This condition rarely persists, due to the increased competition for food, but with a small litter it may become a problem.

Once weaning commences the dam may be less inclined to clean up the faeces. The young should be encouraged to urinate and defecate away from the nest so that cleaning is more easily facilitated. This may hasten toilet training.

Care and management of neonatal foals

A neonatal foal is one that is <4 weeks of age.

The first few days of a foal's life are very important and the newborn foal should be carefully monitored over this time. Foals that appear normal and healthy at birth can develop problems later on. The foal should be observed for the following signs:

- Behavioural changes. Foals should become stronger and more active over the first few days. The first sign of serious trouble may be increased time spent lying down
- Distended abdomen and failure to pass urine within 8 hours of birth
- Failure to pass meconium: the foal strains to defecate and appears uncomfortable
- Decreased nursing or full udder in the mare
- Sleeping standing up
- Lethargy
- Jaundiced appearance
- Diarrhoea
- Any lameness or swelling
- Swelling or pain around the umbilicus.

Basic procedures to maximize foal health and survival include:

- **Umbilical management** – the umbilicus should be dipped immediately and then every 6–8 hours for first 24 hours using 0.5% chlorhexidine (1 part 2% chlorhexidine to 3 parts sterile water – and for every 450 ml of solution 50 ml of surgical spirit is added)
- **Enemas** – all foals should receive an enema to aid the passing of the meconium (see Chapter 17), which should be expelled within 4 hours. There are commercial enemas available that consist of 100 ml phosphate-buffered solution
- **General physical examination** – all foals should undergo a general physical examination to identify whether there are any congenital abnormalities
- **Tetanus prophylaxis** – this is essential for foals, as equids are very sensitive to tetanus toxin. Ideally the mare should be boosted 4–6 weeks prior to birth with tetanus toxoid, in order that her colostrum contains high levels of antibody. The foal can also be injected with tetanus antitoxin, preferably into the largest muscle mass
- **IgG evaluation** – this is important because foals receive all their passive immunity via the colostrum (see below). Concentrations peak at 18 hours postpartum, but a test at 12 hours will still be informative. An IgG concentration of >6–8 g/l is satisfactory; >12 g/l is ideal. If IgG concentration is <6 g/l, the foal has **failure of passive transfer**. This is a very serious condition and must be corrected with a transfusion of plasma. To avoid immune-mediated conditions, such as neonatal isoerythrolysis (discussed below), the plasma should come from a gelding that has no chance of possessing antibodies to the foal's blood group; or a commercially available alternative may be used (e.g. Hypermune Equine Plasma, Veterinary Immunogenics Ltd).

Colostrum

Foals are born essentially without any antibodies and receive all their passive immunity via the **colostrum**. Without sufficient intake of colostrum the foal will have little chance of survival. It is essential that the foal has a sufficient intake (at least 2 litres) of good-quality colostrum in the first 6–8 hours of life. At this time the gut mucosa is said to be 'open' as it can absorb **whole** protein molecules (such as IgG) into the bloodstream. After 12 hours the gut mucosa starts to 'close', meaning protein molecules are broken down using enzymes and used as food. At 24 hours, the gut is completely closed and no whole protein molecules are absorbed.

To assess colostrum quality, a refractometer is used. Good colostrum has a specific gravity (SG) of 1.060. If using a Brix refractometer, the table in Figure 26.29 is used.

Brix %	IgG concentration	Quality
<10–15	0–28	Poor
15–20	28–50	Borderline
20–30	50–80	Adequate
>30	>80	Very good

26.29 Assessing equine colostrum quality with a Brix refractometer.

Care and management of neonatal exotic pets

Small mammals

If disturbed with her young in the first few weeks after parturition, there may be a tendency among small mammals towards cannibalism (or at least abandonment or abuse) of the litter by the dam. For this reason female rats, mice, hamsters, gerbils and rabbits should be left alone with their litters, except for replenishing food and clearing the worst of any cage soiling. Cannibalism is especially common in the hamster, though the female will also protectively place the young in her cheek pouches to move them, which may look like she is 'eating' the young.

Neonatal characteristics in small mammalian species likely to be seen in small animal practice are described in Figure 26.30. Most small mammal species are **altricial** at birth (wholly dependent on the mother for nutrition and survival in the first few weeks of life); they are born blind, deaf, hairless and without teeth. Guinea pigs and chinchillas are **precocial** (relatively mature and mobile) at birth.

Ferrets

The average number of ferret kits in a litter is eight. They are altricial but are born with a prominent fat pad on the dorsum of the neck, which provides some calorific value during the early stages of life. They have a higher calorific requirement than adult ferrets, at 1.5–2 times adult maintenance levels

Rabbits

Rabbits will suckle their kits for only 3–5 minutes at a time and only once or twice in a 24-hour period, but the kits are totally dependent on the doe's milk for up to 21 days. They will begin to take solid foods from the age of 2–3 weeks and they should be weighed at this time. Solid foods offered will increasingly be consumed and weight losses may be seen during this changeover period. Weaning occurs at around 6 weeks of age. The growing kits require higher levels of vitamin D3 and calcium than adult rabbits and should be offered a balanced diet, such as a combination of a pelleted growing-rabbit formulated food along with good-quality grass hay and some greens. The pelleted foods should be chosen carefully; many are nutritionally balanced but it is preferable to use a homogeneous pelleted diet, as rabbits are selective eaters of concentrates and will pick and choose if offered a mixed dry food. They should also be given access to unfiltered natural sunlight, even if for only 15–20 minutes a day, to ensure adequate synthesis of vitamin D.

Birds

After hatching, the chick must be supplied with high levels of energy and protein for the growth phase within 3–4 days. This delay is possible due to the remnants of the yolk sac inside the body cavity still providing some nutrition and immunity for the first few days of life. Failure to internalize the yolk sac prior to hatching is sometimes seen and can lead to septicaemia. Surgical removal of the non-internalized yolk sac is possible but the chick will require immediate supplementary nutritional support due to the removal of this energy/nutrient source.

Species	Terminology	Precocity	Development			Weaning age
			Eyes open	**Ears open**	**Hair and skin**	
Rat	Pups	Altricial	12–15 days	4–5 days	Fur appears at 7–10 days	17–21 days
Mouse	Pups	Altricial	12–14 days	4–5 days	Fur appears at 10 days	21–28 days
Syrian hamster	Pups	Altricial	12–14 days	1.5–3 days	Skin changes from pale pink to darker at 2–3 days	20–28 days
Gerbil	Pups	Altricial	12–14 days	4–5 days	Skin changes from pale pink to darker at 7 days with fur appearing	20–30 days
Guinea pig	Piglets	Precocial	At birth	At birth	Born fully furred	14–28 days (eating solids from day 1)
Chinchilla	Kits	Precocial	At birth	At birth	Born fully furred	36–48 days (eating solids from day 1)
Rabbit	Kits/kittens	Altricial	8–10 days	11–12 days	Fur appears at 5–6 days	6 weeks (eating solids from 2–3 weeks)
Ferret	Kits	Altricial	4–5 weeks	10 days	Fur appears at 2 days, pronounced at 3 weeks	6–8 weeks (ideally 8 weeks)

26.30   Neonatal characteristics of small mammals.

When feathers are produced, a huge demand for protein occurs; there are several feather changes during the first 2 years of life. Young birds also have a large requirement for calcium and vitamin D3 for developing and mineralizing the skeleton. It has been estimated that minimum energy requirements for small psittacine and passerine birds is five times that of adults, with young chicks nearly doubling their weight over 48 hours, with a protein requirement of 15–20% compared with an adult protein need of 10–14%. Diets for chicks have therefore concentrated on preformulated mashes with the desired level of protein, or the use of eggs and dairy products, which have a good broad spectrum of amino acid supplementation and 20% protein levels.

Excessive protein supplementation (>25% of diet) has, however, been shown to lead to behavioural problems and to claw, beak and skeletal deformities, particularly if combined with a lack of calcium.

Reptiles

Once hatched (Figure 26.31), parental neonatal care varies greatly between species, from no care at all to the careful tending of infants in crocodilian species. In some herbivorous species, direct neonatal care is absent but proximity to adults is essential for the development of normal gut flora. Temperature, environmental enrichment and single *versus* group rearing may all affect the behavioural development and survival of reptile neonates. Reptiles initially survive on the nutrients within the yolk sac before moving on to adult type diets.

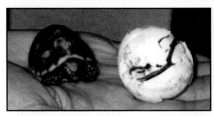

26.31

Healthy hatchling red-footed tortoise and its eggshell

Neonatal reptiles may suffer from retained or infected yolk sacs, often as a result of premature birth or hatching in artificial rearing situations, or where there is suboptimal maternal nutrition. Surgical intervention is usually required in such cases, with subsequent supportive feeding until normal eating commences.

Abnormalities of neonatal puppies and kittens

A number of diseases may affect puppies and kittens early in life. A certain percentage of neonates may die before weaning and it has been suggested that this can be as high as 15–20%. With good management systems (including the avoidance of hypothermia), the number of offspring lost should not be >5%.

Fading puppy or kitten syndrome

The most common problem noted within the neonatal period is that of fading puppies or kittens. Most affected neonates die when <1 week of age. There are numerous factors associated with this loss, but usually it is the inherent susceptibility of the newborn that results in its ultimate demise. Neonates have poor mechanisms of thermoregulation, fluid and energy balance, they are immunologically incompetent, and they may have abnormal lung surfactant composition. When combined with poor management regimes and poor mothering behaviour of the dam, the risk of neonatal mortality can be high. Approximately 50% of neonatal deaths can be attributed to infection, maternal and management-related deficiencies, low birth weight or congenital abnormalities.

Neonatal septicaemia

The inherent vulnerability of the neonate puts it at risk of colonization by a number of bacterial agents. This may result in rapid death after very few initial clinical signs. In some cases ill health results in frequent crying, restlessness and hypothermia, progressing to clinical signs of diarrhoea and/or dyspnoea with resultant dehydration or cyanosis, and ultimately death. Other neonates are more chronically affected and fail to grow as expected prior to the onset of obvious clinical disease.

The majority of passive immunity follows from the intake of colostrum, and gut transfer occurs only during the first 48 hours of life. It is vital, therefore, to ensure an adequate intake of colostrum at this time to protect against these organisms.

Regardless of the cause, rapid and aggressive treatment using intravenous fluid therapy, oral electrolytes, broad-spectrum antimicrobial agents and oxygen administration is essential. Despite such treatment, the mortality rate can be high.

Neonatal viral infection

Viral infections are not common in the neonate, especially when vaccination programmes are used in the adult. Maternally derived antibodies (MDA) frequently provide protection for several weeks.

- Canine herpesvirus may result in the birth of congenitally infected puppies that are weak and die soon after birth. Vaccination of the pregnant bitch can reduce neonatal losses.
- Feline immunodeficiency virus and feline leukaemia virus can infect kittens transplacentally as well as perinatally, and may result in neonatal death after a few weeks of age.
- Neonatal deaths or the birth of kittens with cerebellar hypoplasia are not uncommon following infection with feline panleucopenia virus during pregnancy.
- Feline coronavirus has also been implicated in cases of upper respiratory tract disease and fading kitten syndrome.

Congenital abnormalities

Congenital abnormalities are those that are present at birth. One such problem is a cleft palate, where there is failure of the normal fusion of the palatine arches. The defect may occur anywhere along the length of the hard or soft palate, though most commonly it arises caudal to the incisor ridge. The defect is common in certain breeds and it has been suggested that it is a trait inherited in either a recessive or polygenic manner. In most cases euthanasia of the neonate is advisable, because of problems with sucking and milk aspiration.

Many other congenital abnormalities affect organ systems, such as hernias, fetal 'monsters', hydrocephalus, flat puppies ('swimmers'), microphthalmus, congenital heart disease and atresia of the terminal rectum. A thorough clinical examination of each neonate after birth should allow these abnormalities to be readily detected.

Abnormalities of neonatal foals

Neonatal isoerythrolysis (NI)

This occurs when the mare produces antibodies to the foal's red blood cells; this does not cause a problem until the foal ingests the colostrum and absorbs the antibodies.

The foal inherits blood group antigens from the sire that are not present in the mare. These are strongly antigenic. Antibodies are not produced during gestation, as maternal and fetal circulations are separate; however, a risk of mixing occurs at parturition and antibodies are then produced. This puts subsequent foals at risk. The concentrations of these antibodies rise during the last month of pregnancy. Antibodies to Aa and Qa blood antigens are responsible for 90% of cases of NI. The risk in Thoroughbreds has been calculated at 1%. It is possible to predict the degree of risk if the blood groups of the mare and the sire are known.

Foals with NI become lethargic and weak, spending increased amounts of time recumbent. Heart and respiratory rates are elevated. Icterus is often striking. There may be haemoglobinuria (blood products in the urine). When packed cell volume (PCV) falls below 12% and red blood cell (RBC) count falls below 3×10^{12}/litre a blood transfusion is usually necessary. When the loss of RBCs is rapid, transfusions may be required sooner. Only 20% of transfused RBCs remain in the circulation for >4–7 days after the first transfusion; and after the second transfusion only 20% remain after 48 hours. In the mature horse it takes 4 days for the bone marrow to produce and release new RBCs. Therefore it is essential to continue to monitor RBC parameters in these foals until new RBC production is well established.

Perinatal asphyxia syndrome

Perinatal asphyxia syndrome is also known as 'neonatal maladjustment syndrome', 'neonatal encephalopathy' and 'dummy foal'. The syndrome is associated with signs of cerebral dysfunction, caused by a hypoxic/ischaemic insult during the perinatal period. Although primarily affecting the brain, other organs can be affected, causing ileus/colic, diarrhoea and necrotizing enterocolitis, renal dysfunction and electrolyte imbalances. Clinical signs may include:

- Loss of sucking reflex
- Loss of affinity for the mare
- Disorientation/ incoordination, progressing to loss of righting reflex
- Aimless wandering
- Appearance of blindness
- Sneezing/abnormal vocalization
- Thrashing the limbs in an uncoordinated attempt to rise (may be mistaken for convulsions)
- Abnormal breathing patterns (periods of apnoea or shallow breathing)
- Rapid exhaustion
- Inability to stand or to stay standing.

It is important that other conditions that may cause similar clinical signs are ruled out. These include: septicaemia, immaturity, postnatal trauma, severe electrolyte imbalances, hypoglycaemia, and hepatic or renal disease.

Foals with NE can be subdivided into two categories.

- Category 1:
  - Usually better prognosis (up to 80% survival)
  - Characteristically full term
  - Relative normal delivery
  - Onset of 6–24 hours (have often suckled normally)
  - Clinical pathology normal
  - Usually suffered physical or asphyxial trauma during or immediately after birth. The placenta may be expelled very rapidly, indicating premature placental separation.

- Category 2:
  - Survival rate much lower
  - Abnormal delivery or placenta
  - Abnormalities detected immediately postpartum
  - Show signs of immaturity/sepsis
  - Suffered prenatal insult, such as hypoxia following a placental insufficiency.

Septicaemia

The incidence of this condition shows marked variation; it is seen fairly frequently in the USA but incidence on well managed stud farms in the UK is very low. Although bacteria (including *Escherichia coli*, *Enterobacter*, *Staphylococcus*, *Streptococcus*, *Actinobacillus*, *Klebsiella*, *Pasteurella*, *Salmonella*, *Clostridium* and *Enterococcus*) are the most common cause of septic shock, it can also be triggered by viral or fungal infection, extensive trauma or extensive hypoxic–ischaemic disease. The sites of entry for infection are: the gastrointestinal tract, either by translocation of bacteria through the 'open gut' prior to ingestion of colostrum or following damage to the gastrointestinal mucosal barrier; the respiratory tract; the placenta; and the umbilicus.

There are certain factors that put a neonate at risk of developing septicaemia. These include problems connected with:

- Premises, e.g. heavy environmental challenge, endemic disease
- Pregnancy, e.g. vaginal discharge and placentitis, systemic disease in the mare
- Parturition, e.g. premature placental separation, dystocia, meconium staining of the foal (showing stressful birth)
- The foal, e.g. immaturity, NE, delayed ingestion of colostrum.

Clinical signs often develop within 48 hours postpartum, although they may be seen at any time during the neonatal period. Early signs tend to be subtle and non-specific but can progress very rapidly as the foal goes into septic shock. Signs may include:

- Lethargy
- Loss of sucking reflex
- Sleepiness
- Pyrexia **or** subnormal temperature
- Scleral injection
- Petechiation of mucous membranes
- Convulsion
- Coma.

The foal can deteriorate in a matter of hours; any of these signs in a neonatal foal therefore merits early investigation.

Flexural deformities

Flexural deformities, sometimes incorrectly described as contracted tendons, can occur in foals of any breed as a congenital or acquired condition. Whilst some cases (e.g. mild to moderate carpal flexure) can resolve without specific treatment, other cases (e.g. acquired flexure of the distal interphalangeal (DIP) joint) can be resolved with the help of corrective farriery or, in more severe cases, by surgical release (in this instance of the carpal head of the deep digital flexor tendon). If left uncorrected, acquired DIP contracture can result in a club foot and chronic foot problems in adulthood. Some severe deformities such as those associated with the carpus or fetlock cannot be corrected, and euthanasia may be necessary.

Angular deformities

Angular deformities are quite common, and can be congenital or acquired. Almost any portion of the limb can be involved, but the carpus, fetlock and tarsus are most commonly affected. Both varal and valgal deformities occur. Most cases can be resolved by rest and time, but in severe cases surgical interference may be required after radiological assessment. Temporary physeal bridging using a transphyseal screw can be used on the convex side of the limb at the origin of the deformity, or a periosteal releasing procedure can be used on the concave side of the limb at the same periphyseal location.

Artificial rearing

Puppies and kittens

In some circumstances it may be necessary to rear some or all of the litter artificially. Instances where this may be the case include:

- Death of the dam
- A large litter
- A sick dam
- A dam showing no interest in her litter
- A dam with an inadequate milk supply.

Artificial rearing is best avoided where feasible. In some cases it may be possible to foster the neonates on to another dam. Suitable candidates to foster orphans might include a lactating bitch or queen that has just given birth and lost her litter, one with a pseudopregnancy that is currently lactating, or a dam with a small litter.

In the case of an excessively large litter, it may be possible to rotate some of the neonates between artificial rearing and being reared by the dam. It has been suggested that a small number of neonates should be entirely artificially reared, rather than rotated, but this method is not advocated. In any case, the neonates should, where possible, remain in the nest with the dam to ensure normal socialization.

It is essential that all neonates receive colostrum from the dam to ensure an adequate uptake of immunoglobulins. If the dam has died, it may still be possible to express some colostrum from her, as long as it is not contaminated with drugs or toxins.

Techniques

All the equipment for artificial rearing should be readily available and where possible should be included in the equipment needed in preparation for parturition, so that it is there if needed.

Milk substitutes

There are several commercially available milk substitutes for the artificial rearing of puppies or kittens. It is important that the neonate receives the right formulation. Cow's milk and goat's milk are *not* suitable substitutes, since their composition is very different from the milk of the bitch or queen. It is possible to make up a milk substitute, but this must have the appropriate lactose, fat and protein content, and achieving this is time-consuming. This may be pre-prepared. Milk should be warmed to body temperature (39°C) and fed according to the manufacturer's instructions, with regard to bodyweight and age.

Feeding bottles

Artificial rearing is both demanding and time-consuming, especially if rearing is done entirely without the dam. The neonates normally feed every 2–4 hours during the first 5 days of life, which then reduces to every 4 hours after day 5.

- A commercial feeding kit, which contains a bottle and teat, can be used. This encourages normal feeding, but can be time-consuming. The teat aperture should be large enough to prevent the neonate sucking in air but small enough to prevent excessive volumes of milk flowing through it.
- A dropper bottle or syringe (2 ml) can also be used.

When using either of these methods, care must be taken not to rush the neonate, as this may result in inhalation of milk rather than swallowing, which may cause pneumonia.

Orogastric tube feeding

In some cases it may be beneficial to feed neonates by means of a stomach tube (orogastric tube), especially during the first few days of life, for rapid feeding or for particularly sick neonates. The procedure is relatively simple. A small 2 mm diameter piece of soft polythene tubing should be measured against the neonate's mouth and to the end of the level of the 9th rib. This length should be marked on the tube. The outside of the tube should be lubricated with a small volume of water.

The neonate's head is held in the normal position and the mouth is held just open using a finger and thumb; if the head is extended or flexed, passage of the tube into the trachea is more likely. The tube is directed gently over the tongue into the back of the throat. Swallowing greatly assists passage into the oesophagus, but is not essential. The tube can usually be seen on the left side of the neck as it passes down the oesophagus. There is little resistance as the tube is introduced into the stomach; the length of the tube is the best guide. Once the tube is in position, the syringe can be attached and its contents slowly injected into the stomach. The tube is then gently removed.

General care

When artificial rearing has to take place entirely without the dam, the neonate is fully reliant upon its human carer.

Neonates are unable to open their bladder or bowels voluntarily; normally the mother would stimulate urination or defecation by licking the anogenital region after feeding. In the absence of the mother, this stimulation can be carried out manually by using a moistened piece of cotton wool. This should be performed every 2 hours.

Any spilled milk should be cleaned off the neonate immediately, as this might otherwise result in chilling of very young neonates or cause matting of the coat if allowed to dry.

The neonate's only other need is warmth. This can be achieved by maintaining an environmental temperature of 25°C and ensuring there are no draughts.

Foals

The rearing of foals can be a big commitment; for example in the first few days of life, a foal will require hourly feeds. A newborn foal will need to consume 10–15% of its bodyweight per day (e.g. for a 50 kg foal, 10% is approximately equivalent to 210 ml/h), rising to 25% of bodyweight thereafter. A Thoroughbred foal should have a weight gain of at least 1 kg/day for the first few weeks of its life. Sick foals have a higher demand for nutrition but often consume less.

Bottle-feeding can sometimes be difficult. It is best to offer a bottle with the foal's head under the handler's arm. This mimics the position of the mare's udder, and foals seem to be more willing to take bottles this way. A foal can also be trained to drink from a bucket, which allows the handler to leave milk in a bucket rather than attend every feed. However, it is essential that whatever method is employed to feed the foal, good hygiene must be maintained.

From 1 week of age, foals can receive 'creep feed' (see Chapter 13). This solid food reduces the burden of providing milk at all times. Creep feed can also be used to help wean the orphan foal more quickly than usual. Orphan foals can be weaned at around 3 months once they are consuming sufficient solid food.

Fostering foals

This is common practice and there are agencies in the UK and abroad that provide a database both of mares that can be used as foster mothers and of foals that require help.

Traditionally, the handler would skin a dam's dead foal and lay that skin on the foal to be fostered. This method is reasonably successful but covering a potentially weak and hungry foal in a decomposing skin is less than ideal. Offering a novel odour is a better solution. Peppermint essence can be placed around the mare's nose and on the foal so that when the mare quickly smells the foal it smells familiar. Foals do not seem to mind what shape or colour the foster mare is as long as there is milk. Indeed, foals over the years have been fostered on to goats and donkeys.

Some mares are better at fostering than others, and mares that show aggression towards the foal should be replaced by a more docile mare. Regardless of the mare's temperament, the foal should be introduced to the mare gradually and always with someone holding on to the mare. If all goes well, within a short space of time the foster mare will begin calling and looking for her new foal.

Exotic pets
Small mammals

The basic principles of artificial rearing of small mammal neonates are similar to those described above for dogs and cats; they require suitable feeding, a warm environment and stimulation to urinate and defecate.

Ferrets

Milk replacers for ferret kits have been adapted from puppy or kitten milk replacers, enriched with cream until the fat content reaches 20% (e.g. 3 parts puppy milk replacer to

1 part whipping cream). This can be fed on demand 4–6 times daily and the kits may be weaned on to adult food at 4–5 weeks of age.

Rabbits

Rabbit kits are altricial (see above) and also rely upon the doe for the development of their intestinal microflora. In hand-reared kits this may not occur properly and subsequent deaths from enterotoxaemia are commonplace. It may be possible to prevent this situation by transfaunation of gut flora from a healthy parasite-free adult rabbit to the kits. If hand-rearing is to be tried (Figure 26.32), kitten milk replacers or a home-made formula of 1 part whole full-fat cow's milk to 3 parts condensed milk, adding 6 g skimmed milk powder per 100 ml of the mixture, can be used. Adult foods (including weaning formulated dry foods) should be offered from 2 weeks of age and weaning attempted at 3 weeks, although a naturally reared kit would not be weaned until 6 weeks.

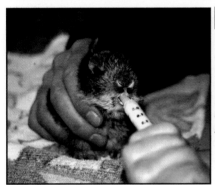

26.32

Hand feeding a rabbit kit. (Reproduced from *BSAVA Manual of Rabbit Medicine and Surgery, 2nd edn*)

Rodents

Hand-rearing of small rodents is challenging and has a high failure rate, owing to the altricial nature of the young of most species (see Figure 26.30). All of the altricial species show evidence of poor thermoregulation and require environmental temperatures of around 35°C while they are hairless, and around 32°C once they are furred. After their eyes open, the temperature may be reduced by 2.5°C per week and a temperature gradient should be provided.

The first concern when providing supportive feeding for orphaned rodents must be to ensure hydration. Initially, oral rehydration solutions suitable for cats and dogs may be used. Once hydration is established, the orphans may be offered dog or cat milk replacers or home-made diets. The milk replacer may be fed from the tip of a paintbrush, or using kitten feeders for older and larger individuals. Feeding should be once every hour during daylight and once every 2 hours overnight. Up to 35–40% of bodyweight may be fed per day.

The precocial young of guinea pigs and chinchillas are able to eat small amounts of solid food within 24 hours of birth, but they are often not hungry for the first 12–24 hours as they are able to make use of brown fat reserves; they should *not* be force-fed during this period. Thereafter, it is important to ensure that high-fibre foods are offered preferentially (to avoid fussy eating in later life). A hand-rearing formula for guinea pigs might be 1 part condensed milk to 2 parts cooled boiled water, fed every 3–4 hours at a rate of 1–3 ml; this may be adapted for chinchillas with the addition of 6 g skimmed milk powder to 100 ml of the formula to help to increase protein levels. Early weaning on to solid adult food is encouraged for both species, and is advised after 7–10 days.

Birds and reptiles

Some information on rearing of birds and reptiles has been given above under 'Care and management of the neonate'; more detailed information can be found in appropriate texts, including the *BSAVA Manual of Psittacine Birds,* the *BSAVA Manual of Raptors, Pigeons and Passerine Birds* and the *BSAVA Manual of Reptiles.*

Weaning

Puppies and kittens

Weaning is a gradual process, which normally starts at about 2.5 weeks for puppies and kittens and will be complete by about 5 weeks. The neonates will still suckle from their mother throughout the process, but once weaning has begun the dam will normally spend an increasing amount of time away from her offspring. She should still be allowed frequent access to them during the day and will normally still spend the night with them.

Until the weaning process begins, the neonate is reliant on the dam for all of its nutritional needs, but once weaning has begun each puppy or kitten should be closely monitored for continued weight gain. Signs associated with undernutrition include crying, inactivity and poor weight gain.

Small quantities of food can be offered to neonates on a finger, allowing them to lick or suck the finger. The range and volume of food can be increased as they get used to feeding. The food offered can be of a proprietary brand specifically designed for weaning. Cooked minced beef can also be offered. Some animals will wean easily, taking solids and lapping straight away, whilst others may take longer. It is therefore especially important to treat each animal individually and to be patient.

Neonates that are weaned directly from the dam should eat a gradually increasing amount of solid food, and should be on five or six feeds per day by the age of 5 weeks. Neonates that are hand-reared should have the volume of milk they receive gradually reduced as the weaning process continues, as if they were being weaned from the dam.

Foals

Foals are usually weaned at approximately 6 months of age. The foal must be nutritionally and emotionally independent of the mare, and so every weaning must be approached on a case-by-case basis.

Box weaning

The foal is placed in a stable and the mare removed. A 'buddy' can be placed in the stable beside the foal to minimize stress. The advantage of this method is that the stable is probably the safest place for the foal when separated from its dam. The disadvantage is that the foal is suddenly isolated from its paddock mates, which can be very stressful.

Paddock weaning

This method involves the mare and foal sharing a paddock with another horse or pony, or other animal such as a sheep, and then removing the mare. The foal will still have the other animal for company and so does not find the situation as stressful. The disadvantage is that if the foal does not tolerate separation from its dam, it may try and escape from the paddock, thereby potentially injuring itself. It may be better to allow mares and foals and brood mares without foals to run together so that the foals develop a relationship with the other foals and the brood mares. They will then more readily tolerate the removal of their dam from the paddock.

Further reading

England GCW (1998) *Allen's Fertility and Obstetrics in the Dog, 2nd edn.* Blackwell Scientific, Oxford

England GCW and Russo M (2011) Reproductive and paediatric emergencies. In: *BSAVA Manual of Canine and Feline Emergency and Critical Care, 2nd edn,* ed. L King and A Boag, pp. 228–240. BSAVA Publications, Gloucester

England GCW and von Heimendahl A (2010) *BSAVA Manual of Canine and Feline Reproduction and Neonatology, 2nd edn.* BSAVA Publications, Gloucester

Girling SJ (2002) *Veterinary Nursing of Exotic Pets.* Blackwell Scientific, Oxford

Hoskins JD (2001) *Veterinary Pediatrics: Dogs and Cats from Birth to Six Months, 2nd edn.* WB Saunders, Philadelphia

McKinnon AO and Voss JL (1993) *Equine Reproduction.* Lea & Febiger, Philadelphia

Meredith A and Johnson-Delaney C (2010) *BSAVA Manual of Exotic Pets, 5th edn.* BSAVA Publications, Gloucester

Munroe GA and Weese JS (2011) *Equine Clinical Medicine, Surgery and Reproduction.* Manson, London

Romagnano A (2005) reproduction and paediatrics. In: *BSAVA Manual of Psittacine Birds, 2nd edn,* ed. N Harcourt-Brown and J Chitty, pp. 222–233. BSAVA Publications, Gloucester

Wright K (2004) Breeding and neonatal care. In: *BSAVA Manual of Reptiles, 2nd edn* (ed. SJ Girling and P Raiti), pp. 40–50. BSAVA Publications, Gloucester

Self-assessment questions

1. Name the four stages of the oestrous cycle in the bitch.
2. How long are the oestrous cycles in the bitch, queen and mare?
3. What is the difference between cryptorchidism and monorchidism?
4. List five advantages of artificial insemination of the mare.
5. Name the three layers of cells that make up the inner cell mass of a conceptus.
6. What are the membranes called that surround an embryo, and what are their four basic components?
7. In the mare, what is an endometrial cup and which hormone(s) do endometrial cups secrete?
8. List three signs of impending parturition in the mare.
9. What are the two main causes of dystocia in the bitch?
10. What are the clinical signs of eclampsia in the bitch?
11. At what age do puppies open their eyes?
12. What is gestation length in guinea pig?
13. What are the three classifications of reptiles in terms of breeding?
14. What are baby ferrets called?

Chapter 27

Dentistry

Cedric Tutt and Sue Vranch

Learning objectives

After studying this chapter, students should be able to:

- **Define the terms used to describe dental disease**
- **Complete a dental chart accurately**
- **Describe how to handle an avulsed tooth**
- **List and describe the power-driven and hand dental instruments used in dentistry in general small animal practice**
- **List the surgical equipment required for extractions**
- **Describe the scale and polish procedure**
- **List the indications for dental radiography**
- **Instruct a client in dental homecare**
- **Describe the common dental conditions in lagomorphs and rodents**

Dental disease

Periodontal disease

The teeth are firmly held in the mouth by the periodontium. This comprises the alveolar bone on one side and the cementum covering the root on the other, with periodontal ligaments anchored in both preventing the tooth from being moved from its normal position. The gingiva (final component of the periodontium) covers the alveolar bone and forms a soft tissue collar around the tooth.

Periodontal disease is one of the most commonly seen diseases in small animal practice (about 85% of dogs and cats >3 years of age may have signs of periodontal disease) and is certainly the most common oral disease. Periodontal disease is the term used for a group of plaque-induced oral diseases. The prevention of this disease is discussed later.

Periodontal disease usually progresses from gingivitis; however, not all patients with gingivitis will go on to develop periodontitis.

- Gingivitis, a reversible condition, is defined as inflammation of the gingiva.
- Periodontitis, an irreversible condition, is inevitably a progression from gingivitis affecting the gingiva, alveolar bone, periodontal ligament and cementum of the tooth.

Aetiology

The primary cause of periodontal disease is the accumulation of dental plaque on the tooth surface. From the time the teeth erupt into the mouth, plaque begins to accumulate on the tooth surface. Plaque consists of desquamated cells, food particles and bacteria. Initially, Gram-positive aerobic bacteria colonize the tooth surface and this population creates conditions that are optimum for Gram-negative anaerobic organisms to thrive. Bacterial toxins cause damage to the gingivae and oral mucosae, which results in damage to the other supporting structures of the teeth. Dental calculus is mineralized plaque, and a layer of plaque always covers the calculus. It has been shown that the surface roughness of calculus is detrimental because of its plaque retentiveness. Therefore, supragingival and subgingival plaque can develop into calculus that hosts the plaque organisms, leading to persistent inflammation.

Gingivitis

The gingiva is made up of an attached part, tightly adhered to the alveolar bone, and a free part that forms the normal gingival sulcus (a collar surrounding the crown of each tooth). Gingivitis is the earliest sign of periodontal disease. Gingivitis presents as redness of the gums and is graded depending on its severity:

- Mild gingivitis (G1) – presents as marginal redness of the gums
- Moderate gingivitis (G2) – the gums bleed when the gingival sulcus is probed
- Severe gingivitis (G3) – the gingivae are swollen and bleed spontaneously.

Gingivitis affects only the gingiva; it does not extend beyond to the deeper supporting tissues and is reversible (as there is no loss of periodontal attachment). When the gingival sulcus is gently probed (see Dental charting below) the severity of gingivitis is scored according to how much bleeding there is (Figure 27.1). In patients with uncomplicated gingivitis there will be normal periodontal sulcus probing depths (with the gingival sulcus in dogs <3 mm and in cats <1 mm). Gingivitis is often accompanied by halitosis. However, accompanying complications to gingivitis such as gingival overgrowth may cause additional problems (see below).

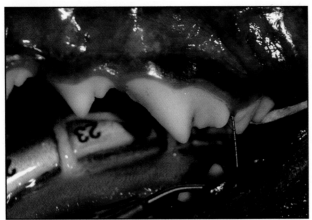

27.1 Gingivitis grade 2 (G2). The gum bleeds when gently probed during the dental examination.

Gingival overgrowth

Gingival overgrowth may be the result of plaque-induced inflammation (e.g. hyperplastic gingivitis); it may be idiopathic or hereditary. Boxers and, to a lesser extent, Border Collies and Labrador Retrievers show a predisposition for the condition.

The significance of gingival overgrowth is the development of a 'pseudo-pocket' due to the altered position of the gingival margin. This 'pocket' is formed due to the enlarged gingiva and not because of the destruction of the periodontal ligament and alveolar bone. In other words, the free gingiva has become taller, giving the impression that there is a pocket. Intraoral radiography helps to confirm the level of the alveolar margin in these cases. The presence of overgrown gingiva compromises normal tooth cleaning from mastication and therefore predisposes to periodontitis.

Periodontitis

Periodontitis *may* develop in an individual with untreated gingivitis. The inflammation seen with periodontitis involves not only the gingiva but also the surrounding periodontal ligament, alveolar bone and cementum (Figure 27.2). The end result of untreated periodontitis is exfoliation of the affected tooth (teeth fall out), due to the destruction of the periodontal ligament and alveolar bone (Figure 27.3). Periodontitis is not site-specific; it may affect one or more sites around one specific tooth or numerous teeth.

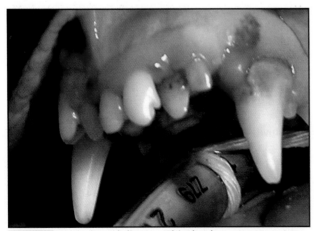

27.2 Periodontal disease. This dog has supernumerary incisors. The incisor set back in the palate has periodontal disease as a result of trapped food and other debris. There is also bony and gingival recession affecting the canine tooth.

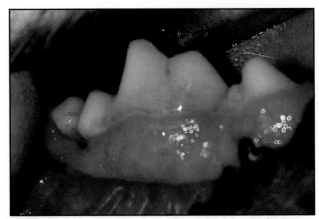

27.3 Periodontal disease. There is a deep pocket between the mandibular right molars 1 and 2. It is often necessary to extract the less important tooth to save the more important tooth.

Periodontitis is not reversible: once the alveolar bone and periodontal ligament have been destroyed it is impossible to replace them without expensive and complicated periodontal surgery. However, it can be managed with the correct treatment and homecare.

Clinical signs of periodontitis include the presence of severe halitosis and large amounts of dental deposits. There may be associated mucosal and glossal ulcers, gingival recession and furcation lesions (loss of alveolar bone between the roots at the neck of the tooth), bleeding from the mouth and/or loose teeth. Patients with severe oral infections develop transient bacteraemia when they eat and groom themselves. This may be associated with distant organ disease affecting the heart, liver, lungs and kidneys.

Periapical periodontitis is usually associated with an exposed pulp that has become necrotic, resulting in inflammation of the tissues surrounding the apex of the root. This may cause a swelling in the jaw or face, and in some cases a draining sinus tract may connect the periapical lesion with the gingival sulcus. Where this occurs there will be a deep narrow pocket extending all the way to the affected root apex. In other cases, the swelling in the jaw may communicate with the oral mucosa or the skin. Blunt trauma to the crown of the tooth can also result in pulp death and periapical periodontitis, even though the tooth crown is intact and has a healthy appearance. These teeth may be treated endodontically (root canal therapy) or extracted.

Other terms defining inflammation of oral tissues

Glossitis

Glossitis is defined as inflammation of the tongue and can be associated with plaque byproducts.

Stomatitis

Stomatitis is inflammation of the oral mucosal surfaces and can be further defined as:

- Buccal stomatitis – inflammation of the cheek mucosa
- Palatitis – inflammation of the palate
- Caudal oral stomatitis – inflammation of the caudal aspects of the oral cavity, rostral to the oropharynx.

The term 'faucitis' is often, incorrectly, used to describe caudal oral inflammation. Caudal oral inflammation describes inflammation of the oral mucosa lateral to the glossopalatine folds. Correctly used, faucitis describes inflammation of the area medial to the glossopalatine folds, which houses the tonsils in their fossae. Inflammation of the lips is termed cheilitis.

Generalized stomatitis is common in cats and is being seen more commonly in dogs, especially Maltese and Cocker Spaniels.

Other dental diseases and conditions

Caries

Caries, or dental decay, occurs in dogs, rabbits, chinchillas and horses. In dogs it usually affects molars (Figure 27.4), as these teeth have occlusal tables that can trap food that is fermented by bacteria, forming acids that induce demineralization of the hard tissues of the tooth. Extensive caries can involve tooth dentine and even invade the pulp tissue. Once the dentine has been destroyed the unsupported enamel crown will fracture; in severe cases, the only remaining tooth remnants may be roots protruding through the gingiva.

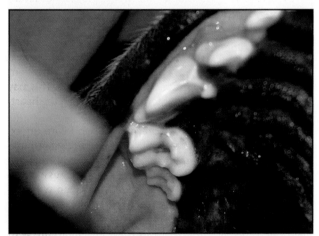

27.4 A typical site for caries in the dog is maxillary molar 1. There is a discoloured carious lesion in the occlusal surface of tooth 109.

Clinically, caries can usually be seen as craters in the dentine that may be filled with soft brown to grey material (although not all lesions are discoloured). A dental explorer will stick into the tooth surface softened by caries. Teeth with carious lesions should be radiographed to reveal the extent of the disease and appropriate treatment can then be carried out.

Teeth with caries need treatment. If the lesion is extensive, with most of the crown lost, the only treatment option is extraction. It is possible to restore a tooth with a small caries lesion. More severely affected teeth, where the lesion involves the pulp, may need endodontic therapy, but this requires referral to a specialist veterinary dentist.

Teeth can become stained for a number of reasons and these lesions should not be confused with caries. Stained teeth usually have intact enamel and dentine, and the surface of these lesions will be hard and smooth when examined with a dental explorer. Tooth staining may be intrinsic, where the dentine is discoloured, or extrinsic, where external pigments affect the tooth colour.

Discoloured teeth

Teeth subjected to trauma, whether in the form of a blunt blow (road traffic accident), as a result of play where teeth have clashed or due to play with certain toys (tug toys), may become discoloured due to pulp inflammation and bleeding. Blood cells permeate the dentine and initially the tooth may appear pink; thereafter, it will progress through the colour changes experienced in bruised soft tissue, ending up being a dull grey. Discoloured teeth may no longer be vital (living). A vital tooth can be distinguished from a non-vital tooth using a bright light source (e.g. auroscope light source). A non-vital tooth will 'absorb' the light, rather than 'transmitting' it as a vital tooth would. This technique of tooth examination is called transillumination (Figure 27.5).

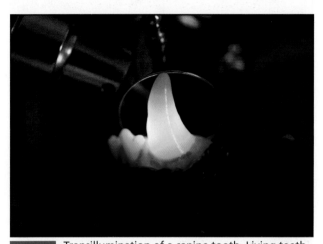

27.5 Transillumination of a canine tooth. Living teeth 'transmit' light and appear 'clear', while 'dead' teeth absorb light and appear dull.

Teeth with enamel defects will become discoloured due to pigments in food and also as a result of gingival bleeding. The use of tetracyclines during odontogenesis (development of the tooth – up to about 3 months of age) may cause discoloration of the tooth, as the substance chelates the calcium laid down in the dental hard tissues and becomes permanently incorporated in the tooth.

Plaque and calculus commonly discolour teeth, but once removed usually a clean crown is revealed. Sometimes calculus formation is associated with demineralization of the crown, leading to discoloration.

Tooth resorption lesions

Tooth resorption lesions (TRs) are common in cats and are being seen more frequently in dogs (Figure 27.6). There are two commonly seen types of tooth resorption:

- Tooth resorption associated with periodontitis
- Idiopathic tooth resorption, not associated with inflammation.

Tooth resorption associated with periodontitis is clinically evident (i.e. the resorptive lesion can be seen on the exposed root) and appears as an 'apple-core' lesion on radiographs. With the idiopathic form there is no associated inflammation and most of the lesions are not visible clinically, with the exception of those that have developed on the crown and have associated hyperplastic gingiva. This gingival overgrowth often bleeds when it is probed with a periodontal probe.

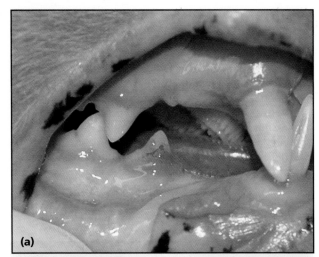

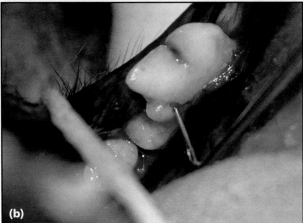

27.6 Tooth resorption lesions. **(a)** TR affecting the mandibular right premolar 3 in a cat. **(b)** TR affecting the mandibular left molar 1 in a dog.

Idiopathic external root resorption begins on the root surface (cementum) and can progress into the root and crown dentine and through the enamel. Often the crowns of affected teeth fracture and remnants may be visible during an oral examination. In some cases roots undergo replacement resorption where the root substance is resorbed and replaced with bone-like material. Some tooth roots may be partially affected by replacement resorption and often fracture during extraction attempts. It is essential to take radiographs of the teeth to be extracted to determine the extent to which the roots are affected by resorption. It does not make sense to try to extract roots that no longer exist. The aetiology of non-inflammatory TRs is unknown; a number of possible causes are currently being investigated, including an excess of vitamin D3 in the diet.

Enamel hypoplasia/dysplasia

Enamel hypoplasia or dysplasia is incomplete or absent enamel formation on the tooth crown and can be caused by systemic disease and infectious, inflammatory, hereditary or traumatic factors. Traumatic injuries to the face and mouth before 3 months of age can damage the enamel organ (enamel-producing and maturing cells), resulting in enamel dysplasia or hypoplasia that is evident when the permanent teeth erupt into the mouth.

Enamel hypoplasia can affect one, several or all of the teeth; it can also affect the primary or secondary teeth

(depending on when the insult occurred). Clinically, the lesions can affect part of the tooth or the whole tooth, depending on when the developing tooth was affected. The longer the noxious cause is present, the greater the area that will be affected (enamel is not produced over the whole crown at the same time). Distemper virus enters the ameloblasts and destroys them, leading to enamel defects. They also affect odontoblasts, dentine production and root development.

Where enamel production has been deficient, dentine will be exposed and can become infected with plaque bacteria, leading to pulp necrosis and periapical pathology (Figure 27.7) that can lead to abscessation.

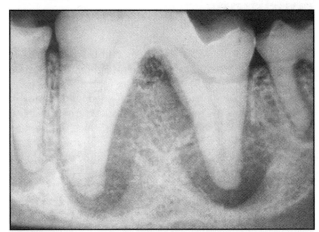

27.7 Radiograph showing periapical pathology due to enamel dysplasia. This resulted in pulpitis and pulp necrosis. (Courtesy of C Gorrel)

Other causes of enamel defects

Fractured deciduous teeth can develop periapical abscesses, which can cause enamel defects in the secondary teeth (the inflammatory reaction as a result of pulpitis and pulp necrosis can damage the enamel organ of the developing secondary tooth).

Pyrexia during amelogenesis (development of tooth enamel) also causes enamel defects that present as bands of malformed enamel. These teeth also have an abnormal shape.

Traumatic tooth injuries

Fractured teeth (Figure 27.8) are commonly found on clinical examination and may require referral to a specialist for treatment. Complicated crown fractures (the pulp is exposed) should be treated either by extraction or by endodontic therapy (root canal therapy). Uncomplicated crown fractures (pulp is not exposed) can also be treated with a restoration if necessary. Immature teeth (those that have not yet developed a root apex) run the risk of pulpitis when the enamel is damaged exposing the dentine, which has wide tubules at this stage. Dentinal sensitivity often occurs after uncomplicated tooth crown fractures and therefore restoration is required to seal the exposed dentinal tubules, eliminating pain and reducing the likelihood of pulp infection.

Fractures that extend below the gum line compromise the periodontium and therefore should be evaluated by a veterinary surgeon who accepts dentistry referrals to determine whether a restoration can be placed or whether the tooth should be extracted or treated endodontically. Subgingival fractures are more plaque retentive than the normal healthy enamel surface and therefore give plaque a foothold.

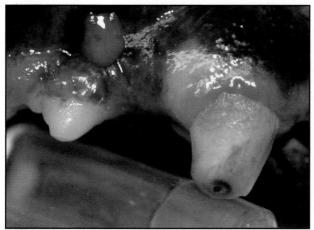

27.8 The pulp in this fractured maxillary right canine tooth has died and caused a root abscess that is draining through the sinus tract just at the mucogingival line caudal to the tooth.

Sometimes teeth are luxated or avulsed as a result of trauma. Avulsed teeth (those wrenched from the alveolus) must be handled by the crown, placed in milk at room temperature and sent with the patient to a veterinary surgeon experienced in orthodontics to be replaced in the mouth. This is a dental emergency and the patient must be attended to within hours if the tooth is to be successfully replanted in the alveolus. Replanted teeth inevitably require endodontic treatment because the communication between the pulp and its neurovascular supply has been severed. Luxated teeth (sometimes seen protruding from beneath the lip) also require urgent attention to reduce and stabilize them. Teeth may be traumatically intruded into the jaw, resulting in destruction of the neurovascular supply to the pulp. Endodontic therapy is inevitably required.

Feline oral cavity disease

Cats with chronic gingivostomatitis are commonly seen. These cats are usually in severe pain and need immediate treatment. The aetiology of this disease complex is unknown (probably multifactorial), but affected animals should always be tested for feline leukaemia virus (FeLV), feline immunodeficiency virus (FIV), feline calicivirus (FCV) and feline herpesvirus (FHV). FCV may be isolated from the majority of cats with chronic gingivostomatitis, but the association between this condition and this virus is at present unknown. In fact, one cat was shown to shed FCV after the oral inflammation had been brought under control.

The oral examination

Dental formulae

Puppy

$$2x \quad \frac{\text{i3 c1 pm3}}{\text{i3 c1 pm3}} = 28 \text{ teeth}$$

Adult dog

$$2x \quad \frac{\text{I3 C1 PM4 M2}}{\text{I3 C1 PM4 M3}} = 42 \text{ teeth}$$

Kitten

$$2x \quad \frac{\text{i3 c1 pm3}}{\text{i3 c1 pm2}} = 26 \text{ teeth}$$

Adult cat

$$2x \quad \frac{\text{I3 C1 PM3 M1}}{\text{I3 C1 PM2 M1}} = 30 \text{ teeth}$$

Where: C = canine; I = incisor; M = molar; PM = premolar. Deciduous teeth are signified by lower case letters.

Dental charting

The oral cavity should be examined thoroughly under general anaesthesia (the conscious examination will reveal only the most superficial and obvious pathology). The animal's head shape, occlusion and each tooth should be examined and the findings recorded on a dental chart; this makes up an essential part of the patient's medical records. The lips, cheeks, tongue, hard and soft palates, oropharynx and larynx, tonsils and the oral mucous membranes should also be examined prior to intubation.

There are many types of dental chart available; examples are shown in Figure 27.9. Each chart has its own system for recording clinical findings and the choice of charting system is a matter of personal preference. It should be noted that dental charts are viewed as if one is looking at the animal face on, i.e. the right side of the mouth is shown (and recorded) on the left of the chart.

Triadan numbering system

On most of the commercially available charts the teeth are numbered using the three-digit Triadan numbering system. The first numeral denotes which quadrant the tooth is in and whether the tooth is part of the permanent or deciduous dentition:

Quadrant	Deciduous dentition numeral	Secondary dentition numeral
Right maxilla	5	1
Left maxilla	6	2
Left mandible	7	3
Right mandible	8	4

The second and third numbers in this system denote the tooth.

Examples

- The tooth numbered 104 is the right maxillary canine tooth
- The tooth numbered 309 is the left mandibular first molar
- The tooth numbered 401 is the right mandibular first incisor.

This system is used for the dog. The cat has fewer teeth and the missing teeth are therefore omitted from the chart (known as the Modified Triadan System of dental nomenclature) (e.g. the mandibular first and second premolars and the second and third molars are not present in the cat) (see Figure 27.9a).

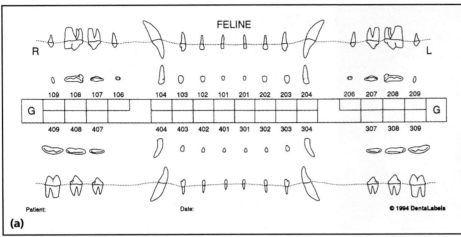

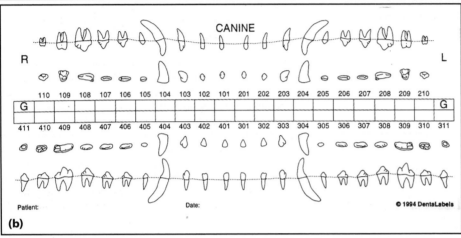

27.9 Examples of dental recording charts used in **(a)** cats and **(b)** dogs. (Reproduced with permission from www.big-o.co.uk, ©DentaLabel.)

When completing dental charts, abbreviations are used to record the information.

Commonly used abbreviations

- Ca = Caries lesion
- CCF = Complicated crown fracture (may be recorded as '#PE')
- ED = Enamel defect
- GH = Gingival overgrowth
- GR = Gingival recession
- NAD = No abnormality detected
- PE = Pulp exposure
- TD = Tertiary dentine
- TR = Tooth resorptive lesion
- UCF = Uncomplicated crown fracture
- WF = Wear facet
- # = Fracture

Tooth fractures are denoted by a line drawn on the chart showing the location of the fracture. For example, if the fracture extends below the gingiva the line should be drawn correspondingly on the chart. Missing teeth are circled. Teeth extracted are crossed through. The patient's occlusion (e.g. scissor bite, short mandibles, short maxillae) should also be recorded on the chart.

The examination and recording procedure

Information to record on the charts for each individual tooth includes the following.

Calculus scores

Gross calculus should be removed prior to examining the teeth and therefore calculus scoring should be carried out first. A slight (CS or 1), moderate (CM or 2) and heavy (CH or 3) scoring method is used. Some veterinary dentists have ceased scoring calculus; however, by scoring and recording calculus at the initial consultation, the examiner is able to compare the teeth against these scores at any subsequent examination. This enables the examiner to monitor the effectiveness of dental homecare programmes. If homecare programmes are correctly implemented the amount of calculus seen at subsequent examinations should be significantly decreased.

Some animals will have heavy calculus on the teeth on one side of the mouth and slight to moderate on the other. There is often a reason for this; for example, there may be a fractured tooth preventing chewing on the side with heavy calculus. Heavy calculus deposits on the teeth on one side of the mouth should also alert the examiner to the possibility of occult disease processes.

Calculus is rough and porous and highly plaque retentive, and although it does not cause periodontitis directly, the fact that it allows the accumulation of plaque often leads to gingivitis.

Gingivitis scores

The modified Löe and Silness gingival index is generally used. It relies on visual inspection and the presence of bleeding on probing of the gingival sulcus (Figure 27.10).

Grade	Gingivitis	Mobility	Furcation
0	Healthy gingiva	No mobility	No furcation involvement
1	Marginal redness with slight thickening of marginal gingiva	Horizontal movement of 1 mm or less in one plane	Probe dips in at the furcation – little bone loss
2	Gingival margin thick and red. Bleeds on probing	Horizontal movement of 1 mm or more in two planes	Probe passes to mid-furcation – significant bone loss
3	Gingiva thickened and red (to bluish). Bleeds spontaneously or when touched	Vertical as well as horizontal movement is possible	Probe passes from buccal to lingual/palatal – no furcation bone remaining

27.10 Grades of gingivitis, tooth mobility and furcation lesions.

Periodontal probing depth

The periodontal probe (see Dental instrumentation and equipment below) should be inserted gently into the gingival sulcus until resistance is encountered at the sulcus base. The depth from the free gingival margin to the base of the sulcus is measured in millimetres. The normal depth of the gingival sulcus is 1–3 mm in dogs and 0.5–1 mm in cats. Measurements that exceed these values indicate the presence of pockets or pseudo-pockets. The measurement should be marked on the dental chart as close to its position on the actual tooth as possible.

Where probing depths are increased, measurements should be made at four sites around the tooth. Some examiners prefer to have one recording per tooth; for example, if the probing depths were as follows: mesiopalatal = 3 mm, mesiobuccal = 3 mm, distobuccal = 5 mm, and distopalatal = 6 mm, they would record a probing depth of 6 mm for the tooth. If the tooth has a single root it may be appropriate to use this scoring system but if there are multiple roots, recording four measurements per tooth is more suitable.

Furcation lesions

In patients with periodontitis, the roots of multirooted teeth can become exposed and the furcation between them becomes visible. Furcation exposure is graded from 0 to 3, depending on severity (see Figure 27.10).

Mobility

Tooth mobility can be tested by using the blunt end of a dental instrument (e.g. the handle of the mirror) in an attempt to move the tooth from its normal position. Using fingers can give a false-positive movement due to the give in the finger. The grading of tooth mobility is shown in Figure 27.10.

Gingival recession

Gingival recession is measured using a periodontal probe (Figure 27.11) and is the distance between the gingival margin and an imaginary line drawn across the normal gingival height

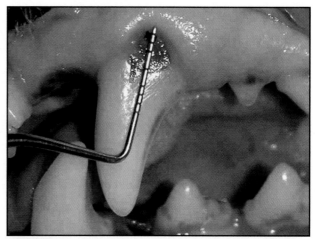

27.11 Gingival recession is measured from the clinical gingival margin to a line joining the normal gingival height mesially and distally on the tooth.

at the mesial and distal edges of the tooth (or mid-buccal surface, depending upon where the defect is). The gingival contour can be drawn on the dental chart, showing the shape of the defect. In some cases the bone will have receded as well and this should also be noted on the chart.

Gingival overgrowth

Overgrown gingiva forms pseudo-pockets as there is an increased probing depth from the margin of the overgrown tissue to the bottom of the sulcus. In some animals with gingival overgrowth, true pockets may also be present in response to plaque on the tooth surface (i.e. they may have concurrent periodontitis). It should be noted that the term gingival overgrowth should be used where the gingiva is enlarged. Gingival hyperplasia is a histopathological/laboratory diagnosis.

Presence of traumatic injuries

This includes, for example, fractured teeth and foreign bodies. Foreign bodies may become lodged across the palate between the maxillary carnassial teeth (Figure 27.12) or longitudinally along the dental arcade, and may cause the jaws to lock closed or prevent the animal from closing its jaws. Patients with oral foreign bodies are often presented with halitosis. This is due to food and other foreign matter around the object becoming necrotic. Some foreign bodies are found during routine oral examinations, without prior clinical signs having been noted.

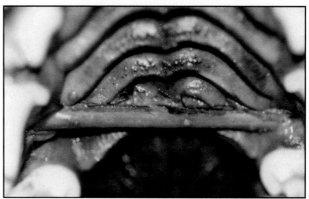

27.12 This foreign body trapped across the palate was an incidental finding in a patient that had a recent history of halitosis.

Exposed pulp

Exposed pulp is denoted on the chart by PE, written adjacent to the affected tooth.

Enamel defects, abrasion and attrition

Enamel defects may be due to trauma or developmental abnormalities.

- Abrasion is the abnormal wear of teeth as a result of the animal's behaviour, e.g. stick or stone chewing, cage biting and playing with a tennis ball (tennis balls are inappropriate toys as they gather sand and grit and abrade the teeth each time they come in contact with them).
- Attrition is abnormal wear due to tooth-to-tooth contact, often seen in dogs with a malocclusion (e.g. brachycephalic dogs with a tight canine–canine–lateral incisor interlock).

Caries

Teeth affected by caries must be differentiated from those that are stained or undergoing resorption. Caries usually present as enamel defects on the tooth surface into which the dental explorer will stick when gently explored. It is often associated with deep dentine craters and halitosis. Surface caries may be seen on carnassial teeth and present as black pits in the enamel.

Stain

Teeth that produce tertiary dentine to protect the pulp as a result of enamel wear may become stained. Tertiary dentine is less structured than secondary dentine and becomes stained by food and other pigments. Arrested caries often also become stained due to the increased permeability of the enamel before remineralization occurs. Surface stain may be removed by polishing, but care must be taken not to damage the pulp as a result of the frictional heat of polishing.

Supernumerary teeth

Supernumerary teeth (teeth in addition to the normal number) may be smaller than their normal counterparts. Some are termed peg teeth, due to their conical shape. These teeth should be drawn on the dental chart. These teeth may require extraction, depending on their relationship to the surrounding secondary dentition.

Mixed dentition

The patient's dentition is considered mixed if there are deciduous and secondary teeth in the mouth at the same time (Figure 27.13). Deciduous teeth that are still present in the mouth when the secondary teeth have come into occlusion are considered persistent deciduous teeth and should be extracted to prevent compromise of the secondary dentition. Radiographs should be taken prior to extraction to help determine which of the teeth are deciduous.

Retained teeth

Retained teeth are those that are found by radiographic examination after they were noted to be clinically missing from

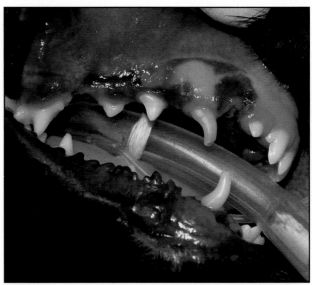

27.13 This puppy has mixed dentition: some secondary teeth have already erupted while some deciduous teeth are still present. None of the deciduous teeth here would be considered persistent as they do not occupy the same location as a secondary tooth.

the mouth. In other words, they have not erupted and remain below the alveolar margin and gingiva. This may be due to impaction where the eruption pathway is obstructed by an adjacent tooth. These teeth may be associated with other pathology (e.g. dentigerous cysts).

Soft tissue injuries

Oral soft tissue injuries should be charted. These include ulcers, lacerations secondary to tooth trauma and degloving injuries.

Dental instrumentation and equipment

It is important that all instruments are clean, sterilized and sharpened before use on each patient. Equipment care and maintenance is of utmost importance. Equally the power equipment should be regularly maintained and serviced to ensure good working order.

The following are essential instruments used regularly in the dental operating room.

Periodontal probe

This is a blunt-ended graduated instrument used to measure gingival sulcus and periodontal pocket depths. It can also be used to measure gingival recession (see Figure 27.11) and overgrowth and for gingivitis scoring, as it is circumscribed around the tooth in the gingival sulcus. It can be used to grade furcation lesions, and the handle (on single-ended instruments) can be used to grade tooth mobility. The graduations on the periodontal probe should be measured so that pocket depth and other measurements are accurate. A Williams 14 periodontal probe (Figure 27.14) is ideal.

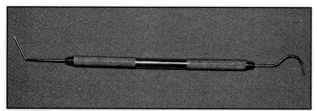

27.14 Williams 14 periodontal probe (left end) combined with a dental explorer (right end). Some clinicians prefer a double-sided instrument, whilst others prefer individual probes and explorers.

Periodontal (dental) explorer

This is a needle-sharp, straight or curved instrument (Figure 27.14) used to explore the tooth surfaces for the presence of caries or other enamel defects (e.g. enamel hypoplasia, fractured teeth and feline TR lesions). It is also possible to explore subgingivally using a dental explorer to examine for residual calculus after the scale and polish procedure. It is important to keep the dental explorer sharp. This instrument should be replaced when damaged, as hand-sharpening produces a roughened sharp tip that is undesirable.

Mirror

A dental mirror is commonly used in human dentistry but not necessarily in veterinary dentistry. It can be used to visualize the palatal and lingual surfaces of teeth (and distal surfaces of caudal teeth) and should be available for each procedure. It can also be used to reflect light into poorly lit areas of the mouth and to examine the nasopharynx. Wiping the surface of the mirror against a moist mucosal surface prevents fogging.

Calculus-removing forceps

Calculus-removing forceps (Figure 27.15) must be correctly used by placing one beak on the gingival extent of the calculus and the other on the incisal tip of the tooth. This generates a shearing force that dislodges the calculus from the tooth surface. Under no circumstances should the tooth surface be 'pinched' between the beaks of the forceps, or the crown may shatter. Care must also be exercised when placing the forceps at the gingival margin, or the gingiva can be damaged as well.

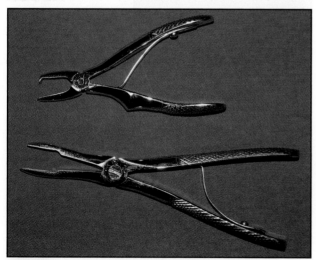

27.15 Calculus-removing forceps are available in numerous patterns. They must be used with care to prevent damage to the tooth and gingiva.

Hand scaler and curette

The dental scale and polish procedure is described in a later section. The scaler and curette (Figure 27.16) are used to remove dental deposits from the tooth surfaces. They consist of a handle, shank and a working tip. The scaler has a sharp, pointed tip that should only be used supragingivally (subgingival use will result in laceration of the gingival tissues). The curette has a blade that ends in a blunt, rounded tip that can be used subgingivally for removal of subgingival deposits and root debridement. Both the scaler and curette should be pulled away from the gingiva towards the crown of the tooth. It is important to maintain the sharpness of these instruments for efficient use.

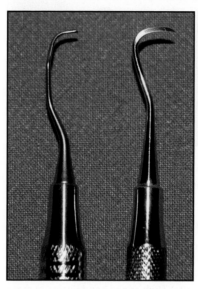

27.16 The hand curette (left) has a blunt end, while the scaler (right) has a sharp tip and is only used above the gum line.

Ultrasonic scaler

The tip of the scaler oscillates at ultrasonic frequencies and is driven by an electromagnetic or piezoelectric handpiece. Ultrasonic tips are manufactured for supragingival and subgingival use. Some subgingival ultrasonic scaler tips are designed to be used on the 'push' rather than 'pull' stroke.

Tip vibration in magnetostrictive scalers is created by an electromagnetic field in the handpiece that surrounds a metal stack or ferrite rod. When an alternating electric current is applied to the handpiece, the insert vibrates. Piezoelectric scaler tips vibrate because of deformation of a crystal in the handpiece when an alternating electric current is applied to it. Sonic scalers are available that are driven by compressed air. Tip vibration is caused when air is driven through an eccentric hole in the shaft to which the tip is attached.

All electromechanical scalers have coolant water directed at their tips and this must be adjusted for optimal function. The water is also responsible for the phenomenon known as cavitation, by which very small bubbles that develop within the coolant liquid implode on the calculus, helping to dislodge it. Cavitation has also been shown to cause disruption of the cell walls of some plaque bacteria (spirochaetes).

Scalers (see Figure 27.24) must never be used with their tips perpendicular to the tooth surface, as the action of the vibrating tip will damage the tooth surface (gouge the enamel). Ultrasonic instruments were first invented to section (cut) teeth prior to extraction but such improper use will damage teeth.

The dental unit (power equipment)

Dental units are available with numerous attachments but the minimum requirements are: high-speed handpiece; low-speed handpiece with contra-angled 'prophy' attachment; (low-speed straight handpiece for rabbit dentistry); three-way air–water syringe; and an ultrasonic scaler (this may be combined into the dental unit or be a separate piece of equipment) (Figure 27.17).

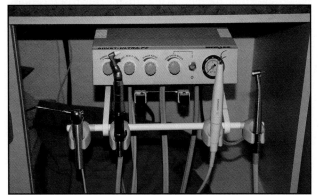

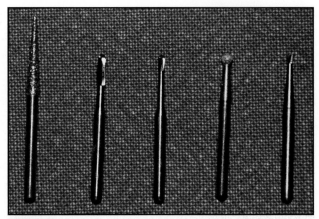

27.18 | A selection of friction grip burs. From left: tapered diamond fissure; round-tipped flat fissure tungsten carbide (TC); pear-shaped TC; round diamond; and small pear-shaped.

27.17 | The dental unit. From left: 3-way syringe; low-speed handpiece with contra-angle polisher; Piezoelectric scaler; and high-speed handpiece.

High-speed handpiece

The high-speed handpiece facilitates tooth extractions by allowing the operator to section multirooted teeth prior to extraction. The bur in the handpiece rotates at about 400,000 rpm (revolutions per minute). High-speed handpieces are more efficient at sectioning teeth but care must be exercised when using them to prevent air emboli and emphysema formation. Some high-speed handpieces have an integrated fibreoptic or LED light that improves visibility in the work field. It is essential that protective eyewear is worn by both the operator and the assistant when this equipment is used.

Low-speed handpiece

The low-speed air motor on the dental unit can accept contra-angle or straight handpieces. It also accepts the contra-angled polishing head. The rotation speed of this air motor is adjustable up to 5500 rpm (but speed-reducing and speed-increasing handpieces may also be used). Straight surgical handpieces are available for use with the low-speed air motor. These can be used for removing and shaping alveolar bone. When being used for sectioning teeth and alveolotomy (incision into the dental alveolus) or alveoloplasty (surgical shaping of the dental alveolus), the tooth or bone must be kept cool by applying sterile coolant to the bur and tooth or bone. This is most effectively carried out by an assistant squirting a gentle stream of polyionic fluid from a syringe on to the operating site. It should be noted that it is not ideal to use a low-speed handpiece to section teeth; however, they are efficient at removing compromised dentine in carious lesions.

Burs

Various burs are available for the high- and low-speed handpieces (Figure 27.18). Generally, fissure burs are used to section teeth and pear-shaped or round burs are used to remove and smooth off alveolar bone. Large round diamond burs are most effective for alveoloplasty and do not damage adjacent soft tissues when used appropriately.

Three-way syringe

The three-way syringe (Figure 27.19) can deliver a jet of water, or a jet of water with air (effectively a water spray), or just air. It is very useful for flushing the mouth during dental procedures. A gentle puff of air will dry the tooth surface, enabling better visualization; residual calculus resembles chalk on the dry tooth surface. The spray or air should not be directed into an open alveolus for fear of causing air emboli or emphysema.

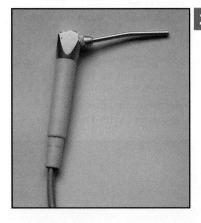

27.19 | Three-way syringe.

Dental Luxator®

The dental Luxator® (Directa Dental AB, Sweden) is used to sever the periodontal ligaments during tooth extraction. It has a fine, sharp tip (Figure 27.20) that is used to cut the epithelial attachment and periodontal ligament, which hold the tooth in the alveolus. An appropriately sized instrument should be used for the root in question (the curvature of the Luxator® blade should approximate that of the root being extracted). When the Luxator® is driven into the periodontal ligament space it causes condensation of the alveolar bone, creating more space that will allow insertion of the dental elevator to further loosen the tooth.

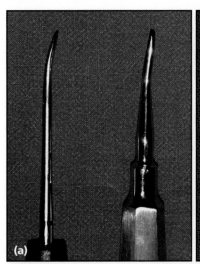
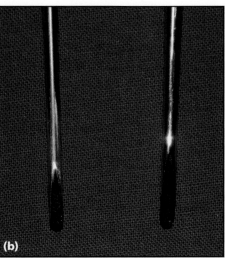
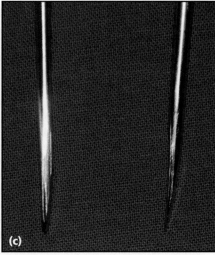

27.20 **(a)** The Luxator® (left) is sharpened to a fine point, whereas elevators are sharpened to about 45 degrees. **(b)** The Luxator Forte® (left) is more robust and has a more abrupt increase in thickness, enabling increased rotational leverage. **(c)** The Luxator® (right) has a fine sharp point that facilitates severing of the periodontal ligament and compression of the alveolar bone, creating space to use the Luxator Forte® (left).

Dental elevator

Once the gingival attachment has been severed and most of the periodontal ligament has been severed and torn and sufficient space has been created by using the Luxator®, the dental elevator (see Figure 27.20) can be worked into the alveolus and used to apply rotational leverage on the root, disrupting its attachment further and leading to it being delivered from the alveolus. The Luxator Forte® (Directa Dental AB, Sweden) can also be used following the Luxator®.

Periosteal elevator

The periosteal elevator (Figure 27.21) is necessary for surgical extraction procedures and other oral surgery. It is used to raise the mucoperiosteal flap to expose the alveolar bone. Once the gingival and alveolar mucosal incisions have been made, the periosteal elevator is inserted below the periosteum beneath the alveolar mucosa and worked along the bone surface, raising the periosteum. Once the alveolar mucosal periosteum has been raised from the bone, the instrument is worked along the bone in the direction of the alveolar margin and then under the attached gingiva. If approached via the gingival sulcus there is a risk that the periosteal elevator will puncture the flap at the mucogingival junction.

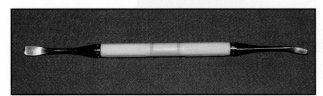

27.21 Periosteal elevator.

Extraction forceps

Extraction forceps should not be used by the veterinary surgeon without extensive training. Extraction forceps must be used appropriately, as incorrect use could fracture the crown of the tooth. There are numerous extraction forceps beak patterns manufactured to fit human teeth. Most of these are inappropriate for use in veterinary dentistry. The beak size used should approximate the size of the root to be extracted to ensure an appropriate fit.

Surgical kit

This should be readily available for surgical extractions and consists of (Figure 27.22):

- Scalpel handle and blades
- Periosteal elevator
- Small scissors (sharp–sharp Metzenbaum and/or iris scissors are ideal)
- Synthetic, monofilament absorbable suture material, 1 metric size (5/0)
- Fine needle holders
- Small rat-toothed tissue forceps (Adsons, Adson Brown)
- Suture cutting scissors.

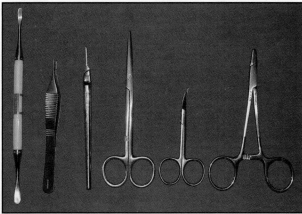

27.22 A surgical kit adequate for raising mucoperiosteal flaps. From left: periosteal elevator (Goldman Fox A&B); fine rat-toothed forceps; No. 3 scalpel holder (No. 15 or 15c scalpel blade not shown); Metzenbaum scissors; suture scissors; comfortable needle holder able to accommodate fine suture material.

Maintenance of instruments and power equipment

When dropped, dental explorers and periodontal probes inevitably bend. Attempts at straightening them may result in their breakage and they should therefore be replaced. Spare periodontal probes and explorers should be kept in case of emergency and replaced as necessary.

The dental unit, handpieces and instruments require daily, weekly, monthly and annual maintenance to ensure that they continue operating at optimum performance. The dental unit will have instructions and a service agreement unique to it. It is recommended that the manufacturer's maintenance guidelines are strictly adhered to.

Handpieces need to be oiled regularly prior to autoclaving and again before use. Over-lubrication can be as detrimental as under-lubrication and the manufacturer's instructions should be followed.

Sharpening instruments

Hand instruments need to be cleaned, sterilized and sharpened. Sharpening these instruments regularly not only increases their useful life but also prevents injuries to the patient and operator due to instrument slippage.

- **Hand scalers** are sharpened by placing the blade of the scaler on a flat sharpening stone (Figure 27.23a). Using the fourth finger as a guide on the table surface to keep the instrument at the correct angle to the sharpening surface, it is drawn towards the operator. Both sides must be sharpened.
- **Dental hand curettes** are sharpened by holding the instrument in the palm grip with the curette tip projecting from the back of the hand. A sharpening stone is held in the other hand, applied to the curette blade and drawn across it in an arc to accommodate the slight curvature of the cutting edge (Figure 27.23b).

- **Luxators** are sharpened on the concave surfaces. The instrument should be placed on a conical or round sharpening stone that is held firmly on a solid surface and then pushed along the stone (Figure 27.23c). This sharpens the tip without forming a 'bur' on the convex side.
- **Dental elevators** are sharpened on a flat sharpening stone. The convex side of the instrument is applied to the stone at the correct inclination (Figure 27.23d) and the instrument is sharpened using a back-and-forth wrist motion.

Health and safety considerations

Dental operating room

The dental operating room should not share airspace with the surgical preparatory room, sterile procedures room or theatres, due to aerosolized plaque and bacteria generated during the dental procedure.

Some dental chemicals contain solvents and the dental operating room should be well ventilated. Ideally it should have an air extraction system that discharges the air outside so that it does not re-enter the building via the clean air supply.

There must be sufficient light in the room and this may be supplemented by an additional light source directed on to the work area. The operating light should not be excessively brighter than the room light or a dazzle effect will be created.

Operator and assistant

To reduce fatigue, both the operator and the assistant should be seated, with the patient, instruments and anaesthetic equipment all within easy reach during the dental procedures.

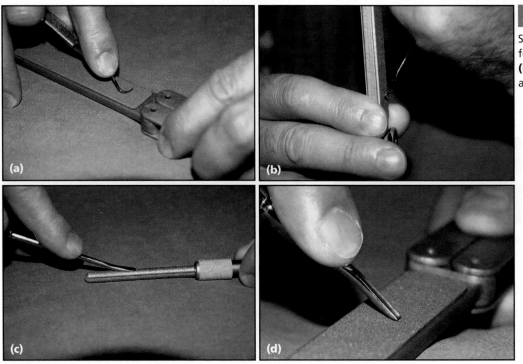

27.23

Sharpening techniques for: **(a)** scaler; **(b)** curette; **(c)** luxator; and **(d)** elevator.

Safety spectacles must be worn by the operator and assistant to prevent injury to the eye from flying debris or a fractured high-speed bur. The bur rotates at approximately 400,000 rpm and will travel at an enormous speed if it fractures. Spectacles also prevent splatter and aerosolized material from landing in the eye.

Examination gloves should be worn, as should protective clothing. It is also recommended that the veterinary surgeon and nurse wear head coverings.

Instruments

All instruments must be kept sharp to prevent accidents that may occur when blunt instruments slip off the tooth or alveolar bone. Care must be exercised when sharpening and washing instruments and the manufacturer's instructions should be followed. Instruments should be sterilized between patients. Disposable 'sharps' must be disposed of correctly (see Chapter 2).

Handling dental instruments

- Correct handling of dental instruments is essential to prevent repetitive strain injury.
- Approximately 300 different bacteria can be cultured from the mouths of cats and dogs. Adequate disinfection of instruments must be performed between patients.
- Instruments must be stored flat, in trays, to prevent damage to the sharp edges.
- Care must be exercised when cleaning dental instruments to prevent iatrogenic injury.
- Hand instruments: scalers, curettes, elevators and luxation instruments must be kept sharp – regular whetting is better than infrequent sharpening and will prolong the useful life of the instrument.

Patient safety

The patient should be placed on a soft surface that will maintain its body heat. Covering the patient with bubble wrap will help maintain body temperature. Adequate provision should be made to remove water delivered from dental equipment in order that the animal does not become wet and cold. The patient's face should be protected from the aerosolized bacteria by a towel or drape. An ocular lubricant should be placed in both eyes to prevent desiccation of the corneas and regularly reapplied throughout the dental procedure.

Scaling and polishing

Tooth scaling and polishing is performed routinely in patients that have slight calculus and mild gingivitis or may be required in the treatment of patients suffering from periodontal disease or in preparation for tooth extraction.

Intubation

Scale-and-polish procedures are performed in animals that are anaesthetized and intubated. The cuff of the endotracheal (ET) tube should be inflated to the correct pressure so as not to cause damage to the trachea or respiratory epithelial lining. Applying a thin layer of sterile water-soluble lubricant will ensure that the ET tube does not adhere to the respiratory epithelium. Inflation of the cuff does not prevent liquid from passing down the trachea and so it is important to keep the mouth lower than the pharynx, enabling liquids to flow from the mouth. It is good practice to place a pharyngeal pack into the pharynx to trap calculus and other debris and prevent blood from accumulating around the ET tube.

The cuffed ET tube ensures that anaesthetic gases are confined to the anaesthetic circuit and disposed of via the scavenging system. It also prevents the anaesthetized animal from inhaling aerosolized bacteria, plaque and calculus.

Scaling

Prior to scaling the teeth, the oral cavity should be flushed with chlorhexidine, as this has been shown to significantly reduce aerosolized bacteria.

After the mouth has been examined and charted, gross calculus can be removed from the teeth using calculus forceps, as described earlier. The remaining calculus can then be removed using hand or electromechanical scalers. When using electromechanical scalers, the scaler tip must be applied side-on to the crown surface (Figure 27.24). If the calculus is tenacious, the operator should move on to an adjacent tooth before returning to complete scaling. This will prevent iatrogenic damage to the tooth by heating. Electromechanical scalers should be applied to the calculus using a brush-stroke technique without applying downward force against the tooth. If the scaler tip is pushed against the tooth, resulting in less vibration, the efficiency of scaling is decreased. Some scaler tips vibrate in an orbital pattern, whilst others oscillate in a longitudinal manner. Knowledge of the scaler tip oscillation pattern will help the operator to use the instrument effectively.

- The point of the ultrasonic scaler tip should never be used against the tooth, as it will etch (engrave) the tooth surface.
- It should be ensured that plenty of water coolant is used to keep the scaler and tooth cool and to flush away debris.

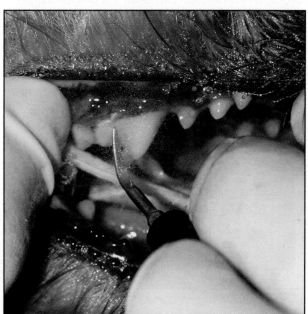

27.24 Piezoelectric scaler being used appropriately with the edge of the scaler against the tooth.

Subgingival scaling and root debridement

Short excursions may be made subgingivally to remove calculus; under ideal circumstances a subgingival scaling tip should be used for this to prevent thermal damage to the crown and gingiva. Hand curettes can be used to remove subgingival calculus, and a dental explorer gently circumscribed around the subgingival crown will reveal residual calculus. Where pockets are deep it may be necessary to debride the root surface, using a curette to remove necrotic cementum. In severe cases, the patient should be referred to a veterinary dentist for open root debridement; a gingival flap is raised to expose the roots and enable debridement before being sutured back in place.

A curette is used for both subgingival scaling and root debridement. It is inserted into the gingival sulcus; the cutting edge should then be engaged against the tooth surface and the curette pulled in a coronal direction. This should be carried out around the whole circumference of the tooth. This procedure also debrides the gingival wall of the pocket. An explorer can then be used to judge the smoothness of the subgingival part of the tooth. Care must be exercised not to denude the root of cementum, as this will expose the dentine and may lead to dentinal hypersensitivity.

Polishing

Polishing removes the remaining plaque that is usually not visible and helps to smooth the tooth surface. If the tooth has been scaled it must be polished, as minor scratches left on the tooth after scaling facilitate plaque retention due to the roughened surface. To minimize the amount of frictional heat generated, the prophylaxis cup or brush, used in a low-speed contra-angle handpiece, should not rotate faster than 1000 rpm. Some prophylaxis cups oscillate (Figure 27.25a) rather than rotate, generating less frictional heat during polishing. In addition, large volumes of prophylaxis paste should be used as it acts as a lubricant during polishing. Using paste and a rubber cup, the tooth surfaces can be polished. When gentle pressure is exerted on the prophylaxis cup against the tooth surface, it flares and can pass under the gingival margin to remove subgingival plaque (Figure 27.25b). 'Prophy' brushes can also be used, although those made of nylon filaments may strip cementum from the root when polishing subgingivally, resulting in dentinal hypersensitivity.

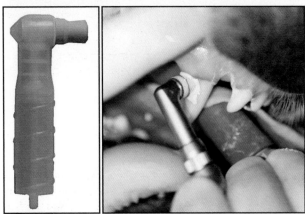

27.25 (a) Reciprocating polisher head. (© IM3 Pty Ltd.)
(b) Subgingival polishing. The 'prophy' cup should be gently pressed on to the tooth to flare out and polish subgingivally.

Radiography of teeth and supporting structures

It is essential to take radiographs when performing veterinary dentistry, as the extent of pathology cannot be seen without them (see Chapter 18). Whereas the clinical examination enables visualization of the tooth crown, radiography reveals the root, which can make up about 75% of the length of the tooth in deciduous canines. Radiographs also show the extent of bone loss in periodontitis and periapical pathology in teeth with inflamed or necrotic pulps.

Indications for radiography

- Missing teeth.
- Fractured teeth.
- Supernumerary teeth (to determine association with adjacent normal teeth).
- Prior to extraction.
- Monitoring treatment progress (e.g. when retrieving root remnants).
- Teeth affected by caries.
- Differentiating teeth with tertiary dentine from those that may have exposed pulps.
- Teeth affected by periodontal disease.
- Persistent deciduous teeth.
- Discoloured teeth.
- Teeth affected by resorption.
- Jaw fractures.
- Investigation of sinus tracts that may be associated with teeth.
- Investigation of nasal discharge.
- Investigation of oral masses.

Good technique is vital; for the radiograph to be diagnostic it must be an accurate representation of the tooth and associated structures. It is therefore best practice to use intraoral radiographic film and techniques or digital dental radiography.

X-ray generators
Medical X-ray machines

Although cumbersome and usually fixed in one room medical X-ray machines (described in detail in Chapter 18) can be used to take diagnostic dental radiographs. The focus–film distance should be adjusted to approximately 40 cm, either by lowering the X-ray tube head or by placing the patient on an object on top of the X-ray table. The kV should be set at 70 and the mAs at 15–25, depending upon the size of the patient. If dental X-ray film is not available, mammography film can be used to good effect but superimposition of structures may be problematic. Using mammography film in flexible cassettes will eliminate superimposition (Figure 27.26).

Dental X-ray machines

A dedicated dental X-ray machine has numerous advantages:

- The machine can be installed in the dental operating area (thus the anaesthetized animal does not need to be

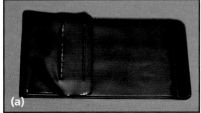

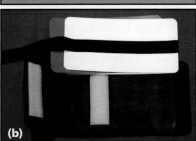

27.26
(a) Flexible intraoral radiography cassette. **(b)** Flexible cassette showing mammograghy film flanked by an intensifying screen.

transported from the dental room to the radiography room each time a radiograph is required)
- The machine can be manoeuvred around the animal
- Cone collimators of a fixed length, reducing scatter radiation
- Using a dedicated dental X-ray machine frees up the radiography room to be used for other patients.

Dental X-ray machines can be attached to a wall, suspended from the ceiling, on castors so they can be wheeled (Figure 27.27a), or portable (Figure 27.27b). Dental X-ray generators usually have a fixed kV and mA, with time being the only adjustable setting on most machines. Modern dental X-ray machines have a fixed kV of 60–80 and mA of 2–8. Time can be adjusted from 0.1 to about 2 seconds.

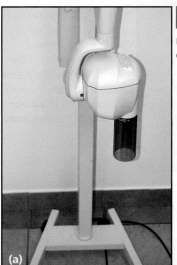

27.27 **(a)** Mobile dental X-ray machine. **(b)** Portable dental X-ray machine.

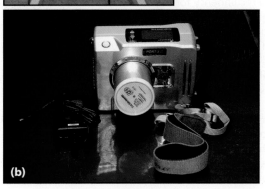

Dental operating room

The dental room should be planned in such a manner that the X-ray machine can be discharged from outside to improve safety for the operator and assistant. The machine may be discharged from outside by depressing a button mounted on the wall or remotely using an extension cable. The door to the dental operating area should be lead-lined, with a window in it permitting constant observation of the patient. Radiation safety advice should be sought before investing in a portable machine.

Dental film

Dental X-ray film is available in a number of sizes. The most commonly used in veterinary dentistry are:

- Adult periapical film: 3 x 4 cm
- Occlusal film: 5 x 7 cm
- Paediatric periapical film: 2 x 3.5 cm.

These X-ray films are non-screen, single emulsion and available in two speeds:

- E (Ekta) – larger crystals, therefore faster (requiring lower exposure settings) but giving poorer resolution
- D (Ultra) – smaller crystals (requiring higher exposure settings) but giving better resolution.

The dental film is packed in envelopes that are backed by a lead insert to reduce scatter (Figure 27.28). Each film has a dot placed in one corner and is packaged in such a way that it faces the incident beam. This allows the picture to be oriented for viewing afterwards.

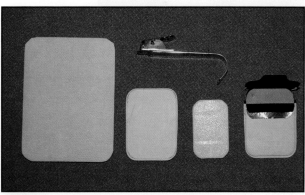

27.28 The dental X-ray films commonly used in practice are from left: occlusal, adult periapical, paediatric periapical. An opened film envelope reveals the film (green), lead backing sheet, and black protective paper. Also shown is an X-ray film clip.

Intraoral techniques
Parallel technique

This is used for the mandibular premolars and molars caudal to premolar 2 in the dog (including this tooth in some animals). The patient is positioned in lateral recumbency and the film is placed adjacent to the tooth or teeth to be radiographed (between the tongue and the mandible) and pushed down so that it becomes palpable beyond the ventral margin of the mandible (Figure 27.29). A piece of scrunched-up paper

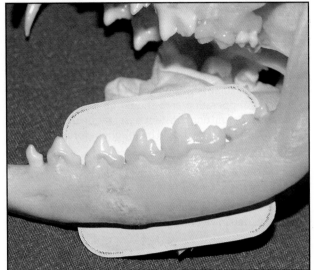

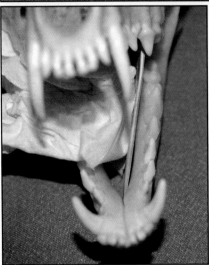

27.29 For the parallel technique, the film is placed between the tongue and teeth/mandible so that the film protrudes past the ventral margin of the mandible. The film should be parallel to the teeth and the incident beam is directed perpendicular to the teeth and film.

towel can be used to keep the film in the correct position. The incident beam is then directed at right angles to the long axis of the tooth and film. The tooth and film are parallel to each other and the incident beam is directed perpendicular to both.

Bisecting angle technique

This technique is used when taking radiographs of the maxillary teeth and the incisors, premolars 1 and 2 and canines in the mandible. The film is placed as close as possible to the tooth or teeth to be radiographed. When maxillary teeth are radiographed, the film spans the palate or is placed on the incisal tips of the canines (Figure 27.30). The tooth axis (an imaginary line joining the tip of the crown and the root tip) is determined and the angle formed by this line and the film axis is bisected. The incident beam is directed perpendicular (at right angles) to the bisecting line, giving a true representation of the tooth on the radiograph. If the incident beam is close to perpendicular to the film axis, the tooth will appear short and the image is termed foreshortened. If the beam is close to perpendicular to the tooth axis, the resultant image will be lengthened and termed elongated.

When radiographing the maxillary carnassial tooth, which has three roots (two mesially (towards the midline) and one distally), the mesial roots are often superimposed on each other. To separate these roots on the radiograph, the incident beam must be directed either rostrally or caudally (maintaining the same bisecting angle). On the resultant image the SLOB (Same Lingual Opposite Buccal) rule is used to identify which root is which. Using the SLOB rule, if the incident beam is directed from rostrally the most mesial root will be the palatal root. If the incident beam is directed from caudally, the more distal of the mesial roots will be the palatal root and the more mesial of the mesial roots will be the buccal root.

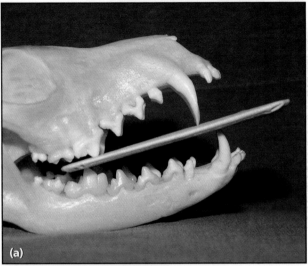

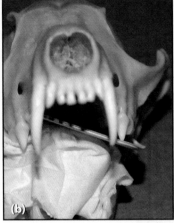

27.30 For the bisecting angle technique, the film is placed as close to the teeth as possible. **(a)** Film positioned for imaging the maxillary incisors including a rostrocaudal view of the maxillary canines. **(b)** Film positioned for imaging maxillary premolars and molars.

Positioning the patient

It may be helpful to position the patient as follows:

- Sternal recumbency for the maxillary incisors
- Lateral or sternal recumbency for the maxillary canines, premolars and molars
- Dorsal recumbency for the mandibular incisors
- Dorsal or lateral recumbency for the mandibular canines
- Lateral recumbency for the mandibular premolars and molars.

When radiographing the maxillary carnassials of a cat, superimposition of the zygomatic arch presents a problem. Lifting the cat's nose or tilting its head in order that the upper dental arch is parallel to the table helps to prevent this superimposition.

Processing intraoral dental film

Intraoral dental film can be processed in a number of ways:

- In a chairside 'darkroom' (Figure 27.31) – a purpose-made enclosure that contains three or four receptacles (developer, rinse water, fixer; or developer, rinse water, fixer, rinse water)
- In the practice darkroom – using a manual processing technique
- Using an automatic film processer suitable for processing dental film.

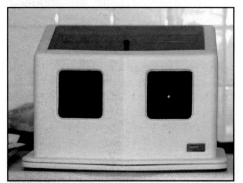

27.31 A chairside 'darkroom' is convenient for processing dental X-ray films.

The film should be held at the edges to prevent fingerprint artefacts. Intraoral radiographs are best viewed in a dark room with the viewing light only coming through the radiograph. The use of magnification is also beneficial. Processed radiographs must be properly dried before being stored in well labelled film holders (envelopes may be used) as part of the animal's clinical records. Dental radiographs can be photographed using a digital camera for archiving and emailing for a second opinion. Transparency scanners can also be used to digitize radiographs.

Digital dental radiography

Veterinary practices are increasingly investing in digital dental radiographic technology (Figure 27.32). The system not only eliminates the need for processing chemicals and takes less space, but also requires lower X-ray exposure settings and the images are visible almost instantaneously. There are two main digital radiographic systems:

- Direct
- Indirect.

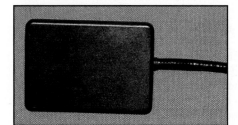

27.32 This transducer is used to take digital dental radiographs using the direct technique. The image is displayed almost immediately on a computer screen.

The direct system uses a digital sensor that is placed in the mouth in the same way as intraoral film. The tooth/teeth are exposed and the image appears on the computer screen within seconds. The sensor may be attached to the computer via a docking station and USB cable, or transmit the captured information via Bluetooth technology. At present there is a limited selection of tranducers, some of which are bulky, making their use in smaller dogs and cats challenging.

Using the indirect system, phosphorescent plates (within protective envelopes) are placed in the mouth in the same way as intraoral film and the tooth/teeth exposed in the usual way. The exposed plate is then placed in a drum reader, which converts the phosphorescent image into a digital image that can be viewed on a computer screen. This system takes slightly longer than the direct system but has a wide range of plate sizes.

Digital radiographs can be manipulated in a number of ways to help produce a clearer image: brightness, contrast, reverse-image, 3D, measurement and magnification can all be altered. Digital radiographs can be appended to the patient record and also emailed to a colleague for a second opinion.

Maintenance of dental health and prevention of dental disease

Disease prevention is vital in the maintenance of dental and oral health. Approximately 85% of dogs and cats >3 years of age suffer from early signs of periodontal disease, probably making dental disease the most common condition seen in general veterinary practice. Periodontitis almost exclusively follows on from gingivitis, a reversible condition; consequently its control is within reach. Treating gingivitis prevents most cases of periodontitis.

In the minority of cases, as a result of periapical root pathology (secondary to necrotic pulp), periodontitis may spread along the root surface in the periodontal space and eventually surface in the gingival sulcus. In these cases gingivitis may be secondary to the periapical lesion, called an endodontic–periodontic lesion.

The causes of gingivitis are discussed above. The treatment is routine dental scale-and-polish followed by thorough dental homecare.

Dental homecare

This consists of daily tooth brushing, feeding an appropriate diet, providing dental chews and encouraging play with tooth-friendly toys. Of these routines, the most important is tooth brushing. As veterinary patients cannot be taught to brush their own teeth, owners must be relied upon to institute and continue dental homecare. Thus, an essential part of professional periodontal therapy is client education.

Pet owners must be aware that, whatever professional treatment is performed, it is only part of the ongoing therapy. Plaque begins to accumulate on tooth surfaces within 24 hours of a scale-and-polish procedure. Where homecare is not implemented, gingivitis scores 3 months after professional periodontal therapy (supra- and subgingival scaling and polishing) have been found to be the same as those prior to treatment. The aim of dental homecare is to minimize the accumulation of plaque and therefore reduce the risk of periodontal disease developing or progressing. Continuous monitoring of dental homecare is essential, to keep owners motivated and to check on the adequacy of the oral hygiene carried out. Nurse-led clinics may be held during which plaque-disclosing solution may be applied to the pet's teeth and gums to show how effective the dental homecare is.

Tooth brushing

Tooth brushing is the most effective method of removing plaque from the tooth surfaces in the conscious animal. Daily tooth brushing can return the gingivae to health, but this will not be maintained if carried out less than daily. In addition, an animal may require professional periodontal therapy at regular intervals, just as some people need to visit the dentist or dental hygienist on a more regular basis. Some animals are more predisposed to plaque accumulation and hence regular professional treatment may be required despite conscientious thorough dental homecare.

The success of plaque control by tooth brushing depends on the owner's ability and the animal's cooperation. Owners should therefore start brushing their pet's teeth as early in its life as possible. Even the youngest puppies and kittens can have their teeth brushed. The primary dentition will be exfoliated but the animal will have become accustomed to the tooth brushing process by the time the secondary dentition has erupted. It is important to brush kittens' teeth, as it is particularly difficult to introduce adult cats to the process.

Most young animals will tolerate tooth brushing as it is begun when the gingivae are healthy and the procedure is not associated with pain (which can lead to negative reinforcement). Pets that have their teeth brushed regularly enjoy increased intervals between professional dental treatments. Tooth brushing (Figure 27.33) should be introduced as part of the daily routine. A treat or a walk can be the reward at the end of a tooth brushing session. In multi-pet households the added individual attention appears to appeal to pets and they will queue to have their turn.

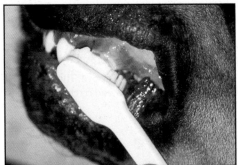

27.33 A medium toothbrush can be used to brush a dog's teeth. Pet toothpaste must be used as human toothpaste can cause fluoride toxicity.

Toothbrushes and toothpaste

Pet toothbrushes are available with double-ended angled heads. A medium texture human toothbrush can also be used (or medium child's toothbrush). Human toothpaste must never be used, due to the high fluoride content, which can cause toxicity when pets swallow it rather than rinsing and spitting. Human toothpastes usually also contain a detergent that causes foaming, a sensation apparently disliked by

animals. Pet toothpastes are available in a variety of flavours and, although not essential, help to familiarize the pet with the tooth brushing process.

Tooth brushing procedure

- Ensure that the animal is comfortable before commencing and introduce the process gradually.
- Start brushing the molars and premolars and brush a few teeth each day until eventually all the teeth can be brushed in one session.
- Gentle circular motions are used to brush the teeth and gingival margin.
- Using a circular movement with the brush at an angle of 45 degrees near the gingival margin, the filaments of the brush can be made to flare slightly into the gingival sulcus, removing subgingival plaque.

Initially it is acceptable to concentrate on brushing the buccal surfaces of the teeth by placing the toothbrush in the animal's cheek, but eventually it is advisable to open the mouth to brush the lingual/palatal surfaces as well. It will take longer for the animal to become accustomed to this.

In patients with periodontal disease, the gums will bleed when tooth brushing is first instituted. The owners should be informed that this will happen and that they should continue brushing. As the gingivae return to health there will be less bleeding, until brushing does not elicit any blood at all.

Diet, chews and toys

There are numerous diets formulated to be tooth friendly. Some have a structure that ensures that the food is chewed and the tooth surface is mechanically cleaned. Other diets contain minerals that prevent mineralization of plaque to calculus by binding with calcium.

Some dental chews contain enzymes that prevent calculus formation with or without a physical cleansing effect (e.g. raw hide).

Tooth-friendly toys may have a 'window-wiper blade' effect or have projections that clean the tooth surface. Some also dispense toothpaste as the animal plays with the toy.

Dentistry in rabbits and rodents

Definitions

- **Brachyodont** – short crown:root ratio with a true root. The mature tooth has a closed root apex (e.g. humans, dogs, cats, ferrets and some rodents).
- **Hypsodont** – tooth with a long crown and comparatively short or no true root. The subgingival part is called the reserve crown. The dentition or part thereof is radicular or aradicular:
  - Radicular hypsodont – true tooth root develops later in the life of the animal (e.g. horses, cattle)
  - Aradicular hypsodont – tooth never forms a true root with an apex, and continues to grow throughout life (e.g. rabbits, hares, guinea pigs, chinchillas).

Normal dentition

Rodents have aradicular hypsodont incisors and either aradicular hypsodont or brachyodont cheek teeth. Rodents have only one pair of upper and lower incisors. Guinea pigs and chinchillas have aradicular hypsodont dentition, whilst rats and mice have aradicular hypsodont incisors and brachyodont cheek teeth.

Lagomorphs (hares and rabbits) have aradicular hypsodont dentition. They have four incisors in the maxillae in two rows, two large central incisors labially and two peg teeth palatally. They have no canine teeth. The teeth grow at a rate of about 2 mm per week.

The teeth of rabbits, hares, chinchillas and guinea pigs grow continuously. An abrasive diet, such as grass supplemented with hay, keeps the teeth worn to a physiological length. Commercial mixes, whilst providing a nutritionally balanced diet, do not provide the wear required for dental health.

In lagomorphs the incisors are in occlusion (touching each other) at rest and the cheek teeth are apart. This is in contrast to rodents, where the cheek teeth are in occlusion at rest and the incisors are apart. Rodents gnaw with their incisors, whereas lagomorphs use their incisors in a sideways cutting action. As with many other species, the jaws of rabbits and rodents are anisognathic (upper and lower jaws of unequal width). In rabbits the mandibular arcades are narrower than the maxillary arcades, while in guinea pigs the mandibular arcades are wider than the maxillary arcades (Figure 27.34).

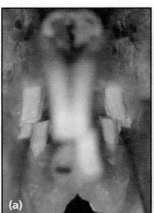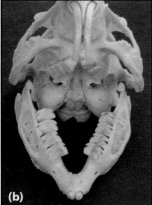

27.34 (a) Rabbit skull, showing mandibular cheek teeth arcades set narrower than maxillary cheek teeth arcades. (b) Guinea pig skull, showing mandibular cheek teeth arcades set wider apart than the maxillary cheek teeth arcades.

Malocclusion

This is the most common presentation of dental disease. It may be caused by:

- Incorrect diet leading to lack of wear and tooth overgrowth
- Congenital deformity of the maxillae – seen most commonly in brachycephalic rabbits (e.g. dwarf rabbits)
- Tooth or mandibular trauma
- Tooth apex infection
- Neoplasia.

Incisor malocclusion

Incisor malocclusion may be primary or secondary. In brachycephalic breeds the malocclusion is primary, as a result of the maxillae being short and the mandibular incisors consequently protruding rostrally.

Secondary incisor malocclusion occurs in animals whose diet lacks fibre, resulting in cheek tooth overgrowth. As the cheek teeth do not undergo normal wear, they come into occlusion, and the force of occlusion causes the jaws to be pushed apart and the mandibular incisors to lose occlusal contact with the maxillary incisors and protrude rostrally. The maxillary incisors may come to occlude on the lingual surface of the mandibular incisors, causing them to curl back into the mouth and in severe cases they may impinge on the palate.

Maloccluding incisors cannot prehend food. Rabbits that chew in one direction (normally they will chew clockwise and anticlockwise alternately) develop an inclination in the occlusal surfaces of the incisor teeth. Clinical signs include anorexia and weight loss, lack of grooming, grinding of the teeth and slobbering (wet chin and neck). Treatment involves tooth trimming or in some cases incisor extraction.

Molar malocclusion

This may occur as a result of one of the factors listed above. An important cause of the acquired condition is abnormal tooth wear. Rabbit teeth erupt at about 2 mm per week and if normal wear does not occur the cheek teeth develop sharp spikes. The mandibular cheek teeth form sharp spikes that protrude lingually and can lacerate the tongue, whilst the maxillary cheek teeth develop spikes that protrude buccally often lacerating the cheeks. Spikes can be so long that they entrap the soft tissues.

When the overgrowing cheek teeth come into occlusion, the force exerted by the opposing cheek teeth prevents normal tooth eruption, resulting in retrograde eruption of the teeth into the mandibles and maxillae. This causes periosteal pain. Irreversible changes occur if the growth tip penetrates the jaw and the ventral mandibular margin or the orbit is perforated. Swellings may be palpated on the upper and lower jaws. Retrograde eruption of maxillary cheek and incisor teeth may cause obstruction of the nasolacrimal duct, leading to lacrimation and/or dacryocystitis. This may progress to tooth root-associated abcessation and osteomyelitis.

Selective feeding may be the initial clinical sign, progressing to anorexia, weight loss, excessive salivation and difficulty in eating. Signs of pain include slobbering (wet chin and neck), teeth grinding, aggression and depression. An animal with tooth root abcessation will present with facial swelling, by which time the prognosis is grave. Diagnosis is confirmed by a lateral extraoral radiograph of the patient's jaws, and the condition can be monitored by dental radiography.

Analgesia is essential. If the ventral mandibular margin and the orbit are intact, recreating the normal occlusal surfaces is advised. Following treatment the normal abrasive diet of fresh grass or hay (less effective than fresh grass) should be fed to help prevent recurrence. Commercial mixes do not provide the tooth wear required.

Regular weighing is an ideal method of monitoring patients that may be affected by this form of dental disease. A 5% reduction in body mass is a good indication of dental disease. Owner education is essential.

Chinchillas are often presented with advanced dental disease and euthanasia may be the only option. Radiographs should be taken to confirm the diagnosis and aid in treatment planning or the decision to euthanase the animal.

Guinea pigs are often presented with cheek teeth overgrowth to the extent that the premolars bridge the tongue, limiting its function. The tongue of a guinea pig has both a movable and an attached part. The jaw configuration of the guinea pig is different to that of the rabbit – the mandibles are at a wider angle than the maxillae and, therefore, the mandibular cheek teeth overlap the maxillary cheek teeth in the normal animal.

Tooth trimming

Teeth should not be clipped, as the uneven pressure applied to the tooth surfaces can cause the tooth to shatter. Clipping can cause damage to the periapical tissues, affecting future tooth growth, or fissures may be produced, leading to periodontal problems and pulp infection. In addition, sharp edges are caused, leading to oral discomfort.

The incisors are effectively trimmed using a high-speed dental fissure bur (this can be performed in the conscious animal if it is properly restrained). Care should be exercised to prevent thermal damage to the teeth. While trimming and reshaping is performed, the soft tissues should be protected by placing a tongue depressor or empty syringe case behind the incisors. The cheek teeth can be trimmed using a long-shank fissure bur in a soft tissue protective shroud or using an acrylic bur. Cheek teeth are trimmed when the animal is anaesthetized. Care must be exercised to ensure the soft tissues are kept well away from the rotating instruments or severe extensive trauma may result.

Extraction of maloccluding incisor teeth should be performed by an experienced veterinary surgeon.

Lagomorphs and rodents undergoing dental treatment should be treated with analgesics to relieve existing and postoperative pain and discomfort. Gut motility modifiers are useful in animals that have been anorexic and fluid administration is also indicated.

Equipment

Equipment for lagomorph and rodent dentistry includes the following (Figure 27.35a):

- High-speed handpiece and fissure burs
- Low-speed straight handpiece with acrylic or long-shank fissure bur
- Cheek dilator
- Mouth gag
- Cheek protector
- Cheek tooth luxator
- Incisor luxator
- Molar extraction forceps
- Good light source
- Cotton buds to remove tooth dust from the mouth.

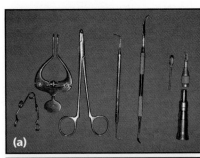

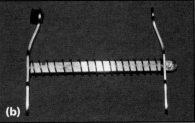

27.35 **(a)** Rabbit dental kit. From left: cheek dilator; mouth opener; cheek teeth extraction forceps; cheek teeth luxators; incisor luxators; acrylic bur for shortening cheek teeth; straight surgical fissure bur and soft tissue guard with a straight low-speed handpiece. **(b)** Sprung mouth opener, which must **NOT** be used.

It should be noted that damage to the temporomandibular joint (TMJ) capsules may occur if the mouth is opened excessively using the mouth gag. Using sprung mouth gags (Figure 27.35b) is not recommended as they keep the TMJs under continuous tension.

Further reading

Capello V (2005) *Rabbit and Rodent Dentistry Handbook.* Zoological Education Network, Florida

Gorrel C and Derbyshire S (2005) *Veterinary Dentistry for the Nurse and Technician.* Elsevier Butterworth Heinemann, Oxford

Hobson P (2006) Dentistry. In: *BSAVA Manual of Rabbit Medicine and Surgery, 2nd edn,* ed. A Meredith and P Flecknell, pp. 184–196. BSAVA Publications, Gloucester

Tutt C (2006) *Small Animal Dentistry: A Manual of Techniques.* Blackwell Publishing, Oxford

Tutt C, Deeprose J and Crossley D (2007) *BSAVA Manual of Canine and Feline Dentistry, 3rd edn.* BSAVA Publications, Gloucester

Self-assessment questions

1. **Write the dental formula of a kitten.**
2. **Write the dental formula of an adult dog.**
3. **Describe the bisecting angle technique used to radiograph most teeth in dogs.**
4. **List the abbreviations used during charting.**
5. **The upper and lower jaws of rabbits and guinea pigs are of unequal size. What term describes this phenomenon and what is the difference between rabbits and guinea pigs?**
6. **Describe periodontitis. How does it differ from gingivitis?**
7. **Describe why scaling a tooth with an ultrasonic scaler for more than 8–10 seconds continuously is detrimental to the tooth.**
8. **Why should the tip of an ultrasonic scaler not be applied at right angles (perpendicular) to the tooth surface?**
9. **Formulate a dental homecare programme for a 6-week-old Golden Retriever puppy.**
10. **List the advantages of using a reciprocating polisher head.**

Appendix 1

Some common breeds

Dogs

The Kennel Club website (www.thekennelclub.org.uk) lists seven Dog Groups. Individual breeds, with their own specified Breed Standards, are placed within these Groups.

Hound Group

Includes: Afghan Hound, Beagle, Whippet, Wire-haired Dachshund

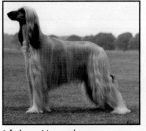

Afghan Hound

Gundog Group

Includes: English Setter, Labrador Retriever, Cocker Spaniel, Weimaraner

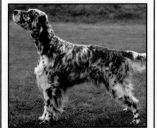

English Setter

Terrier Group

Includes: Bedlington Terrier, Norfolk Terrier, West Highland White Terrier

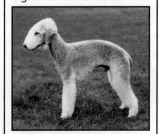

Bedlington Terrier

Utility Group

Includes: Chow Chow, Dalmatian, Shih Tzu, Standard Poodle

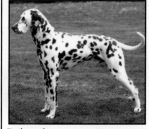

Dalmatian

Working Group

Includes: Boxer, Mastiff, Great Dane, Newfoundland, St Bernard

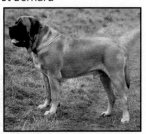

Mastiff

Pastoral Group

Includes: Border Collie, Old English Sheepdog, Pembroke Welsh Corgi

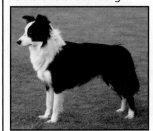

Border Collie

Toy Group

Includes: Bichon Frise, Cavalier King Charles Spaniel, Yorkshire Terrier

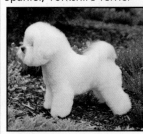

Bichon Frise

(Photographs © The Kennel Club)

Cats

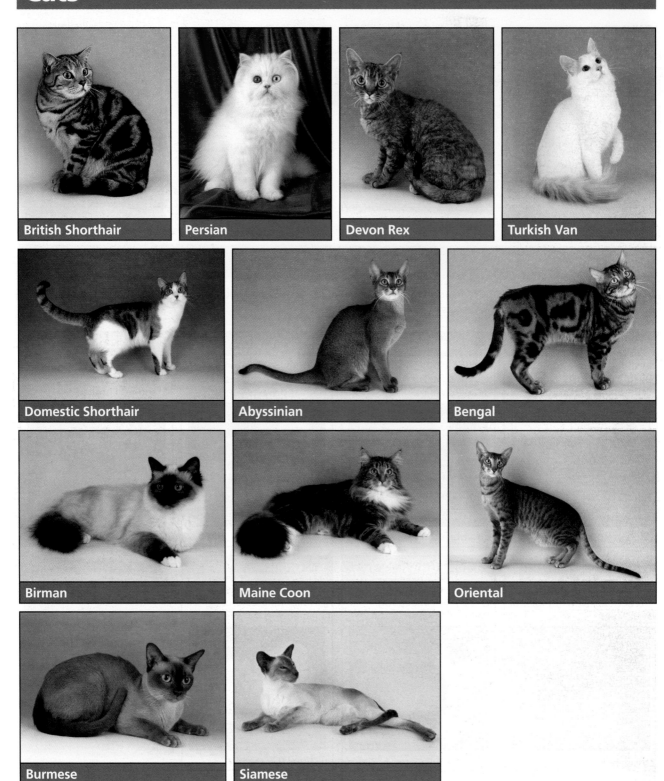

British Shorthair

Persian

Devon Rex

Turkish Van

Domestic Shorthair

Abyssinian

Bengal

Birman

Maine Coon

Oriental

Burmese

Siamese

(Photographs © Alan Robinson)

Horses

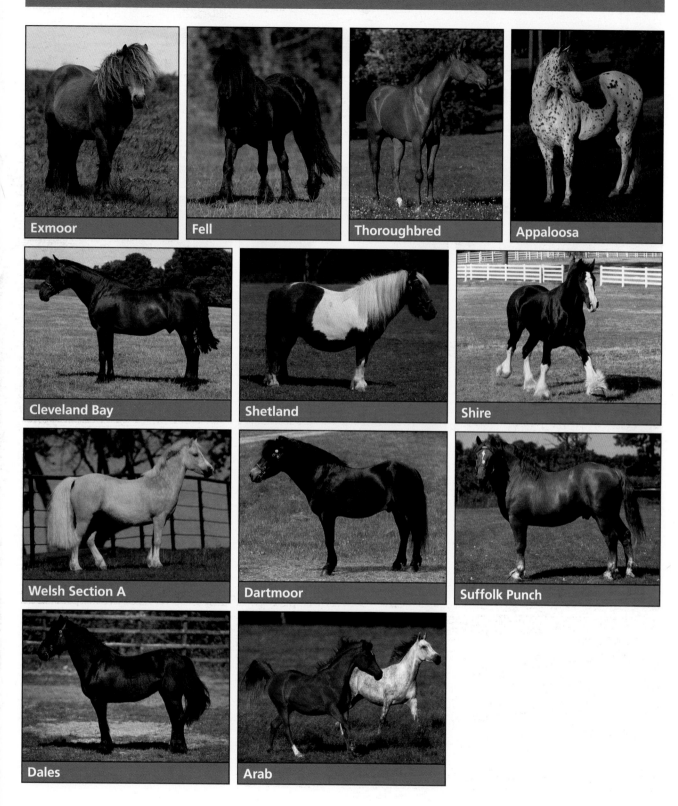

Exmoor

Fell

Thoroughbred

Appaloosa

Cleveland Bay

Shetland

Shire

Welsh Section A

Dartmoor

Suffolk Punch

Dales

Arab

(Photographs © Bob Langrish)

Rabbits

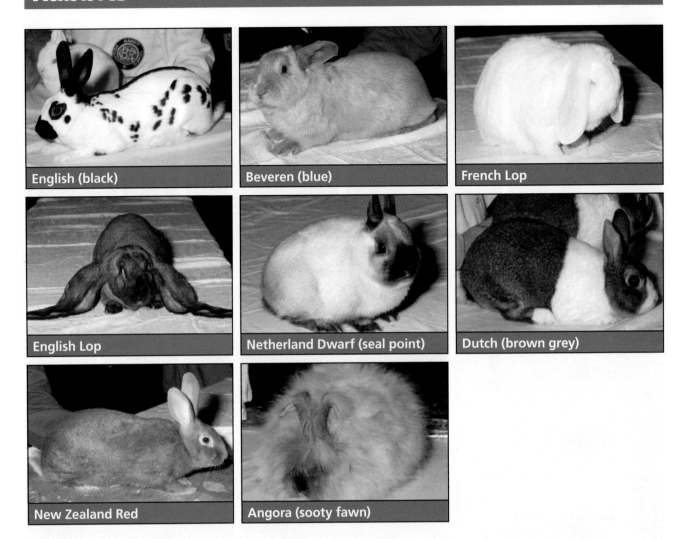

English (black)

Beveren (blue)

French Lop

English Lop

Netherland Dwarf (seal point)

Dutch (brown grey)

New Zealand Red

Angora (sooty fawn)

(Photographs © CBC, University of Newcastle)

Appendix 2

A summary of normal parameters in dogs, cats, horses and rabbits

Parameter	Normal range	Comments
Dogs		
Body temperature	38.3–39.2 °C	Depends on individual physiology and environmental effects
Pulse/heart rate	70–140 beats/min	Depends on individual physiology and excitement/stress
Respiration rate	10–30 breaths/min	Depends on individual physiology and excitement/stress
Water intake	40–60 ml/kg/day	Depends on individual physiology
Urine production	24–48 ml/kg/day	Depends on intake
Cats		
Body temperature	38.2–38.6 °C	Depends on individual physiology and environmental effects
Pulse/heart rate	100–200 beats/min	Depends on individual physiology and excitement/stress
Respiration rate	20–30 breaths/min	Depends on individual physiology and excitement/stress
Water intake	40–60 ml/kg/day	Depends on individual physiology
Urine production	24–48 ml/kg/day	Depends on intake
Horses		
Body temperature	37.2–38.9 °C	Depends on individual physiology and environmental effects
Pulse/heart rate	30–40 beats/min	Depends on individual physiology and excitement/stress
Respiration rate	12–20 breaths/min	Depends on individual physiology and excitement/stress
Water intake	50–60 ml/kg/day	Depends on individual physiology
Urine production	24–48 ml/kg/day	Depends on intake
Rabbits		
Body temperature	38.5–40.0 °C	Depends on individual physiology and environmental effects
Pulse/heart rate	130–325 beats/min	Depends on individual physiology and excitement/stress
Respiration rate	30–60 breaths/min	Depends on individual physiology and excitement/stress
Water intake	50–150 ml/kg/day	Very variable
Urine production	12–48 ml/kg/day	Very variable

Appendix 3

Conversion tables

Biochemistry

	SI unit	Conversion	Non-SI unit
Alanine aminotransferase	IU / l	x 1	IU / l
Albumin	g / l	x 0.1	g / dl
Alkaline phosphatase	IU / l	x 1	IU / l
Aspartate aminotransferase	IU / l	x 1	IU / l
Bilirubin	µmol / l	x 0.0584	mg / dl
Calcium	mmol / l	x 4	mg / dl
Carbon dioxide (total)	mmol / l	x 1	mEq / l
Cholesterol	mmol / l	x 38.61	mg / dl
Chloride	mmol / l	x 1	mEq / l
Cortisol	nmol / l	x 0.362	ng / ml
Creatine kinase	IU / l	x 1	IU / l
Creatinine	µmol / l	x 0.0113	mg / dl
Glucose	mmol / l	x 18.02	mg / dl
Insulin	pmol / l	x 0.1394	µIU / ml
Iron	µmol / l	x 5.587	µg / dl
Magnesium	mmol / l	x 2	mEq / l
Phosphorus	mmol / l	x 3.1	mg / dl
Potassium	mmol / l	x 1	mEq / l
Sodium	mmol / l	x 1	mEq / l
Total protein	g / l	x 0.1	g / dl
Thyroxine (T4) (free)	pmol / l	x 0.0775	ng / dl
Thyroxine (T4) (total)	nmol / l	x 0.0775	µg / dl
Tri-iodothyronine (T3)	nmol / l	x 65.1	ng / dl
Triglycerides	mmol / l	x 88.5	mg / dl
Urea	mmol / l	x 2.8	mg of urea nitrogen / dl

Temperature

	SI unit	Conversion	Conventional unit
	°C	(x 9/5) + 32	°F
To convert from °F to °C, subtract 32 and then multiply by 5 and divide by 9			

Haematology

	SI unit	Conversion	Non-SI unit
Red blood cell count	10^{12} / l	x 1	10^6 / µl
Haemoglobin	g / l	x 0.1	g / dl
MCH	pg / cell	x 1	pg / cell
MCHC	g / l	x 0.1	g / dl
MCV	fl	x 1	µm³
Platelet count	10^9 / l	x 1	10^3 / µl
White blood cell count	10^9 / l	x 1	10^3 / µl

Hypodermic needles

	Metric	Non-metric
External diameter	0.8 mm	21 G
	0.6 mm	23 G
	0.5 mm	25 G
	0.4 mm	27 G
Needle length	12 mm	$^1/_2$ inch
	16 mm	$^5/_8$ inch
	25 mm	1 inch
	30 mm	$1^1/_4$ inch
	40 mm	$1^1/_2$ inch

Suture material sizes

Metric	USP
0.1	11/0
0.2	10/0
0.3	9/0
0.4	8/0
0.5	7/0
0.7	6/0
1	5/0
1.5	4/0
2	3/0
3	2/0
3.5	0
4	1
5	2
6	3

Appendix 4

Study skills

Beverley Crawford

Introduction

Study skills are the strategies and approaches that can be used to improve the ability to learn. Possessing good study skills will improve your ability to gain and apply new knowledge. A range of methods may be used and adapted to enable more efficient and effective study.

Studying to gain a qualification will almost certainly involve a great deal of reading and writing – both complex activities made easier by knowing shortcuts and purposeful methods. There will be lectures to attend, notes to be taken and learnt from, and almost certainly you will need to know how to prepare for, take and pass examinations. Possessing successful study skills will also help in everyday life, as they are transferable and useful when approaching all work and life tasks.

Different study skills work for different people, as the process of learning is very personal. It is important to be familiar with a range of techniques, in order to work out which is best for you.

Purpose, Organization, Place, Planning: the POPP approach

As you embark on your studies, it may be beneficial to take a few moments to answer the following questions:

- **Purpose – why am I undertaking this course and what do I hope to gain from it in the short and long term?**
  (*Keeping this at the forefront of your mind will help you to persevere when the going gets tough*)
- **Organization – how will I organize my learning materials?**
  You may have a large ring binder with dividers or you may prefer separate folders for each subject area. Whichever you choose, the key to successful organization is to take the time to organize and file your notes. Where will you store your textbooks?
  (*Organized materials will be easier to access and so more inviting to look at. It will also enable time to be spent on learning rather than searching for materials*)
- **Place – where will I study?**
  Having a designated study area can ensure study time is not used up by other activities. Whether you have a home study, or work at the kitchen table or at the local coffee shop is largely irrelevant. Studying is a ▶

state of mind and it is *your* mind you have to prepare. Having a designated place will help you to stay focussed.
(*Having a predetermined place devoted to studying may help avoid the common pitfall of not being able to start studying – i.e. if we always sit here to study we are less likely to be distracted by the TV, a magazine, the need to call a friend for a chat or clean the bathroom*)
- **Planning – when will I study and how will I divide this time?**
  You may be at your best in the mornings – in which case you could arrange to rise an hour earlier and study then, whereas others prefer to study in the evening or late at night. However, it is useful to decide your preference and then adopt a routine. Begin each session by going over your lecture notes/revising what you have already covered before tackling new learning, leaving time to summarize this.
  (*Starting with the familiar can help us to get started – it feels comfortable and can ease us into the idea of studying*)

Planning skills

For most people embarking on a course of study, using the time they already have in a more effective and productive way will be easier than finding more time. Much has been written about the techniques for effective 'time management' and a half hour search on the internet will furnish the student with various tips and techniques, from learning to say 'No' to delegating tasks to others. Good time management requires **proper planning**.

The 'golden rules' of proper planning
Plan your time

- Identify the important and urgent tasks, which are to be completed as your **priority**.
- Note the **end date** of the work (assignment due date, examination date).

- **Count back** the number of days/weeks/months you have to prepare.
- Note any **other important dates** you have within this period that may reduce your study time.
- Identify and count the **study periods** you have.
- Draw up a **study programme** with your study times identified – perhaps use a calendar to do this.

Break the task into smaller chunks

- If revising for an examination, break the revision into **subject areas** – decide on the number of sessions each will require, allocating more sessions to the subjects you find most difficult.
- If writing an assignment, your plan will need to include the time allocated for **different elements**:
  - Planning the assignment
  - Writing the first draft
  - Editing and re-writing
  - Checking the final version
  - Delivery.

Avoid distractions

- **Recognize** non-urgent tasks as distractions. These may include day-to-day activities such as washing-up, ironing, talking to friends or rearranging your bedroom, which seem to take on greater urgency every time you sense the need to begin studying.
- Plan your study start and finish **times**. Consign non-urgent tasks (e.g. household chores) to set times that do not impact on your study time.
- Set yourself a **reward** – e.g. study from 6–8 pm, then reward yourself by calling a friend for a catch-up or watching TV.

Get started

Recognize distractions and excuses for what they are, and start now.

Complete

- Complete each task by the planned end date.
- Take a moment to reflect on what you achieved – after each session and at the end date. Congratulate yourself when you did well.

Reading skills

There are many different ways to read. If reading a novel, you would usually start on the first page and read every word on every page until you reached the last word on the last page. In contrast, with a magazine you are far more likely to flick through the pages, stopping to read in detail any article that attracts your attention. You may look up specific articles – perhaps those detailed on the front cover, or those in the list of contents that look interesting. Now contrast this with reading a textbook when, to be effective, yet another approach is called for.

To study effectively from an academic textbook you will need to use a combination of the following methods:

- **Scanning** through the chapter to look for subheadings/

pictures or images that you want to examine in more detail

- **Skimming** or reading quickly through the text to see if there is anything of interest. You might run your finger down the centre of the page and sweep your eyes quickly from one side of the finger to the other and thus see the text without tackling it in any deep or memorable way. Until, that is, you notice something of interest
- **Using the contents page**. The list of chapter titles might be the best place to start – e.g. if you are looking for information on muscles, you may start by looking in a chapter on this subject
- **Using the index** at the back of the book. This enables you to locate specific references to a topic. There may be several entries with several page references
- **Close reading of the text**. This means reading every word, thinking about it, considering what you are being told, then attaching this new information to what you already know. It may involve re-reading a particularly difficult or important section.

How to remember what you have read

- **Take notes as you read.** Select the main points; do not rewrite the whole page, or write without thinking about what you are actually reading.
- **Write a summary of the piece.** Think about what you have read and note the main points. Use subheadings and bullet points as this will stop you from copying what you have read.
- **Draw a chart or table of the information you have learned.** This will enable you to organize the information so you are clear what you have learnt and will help you attach significance to it. This gives the same information as the mind map. As an example, this might be how we would organize information about the liver:

Functions of the liver	Diseases of the liver	Clinical signs of liver disease

- **Draw a 'mind map' of the information.** This technique will suit visual learners, enabling links to be made between pieces of information. Use a large sheet of paper and spread your map out, so that extra information can be added over time. As an example, Figure A4.1 shows how a mind map might be used to organize information about the liver.

Whichever method you prefer, and this may vary according to the type of reading you are doing, ask yourself these questions:

- Have I noted all the main points?
- Do my notes make sense?
- Will I understand them in a few months?

If you have not answered 'yes' to all of these questions, adjust your notes and then ask yourself the questions again.

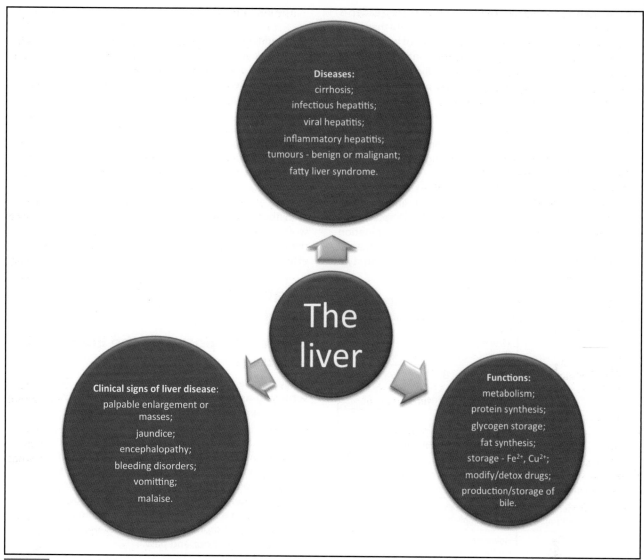

| A4.1 | A mind map can be used to display information about the liver. |

Writing skills

The first question to ask before beginning a piece of writing is, 'What is its intended purpose?' Writing a text message or an email to a friend requires a very different style to writing a report for work or instructions for a colleague to follow. All writing seeks to communicate, but exactly what is to be communicated and to whom will determine the structure of the writing and how formal it is to be.

Planning for writing

Writing must be divided into paragraphs. This is both a convention and a good device for organizing and prioritizing information, ensuring all points are fully explained and supported with evidence, and encouraging the reader to read your work. As you begin to plan what information you need to communicate, you can begin to decide the paragraphs; there are different ways in which to tackle this, depending on your preference.

A **paragraph** is a group of sentences all based on the same idea. You may begin by making a point and then provide supportive evidence, followed by an example. A further or contrary point may then be covered in a new paragraph, again with supporting evidence and an example.

You may plan the paragraphs for your piece in the following ways:

- 'Post-it' planning:
  - Write the titles of the paragraphs you will need to cover on sticky notes or pieces of paper
  - Rearrange these until you are happy with the order of paragraphs
  - Combine paragraphs if, on reflection, they seem to be making the same point, only in different words.
- 'Mind map' planning:
  - Often called a 'spider diagram'
  - This is a visual tool that shows links between ideas
  - It can be used to plan work or to aid revision.

Connectives

Without doubt, the difference between a passable piece of writing and a really good piece can be as simple as the use of connectives. Essentially, connectives are words or short phrases used to join ideas seamlessly so that the reader is guided to continue reading through the piece until they have reached the end. Without connectives a piece of writing may resemble a shopping list of unconnected points. The writing is staccato and the ideas are presented individually, often in an abrupt or disjointed way. The ideal is to present your facts, ideas and arguments as part of a whole.

Paragraphs can begin with a connective, and ideas within the paragraph can be linked with other connectives. There are several of these to choose from, depending on what you are writing and what your writing is hoping to achieve. Some examples are given in Figure A4.2.

There are occasions, however, when time constraints (e.g. in an exam) or editorial considerations (e.g. limited space available within a magazine article or book chapter) may necessitate a different, more punchy style. In an examination setting in particular it is more important to make sure that all the relevant facts are in place rather than spend time on style at the expense of substance.

Purpose	Examples
To put ideas into order	First... Secondly... Finally...
To add information	Another point is... In addition... Another point to note is...
To explain ideas	For instance... In other words... A further example of this is...
To conclude the writing	In summary... In conclusion... To sum up...
General statements to introduce a paragraph	Some people think... Many people believe...
To introduce the idea that contrasting evidence will be presented	However... On the other hand... Many people would disagree...

A4.2 Using connectives.

Editing

Veterinary nurses need to be good at checking. During the course of a day, veterinary nurses check a number of things; these may include:

- Checking on an animal in postoperative care (temperature, blood pressure, respiration, etc.)
- Checking on stock levels to ensure they are sufficient to meet all needs
- Checking that a client understands the instructions he/she has been given
- Checking an invoice
- Checking a bill has been paid
- Checking the content of an assignment completed by a student veterinary nurse.

Editing a piece of written work involves various stages of **checking**. Each of these checks should be done separately, either on the same day, or separated by a day or two. Re-editing work after a gap of a day or two means we are far more likely to read the words we have actually written and far less likely to 'read' what we meant to write.

The editing sequence:

- 1st edit: Read through your work and check that it meets the task you were set, by carefully re-reading the question or assignment brief
- 2nd edit: Read through the work and check that every sentence makes sense and that the tense is consistent (i.e. doesn't swing between past, present and future)
- 3rd edit: Read through the work and check punctuation and spelling
- 4th edit: Read through the work from start to finish and check that it holds together well as a piece of writing.

Without doubt, editing is an important activity and yet so many people neglect it. It requires discipline, as it is not the most exciting part of the writing process. However, the effort you expend on editing is always worthwhile.

Learning to spell more confidently
Challenges posed by the English language

Many people lack confidence with spelling. This is hardly surprising as the English language provides several challenges, even for those who consider themselves to be competent spellers.

- Many words contain different sounds for the same strings of letters. For example, there are many different sounds for the -ough string of letters – e.g. in cough, rough, thought, through, although and bough.
- Many words also change spelling according to the meaning, but sound the same. For example, to, too and two and pour, poor and paw.

How to become a better speller

Although a good place to start, computer spellcheckers are only useful up to a point. Most are not yet sufficiently sophisticated to identify errors in the use of 'there', 'their' and 'they're', for example.

A popular method of learning a particular spelling is to use a chart:

Word list	Day 1	Day 2	Day 4	Day 7
separate				

1. Make a list of the words you wish to spell.
2. Look at each word in turn, cover it over and write it from memory. Check back to ensure it is correct.
3. As the chart suggests, the time period between attempts should be gradually increased from a day to a few days, to take the words from short- to long-term memory.

Grouping words to learn them is another effective technique. For example, to learn the word 'veterinary' you might group it like this:

Word list	Day 1	Day 2	Day 4	Day 7
veterinary				
dictionary				
contemporary				
library				

This would help you to learn the word veterinary if the 'ary' part is giving you the problem. However, if it is the 'er' part you would look for words with 'er' in them, e.g. consideration.

The key is to find words that contain the part of the word pattern you are struggling with. Devising and learning a saying can help, e.g. *veterinary nurses should be shown consideration*. So useful is this process of association that it is unimportant if you add a word to the list that you can already spell. In fact, it is helpful to link words that you have problems spelling to those you can spell confidently and with ease. This practice enables you to attach a difficult spelling to one you already know and thus learn the new word. This process also assists the learning of technical vocabulary, as does looking at the meaning of words.

Punctuation

The purpose of punctuation is to help the reader understand what you are trying to communicate. You should aim to use the punctuation shown in Figure A4.3 proficiently within your work.

Capital letters should be used:

- To begin a sentence
- To show that a noun is a proper noun, e.g. a name.

Using the above information, identify why each capital letter is used in the following piece:

For the last two years Julie Brown has worked at Country Vets in Kent. She has, however, recently been offered a new job in York by the Sunnyside Veterinary Practice. She will take Tim, her Great Dane, with her and has already found a small house in Lion Street to rent. She will move on Monday 15th November and so will be settled there before Christmas. Although it is not ideal to move in the winter, she has a lot of friends who will help her to settle in.

Plagiarism

Plagiarism is the practice of copying the work of another without crediting them as the source. This can be from published or unpublished texts. To avoid being accused, or indeed guilty, of plagiarism, ensure you list all the sources of your research so that these can be referenced. Read widely around a topic so that you are exposed to the ideas and research of a range of people. Note that the crime here is not that the work of others has been used, but that this has not been acknowledged, and you are therefore trying to pass these ideas off as your own.

Referencing

To avoid any unintentional plagiarism and to show the extent of your reading around the topic, you will need to reference the books, journals, diagrams and websites you have used to gather your information. Each reference must be in the text in a shortened form after you have referred to it, as well as in the list of references at the end of the piece. Typically, the Harvard Referencing System is used.

Punctuation mark		What it is for	An example of how this punctuation is used
Full stop	.	Goes at the end of a sentence	I work hard on my assignments.
Comma	,	Separates items in a list.	Bread, sugar, tea, coffee and milk... (note there is no comma between the last two items – use 'and' instead)
		Separates extra information from the rest of the sentence. In this case the sentence is about the car and dog – where the car is parked is extra information that is not needed in order for the sentence to make sense	The car, which was parked in the sun, had a dog on the back seat.
Question mark	?	Goes at the end of any sentence that asks a question	Shall I clean the kennel?
Exclamation mark	!	Used in place of a full stop to end a sentence. It shows surprise, shock or horror. Only one is needed	Stop! Fantastic! That was amazing!
Semi-colon	;	Used to join two sentences in place of 'and', 'because', 'since', or 'while'	My dog seems happy at puppy training classes; he likes being with the other dogs.
Colon	:	Comes before a list or example	To clean the kennel you will need: a bucket of water, a broom, brushes and disinfectant.
Apostrophe	'	Used to show ownership of something	Helen's cat David's coffee Note: the dogs' barking woke everyone up. This shows there was more than one dog barking – for plurals the apostrophe goes after the 's'
		Used to shorten words in informal writing – the apostrophe shows where the letters are missing	Wasn't – from was not Weren't – from were not I'll – from I will He'll – from he will

A4.3   Punctuation and its uses.

In-text referencing

This reference should come immediately before or after the material to be referenced and should only include the author's name and the year of publication; for example, (Brown, 2009). Page numbers are needed only if you have included a direct quote; for example, (Brown, 2009, p16).

Reference list

This list should come at the end of your piece of writing and should be set out according to the referencing system you are using (e.g. the Harvard Referencing System).

Revision skills

Revising for examinations is vitally important – it can make the difference between success and failure. Start revision early. Accept that at times you will feel anxiety. Don't let the anxiety rule you; keep going, stay steady and stick to your timetable. Believe that you can pass if you study.

Use your learning style as a guide to how to revise.

- **Visual learners** may find mind maps/diagrams/sketches/colour coding useful.
- **Auditory learners** may find reading notes aloud/revising with others/recording notes and listening to them useful.
- **Theorists** may prefer to copy out notes and/or rewrite the key points.
- **Active learners** may prefer to take regular

activity-fuelled breaks or to think through learning while walking.

You will most likely find a combination of these techniques useful (Figure A4.4).

References and further reading

Burns T and Sinfield S (2008) *Essential Study Skills: The Complete Guide to Success at University, 2nd edn.* Sage, London

Cottrell S (2008) *The Study Skills Handbook, 3rd edn.* Palgrave Macmillan, UK

Useful websites

For general study skills information: www.bbc.co.uk/skillswise and www.learndirect.co.uk

Grammar: www.bbc.co.uk/skillswise/words/grammar/ and www.learnenglish.de/grammarpage.htm

Time management: www.teal.org.uk/sv/timemgnt.htm

Spelling: www.bbc.co.uk/skillswise/words/spelling/waystolearn/lookcover/factsheet.shtml

Mind maps: www.imindmap.com/

Harvard referencing: http://libweb.anglia.ac.uk/referencing/harvard.htm?harvard_id=63#63

Revision techniques: www.studyskills.soton.ac.uk/studytips/exams.htm

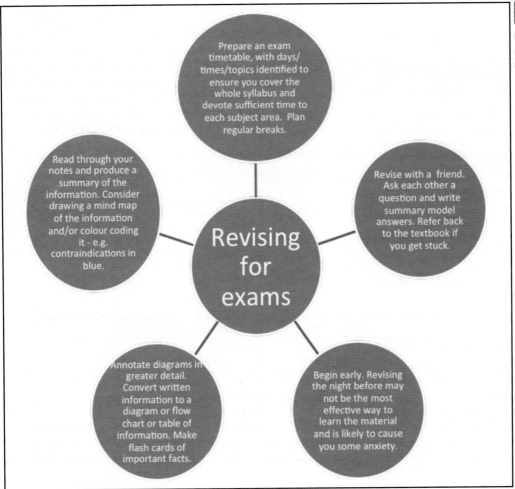

A4.4

Revision mind map: making revision manageable.

Appendix 5

Personal and professional development: reflective insight

Barbara Cooper

Introduction

Reflective insight explains why we react and think in certain ways, and provides possibilities for development and change. It also helps us to identify the resources that are available to us, in the form of colleagues, family, friends and personal knowledge. Developing reflective insight is an important starting point for any professional, including veterinary nurses. Questions of context, feelings and knowledge base are important features of all types of reflection.

Integrating personal and professional experience

Personal experience is a rich resource that may not always be seen as relevant to professional life, or professional experience. Nevertheless, the skills and knowledge developed within *personal* experience are the foundation upon which the person builds their *professional* identity and skills. Some of the roles that veterinary nurses play within their lives, such as being a parent, a member of a group or a clinical coach, bring valuable experiences that can be integrated with professional experience to advance knowledge and practice in different ways. For example, if you have volunteered for a local charity, you may have developed skills in leadership and organization.

Integrating personal and professional experience involves reflecting upon what your personal experience has taught you and identifying how this relates to your professional experience. For example, some of the knowledge developed through a parenting role is likely to include lifespan development, disease management, communication and negotiation, leadership, organization, nutrition, first aid, and learning. **Integration** involves connecting this knowledge with what is learned through the professional/student veterinary nurse role.

Self-evaluation

It is important to evaluate your performance as soon as possible after every activity you undertake. You must be able to demonstrate that you can analyse your practice in enough depth to identify both your strengths and areas for improvement. Self-evaluation is a skill you will need to use throughout your life. Keeping a reflective diary can be helpful.

References and further reading

Boud D, Keogh R and Walker D (1985) *Reflection: Turning Experience into Learning*. Kogan Page, London

Reflective questions to consider upon completion of an assessment activity

1. What were you aiming to achieve when you started out?
2. Did your aims change? Why?
3. What did you want to get out of the assessment? How do you know this?
4. Did you notice anything about a person's body language? How did you tackle this?
5. What questions were you asked? When were you asked? How did you tackle this?
6. Who did you liaise with before the assessment? Was this helpful? Why/why not?
7. Do you think that you managed to collect all the information you needed to carry out a particular task? If yes, what strategies helped you in this case? (Was it that the assessment was straightforward? Did you use a particular type of questioning – open, closed, probing, rhetorical, hypothetical? Did you prepare in a particular way?) If you didn't get the information you needed, what got in your way?

continues ▶

continued

8. What, if any, were the barriers to change? How do you know this? How did you tackle them? Was your strategy successful? How do you know this?

9. Did you give any advice? Do you think this helped? How do you know this? Did you help other staff/clients? How do you know this?

10. Do you think your knowledge was adequate in this case? Do you have evidence (this could be from books or journals or from your experience of practice) to back up your advice? What was your rationale for each action you took? Was there anything you were unsure about? If yes, what could you do about this?

11. Does your record of an assessment represent all the information someone would need to follow this up? How do you know this? Summarize the assessment out loud to yourself. Does the record fully reflect this summary? Why/why not? Have you used abbreviations?

12. Have you seen a similar problem before? How did this assessment differ? Were you prepared for this?

13. Did you liaise with anyone after the assessment? Do you feel this communication was helpful to the other person/clinical coach/yourself, and how do you know this?

14. How did your communication with the person you dealt with differ from that with the other professionals or students? Do you feel that you used an appropriate communication style? What sort of terminology did you use? How would you describe your manner (formal, informal, chatty, serious)? Was this appropriate? How do you know?

15. Are you aware of any issues relating to:

   - Antidiscriminatory practice?
   - Professionalism
   - Team working
   - Veterinary Surgeons Act or guides to professional conduct?

   If yes, think about how your practice demonstrates competence (or not) and make a record in your reflective diary.

16. What actions do you need to take after the assessment? Do you feel competent to tackle these?

17. Did you keep to time? If not, what delayed you? How could you tackle this if it happened again?

18. What pleased you most about this assessment and why? What troubled you most about this assessment and why?

Index